NCLEX-RN®
Questions & Answers

made
Incredibly
Easy!®

Sixth Edition

Susan Lisko, DNP, RN, CNE
Associate Professor of Nursing
Scheduling Coordinator
Youngstown State University
Youngstown, OH

6,500 + Questions!

Wolters Kluwer | Lippincott Williams & Wilkins
Health

Philadelphia · Baltimore · New York · London
Buenos Aires · Hong Kong · Sydney · Tokyo

Staff

Acquisitions Editor
Bill Lamsback

Project Manager
Priscilla Crater

Manufacturing Manager
Beth Welsh

Marketing Manager
Sara Schuessler

Creative Director
Doug Smock

Design Coordinator
Joan Wendt

Production Services
Absolute Service, Inc.

Sixth Edition
Copyright © 2014, 2011, 2008 Wolters Kluwer Health | Lippincott
Williams & Wilkins

Two Commerce Square
2001 Market Street
Philadelphia, PA 19103 USA
LWW.com

Printed in China

Care has been taken to confirm the accuracy of the information
presented and to describe generally accepted practices. However,
the authors, editors, and publisher are not responsible for errors or
omissions or for any consequences from application of the information
in this book and make no warranty, expressed or implied, with respect
to the currency, completeness, or accuracy of the contents of the publication. Application of this information in a particular situation remains
the professional responsibility of the practitioner.

The authors, editors, and publisher have exerted every effort to ensure
that drug selection and dosage set forth in this text are in accordance
with current recommendations and practice at the time of publication.
However, in view of ongoing research, changes in government regulations, and the constant flow of information relating to drug therapy
and drug reactions, the reader is urged to check the package insert
for each drug for any change in indications and dosage and for added
warnings and precautions. This is particularly important when the
recommended agent is a new or infrequently employed drug.

Some drugs and medical devices presented in this publication have
Food and Drug Administration (FDA) clearance for limited use in
restricted research settings. It is the responsibility of health care
providers to ascertain the FDA status of each drug or device planned
for use in their clinical practice.

The publishers have made every effort to trace copyright holders
for borrowed material. If they have inadvertently overlooked any,
they will be pleased to make the necessary arrangements at the first
opportunity.

To purchase additional copies of this book, call our customer service
department at (800) 638-3030 or fax orders to (301) 223-2320. International customers should call (301) 223-2300.

Visit Lippincott Williams & Wilkins on the Internet at LWW.com.
Lippincott Williams & Wilkins customer service representatives are
available from 8:30 am to 6 pm, EST.

10 9 8 7 6 5 4 3 2 1

Library of Congress Cataloging-in-Publication Data
Lisko, Susan, author.
 NCLEX-RN questions & answers made incredibly easy /
Susan Lisko. — Sixth edition.
   p. ; cm.
 NCLEX-RN questions and answers made incredibly easy!
 Includes index.
 Preceded by (work): NCLEX-RN questions & answers made
incredibly easy!. 5th ed. c2011.
 ISBN 978-1-4511-8549-2
 I. NCLEX-RN questions & answers made incredibly easy!. Preceded
by (work): II. Title. III. Title: NCLEX-RN questions and answers made
incredibly easy!
 [DNLM: 1. Nursing Care—Examination Questions. 2. Nursing—
Examination Questions. WY 18.2]
 RT55
 610.73076—dc23
                                                      2013023353

Contents

Contributors

Judith Alexander, RN, PhD
Associate Professor
Armstrong Atlantic State University
Savannah, GA

Dometrives Armstrong, MSN, FNP, PHN, RN
Associate Professor
San Diego City College, Nursing Education
San Diego, CA

Peggy Baikie, DNP, RN, PNP-BC, NNP-BC
Program Manager/Nurse Practitioner
Denver Health
Affiliate Professor
Metropolitan State University of Denver
Denver, CO

Catherine A. Bailey, DNP, RN, CNE
Associate Professor
Shawnee State University
Portsmouth, OH

Vicky H. Becherer, PhD, RN
Adjunct Assistant Teaching Professor
College of Nursing at UM-St. Louis
St. Louis, MO

Cheryl L. Brady, RN, MSN, CNE
Associate Lecturer
Kent State University
Salem, OH

Kim Cooper, RN, MSN
Dean, School of Nursing
Ivy Tech Community College
Terre Haute, IN

Linda Carman Copel, PhD, RN, PMHCNS, BC, CNE, NCC, FAPA
Professor
Villanova University
Villanova, PA

Lillian Craig, MSN, RN, FNP-C
Adjunct Faculty
Oklahoma Panhandle State University
Goodwell, OK

Kelly J. Gosnell, RN, MSN
Associate Professor of Nursing
Ivy Tech Community College
Terre Haute, IN

Corlis Hayden, MSN, RN
Assistant Professor
Nebraska Methodist College
Omaha, NE

Connie S. Heflin, MSN, RN
Professor
Dean of Online Learning
West Kentucky Community and Technical College
Paducah, KY

Karla Jones, MS, RN
Nursing Faculty
College of Western Idaho
Nampa, ID

Susan Joseph, RN, MS, CNE
Instructor
Cochran School of Nursing
Yonkers, NY

CJ Kingston, RN, MSN
Instructor
Saint Francis Medical Center College of Nursing
Peoria, IL

Kathleen Lehmann, RN-BC, EdS, MEd, BSN, BA
Charge Nurse
Edith Nourse Rogers Memorial Veterans Hospital
Bedford, MA

Noel C. Piano, RN, MS
Instructor/Director
Lafayette School of Practical Nursing
Williamsburg, VA

Nan C. Riedé, RN, MSN, CPN
Assistant Professor
Baptist College of Health Sciences
Memphis, TN

Ora V. Robinson, RN, CNE, PhD
Assistant Professor of Nursing
California State University
San Bernardino, CA

Allison J. Terry, PhD, MSN, RN
Associate Professor of Nursing
Auburn University Montgomery
Montgomery, AL

Mary Terwilliger, PhD, RN
Assistant Professor
Simulation Lab Coordinator
Venango College of Clarion University
Oil City, PA

Becky A. Thiel, DNP, RN, CNE
Professor of Nursing
Chair, Department of Nursing
Shawnee State University
Portsmouth, OH

Sandra K. Voll, MS, NP, CNM
Clinical Assistant Professor
Virginia Commonwealth University School of Nursing
Richmond, VA

Polly Gerber Zimmermann, RN, MS, MBA, CEN, FAEN
Associate Professor
Harry S Truman College
Chicago, IL

Patricia Zrelak, RN, PhD, NEA-BC, CNRN
Nurse Researcher
University of California Davis
Davis, CA

Advisory board

Preface

As a Nurse Educator for more than 28 years, my goal has been to inspire students to aspire to be the best nurse possible. To achieve that goal, many hours of instruction have been dedicated to providing students with a strong foundation of core concepts. Lectures, quizzes, theory examinations, case studies, clinical experiences, and simulations prepare them to complete the final phase of the educational process: passing the NCLEX® licensure exam. Many students reach the final phase and are in search of a resource to guide their preparation for success on the NCLEX. The sixth edition of *NCLEX–RN Questions & Answers Made Incredibly Easy* has been developed to assist in achieving that goal. This book provides you with more than 6,500 exemplary questions and answers designed to help you discover those areas in which you are strong and those areas in which some degree of review might be in order.

You will find questions written at the Analysis and Application level reflecting the most current changes to the NCLEX test plan, including alternative formats: select all, drag and drop, hot spot, chart exhibit, calculation, audio (online), and graphic option. Each answer includes not only the rationale for the correct and incorrect responses but also information as to which aspects of nursing are being evaluated by that question. Thus, you will discover which parts of the nursing process are more problematic for you and which client needs categories are most challenging for you. Knowing this can help you focus on the further review needed for you to be successful.

Remember knowledge is power! To be successful on the NCLEX exam, plan your time, think positive, and practice, practice, practice! I wish you NCLEX SUCCESS.

Susan Lisko, DNP, RN, CNE

About the author

Dr. Susan Lisko is an established nurse educator and NCLEX instructor with a passion for nursing. She earned a diploma in Nursing from St. Elizabeth Hospital Medical Center in Youngstown, Ohio, and then a BSN in Nursing from Youngstown State University, an MSN with a specialty in Nursing Education from Gannon University, and a Doctorate of Nursing Practice (DNP) from The Frances Payne Bolton School of Nursing, Case Western Reserve University. Most recently, she achieved certification as a Nurse Educator (CNE) from the National League for Nursing. The certification recognizes *excellence in the advanced specialty role of the academic nurse educator*. Dr. Lisko's awards for recognition of expertise and contribution to nursing education include being named a 2011 Distinguished Professor of Teaching at Youngstown State University and Educator of the Year in Ohio. Throughout her career, she has published in refereed journals and in textbooks, and she has presented her scholarly research at nursing conferences throughout the country. She continues to teach at the undergraduate and graduate level and she travels throughout the country teaching NCLEX-RN review courses.

Part I   Surviving the NCLEX®

Chapter 1
Preparing for the NCLEX®

Just the facts

In this chapter, you'll learn:

- about the NCLEX® and why you must take it
- what you need to know about taking the NCLEX by computer
- strategies to use when answering NCLEX questions
- how to recognize and answer alternate-format questions
- how to avoid common mistakes when taking the NCLEX.

NCLEX® basics

All your experience with testing means you're ready to do battle with this exam!

Passing the National Council Licensure Examination (NCLEX®) is an important landmark in your career as a nurse. The first step on your way to passing the NCLEX is to understand what it is and how it's administered.

NCLEX® structure

The NCLEX is a test written by nurses who, like most of your nursing instructors, have an advanced degree and clinical expertise in a particular area. Only one small difference distinguishes nurses who write NCLEX questions: They're trained to write questions in a style particular to the NCLEX.

If you've completed an accredited nursing program, you've already taken numerous tests written by nurses with backgrounds and experiences similar to those of the nurses who write for the NCLEX. The test-taking experience you've already gained will help you pass the NCLEX. So your NCLEX review should be just that—a review.

What's the point of it all?

The NCLEX is designed for one purpose: to determine whether it's appropriate for you to receive a license to practice as a nurse. By passing the NCLEX, you demonstrate that you possess the minimum level of knowledge necessary to practice nursing safely.

Studying abroad

If you completed your nursing education in a foreign country, you must follow certain guidelines to be eligible to work as a registered nurse in the United States. (See *Guidelines for international nurses*, page 5.)

Mix 'em up

In nursing school, you probably took courses that were separated into such subjects as pharmacology; nursing leadership; health assessment; adult health; and pediatric, maternal-neonatal, and psychiatric nursing. In contrast, the NCLEX is integrated, meaning that different subjects are mixed together.

As you answer NCLEX questions, you may encounter patients in any stage of life, from neonatal to geriatric. These patients—clients, in NCLEX terminology—may be of any background, and may be completely well or extremely ill, and may have any of a variety of disorders.

Client needs, front and center

The NCLEX draws questions from four categories of client needs that were developed by the *National Council of State Boards of Nursing* (NCSBN), the organization that sponsors and manages the NCLEX. *Client needs categories* ensure that a wide variety of topics appears on every NCLEX examination.

The NCSBN developed client needs categories after conducting a practice analysis of new nurses. All aspects of nursing care observed in the study were broken down into four main categories, some of which were broken down further into subcategories. (See *Client needs categories*, page 6.)

What's the plan?

The categories and subcategories are used to develop the *NCLEX test plan*, the content guidelines for the distribution of test questions. Question writers and the people who put the NCLEX together use the test plan and client needs categories to make sure that a full spectrum of nursing activities is covered in the NCLEX. Client needs categories appear in most NCLEX review and question-and-answer books, including this one. As a test-taker, you don't have to concern yourself with client needs categories. You'll see those categories for each question and answer in this book, but they'll be invisible on the actual NCLEX.

Guidelines for international nurses

In order to become eligible to work as a registered nurse (RN) in the United States, you will need to complete several steps. In addition to passing the NCLEX-RN, you may need to obtain a certificate and credentials evaluation from the Commission on Graduates of Foreign Nursing Schools (CGFNS®) and acquire a visa. Since requirements differ from state to state, it's important that you first contact the Board of Nursing in the state where you want to practice nursing.

CGFNS Certification Program

Most states require that you obtain CGFNS certification. This certification requires:

- a review and authentication of your credentials, including your nursing education, registration, and licensure
- a passing score on the CGFNS Qualifying Examination of nursing knowledge
- a passing score on an English language proficiency test.

In order to be eligible to take the CGFNS Qualifying Examination, you must complete a minimum number of classroom and clinical practice hours in medical-surgical nursing, maternal-neonatal nursing, pediatric nursing, and psychiatric and mental health nursing from a government-approved nursing school. You must also be registered as a first-level nurse in your country of education and currently hold a license as an RN in some jurisdiction.

The CGFNS Qualifying Examination is a paper and pencil test that includes 260 multiple-choice questions. It's administered under controlled testing conditions. Because the test is designed to predict your likelihood of successfully passing the NCLEX-RN exam, it's based on the NCLEX-RN test plan.

You may select from three English proficiency examinations: Test of English as a Foreign Language (TOEFL®), Test of English for International Communication (TOEIC®), or International English Language Testing System (IELTS). Each test has different passing scores, and the scores are valid for up to 2 years.

CGFNS credentials evaluation service

This evaluation is a comprehensive report that analyzes and compares your education and licensure with U.S. standards. It's prepared by the CGFNS for a state board of nursing, an immigration office, an employer, or a university. It requires that you complete an application, submit appropriate documentation, and pay a fee.

More information about the CGFNS certification program and credentials evaluation service is available at *www.cgfns.org*.

Visa

You can't legally immigrate to work in the United States without an occupational visa (temporary or permanent) from the U.S. Citizenship and Immigration Services (USCIS). The visa process is separate from the CGFNS certification process, although some of the same steps are involved. Some visas require prior CGFNS certification and a *VisaScreen*™ Certificate from the International Commission on Healthcare Professions. The *VisaScreen* program involves:

- a credentials review of your nursing education and current registration or licensure
- successful completion of either the CGFNS certification program or the NCLEX-RN to provide proof of nursing knowledge
- a passing score on an approved English language proficiency examination.

Once you successfully complete all parts of the *VisaScreen* program, you will receive a certificate to present to the USCIS. The visa-granting process can take up to a year.

You can obtain more detailed information about visa application at *www.uscis.gov*.

Client needs categories

Each question on the NCLEX is assigned a category based on client needs. This chart lists client needs categories and subcategories and the percentages of each type of question that appears on an NCLEX examination.

Category	Subcategories	Percentage of NCLEX questions
Safe, effective care environment	• Management of care • Safety and infection control	17% to 23% 9% to 15%
Health promotion and maintenance		6% to 12%
Psychosocial integrity		6% to 12%
Physiological integrity	• Basic care and comfort • Pharmacological and parenteral therapies • Reduction of risk potential • Physiological adaptation	6% to 12% 12% to 18% 9% to 15% 11% to 17%

Testing by computer

Like many standardized tests today, the NCLEX is administered by computer. That means you won't be filling in empty circles, sharpening pencils, or erasing frantically. It also means that you must become familiar with computer tests, if you aren't already. Fortunately, the skills required to take the NCLEX on a computer are simple enough to allow you to focus on the questions, not the keyboard.

Q&A

When you take the test, depending on the question format, you'll be presented with a question and four or more possible answers, a blank space in which to enter your answer, a figure on which you'll click the mouse to select the correct area of the figure, a series of charts or exhibits to view in order to select the correct response, items you must prioritize by dragging and dropping them in place, an audio recording to listen to in order to select the correct response, or a question and four graphic options.

Feeling smart? Think hard!

The NCLEX is a *computer-adaptive test*, meaning that the computer reacts to the answers you give, supplying more difficult questions if you answer correctly and slightly easier questions if you answer incorrectly. Each test is thus uniquely adapted to the individual test-taker.

I react to you!

A matter of time

You have a great deal of flexibility with the amount of time you spend on individual questions. The examination lasts a maximum of 6 hours, however, so don't waste time. If you fail to answer a set number of questions within 6 hours, the computer will determine that you lack minimum competency.

Most students have plenty of time to complete the test, so take as much time as you need to get the question right without wasting time. Keep moving at a decent pace to help maintain concentration.

Difficult items = Good news

If you find as you progress through the test that the questions seem to be increasingly difficult, it's a good sign. The more questions you answer correctly, the more difficult the questions become.

Some students, though, knowing that questions get progressively harder, focus on the degree of difficulty of subsequent questions to try to figure out if they're answering questions correctly. Avoid the temptation to do this, as this may get you off track.

The finish line

The computer test finishes when one of these events occurs:
- You demonstrate minimum competency, according to the computer program, which does so with 95% certainty that your ability exceeds the passing standard.
- You demonstrate a lack of minimum competency, according to the computer program.
- You've answered the maximum number of questions (265 total questions).
- You've used the maximum time allowed (6 hours).

The harder it gets, the better I do.

Unlocking the NCLEX® mystery

During the exam, the candidate will be required to respond to a variety of formats. These items may include multiple-choice, multiple-response, fill-in-the-blank calculations, drag-and-drop, and hotspots. All items may include multimedia, charts, tables, graphics, sound, or visuals. Certain strategies can help you understand and answer any type of NCLEX question.

Alternate formats

The first type of alternate-format item is the *multiple-response, multiple-choice question*. Unlike a traditional multiple-choice question, each multiple-response, multiple-choice question has more than one correct answer for every question, and it may contain more than four possible answer options. You'll recognize this type of question because it will ask you to select *all* answers that apply—not just the best answer (as may be requested in the more traditional multiple-choice questions).

No points for partials

Keep in mind that for each multiple-response, multiple-choice question, you must select at least one answer and you must select all correct answers for the item to be counted as correct. On the NCLEX, there's no partial credit in the scoring of these items.

Don't go blank!

The second type of alternate-format item is the *fill-in-the-blank*. These questions require you to provide the answer yourself, rather than select it from a list of options. You will perform a calculation, and then type your answer (a number without any words, units of measurement, commas, or spaces) in the blank space provided after the question. Rules for rounding are included in the question stem if appropriate. A calculator button is provided so you can easily do your calculations electronically.

Master that mouse!

The third type of alternate-format item is a question that asks you to identify an area on an illustration or graphic. For these so-called *"hotspot"* questions, the computerized exam will ask you to place your cursor and click over the correct area on an illustration. Try to be as precise as possible when marking the location. As with the fill-in-the-blanks, the identification questions on the computerized exam may require extremely precise answers to be considered correct.

Chart smarts

The fourth type of alternate-format item is the *chart/exhibit* format. Here you'll be given a problem, then a series of small screens containing additional information you'll need in order to answer the question. By clicking on the Tab button, you can access each screen in turn. Your answer can then be chosen from four multiple-choice answer options.

All in order

The fifth type of alternate-format item involves prioritizing or placing in correct order a series of statements, using a *drag-and-drop* technique. You'll decide which of the given options is first, click and hold it with the mouse, and then drag it into the first box given underneath and drop it into place. You'll repeat this process until you've placed all the available options in the lower boxes.

Now hear this!

The sixth alternate-format item type is the *audio item* format. You'll be given a set of headphones and you'll be asked to listen to an audio clip and select the correct answer from four options. You'll need to select the correct answer on the computer screen as you would with the traditional multiple-choice questions.

Picture perfect

The final alternate-format item type is the *graphic option* question. This varies from the exhibit format type because in the graphic option, your answer choices will be graphics, such as ECG strips. You'll have to select the appropriate graphic to answer the question presented.

The standard's still the standard

The NCSBN hasn't yet established a percentage of alternate-format items to be administered to each candidate. So relax; the standard, four-option, multiple-choice format questions compose the bulk of the test. (See *Sample NCLEX questions*, pages 10–12.)

Understanding the question

NCLEX questions are usually long. As a result, it's easy to feel overwhelmed with information. To focus on the question, apply proven strategies for answering NCLEX questions, including:
- determining what the question is asking
- determining relevant facts about the client
- rephrasing the question in your mind
- choosing the best option(s) before entering your answer.

Determine what the question is asking

Read the question twice. If the answer isn't apparent, rephrase the question in simpler, more personal terms. Breaking down the question into easier, less intimidating terms may help you to focus more accurately on the correct answer.

Give it a try

For example, a question might be, "A 74-year-old client with a history of heart failure is admitted to the coronary care unit with pulmonary edema. He's intubated and placed on a mechanical ventilator. Which parameter should the nurse monitor closely to assess the client's response to a bolus dose of furosemide (Lasix) I.V.?"

The options for this question—numbered from 1 to 4—may be:
1. Daily weight
2. 24-hour intake and output
3. Serum sodium levels
4. Hourly urine output

Sample NCLEX® questions

Sometimes, getting used to the test format is as important as knowing the material covered. Try your hand at these sample questions and you'll have a leg up when you take the real test!

Sample four-option, multiple-choice question

A client's arterial blood gas (ABG) results are as follows: pH, 7.16; $Paco_2$, 80 mm Hg; Pao_2, 46 mm Hg; HCO_3^-, 24 mEq/L; Sao_2, 81%. This ABG result represents which condition?

1. Metabolic acidosis
2. Metabolic alkalosis
3. Respiratory acidosis
4. Respiratory alkalosis

Correct answer: 3

Sample multiple-response, multiple-choice question

The nurse is caring for a 45-year-old married client who has undergone hemicolectomy for colon cancer. The client has two children. Which concepts about families should the nurse keep in mind when providing care for this client? Select all that apply.

1. Illness in one family member can affect all members.
2. Family roles don't change because of illness.
3. A family member may have more than one role in the family.
4. Children typically aren't affected by adult illness.
5. The effects of an illness on a family depend on the stage of the family's life cycle.
6. Changes in sleeping and eating patterns may be signs of stress in a family.

Correct answer: 1, 3, 5, 6

Sample fill-in-the-blank calculation question

An infant who weighs 8 kg is to receive ampicillin 25 mg/kg I.V. every 6 hours. How many milligrams should the nurse administer per dose? Record your answer using a whole number.

_____ milligrams

Correct answer: 200

Sample hotspot question

A client has a history of aortic stenosis. Identify the area where the nurse should place the stethoscope to best hear the murmur.

Correct answer:

Sample NCLEX® questions (continued)

Sample chart/exhibit question

A 3-year-old client is being treated for severe status asthmaticus. After reviewing the progress notes (shown below), the nurse should determine that this client is being treated for which condition?

Progress notes	
4/5/10	Pt. was acutely restless, diaphoretic, and with
0600	dyspnea at 0530. Dr. T. Smith notified and
	ordered ABG analysis. ABG drawn from ⓡ
	radial artery. Stat results as follows: pH 7.28,
	Paco2 55 mm Hg, HCO₃- 26 mEg/L. Dr. Smith
	with pt. now. ————— J. Collins, R.N.

1. Metabolic acidosis
2. Respiratory alkalosis
3. Respiratory acidosis
4. Metabolic alkalosis

Correct answer: 3

Sample drag-and-drop question

When teaching an antepartal client about the passage of the fetus through the birth canal during labor, the nurse describes the cardinal mechanisms of labor. Place these events in the sequence in which they occur. Use all the options.

1. Flexion
2. External rotation
3. Descent
4. Expulsion
5. Internal rotation
6. Extension

Correct answer:

3. Descent
1. Flexion
5. Internal rotation
6. Extension
2. External rotation
4. Expulsion

continued

Sample NCLEX® questions *(continued)*

Sample audio item question

Listen to the audio clip. What sound do you hear in the bases of this client with heart failure?

1. Crackles
2. Rhonchi
3. Wheezes
4. Pleural friction rub

Correct answer: 1

Sample graphic option question

Which electrocardiogram strip should the nurse document as sinus tachycardia?

Correct answer: 3

Hocus, focus on the question

Read the question again, ignoring all details except what's being asked. Focus on the last line of the question. It asks you to select the appropriate assessment for monitoring a client who received a bolus of furosemide I.V.

Determine what facts about the client are relevant

Next, sort out the relevant client information. Start by asking whether any of the information provided about the client isn't relevant. For instance, do you need to know that the client has been admitted to the coronary care unit? Probably not; his reaction to I.V. furosemide won't be affected by his location in the hospital.

Determine what you do know about the client. In the example, you know that:

- he just received an I.V. bolus of furosemide, a crucial fact
- he has pulmonary edema, the most fundamental aspect of the client's underlying condition
- he's intubated and placed on a mechanical ventilator, suggesting that his pulmonary edema is serious
- he's 74 years old and has a history of heart failure, a fact that may or may not be relevant.

Focusing on what the question is really asking can help you choose the correct answer.

Rephrase the question

After you've determined relevant information about the client and the question being asked, consider rephrasing the question to make it more clear. Eliminate jargon and put the question in simpler, more personal terms. Here's how you might rephrase the question in the example: "My client has pulmonary edema. He requires intubation and mechanical ventilation. He's 74 years old and has a history of heart failure. He received an I.V. bolus of furosemide. What assessment parameter should I monitor?"

Choose the best option

Armed with all the information you now have, it's time to select an option. You know that the client received an I.V. bolus of furosemide, a diuretic. You know that monitoring fluid intake and output is a key nursing intervention for a client taking a diuretic, a fact that eliminates options 1 and 3 (daily weight and serum sodium levels), narrowing the answer down to option 2 or 4 (24-hour intake and output or hourly urine output).

You also know that the drug was administered by I.V. bolus, suggesting a rapid effect. (In fact, furosemide administered by I.V. bolus takes effect almost immediately.) Monitoring the client's 24-hour intake and output would be appropriate for assessing the effects of repeated doses of furosemide. Hourly urine output, however, is most appropriate in this situation because it monitors the immediate effect of this rapid-acting drug.

Key strategies

Regardless of the type of question, four key strategies will help you determine the correct answer for each question. These strategies are:

- considering the nursing process
- referring to Maslow's hierarchy of needs
- reviewing patient safety
- reflecting on principles of therapeutic communication.

Nursing process

One of the ways to answer a question is to apply the nursing process. Steps in the nursing process include:
- assessment
- diagnosis
- planning
- implementation
- evaluation.

Say it 1,000 times: Studying for the NCLEX is fun... studying for the NCLEX is fun...

Process pointers

The nursing process may provide insights that help you analyze a question. According to the nursing process, assessment comes before analysis, which comes before planning, which comes before implementation, which comes before evaluation.

You're halfway to the correct answer when you encounter a four-option, multiple-choice question that asks you to assess the situation and then provides two assessment options and two implementation options. You can immediately eliminate the implementation options, which then gives you, at worst, a 50-50 chance of selecting the correct answer. Use the following sample question to apply the nursing process:

A client returns from an endoscopic procedure during which he was sedated. Before offering the client food, which action should the nurse take?
1. Assess the client's respiratory status.
2. Check the client's gag reflex.
3. Place the client in a side-lying position.
4. Have the client drink a few sips of water.

Assess before intervening

According to the nursing process, the nurse must assess a client before performing an intervention. Does the question indicate that the client has been properly assessed? No, it doesn't. Therefore, you can eliminate options 3 and 4 because they're both interventions.

That leaves options 1 and 2, both of which are assessments. Your nursing knowledge should tell you the correct answer—in this case, option 2. The sedation required for an endoscopic procedure may impair the client's gag reflex, so you would assess the gag reflex before giving food to the client to reduce the risk of aspiration and airway obstruction.

Watch phrasing

Why not select option 1, assessing the client's respiratory status? You might select this option, but the question is specifically asking about offering the client food, an action that wouldn't be taken if the client's respiratory status was at all compromised. In this case, you're making a judgment based on the phrase, "Before offering the client food." If the question was trying to test your knowledge of respiratory depression following an endoscopic procedure, it probably wouldn't mention a function—such as giving food to a client—that clearly occurs only after the client's respiratory status has been stabilized.

Maslow's hierarchy

Knowledge of Maslow's hierarchy of needs can be a vital tool for establishing priorities on the NCLEX. Maslow's theory states that physiological needs are the most basic human needs of all. Only after physiological needs have been met can safety concerns be addressed. Only after safety concerns are met can concerns involving love and belonging be addressed, and so forth. Apply the principles of Maslow's hierarchy of needs to the following sample question:

A client complains of severe pain 2 days after surgery. Which action should the nurse perform first?
1. Offer reassurance to the client that he will feel less pain tomorrow.
2. Allow the client time to verbalize his feelings.
3. Check the client's vital signs.
4. Administer an analgesic.

Phys before psych

In this example, two of the options—3 and 4—address physiological needs. Options 1 and 2 address psychosocial concerns. According to Maslow, physiological needs must be met before psychosocial needs, so you can eliminate options 1 and 2.

Final elimination

Now, use your nursing knowledge to choose the best answer from the two remaining options. In this case, option 3 is correct because the client's vital signs should be checked before administering an analgesic (assessment before intervention). When prioritizing according to Maslow's hierarchy, remember your ABCs—airway, breathing, circulation—to help you further prioritize. Check for a patent airway before addressing breathing. Check breathing before checking the health of the cardiovascular system.

Tricky, tricky

Just because an option appears on the NCLEX doesn't mean it's a viable choice for the client referred to in the question. Always examine your choice in light of your knowledge and experience. Ask yourself, "Does this choice make sense for this client?" Allow yourself to eliminate choices—even ones that might normally take priority—if they don't make sense for a particular client's situation.

Patient safety

As you might expect, patient safety takes high priority on the NCLEX. You'll encounter many questions that can be answered by asking yourself, "Which answer will best ensure the safety of this client?" Use patient safety criteria for situations involving laboratory values, drug administration, activities of daily living, or nursing care procedures.

Patient safety takes high priority on the NCLEX.

Client first, equipment second

You may encounter a question in which some options address the client and others address the equipment. When in doubt, select an option relating to the client; never place equipment before a client.

For instance, suppose a question asks what the nurse should do first when entering a client's room where an infusion pump alarm is sounding. If two options deal with the infusion pump, one with the infusion tubing, and another with the client's catheter insertion site, select the one relating to the client's catheter insertion site. Always check the client first; the equipment can wait.

Therapeutic communication

Some NCLEX questions focus on the nurse's ability to communicate effectively with the client. Therapeutic communication incorporates verbal or nonverbal responses and involves:
• listening to the client
• understanding the client's needs
• promoting clarification and insight about the client's condition.

Room for improvement

Like other NCLEX questions, those dealing with therapeutic communication require choosing the best response. First, eliminate options that indicate the use of poor therapeutic communication techniques, such as those in which the nurse:
• tells the client what to do without regard to the client's feelings or desires (the "do this" response)
• asks a question that can be answered "yes" or "no," or with another one-syllable response
• seeks reasons for the client's behavior
• implies disapproval of the client's behavior
• offers false reassurances
• attempts to interpret the client's behavior rather than allowing the client to verbalize his own feelings
• offers a response that focuses on the nurse, not the client.

I said that some exam questions will focus on good therapeutic COMMUNICATION!

Ah, that's better!

When answering NCLEX questions, look for responses that:
• allow the client time to think and reflect
• encourage the client to talk
• encourage the client to describe a particular experience
• reflect that the nurse has listened to the client, such as through paraphrasing the client's response.

Avoiding pitfalls

Even the most knowledgeable students can get tripped up on certain NCLEX questions. (See *A tricky question*.) Students commonly cite three areas that can be difficult for unwary test-takers:

👆 knowing the difference between the NCLEX and the "real world"

✌️ delegating care

🤟 knowing laboratory values.

Remember, this is the real world. The NCLEX may not always reflect what happens in it.

NCLEX® versus the real world

Some students who take the NCLEX have extensive practical experience in health care. For example, many test-takers have worked as licensed practical nurses or nursing assistants. In one of those capacities, test-takers might have been exposed to less than optimum clinical practice and may carry those experiences over to the NCLEX.

However, the NCLEX is a textbook examination—not a test of clinical skills. Take the NCLEX with the understanding that what happens in the real world may differ from what the NCLEX and your nursing school say should happen.

Advice from the experts

A tricky question

The NCLEX occasionally asks a particular kind of question called the "further teaching" question, which involves patient-teaching situations. These questions can be tricky. You'll have to choose the response that suggests that the patient has *not* learned the correct information. Here's an example:

> 37. A client undergoes a total hip replacement. Which statement by the client indicates that he requires further teaching?
>
> 1. "I'll need to keep several pillows between my legs at night."
> 2. "I'll need to remember not to cross my legs. It's such a bad habit."
> 3. "The occupational therapist is showing me how to use a 'sock puller' to help me get dressed."
> 4. "I don't know if I'll be able to get off that low toilet seat at home by myself."

The answer you should choose here is option 4 because it indicates that the client has a poor understanding of the precautions required after a total hip replacement and that he needs further teaching. *Remember:* If you see the phrase *further teaching* or *further instruction*, you're looking for a wrong answer by the patient.

Don't take shortcuts

If you've had practical experience in health care, you may know a quicker way to perform a procedure or tricks to get by when you don't have the right equipment. Situations such as staff shortages may force you to improvise. On the NCLEX, such scenarios can lead to trouble. Always check your practical experiences against textbook nursing care, taking care to select the response that follows the textbook.

Delegating care

On the NCLEX, you may encounter questions that assess your ability to delegate care. Delegating care involves coordinating the efforts of other health care workers to provide effective care for your client. On the NCLEX, you may be asked to assign duties to:
• licensed practical nurses or licensed vocational nurses
• direct care workers, such as nursing assistants and personal care aides
• other support staff, such as nutrition assistants and housekeepers.
    In addition, you'll be asked to decide when to notify a physician, a social worker, or another hospital staff member. In each case, you'll have to decide when, where, and how to delegate.

Shoulds and shouldn'ts

As a general rule, it's okay to delegate actions that involve stable clients or standard, unchanging procedures. Bathing, feeding, dressing, and transferring clients are examples of procedures that can be delegated.
    Be careful not to delegate complicated or complex activities. In addition, don't delegate activities that involve assessment, evaluation, or your own nursing judgment. On the NCLEX and in the real world, these duties fall squarely on your shoulders. Make sure that you take primary responsibility for assessing and evaluating the client and for making decisions about the client's care. Never hand off those responsibilities to someone with less training.

Calling in reinforcements

Deciding when to notify a physician, a social worker, or another hospital staff member is an important element of nursing care. On the NCLEX, however, choices that involve notifying the physician are usually incorrect. Remember that the NCLEX wants to see you, the nurse, at work.
    If you're sure the correct answer is to notify the physician, though, make sure the client's safety has been addressed before notifying a physician or another staff member. On the NCLEX, the client's safety has a higher priority than notifying other health care providers.

Knowing laboratory values

Some NCLEX questions supply laboratory results without indicating normal levels. As a result, answering questions involving laboratory values requires you to have the normal range of the most common laboratory values memorized to make an informed decision. (See *Normal laboratory values*.)

Normal laboratory values

• Blood urea nitrogen: 10 to 20 mg/dl

• Creatinine: 0.6 to 1.5 mg/dl

• Sodium: 135 to 145 mmol/L

• Potassium: 3.5 to 5.5 mEq/L

• Chloride: 97 to 110 mmol/L

• Glucose (fasting plasma): 60 to 110 mg/dl

• Hemoglobin
  Male: 13.8 to 17.2 g/dl
  Female: 12.1 to 15.1 g/dl

• Hematocrit
  Male: 40.7% to 50.3%
  Female: 36.1% to 44.3%

As you count down the weeks, days, and finally hours to the NCLEX, refer back to the information in this chapter. It's a recipe for NCLEX success!

Chapter 2
Passing the NCLEX®

Just the facts

In this chapter, you'll learn:

• how to properly prepare for the NCLEX®

• how to concentrate during difficult study times

• ways to make more effective use of your time

• why creative studying strategies can enhance learning

• how to get the most out of NCLEX practice tests.

Most students pass the NCLEX on the first try. I know you can, too!

Study preparations

If you're like most people preparing to take the test, you're probably feeling nervous, anxious, or concerned. Keep in mind that most test-takers pass the NCLEX® the first time around.

Passing the test won't happen by accident, though; you'll need to prepare carefully and efficiently. To help jump-start your preparations:

• determine your strengths and weaknesses

• create a study schedule

• set realistic goals

• find an effective study space

• think positively

• start studying sooner rather than later.

Strengths and weaknesses

Most students recognize that, even at the end of their nursing studies, they know more about some topics than others. Because the NCLEX covers a broad range of material, you should make some decisions about how intensively you'll review each topic.

Make a list

Base those decisions on a list. Divide a sheet of paper in half vertically. On one side, list topics you think you know well. On the other side, list topics you need to review. Pay no attention if one side is longer than the other. When you're done studying, you'll feel strong in every area.

Where the list comes from

To make sure your list reflects a comprehensive view of all the areas you studied in school, look at the contents page in the front of this book. For each topic listed, place it in the "know well" column or "needs review" column. Separating content areas this way shows immediately which topics need less study time and which need more time.

Scheduling study time

Study when you're most alert. Most people can identify a period of the day when they feel most alert. If you feel most alert and energized in the morning, for example, set aside sections of time in the morning for topics that need a lot of review. Then you can use the evening, a time of lesser alertness, for topics that need some refreshing. The opposite is true as well; if you're more alert in the evening, study difficult topics at that time.

I'll cover difficult topics in the morning when I'm more alert.

What and when

Set up a basic schedule for studying. Using a calendar or organizer, determine how much time remains before you'll take the NCLEX. (See *2 to 3 months before the NCLEX*, page 21.) Fill in the remaining days with specific times and topics to be studied. For example, you might schedule the respiratory system on a Tuesday morning and the GI system that afternoon. Remember to schedule difficult topics during your most alert times.

Keep in mind that you shouldn't fill each day with studying. Be realistic and set aside time for normal activities. Try to create ample study time before the NCLEX and then stick to the schedule. Allow some extra time in the schedule in case you get behind or come across a topic that requires extra review.

Keep goals manageable

Part of creating a schedule means setting goals you can accomplish. You no doubt studied a great deal in nursing school, and by now you have a sense of your own capabilities. Ask yourself, "How much can I cover in a day?" Set that amount of time aside and then stay on

To-do list
2 to 3 months before the NCLEX®

With 2 to 3 months remaining before you plan to take the examination, take these steps:
- Establish a study schedule. Set aside ample time to study but also leave time for social activities, exercise, family or personal responsibilities, and other matters.
- Become knowledgeable about the NCLEX-RN examination, its content, the types of questions it asks, and the testing format.
- Begin studying your notes, texts, and other study materials.
- Take some NCLEX practice questions to help you diagnose strengths and weaknesses as well as to become familiar with NCLEX-style questions.

This chair invites slacking, not studying! You should find a chair that encourages good posture instead.

task. You'll feel better about yourself—and your chances of passing the NCLEX—when you meet your goals regularly.

Study space

Find a space conducive to effective learning and then study there. Whatever you do, don't study with a television on in the room. Instead, find a quiet, inviting study space that:
- is located in a quiet, convenient place, away from normal traffic patterns
- contains a solid chair that encourages good posture (Avoid studying in bed; you'll be more likely to fall asleep and not accomplish your goals.)
- uses comfortable, soft lighting with which you can see clearly without eye strain
- has a temperature between 65° and 70° F
- contains flowers or green plants, familiar photos or paintings, and easy access to soft, instrumental background music.

Accentuate the positive

Consider taping positive messages around your study space. Make signs with words of encouragement, such as, "You can do it!" "Keep studying!" and "Remember the goal!" These upbeat messages can help keep you going when your attention begins to waver.

Maintaining concentration

When you're faced with reviewing the amount of information covered by the NCLEX, it's easy to become distracted and lose your concentration. When you lose concentration, you make less effective use of valuable study time. To help stay focused, keep these tips in mind:

- Alternate the order of the subjects you study during the day to add variety to your study.
- Approach your studying with enthusiasm, sincerity, and determination.
- Once you've decided to study, begin immediately. Don't let anything interfere with your thought processes once you've begun.
- Concentrate on accomplishing one task at a time to the exclusion of everything else.
- Don't try to do two things at once, such as studying and watching television or conversing with friends.
- Work continuously without interruption for a while but don't study for such a long period that the whole experience becomes grueling or boring.
- Allow time for periodic breaks to give yourself a change of pace. Use these breaks to ease your transition into studying a new topic.
- When studying in the evening, wind down from your studies slowly. Don't progress directly from studying to sleeping.

Taking care of yourself

Never neglect your physical and mental well-being in favor of longer study hours. Maintaining physical and mental health is critical for success in taking the NCLEX. (See *4 to 6 weeks before the NCLEX*.)

A few simple rules

You can increase your likelihood of passing the test by following these simple health rules:

- Get plenty of rest. You can't think deeply or concentrate for long periods when you're tired.
- Drink enough noncaffeinated beverages. Mild dehydration increases the effort required to concentrate and reason while distracting attention through feelings of fatigue and thirst.
- Eat nutritious meals. Maintaining your energy level is impossible when you're undernourished.

To-do list

4 to 6 weeks before the NCLEX®

With 4 to 6 weeks remaining before you plan to take the examination, take these steps:

- Focus on your areas of weakness. That way, you'll have time to review these areas again before the test date.
- Find a study partner or form a study group.
- Take a practice test to gauge your skill level early.
- Take time to eat, sleep, exercise, and socialize to avoid burnout.

• Exercise regularly. Regular exercise, preferably 30 minutes daily, helps you work harder and think more clearly. As a result, you'll study more efficiently and increase the likelihood of success.

Memory powers, activate!

If you're having trouble concentrating but would rather push through than take a break, try making your studying more active by reading out loud. Active studying can renew your powers of concentration. By reading review material out loud to yourself, you're engaging your ears as well as your eyes—and making your studying a more active process. Hearing the material out loud also fosters memory and subsequent recall.

You can also rewrite in your own words a few of the more difficult concepts you're reviewing. Explaining these concepts in writing forces you to think through the material and can jump-start your memory.

A short jog now will help us concentrate later.

Study schedule

When you were creating your schedule, you might have asked yourself, "How long should I study? One hour at a stretch? Two hours? Three?" To make the best use of your study time, you'll need to answer those questions.

Optimum study time

Consider studying in 20- to 30-minute intervals with a short break in between. You remember the material you study at the beginning and end of a session best and tend to remember less material studied in the middle of the session. The total length of time in each study session depends on you and the amount of material you need to cover.

To thine own self be true

So what's the answer? It doesn't matter as long as you determine what's best for *you*. At the beginning of your NCLEX study schedule, try study periods of varying lengths. Pay close attention to those that seem more successful.

Remember that you're a trained nurse who is competent at assessment. Think of yourself as a patient, and assess your own progress. Then implement the strategy that works best for you.

I've found that hour-and-a-half sessions work best for me.

Finding time to study

So does that mean that short sections of time are useless? Not at all. We all have spaces in our day that might otherwise be dead time. (See *1 week before the NCLEX*.) These are perfect times to review for the NCLEX but not to cover new material because by the time you get deep into new material, your time will be over. Always keep some flash cards or a small notebook handy for situations when you have a few extra minutes.

You'll be amazed how many short sessions you can find in a day and how much reviewing you can do in 5 minutes. The following places offer short stretches of time you can use:

- eating breakfast
- waiting for, or riding on, a train or bus
- waiting in line at the bank, post office, bookstore, or other places
- using exercise equipment, such as a treadmill.

Creative studying

Even when you study in a perfect study space and concentrate better than ever, studying for the NCLEX can get a little, well, dull. Even people with terrific study habits occasionally feel bored or sluggish. That is why it's important to have some creative tricks in your study bag to liven up your studying during those down times.

Creative studying doesn't have to be hard work. It involves making efforts to alter your study habits a bit. Some techniques that might help include studying with a partner or group and creating flash cards or other audiovisual study tools.

Study partners

Studying with a partner or group of students (3 or 4 students at most) can be an excellent way to energize your studying. Working with a partner allows you to test each other on the material you've reviewed. Your partner can give you encouragement and motivation. Perhaps most important, working with a partner can provide a welcome break from solitary studying.

Be choosy

Exercise some care when choosing a study partner or assembling a study group. A partner who doesn't

To-do list

1 week before the NCLEX®

With 1 week remaining before the NCLEX examination, take these steps:
- Take a review test to measure your progress.
- Record key ideas and principles on note cards or audiotapes.
- Rest, eat well, and avoid thinking about the examination during nonstudy times.
- Treat yourself to one special event. You've been working hard, and you deserve it!

Find a partner with similar goals and strengths. But remember to stay focused!

fit your needs won't help you make the most of your study time. Look for a partner who:

- possesses similar goals to yours. For example, someone taking the NCLEX at approximately the same date who feels the same sense of urgency as you do might make an excellent partner.
- possesses about the same level of knowledge as you. Tutoring someone can sometimes help you learn, but partnering should be give-and-take so both partners can gain knowledge.
- can study without excess chatting or interruptions. Socializing is an important part of creative study, but remember, you've still got to pass the NCLEX—so stay serious!

Audiovisual tools

Flash cards and other audiovisual tools foster retention and make learning and reviewing fun.

Flash Gordon? No, it's Flash Card!

Flash cards can provide you with an excellent study tool. The process of writing material on a flash card will help you remember it. In addition, flash cards are small and easily portable, perfect for those 5-minute slivers of time that show up during the day.

Creating a flash card should be fun. Use magic markers, highlighters, and other colorful tools to make them visually stimulating. The more effort you put into creating your flash cards, the better you'll remember the material contained on the cards.

Other visual tools

Flowcharts, drawings, diagrams, and other image-oriented study aids can also help you learn material more effectively. Substituting images for text can be a great way to give your eyes a break and recharge your brain. Remember to use vivid colors to make your creations visually engaging.

Charts, drawings, and diagrams make concepts less puzzling.

Hear's the thing

If you learn more effectively when you hear information rather than see it, consider recording key ideas using a handheld tape recorder. Recording information helps promote memory because you say the information aloud when taping and then listen to it when playing it back. Like flash cards, tapes are portable and perfect for those short study periods during the day. (See *The day before the NCLEX.*)

To-do list

The day before the NCLEX®

With 1 day before the NCLEX examination, take these steps:

- Drive to the test site, review traffic patterns, and find out where to park. If your route to the test site occurs during heavy traffic or if you're expecting bad weather, set aside extra time to ensure prompt arrival.
- Do something relaxing during the day.
- Avoid concentrating on the test.
- Eat and drink well and avoid dwelling on the NCLEX during nonstudy periods.
- Call a supportive friend or relative for some last-minute words of encouragement.
- Get plenty of rest the night before and allow for plenty of time in the morning.

Practice tests

Practice questions should constitute an important part of your NCLEX study strategy. Practice questions can improve your studying by helping you review material and familiarizing yourself with the exact style of questions you'll encounter on the NCLEX.

Practice at the beginning

Consider working through some practice questions as soon as you begin studying for the NCLEX. For example, you might try a half-dozen questions from each chapter in this book.

If you score well, you probably know the material contained in that chapter fairly well and can spend less time reviewing that particular topic. If you have trouble with the questions, spend extra study time on that topic.

You're getting there

Practice questions can also provide an excellent means of marking your progress. Don't worry if you have trouble answering the first few practice questions you take; you'll need time to adjust to the way the questions are asked. Eventually, you'll become accustomed to the question format and begin to focus more on the questions themselves.

If you make practice questions a regular part of your study regimen, you'll be able to notice areas in which you're improving. You can then adjust your study time accordingly.

Practice makes perfect

As you near the examination date, continue to answer practice questions, but also set aside time to take an entire NCLEX practice test. (We've included six at the back of this book.) That way, you'll know exactly what to expect. (See *The day of the NCLEX*.) The more you know ahead of time, the better you're likely to do on the NCLEX.

Taking an entire practice test is also a way to gauge your progress. When you find yourself answering questions correctly, it will give you the confidence you need to conquer the real NCLEX.

Because I've taken lots of practice tests, I understand how the questions work.

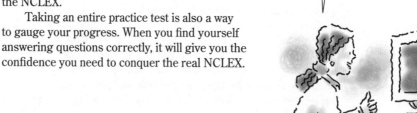

To-do list

The day of the NCLEX®

On the day of the NCLEX examination, take these steps:
- Get up early.
- Wear comfortable clothes, preferably with layers you can adjust to fit the room temperature.
- Drink a glass of water and eat a small nutritious breakfast.
- Leave your house early.
- Arrive at the test site early with the required paperwork in hand.
- Avoid looking at your notes as you wait for your computer test.
- Listen carefully to the instructions given before entering the test room.
- Succeed, succeed, *succeed!*

Quick quiz

1. The best time to study is:
   A. in the morning.
   B. early in the evening.
   C. after eating a full meal.
   D. when you feel most alert.

Answer: D. Study when you're most alert. If you feel most alert and energized in the morning, for example, set aside sections of time in the morning for topics that need a lot of review.

2. The temperature of the ideal study area should be between:
   A. 60° and 65° F.
   B. 65° and 70° F.
   C. 70° and 75° F.
   D. 75° and 80° F.

Answer: B. The ideal study area has a temperature between 65° and 70° F.

3. To help you maintain concentration durin g long study periods, recommended study strategies include:
   A. Study the topics you find most interesting first, followed by the topics you find least interesting.
   B. Study the topics you find least interesting first, followed by the topics you find most interesting.
   C. Alternate the order of the subjects you study during the day.
   D. Study only the topics you find least interesting; you'll remember the others.

Answer: C. Alternating the order of the subjects you study during the day adds variety to your study and helps you remain focused and make the most of your study time.

4. When selecting a study partner, choose one who:
   A. possesses similar goals as you.
   B. is highly social and will keep you entertained.
   C. isn't as knowledgeable as you so you can tutor him.
   D. likes to take a lot of breaks.

Answer: A. A partner who doesn't fit your needs won't help you make the most of your study time. Look for a partner who has similar goals to yours, possesses about the same level of knowledge as you, and won't spend too much time socializing.

Scoring

 If you answered all four questions correctly, wow! We hope the exam is ready for *you*!

⭐⭐ If you answered three questions correctly, terrific! You're cruising toward an exam day victory!

⭐ If you answered fewer than three questions correctly, fear not. By the time you're done practicing, you'll be an NCLEX success!

Part II   Care of the adult

If you'd like to rummage through a Web site dedicated to cardiovascular disorders, check out the American Heart Association's at **www.americanheart.org**.

1. A client's electrocardiogram (ECG) is showing ST elevation in leads V_2, V_3, and V_4. Which artery is most likely to be occluded?
1. Circumflex artery
2. Internal mammary artery
3. Left anterior descending artery
4. Right coronary artery

2. A nurse on a telemetry unit teaches a client diagnosed with acute coronary syndrome about coronary blood flow. Which of the following statements made by the nurse is correct?
1. Most of the blood flow to coronary arteries is supplied during inspiration.
2. Most of the blood flow to coronary arteries is supplied during diastole.
3. Blood flow to coronary arteries is related to breathing patterns.
4. A large portion of blood flow occurs to coronary arteries during systole.

3. Which of the following illnesses, if stated by a client, would indicate that he understands the leading cause of death in the United States?
1. Cancer
2. Coronary artery disease (CAD)
3. Liver failure
4. Renal failure

4. A client is admitted to the telemetry floor with acute chest pain radiating down his left arm. The nurse anticipates that which of the following laboratory studies would be ordered to evaluate myocardial damage? Select all that apply.
1. Hemoglobin and hematocrit
2. Serum glucose
3. Creatinine phosphokinase (CPK)
4. Troponin T and troponin I
5. Myoglobin
6. Blood urea nitrogen (BUN)

Different arteries supply my different sections with the blood I need to stay healthy.

Stop and think! Although all of the answers relate to CAD, only one answer is correct.

1. 3. The left anterior descending artery is the primary source of blood for the anterior wall of the heart. The circumflex artery supplies the lateral wall, the internal mammary artery supplies the mammary, and the right coronary artery supplies the inferior wall of the heart. The ST elevation in leads V_2, V_3, and V_4 suggests an anterior-wall myocardial infarction.

CN: Physiological integrity; CNS: Physiological adaptation; CL: Analysis

2. 2. Although the coronary arteries may receive a minute portion of blood during systole, most of the blood flow to coronary arteries is supplied during diastole. Breathing patterns are irrelevant to blood flow.

CN: Physiological integrity; CNS: Physiological adaptation; CL: Application

3. 2. CAD accounts for 30% of all deaths in the United States. Cancer accounts for approximately 20%. Liver failure and renal failure account for less than 10% of all deaths in the United States.

CN: Health promotion and maintenance; CNS: None; CL: Analysis

4. 3, 4, and 5. Levels of CPK, troponin T, and troponin I rise because of cellular damage. Myoglobin elevation is an early indicator of myocardial damage. Hemoglobin, hematocrit, and BUN levels do not provide information related to myocardial ischemia.

CN: Health promotion and maintenance; CNS: Prevention and early detection of disease; CL: Application

5. A nurse is teaching a client about atherosclerosis. The nurse determines further teaching is necessary when the client makes which of the following statements?
1. Plaques obstruct the coronary artery.
2. Plaques obstruct the vein.
3. Hardened vessels can't dilate to allow blood to flow through.
4. Atherosclerosis can cause angina.

6. The nurse is assessing a client with angina pectoris. Which of the following are characteristics of the substernal chest pain that occurs with this condition? Select all that apply.
1. Occurs without cause
2. Radiates to the left arm
3. Lasts less than 15 minutes
4. Usually occurs in the morning
5. Is relieved by rest and nitroglycerine
6. Is precipitated by exertion or stress

> Exercise does wonders for me!

7. The nurse is reviewing a client's lab work to determine if a risk for coronary artery disease (CAD) is present. The nurse is most concerned when the results identify which of the following?
1. HDL = 100 mg/dl
2. LDL = 140 mg/dl
3. VLDL = 20%
4. Total cholesterol = 240 mg/dl

8. A client is experiencing signs and symptoms of coronary artery disease. What should be the nurse's <u>first</u> priority?
1. Decrease anxiety.
2. Enhance myocardial oxygenation.
3. Administer sublingual nitroglycerin.
4. Educate the client about his symptoms.

> Conservative methods of treatment should always be your first course of action.

9. Medical management of coronary artery disease (CAD) has been discussed with a client. The nurse anticipates that management will include which of the following?
1. Cardiac catheterization
2. Coronary artery bypasses surgery
3. Oral medication administration
4. Percutaneous transluminal coronary angioplasty

5. 2. Arteries, not veins, supply the coronary arteries with oxygen and other nutrients. Atherosclerosis is a direct result of plaque formation in the artery. Hardened vessels can't dilate properly and, therefore, constrict blood flow and oxygen, causing angina.
CN: Physiological integrity; CNS: Physiological adaptation; CL: Analysis

6. 2, 3, 5, and 6. Angina pectoris is a temporary imbalance between the coronary artery's ability to supply oxygen and the cardiac muscle's demand for oxygen. The substernal chest pain that occurs in angina radiates to the left arm, is precipitated by exertion or stress, is relieved by rest or nitroglycerin, and lasts less than 15 minutes. Myocardial infarction occurs when myocardial tissue is abruptly and severely deprived of oxygen. The substernal chest pain that occurs in myocardial infarction radiates to the left arm, back, or jaw; occurs without cause, usually in the morning; is relieved only by opioids; and lasts 30 minutes or longer.
CN: Physiological integrity; CNS: Physiological adaptation; CL: Analysis

7. 4. Cholesterol levels above 240 mg/dl are considered excessive. They require dietary restriction and perhaps medication. Exercise also helps reduce cholesterol levels. The other levels listed are all nationally accepted levels for cholesterol and carry a lesser risk of CAD.
CN: Physiological integrity; CNS: Reduction of risk potential; CL: Comprehension

8. 2. Enhancing myocardial oxygenation is always the first priority when a client exhibits signs or symptoms of cardiac compromise. Without adequate oxygen, the myocardium suffers damage. Sublingual nitroglycerin is administered to treat acute angina, but its administration isn't the first priority. Although educating the client and decreasing anxiety are important in care delivery, neither are priorities when a client is compromised.
CN: Physiological integrity; CNS: Physiological adaptation; CL: Application

9. 3. Oral medication administration is a non-invasive medical management for CAD. Cardiac catheterization isn't a treatment but a diagnostic tool. Coronary artery bypass surgery and percutaneous transluminal coronary angioplasty are invasive, surgical treatments.
CN: Physiological integrity; CNS: Physiological adaptation; CL: Analysis

10. A client's electrocardiogram shows ST elevation in leads II, III, and aV$_F$, suggesting occlusion of the right coronary artery. The client asks the nurse what area of the heart this has affected. What is the nurse's best response?
1. Anterior
2. Apical
3. Inferior
4. Lateral

11. A client with no history of cardiovascular disease comes to the ambulatory clinic with flu-like symptoms. The client suddenly complains of chest pain. What is the most important question for the nurse to ask the client?
1. "Can you describe the pain to me?"
2. "Have you ever had this pain before?"
3. "Does the pain get worse when you breathe in?"
4. "Can you rate the pain on a scale of 1 to 10, with 10 being the worst?"

12. Prior to administration of Lanoxin (digoxin), the nurse must obtain the apical pulse. Where does the nurse place the stethoscope?
1. Left fifth intercostal space, midaxillary line
2. Left fifth intercostal space, midclavicular line
3. Left second intercostal space, midclavicular line
4. Left seventh intercostal space, midclavicular line

13. A client describes knifelike chest pain that increases in intensity with inspiration to the nurse. The nurse is aware that the most likely origin of pain is:
1. cardiac
2. gastrointestinal
3. musculoskeletal
4. pulmonary

14. While assessing a client's heart sounds, the nurse auscultates a murmur at the second left intercostal space along the left sternal border. Which valve is most likely involved?
1. Aortic
2. Mitral
3. Pulmonic
4. Tricuspid

Did someone murmur something?

10. 3. The right coronary artery supplies the right ventricle, or the inferior portion of the heart. Therefore, occlusion could produce an infarction in that area. The right coronary artery doesn't supply the anterior portion (left ventricle), lateral portion (some of the left ventricle and the left atrium), or apical portion (left ventricle) of the heart.
CN: Physiological integrity; CNS: Physiological adaptation; CL: Application

11. 3. Chest pain is assessed by using the standard pain assessment parameters such as characteristics, location, duration, intensity, precipitating factors, and associated symptoms. Options 1, 2, and 4 may or may not help discriminate the cause of pain. If the pain is pleural, it usually worsens on inspiration.
CN: Physiological integrity; CNS: Physiological adaptation; CL: Analysis

12. 2. The correct landmark for obtaining an apical pulse is the left fifth intercostal space in the midclavicular line. This is the point of maximum impulse and the location of the left ventricular apex. The left second intercostal space in the midclavicular line is where pulmonic sounds are auscultated. Normally, heart sounds aren't heard in the midaxillary line or the seventh intercostal space in the midclavicular line.
CN: Physiological integrity; CNS: Basic care and comfort; CL: Application

13. 4. Pulmonary pain is generally described by these symptoms. Musculoskeletal pain only increases with movement. Cardiac and gastrointestinal pains don't change with respiration.
CN: Physiological integrity; CNS: Physiological adaptation; CL: Analysis

14. 3. Abnormalities of the pulmonic valve are auscultated at the second left intercostal space along the left sternal border. Aortic valve abnormalities are heard at the second intercostal space, to the right of the sternum. Mitral valve abnormalities are heard at the fifth intercostal space in the midclavicular line. Tricuspid valve abnormalities are heard at the third and fourth intercostal spaces along the sternal border.
CN: Physiological integrity; CNS: Physiological adaptation; CL: Application

15. The nurse is caring for a client receiving digoxin (Lanoxin). Which of the following manifestations correlate with a digoxin level of 2.3 ng/dl? Select all that apply.
1. Nausea
2. Drowsiness
3. Photophobia
4. Increased appetite
5. Increased energy level
6. Seeing halos around bright objects

15. 1, 2, 3, and 6. Digoxin is a cardiac glycoside used to manage and treat heart failure, control ventricular rate in clients with atrial fibrillation, and treat and prevent recurrent paroxysmal atrial tachycardia. The therapeutic range of digoxin is 0.8 to 2.0 ng/dl. Signs of toxicity include gastrointestinal disturbances, including anorexia, nausea, and vomiting; neurological abnormalities such as fatigue, headache, depression, weakness, drowsiness, confusion, and nightmares; facial pain; personality changes; and ocular disturbances such as photophobia, halos around bright lights, and yellow or green color perception.
CN: Physiological integrity; CNS: Physiological adaptation; CL: Analysis

16. A client with a myocardial infarction asks the nurse why he is receiving morphine. What is the best response by the nurse?
1. To sedate the client
2. To decrease the client's pain
3. To decrease the client's anxiety
4. To decrease oxygen demand on the client's heart

16. 4. Morphine is administered because it decreases myocardial oxygen demand. Morphine will also decrease pain and anxiety while causing sedation, but it isn't primarily given for those reasons.
CN: Physiological integrity; CNS: Pharmacological and parenteral therapies; CL: Application

17. In caring for a client with cardiac problems, the nurse must know that the condition most likely responsible for myocardial infarction (MI) is which of the following?
1. Aneurysm
2. Heart failure
3. Coronary artery thrombosis
4. Renal failure

17. 3. Coronary artery thrombosis causes an occlusion of the artery, leading to myocardial death. An aneurysm is an outpouching of a vessel and doesn't cause an MI. Heart failure is usually the result of an MI. Renal failure can be associated with MI but isn't a direct cause.
CN: Physiological integrity; CNS: Physiological adaptation; CL: Analysis

18. The nurse is aware that the supplemental medication most frequently ordered in conjunction with furosemide (Lasix) is:
1. chloride.
2. digoxin.
3. potassium.
4. sodium.

18. 3. Supplemental potassium is given with furosemide because of the potassium loss that occurs as a result of this diuretic. Chloride and sodium aren't lost during diuresis. Digoxin acts to increase contractility but isn't given routinely with furosemide.
CN: Physiological integrity; CNS: Pharmacological and parenteral therapies; CL: Analysis

19. In order to anticipate problems in a client following a myocardial infarction (MI), the nurse should understand that which type of physiological changes will increase serum glucose levels and free fatty acid production?
1. Electrophysiological
2. Hematological
3. Mechanical
4. Metabolic

It's important to know what physiologic changes occur in your client after a heart attack.

19. 4. Both glucose and fatty acids are metabolites whose levels increase after an MI. Mechanical changes are those that affect the pumping action of the heart, and electrophysiological changes affect conduction. Hematological changes would affect the blood.
CN: Physiological integrity; CNS: Physiological adaptation; CL: Application

CN: Client needs category   CNS: Client needs subcategory   CL: Cognitive level

20. The nurse auscultates a third heart sound (S_3) while assessing her client. The nurse is aware that this results from:
1. ventricular dilation.
2. systemic hypertension.
3. aortic valve malfunction.
4. increased atrial contractions.

21. After an anterior-wall myocardial infarction (MI), which problem is indicated by auscultation of crackles in the lungs?
1. Left-sided heart failure
2. Pulmonic valve malfunction
3. Right-sided heart failure
4. Tricuspid valve malfunction

Twenty questions done! Good job!

22. A client who is being evaluated for myocardial infarction (MI) asks the nurse which diagnostic tool is <u>most commonly</u> used to determine the location of myocardial damage. The best response by the nurse is:
1. cardiac catheterization.
2. cardiac enzymes.
3. echocardiogram.
4. electrocardiogram (ECG).

Prioritize!

23. What is the <u>first</u> intervention for the nurse to implement for a client experiencing myocardial infarction (MI)?
1. Administer morphine.
2. Administer oxygen.
3. Administer sublingual nitroglycerin.
4. Obtain an electrocardiogram (ECG).

20. 1. Rapid filling of the ventricle causes vasodilation that is auscultated as S_3. Systemic hypertension or increased atrial contraction can result in a fourth heart sound. Aortic valve malfunction is heard as a murmur.
CN: Health promotion and maintenance; CNS: None; CL: Analysis

21. 1. The left ventricle is responsible for most of the cardiac output. An anterior-wall MI may result in a decrease in left ventricular function. When the left ventricle doesn't function properly, resulting in left-sided heart failure, fluid accumulates in the interstitial and alveolar spaces in the lungs and causes crackles. Pulmonic and tricuspid valve malfunction causes right-sided heart failure.
CN: Physiological integrity; CNS: Physiological adaptation; CL: Analysis

22. 4. The ECG is the quickest, most accurate, and most widely used tool to determine the location of myocardial infarction (MI). Cardiac catheterization is an invasive study for determining coronary artery disease and may also indicate the location of myocardial damage, but the study may not be performed immediately. Cardiac enzymes are used to diagnose MI but can't determine the location. An echocardiogram is used most widely to view myocardial wall function after an MI has been diagnosed.
CN: Physiological integrity; CNS: Reduction of risk potential; CL: Application

23. 2. Administering supplemental oxygen to the client is the first priority of care. The myocardium is deprived of oxygen during an infarction, so additional oxygen is administered to assist in oxygenation and prevent further damage. Morphine and sublingual nitroglycerin are also used to treat MI, but they're more commonly administered after the oxygen. An ECG is the most common diagnostic tool used to evaluate MI.
CN: Safe, effective care environment; CNS: Management of care; CL: Analysis

24. A client who experienced a myocardial infarction (MI) tells the nurse he is fearful of dying. The <u>most appropriate</u> response by the nurse is:
1. "Tell me about your feelings right now."
2. "When the doctor arrives, everything will be fine."
3. "This is a bad situation, but you'll feel better soon."
4. "Please be assured we're doing everything we can to make you feel better."

Be sensitive to your client's feelings during an emergency.

25. What is the class of medications that protects the ischemic myocardium by blocking catecholamines and sympathetic nerve stimulation?
1. Beta-adrenergic blockers
2. Calcium channel blockers
3. Opioids
4. Nitrates

26. The nurse is aware that a client who has just experienced a myocardial infarction (MI) is most at risk for developing:
1. cardiogenic shock.
2. heart failure.
3. arrhythmias.
4. pericarditis.

27. A hospitalized client with heart failure suddenly develops dyspnea at rest, disorientation, confusion, and crackles in the lung bases on auscultation. The most important intervention(s) by the nurse would be? Select all that apply.
1. Insert a Foley catheter.
2. Monitor urinary output.
3. Administer nasal oxygen.
4. Administer a rapid-acting diuretic.
5. Place the client in a modified Trendelenburg position.
6. Administer a 500-ml intravenous (I.V.) normal saline solution bolus.

24. 1. Validation of a client's feelings is the most appropriate response. It gives the client a feeling of comfort and safety. The other three responses give the client false hope. No one can determine if a client experiencing an MI will feel or get better, and therefore, these responses are inappropriate.
CN: Psychosocial integrity; CNS: None; CL: Comprehension

25. 1. Beta-adrenergic blockers work by blocking beta receptors in the myocardium, reducing the response to catecholamines and sympathetic nerve stimulation. They protect the myocardium, helping to reduce the risk of another infarction by decreasing the workload of the heart and decreasing myocardial oxygen demand. Calcium channel blockers reduce the workload of the heart by decreasing the heart rate. Opioids reduce myocardial oxygen demand, promote vasodilation, and decrease anxiety. Nitrates reduce myocardial oxygen consumption by decreasing left ventricular end-diastolic pressure (preload) and systemic vascular resistance (afterload).
CN: Physiological integrity; CNS: Pharmacological and parenteral therapies; CL: Application

26. 3. Arrhythmias, caused by oxygen deprivation to the myocardium, are the most common complication of an MI. Cardiogenic shock, another complication of MI, is defined as the end stage of left ventricular dysfunction. The condition occurs in approximately 15% of clients with MI. Because the pumping function of the heart is compromised by an MI, heart failure is the second most common complication. Pericarditis most commonly results from a bacterial or viral infection but may occur after MI.
CN: Physiological integrity; CNS: Physiological adaptation; CL: Application

27. 1, 2, 3, and 4. Acute pulmonary edema is a life-threatening event in which the left ventricle of the heart fails to eject sufficient blood. The pressure in the lungs increases because of the accumulated blood. Interventions should be done to decrease this pressure. The client is placed in a high Fowler's position to assist in breathing. The nurse ensures that vascular access is present, but I.V. fluids are not administered because this will increase body fluid. Oxygen is administered, and the physician prescribes a rapid-acting diuretic to eliminate body fluid. A Foley catheter is inserted to assess urinary output after diuretic administration and to minimize exertion related to voiding.
CN: Physiological integrity; CNS: Pharmacological and parenteral therapies CL: Application

28. The nurse is preparing to assess a client for jugular vein distention. How should the nurse position the head of the client's bed?
  1. High Fowler's
  2. Raised 10 degrees
  3. Raised 30 degrees
  4. Supine

Keep in mind that digoxin strengthens myocardial contraction.

29. A client is ordered to start receiving digoxin 0.25 mg P.O. What is the priority assessment by the nurse administering the medication?
  1. Apical pulse
  2. Blood pressure
  3. Radial pulse
  4. Respiratory rate

30. The nurse is performing an admission assessment on a client who has been diagnosed with a cardiovascular disease. The nurse would anticipate the data to include which of the following? Select all that apply.
  1. Fatigue
  2. Chest pain
  3. Weight loss
  4. Light-headedness
  5. Dependent edema
  6. Difficulty breathing in an upright position

You're doing great! Keep going!

31. A nurse is monitoring a client for manifestations of cardiac tamponade. It is important for the nurse to assess the client for which of the following? Select all that apply.
  1. Bradycardia
  2. Hypertension
  3. Kussmaul's sign
  4. Muffled heart sounds
  5. Widened pulse pressure
  6. Distended neck veins on inspiration

28. 3. Jugular venous pressure is measured with a centimeter ruler to obtain the vertical distance between the sternal angle and the point of highest pulsation with the head of the bed inclined between 15 and 30 degrees. Increased pressure can't be seen when the client is supine or when the head of the bed is raised 10 degrees because the point that marks the pressure level is above the jaw (therefore, not visible). In high Fowler's position, the veins would be barely discernible above the clavicle.
CN: Physiological integrity; CNS: Reduction of risk potential; CL: Analysis

29. 1. An apical pulse is essential for accurately assessing the client's heart rate before administering digoxin. The apical pulse is the most accurate pulse point in the body. Blood pressure is usually only affected if the heart rate is too low, in which case the nurse would withhold digoxin. The radial pulse can be affected by cardiac and vascular disease and, therefore, won't always accurately depict the heart rate. Digoxin has no effect on respiratory function.
CN: Physiological integrity; CNS: Pharmacological and parenteral therapies; CL: Application

30. 1, 2, 4, and 5. Cardiovascular disease is any abnormal condition characterized by dysfunction of the heart and blood vessels. Common clinical manifestations of cardiovascular disease include chest pain, irregularities of the heart rhythm, cyanosis, fatigue, light-headedness, weight gain, dependent edema, and respiratory manifestations such as dyspnea. The client complains of difficulty breathing when lying in a flat position, not when in an upright position.
CN: Physiological integrity; CNS: Physiological adaptation; CL: Analysis

31. 3, 4, and 6. Cardiac tamponade is a life-threatening condition caused by the accumulation of fluid in the pericardium. This fluid, which can be blood, pus, or air in the pericardial sac, accumulates fast and in sufficient quantity to compress the heart and restrict blood flow in and out of the ventricles. The following are manifestations of cardiac tamponade and should be reported immediately: elevated venous pressure, distended neck veins, and Kussmaul's sign (distended neck veins on inspiration); hypotension and narrowed pulse pressure; tachycardia; dyspnea, restlessness, and anxiety; cyanosis of the lips and nails; diaphoresis; muffled heart sounds; pulsus paradoxus; decreased friction rub; decreased QRS voltage; and electrical alternans.
CN: Physiological integrity; CNS: Physiological adaptation; CL: Analysis

32. A nurse is assessing a bedridden client and notes sacral edema. The nurse determines that the edema is most likely the result of which of the following?
1. Diabetes mellitus
2. Pulmonary emboli
3. Chronic kidney disease
4. Right-sided heart failure

33. The nurse anticipates that a client with right-sided heart failure will exhibit which of the following?
1. Adequate urine output
2. Polyuria
3. Oliguria
4. Polydipsia

34. Which of the following drug classes should be administered to a client with heart failure to maximize cardiac performance?
1. Beta-adrenergic blockers
2. Calcium channel blockers
3. Diuretics
4. Inotropic agents

35. The heart rhythm of a client who has experienced cardiac arrest and is receiving cardiopulmonary resuscitation (CPR) deteriorates to ventricular fibrillation. What is the most important action of the nurse?
1. Administer 1 mg of epinephrine I.V.
2. Defibrillate with 360 joules.
3. Continue CPR.
4. Administer vasopressin 40 units I.V.

36. Which condition is most closely associated with weight gain, nausea, and a decrease in urine output?
1. Angina pectoris
2. Cardiomyopathy
3. Left-sided heart failure
4. Right-sided heart failure

Make sure you understand how these different drugs work to benefit the heart.

This question asks you to distinguish between symptoms of left- and right-sided heart failure.

32. 4. The most accurate area on the body to assess dependent edema in a bedridden client is the sacral area. Sacral, or dependent, edema is secondary to right-sided heart failure. Diabetes mellitus, pulmonary emboli, and chronic kidney disease aren't directly linked to sacral edema.
CN: Physiological integrity; CNS: Physiological adaptation; CL: Analysis

33. 3. Inadequate deactivation of aldosterone by the liver after right-sided heart failure leads to fluid retention, which causes oliguria. Adequate urine output, polyuria, and polydipsia aren't associated with right-sided heart failure.
CN: Physiological integrity; CNS: Physiological adaptation; CL: Application

34. 4. Inotropic agents are administered to increase the force of the heart's contractions, thereby increasing ventricular contractility and ultimately increasing cardiac output. Beta-adrenergic blockers and calcium channel blockers decrease the heart rate and ultimately decrease the workload of the heart. Diuretics are administered to decrease the overall vascular volume, also decreasing the workload of the heart.
CN: Physiological integrity; CNS: Pharmacological and parenteral therapies; CL: Application

35. 2. To attempt to convert the rhythm, the nurse should first defibrillate the client with 360 joules. If this is unsuccessful, she would then continue CPR for five cycles and attempt to defibrillate again. Epinephrine and vasopressin may be given but not until after the first two defibrillation attempts.
CN: Physiological integrity; CNS: Physiological adaptation; CL: Analysis

36. 4. Weight gain, nausea, and a decrease in urine output are secondary effects of right-sided heart failure. Cardiomyopathy is usually identified as a symptom of left-sided heart failure. Left-sided heart failure causes primarily pulmonary symptoms rather than systemic ones. Angina pectoris doesn't cause weight gain, nausea, or a decrease in urine output.
CN: Physiological integrity; CNS: Physiological adaptation; CL: Application

37. A client's rhythm strip shows a regular rhythm with atrial and ventricular rates of 70 beats/minute, a PR interval of 0.24 seconds, and a QRS duration of 0.08 seconds. The nurse interprets this rhythm as:
1. normal sinus rhythm (NSR).
2. NSR with 1-degree atrioventricular (AV) block.
3. sinus arrhythmia.
4. accelerated junctional rhythm.

38. A client with abdominal aortic aneurysm asks the nurse in which area are abdominal aortic aneurysms <u>most commonly</u> located. The best response by the nurse is:
1. distal to the iliac arteries.
2. distal to the renal arteries.
3. adjacent to the aortic arch.
4. proximal to the renal arteries.

39. While palpating a client's abdomen, the nurse notes a pulsating abdominal mass. This may indicate which condition?
1. Abdominal aortic aneurysm
2. Enlarged spleen
3. Gastric distention
4. Gastritis

40. What is the most common symptom in a client with abdominal aortic aneurysm?
1. Abdominal pain
2. Diaphoresis
3. Headache
4. Upper back pain

Looking good! Keep at it!

37. 2. An increased PR interval is indicative of a 1-degree AV block. NSR and sinus arrhythmia have normal PR intervals. The PR interval (if present) is less than 0.12 seconds in accelerated junctional rhythm.
CN: Physiological integrity; CNS: Reduction of risk potential; CL: Analysis

38. 2. The portion of the aorta distal to the renal arteries is more prone to an aneurysm because the vessel isn't surrounded by stable structures, unlike the proximal portion of the aorta. Distal to the iliac arteries, the vessel is again surrounded by stable vasculature, making this an uncommon site for an aneurysm. There is no area adjacent to the aortic arch, which bends into the thoracic (descending) aorta.
CN: Physiological integrity; CNS: Physiological adaptation; CL: Application

39. 1. The presence of a pulsating mass in the abdomen is an abnormal finding, usually indicating an outpouching in a weakened vessel, as in abdominal aortic aneurysm. The finding, however, can be normal on a thin person. An enlarged spleen, gastric distention, and gastritis do not cause pulsation.
CN: Health promotion and maintenance; CNS: None; CL: Application

40. 1. Abdominal pain in a client with an abdominal aortic aneurysm results from the disruption of normal circulation in the abdominal region. Diaphoresis and headache aren't associated with abdominal aortic aneurysm. Lower back pain, not upper, is a common symptom, usually signifying expansion and impending rupture of the aneurysm.
CN: Physiological integrity; CNS: Basic care and comfort; CL: Application

41. A client is admitted to the step-down unit with an abdominal aortic aneurysm. The nurse would be most concerned if the client experienced:
1. hypotension.
2. cramping in the legs.
3. sudden, severe back pain.
4. diaphoresis.

42. A client is scheduled for testing to diagnose an abdominal aortic aneurysm. The most definitive test would be?
1. Abdominal X-ray
2. Aortogram
3. Computed tomography (CT) scan
4. Ultrasound

Knowing which symptom relates to which complication will help you to make a more accurate diagnosis.

43. The nurse is caring for a preoperative client with an abdominal aortic aneurysm. The client is <u>most</u> at risk for:
1. hypertension.
2. aneurysm rupture.
3. cardiac arrhythmias.
4. diminished pedal pulses.

This question is asking you to prioritize, once again.

44. A client with a myocardial infarction has received a thrombolytic agent. What is the most important intervention by the nurse?
1. Avoid puncture wounds.
2. Monitor potassium levels.
3. Maintain a supine position.
4. Encourage fluids.

41. 3. If expansion and impending rupture of an abdominal aneurysm is suspected, the nurse assesses for onset of sudden and severe pain in the back or lower abdomen, which may radiate to the groin.
CN: Physiological integrity; CNS: Basic care and comfort; CL: Application

42. 2. An aortogram accurately and directly depicts the vasculature; therefore, it clearly delineates the vessels and any abnormalities. An abdominal aneurysm would only be visible on an X-ray if it were calcified. CT scan and ultrasound don't give a direct view of the vessels and don't yield as accurate a diagnosis as the aortogram.
CN: Health promotion and maintenance; CNS: None; CL: Application

43. 2. Rupture of the aneurysm is a life-threatening emergency and is of the greatest concern for the nurse caring for this type of client. Hypertension should be avoided and controlled because it can cause the weakened vessel to rupture. Cardiac arrhythmias aren't directly linked to an aneurysm. Diminished pedal pulses, a sign of poor circulation to the lower extremities, are associated with an aneurysm but aren't life threatening.
CN: Physiological integrity; CNS: Basic care and comfort; CL: Analysis

44. 1. Thrombolytic agents are declotting agents that place the client at risk for hemorrhage from puncture wounds. All unnecessary needle sticks and invasive procedures should be avoided. The potassium level should be monitored in all cardiac clients, not just those receiving a thrombolytic agent. Although no specific position is required, most cardiac clients seem more comfortable in semi-Fowler's position. The client's fluid balance must be carefully monitored, so it may be inappropriate to encourage fluids at this time.
CN: Physiological integrity; CNS: Reduction of risk potential; CL: Application

45. The nurse is assessing a client for an abdominal aortic aneurysm. Which area does the nurse palpate?
1. Right upper quadrant
2. Directly over the umbilicus
3. Middle lower abdomen to the left of the midline
4. Middle lower abdomen to the right of the midline

46. Which condition is linked to more than 50% of clients with abdominal aortic aneurysms?
1. Diabetes mellitus
2. Hypertension
3. Peripheral vascular disease
4. Syphilis

47. When auscultating the abdominal region of a client with abdominal aortic aneurysm, the nurse hears a bruit. How does the nurse interpret this finding?
1. It is a normal finding.
2. It reflects a partial arterial occlusion.
3. It indicates a collection of fluid in the lungs.
4. It shows an inflammation of the peritoneal surface.

48. The nurse assesses a client with an abdominal aortic aneurysm and is most concerned when the client presents with which of the following?
1. Lower back pain, increased blood pressure, decreased red blood cell (RBC) count, and increased white blood cell (WBC) count
2. Severe lower back pain, decreased blood pressure, decreased RBC count, increased WBC count
3. Severe lower back pain, decreased blood pressure, decreased RBC count, decreased WBC count
4. Intermittent lower back pain, decreased blood pressure, decreased RBC count, increased WBC count

I'm suddenly feeling a little tense, a little hyper. (Get it?)

This is a real bruit of a question.

45. 3. The aorta lies directly left of the umbilicus; therefore, any other region is inappropriate for palpation.
CN: Physiological integrity; CNS: Basic care and comfort; CL: Application

46. 2. Continuous pressure on the vessel walls from hypertension causes the walls to weaken and an aneurysm to occur. Diabetes mellitus doesn't have a direct link to aneurysm. Atherosclerotic changes can occur with peripheral vascular diseases and are linked to aneurysms, but the link isn't as strong as it is with hypertension. Only 1% of clients with syphilis experience an aneurysm.
CN: Health promotion and maintenance; CNS: None; CL: Application

47. 2. A bruit is a vascular sound that reflects partial arterial occlusion. It is not a normal finding. Fluid in the lungs is called crackles, and inflammation of the peritoneal surface produces a friction rub.
CN: Physiological integrity; CNS: Basic care and comfort; CL: Analysis

48. 2. Severe lower back pain indicates an aneurysm rupture, secondary to pressure being applied within the abdominal cavity. When rupture occurs, the pain is constant because it can't be alleviated until the aneurysm is repaired. Blood pressure decreases due to the loss of blood. After the aneurysm ruptures, the vasculature is interrupted and blood volume is lost, so blood pressure wouldn't increase. For the same reason, the RBC count is decreased. The WBC count increases as cells migrate to the site of injury.
CN: Physiological integrity; CNS: Physiological adaptation; CL: Application

49. During the assessment of a client who had an abdominal aortic repair, the nurse notes a hematoma in the perineal area. The nurse interprets this as:
1. hernia.
2. stage 1 pressure ulcer.
3. retroperitoneal rupture at the repair site.
4. rapid expansion of the aneurysm.

50. A client who was recently diagnosed with an aneurysm asks the nurse if any genetic disease is closely linked to an aneurysm. What is the best response by the nurse?
1. Cystic fibrosis
2. Hemophilia
3. Marfan's syndrome
4. Sickle cell anemia

51. A client's aneurysm has ruptured. What is the priority intervention?
1. Antihypertensive medication administration
2. Aortogram
3. Beta-adrenergic blocker administration
4. Surgical intervention

52. A nurse is teaching a client about cardiomyopathy and determines further teaching is needed when the client states:
1. "It is caused by a plaque in the arteries."
2. "It is caused by a virus."
3. "It is caused by bacteria."
4. "It is caused by certain drugs."

53. The nurse is counseling a client on types of cardiomyopathy associated with childbirth. The nurse should teach the client about which of the following?
1. Dilated
2. Hypertrophic obstructive
3. Myocarditis
4. Restrictive

You've finished 50 questions! Good job!

Think! This question is asking for a treatment, not a preventive measure.

49. 3. Blood collects in the retroperitoneal space and is exhibited as a hematoma in the perineal area. This rupture is most commonly caused by leakage at the repair site. A hernia doesn't cause vascular disturbances, nor does a pressure ulcer. Because no bleeding occurs with rapid expansion of the aneurysm, a hematoma won't form.
CN: Physiological integrity; CNS: Physiological adaptation; CL: Application

50. 3. Marfan's syndrome results in the degeneration of the elastic fibers of the aortic media. Therefore, clients with this syndrome are more likely to develop an aneurysm. Although cystic fibrosis, hemophilia, and sickle cell anemia are all genetic diseases, they haven't been linked to aneurysms.
CN: Health promotion and maintenance; CNS: None; CL: Application

51. 4. When the vessel ruptures, surgery is the only intervention that can repair it. Administration of antihypertensive medications and beta-adrenergic blockers can help control hypertension, reducing the risk of rupture. An aortogram is a diagnostic tool used to detect an aneurysm.
CN: Physiological integrity; CNS: Basic care and comfort; CL: Application

52. 1. Cardiomyopathy isn't usually caused by plaque in the arteries or atherosclerosis. The etiology in most cases is viral or bacterial infection or cardiotoxic effects of drugs or alcohol.
CN: Physiological integrity; CNS: Physiological adaptation; CL: Application

53. 1. Although the cause isn't entirely known, cardiac dilation and heart failure may develop during the last month of pregnancy or the first few months after birth. The condition may result from a preexisting cardiomyopathy not apparent prior to pregnancy. Hypertrophic obstructive cardiomyopathy is an abnormal symmetry of the ventricles that has an unknown etiology but a strong familial tendency. Myocarditis isn't a form of cardiomyopathy; it's an inflammation of the cardiac muscle. Restrictive cardiomyopathy indicates constrictive pericarditis; the underlying cause is usually myocardial.
CN: Physiological integrity; CNS: Physiological adaptation; CL: Application

CN: Client needs category   CNS: Client needs subcategory   CL: Cognitive level

54. The nurse is reviewing a client's echocardiogram report, which states, "hypertrophy of the ventricular septum." The client should be further evaluated for which type of cardiomyopathy?
1. Congestive
2. Dilated
3. Hypertrophic obstructive
4. Restrictive

55. A nurse is caring for a client with cardiomyopathy and is aware that the client is at high risk for developing:
1. heart failure.
2. diabetes mellitus.
3. myocardial infarction (MI).
4. pericardial effusion.

56. While assessing a client with dilated cardiomyopathy, the nurse notices that the electrocardiogram (ECG) rhythm no longer has any P waves, only a fine wavy line. The ventricular rhythm is irregular with a QRS duration of 0.08 seconds. The heart rate is 110 beats/minute. The nurse interprets this rhythm as:
1. atrial fibrillation.
2. ventricular fibrillation.
3. atrial flutter.
4. sinus tachycardia.

57. The nurse performs an assessment on a newly admitted client. The data include dyspnea, cough, weight gain, weakness, and edema. The nurse interprets these as <u>signs and symptoms</u> of:
1. pericarditis.
2. hypertension.
3. myocardial infarction (MI).
4. heart failure.

This is a tough one! Keep plugging along!

I don't know about you, but along about now, I'm getting kinda fried.

This question is a classic one, if you catch my drift.

54. 3. In hypertrophic obstructive cardiomyopathy, hypertrophy of the ventricular septum—not the ventricle chambers—is apparent. This abnormality isn't seen in other types of cardiomyopathy. Congestive isn't a form of cardiomyopathy.
CN: Physiological integrity; CNS: Physiological adaptation; CL: Analysis

55. 1. Because the structure and function of the heart muscle are affected, heart failure most commonly occurs in clients with cardiomyopathy. Diabetes mellitus is unrelated to cardiomyopathy. MI results from prolonged myocardial ischemia due to reduced blood flow through one of the coronary arteries. Pericardial effusion is most predominant in clients with pericarditis.
CN: Physiological integrity; CNS: Physiological adaptation; CL: Comprehension

56. 1. Atrial fibrillation is defined as chaotic, asynchronous, electrical activity in the atrial tissue. On an ECG, uneven baseline fibrillating waves appear rather than distinguishable P waves. Ventricular fibrillation is a chaotic rhythm with no QRS complexes. In atrial flutter, there are flutter waves that are "sawtooth" in appearance. P waves are present in sinus tachycardia.
CN: Physiological integrity; CNS: Physiological adaptation; CL: Analysis

57. 4. These are the classic symptoms of heart failure. Pericarditis is exhibited by a feeling of fullness in the chest and auscultation of a pericardial friction rub. Hypertension is usually exhibited by headaches, visual disturbances, and a flushed face. MI is usually exhibited by chest pain and diaphoresis.
CN: Physiological integrity; CNS: Reduction of risk potential; CL: Application

58. The nurse determines further teaching is necessary when a client with cardiomyopathy states:
1. dilated cardiomyopathy decreases cardiac output.
2. cardiac output increases in hypertrophic obstructive cardiomyopathy.
3. cardiac output is not affected by hypertrophic obstructive cardiomyopathy.
4. restrictive cardiomyopathy decreases cardiac output.

59. The nurse is performing a cardiac assessment on her client and auscultates a fourth heart sound (S_4). The nurse interprets this as indicative of which of the following?
1. Dilated aorta
2. Normally functioning heart
3. Decreased myocardial contractility
4. Failure of the ventricle to eject all the blood during systole

60. Which class of drugs is most widely used in the treatment of cardiomyopathy?
1. Anticoagulants
2. Beta-adrenergic blockers
3. Calcium channel blockers
4. Nitrates

61. If medical treatment for cardiomyopathy fails, the nurse should prepare the client for which of the following procedures?
1. Cardiac catheterization
2. Coronary artery bypass graft (CABG)
3. Heart transplantation
4. Intra-aortic balloon pump (IABP)

It's important to know what the different sounds I make indicate.

58. 2. Cardiac output isn't affected by hypertrophic obstructive cardiomyopathy because the size of the ventricle remains relatively unchanged. Dilated cardiomyopathy and restrictive cardiomyopathy decrease cardiac output.

CN: Physiological integrity; CNS: Physiological adaptation; CL: Application

59. 4. An S_4 occurs as a result of increased resistance to ventricular filling after atrial contraction. This increased resistance is related to decreased compliance of the ventricle. A dilated aorta doesn't cause an extra heart sound, though it does cause a murmur. Decreased myocardial contractility is heard as a third heart sound. An S_4 isn't heard in a normally functioning heart.

CN: Physiological integrity; CNS: Physiological adaptation; CL: Application

60. 2. By decreasing the heart rate and contractility, beta-adrenergic blockers improve myocardial filling and cardiac output, which are primary goals in the treatment of cardiomyopathy. Anticoagulants may sometimes be used to reduce the risk of emboli, but this practice is considered controversial. Calcium channel blockers are sometimes used for the same reasons as beta-adrenergic blockers; however, they aren't as effective as beta-adrenergic blockers and cause increased hypotension. Nitrates aren't used because of their dilating effects, which would further compromise the myocardium.

CN: Physiological integrity; CNS: Pharmacological and parenteral therapies; CL: Comprehension

61. 3. The only definitive treatment for cardiomyopathy that can't be controlled medically is a heart transplant because the damage to the heart muscle is irreversible. Cardiac catheterization is an invasive diagnostic procedure for coronary artery disease. CABG is a surgical intervention used for atherosclerotic vessels. An IABP is an invasive treatment that assists the failing heart; however, it's only a temporary solution.

CN: Physiological integrity; CNS: Physiological adaptation; CL: Application

62. Which condition is associated with a predictable level of pain that occurs as a result of physical or emotional stress?
1. Anxiety
2. Stable angina
3. Unstable angina
4. Variant angina

63. After undergoing a cardiac catheterization, a client has a large puddle of blood under his buttocks. The <u>most important</u> intervention by the nurse is:
1. call for help.
2. obtain vital signs.
3. ask the client to "lift up."
4. apply gloves and assess the groin site.

64. A client with angina pectoris has a stat electrocardiogram (ECG) performed during an episode of chest pain. The nurse reviews the ECG and notes myocardial ischemia. This would be displayed as:
1. increased QRS duration.
2. shortened PR interval.
3. pathological Q-wave formation.
4. T-wave inversion.

65. A client with an impending myocardial infarction (MI) is experiencing angina. The nurse would document the angina as?
1. Variant angina
2. Chronic stable angina
3. Microvascular angina
4. Unstable angina

Stress can be a real pain in the heart.

You've finished 65 questions! Keep going!

62. 2. The pain of stable angina is predictable in nature, builds gradually, and quickly reaches maximum intensity. Anxiety generally isn't described as painful. Unstable angina doesn't always need a trigger, is more intense, and lasts longer than stable angina. Variant angina usually occurs at rest—not as a result of exertion or stress.

CN: Physiological integrity; CNS: Physiological adaptation; CL: Analysis

63. 4. Observing standard precautions is the first priority when dealing with any body fluid. Assessment of the groin site is the second priority. This establishes where the blood is coming from and determines how much blood has been lost. The goal in this situation is to stop the bleeding. The nurse would call for help if it were warranted after the assessment of the situation. After determining the extent of the bleeding, vital signs assessment is important. The nurse should never move the client, in case a clot has formed. Moving can disturb the clot and cause rebleeding.

CN: Safe, effective care environment; CNS: Management of care; CL: Analysis

64. 4. Ischemic changes are represented on an ECG by T-wave inversion. An increased QRS duration suggests a bundle-branch block. A shortened PR interval indicates a junctional rhythm. Pathological Q waves are present with myocardial infarction.

CN: Physiological integrity; CNS: Physiological adaptation; CL: Analysis

65. 4. Unstable angina progressively increases in frequency, intensity, and duration and is related to an increased risk of MI within 3 to 18 months. Variant angina is related to coronary artery spasm, chronic stable angina is predictable and relieved by rest and nitrates, and microvascular angina is related to impairment of vasodilator reserve in normal coronary arteries.

CN: Physiological integrity; CNS: Physiological adaptation; CL: Application

66. A client with angina pectoris comes to the emergency room. Which of the following drugs can the nurse expect to administer?
1. Aspirin
2. Furosemide (Lasix)
3. Nitroglycerin
4. Nifedipine (Procardia)

67. While assessing a client diagnosed with angina, the client asks what causes it. Which of the following responses by the nurse would be the <u>most appropriate</u>?
1. Increased preload
2. Decreased afterload
3. Coronary artery spasm
4. Inadequate oxygen supply to the myocardium

68. A nurse is preparing a client for cardiac catheterization. What is the priority assessment for the nurse to obtain?
1. Weight and height
2. Allergy to iodine or shellfish
3. Apical heart rate
4. Cardiac rhythm

69. The nurse is teaching a client about angina. Which statement by the nurse would be <u>most accurate</u> regarding the <u>primary</u> treatment goal?
1. Reversal of ischemia
2. Reversal of infarction
3. Reduction of stress and anxiety
4. Reduction of associated risk factors

70. A 59-year-old female client is experiencing chest pain at rest that is unresponsive to nitroglycerine. The physician diagnoses unstable angina and alerts the nurse that the client will require treatment with immediate <u>surgical</u> intervention. Which treatment is most appropriate?
1. Cardiac catheterization
2. Echocardiogram
3. Heart transplantation
4. Percutaneous transluminal coronary angioplasty (PTCA)

Remember: This question is asking for the *primary* treatment goal.

66. **3.** Nitroglycerin is administered to reduce the myocardial demand, which decreases ischemia and relieves pain. In addition, nitroglycerin dilates the vasculature, thereby reducing preload. Aspirin is administered to reduce the risk of myocardial infarction in clients with unstable angina. Furosemide is a loop diuretic that won't directly reduce pain or prevent angina. Nifedipine is a calcium channel blocker primarily used to decrease coronary artery spasm, as in variant angina.
CN: Physiological integrity; CNS: Pharmacological and parenteral therapies; CL: Analysis

67. **4.** Inadequate oxygen supply to the myocardium is responsible for the pain accompanying angina. Increased preload would be responsible for right-sided heart failure. Decreased afterload causes increased cardiac output. Coronary artery spasm is responsible for variant angina.
CN: Physiological integrity; CNS: Physiological adaptation; CL: Analysis

68. **2.** Since cardiac catheterization involves the injection of a radiopaque dye, it's most important for the nurse to determine if the client has allergies to iodine or shellfish. The other three parameters are also part of the assessment, but none is the most critical assessment.
CN: Physiological integrity; CNS: Reduction of risk potential; CL: Analysis

69. **1.** Reversal of the ischemia is the primary goal, achieved by reducing oxygen consumption and increasing oxygen supply. An infarction is permanent and can't be reversed. Reduction of associated risk factors, such as stress and anxiety, is a progressive, long-term treatment goal that has cumulative effects. Reduction of these factors will decrease the risk for angina, but this usually isn't an immediate goal.
CN: Physiological integrity; CNS: Physiological adaptation; CL: Application

70. **4.** PTCA can alleviate the blockage and restore blood flow and oxygenation. Cardiac catheterization is a diagnostic tool—not a treatment. An echocardiogram is a noninvasive diagnostic test. Heart transplantation involves replacing the client's heart with a donor heart and is the treatment for end-stage cardiac disease.
CN: Physiological integrity; CNS: Physiological adaptation; CL: Application

71. The nurse is ambulating a client. After ambulating 50 feet, the client experiences chest pain. What should be the <u>priority</u> intervention by the nurse?
1. Sit the client down.
2. Get the client back to bed.
3. Obtain an electrocardiogram (ECG).
4. Administer sublingual nitroglycerin.

72. The nurse is assessing a client with heart failure. The client is experiencing tachycardia, decreased blood pressure, and decreased peripheral pulses. The nurse interprets these symptoms as indicative of what?
1. Anaphylactic shock
2. Cardiogenic shock
3. Distributive shock
4. Myocardial infarction (MI)

73. The nurse in the cardiac unit is reviewing the conditions of the assigned clients to determine if a risk for cardiogenic shock is present. The client most at risk presents with which condition?
1. Acute myocardial infarction (MI)
2. Coronary artery disease (CAD)
3. Decreased hemoglobin level
4. Hypotension

74. Four clients have been admitted to the cardiac intensive care unit after experiencing acute myocardial infarctions. The nurse reviews each client's chart to determine the assessment of cardiac damage and risk for development of cardiogenic shock. What is the percentage of damage that places the client at risk for the development of shock?
1. 10%
2. 25%
3. 40%
4. 90%

75. Which of the following parameters increases as myocardial oxygen consumption increases?
1. Preload, afterload, and cerebral blood flow
2. Preload, afterload, and renal blood flow
3. Preload, afterload, contractility, and heart rate
4. Preload, afterload, cerebral blood flow, and heart rate

Pay attention. This info could really shock you!

71. 1. The initial priority is to decrease the oxygen consumption; this would be achieved by sitting the client down. When the client's condition is stabilized, he can be returned to bed. An ECG can be obtained after the client is sitting down. After the ECG, sublingual nitroglycerin would be administered.
CN: Physiological integrity; CNS: Basic care and comfort; CL: Analysis

72. 2. Cardiogenic shock is shock related to reduced cardiac output and ineffective pumping of the heart. Anaphylactic shock results from an allergic reaction. Distributive shock results from changes in the intravascular volume distribution and is usually associated with increased cardiac output. MI isn't a shock state, although a severe MI can lead to shock.
CN: Physiological integrity; CNS: Physiological adaptation; CL: Analysis

73. 1. Of all clients with an acute MI, 15% suffer cardiogenic shock secondary to the myocardial damage and decreased function. CAD causes MI. A decreased hemoglobin level is a result of bleeding. Hypotension is the result of a reduced cardiac output produced by the shock state.
CN: Physiological integrity; CNS: Reduction of risk potential; CL: Analysis

74. 3. At least 40% of the heart muscle must be involved for cardiogenic shock to develop. In most circumstances, the heart can compensate for up to 25% damage. An infarction involving 90% of the heart would result in death.
CN: Physiological integrity; CNS: Physiological adaptation; CL: Comprehension

75. 3. Myocardial oxygen consumption increases as preload, afterload, contractility, and heart rate increase. Cerebral blood flow and renal blood flow don't directly affect myocardial oxygen consumption.
CN: Physiological integrity; CNS: Physiological adaptation; CL: Application

76. The nurse determines that a client at risk for the development of cardiogenic shock would present with which of the following?
1. Decreased heart rate
2. Decreased cardiac index
3. Decreased blood pressure
4. Decreased cerebral blood flow

Pay attention. This question involves assessing the order of symptoms.

77. The nurse is assessing a client who is displaying the <u>earliest</u> sign of cardiogenic shock. The nurse would document this assessment finding as:
1. cyanosis.
2. decreased urine output.
3. presence of fourth heart sound (S_4).
4. altered level of consciousness.

78. Which diagnostic study can determine when cellular metabolism becomes anaerobic and when pH decreases?
1. Arterial blood gas (ABG) levels
2. Complete blood count (CBC)
3. Electrocardiogram (ECG)
4. Lung scan

79. The nurse is planning care for a client in cardiogenic shock. What is the <u>priority</u> goal?
1. Correct hypoxia.
2. Prevent infarction.
3. Correct metabolic acidosis.
4. Increase myocardial oxygen supply.

80. Which drug is <u>most commonly</u> used to treat cardiogenic shock?
1. Dopamine
2. Enalapril (Vasotec)
3. Furosemide (Lasix)
4. Metoprolol (Lopressor)

When answering questions, look for phrases such as most commonly. These are often clues.

76. 2. The cardiac index, a figure derived by dividing the cardiac output by the client's body surface area, is used for identifying whether the cardiac output is meeting a client's needs. Heart rate, blood pressure, and decreased cerebral blood flow are less useful in detecting the risk of cardiogenic shock.

CN: Physiological integrity; CNS: Physiological adaptation; CL: Analysis

77. 4. Initially, the decrease in cardiac output results in a decrease in cerebral blood flow that causes restlessness, agitation, or confusion. Cyanosis, decreased urine output, and presence of an S_4 are all later signs of shock.

CN: Physiological integrity; CNS: Basic care and comfort; CL: Application

78. 1. ABG levels reflect cellular metabolism and indicate hypoxia. A CBC is performed to determine various constituents of venous blood. An ECG shows the electrical activity of the heart. A lung scan is performed to view functionality of the lungs.

CN: Health promotion and maintenance; CNS: None; CL: Analysis

79. 4. A balance must be maintained between oxygen supply and demand. In a shock state, the myocardium requires more oxygen. If it can't get more oxygen, the shock worsens. Increasing the oxygen will also play a large role in correcting metabolic acidosis and hypoxia. Infarction typically causes the shock state, so prevention isn't an appropriate goal for this condition.

CN: Physiological integrity; CN: Physiological adaptation; CL: Analysis

80. 1. Dopamine, a sympathomimetic drug, improves myocardial contractility and blood flow through vital organs by increasing perfusion pressure. Enalapril is an angiotensin-converting enzyme inhibitor that directly lowers blood pressure. Furosemide is a diuretic and doesn't have a direct effect on contractility or tissue perfusion. Metoprolol is a beta-adrenergic blocker that slows heart rate and lowers blood pressure; neither is a desired effect in the treatment of cardiogenic shock.

CN: Physiological integrity; CNS: Pharmacological and parenteral therapies; CL: Application

81. Which is the most important instrument used as a diagnostic and monitoring tool for determining the severity of a shock state?
1. Arterial line
2. Indwelling urinary catheter
3. Electrocardiogram (ECG) monitor
4. Pulmonary artery catheter

82. A client has a continuous blood pressure reading of 142/90 mm Hg. The reading is interpreted as indicative of what?
1. Stage 2 hypertension
2. Prehypertension
3. Stage 1 hypertension
4. Normal

83. Which sound will be heard during the first phase of Korotkoff's sounds?
1. Disappearance of sounds
2. Faint, clear tapping sounds
3. A murmur or swishing sounds
4. Soft, muffling sounds

How would I respond to a rise in blood pressure?

84. When hypertension occurs, which responses by the kidneys help normalize blood pressure?
1. The kidneys retain sodium and excrete water.
2. The kidneys excrete sodium and excrete water.
3. The kidneys retain sodium and retain water.
4. The kidneys excrete sodium and retain water.

85. Which physiological change would indicate that the baroreceptors in the carotid artery walls and aorta are functioning?
1. Changes in blood pressure
2. Changes in arterial oxygen tension
3. Changes in arterial carbon dioxide tension
4. Changes in heart rate

81. 4. A pulmonary artery catheter is used to give accurate pressure measurements within the heart, which aids in determining the course of treatment. An arterial line, an indwelling urinary catheter, and an ECG monitor all provide valuable information related to the severity of a shock state but aren't the most important instrument.
CN: Physiological integrity; CNS: Pharmacological and parenteral therapies; CL: Analysis

82. 3. According to the Seventh Joint National Committee (JNC 7), a systolic blood pressure of 140 to 159 mm Hg or a diastolic pressure of 90 to 99 mm Hg represents stage 1 hypertension. A systolic pressure greater than or equal to 160 mm Hg or diastolic pressure greater than or equal to 100 mm Hg represents stage 2 hypertension. A systolic pressure of 120 to 139 mm Hg or diastolic pressure of 80 to 89 mm Hg represents prehypertension. A systolic pressure less than 120 mm Hg and diastolic pressure less than 80 mm Hg are considered normal.
CN: Health promotion and maintenance; CNS: None; CL: Application

83. 2. In phase I, auscultation produces a faint, clear tapping sound that gradually increases in intensity. Phase II produces a murmur sound and precedes phase III, the phase marked by an increased intensity of sound. Phase IV produces a muffling sound that gives a soft blowing noise. Phase V, the final phase, is marked by the disappearance of sounds.
CN: Physiological integrity; CNS: Basic care and comfort; CL: Application

84. 2. The kidneys respond to a rise in blood pressure by excreting sodium and excess water. This response ultimately affects systolic blood pressure by regulating blood volume. Sodium or water retention would only further increase blood pressure. Sodium and water travel together across the membrane in the kidneys; one can't travel without the other.
CN: Physiological integrity; CNS: Physiological adaptation; CL: Application

85. 1. Baroreceptors located in the carotid arteries and aorta sense pulsatile pressure. Peripheral chemoreceptors in the aorta and carotid arteries are primarily stimulated by oxygen. Chemoreceptors in the medulla are primarily stimulated by carbon dioxide. Decreases in pulsatile pressure cause a reflex increase in heart rate.
CN: Physiological integrity; CNS: Physiological adaptation; CL: Analysis

86. The nurse is teaching a client about blood pressure and hormones. Which of the following responses indicates the client understands which hormone raises arterial pressure and promotes venous return?
1. Angiotensin I
2. Angiotensin II
3. Thyroid hormone
4. Insulin

87. Which term would the nurse use to describe persistently elevated blood pressure with an unknown cause?
1. Accelerated hypertension
2. Malignant hypertension
3. Primary hypertension
4. Secondary hypertension

88. Prioritize the steps for performing an electrocardiogram (ECG).
1. Wash hands.
2. Clean the gel from the client's skin.
3. Apply conductive gel to the client's skin.
4. Disconnect the electrodes from the client.
5. Attach electrodes to the client's skin and obtain a reading.
6. Explain the importance of lying still, breathing normally, and refraining from talking during the test.

89. The nurse is evaluating the following telemetry strip from one of her clients. Which of the following would the nurse document?

Rate = 86

1. Sinus tachycardia with a heart rate of 86 to 100
2. Normal sinus rhythm with heart rate of about 80
3. First-degree heart block with PR interval greater than 0.20 seconds
4. Pacemaker beat with a 1:1 capture

Don't get two tense to answer this question. (Oh, I am just two, er, too clever for words.)

86. 2. Angiotensin II is a potent vasoconstrictor, thereby promoting venous return. Angiotensin I is a precursor that is converted in the pulmonary vasculature to angiotensin II. Neither thyroid hormone nor insulin has vasoconstrictive properties.
CN: Physiological integrity; CNS: Physiological adaptation; CL: Analysis

87. 3. Characterized by a progressive, usually asymptomatic blood pressure increase over several years, primary hypertension is the most common type. Malignant hypertension, also known as accelerated hypertension, is rapidly progressive, uncontrollable, and causes a rapid onset of complications. Secondary hypertension occurs secondary to a known, correctable cause.
CN: Physiological integrity; CNS: Reduction of risk potential; CL: Analysis

88. 1, 6, 3, 5, 4, and 2. The ECG is a noninvasive tool for evaluating the heart rhythm and displays the electrical activity of the heart. The nurse first washes the hands and then explains the procedure to the client, including the importance of lying still, breathing normally, and refraining from talking during the test. The nurse next applies conductive gel to the client's skin, attaches electrodes to the client's skin, and adjusts the monitor to obtain a reading. Once the reading is obtained, the nurse disconnects the electrodes from the client and cleans the gel from the client's skin.
CN: Physiological integrity; CNS: Physiological adaptation; CL: Application

89. 2. Characteristics of normal sinus rhythm include the presence of uniform P waves preceding each QRS complex, a heart rate between 60 and 100 beats/minute, and regular rhythm. This is not sinus tachycardia because the heart rate is below 100; not first-degree block because the PR interval is 0.20 seconds, which is in the normal range, and not pacemaker beat because it has uniform P waves, not spikes.
CN: Physiological integrity; CNS: Physiological adaptation; CL: Analysis

90. Which of the following statements, if made by the client, indicates an understanding of why furosemide (Lasix) is administered to treat hypertension?
1. It dilates peripheral blood vessels.
2. It decreases sympathetic cardioacceleration.
3. It inhibits the angiotensin-converting enzyme.
4. It inhibits reabsorption of sodium and water in the loop of Henle.

This question is asking for the mechanism of action of furosemide.

91. A 52-year-old client with a history of hypertension has just had a total hip replacement. The physician orders hydrochlorothiazide 35 mg oral solution by mouth, once per day. The label on the solution reads hydrochlorothiazide 50 mg/5 ml. To administer the correct dose, how many milliliters should the nurse pour? Record your answer using one decimal place. _____ milliliters

92. Which statement by the nurse accurately explains the need for a client with hypertension to obtain an annual eye exam?
1. "By examining your corneas, an ophthalmologist can visualize microvascular hemorrhages in your eyes."
2. "By examining the fovea in your eyes, an ophthalmologist can visualize microvascular venous occlusions in your eyes."
3. "By examining the retina in your eyes, an ophthalmologist can detect changes in the arteries in your eyes."
4. "By examining the sclera of your eyes, an ophthalmologist can detect changes in the arteries in your eyes."

93. What clinical manifestations would the nurse expect to find in a client who has superficial thrombophlebitis? Select all that apply.
1. Redness noted along the vein
2. Induration noted along the vein
3. Warmth palpated along the vein
4. Tenderness on palpation of the vein
5. Diminished pulses in the affected extremity
6. Dilated blue-colored veins noted along the length of the extremity

90. 4. Furosemide is a loop diuretic that inhibits sodium and water reabsorption in the loop of Henle, thereby causing a decrease in blood pressure. Vasodilators cause dilation of peripheral blood vessels, directly relaxing vascular smooth muscle and decreasing blood pressure. Adrenergic blockers decrease sympathetic cardioacceleration and decrease blood pressure. Angiotensin-converting enzyme inhibitors decrease blood pressure due to their action on angiotensin.
CN: Physiological integrity; CNS: Pharmacological and parenteral therapies; CL: Analysis

91. 3.5. The correct formula to calculate a drug dosage is:
Dose on hand/quantity on hand
    = dose desired/X.
In this example, the equation is:
    50 mg/5 ml = 35 mg/X
    X = 3.5 ml.
CN: Physiological integrity; CNS: Pharmacological and parenteral therapies; CL: Application

92. 3. The retina is the only site in the body where arteries can be seen without invasive techniques. Changes in the retinal arteries signal similar damage to vessels elsewhere. The cornea is the nonvascular, transparent fibrous coat where the iris can be seen. The fovea is the point of central vision. The sclera is the fibrous tissue that forms the outer protective covering over the eyeball.
CN: Health promotion and maintenance; CNS: None; CL: Application

93. 1, 2, 3, and 4. Superficial thrombophlebitis is an inflammation of a superficial vein accompanied by the formation of a clot. Clinical manifestations of superficial thrombophlebitis include redness, induration, warmth, and tenderness along a vein. Discomfort may be relieved by applying heat. Activity is encouraged as prescribed, and a supportive wrap or stocking should be applied. Diminished pulses and dilated blue-colored veins are not manifestations of superficial thrombophlebitis.
CN: Physiological integrity; CNS: Physiological adaptation; CL: Application

94. A nurse determines that a client with varicose veins understands the cause of <u>primary</u> varicose veins when the client states which cause?
1. Hypertension
2. Pregnancy
3. Thrombosis
4. Trauma

I love babies, but not the varicose veins that go with them!

94. 2. Primary varicose veins have a gradual onset and progressively worsen. In pregnancy, the expanding uterus and increased vascular volume impede blood return to the heart. The pressure places increased stress on the veins. Hypertension has no role in varicose vein formation. Thrombosis and trauma cause valvular incompetence and so are secondary causes of varicosities—not primary.
CN: Health promotion and maintenance; CNS: None; CL: Analysis

95. The nurse would assess a client with varicose veins for which symptoms?
1. Fatigue and pressure
2. Fatigue and cool feet
3. Sharp pain and fatigue
4. Sharp pain and cool feet

95. 1. Fatigue and pressure are classic signs of varicose veins, secondary to increased blood volume and edema. Sharp pain and cool feet are symptoms of alteration in arterial blood flow.
CN: Physiological integrity; CNS: Physiological adaptation; CL: Application

96. A nurse monitors a client with a tumor of the esophagus for signs of superior vena cava (SVC) syndrome. The nurse would assess the client for which of the following? Select all that apply.
1. Nosebleeds
2. Edema in the eyes
3. Edema in the hands
4. Difficulty breathing
5. Mental status changes
6. Weight loss with complaints of looseness of clothing, especially around the neck

96. 1, 2, 3, 4, and 5. SVC syndrome occurs when the SVC is compressed or obstructed by tumor growth. The manifestations result from the blockage of blood flow in the venous system of the head, neck, and upper trunk. Early manifestations occur when the client arises after a night's sleep and include edema of the face, especially around the eyes, and tightness of the shirt or blouse collar (Stokes' sign). As the compression worsens, edema in the hands and arms, dyspnea, erythema of the upper body, and epistaxis occur. Late manifestations include hemorrhage, cyanosis, mental status changes, decreased cardiac output, and hypotension.
CN: Physiological integrity; CNS: Physiological adaptation; CL: Analysis

97. Which condition is caused by increased hydrostatic pressure and chronic venous stasis?
1. Venous occlusion
2. Cool extremities
3. Nocturnal calf muscle cramps
4. Diminished blood supply to the feet

97. 3. Calf muscle cramps result from increased pressure and venous stasis secondary to varicose veins. An occlusion is a blockage of blood flow. Cool extremities and diminished blood supply to the feet are symptoms of arterial blood flow changes.
CN: Health promotion and maintenance; CNS: None; CL: Analysis

98. The nurse is providing discharge instructions for a client with varicose veins. The nurse determines the need for further teaching when the client makes which statement?
1. "Exercise will make me feel better."
2. "I have to elevate my legs."
3. "Lying down can relieve my symptoms."
4. "Wearing tight clothes will not affect me."

Be careful. This question could put you in a tight squeeze.

98. 4. Tight clothing, especially below the waist, increases vascular volume and impedes blood return to the heart. Exercise, leg elevations, and lying down usually relieve symptoms of varicose veins.
CN: Health promotion and maintenance; CNS: None; CL: Analysis

99. A client is suspected of having deep venous thrombosis (DVT). The nurse anticipates that which diagnostic studies will be prescribed? Select all that apply.
1. Platelet count
2. D-dimer blood test
3. Electrocardiography
4. Venous duplex scanning
5. Magnetic resonance imaging (MRI)
6. International normalized ratio (INR)

99. 2 and 4. DVT is a disorder involving a thrombus in one of the deep veins of the body, most commonly the iliac or femoral veins. Venous duplex scanning is a primary diagnostic test for DVT because it allows visualization of the vein, which provides a reliable diagnosis of venous thrombus. The D-dimer blood test is also used in evaluation of DVT. The D-dimer is a product of fibrin degradation and is indicative of fibrinolysis, which occurs with thrombosis. A platelet count will not provide information related to the presence of DVT. An INR is a blood test used to evaluate the effectiveness of warfarin (Coumadin) therapy. Electrocardiography evaluates the electrical activity of the heart. An MRI may be used for a variety of reasons, such as to detect the presence of a tumor. It will not diagnose DVT.

CN: Physiological integrity; CNS: Physiological adaptation; CL: Analysis

100. The nurse should assess a client with <u>secondary</u> varicose veins for which signs and symptoms?
1. Pallor and severe pain
2. Severe pain and edema
3. Edema and pigmentation
4. Absent hair growth and pigmentation

100. 3. Secondary varicose veins result from an obstruction of the deep veins. Incompetent valves lead to impaired blood flow, and edema and pigmentation result from venous stasis. Severe pain, pallor, and absent hair growth are symptoms of an altered arterial blood flow.

CN: Physiological integrity; CNS: Physiological adaptation; CL: Application

101. The nurse should prepare a client for which treatment to eliminate varicose veins?
1. Ablation therapy
2. Cold therapy
3. Ligation and stripping
4. Radiation

Congratulations! You've finished 100 questions! You're almost there!

101. 3. Ligation and stripping of the vein can rid the vein of varicosity. This invasive procedure will take care of current varicose veins only; it won't prevent others from forming. The other procedures aren't used for varicose veins.

CN: Physiological integrity; CNS: Pharmacological and parenteral therapies; CL: Application

102. A client has undergone ligation and stripping. What is the best intervention for the nurse to implement postoperatively?
1. Sitting
2. Bed rest
3. Ice packs
4. Elastic leg compression

102. 4. Elastic leg compression helps venous return to the heart, thereby decreasing venous stasis. Sitting and bed rest are contraindicated because both promote decreased blood return to the heart and venous stasis. Although ice packs would help reduce edema, they would also cause vasoconstriction and impede blood flow.

CN: Physiological integrity; CNS: Basic care and comfort; CL: Application

103. Which client is <u>most</u> at risk for developing deep vein thrombosis (DVT)?
1. A 62-year-old female recovering from a total hip replacement
2. A 35-year-old female 2 days postpartum
3. A 33-year-old male runner with Achilles tendonitis
4. An ambulatory 70-year-old male who is recovering from pneumonia

I'll answer this question after I've had my nap.

103. 1. DVT is more common in immobilized clients who have had surgical procedures such as total hip replacement. Pregnancy can cause varicose veins, which can lead to venous stasis, but it isn't a primary cause of DVT. Clients who are recovering from an injury or pneumonia may have decreased mobility, but these clients don't have the highest risk of developing DVT.

CN: Physiological integrity; CNS: Reduction of risk potential; CL: Analysis

104. A client admitted for a lower extremity deep vein thrombosis is experiencing dyspnea, chest pain, and diminished breath sounds. The nurse suspects this client may be developing which condition?
1. Hemothorax
2. Pneumothorax
3. Pulmonary embolism
4. Pulmonary hypertension

105. Which term refers to the condition of blood coagulating faster than normal, causing thrombin and other clotting factors to multiply?
1. Embolus
2. Hypercoagulability
3. Venous stasis
4. Venous wall injury

106. A client with a newly developed deep vein thrombosis (DVT) complains of pain. How does the nurse expect the client to describe the pain?
1. Dull ache
2. No pain
3. Sudden onset
4. Tingling

107. A client is admitted with deep vein thrombosis (DVT). Which of the following interventions would be <u>most</u> appropriate to relieve the pain?
1. Application of heat
2. Bed rest
3. Exercise
4. Leg elevation

108. Which term best describes the findings on cautious palpation of the vein in typical superficial thrombophlebitis?
1. Dilated
2. Knotty
3. Smooth
4. Tortuous

I see ... This question is asking you to characterize the type of pain experienced during deep vein thrombosis.

104. 3. A pulmonary embolism is a blood clot that forms in a vein, travels to the lungs, and lodges in the pulmonary vasculature. A hemothorax refers to blood in the pleural space. A pneumothorax is caused by an opening in the pleura. Pulmonary hypertension is an increase in pulmonary artery pressure, which increases the workload of the right ventricle.
CN: Physiological integrity; CNS: Physiological adaptation; CL: Analysis

105. 2. Hypercoagulability is the condition of blood coagulating faster than normal, causing thrombin and other clotting factors to multiply. This condition, along with venous stasis and venous wall injury, accounts for the formation of deep vein thrombosis. An embolus is a blood clot or fatty globule that formed in one area and is carried through the bloodstream to another area.
CN: Physiological integrity; CNS: Physiological adaptation; CL: Application

106. 3. DVT is associated with deep leg pain of sudden onset, which occurs secondary to the occlusion. A dull ache is more commonly associated with varicose veins. If the thrombus is large enough, it will cause pain. A tingling sensation is associated with an alteration in arterial blood flow.
CN: Physiological integrity; CNS: Basic care and comfort; CL: Analysis

107. 4. Leg elevation alleviates the pressure caused by thrombosis and occlusion by assisting venous return. The application of heat would dilate the vessels and pool blood in the area of the thrombus, increasing the risk of further thrombus formation. Bed rest adds to venous stasis by increasing the risk of thrombosis formation. When DVT is diagnosed, exercise isn't recommended until the clot has dissolved.
CN: Physiological integrity; CNS: Basic care and comfort; CL: Application

108. 2. The knotty feeling is secondary to the emboli adhering to the vein wall. Varicose veins may be described as dilated and tortuous. Normal veins feel smooth.
CN: Physiological integrity; CNS: Physiological adaptation; CL: Application

CN: Client needs category   CNS: Client needs subcategory   CL: Cognitive level

109. While assessing a client with deep vein thrombosis (DVT), which of the following terms indicates calf pain experienced by the client due to sharp dorsiflexion of the foot?
1. Dyskinesia
2. Eversion
3. Positive Babinski's reflex
4. Positive Homans' sign

110. A client is admitted to the unit with intermittent claudication. Which of the following responses by the nurse would <u>most</u> accurately explain the cause of the condition to the client?
1. Inadequate blood supply
2. Elevated leg position
3. Dependent leg position
4. Inadequate muscle oxygenation

111. The nurse anticipates that a client with intermittent claudication will receive which medication?
1. Analgesics
2. Warfarin (Coumadin)
3. Heparin
4. Pentoxifylline (Trental)

112. Which <u>oral</u> medication is administered to prevent further thrombus formation?
1. Warfarin (Coumadin)
2. Heparin
3. Furosemide (Lasix)
4. Metoprolol (Lopressor)

113. A client is experiencing acute pulmonary edema. What is the best position for the nurse to place the client in?
1. Lying flat in bed
2. Left side-lying
3. High Fowler's position
4. Semi-Fowler's position

I have a pain in my foot. I'm going to go Homan rest it.

This question requires you to know how certain drugs are administered.

109. 4. A positive Homans' sign (elicited by quickly dorsiflexing the foot), when accompanied by other findings, is diagnostic of DVT. Alone, however, Homans' sign can't be used to diagnose DVT because other conditions of the calf can produce a positive Homans' sign. Dyskinesia is the inability to perform voluntary movement. Eversion is the outward movement of the transverse tarsal joint. A positive Babinski's reflex is an extensor plantar response.
CN: Health promotion and maintenance; CNS: None; CL: Application

110. 4. When a muscle is starved of oxygen, it produces pain much like that of angina. Inadequate blood supply would cause necrosis. Leg position either alleviates or aggravates the condition.
CN: Physiological integrity; CNS: Physiological adaptation; CL: Application

111. 4. Pentoxifylline decreases blood viscosity, increases red blood cell flexibility, and improves flow through small vessels. Analgesics are administered for pain relief. Warfarin and heparin are anticoagulants.
CN: Physiological integrity; CNS: Pharmacological and parenteral therapies; CL: Analysis

112. 1. Warfarin prevents vitamin K from synthesizing certain clotting factors. This oral anticoagulant can be given long term. Heparin is a parenteral anticoagulant that interferes with coagulation by readily combining with antithrombin; it can't be given by mouth. Neither furosemide nor metoprolol affects anticoagulation.
CN: Physiological integrity; CNS: Pharmacological and parenteral therapies; CL: Application

113. 3. A high Fowler's position promotes ventilation and facilitates breathing by reducing venous return. Lying flat and side-lying positions worsen the breathing and increase workload of the heart. Semi-Fowler's position won't reduce the workload of the heart as well as high Fowler's position will.
CN: Physiological integrity; CNS: Basic care and comfort; CL: Application

114. Which blood gas abnormality is initially most suggestive of pulmonary edema?
1. Anoxia
2. Hypercapnia
3. Hyperoxygenation
4. Hypocapnia

115. A nurse is caring for a 78-year-old female client with sick sinus syndrome who is awaiting permanent pacemaker placement. The nurse is aware that which assessment finding indicates that the client is experiencing an initial drop in cardiac output?
1. Decreased blood pressure
2. Alteration in level of consciousness (LOC)
3. Decreased blood pressure and diuresis
4. Increased blood pressure and fluid volume

116. What is the most appropriate <u>initial</u> action by the nurse for a client coughing up pink, frothy sputum?
1. Call for help.
2. Call the physician.
3. Start an I.V. line.
4. Suction the client.

117. The nurse is providing teaching for a client who experienced an acute episode of pulmonary edema. What is the most important instruction for the nurse to provide?
1. Limit caloric intake.
2. Restrict carbohydrates.
3. Measure weight twice per day.
4. Call the physician if there is weight gain of more than 3 lb (1.5 kg) in 1 day.

Don't panic! Just think about what to do first.

114. 4. In an attempt to compensate for increased work of breathing due to hyperventilation, carbon dioxide (CO_2) decreases, causing hypocapnia. If the condition persists, CO_2 retention occurs and hypercapnia results. Although oxygenation is relatively low, the client isn't anoxic. Hyperoxygenation would result if the client was given oxygen in excess. However, secondary to fluid buildup, the client would have a low oxygenation level.
CN: Physiological integrity; CNS: Physiological adaptation; CL: Analysis

115. 4. The body compensates for a decrease in cardiac output with a rise in blood pressure, due to the stimulation of the sympathetic nervous system and an increase in blood volume as the kidneys retain sodium and water. Blood pressure doesn't initially drop in response to the compensatory mechanism of the body. Alteration in LOC will occur only if the decreased cardiac output persists.
CN: Physiological integrity; CNS: Physiological adaptation; CL: Analysis

116. 1. Production of pink, frothy sputum is a classic sign of acute pulmonary edema. Because the client is at high risk for decompensation, the nurse should call for help but not leave the room. The other three interventions should immediately follow.
CN: Physiological integrity; CNS: Physiological adaptation; CL: Analysis

117. 4. Gaining 3 lb in 1 day is indicative of fluid retention that would increase the workload of the heart, thereby putting the client at risk for acute pulmonary edema. Limiting caloric intake doesn't influence fluid status. Restricting carbohydrates wouldn't affect fluid status. The body needs carbohydrates for energy and healing. The client must be weighed in the morning after the first urination. If the client is weighed later in the day, the finding wouldn't be accurate because of fluid intake during the day.
CN: Physiological integrity; CNS: Reduction of risk potential; CL: Application

118. The nurse knows that a 45-year-old client with severe hypertension will experience increased workload of the heart due to which of the following?
1. Increased afterload
2. Increased cardiac output
3. Overload of the heart
4. Increased preload

119. A client with acute pulmonary edema has been taking an angiotensin-converting enzyme (ACE) inhibitor. The nurse teaches him that this medication has been ordered for which reason?
1. To promote diuresis
2. To increase contractility
3. To decrease contractility
4. To reduce blood pressure

This is another question that tests your knowledge of what certain drugs do.

120. A client with acute pulmonary edema caused by heart failure asks the nurse which area of the heart is usually damaged. What is the best response by the nurse?
1. Left atrium
2. Right atrium
3. Left ventricle
4. Right ventricle

121. Which statement by a nurse to the health care aide <u>best</u> explains the need to promptly report changes in respiratory rate for a client diagnosed with heart failure?
1. "Pulmonary edema, a life-threatening condition, can develop in minutes."
2. "Severe acute respiratory syndrome (SARS) is a complication of heart failure."
3. "Pneumonia is a consequence of inadequate ventilation with heart failure."
4. "Pneumothorax, a life-threatening condition, can develop in minutes."

118. 1. Afterload refers to the resistance normally maintained by the aortic and pulmonic valves, the condition and tone of the aorta, and the resistance offered by the systemic and pulmonary arterioles. Hypertension increases afterload, as the left ventricle has to work harder to eject blood against vasoconstriction. Cardiac output is the amount of blood expelled from the heart per minute. Overload refers to an abundance of circulating volume. Preload is the volume of blood in the ventricle at the end of diastole.
CN: Physiological integrity; CNS: Physiological adaptation; CL: Analysis

119. 4. ACE inhibitors are given to reduce blood pressure by inhibiting aldosterone production, which in turn decreases sodium and water reabsorption. ACE inhibitors also reduce production of angiotensin II, a potent vasoconstrictor. Diuretics are given to promote diuresis. Inotropic agents increase contractility. Negative inotropic agents decrease contractility.
CN: Physiological integrity; CNS: Pharmacological and parenteral therapies; CL: Application

120. 3. The left ventricle is responsible for the majority of force for cardiac output. If the left ventricle is damaged, the output decreases and fluid accumulates in the interstitial and alveolar spaces, causing pulmonary edema. Damage to the left atrium would contribute to heart failure but wouldn't affect cardiac output or, therefore, the onset of pulmonary edema. If the right atrium and right ventricle were damaged, right-sided heart failure would result.
CN: Physiological integrity; CNS: Physiological adaptation; CL: Application

121. 1. Pulmonary edema, a life-threatening complication of heart failure, can develop in minutes, secondary to a sudden fluid shift from the pulmonary vasculature to the lung interstitial alveoli. SARS and pneumonia are caused by infections. Pneumothorax is a collection of air or gas in the pleural space, causing the lung to collapse.
CN: Physiological Integrity; CNS: Reduction of risk potential; CL: Application

122. The nurse evaluates her teaching by asking the student nurse which term is used to describe the amount of stretch on the myocardium at the end of diastole. Which is the most accurate response?
1. Afterload
2. Cardiac index
3. Cardiac output
4. Preload

123. What is the most appropriate action for a nurse to take when administering a new blood pressure medication to a client?
1. Administer the medication to the client without explanation.
2. Inform the client of the new drug only if he asks about it.
3. Inform the client of the new medication, its name and use, and the reason for the change in medication.
4. Administer the medication, and inform the client that the physician will later explain the medication.

124. The nurse is aware that antihypertensives should be used cautiously in clients already taking which other drug?
1. Ibuprofen (Advil)
2. Diphenhydramine (Benadryl)
3. Thioridazine
4. Vitamins

125. A 57-year-old client with a history of bronchial asthma is prescribed propranolol (Inderal) to control hypertension. Before administering propranolol, which action should the nurse take first?
1. Monitor apical pulse rate.
2. Instruct the client to take the medication with food.
3. Question the physician about the order.
4. Caution the client to rise slowly when standing.

Which answer best promotes compliance?

Note the first in question 125. It's the key to the right answer.

122. 4. Preload is the amount of stretch of the cardiac muscle fibers at the end of diastole. The volume of blood in the ventricle at the end of diastole determines preload. Afterload is the force against which the ventricle must expel blood. Cardiac index is the individualized measurement of cardiac output, based on the client's body surface area. Cardiac output is the amount of blood the heart is expelling per minute.
CN: Physiological integrity; CNS: Physiological adaptation; CL: Application

123. 3. Informing the client of the medication, its use, and the reason for the medication change is important to the care of the client. Teaching the client about his treatment regimen promotes compliance. The other responses are inappropriate.
CN: Safe, effective care environment; CNS: Management of care; CL: Application

124. 3. Thioridazine affects the neurotransmitter norepinephrine, which causes hypotension and other cardiovascular effects. Administering an antihypertensive to a client who already has hypotension could have serious adverse effects. Ibuprofen is an anti-inflammatory that doesn't interfere with the cardiovascular system. Although diphenhydramine does have histaminic effects such as sedation, it isn't known to decrease blood pressure. Vitamins aren't drugs and don't interfere with cardiovascular function.
CN: Physiological integrity; CNS: Pharmacological and parenteral therapies; CL: Application

125. 3. Propranolol and other beta-adrenergic blockers are contraindicated in a client with bronchial asthma, so the nurse should question the physician before giving the dose. The other responses are appropriate actions for a client receiving propranolol, but questioning the physician takes priority. The client's apical pulse should always be checked before giving propranolol; if the pulse rate is extremely low, the nurse should withhold the drug and notify the physician. Taking propranolol with food enhances its absorption. Because propranolol can cause light-headedness, the client should be told to rise slowly when standing.
CN: Physiological integrity; CNS: Pharmacological and parenteral therapies; CL: Application

126. One hour after I.V. furosemide (Lasix) is administered to a client with heart failure, a short burst of ventricular tachycardia appears on the cardiac monitor. Which electrolyte imbalance should the nurse suspect?
1. Hypocalcemia
2. Hypermagnesemia
3. Hypokalemia
4. Hypernatremia

127. A client has a reduced serum high-density lipoprotein (HDL) level and an elevated low-density lipoprotein (LDL) level. Which dietary modification is appropriate for this client?
1. Fiber intake of less than 10% of total calories daily
2. Less than 40% of calories from fat
3. Cholesterol intake of less than 300 mg daily
4. Less than 7% of calories from saturated fat

128. A paradoxical pulse occurs in a client who had coronary artery bypass graft (CABG) surgery 2 days ago. Which surgical complication should the nurse suspect?
1. Left-sided heart failure
2. Aortic regurgitation
3. Complete heart block
4. Pericardial tamponade

Just as I suspected—a pericardial paradox!

129. A 35-year-old client was admitted to the coronary care unit (CCU) 2 days ago with an acute myocardial infarction. Which action would breach client confidentiality?
1. The CCU nurse gives a verbal report to the nurse on the telemetry unit before transferring the client to that unit.
2. The CCU nurse notifies the on-call physician about a change in the client's condition.
3. The emergency department (ED) nurse calls up the latest electrocardiogram results to check the client's progress.
4. At the client's request, the CCU nurse updates the client's wife on his condition.

126. 3. Furosemide is a potassium-depleting diuretic that can cause hypokalemia. In turn, hypokalemia increases myocardial excitability, leading to ventricular tachycardia. Hypocalcemia, which slows conduction through the atrioventricular junction, can cause such bradyarrhythmias as atrioventricular block. Hypermagnesemia may lead to bradycardia, not tachycardia. Hypernatremia may cause sinus tachycardia as a result of water loss.
CN: Physiological integrity; CNS: Physiological adaptation; CL: Analysis

127. 4. A client with low serum HDL and high serum LDL levels should get less than 7% of daily calories from saturated fat. Fiber intake should be at least 15% of total daily calories, total fat intake should be only 25% to 35% of daily calories, and cholesterol intake should be less than 200 mg daily.
CN: Physiological integrity; CNS: Reduction of risk potential; CL: Application

128. 4. A paradoxical pulse (a palpable decrease in pulse amplitude on quiet inspiration) signals pericardial tamponade, a complication of CABG surgery. Left-sided heart failure can cause pulsus alternans (pulse amplitude alternation from beat to beat, with a regular rhythm). Aortic regurgitation may cause bisferious pulse (an increased arterial pulse with a double systolic peak). Complete heart block may cause a bounding pulse (a strong pulse with increased pulse pressure).
CN: Physiological integrity; CNS: Physiological adaptation; CL: Application

129. 3. The ED nurse is no longer directly involved with the client's care and thus has no legal right to information about his present condition. Anyone directly involved in his care (such as the telemetry nurse and the on-call physician) has the right to information about his condition. Because the client requested that the nurse update his wife on his condition, doing so doesn't breach confidentiality.
CN: Safe, effective care environment; CNS: Management of care; CL: Application

130. A client arriving in the emergency department (ED) is receiving cardiopulmonary resuscitation from paramedics, who are giving ventilations through an endotracheal (ET) tube that they placed in the client's home. During a pause in compressions, the cardiac monitor shows narrow QRS complexes and a heart rate of 55 beats/minute with a palpable pulse. Which action should the nurse take <u>first</u>?
1. Start an I.V. line and administer amiodarone, 300 mg I.V. over 10 minutes.
2. Check ET tube placement.
3. Obtain an arterial blood gas (ABG) sample.
4. Administer atropine, 1 mg I.V.

Hint! Hint!
It's the first action.

131. After unsuccessful cardiopulmonary resuscitation efforts, the nurse must prepare an Islamic client for the morgue. Which nursing action should the nurse take?
1. Allowing the client's family to perform the ritualistic washing
2. Doing nothing; the Burial Society will perform a ritual cleansing
3. Doing nothing; only the family and close friends may touch the body
4. Providing routine postmortem care

132. A 63-year-old client has Prinzmetal's angina. To reduce the risk of coronary artery spasms, which type of medication is the physician <u>most</u> likely to prescribe?
1. Beta-adrenergic blocker
2. Angiotensin-converting enzyme (ACE) inhibitor
3. Inotropic vasodilator
4. Calcium channel blocker

One of these medications will reduce the risk of coronary artery spasms.

133. An 86-year-old client with heart failure is receiving furosemide (Lasix), 40 mg I.V. The physician orders 40 mEq of potassium chloride in 100 ml of dextrose 5% in water, to infuse over 4 hours. The client's most recent serum potassium level is 3.0 mEq/L. At which infusion rate should the nurse set the I.V. pump?
1. 25 ml/hour
2. 10 ml/hour
3. 100 ml/hour
4. 50 ml/hour

130. 2. ET tube placement should be confirmed as soon as the client arrives in the ED. Once the airway is secured, oxygenation and ventilation should be confirmed using an end-tidal carbon dioxide monitor and pulse oximetry. Next, the nurse should make sure I.V. access is established. If the client experiences symptomatic bradycardia, atropine is administered as ordered, 0.5 to 1 mg every 3 to 5 minutes to a total of 3 mg. Then the nurse should try to find the cause of the client's arrest by obtaining an ABG sample. Amiodarone is indicated for ventricular tachycardia, ventricular fibrillation, and atrial flutter—not symptomatic bradycardia.
CN: Physiological integrity; CNS: Physiological adaptation; CL: Application

131. 1. Physical care at death for a person of the Islamic faith consists of ritualistic washing by the family, with the client's body positioned toward Mecca. The Burial Society may perform ritual cleansing for clients of the Jewish faith. Hindu clients believe that only family and close friends should touch the body. Routine postmortem care is appropriate for Christian clients.
CN: Psychosocial integrity; CNS: None; CL: Application

132. 4. A calcium channel blocker, such as diltiazem (Cardizem), is indicated in managing Prinzmetal's angina because it reduces the incidence of coronary artery spasm. A beta-adrenergic blocker, such as metoprolol (Lopressor), treats angina by decreasing myocardial oxygen needs and has no effect on coronary artery spasms. An ACE inhibitor, such as enalapril (Vasotec), is used to manage hypertension. An inotropic vasodilator, such as milrinone, is indicated for short-term I.V. therapy in heart failure.
CN: Physiological integrity; CNS: Pharmacological and parenteral therapies; CL: Application

133. 1. Use this formula to determine the infusion rate:

$$ml/hour = \frac{total\ volume\ (in\ ml)\ to\ be\ infused}{total\ time\ of\ infusion\ in\ hours}$$

$$ml/hour = \frac{100\ ml}{4\ hours}$$

$$ml/hour = 25$$

CN: Physiological integrity; CNS: Pharmacological and parenteral therapies; CL: Application

134. A nurse is planning discharge instructions for a client who is being treated for ventricular tachycardia. Which of the following rationales for including bananas in the client's diet is <u>most</u> accurate?
1. Bananas are high in carbohydrate.
2. Bananas are high in potassium.
3. Bananas are low in sodium.
4. Bananas are high in fiber.

135. After cardiac surgery, a client's blood pressure measures 126/80 mm Hg. The nurse determines that mean arterial pressure (MAP) is:
1. 46 mm Hg.
2. 80 mm Hg.
3. 95 mm Hg.
4. 90 mm Hg.

I'm good for the heart. Can you guess why?

136. A charge nurse is preparing client care assignments for the next shift. A client who underwent femoral-popliteal bypass surgery is scheduled to return from the postanesthesia care unit. Which staff member should receive this client?
1. Registered nurse with 1 year of experience
2. Licensed practical nurse (LPN) with 5 years of experience
3. Nursing assistant with 15 years of experience
4. Charge nurse with 10 years of experience

137. An 18-year-old client who recently had an upper respiratory infection is admitted with suspected rheumatic fever. Which assessment findings confirm this diagnosis?
1. Erythema marginatum, subcutaneous nodules, and fever
2. Tachycardia, finger clubbing, and a loud second heart sound (S_2)
3. Dyspnea, cough, and palpitations
4. Dyspnea, fatigue, and syncope

There are several findings here. Which answer confirms the diagnosis?

134. 2. A low serum potassium level increases the risk of ventricular tachycardia. Therefore, the client should be instructed to eat potassium-rich foods such as bananas.

CN: Health promotion and maintenance; CNS: None; CL: Analysis

135. 3. Use this formula to calculate MAP:

$$MAP = \frac{systolic + 2\ (diastolic)}{3}$$

$$MAP = \frac{126\ mm\ Hg + 2\ (80\ mm\ Hg)}{3}$$

$$MAP = \frac{286\ mm\ Hg}{3}$$

$$MAP = 95\ mm\ Hg$$

CN: Physiological integrity; CNS: Reduction of risk potential; CL: Analysis

136. 1. Because this client requires frequent neurovascular assessments, a registered nurse should receive him. An LPN, although she's experienced and can collect data, doesn't have the education to perform the physical assessment required by this client. The nursing assistant lacks the necessary assessment skills. The charge nurse needs to be available to direct the care of other clients.

CN: Safe, effective care environment; CNS: Management of care; CL: Analysis

137. 1. Diagnosis of rheumatic fever requires that the client have either two major Jones criteria or one minor criterion plus evidence of a previous streptococcal infection. Major criteria include carditis, polyarthritis, Sydenham's chorea, subcutaneous nodules, and erythema marginatum (transient, nonpruritic macules on the trunk or inner aspects of the upper arms or thighs). Minor criteria include fever, arthralgia, elevated levels of acute phase reactants, and a prolonged PR interval on electrocardiography. Tachycardia, finger clubbing, and a loud S_2 suggest transposition of the great arteries (a cyanotic congenital heart defect). Dyspnea, cough, and palpitations occur with mitral insufficiency. Dyspnea, fatigue, and syncope indicate aortic insufficiency.

CN: Physiological integrity; CNS: Physiological adaptation; CL: Application

138. A client with new onset of atrial fibrillation is receiving warfarin (Coumadin) to help prevent thromboemboli. The warfarin dosage will reach therapeutic levels when the international normalized ratio (INR) falls within which range?
1. 1 to 2
2. 1.5 to 2.5
3. 2 to 3
4. 2.5 to 3.5

139. A 38-year-old client comes to the emergency department complaining that his heart "suddenly began to race." After attaching him to the cardiac monitor, the nurse observes atrial tachycardia. Which rhythm strip characteristics indicate this arrhythmia?
1. Atrial rate greater than the ventricular rate, sawtooth P waves
2. Irregular rhythm, indiscernible atrial rate, absent P waves
3. Regular atrial and ventricular rhythms, rate of 123 beats/minute
4. Regular atrial and ventricular rhythms, P wave hidden in the T wave, rate of 210 beats/minute

140. A client is receiving spironolactone to treat hypertension. Which instruction should the nurse provide?
1. "Eat foods high in potassium."
2. "Take daily potassium supplements."
3. "Discontinue sodium restrictions."
4. "Avoid salt substitutes."

141. A 23-year-old client develops cardiac tamponade when the car he was driving hits a telephone pole; he wasn't wearing a seat belt. The nurse helps the physician perform a pericardiocentesis. Which outcome would indicate that the treatment has been effective?
1. Neck vein distention
2. Pulsus paradoxus
3. Increased blood pressure
4. Muffled heart sounds

142. A client admitted with angina complains of severe chest pain and suddenly becomes unresponsive. After establishing unresponsiveness, which action should the nurse take <u>first</u>?
1. Activate the resuscitation team.
2. Open the client's airway.
3. Check for breathing.
4. Check for signs of circulation.

Your first hint is the word first.

138. 3. In a client with atrial fibrillation, warfarin reaches therapeutic levels when the INR is 2 to 3. Lower ratios are below the therapeutic range. A range of 2.5 to 3.5 is too high for a client on warfarin and increases the hemorrhage risk.
CN: Physiological integrity; CNS: Reduction of risk potential; CL: Application

139. 4. With atrial tachycardia, the rhythm is regular, the P wave is hidden in the preceding T wave, and the rate ranges from 140 to 250 beats/ minute. A ventricular rate that varies with the degree of atrioventricular block, along with saw-tooth P waves, characterizes atrial flutter. Irregular ventricular response and absent P waves character- ize atrial fibrillation. Regular and equal atrial and ventricular rhythms and a rate of 100 to 160 beats/ minute characterize sinus tachycardia.
CN: Physiological integrity; CNS: Physiological adaptation; CL: Application

140. 4. Because spironolactone is a potassium- sparing diuretic, the client should avoid salt substi- tutes because of their high potassium content. The client should also avoid potassium-rich foods and potassium supplements. To reduce fluid volume overload, sodium restrictions should continue.
CN: Physiological integrity; CNS: Pharmacological and parenteral therapies; CL: Application

141. 3. Cardiac tamponade is associated with decreased cardiac output, which in turn reduces blood pressure. By removing a small amount of blood, pericardiocentesis increases blood pressure. Neck vein distention, pulsus paradoxus, and muffled heart sounds indicate persistent car- diac tamponade, meaning that pericardiocentesis hasn't been effective.
CN: Physiological integrity; CNS: Physiological adaptation; CL: Application

142. 1. Immediately after establishing unrespon- siveness, the nurse should activate the resuscita- tion team. The next step is to open the airway using the head-tilt, chin-lift maneuver and check for breathing (looking, listening, and feeling for no more than 10 seconds). If the client isn't breathing, give two slow breaths using a bag mask or pocket mask. Next, check for signs of circulation by palpating the carotid pulse.
CN: Physiological integrity; CNS: Physiological adaptation; CL: Application

143. A 54-year-old client is admitted with an acute inferior-wall myocardial infarction (MI). During the admission interview, he says he stopped taking his metoprolol (Lopressor) 5 days ago because he was feeling better. Which nursing diagnosis takes <u>priority</u> for this client?
1. Anxiety
2. Risk for decreased cardiac tissue perfusion
3. Acute pain
4. Ineffective family therapeutic regimen management

144. A client comes to the emergency department with acute shortness of breath and a cough that produces pink, frothy sputum. Admission assessment reveals crackles and wheezes, a blood pressure of 82/45 mm Hg, a heart rate of 120 beats/minute, and a respiratory rate of 38 breaths/minute. The client's medical history includes diabetes mellitus, hypertension, and heart failure. Which disorder should the nurse suspect?
1. Pulmonary edema
2. Pneumothorax
3. Cardiac tamponade
4. Pulmonary embolus

145. A 57-year-old client with acute arterial occlusion of the left leg undergoes an emergency embolectomy. Six hours later, the nurse isn't able to obtain pulses in his left foot using Doppler ultrasound. She immediately notifies the physician, who asks her to prepare the client for surgery. As the nurse enters the client's room to prepare him, he states that he won't have any more surgery. What is the most appropriate <u>initial</u> action of the nurse?
1. Explaining the risks of not having the surgery
2. Notifying the physician immediately
3. Notifying the nursing supervisor
4. Recording the client's refusal in the nurses' notes

Here you're looking for the best *initial* response.

146. The nurse coming on duty receives the report from the nurse going off duty. Which client should the on-duty nurse assess <u>first</u>?
1. The 58-year-old client who was admitted 2 days ago with heart failure, blood pressure of 126/76 mm Hg, and a respiratory rate of 22 breaths/minute
2. The 89-year-old client with end-stage right-sided heart failure, blood pressure of 78/50 mm Hg, and a "do not resuscitate" order
3. The 62-year-old client who was admitted 1 day ago with thrombophlebitis and is receiving I.V. heparin
4. The 75-year-old client who was admitted 1 hour ago with new-onset atrial fibrillation and is receiving I.V. diltiazem (Cardizem)

143. **2.** MI results from prolonged myocardial ischemia caused by reduced blood flow through the coronary arteries. Therefore, the priority nursing diagnosis for this client is risk for decreased cardiac tissue perfusion. Anxiety, acute pain, and ineffective family therapeutic regimen management are appropriate but don't take priority.
CN: Safe, effective care environment; CNS: Management of care; CL: Analysis

144. **1.** Shortness of breath, tachypnea, low blood pressure, tachycardia, diffuse crackles, and a cough producing pink, frothy sputum are late signs of pulmonary edema. Pneumothorax causes sudden, sharp pleuritic pain exacerbated by chest movement, breathing, and coughing; shortness of breath; and absent breath sounds on the affected side. Cardiac tamponade produces muffled heart sounds, pulsus paradoxus, and jugular vein distention. Pulmonary embolus may cause fever, cough, hemoptysis, and a pleural friction rub.
CN: Physiological integrity; CNS: Physiological adaptation; CL: Application

145. **1.** The best initial response is to explain the risks of not having the surgery. If the client understands the risks but still refuses, the nurse should notify the physician and the nursing supervisor and then record the client's refusal in the nurses' notes.
CN: Safe, effective care environment; CNS: Management of care; CL: Analysis

146. **4.** The client with atrial fibrillation has the greatest potential to become unstable and is on I.V. medication that requires close monitoring. After assessing this client, the nurse should assess the 62-year-old client with thrombophlebitis who is receiving a heparin infusion, and then the 58-year-old client admitted 2 days ago with heart failure (his signs and symptoms are resolving and don't require immediate attention). The lowest priority is the 89-year-old with end-stage right-sided heart failure, who requires time-consuming supportive measures.
CN: Safe, effective care environment; CNS: Management of care; CL: Analysis

147. A client's blood pressure is being checked at a health clinic. Which statement by the client demonstrates awareness of having a risk factor for hypertension?
  1. "My doctor told me my body mass index is 23."
  2. "I usually have a glass of wine or two to unwind when I come home from work."
  3. "I should get my blood pressure checked more often because I am African American."
  4. "I have colds during the winter, so I see my doctor to get the flu shot every year."

148. Which finding suggests to the nurse that fluid resuscitation has been effective for a 23-year-old client admitted in hypovolemic shock?
  1. Urine output of 15 ml/hour
  2. Urine output of 20 ml/hour
  3. Urine output of 25 ml/hour
  4. Urine output of 30 ml/hour

149. A client is being monitored via telemetry using a 3-lead system. Which graphic shows the correct electrode positions to monitor modified chest lead 1 (MCL1)?

1.

2.

3.

4.

147. 3. Research studies have shown that clients who are aware of their personal risk factors are more motivated to achieve adequate control of blood pressure. African Americans are at risk for hypertension.
CN: Health promotion and maintenance; CNS: Management of care; CL: Application

148. 4. In an adult, urine output below 30 ml/hour indicates inadequate blood flow to the kidneys. Therefore, urine output of 30 ml/hour or greater reflects adequate fluid resuscitation.
CN: Physiological integrity; CNS: Physiological adaptation; CL: Analysis

149. 4. Option 4 shows the correct electrode placement for MCL1. Option 1 shows the correct placement to monitor lead III. Option 2 shows the correct placement to monitor MCL6. Option 3 shows the correct placement to monitor lead II.
CN: Physiological integrity; CNS: Reduction of risk potential; CL: Application

150. An elderly client has a history of aortic stenosis. Identify the area where the nurse should place the stethoscope to best hear the murmur.

150. The murmur of aortic stenosis is low-pitched, rough, and rasping. It's heard loudest in second intercostal space to right of sternum.
CN: Physiological integrity; CNS: Physiological adaptation; CL: Application

151. A client with deep vein thrombosis has an I.V. infusion of heparin sodium infusing at 1,500 units/hour. The concentration in the bag is 25,000 units/500 ml. How many milliliters should the nurse document as intake from this infusion for an 8-hour shift? Record your answer using a whole number.

_____ milliliters

151. 240. First, calculate how many units are in each milliliter of the medication: 25,000 units/500 ml = 50 units/ml. Next, calculate how many milliliters the client receives each hour: 1 ml/50 units × 1,500 units/hour = 30 ml/hour. Lastly, multiply by 8 hours: 30 ml × 8 hours = 240 ml.
CN: Physiological integrity; CNS: Pharmacological and parenteral therapies; CL: Application

152. The nurse suspects that her client is in cardiac arrest. According to the American Heart Association (AHA), she should perform the actions listed below. Order these actions in the sequence that the nurse should perform them.

| 1. Activate the emergency response team. |
| 2. Assess responsiveness. |
| 3. Call for a defibrillator. |
| 4. Provide two slow breaths. |
| 5. Assess pulse. |
| 6. Assess breathing. |

152. According to the AHA, the nurse should first assess responsiveness. If the client is unresponsive, she should activate the emergency response system, and then call for a defibrillator. Next, she should assess breathing by opening the airway and then look, listen, and feel for respirations. If respirations aren't present, she should administer two slow breaths, and then assess carotid pulse. If no pulse is present, she should start chest compressions.
CN: Physiological integrity; CNS: Physiological adaptation; CL: Application

| 2. Assess responsiveness. |
| 1. Activate the emergency response team. |
| 3. Call for a defibrillator. |
| 6. Assess breathing. |
| 4. Provide two slow breaths. |
| 5. Assess pulse. |

Congratulations! You did it!

Chapter 4
Hematologic & immune disorders

1. A 27-year-old male who is an established client in the in the Family Medicine Clinic was recently diagnosed with acquired immunodeficiency syndrome (AIDS). When reviewing his chart, what does the nurse expect to find with this diagnosis?
1. Infection with human immunodeficiency virus (HIV), tuberculosis, and cytomegalovirus
2. Infection with HIV, an alternative lifestyle, and a T-cell count above 200 cells/μl
3. Infection with HIV, CD4+ count below 200 cells/μl, and a T-cell count above 400 cells/μl
4. Infection with HIV, a history of acute HIV infection, and a CD4+ T-cell count below 200 cells/μl

2. A nurse has volunteered for a mission trip to an area with a high incidence of HIV. Part of the responsibility will be teaching a class about HIV. The next question in the PowerPoint presentation is, "Which body substances <u>most easily</u> transmit human immunodeficiency virus (HIV)?" Which of the following options would you include in your next PowerPoint slide to answer that question?
1. Feces and saliva
2. Blood and semen
3. Breast milk and tears
4. Vaginal secretions and urine

3. Immediately after giving an injection, a nurse is accidentally stuck with the needle. The nurse is aware that testing for human immunodeficiency virus (HIV) antibodies should occur:
1. immediately and then again in 6 weeks.
2. immediately and then again in 3 months.
3. in 2 weeks and then again in 6 months.
4. in 2 weeks and then again in 1 year.

More than one answer may seem correct. Be careful to choose the best answer.

Time is often a crucial element in testing for HIV.

1. 4. Three criteria must be met for an adult client to be diagnosed with AIDS. He must be HIV-positive, have a CD4+ T-cell count below 200 cells/μl, and have one or more specific conditions that include acute infection with HIV. Because HIV attaches to the CD4+ receptor sites of the T cell, a T-cell value alone is incorrect.
CN: Physiological integrity; CNS: Physiological adaptation; CL: Application

2. 2. HIV is most easily transmitted in blood, semen, and vaginal secretions. However, it has also been found in urine, feces, saliva, tears, and breast milk.
CN: Health promotion and maintenance; CNS: None; CL: Analysis

3. 2. The employer will want to test the nurse immediately to determine whether a preexisting infection is present, and then again in 3 months to detect seroconversion as a result of the needle stick. Waiting 2 weeks to perform the first test is too late to detect preexisting infection. Testing sooner than 3 months may yield false-negative results.
CN: Health promotion and maintenance; CNS: None; CL: Analysis

CN: Client needs category   CNS: Client needs subcategory   CL: Cognitive level

4. The nurse determines that the <u>initial</u> blood test used to identify a response to human immunodeficiency virus (HIV) infection would be?
1. Western blot
2. CD4+ T-cell count
3. Erythrocyte sedimentation rate
4. Enzyme-linked immunosorbent assay (ELISA)

Question 4 is asking you to prioritize.

5. A client with HIV experiences frequent bouts of diarrhea. The nurse determines dietary teaching is effective when the client states the need to avoid:
1. milk.
2. red licorice.
3. chicken soup.
4. broiled meat.

6. A nurse is preparing a dietary teaching plan for a client with rheumatoid arthritis. Select the recommended supplement that will reduce inflammation for the client.
1. Fish oil
2. Vitamin D
3. Iron-rich foods
4. Calcium carbonate

7. A client is diagnosed with uncomplicated rheumatoid arthritis. The nurse explains to the client that nonsteroidal anti-inflammatory drugs (NSAIDs) are used in the treatment plan. Which NSAID medication is used to treat rheumatoid arthritis?
1. Furosemide
2. Haloperidol
3. Ibuprofen
4. Methotrexate

4. 4. The ELISA is the first screening test for HIV. A Western blot test confirms a positive ELISA test. Other blood tests that support the diagnosis of HIV include CD4+ and CD8+ counts, complete blood counts, immunoglobulin levels, p24 antigen assay, and quantitative ribonucleic acid assays.
CN: Health promotion and maintenance; CNS: None; CL: Analysis

5. 1. Clients with chronic diarrhea may develop intolerance to lactose, which may worsen the diarrhea. Although red licorice may be eaten, black licorice should be avoided. Other foods that the client should avoid include fatty foods, other lactose-containing foods, caffeine, and sugar. Chicken soup and broiled meat may be consumed.
CN: Physiological integrity; CNS: Reduction of risk potential; CL: Application

6. 1. The therapeutic effect of fish oil suppresses inflammatory mediator production (such as prostaglandins); how it works is unknown. Iron-rich foods are recommended to decrease the anemia associated with rheumatoid arthritis. Vitamin D and calcium supplements may help reduce bone resorption.
CN: Physiological integrity; CNS: Physiological adaptation; CL: Application

7. 3. Ibuprofen, fenoprofen, naproxen, piroxicam, and indomethacin are NSAIDs used for clients with rheumatoid arthritis. Furosemide is a loop diuretic and haloperidol is an antipsychotic agent, neither of which is used to treat rheumatoid arthritis. Methotrexate is an immunosuppressant used in the early treatment of rheumatoid arthritis.
CN: Physiological integrity; CNS: Pharmacological and parenteral therapies; CL: Application

8. The nurse is teaching a client about the method of human immunodeficiency virus (HIV) transmission that carries the <u>most</u> risk. The client demonstrates understanding of exposure risks by making which of the following statements?
1. "I can have routine teeth cleaning at the dentist's office."
2. "I may have intercourse with my spouse."
3. "I may engage in unprotected, noninsertive sexual contact."
4. "I should not engage in intercourse with a new partner without a condom."

The key word in question 8 is most.

9. While preparing a case study, the nurse notes that which client is most likely to develop rheumatoid arthritis?
1. A 25-year-old woman
2. A 40-year-old man
3. A 65-year-old woman
4. A 70-year-old man

10. A nurse is caring for a client with acquired immunodeficiency syndrome (AIDS) who is receiving Retrovir (zidovudine). The client asked the nurse, "How does this drug work?" The nurse determines that teaching was effective when the client makes which statement?
1. "It kills the human immunodeficiency (HIV) virus."
2. "It suppresses the HIV virus."
3. "I won't infect anyone else when I take this drug."
4. "It's the only drug for HIV I need to take."

11. A nursing student is assigned an HIV-positive client. The student asks the staff nurse what precautions are necessary when taking the clients blood pressure. The nurse instructs the student to:
1. wear gloves.
2. wear a gown.
3. use contact precautions.
4. wash hands.

12. A nurse is teaching a community education class on human immunodeficiency virus (HIV). The nurse explains to her clients that the group or factor linked to higher morbidity and mortality in HIV-infected clients is:
1. homosexual men.
2. lower socioeconomic status.
3. treatment in a large teaching hospital.
4. treatment by a physician who specializes in HIV infection.

8. **4.** Having intercourse with a new partner is risky because of the unknown I.V. drug use and sexual history. Use of a condom may increase the protection against HIV exposure. Absolutely safe sex practices include autosexual activities, abstinence, and intercourse within a monogamous, uninfected couple. Very safe practices include noninsertive sexual contact. Having your teeth cleaned isn't a risk factor if the dental office properly sterilizes the equipment.
CN: Health promotion and maintenance; CNS: None; CL: Analysis

9. **3.** Rheumatoid arthritis affects women three times more often than men. The average age of onset is 55.
CN: Health promotion and maintenance; CNS: None; CL: Analysis

10. **2.** Zidovudine is an antiviral drug that suppresses the replication of the HIV virus. It is most commonly used for HIV clients in conjunction with other antiretroviral drugs. It also helps prevent maternal–fetal transmission of HIV. However, it is not a cure, it doesn't kill the HIV virus, and clients taking this medication remain infectious.
CN: Physiological integrity; CNS: Pharmacological therapies; CL: Analysis

11. **4.** Since taking a client's blood pressure doesn't involve contact with his blood or secretions, washing hands is all that is necessary.
CN: Safe, effective care environment; CNS: Safety and infection control; CL: Application

12. **2.** Morbidity and mortality have been associated with lower socioeconomic status, receiving care in a community hospital or by a physician without much experience with HIV infections, and lack of access to adequate health care.
CN: Physiological integrity; CNS: Physiological adaptation; CL: Analysis

13. The nurse determines that teaching a client about rheumatoid arthritis was successful when the client makes which statement?
1. "It will get better and worse again."
2. "Once it clears up, it will never come back."
3. "I will definitely have to have surgery for this."
4. "It will never get any better than it is right now."

14. The nurse is reviewing <u>first</u>-line therapy medications of a client recently diagnosed with rheumatoid arthritis. Which medication does the nurse anticipate will be included?
1. Aspirin
2. Cytoxan
3. Ferrous sulfate
4. Prednisone

15. The nurse is reviewing a client's complete blood count and notes a decreased number of erythrocytes, leukocytes, and platelets. The nurse interprets this as indicative of what condition?
1. Pernicious anemia
2. Aplastic anemia
3. Sickle cell anemia
4. Polycythemia

16. A nurse is reviewing the laboratory results of a client with anemia and anticipates which lab value would be decreased?
1. Erythrocytes
2. Granulocytes
3. Leukocytes
4. Platelets

17. The nurse is assessing a client in the emergency room who has been experiencing black stools for the past month. The client suddenly complains of chest and stomach pain. What is the <u>most important</u> action for the nurse to perform?
1. Give nasal oxygen.
2. Take vital signs.
3. Begin cardiac monitoring.
4. Draw blood for laboratory analysis.

The word *first* should shed some light on the answer.

Put your thinking cap on! Remember: assessment before intervention.

13. 1. The client with rheumatoid arthritis needs to understand it is a somewhat unpredictable disease characterized by periods of exacerbation and remission. There's no cure, but symptoms can be managed at times. Surgery may be indicated in some cases but not always.
CN: Psychosocial integrity; CNS: None; CL: Application

14. 1. Nonsteroidal anti-inflammatory drugs (NSAIDs) such as aspirin are considered first-line therapy by some physicians. Cytoxan may be used in cases of severe synovitis, rather than as first-line therapy. Ferrous sulfate isn't used to treat rheumatoid arthritis. Prednisone may be used to control inflammation when NSAIDs aren't tolerated.
CN: Physiological integrity; CNS: Pharmacological and parenteral therapies; CL: Application

15. 2. Aplastic anemia is a pathology of bone marrow dysfunction. Red blood cells, white blood cells, and platelets are decreased.
CN: Physiological integrity; CNS: Physiological adaptation; CL: Application

16. 1. Anemia is defined as a decreased number of erythrocytes (red blood cells). Leukopenia is a decreased number of leukocytes (white blood cells [WBCs]). Thrombocytopenia is a decreased number of platelets. Lastly, granulocytopenia is a decreased number of granulocytes (a type of WBC).
CN: Health promotion and maintenance; CNS: None; CL: Application

17. 2. The client's vital signs will show hemodynamic stability, and monitoring his heart rhythm may be indicated based on assessment findings. Giving nasal oxygen and drawing blood require a physician's order and shouldn't be part of a screening evaluation.
CN: Safe, effective care environment; CNS: Management of care; CL: Analysis

18. A client arrives at the emergency department complaining of chest and stomach pain and a report of black, tarry stools for the past 2 months. Which orders should the nurse anticipate?
1. Cardiac monitor, oxygen, creatine kinase, and lactate dehydrogenase (LD) levels
2. Prothrombin time (PT), partial thromboplastin time (PTT), fibrinogen, and fibrin split product values
3. ECG, complete blood count, testing for occult blood, and comprehensive serum metabolic panel
4. EEG, alkaline phosphatase and aspartate aminotransferase levels, and basic serum metabolic panel

19. The nurse is developing a plan of care for a client diagnosed with rheumatoid arthritis. What is the goal of treatment?
1. To cure the disease
2. To prevent osteoporosis
3. To control inflammation
4. To encourage bone regeneration

20. A client diagnosed with anemia asks the nurse to explain the difference between anemia and fatigue. The nurse explains that anemia stems from a decreased number of red blood cells and that fatigue results from a/an:
1. increase in carbon dioxide.
2. absence of factor VIII.
3. decrease in oxygen.
4. generation of T-cell antibodies.

21. The nurse determines that a client is at risk for developing anemia if which of the following predisposing factors is identified?
1. Colostomy following colon resection
2. Gastroesophageal reflux disease (GERD)
3. Gastrectomy
4. Bouts of dumping syndrome

22. The nurse is developing a dietary care plan for a client diagnosed with microcytic anemia. Which foods, if selected by the client, would indicate to the nurse that teaching was effective?
1. Enriched breakfast cereal and hot tea
2. Eggs and yogurt
3. Chicken and brown rice
4. Split pea soup with ham

Make sure you know the action of the drug before you administer it.

So, where do you stem from?

18. **3.** An ECG evaluates the complaint of chest pain, laboratory tests determine anemia, and the test for occult blood determines blood in the stool. Cardiac monitoring, oxygen, creatine kinase, and LD levels are appropriate for a cardiac primary problem. A basic metabolic panel and alkaline phosphatase and aspartate aminotransferase levels assess liver function. PT, PTT, fibrinogen, and fibrin split products are measured to verify bleeding dyscrasias. An EEG evaluates brain electrical activity.

CN: Physiological integrity; CNS: Reduction of risk potential; CL: Analysis

19. **3.** The primary goal in the treatment of rheumatoid arthritis is to control inflammation and slow the progression of the disease. There is no cure for rheumatoid arthritis. Rheumatoid arthritis causes bone erosion at the joints, not osteoporosis. Medications aren't available to replace bone lost through erosion.

CN: Physiological integrity; CNS: Pharmacological and parenteral therapies; CL: Application

20. **3.** Anemia stems from a decreased number of red blood cells. Red blood cells carry hemoglobin and oxygen. The lack of red blood cells results in a deficiency of oxygen in body tissues. Clotting factors, such as factor VIII, relate to the body's ability to form blood clots and aren't related to anemia, nor is carbon dioxide or T-cell antibodies.

CN: Physiological integrity; CNS: Physiological adaptation; CL: Application

21. **3.** Lack of intrinsic factor following gastrectomy would cause pernicious anemia due to the client's inability to absorb vitamin B_{12}. The presence of a colostomy, GERD, or dumping syndrome would not place a client at risk for developing anemia.

CN: Physiological integrity; CNS: Physiological adaptation; CL: Application

22. **4.** Combining a nonheme iron source (split pea soup) with a heme iron source (ham) increases absorption of nonheme iron. Tea, calcium (in yogurt), and phytates (brown rice) block iron absorption.

CN: Physiological integrity; CNS: Basic care and comfort; CL: Analysis

23. A client is admitted with a possible diagnosis of rheumatoid arthritis (RA). Which of the following screening tests should the nurse expect to be ordered?
1. Antinuclear antibody (ANA) titer
2. Complete blood count (CBC)
3. Erythrocyte sedimentation rate (ESR)
4. Rheumatoid factor (RF)

24. The nurse reviews lab results of a second-day postoperative client and notes a hemoglobin level of 10 g/dl. During assessment of the client, the nurse would expect to see which of the following?
1. No clinical sign
2. Pallor
3. Palpitations
4. Shortness of breath

25. A client asks the nurse about what <u>commonly</u> causes anemia. The best response by the nurse would be?
1. Lack of dietary iron
2. Vitamin C deficiency
3. Virus
4. Hereditary disorders of the red blood cells

26. The nurse is reviewing client's charts. Select the client who would be <u>most</u> at risk for developing anemia.
1. A 2-year old in day care
2. A 22-year-old college student
3. A 55-year-old neighbor
4. An elderly nursing home resident

The word *most* is a hint!

27. A client has received an antibiotic infusion and is now experiencing an anaphylactic reaction. What is the <u>most important</u> intervention by the nurse?
1. Administer a bolus of normal saline solution.
2. Maintain a patent airway.
3. Administer epinephrine.
4. Monitor vital signs.

28. The nurse is assessing a postoperative client who is recovering from a partial gastrectomy. The nurse is aware that the client is at risk for developing:
1. anemia.
2. polycythemia.
3. purpura.
4. thrombocytopenia.

23. 1. ANA is commonly used as a screening tool rather than a diagnostic tool for RA because many people without RA can have elevated titers. CBC, ESR, and RF are all used as diagnostic tools and to monitor progress of the disease or response to therapy.
CN: Health promotion and maintenance; CNS: None; CL: Analysis

24. 1. Mild anemia usually has no clinical signs. Pallor, palpitations, and shortness of breath are associated with severe anemia.
CN: Physiological adaptation; CNS: Reduction of risk potential; CL: Application

25. 1. Anemia can commonly be caused by a lack of vitamin B_{12}, iron, and folic acid as well as inflammation caused by some chronic diseases. Vitamin C deficiency doesn't cause anemia. Viruses and hereditary disorders are less common causes of anemia.
CN: Physiological integrity; CNS: Physiological adaptation; CL: Analysis

26. 4. Elderly people are most at risk for developing anemia, often due to financial concerns affecting protein intake or poor dentition that interferes with chewing meat.
CN: Health promotion and maintenance; CNS: None; CL: Analysis

27. 2. The first priority is to maintain a patent airway. The client will require an epinephrine injection next. If hypotension develops, a saline bolus may be given. His vital signs should be monitored but not as the first action.
CN: Safe, effective care environment; CNS: Management of care; CL: Analysis

28. 1. Surgery is a risk factor for anemia. Polycythemia can occur from severe hypoxia due to congenital heart and pulmonary disease. Purpura and thrombocytopenia may result from decreased bone marrow production of platelets and do not result from surgery.
CN: Physiological integrity; CNS: Reduction of risk potential; CL: Analysis

29. The nurse is reviewing a 52-year-old client's laboratory values. The platelet count is 75,000/µl. How would the nurse interpret this value?
1. Normal platelet count
2. Thrombocytopenia
3. Thrombocytopathy
4. Thrombocytosis

30. The nurse is aware that a client with a diagnosis of thrombocytopenia would be likely to complain of which of the following?
1. Weakness and fatigue
2. Dizziness and vomiting
3. Bruising and petechiae
4. Light-headedness and nausea

31. The nurse is planning care for a 67-year-old client who recently had abdominal aortic aneurysm repair surgery. The client has developed disseminated intravascular coagulation (DIC). The nurse is aware that the client has an <u>increased risk</u> for what?
1. Ineffective breathing pattern
2. Risk for aspiration
3. Risk for infection
4. Risk for ineffective cerebral tissue perfusion

32. A client had coronary artery bypass graft (CABG) surgery 3 days ago. The nurse notes a decrease in the client's platelet count from 230,000/µl to 5,000/µl. The nurse determines the client may be developing:
1. pancytopenia.
2. idiopathic thrombocytopenic purpura (ITP).
3. disseminated intravascular coagulation (DIC).
4. heparin-associated thrombosis and thrombocytopenia (HATT).

33. The nurse has instructed the client on self-administration of heparin injections. The nurse determines teaching is effective when the client makes which statement?
1. Heparin slows the time it takes for the blood to clot.
2. Heparin stops the blood from clotting.
3. Heparin thins the blood.
4. Heparin dissolves clots in the arteries of the heart.

Pay close attention to the word increased risk before choosing an answer.

29. 2. Thrombocytopenia is a decreased number of platelets. In adults, this would be less than 100,000/µl. Normal platelet count ranges from 140,000/µl to 400,000/µl. Thrombocytopathy is platelet dysfunction, and thrombocytosis is an excess number of platelets.
CN: Physiological integrity; CNS: Reduction of risk potential; CL: Application

30. 3. Platelets are necessary for clot formation, so petechiae and bruising are classic signs of a decreased number of platelets. Weakness and fatigue are signs of anemia. Light-headedness, nausea, dizziness, and vomiting are not classic signs of thrombocytopenia.
CN: Physiological integrity; CNS: Physiological adaptation; CL: Analysis

31. 4. DIC affects cerebral, cardiopulmonary, and peripheral tissues with clotting that obstructs tissue perfusion. This can result in damage to these tissues. Although risk for infection is a problem for this client following surgery, it is not the most critical diagnosis. Ineffective breathing pattern and risk for aspiration would not be problems initially.
CL: Physiological integrity; CNS: Reduction of risk potential; CL: Analysis

32. 4. HATT may occur after CABG surgery due to heparin use during surgery. Pancytopenia is a reduction in all blood cells. Although ITP and DIC cause platelet aggregation and bleeding, neither is common in a client after revascularization surgery.
CN: Physiological integrity; CNS: Physiological adaptation; CL: Application

33. 1. Heparin prolongs the time needed for blood to clot; however, it doesn't thin the blood. If given in large doses, heparin may stop the blood from clotting; however, this isn't why heparin is usually given. Heparin doesn't dissolve clots.
CN: Physiological integrity; CNS: Pharmacological and parenteral therapies; CL: Application

34. A pregnant client arrives at the emergency department with abruptio placentae at 34 weeks' gestation. The nurse is aware that the client is at risk for developing:
1. thrombocytopenia.
2. idiopathic thrombocytopenic purpura (ITP).
3. disseminated intravascular coagulation (DIC).
4. heparin-associated thrombosis and thrombocytopenia (HATT).

35. While assessing a client with disseminated intravascular coagulation (DIC), the nurse suspects the client has developed internal bleeding. The nurse should assess the client for:
1. hypertension.
2. petechiae.
3. increasing abdominal girth.
4. bradycardia.

36. A 36-year-old client complains of fatigue, weight loss, and a low-grade fever. He also has pain in his fingers, elbows, and ankles. The nurse identifies these symptoms as indicative of:
1. anemia.
2. leukemia.
3. rheumatic arthritis.
4. systemic lupus erythematosus (SLE).

37. The nurse is aware that in addition to the client's platelet count, the <u>best</u> test to confirm the diagnosis of essential thrombocytopenia would be?
1. Bleeding time
2. White blood cell (WBC) count
3. Immunoglobulin (Ig) G level
4. Prothrombin time (PT) and international normalized ratio (INR)

38. The nurse is caring for a client with idiopathic thrombocytopenic purpura. The client asks the nurse what medication the doctor ordered to improve his platelet count. What is the best response by the nurse?
1. Acetylsalicylic acid (ASA)
2. Corticosteroids
3. Methotrexate
4. Vitamin K

So many tests! Which is the best?

34. 3. Abruptio placentae is a cause of DIC because of activation of the clotting cascade after hemorrhage. Thrombocytopenia results from decreased bone marrow production. ITP can result in DIC but isn't associated with abruptio placentae. A client with abruptio placentae wouldn't receive heparin and, as a result, wouldn't be at risk for HATT.
CN: Physiological integrity; CNS: Reduction of risk potential; CL: Application

35. 3. As blood collects in the peritoneal cavity, dilation and distention of the abdomen occur. This is reflected by an increase in abdominal girth. The client with DIC would have hypotension and tachycardia. Petechiae are a result of the leaking of blood from tiny blood vessels into the skin.
CN: Physiological integrity; CNS: Physiological adaptation; CL: Analysis

36. 3. Fatigue, weight loss, and a low-grade fever are all early signs of many immune system diseases, including anemia, leukemia, and SLE. However, only rheumatic arthritis is associated with pain in the fingers, elbows, wrists, ankles, and knees.
CN: Physiological integrity; CNS: Physiological adaptation; CL: Application

37. 1. After a platelet count, the best test to determine thrombocytopenia is a bleeding time. The platelet count is decreased, and bleeding time is prolonged. IgG assays are nonspecific but may help determine the diagnosis. A WBC count shows WBC values, and the PT and INR evaluate the effect of warfarin therapy.
CN: Physiological integrity; CNS: Reduction of risk potential; CL: Application

38. 2. Corticosteroid therapy can decrease antibody production and phagocytosis of the antibody-coated platelets, retaining more functioning platelets. ASA decreases platelet aggregation. Methotrexate can cause thrombocytopenia. Vitamin K is used to treat an excessive anticoagulable state from warfarin overload.
CN: Physiological integrity; CNS: Pharmacological and parenteral therapies; CL: Application

39. A client with sickle cell disease is discussing his therapeutic regimen. Which statement by the client indicates further teaching is needed?
1. "I should avoid vacationing or traveling in areas of high altitude."
2. "Cigarette smoking can cause a sickle cell crisis."
3. "I should drink 4 to 6 L of fluid each day."
4. "I should take one baby aspirin daily to help prevent sickle cell crisis."

40. A nurse is preparing to teach a client about the immune system. The nurse explains that the thymus gland is:
1. a reservoir for blood cells.
2. stores blood cells until they mature.
3. protects the body against ingested pathogens.
4. removes bacteria and toxins from the circulatory system.

41. A client with thrombocytopenia, secondary to leukemia, develops epistaxis. The nurse would instruct the client to:
1. lie supine with his neck extended.
2. sit upright, leaning slightly forward.
3. blow his nose and then put lateral pressure on it.
4. hold his nose while bending forward at the waist.

42. The nurse is providing preoperative teaching for a client scheduled to receive a porcine heart valve replacement. The nurse determines that the client has an understanding of the type of replacement he will receive when the client describes the replacement as what?
1. Allogeneic
2. Autologous
3. Syngeneic
4. Xenogeneic

Don't quit now! You're getting there!

39. 4. Aspirin inhibits platelet aggregation and won't help prevent sickle cell crisis. Hydroxyurea is prescribed for some people to help prevent sickle cell crisis. High altitude increases oxygen demand and therefore can also precipitate a crisis. Tobacco, alcohol, and dehydration can precipitate a sickle cell crisis and should be avoided.
CN: Health promotion and maintenance; CNS: None; CL: Analysis

40. 2. Bone marrow produces immature blood cells (stem cells). Those that become lymphocytes migrate to the bone marrow for maturation (to B lymphocytes) or to the thymus for maturation (to T lymphocytes). These lymphocytes are responsible for cell-mediated immunity. The spleen is a reservoir for blood cells. The tonsils shield against airborne and ingested pathogens, and the lymph nodes remove bacteria and toxins from the bloodstream.
CN: Physiological integrity; CNS: Physiological adaptation; CL: Application

41. 2. The upright position, leaning slightly forward, avoids increasing the vascular pressure in the nose and helps the client avoid aspirating blood. Lying supine won't prevent aspiration of blood. Nose blowing can dislodge any clotting that has occurred. Bending at the waist increases vascular pressure and promotes bleeding rather than stopping it.
CN: Physiological integrity; CNS: Physiological adaptation; CL: Application

42. 4. A xenogeneic transplant is between humans and another species. An allogeneic transplant is between two humans, a syngeneic transplant is between identical twins, and autologous is a transplant from the same individual.
CN: Physiological integrity; CNS: Physiological adaptation; CL: Analysis

43. The nurse is reviewing assessment data of clients who may be at risk for developing malignant lymphoma. The nurse determines that the client at <u>highest</u> risk would be?
1. A 22-year-old man with a history of mononucleosis
2. A 25-year-old man who smokes a pack of cigarettes a day
3. A 33-year-old man with a cousin with Hodgkin's lymphoma
4. A 40-year-old woman with a history of human immunodeficiency virus (HIV) infection

44. A nurse is teaching a client about idiopathic thrombocytopenia and explains that the average normal life span of a platelet is:
1. 1 to 3 days.
2. 3 to 5 days.
3. 7 to 10 days.
4. 3 to 4 months.

45. A nurse is documenting care for a client with iron deficiency anemia. What is the <u>most appropriate</u> nursing diagnosis?
1. Impaired gas exchange
2. Deficient fluid volume
3. Ineffective airway clearance
4. Ineffective breathing pattern

46. The nurse determines that teaching was effective when the client with thrombocytopenia makes which statement?
1. "Platelets regulate acid–base balance."
2. "Platelets regulate the immune response."
3. "Platelets protect the body from infection."
4. "Platelets stop the bleeding when arteries and veins are injured."

47. A 43-year-old client undergoing colon cancer treatment has developed thrombocytopenia. The nurse should assess the client for:
1. diarrhea.
2. thin, brittle hair.
3. bruises on the skin.
4. urinary urgency.

Make sure you observe.

43. 1. Malignant lymphoma has a peak incidence between ages 20 and 30 and after age 50. It's more common in men than women and is associated with a history of Epstein-Barr virus (which causes mononucleosis). There is also an increased incidence of the disease among siblings. There is no reported association between malignant lymphoma and smoking or HIV infection.
CN: Health promotion and maintenance; CNS: None; CL: Application

44. 3. The normal life span of a platelet is 7 to 10 days. However, in idiopathic thrombocytopenia, the platelet life span is reduced to 1 to 3 days.
CN: Physiological integrity; CNS: Physiological adaptation; CL: Application

45. 1. Iron is necessary for hemoglobin synthesis. Hemoglobin is responsible for oxygen transport in the body. Iron deficiency anemia causes subnormal hemoglobin levels, which impair tissue oxygenation and warrant a nursing diagnosis of impaired gas exchange. Iron deficiency anemia doesn't cause a deficient fluid volume and is less directly related to ineffective airway clearance and ineffective breathing pattern than it is to ineffective gas exchange.
CN: Physiological integrity; CNS: Physiological adaptation; CL: Analysis

46. 4. Platelets clump together to plug small breaks in blood vessels. They also initiate the clotting cascade by releasing thromboplastin, which (in the presence of calcium) converts prothrombin into thrombin. Platelets don't perform the other functions listed.
CN: Physiological integrity; CNS: Reduction of risk potential; CL: Application

47. 3. With thrombocytopenia, there's an abnormal decrease in the number of blood platelets, which can result in bruises and bleeding. The client may have constipation but usually not diarrhea. Thin, brittle hair isn't a sign of thrombocytopenia but could be a sign of hypothyroidism. Urinary urgency could be a sign of urinary tract infection but not thrombocytopenia.
CN: Physiological integrity; CNS: Reduction of risk potential; CL: Application

48. A 16-year-old client involved in a motor vehicle collision arrives in the emergency department unconscious and severely hypotensive. He has several possible fractures of the pelvis and legs. Which parenteral fluid would the nurse expect to administer to this client?
1. Fresh frozen plasma
2. Normal saline solution
3. Lactated Ringer's solution
4. Packed red blood cells (RBCs)

49. The nurse is providing information to a client diagnosed with systemic lupus erythematosus (SLE). The client asks the nurse if any type of blood dyscrasia may develop. What is the best response by the nurse?
1. Dressler's syndrome
2. Polycythemia
3. Essential thrombocytopenia
4. von Willebrand's disease

50. The nurse is attending the annual neighborhood picnic. A neighbor tells the nurse that a friend was recently diagnosed with systemic lupus erythematosus (SLE) and she is afraid she will contract it. Which of the following clients is <u>most</u> at risk for SLE?
1. A 20-year-old White man
2. A 25-year-old Black woman
3. A 45-year-old Hispanic man
4. A 65-year-old Black woman

51. The nurse is caring for a client newly diagnosed with systemic lupus erythematosus (SLE). Which system is <u>most affected</u> by the disease?
1. Connective
2. Heart
3. Lung
4. Nerve

52. The nurse is assessing a client with an early diagnosis of stage I Hodgkin's disease. Which finding is the nurse likely to document?
1. Pericarditis
2. Night sweats
3. Splenomegaly
4. Persistent hypothermia

Client teaching is important.

48. 4. In a trauma situation, the first blood product given is unmatched (O negative) packed RBCs. Fresh frozen plasma is often used to replace clotting factors. Normal saline or lactated Ringer's solution is used to increase volume and blood pressure, but too much colloid will hemodilute the blood and won't improve oxygen-carrying capacity as RBCs would.
CN: Physiological integrity; CNS: Physiological adaptation; CL: Application

49. 3. Essential thrombocytopenia is linked to immunological disorders, such as SLE and human immunodeficiency virus. Dressler's syndrome is pericarditis that occurs after a myocardial infarction and isn't linked to SLE. Moderate to severe anemia is associated with SLE, not polycythemia. The disorder known as von Willebrand's disease is a type of hemophilia and isn't linked to SLE.
CN: Health promotion and maintenance; CNS: None; CL: Application

50. 2. SLE affects women eight times more often than men and usually strikes during childbearing age. It's three times more common in Black women than in White women.
CN: Health promotion and maintenance; CNS: None; CL: Analysis

51. 1. SLE is a chronic, inflammatory, autoimmune disorder that primarily affects connective tissue. It also affects the skin and kidneys and may affect the pulmonary, cardiac, neural, and renal systems.
CN: Physiological integrity; CNS: Physiological adaptation; CL: Application

52. 2. In stage I, symptoms include a single enlarged lymph node (usually), unexplained fever, night sweats, malaise, and generalized pruritus. Although splenomegaly may be present in some clients, night sweats are generally more prevalent. Pericarditis isn't associated with Hodgkin's disease. Moreover, splenomegaly and pericarditis aren't symptoms. Persistent hypothermia is associated with Hodgkin's but isn't an early sign of the disease.
CN: Health promotion and maintenance; CNS: None; CL: Application

53. A client has experienced an exacerbation of systemic lupus erythematosus (SLE). The nurse determines further teaching is necessary when the client makes which statement?
1. "I need to stay away from sunlight."
2. "I don't have to worry if I get a strep throat."
3. "I need to work on managing stress in my life."
4. "I don't have to worry about changing my diet."

54. The nurse explains to the client that a <u>common</u> but <u>life-threatening</u> complication of systemic lupus erythematosus (SLE) is:
1. arthritis.
2. nephritis.
3. pericarditis.
4. pleural effusion.

55. The nurse is caring for a client with systemic lupus erythematosus (SLE). The nurse is aware that a sign of neurologic involvement in SLE would be?
1. Facial tic
2. Psychosis
3. Extremity weakness
4. Cerebrovascular accidents

56. A nurse is reviewing the physician's orders for a client with systemic lupus erythematosus (SLE). The nurse determines that the medication most appropriate for the treatment plan is:
1. morphine.
2. ketoconazole.
3. hydroxychloroquine.
4. dimenhydrinate.

57. A nurse is aware that which of the following is a <u>classic</u> symptom of systemic lupus erythematosus (SLE)?
1. Fatigue and fever
2. Weight loss
3. Shortness of breath
4. Superficial lesions over the cheeks and nose

Hmm... I think some more teaching is in order.

This question is a classic.

53. 2. Infection may cause an exacerbation of SLE. Other factors that can precipitate an exacerbation are immunizations, sunlight exposure, and stress.

CN: Health promotion and maintenance; CNS: None; CL: Application

54. 2. About 50% of the clients with SLE have some type of nephritis, and kidney failure is the most common cause of death for clients with SLE. Pericarditis is the most common cardiovascular manifestation of SLE, but it isn't usually life threatening. Arthritis is very common (95%), as are pleural effusions (50%), but neither is life threatening.

CN: Physiological integrity; CNS: Physiological adaptation; CL: Analysis

55. 2. Neurologic involvement may be shown by psychosis, seizures, and headaches. Tics and cerebrovascular accidents aren't related to SLE. Weakness may be present, but it's usually related to muscle atrophy, not neurologic involvement.

CN: Physiological integrity; CNS: Physiological adaptation; CL: Application

56. 3. Hydroxychloroquine is used in the treatment of SLE to prevent inflammation. Pharmacological treatment of SLE also involves nonsteroidal anti-inflammatory drugs, corticosteroids, and immunosuppressive agents. Morphine is an opioid analgesic, ketoconazole is an antifungal agent, and dimenhydrinate is an antiemetic.

CN: Physiological integrity; CNS: Pharmacological and parenteral therapies; CL: Analysis

57. 4. Although all of these symptoms can be signs of SLE, the classic sign is the butterfly rash over the cheeks and nose.

CN: Physiological integrity; CNS: Physiological adaptation; CL: Application

58. A nurse suspects a diagnosis of systemic lupus erythematosus (SLE). The nurse is most concerned when lab results identify:
1. elevated serum complement level.
2. thrombocytosis, elevated sedimentation rate.
3. pancytopenia, elevated antinuclear antibody (ANA) titer.
4. leukocytosis, elevated blood urea nitrogen (BUN) and creatinine levels.

59. The nurse is reviewing laboratory values of a client recently diagnosed with chronic lymphocytic leukemia. The nurse would anticipate the results to include which of the following?
1. Elevated sedimentation rate
2. Uncontrolled proliferation of granulocytes
3. Thrombocytopenia and increased lymphocytes
4. Elevated aspartate aminotransferase and alanine aminotransferase levels

60. A nurse is assessing a client newly diagnosed with stage I Hodgkin's lymphoma. Which area of the body is <u>most likely</u> to be involved?
1. Back
2. Chest
3. Groin
4. Neck

61. According to a standard staging classification of Hodgkin's disease, which criterion reflects stage II?
1. Involvement of extralymphatic organs or tissues
2. Involvement of a single lymph node region or structure
3. Involvement of two or more lymph node regions or structures
4. Involvement of lymph node regions or structures on both sides of the diaphragm

58. 3. Laboratory findings for clients with SLE usually show pancytopenia, elevated ANA titer, and decreased serum complement levels. Clients may have elevated BUN and creatinine levels from nephritis, but the increase does not indicate SLE.
CN: Physiological integrity; CNS: Reduction of risk potential; CL: Application

59. 3. Chronic lymphocytic leukemia shows a proliferation of small abnormal mature B lymphocytes and decreased antibody response. Thrombocytopenia also is often present. Uncontrolled proliferation of granulocytes occurs in myelogenous leukemia. Aspartate aminotransferase, alanine aminotransferase, and erythrocyte sedimentation rate values are not affected.
CN: Physiological integrity; CNS: Reduction of risk potential; CL: Application

60. 4. At the time of diagnosis of stage I Hodgkin's lymphoma, a painless cervical lesion is often present. The back, chest, and groin areas may be involved in later stages.
CN: Physiological integrity; CNS: Physiological adaptation; CL: Application

61. 3. Stage II involves two or more lymph node regions. Stage I involves only one lymph node region; stage III involves nodes on both sides of the diaphragm; and stage IV involves extralymphatic organs or tissues.
CN: Physiological integrity; CNS: Physiological adaptation; CL: Analysis

You're doing great! Don't quit now!

62. A client diagnosed with acute lymphocytic leukemia is about to begin chemotherapy. The nurse recognizes that further teaching is necessary when the client makes which statement?
1. "I'll have treatments only once a month."
2. "I'll be getting high doses of chemotherapy."
3. "I won't get sick at this stage of the treatment."
4. "The purpose of these treatments is to induce a remission."

63. Which statement is correct about the rate of cell growth in relation to chemotherapy?
1. Faster growing cells are less susceptible to chemotherapy.
2. Nondividing cells are more susceptible to chemotherapy.
3. Faster growing cells are more susceptible to chemotherapy.
4. Slower growing cells are more susceptible to chemotherapy.

64. A client receiving chemotherapy is considered at high risk for developing lysis syndrome. The nurse would anticipate monitoring the client 48 to 72 hours after the infusion and assessing which laboratory values?
1. Complete blood count, prothrombin time, and partial thromboplastin time
2. Myoglobin, troponin, and creatine kinase
3. Glucose, bilirubin, and alanine aminotransferase
4. Electrolytes, blood urea nitrogen (BUN), and creatinine

65. The nurse recognizes that the most appropriate treatment for clients with tumor lysis syndrome is:
1. antibiotics.
2. I.V. hydration.
3. packed red blood cells (RBCs).
4. potassium chloride I.V.

66. A client with leukemia has developed neutropenia. The nurse informs the client to avoid which food?
1. White bread
2. Carrot sticks
3. Stewed apples
4. Medium rare steak

Would this meal affect a neutropenic leukemia patient in any way?

62. 1. The initial phase of chemotherapy is called the induction phase and is designed to put the client into remission by giving high doses of the drugs; however, treatments will be closer together than once each month. Monthly treatments usually occur during the maintenance phase of chemotherapy. The other options indicate that the client understands chemotherapy.

CN: Physiological integrity; CNS: Basic care and comfort; CL: Application

63. 3. The faster the cell grows, the more susceptible it is to chemotherapy and radiation therapy. Slow-growing and nondividing cells are less susceptible to chemotherapy. Repeated cycles of chemotherapy are used to destroy nondividing cells as they begin active cell division.

CN: Physiological integrity; CNS: Physiological adaptation; CL: Application

64. 4. Because the client is at high risk for electrolyte imbalances and acute renal failure, electrolyte, BUN, and creatinine levels should be measured prior to treatment and for 48 to 72 hours afterward. The other tests wouldn't be indicated.

CN: Physiological integrity; CNS: Reduction of risk potential; CL: Application

65. 2. The treatment for tumor lysis syndrome is I.V. hydration, allopurinol, and alkalizing the urine. Antibiotics are given when infection is first detected. Transfusions of RBCs aren't given until the body can produce mature cells. The potassium level is often elevated in tumor lysis syndrome, so potassium chloride wouldn't be indicated.

CN: Physiological integrity; CNS: Pharmacological and parenteral therapies; CL: Analysis

66. 2. A low-bacteria diet would be indicated, which excludes raw fruits and vegetables.

CN: Safe, effective care environment; CNS: Safety and infection control; CL: Application

67. A client diagnosed with leukemia is now experiencing neutropenia. Which of the following is a priority assessment by the nurse?
1. Blood pressure
2. Bowel sounds
3. Heart sounds
4. Breath sounds

68. The nurse is planning care for a client undergoing chemotherapy. What is the most important instruction for the nurse to give the client?
1. "Maintain bed rest."
2. "Perform activity as tolerated."
3. "Walk to the bathroom only."
4. "Get out of bed for brief periods."

69. The nurse is examining charts to identify clients at risk for developing multiple myeloma. The client who is most at risk would be?
1. A 20-year-old Asian woman
2. A 30-year-old White man
3. A 50-year-old Hispanic woman
4. A 60-year-old Black man

70. The nurse is monitoring the lab values of a client diagnosed with multiple myeloma early in the disease course. The nurse would anticipate the lab values to identify abnormal:
1. immunoglobulins.
2. platelets.
3. red blood cells (RBCs).
4. white blood cells (WBCs).

71. A client has been diagnosed with multiple myeloma. The nurse should assess the client for:
1. hypercalcemia.
2. hyperkalemia.
3. hypernatremia.
4. hypermagnesemia.

72. A client is admitted to the hospital with hypercalcemia. The nurse is aware that the client is at risk for what?
1. Tremors
2. Headache
3. Confusion
4. Muscle weakness

Forget the weights. Keep an eye on those "abs."

Don't get confused by this prefix! (Tee-hee!)

67. **4.** Pneumonia, both viral and fungal, is a common cause of death in clients with neutropenia, so frequent assessment of respiratory rate and breath sounds is required. Although assessing blood pressure, bowel sounds, and heart sounds is important, it won't help detect pneumonia.
CN: Physiological integrity; CNS: Physiological adaptation; CL: Application

68. **2.** It's important that the client be able to engage in activities that are of interest and to maintain as much independence and autonomy as possible. Bed rest isn't necessary, nor is it necessary to limit the client's activity to only walking to the bathroom or to getting out of bed for brief periods.
CN: Health promotion and maintenance; CNS: None; CL: Application

69. **4.** Multiple myeloma is more common in middle-aged and older clients (the median age at diagnosis is 60 years) and is twice as common in Blacks as Whites. It occurs most often in Black men.
CN: Health promotion and maintenance; CNS: None; CL: Analysis

70. **1.** Multiple myeloma is characterized by malignant plasma cells that produce an increased amount of immunoglobulin that isn't functional. As more malignant plasma cells are produced, there's less space in the bone marrow for RBC production. In late stages, platelets and WBCs are reduced as the bone marrow is infiltrated by malignant plasma cells.
CN: Health promotion and maintenance; CNS: None; CL: Analysis

71. **1.** Calcium is released when bone is destroyed. This causes an increase in serum calcium levels. Multiple myeloma doesn't affect potassium, sodium, or magnesium levels.
CN: Physiological integrity; CNS: Physiological adaptation; CL: Application

72. **3.** Signs of hypercalcemia include confusion, anorexia, nausea, vomiting, abdominal pain, ileus, constipation, and eventually impaired renal function. Tremors, headache, and muscle weakness aren't common symptoms of hypercalcemia.
CN: Physiological integrity; CNS: Physiological adaptation; CL: Application

73. A client with multiple myeloma has developed hypercalcemia. The nurse is aware that the client is at risk for what <u>secondary</u> complication?
1. Pneumonia
2. Muscle spasms
3. Renal insufficiency
4. Myocardial irritability

74. Neurologic complications of multiple myeloma usually involve the:
1. brain.
2. spinal column.
3. autonomic nervous system.
4. parasympathetic nervous system.

75. The nurse is teaching the family of a client newly diagnosed with multiple myeloma. The nurse determines that teaching has been effective when the family states the importance of:
1. maintaining bed rest.
2. enforcing fluid restriction.
3. drinking 3 qt (3 L) of fluid daily.
4. keeping the lower extremities elevated.

76. The nurse is aware that a client's physiological response to a health crisis is important to the health outcome. Which nursing intervention <u>must</u> also be addressed?
1. Teaching the family how to care for the client
2. Helping the client effectively cope with the crisis
3. Maintaining I.V. access, medications, and diet
4. Teaching the client basic information about the illness

Wait a second! Here's a hint for you!

Here's a question that uses a clever little technique—must—to get you to prioritize.

73. 3. Twenty percent of multiple myeloma clients with hypercalcemia and hyperuricemia develop renal insufficiency. Pneumonia doesn't result from hypercalcemia. Hypocalcemia causes muscle spasms, and hypokalemia causes myocardial irritability.
CN: Physiological integrity; CNS: Physiological adaptation; CL: Application

74. 2. Back pain or paresthesia in the lower extremities may indicate impending spinal cord compression from a spinal tumor. This should be recognized and treated promptly as progression of the tumor may result in paraplegia. The other options, which reflect parts of the nervous system, aren't usually affected by multiple myeloma.
CN: Physiological integrity; CNS: Physiological adaptation; CL: Application

75. 3. The client needs to drink 3 to 5 qt (3 to 5 L) of fluid each day to dilute calcium and uric acid to try to reduce the risk of renal dysfunction. Walking is encouraged to prevent further bone demineralization. The lower extremities don't need to be elevated.
CN: Physiological integrity; CNS: Basic care and comfort; CL: Application

76. 2. Although all of the answers are important in the care of the client, if the individual isn't able to cope with the emotional, spiritual, and psychological aspects of his crisis, the other components of care may be ineffective as well.
CN: Psychosocial integrity; CNS: None; CL: Application

77. What is the most appropriate nursing intervention to promote healing of a laceration?
1. Elevate the body part.
2. Monitor blood pressure.
3. Apply a pressure dressing and heat.
4. Apply a pressure dressing and ice pack.

Only 29 more questions! You're a whiz at this!

77. 4. Pressure dressings help clotting by promoting the localization of microorganisms and the development of meshwork for repair and healing. Ice decreases blood flow to the site, slowing the bleeding. Elevating the body part helps reduce edema but doesn't directly promote healing. Monitoring blood pressure is important when the individual is bleeding but does nothing to promote clotting. Heat increases blood flow to the site, increasing the bleeding.

CN: Physiological integrity; CNS: Physiological adaptation; CL: Application

78. A mother brings her 12-month-old, African-American female child to the emergency department. The mother states the child's eyes are yellow. The nurse assesses the child and notes tachycardia and shortness of breath. The nurse anticipates a diagnosis of:
1. thalassemia.
2. hemophilia A.
3. sickle cell anemia.
4. leukemia.

78. 3. Clinical signs of sickle cell anemia may not appear until the child is 12 months old after fetal hemoglobin has been replaced.

CN: Physiological integrity; CNS: Physiological adaptation; CL: Application

79. Which response to an antigen is an <u>appropriate</u> therapeutic immune system response?
1. Widespread histamine release
2. Autoimmune response
3. Inflammation and increased body temperature
4. Antibody production by T cells

Is this question appropriate, or is it just me?

79. 3. Inflammation and increased body temperature are normal immune responses to detected antigens. Allergies are heightened responses to antigens. Widespread histamine release is an exaggerated response that can lead to anaphylaxis. Autoimmune response is one in which the immune system forms antibodies against the body's own tissues, resulting in disease. Antibodies are produced by B cells, not T cells.

CN: Physiological integrity; CNS: Reduction of risk potential; CL: Analysis

80. Which intervention has the <u>most</u> impact in delaying the development of acquired immunodeficiency syndrome (AIDS) once a client has been infected with human immunodeficiency virus (HIV)?
1. Monthly plasmapheresis
2. Eating a balanced, nutritious diet
3. Compliance with complete therapeutic regimen
4. Getting adequate rest and sleep

80. 3. Compliance with the complete therapeutic regimen includes adhering to a healthy lifestyle, taking prescribed medications, and reducing risks from other infections and is the most important intervention in delaying the onset of AIDS. Eating a balanced diet and getting adequate rest and sleep are part of the overall therapeutic regimen. Plasmapheresis isn't a treatment for HIV/AIDS.

CN: Health promotion and maintenance; CNS: None; CL: Analysis

81. A child has developed chickenpox. The mother asks the nurse if the child has immunity. What is the best response by the nurse?
1. The child has passive immunity.
2. The child has immunological immunity.
3. The child has active immunity.
4. The child has adaptive immunity.

82. The nurse is teaching a client about stress management. Which rationale by the nurse <u>best</u> explains the reason for using stress management?
1. Everyone is stressed.
2. It has become an accepted practice.
3. Eastern health practices have shown its effectiveness.
4. Prolonged psychological stress may contribute to the development of physical illness.

83. A client asks the nurse what corticosteroid drugs suppress. What is the <u>most</u> appropriate response by the nurse?
1. Sympathetic response
2. Pain receptors
3. Immune response
4. Neural transmission

Don't suppress your response here.

84. The nurse determines that teaching was successful when a client with a negative human immunodeficiency virus (HIV) antibody test makes which statement?
1. "I'm not infected with HIV."
2. "I haven't produced antibodies to HIV."
3. "I'm immune to HIV."
4. "I have antibodies to HIV."

81. 3. Active immunity results from the development of antibodies in response to the presence of antigens from a vaccination or an exposure to an infectious disease.
CN: Health promotion and maintenance; CNS: None; CL: Analysis

82. 4. Psychological and emotional stress stimulate the central nervous system, increasing the levels of corticotropin and cortisol, which results in harmful effects on immune, cardiac, neural, and endocrine function. Many people report high levels of stress but not everyone would claim to be stressed. Although stress management may be a common therapy for stressed individuals and Eastern countries may promote its use, nursing interventions must have research-based rationales.
CN: Psychosocial integrity; CNS: None; CL: Application

83. 3. Corticosteroids suppress eosinophils, lymphocytes, natural-killer cells, and other microorganisms, inhibiting the natural inflammatory process in an infected or injured part of the body. This promotes resolution of inflammation, stabilizes lysosomal membranes, decreases capillary permeability, and depresses phagocytosis of tissues by white blood cells, thus blocking the release of more inflammatory materials. Corticosteroids don't affect the sympathetic response, pain receptors, or neural transmission.
CN: Physiological integrity; CNS: Pharmacological and parenteral therapies; CL: Application

84. 2. A negative HIV antibody test means that HIV antibodies weren't in the client's blood at the time the test was performed. Antibodies may take 3 weeks to 6 months or longer to develop. A negative test result doesn't indicate immunity. If antibodies to HIV are present, the test result is positive.
CN: Physiological integrity; CNS: Reduction of risk potential; CL: Application

85. In community health and epidemiologic studies, which definition of disease prevalence is correct?
1. The number of individuals affected by a particular disease at a specific time
2. The rate at which individuals without a specific disease develop that disease
3. The proportion of individuals affected by the disease who live for a particular period of time
4. The proportion of individuals without the disease who eventually develop the disease within a specific period of time

86. A 73-year-old client is about to receive a blood transfusion to treat severe anemia and asks the nurse how long the procedure will take. What is the <u>most appropriate</u> response?
1. 8 hours
2. At least 12 hours
3. At least 24 hours
4. No longer than 4 hours

87. A nurse anticipates that a client who has been prescribed corticosteroids would also have an order for:
1. blood glucose checks every 6 hours.
2. restriction of fluids to 1,000 ml in 24 hours.
3. administer lactulose 40 g in 4 oz. of water daily.
4. obtain serum platelet counts with hemoglobin and hematocrit levels every 12 hours.

88. A 32-year-old client is admitted with a tentative diagnosis of acquired immunodeficiency syndrome (AIDS). The preliminary report of biopsies done on his facial lesions indicates Kaposi's sarcoma. What is the <u>most appropriate</u> response by the nurse?
1. Tell the client that Kaposi's sarcoma is common in people with AIDS.
2. Pretend not to notice the lesions on the client's face.
3. Inform the client of the biopsy results and support him emotionally.
4. Explore the client's feelings about his facial disfigurement.

"Note" the words *most appropriate* in question 88. They're a key to the right answer.

85. **1.** Prevalence is the number of individuals affected by the disease at a specific time. Incidence rate is the rapidity with which individuals without the disease contract it. Survival is the proportion of individuals affected by the disease who live for a particular length of time. Risk is the proportion of individuals without the disease who develop the disease within a particular time period.

CN: Health promotion and maintenance; CNS: None; CL: Analysis

86. **4.** The American Association of Blood Banks recommends that blood or blood components should be transfused within 4 hours. If they aren't, they should be divided and stored appropriately in the blood bank. Any length of time over 4 hours would compromise the integrity of the transfusion components.

CN: Safe, effective care environment; CNS: Safety and infection control; CL: Application

87. **1.** Corticosteroids cause elevated blood glucose levels; insulin may be necessary to maintain normal blood glucose levels. Corticosteroids can cause edema, but fluid restrictions are generally unnecessary unless the client also has renal or cardiac disease. Lactulose is given for constipation and to treat hepatic encephalopathy. Hematologic studies, such as platelet counts, hemoglobin, and hematocrit levels, aren't usually necessary when monitoring clients undergoing corticosteroid therapy.

CN: Physiological integrity; CNS: Pharmacological therapies; CL: Application

88. **4.** Facial lesions can contribute to decreased self-esteem and an altered body image. Discussing AIDS with a client whose diagnosis isn't final may be inappropriate and doesn't provide emotional support. Pretending not to notice visible lesions ignores the client's concerns. The physician—not the nurse—should inform the client of the biopsy results.

CN: Psychosocial integrity; CNS: None; CL: Application

89. The nurse is reviewing lab results on a postoperative client. Upon analysis of the lab work, the nurse notes the client is immunocompromised. The nurse should assess the client for which of the following?
1. Nutrition
2. Acquired immune disorder
3. Family history of immune problems
4. Personal history of substance abuse or use

90. The nurse is performing mouth care on a client with acquired immunodeficiency syndrome (AIDS). The most appropriate nursing intervention is:
1. use reverse isolation.
2. place the client in a private room.
3. put on a mask, gloves, and a gown.
4. wear gloves.

91. The nurse is reviewing a client's laboratory values and recognizes that the lab changes <u>most consistent</u> with a diagnosis of aplastic anemia would be?
1. Decreased production of T-helper cells
2. Decreased levels of white blood cells (WBCs), red blood cells (RBCs), and platelets
3. Increased levels of WBCs, RBCs, and platelets
4. Reed-Sternberg cells and lymph node enlargement

92. The nurse is providing discharge instructions for a client with iron deficiency anemia. What is the most important information for the nurse to include about the prescribed ferrous gluconate therapy?
1. "Take the medication with an antacid."
2. "Take the medication with a glass of milk."
3. "Take the medication with whole-grain cereal."
4. "Take the medication on an empty stomach."

Don't get puzzled; you're looking for the most consistent answer.

89. 4. Substance abuse, including alcohol consumption and tobacco or marijuana use, influences immunocompetence and overall health status. Although nutrition is important for immunocompetence, it would be part of the client's daily assessment. A family history would have been assessed initially. Assessing the client for an acquired immune disorder would be a joint effort with the physician and wouldn't be conducted independently.

CN: Health promotion and maintenance; CNS: None; CL: Application

90. 4. Standard precautions stipulate that a health care worker who anticipates coming into contact with a client's blood or body fluids must wear gloves. Reverse isolation is used to protect the client from the health care worker, not the other way around. A private room doesn't provide barrier protection, an essential step in standard precautions. A mask and gloves are needed only for anticipated contact with airborne droplets of blood or body fluids; a gown is needed only for anticipated contact with splashes of blood or body fluids. Neither is the case when performing oral hygiene.

CN: Safe, effective care environment; CNS: Safety and infection control; CL: Application

91. 2. In aplastic anemia, the diagnostic findings are decreased levels of all the cellular elements of the blood (pancytopenia). T-helper cell production doesn't decrease in aplastic anemia. Reed-Sternberg cells and lymph node enlargement occur with Hodgkin's disease.

CN: Physiological integrity; CNS: Physiological adaptation; CL: Analysis

92. 4. Preferably, ferrous gluconate should be taken on an empty stomach. Ferrous gluconate shouldn't be taken with antacids, milk, or whole-grain cereals because these foods reduce iron absorption.

CN: Physiological integrity; CNS: Pharmacological and parenteral therapies; CL: Application

93. A nurse is working on a medical/surgical unit and notes that one of the client's assigned has a diagnosis of ankylosing spondylitis. The nurse would assess this client for:
1. red, painful, swollen joints
2. fatigue and night sweats
3. low back pain
4. neck pain and stiffness

94. A female client with the beta-thalassemia trait plans to marry a man of Italian ancestry who also has the trait. The nurse determines teaching is successful when the client makes which statement?
1. "Thalassemia is treated with iron supplements."
2. "I need to learn how to give myself vitamin B_{12} injections."
3. "I'll see a genetic counselor before starting a family."
4. "If my fiancé were of Middle Eastern descent, I wouldn't be worried about having children."

95. A young, African-American, female client with a history of sickle cell disease is complaining of severe abdominal pain. What is the <u>priority</u> intervention by the nurse?
1. Obtaining a history of the sequence of symptoms
2. Keeping the client nothing by mouth (NPO)
3. Administering I.V. fluids
4. Preparing the client for a computed tomography (CT) scan of the abdomen

Here come those priorities again!

96. A nurse is developing a care plan for a neutropenic client with lymphoma. Appropriate nursing interventions for this client would include?
1. Have the client use a soft toothbrush and electric razor, avoid using enemas, and watch for signs of bleeding.
2. Put on a mask, gown, and gloves when entering the client's room.
3. Provide a clear liquid, low-sodium diet.
4. Eliminate fresh fruits and vegetables, avoid using enemas, and practice frequent hand washing.

Which precautions should the nurse include in her care plan?

Caution

93. 3. Typically, intermittent low back pain is the first indication of ankylosing spondylitis. Red, painful, swollen joints occur with rheumatoid arthritis. Although ankylosing spondylitis may cause fatigue, it rarely produces night sweats. Neck pain and stiffness from involvement of the cervical spine are relatively late manifestations.

CN: Physiological integrity; CNS: Physiological adaptation; CL: Analysis

94. 3. Two people with the beta-thalassemia trait have a 25% chance of having a child with thalassemia major, a potentially life-threatening disease. Iron supplements aren't used to treat thalassemia; in fact, they could contribute to iron overload. Vitamin B_{12} injections are used to treat pernicious anemia, not thalassemia. Thalassemia occurs primarily in people of Italian, Greek, African, Asian, Middle Eastern, East Indian, and Caribbean descent.

CN: Health promotion and maintenance; CNS: None; CL: Application

95. 1. Although the client may be in a sickle cell crisis and experiencing acute abdominal pain caused by sickling in the mesenteric circulation, it's important to remember that clients with sickle cell disease aren't spared from appendicitis or other intra-abdominal events. The history obtained from the client outlining the sequence of symptoms provides the most important assessment information. Other nursing interventions would include preparing the client for possible surgery by keeping her NPO and for diagnostic studies such as CT scanning. Administering I.V. fluids will help replenish fluid volume.

CN: Physiological integrity; CNS: Reduction of risk potential; CL: Application

96. 4. Neutropenia occurs when the absolute neutrophil count falls below 1,000/mm³, reflecting a severe risk for infection. The nurse should provide a low-bacterial diet, which means eliminating fresh fruits and vegetables; avoid invasive procedures, such as enemas, because they increase the infection risk; and practice frequent hand washing to lower the infection risk. Using a soft toothbrush, avoiding straight-edged razors and enemas, and monitoring for bleeding are thrombocytopenia precautions. Putting on a mask, gown, and gloves when entering the client's room are reverse isolation measures. A neutropenic client doesn't need a clear liquid diet or sodium restrictions.

CN: Safe, effective care environment; CNS: Safety and infection control; CL: Application

97. The nurse is reviewing a client's laboratory values and notes a deficiency of factor VIII. What diagnosis does the nurse suspect?
1. Sickle cell disease
2. Christmas disease
3. Hemophilia A
4. Hemophilia B

98. A 19-year-old client admitted with heat stroke begins to show signs of disseminated intravascular coagulation (DIC). The nurse analyzes the laboratory findings and identifies which finding as <u>most consistent</u> with DIC?
1. Low platelet count
2. Elevated fibrinogen levels
3. Low levels of fibrin degradation products
4. Reduced prothrombin time (PT)

99. A client comes to the clinic complaining of fever, drenching night sweats, and unexplained weight loss over the past 3 months. Physical examination reveals a single enlarged supraclavicular lymph node. The nurse suspects which <u>probable</u> diagnosis?
1. Influenza
2. Sickle cell anemia
3. Leukemia
4. Hodgkin's disease

100. A client has been informed by the physician that he has Hodgkin's disease. After the physician leaves the room, the client tells the nurse he's afraid of dying. What is the most appropriate response by the nurse?
1. "Don't worry, many people survive this disease."
2. "Hodgkin's disease is very treatable."
3. "You're afraid of dying?"
4. "You should speak with your minister."

101. Before starting treatment for leukemia, a client receives I.V. fluids and allopurinol (Zyloprim). The goal of these interventions is to reduce the risk of:
1. disseminated intravascular coagulation (DIC).
2. pancytopenia.
3. tumor lysis syndrome.
4. mucositis.

We're most consistent with these hints, aren't we?

97. 3. Hemophilia A results from a deficiency of factor VIII. Sickle cell disease is caused by a defective hemoglobin molecule. Christmas disease, also called hemophilia B, results from a factor IX deficiency.
CN: Physiological integrity; CNS: Physiological adaptation; CL: Analysis

98. 1. In DIC, platelets and clotting factors are consumed, resulting in microthrombi and excessive bleeding. As clots form, fibrinogen levels decrease and the PT increases. Fibrin degradation products increase as fibrinolysis takes place.
CN: Physiological integrity; CNS: Physiological adaptation; CL: Analysis

99. 4. Hodgkin's disease typically causes fever, night sweats, weight loss, and lymph node enlargement. Influenza doesn't last for months. Clients with sickle cell anemia manifest signs and symptoms of chronic anemia with pallor of the mucous membranes, fatigue, and decreased tolerance for exercise; they don't show fever, night sweats, weight loss, or lymph node enlargement. Leukemia doesn't cause lymph node enlargement.
CN: Health promotion and maintenance; CNS: None; CL: Application

100. 3. Repeating what the client has said (or describing his feelings) encourages the client to elaborate on his thoughts and feelings. Telling him not to worry and saying that Hodgkin's disease is very treatable ignores his feelings and offers false reassurance. Telling a client what to do, such as calling his minister, also ignores his feelings.
CN: Psychosocial integrity; CNS: None; CL: Application

101. 3. During chemotherapy for leukemia, tumor lysis syndrome may occur as cell destruction releases intracellular components, resulting in hyperuricemia. Large fluid quantities and allopurinol therapy help reduce the amount of uric acid as a result of tumor lysis syndrome but don't stop the cell lysis. Although DIC, pancytopenia, and mucositis are possible chemotherapy complications, they're not treated with I.V. fluids and allopurinol.
CN: Physiological integrity; CNS: Pharmacological and parenteral therapies; CL: Application

102. A client with a gunshot wound requires an emergency blood transfusion. His blood type is AB negative. The nurse is aware that the <u>safest</u> blood type for the client to receive would be?
1. AB Rh-positive
2. A Rh-positive
3. A Rh-negative
4. O Rh-positive

Be on the safe side and choose the safest type.

103. Which client is <u>most</u> at risk for developing acute lymphocytic leukemia?
1. 25-year-old Black male
2. 4-year-old White female
3. 44-year-old White male
4. 51-year-old Asian female

104. A client with Hodgkin's disease who weighs 143 lb is to receive vincristine 25 mcg/kg I.V. The nurse computes the correct dose in micrograms. How many micrograms should the client receive? Record your answer using a whole number.

_____ micrograms

105. The nurse initiates the treatment for a delayed hypersensitivity reaction. What is the most appropriate treatment?
1. Intravenous epinephrine
2. Breathing treatment with albuterol
3. Corticosteroids
4. Benadryl

106. Which nonpharmacologic interventions are included in the care plan for a client who has moderate rheumatoid arthritis? Select all that apply.
1. Massaging inflamed joints
2. Avoiding range-of-motion (ROM) exercises
3. Applying splints to inflamed joints
4. Using assistive devices at all times
5. Selecting clothing that has Velcro fasteners
6. Applying moist heat to joints

Success! You did it!

102. 3. Human blood can sometimes contain an inherited D antigen. Persons with the D antigen have Rh-positive blood type; those lacking the antigen have Rh-negative blood. It's important that a person with Rh-negative blood receives Rh-negative blood. If Rh-positive blood is administered to an Rh-negative person, the recipient develops anti-Rh agglutinins, and subsequent transfusions with Rh-positive blood may cause serious reactions with clumping and hemolysis of red blood cells.

CN: Physiological integrity; CNS: Pharmacological and parenteral therapies; CL: Application

103. 2. Acute lymphocytic leukemia is most common in young children and in adults age 65 and older. It's also more common in Whites than in Blacks or Asians.

CN: Health promotion and maintenance; CNS: None; CL: Analysis

104. 1,625. First, convert the client's weight from pounds to kilograms:
    1 lb = 2.2 kg;
    143 lb = X kg; 143 lb/2.2 kg = 65 kg.
Next, multiply the weight in kilograms by the number of micrograms desired per kilogram:
    65 kg × 25 = 1,625 mcg.

CN: Physiological integrity; CNS: Pharmacological and parenteral therapies; CL: Application

105. 3. Delayed hypersensitivity reactions are inflammatory reactions not histamine reactions.

CN: Physiological integrity; CNS: Physiological adaptation; CL: Application

106. 3, 5, and 6. Supportive, nonpharmacologic measures for the client with rheumatoid arthritis include applying splints to rest inflamed joints, using Velcro fasteners on clothes to aid dressing, and applying moist heat to joints to relax muscles and relieve pain. Inflamed joints should never be massaged because doing so can aggravate inflammation. A physical therapy program including ROM exercises and carefully individualized therapeutic exercises prevents loss of joint function. Assistive devices should be used only when marked loss of ROM occurs.

CN: Physiological integrity; CNS: Basic care and comfort; CL: Application

Looking for the latest information about respiratory disorders? Check out the American Association for Respiratory Care's Web site at **www.aarc.org.** It will respire—er, inspire—you.

Chapter 5
Respiratory disorders

1. A client who has been experiencing a chronic illness develops pneumonia. The nurse is aware that the factor <u>most likely contributing</u> to the client's development of pneumonia is:
1. dehydration.
2. group living.
3. malnutrition.
4. severe periodontal disease.

In question 1, the terms *most likely contributing* are a hint for finding the correct answer.

1. 2. Clients with chronic illnesses generally have poor immune systems. Often, residing in group living situations increases the chance of disease transmission. Adequate fluid intake, adequate nutrition, and proper oral hygiene help maintain normal defenses and can reduce the incidence of getting such diseases as pneumonia.

CN: Physiological integrity; CNS: Physiological adaptation; CL: Analysis

2. A client develops pneumonia. The nurse can expect which pathophysiological mechanism to develop as a secondary response to the pneumonia?
1. Atelectasis
2. Bronchiectasis
3. Effusion
4. Inflammation

2. 4. The common feature of all types of pneumonia is an inflammatory pulmonary response to the offending organism or agent. Atelectasis and bronchiectasis indicate a collapse of a portion of the airway that doesn't occur in pneumonia. An effusion is an accumulation of excess pleural fluid in the pleural space, which may be a secondary response to pneumonia.

CN: Physiological integrity; CNS: Physiological adaptation; CL: Application

3. The nurse is reviewing the chart of a 58-year-old male client with community-acquired pneumonia and determines that which of the following is the <u>most likely</u> causative organism?
1. *Haemophilus influenzae*
2. *Klebsiella pneumoniae*
3. *Streptococcus pneumoniae*
4. *Staphylococcus aureus*

Pssst. Yeah, I'm talking to you. You'd better strep lively—er, I mean, step lively. Got it?

3. 3. Pneumococcal or streptococcal pneumonia, caused by *Streptococcus pneumoniae*, is the most common cause of community-acquired pneumonia. *Haemophilus influenzae* is the most common cause of infection in children. *Klebsiella* species is the most common gram-negative organism found in the hospital setting. *Staphylococcus aureus* is the most common cause of hospital-acquired pneumonia.

CN: Physiological integrity; CNS: Reduction of risk potential; CL: Application

4. An elderly client developed pneumonia. The nurse is aware that the <u>initial</u> symptom the client may manifest is:
1. altered mental status and dehydration.
2. fever and chills.
3. hemoptysis and dyspnea.
4. pleuritic chest pain and cough.

4. 1. Fever, chills, hemoptysis, dyspnea, cough, and pleuritic chest pain are the common symptoms of pneumonia, but elderly clients may first appear with only an altered mental status and dehydration due to a blunted immune response.

CN: Physiological integrity; CNS: Physiological adaptation; CL: Application

CN: Client needs category   CNS: Client needs subcategory   CL: Cognitive level

5. When auscultating the chest of a client with pneumonia, the nurse should expect to hear which type of sounds over areas of consolidation?
1. Bronchial
2. Bronchovesicular
3. Tubular
4. Vesicular

For question 5, think of where you normally hear each type of breath sound.

6. The client is exhibiting symptoms indicative of pneumonia. The nurse anticipates that which diagnostic test will be orders to confirm the diagnosis?
1. Arterial blood gas (ABG) analysis
2. Chest X-ray
3. Blood cultures
4. Sputum culture and sensitivity

7. A 78-year-old client is admitted with a diagnosis of dehydration and change in mental status. He's being hydrated with I.V. fluids. When the nurse takes his vital signs, she notes he has a fever of 103.7° F (39.47° C), a cough producing yellow sputum, and pleuritic chest pain. The nurse suspects this client may have developed:
1. acute respiratory distress syndrome (ARDS).
2. myocardial infarction (MI).
3. pneumonia.
4. tuberculosis (TB).

The nurse can give oxygen without a physician's order to help her client breathe easier.

8. A client with pneumonia develops dyspnea, a respiratory rate of 32 breaths/minute, and difficulty expelling secretions. The nurse auscultates the lung fields and hears bronchial sounds in the left lower lobe. Which action should the nurse take <u>first</u>?
1. Administer antibiotics.
2. Encourage bed rest.
3. Apply oxygen.
4. Assess nutritional intake.

5. **1.** Chest auscultation reveals bronchial breath sounds over areas of consolidation. Bronchovesicular breath sounds are normal over midlobe lung regions, tubular sounds are commonly heard over large airways, and vesicular breath sounds are commonly heard in the bases of the lung fields.
CN: Physiological integrity; CNS: Reduction of risk potential; CL: Application

6. **4.** Sputum culture and sensitivity is the best way to identify the organism causing the pneumonia. ABG analysis will determine the extent of hypoxia present due to the pneumonia. Chest X-ray will show the area of lung consolidation. Blood cultures will help determine if the infection is systemic.
CN: Physiological integrity; CNS: Reduction of risk potential; CL: Application

7. **3.** Fever, productive cough, and pleuritic chest pain are common signs and symptoms of pneumonia. The client with ARDS has dyspnea and hypoxia, with worsening hypoxia over time if not treated aggressively. Pleuritic chest pain varies with respiration, unlike the constant chest pain during an MI, so this client most likely isn't having an MI. The client with TB typically has a cough producing blood-tinged sputum. A sputum culture should be obtained to confirm the nurse's suspicions.
CN: Physiological integrity; CNS: Physiological adaptation; CL: Analysis

8. **3.** The client is having difficulty breathing and is probably becoming hypoxic. As an emergency measure, the nurse can provide oxygen without waiting for a physician's order. Antibiotics may be warranted, but this isn't a nursing decision. The client should be maintained on bed rest if he's dyspneic to minimize his oxygen demands, but providing additional oxygen will deal more immediately with his problem. The client will need nutritional support, but while dyspneic, he may be unable to spare the energy needed to eat and at the same time maintain adequate oxygenation.
CN: Safe, effective care environment; CNS: Management of care; CL: Analysis

9. A client has been treated with a 10-day course of antibiotic therapy for right lower lobe pneumonia and is scheduled to be discharged today. Select the assessment finding that indicates the client is ready to be discharged.
1. Continued dyspnea
2. Fever of 102.7° F (38.97° C)
3. Respiratory rate of 32 breaths/minute
4. Vesicular breath sounds in right base

10. A 20-year-old client is being treated for pneumonia. He has a persistent cough and complains of severe pain when coughing. The most appropriate instruction the nurse would give the client to reduce discomfort is:
1. "Hold in your cough as much as possible."
2. "Place the head of your bed flat to help with coughing."
3. "Restrict fluids to help decrease the amount of sputum."
4. "Splint your chest wall with a pillow for comfort."

All this coughing is so uncomfortable.

11. A client in a long-term care facility has been receiving continuous tube feedings. The nurse notes the client has a cough producing tan sputum and is now febrile to 102.7° F (38.9° C). The nurse auscultates the client's lung fields and hears bronchial breath sounds in the right middle lobe. The nurse suspects the client may have developed:
1. atelectasis.
2. bronchitis.
3. pneumonia.
4. pulmonary embolism.

Asking a client questions will help determine his degree of risk.

12. A nurse working in a rural county's Public Health Department has been alerted that there is an outbreak of tuberculosis (TB) in the area. The client most at risk for developing TB would be?
1. A 16-year-old female high school student
2. A 33-year-old day-care worker
3. A 43-year-old homeless man with a history of alcoholism
4. A 54-year-old businessman

9. 4. If the client is to be discharged after receiving treatment for pneumonia, he should have stable vital signs, have clear breath sounds bilaterally, and have no evidence of shortness of breath.
CN: Physiological integrity; CNS: Physiological adaptation; CL: Analysis

10. 4. Showing this client how to splint his chest wall will help decrease discomfort when coughing. Holding in his coughs will only increase the amount of pain he has. Placing the head of the bed flat may increase the frequency of his cough and require more work; a 45-degree angle may help him cough more efficiently and with less pain. Increasing fluid intake will help thin his secretions, making it easier for him to clear them. Promoting fluid intake is appropriate in this situation.
CN: Physiological integrity; CNS: Basic care and comfort; CL: Application

11. 3. The client probably has aspirated the contents of his tube feedings and developed aspiration pneumonia. This is the most common cause of pneumonia in clients with tube feedings. Atelectasis wouldn't be associated with a productive cough, and breath sounds would be decreased in the areas of atelectasis. The client most likely hasn't developed bronchitis because in that condition, he may have a nonproductive or productive cough but secretions are usually clear. A client with a pulmonary embolism wouldn't have a cough producing tan sputum, and pulmonary embolisms aren't typically associated with high fever.
CN: Physiological integrity; CNS: Physiological adaptation; CL: Analysis

12. 3. Clients who are economically disadvantaged, malnourished, and have reduced immunity, such as a client with a history of alcoholism, are at extremely high risk for developing TB. A high school student, day-care worker, and businessman probably have a much lower risk of contracting TB.
CN: Physiological integrity; CNS: Physiological adaptation; CL: Application

13. The nurse is conducting a class for family members of clients diagnosed with tuberculosis (TB). The nurse determines that teaching is effective when the family member states:
1. "The disease is transmitted by sexual contact."
2. "The disease is transmitted by contaminated needles."
3. "The disease is transmitted through contaminated eating utensils."
4. "The disease is transmitted by droplets exhaled from an infected person."

14. The nurse performs a purified protein derivative (PPD) test on an adult client being screened for TB. The client reports having negative PPD test results in the past. The nurse instructs the client to return and have the results interpreted:
1. immediately after performing the test.
2. 24 hours after performing the test.
3. 48 hours after performing the test.
4. 1 week after performing the test.

15. A client received a purified protein derivative (PPD) test for tuberculosis (TB) on the right forearm. The site is reddened and raised about 3 mm. The nurse interprets this result as:
1. indeterminate.
2. needs to be redone.
3. negative.
4. positive.

16. A client has recently been diagnosed with tuberculosis (TB). The nurse caring for the client anticipates that the client will develop:
1. active TB within 2 weeks.
2. active TB within 1 month.
3. a fever that requires hospitalization.
4. a positive skin test.

This droplet transmission stuff sure beats the subway! Wheeee!

The timing is the clue!

13. 4. The TB bacillus is airborne and carried in droplets exhaled by an infected person who is coughing, sneezing, laughing, or singing. Sexual contact and contaminated needles don't spread the TB bacillus but may spread other communicable diseases. It's never advisable to use contaminated utensils, but if they're cleaned normally, it isn't necessary to dispose of eating utensils used by someone infected with TB.
CN: Safe, effective care environment; CNS: Safety and infection control; CL: Application

14. 3. PPD tests should be read in 48 to 72 hours. If read too early or too late, the results won't be accurate.
CN: Physiological integrity; CNS: Reduction of risk potential; CL: Application

15. 3. This test would be classed as negative. A 3-mm raised area would be a positive result if the client had recent close contact with someone diagnosed with or suspected of having infectious TB. Follow-up should be done with this client, and a chest X-ray should be ordered. Indeterminate isn't a term used to describe results of a PPD test. The test can be redone in 6 months to see if the client's test results change. If the PPD test is reddened and raised 10 mm or more, it's considered positive according to the Centers for Disease Control and Prevention.
CN: Physiological integrity; CNS: Reduction of risk potential; CL: Analysis

16. 4. A primary TB infection occurs when the bacillus has successfully invaded the entire body after entering through the lungs. At this point, the bacilli are walled off and skin tests read positive. The general population has a 10% risk of developing active TB over their lifetime, in many cases because of a break in the body's immune defenses. The active stage shows the classic symptoms of TB: fever, hemoptysis, and night sweats.
CN: Physiological integrity; CNS: Physiological adaptation; CL: Analysis

17. A client was infected with tuberculosis (TB) bacillus 10 years ago but never developed the disease. He's now being treated for cancer. The client begins to develop signs of TB. The nurse suspects the client is exhibiting:
1. active infection.
2. latent infection.
3. superinfection.
4. tertiary infection.

Think: How does cancer affect the immune system?

18. A client has been diagnosed with active tuberculosis (TB). The nurse should assess the client for:
1. chest and lower back pain.
2. chills, fever, night sweats, and hemoptysis.
3. fever of more than 104.7° F (40.7° C) and nausea.
4. headache and photophobia.

19. A client has received a preliminary diagnosis of tuberculosis. In order to obtain a definitive diagnosis, the nurse anticipates that the physician will order which test?
1. Chest X-ray
2. Mantoux test
3. Sputum culture
4. Tuberculin test

20. A client has a positive Mantoux test, and a chest X-ray is ordered. The client asks the nurse the reason for the X-ray. What is the best response by the nurse?
1. To confirm the diagnosis
2. To determine if a repeat skin test is needed
3. To determine the extent of lesions
4. To determine if this is a primary or secondary infection

Remember what a positive skin test means.

21. A chest X-ray shows a client's lungs to be clear; however, the Mantoux test is positive with 10 mm of induration, and the previous test was negative. The nurse explains to the client that these test results are possible because:
1. he had tuberculosis (TB) in the past and no longer has it.
2. he was successfully treated for TB, but skin tests always stay positive.
3. he's a "seroconverter," meaning the TB has gotten to his bloodstream.
4. he's a "tuberculin converter," which means he has been infected with TB since his last skin test.

17. 1. Some people carry dormant TB infections that may develop into active disease. If there's no active infection, it's called a latent infection. The TB bacilli may remain latent for years and then activate when the client's resistance is lowered, as when a client is being treated for cancer. Superinfection doesn't apply in this case, and there's no such thing as tertiary infection.
CN: Physiological integrity; CNS: Physiological adaptation; CL: Application

18. 2. Typical signs and symptoms are chills, fever, night sweats, and hemoptysis. Chest pain may be present from coughing but isn't usual. Clients with TB typically have low-grade fevers, not higher than 102.7° F (38.97° C). Nausea, headache, and photophobia aren't usual TB symptoms.
CN: Physiological integrity; CNS: Physiological adaptation; CL: Application

19. 3. The sputum culture for *Mycobacterium tuberculosis* is the only method of confirming the diagnosis. Lesions in the lung may not be big enough to be seen on X-ray. Skin tests may be falsely positive or falsely negative.
CN: Physiological integrity; CNS: Reduction of risk potential; CL: Application

20. 3. If the lesions are large enough, the chest X-ray will show their presence in the lungs. Sputum culture confirms the diagnosis. There can be false-positive and false-negative skin test results. A chest X-ray can't determine if this is a primary or secondary infection.
CN: Physiological integrity; CNS: Reduction of risk potential; CL: Application

21. 4. A tuberculin converter's skin test will be positive, meaning he has been exposed to and infected with TB and now has a cell-mediated immune response to the skin test. The client's blood and X-ray results may stay negative. It doesn't mean the infection has advanced to the active stage. Because his X-ray is negative, he should be monitored every 6 months to see if he develops changes in his chest X-ray or pulmonary examination. Being a seroconverter doesn't mean the TB has gotten into his bloodstream; it means it can be detected by a blood test.
CN: Physiological integrity; CNS: Physiological adaptation; CL: Analysis

22. A client with a positive skin test for tuberculosis (TB) is not showing signs of active disease and is treated with isoniazid, 300 mg daily. The nurse explains to the client that the medication should be taken for how long?
1. 10 to 14 days
2. 2 to 4 weeks
3. 3 to 6 months
4. 9 to 12 months

23. A client with a productive cough, chills, and night sweats is suspected of having active tuberculosis (TB). The most important intervention by the nurse would be?
1. Maintain the client on respiratory isolation.
2. Prepare the client to be discharged on bed rest.
3. Administer the tuberculin test ordered by the physician.
4. Administer the isoniazid ordered by the physician immediately before discharge.

24. A client is diagnosed with active tuberculosis and started on triple antibiotic therapy. The nurse would be concerned if the client demonstrates which of the following?
1. Decreased shortness of breath
2. Improved chest X-ray
3. Nonproductive cough
4. Positive acid-fast bacilli in a sputum sample after 2 months of treatment

25. What is the priority instruction the nurse should give a client about his active tuberculosis (TB)?
1. "It's OK to miss a dose every day or two."
2. "If side effects occur, stop taking the medication."
3. "Only take the medication until you feel better."
4. "You must comply with the medication regimen to treat TB."

22. 4. Because of the increasing incidence of resistant strains of TB, the disease must be treated for up to 24 months in some cases, but treatment typically lasts from 9 to 12 months. Isoniazid is the most common medication used for the treatment of TB, but other antibiotics are added to the regimen to obtain the best results.

CN: Physiological integrity; CNS: Pharmacological and parenteral therapies; CL: Application

23. 1. This client is showing signs and symptoms of active TB and, because of the productive cough, is highly contagious. He should be admitted to the hospital and placed in respiratory isolation, and three sputum cultures should be obtained to confirm the diagnosis. He would most likely be given isoniazid and two or three other antitubercular antibiotics until the diagnosis is confirmed, and then isolation and treatment would continue if the cultures were positive for TB. After 7 to 10 days, three more consecutive sputum cultures will be obtained. If they're negative, he would be considered noncontagious and may be sent home, although he'll continue to take the antitubercular drugs for 9 to 12 months.

CN: Physiological integrity; CNS: Physiological adaptation; CL: Application

24. 4. Continuing to have acid-fast bacilli in the sputum after 2 months indicates continued infection. The other choices would all indicate improvement with therapy.

CN: Physiological integrity; CNS: Physiological adaptation; CL: Application

25. 4. The regimen may last up to 24 months. It's essential that the client comply with therapy during that time or resistance will develop. At no time should he stop taking the medications before his physician tells him to.

CN: Safe, effective care environment; CNS: Management of care; CL: Analysis

CN: Client needs category   CNS: Client needs subcategory   CL: Cognitive level

26. A client has been diagnosed with active tuberculosis (TB) and asks the nurse if he will be admitted to the hospital. The nurse responds that hospitalization would be most likely to occur:
1. to evaluate his condition.
2. to determine his compliance.
3. to prevent spread of the disease.
4. to determine the need for antibiotic therapy.

27. A 7-year-old who recently had a cold is brought to the emergency department. The nurse assesses the child and finds he is afebrile, has a respiratory rate of 36 breaths/minute, and has a nonproductive cough. The nurse suspects that the child may be experiencing what?
1. Acute asthma
2. Bronchial pneumonia
3. Chronic obstructive pulmonary disease (COPD)
4. Emphysema

28. The nurse is performing an assessment on a client with a suspected diagnosis of asthma. Which assessment finding supports the diagnosis?
1. Circumoral cyanosis
2. Increased forced expiratory volume
3. Inspiratory and expiratory wheezing
4. Normal breath sounds

29. A client recently experienced a common cold and a subsequent asthma attack. Based on the assessment findings, the nurse determines that the client is experiencing which type of asthma?
1. Emotional
2. Allergic
3. Nonallergic
4. Mediated

30. A client with acute asthma is experiencing inspiratory and expiratory wheezes and a decreased forced expiratory volume. What is the <u>priority</u> intervention by the nurse?
1. Beta-adrenergic blockers
2. Bronchodilators
3. Inhaled steroids
4. Oral steroids

You're doing great! Keep it up!

Listen to how we sound—any changes from normal are clues.

26. 3. The client with active TB is highly contagious until three consecutive sputum cultures are negative, so he's put in respiratory isolation in the hospital. Neither assessment of physical condition, determinations of compliance, nor antibiotic therapy is a primary reason for hospitalization in this case.

CN: Safe, effective care environment; CNS: Safety and infection control; CL: Application

27. 1. Based on the child's history and symptoms, acute asthma is the most likely diagnosis. He's unlikely to have bronchial pneumonia without a productive cough and fever, and he's too young to have developed COPD and emphysema.

CN: Physiological integrity; CNS: Physiological adaptation; CL: Analysis

28. 3. Inspiratory and expiratory wheezes are typical findings in asthma. Circumoral cyanosis may be present in extreme cases of respiratory distress. The nurse would expect the client to have a decreased forced expiratory volume because asthma is an obstructive pulmonary disease. Breath sounds will be "tight" sounding or markedly decreased; they won't be normal.

CN: Physiological integrity; CNS: Physiological adaptation; CL: Analysis

29. 3. Nonallergic asthma doesn't have an easily identifiable allergen and can be triggered by the common cold. Asthma caused by emotional reasons is considered to be in the extrinsic category. Allergic asthma is caused by dust, molds, and pets—easily identifiable allergens. Mediated asthma doesn't exist.

CN: Physiological integrity; CNS: Physiological adaptation; CL: Analysis

30. 2. Bronchodilators are the first line of treatment for asthma because bronchoconstriction is the cause of reduced airflow. Beta-adrenergic blockers aren't used to treat asthma and can cause bronchoconstriction. Inhaled or oral steroids may be given to reduce the inflammation but aren't used for emergency relief.

CN: Physiological integrity; CNS: Pharmacological and parenteral therapies; CL: Application

31. A 19-year-old client comes to the emergency department with acute asthma. His respiratory rate is 44 breaths/minute, and he appears in acute respiratory distress. What is the <u>most important</u> action for the nurse to take?
1. Take a full medical history.
2. Give a bronchodilator by nebulizer.
3. Apply a cardiac monitor to the client.
4. Provide emotional support to the client.

32. A client tells the nurse that he was recently diagnosed with an allergy to Chinese food after he experienced an asthmatic attack. The nurse determines that teaching is successful when the client makes which statement?
1. "I should only eat Chinese food once per month."
2. "I should use my inhalers before eating Chinese food."
3. "I should avoid Chinese food because this is a trigger for me."
4. "I should determine other causes because Chinese food wouldn't cause such a violent reaction."

33. A 58-year-old client with a 40-year history of smoking one to two packs of cigarettes per day has a chronic cough producing thick sputum, peripheral edema, and cyanotic nail beds. Based on this assessment, the nurse suspects the client may be experiencing:
1. acute respiratory distress syndrome (ARDS).
2. asthma.
3. chronic obstructive bronchitis.
4. emphysema.

34. The nurse hears a physician refer to a client as a "blue bloater." The nurse is aware that this term refers to:
1. acute respiratory distress syndrome (ARDS).
2. asthma.
3. chronic obstructive bronchitis.
4. emphysema.

31. 2. The client having an acute asthma attack needs to increase oxygen delivery to the lung and body. Nebulized bronchodilators open airways and increase the amount of oxygen delivered. First, resolve the acute phase of the attack, and then obtain a full medical history to determine the cause of the attack and how to prevent attacks in the future. It may not be necessary to place the client on a cardiac monitor because he's only 19 years old, unless he has a past medical history of cardiac problems.
CN: Physiological integrity; CNS: Physiological adaptation; CL: Application

32. 3. If the trigger of an acute asthma attack is known, this trigger should be avoided at all times. Using an inhaler before eating wouldn't prevent the attack, and food is commonly a trigger for an acute asthma attack.
CN: Physiological integrity; CNS: Physiological adaptation; CL: Application

33. 3. Because of his extensive smoking history and symptoms, the client most likely has chronic obstructive bronchitis. Clients with ARDS have acute symptoms of hypoxia and typically need large amounts of oxygen. Clients with asthma and emphysema tend not to have a chronic cough or peripheral edema.
CN: Physiological integrity; CNS: Physiological adaptation; CL: Application

34. 3. Clients with chronic obstructive bronchitis appear bloated; they have large barrel chests and peripheral edema, cyanotic nail beds, and, at times, circumoral cyanosis. Clients with ARDS are acutely short of breath and frequently need intubation for mechanical ventilation and large amounts of oxygen. Clients with asthma don't exhibit characteristics of chronic disease, and clients with emphysema appear pink and cachectic.
CN: Physiological integrity; CNS: Physiological adaptation; CL: Application

---

CN: Client needs category   CNS: Client needs subcategory   CL: Cognitive level

35. The nurse views the term "pink puffer" on a client's chart. This assessment finding leads the nurse to suspect that the client may be experiencing:
1. acute respiratory distress syndrome (ARDS).
2. asthma.
3. chronic obstructive bronchitis.
4. emphysema.

36. A 66-year-old client has marked dyspnea at rest, is thin, and uses accessory muscles to breathe. He's tachypneic, with a prolonged expiratory phase and has no cough. He leans forward with his arms braced on his knees to support his chest and shoulders for breathing. Based on the assessment findings, the nurse suspects that the client is experiencing which condition?
1. Acute respiratory distress syndrome (ARDS)
2. Asthma
3. Chronic obstructive bronchitis
4. Emphysema

37. The community health nurse is administering Pneumovax and flu vaccinations to clients with asthma, chronic bronchitis, and emphysema. A client asks the nurse why these vaccines are recommended. What is the best response by the nurse?
1. "These vaccines are recommended for all clients."
2. "These vaccines produce bronchodilation and improve oxygenation."
3. "These vaccines help reduce the tachypnea these clients experience."
4. "Respiratory infections can cause severe hypoxia and possibly death in these clients."

38. The nurse is conducting a weekly support group for clients diagnosed with asthma, chronic bronchitis, and emphysema. The topic of today's class is exercise. The nurse determines teaching is effective when the clients states that exercise:
1. enhances cardiovascular fitness.
2. improves respiratory muscle strength.
3. reduces the number of acute attacks.
4. worsens respiratory function and is discouraged.

Terms like these make remembering symptoms a snap!

SNAP

Think of illnesses we're susceptible to.

35. 4. Because of the large amount of energy it takes to breathe, clients with emphysema are usually cachectic. They're pink and usually breathe through pursed lips, hence the term "puffer." Clients with ARDS are usually acutely short of breath. Clients with asthma don't have any particular characteristics, and clients with chronic obstructive bronchitis are bloated and cyanotic in appearance.
CN: Physiological integrity; CNS: Physiological adaptation; CL: Application

36. 4. These are classic signs and symptoms of a client with emphysema. Clients with ARDS are acutely short of breath and require emergency care; those with asthma are also acutely short of breath during an attack and appear very frightened. Clients with chronic obstructive bronchitis are bloated and cyanotic in appearance.
CN: Physiological integrity; CNS: Physiological adaptation; CL: Application

37. 4. It's highly recommended that clients with respiratory disorders be given vaccines to protect against respiratory infection. Infections can cause these clients to need intubation and mechanical ventilation, and it may be difficult to wean these clients from the ventilator. The vaccines have no effect on bronchodilation or respiratory rate.
CN: Health promotion and maintenance; CNS: None; CL: Application

38. 1. Exercise can improve cardiovascular fitness and help the client tolerate periods of hypoxia better, perhaps reducing the risk of heart attack. Most exercise has little effect on respiratory muscle strength, and these clients can't tolerate the type of exercise necessary to do this. Exercise won't reduce the number of acute attacks. In some instances, exercise may be contraindicated, and the client should check with his physician before starting any exercise program.
CN: Health promotion and maintenance; CNS: None; CL: Application

39. A client with chronic obstructive bronchitis asks the nurse why he is receiving diuretic therapy. What is the <u>best</u> response by the nurse?
1. Reducing fluid volume reduces oxygen demand.
2. Reducing fluid volume improves clients' mobility.
3. Reducing fluid volume reduces sputum production.
4. Reducing fluid volume improves respiratory function.

40. The nurse is assessing a 69-year-old client who appears thin and cachectic. The client is short of breath at rest, dyspneic with the slightest exertion, and has diminished breath sounds with deep inspiration. The nurse interprets these assessment findings as indicative of:
1. acute respiratory distress syndrome (ARDS).
2. asthma.
3. chronic obstructive bronchitis.
4. emphysema.

41. A student nurse is asking the staff nurse why a client with emphysema should receive only 1 to 3 L/minute of oxygen, if needed. The nurse determines that teaching was effective when the student makes which statement?
1. "The client doesn't notice he needs to breathe."
2. "The client breathes only when his oxygen levels climb above a certain point."
3. "The client breathes only when his oxygen levels dip below a certain point."
4. "The client breathes only when his carbon dioxide level dips below a certain point."

42. What is the most important information for a nurse to teach a client with chronic obstructive pulmonary disease?
1. How to assess his own pulse and respiratory rates
2. How to recognize when a change is needed in his oxygen therapy
3. How to treat respiratory infections without use of antibiotics
4. How to recognize the signs of an impending respiratory infection

39. 1. Reducing fluid volume reduces the workload of the heart, which reduces oxygen demand and, in turn, reduces the respiratory rate. It also may reduce edema and improve mobility a little, but exercise tolerance will still be poor. Sputum may get thicker and make it harder to clear airways. Reducing fluid volume won't improve respiratory function but may improve oxygenation.
CN: Physiological integrity; CNS: Physiological adaptation; CL: Application

40. 4. In emphysema, the wall integrity of the individual air sacs is damaged, reducing the surface area available for gas exchange. Very little air movement occurs in the lungs because of bronchiole collapse as well. In ARDS, the client's condition is more acute and typically requires mechanical ventilation. In asthma and bronchitis, wheezing is prevalent.
CN: Physiological integrity; CNS: Physiological adaptation; CL: Application

41. 3. Clients with emphysema breathe when their oxygen levels drop to a certain level; this is known as the hypoxic drive. They don't take a breath when their levels of carbon dioxide are higher than normal, as do those with healthy respiratory physiology. If too much oxygen is given, the client has little stimulus to take another breath. In the meantime, his carbon dioxide levels continue to climb, and the client will pass out, leading to respiratory arrest.
CN: Physiological integrity; CNS: Physiological adaptation; CL: Analysis

42. 4. Respiratory infection in clients with a respiratory disorder can be fatal. It's important that the client understands how to recognize the signs and symptoms of an impending respiratory infection. It isn't appropriate to teach a client how to listen to his own lungs or change his oxygen therapy regimen. If the client has signs and symptoms of an infection, he should contact his physician at once.
CN: Health promotion and maintenance; CNS: None; CL: Application

43. The nurse is caring for a client in the immediate postoperative period. The priority of care would include interventions to prevent:
1. atelectasis.
2. bronchitis.
3. pneumonia.
4. pneumothorax.

What's the most important thing to prevent?

43. 1. Atelectasis develops when there's interference with the normal negative pressure that promotes lung expansion. Clients in the postoperative phase often splint their breathing because of pain and positioning, which causes hypoxia. It's uncommon for any of the other respiratory disorders to develop.
CN: Physiological integrity; CNS: Reduction of risk potential; CL: Application

44. The nurse is preparing a plan of care for a postoperative client. What is the most appropriate nursing intervention to prevent the development of atelectasis?
1. Chest physiotherapy
2. Mechanical ventilation
3. Reducing oxygen requirements
4. Use of an incentive spirometer

44. 4. Using an incentive spirometer requires the client to take deep breaths and promotes lung expansion. Chest physiotherapy helps mobilize secretions but won't prevent atelectasis. Reducing oxygen requirements or placing someone on mechanical ventilation doesn't affect the development of atelectasis.
CN: Physiological integrity; CNS: Reduction of risk potential; CL: Application

45. A client is experiencing status asthmaticus. What is the nurse's priority intervention for this client?
1. Inhaled beta-adrenergic agents
2. Inhaled corticosteroids
3. I.V. beta-adrenergic agents
4. Oral corticosteroids

For question 46, you need to choose the highest priority out of several possible goals.

45. 1. Inhaled beta-adrenergic agents help promote bronchodilation, which improves oxygenation. I.V. beta-adrenergic agents can be used but have to be monitored because of their greater systemic effects. They're typically used when the inhaled beta-adrenergic agents don't work. Corticosteroids are slow-acting, so their use won't reduce hypoxia in the acute phase.
CN: Physiological integrity; CNS: Physiological adaptation; CL: Application

46. Which treatment goal is the nurse's <u>highest priority</u> for a client with status asthmaticus?
1. Avoiding intubation
2. Determining the cause of the attack
3. Improving exercise tolerance
4. Reducing secretions

46. 1. Inhaled beta-adrenergic agents, I.V. corticosteroids, and supplemental oxygen are used to reduce bronchospasm, improve oxygenation, and avoid intubation. Determining the trigger for the client's attack and improving exercise tolerance are later goals. Typically, secretions aren't a problem in status asthmaticus.
CN: Physiological integrity; CNS: Physiological adaptation; CL: Application

47. A client was given morphine for pain at 9:00 am. At 9:45 a.m., the nurse assesses the client and notes a respiratory rate of 4 breaths/minute. The nurse recognizes that the client is at highest risk for which of the following?
1. Asthma attack
2. Respiratory arrest
3. Seizure
4. Arousal

47. 2. Opioids such as morphine can cause respiratory arrest if given in large quantities. It's unlikely the client will have an asthma attack or a seizure or wake up on his own.
CN: Physiological integrity; CNS: Pharmacological and parenteral therapies; CL: Analysis

48. A client has a respiratory rate of 4 breaths/minute. The <u>most important</u> assessments for the nurse to obtain would be?
1. Arterial blood gas (ABG) and breath sounds
2. Level of consciousness and a pulse oximetry value
3. Breath sounds and reflexes
4. Pulse oximetry value and heart sounds

48. **2.** First, the nurse should attempt to rouse the client because this should increase the client's respiratory rate. If available, a spot pulse oximetry check should be done and breath sounds should be checked. The physician should be notified immediately of the findings. He'll probably order ABG analysis to determine specific carbon dioxide and oxygen levels, which will indicate the effectiveness of ventilation. Reflexes and heart sounds will be part of the more extensive examination done after these initial actions are completed.

CN: Physiological integrity; CNS: Physiological adaptation; CL: Application

49. The nurse assesses a client who has been given an opioid analgesic and determines that the client is at risk for developing respiratory arrest. An arterial blood gas (ABG) is obtained. The nurse reviews blood gas results and determines which $Paco_2$ value places the client at highest risk?
1. 15 mm Hg
2. 30 mm Hg
3. 40 mm Hg
4. 80 mm Hg

49. **4.** A client about to go into respiratory arrest will have inefficient ventilation and will be retaining carbon dioxide. The value expected would be around 80 mm Hg. All other values are lower than expected.

CN: Physiological integrity; CNS: Physiological adaptation; CL: Analysis

50. A client's arterial blood gas (ABG) results are as follows: pH, 7.16; $Paco_2$, 80 mm Hg; Pao_2, 46 mm Hg; HCO_3^-, 24 mEq/L; Sao_2, 81%. The nurse would interpret the results as indicating:
1. metabolic acidosis.
2. metabolic alkalosis.
3. respiratory acidosis.
4. respiratory alkalosis.

50. **3.** Because the $Paco_2$ is high at 80 mm Hg and the metabolic measure, HCO_3^-, is normal, the client has respiratory acidosis. The pH is less than 7.35, acidemic, which eliminates metabolic and respiratory alkalosis as possibilities. If the HCO_3^- was below 22 mEq/L, the client would have metabolic acidosis.

CN: Physiological integrity; CNS: Physiological adaptation; CL: Application

Which condition would most likely cause us to fail?

51. Which client would be considered to be at the <u>highest risk</u> for respiratory failure?
1. A client with breast cancer
2. A client with cervical sprains
3. A client with a fractured hip
4. A client with Guillain-Barré syndrome

51. **4.** Guillain-Barré syndrome is a progressive neuromuscular disorder that can affect the respiratory muscles and cause respiratory failure. The other conditions typically don't affect the respiratory system.

CN: Physiological integrity; CNS: Physiological adaptation; CL: Analysis

52. A client has started a new drug for hypertension. Thirty minutes after he takes the drug, he develops chest tightness, shortness of breath, tachypnea, and decreased level of consciousness. The nurse interprets this assessment data as indicating:
1. asthma attack.
2. pulmonary embolism.
3. respiratory failure.
4. rheumatoid arthritis.

53. A client is experiencing an anaphylactic reaction to a drug. What is the most important intervention for the nurse to perform?
1. Administering oxygen
2. Inserting an I.V. catheter
3. Obtaining a complete blood count (CBC)
4. Taking vital signs

54. A client diagnosed with asthma is experiencing an anaphylactic reaction to a drug. After administering initial emergency care, the nurse would:
1. administer beta-adrenergic blockers.
2. administer bronchodilators.
3. obtain serum electrolyte levels.
4. have the client lie flat in the bed.

55. A 19-year-old client went to a party, took "some pills," and drank beer. He is brought to the emergency department because he won't wake up. When assessing the client, the nurse would anticipate which of the following?
1. Hyperreflexive reflexes
2. Muscle spasms
3. Shallow respirations
4. Tachypnea

56. The nurse's initial assessment of the client is indicative of probable opioid overdose complicated by alcohol ingestion. What is the most important intervention for the nurse to perform?
1. Administer I.V. fluids.
2. Administer I.V. naloxone (Narcan).
3. Continue close monitoring of vital signs.
4. Draw blood for a drug screen.

> Set your priorities properly. What should be done first?

> In a drug overdose, you'll want to do only one of these first. Which one?

52. 3. The client was reacting to the drug with respiratory signs of impending anaphylaxis, which could lead to eventual respiratory failure. Although the signs are also related to an asthma attack or a pulmonary embolism, consider the new drug first. Rheumatoid arthritis doesn't manifest these signs.
CN: Physiological integrity; CNS: Pharmacological and parenteral therapies; CL: Analysis

53. 1. Giving oxygen would be the best first action in this case. Vital signs should then be checked and the physician immediately notified. If the client doesn't already have an I.V. catheter, one may be inserted now if anaphylactic shock is developing. Obtaining a CBC wouldn't help the emergency situation.
CN: Physiological integrity; CNS: Physiological adaptation; CL: Analysis

54. 2. Bronchodilators would help open the client's airway and improve his oxygenation status. Beta-adrenergic blockers aren't indicated in the management of asthma because they may cause bronchospasm. Obtaining laboratory values wouldn't be done on an emergency basis, and having the client lie flat in bed could worsen his ability to breathe.
CN: Physiological integrity; CNS: Physiological adaptation; CL: Analysis

55. 3. The client probably can't be roused from the combination of pills and alcohol he has taken. This has probably caused him to breathe shallowly, which, if not monitored closely, could lead to respiratory arrest. The nurse wouldn't expect to find tachypnea and doesn't have enough information about which drugs he took to expect muscle spasms or hyperreflexia.
CN: Physiological integrity; CNS: Physiological adaptation; CL: Application

56. 2. If the client took opioids, giving naloxone could reverse the effects and awaken the client. I.V. fluids will most likely be administered, and he'll be closely monitored over a period of several hours to several days. A drug screen should be drawn, but results may not come back for several hours.
CN: Physiological integrity; CNS: Physiological adaptation; CL: Analysis

57. An unconscious client who overdosed on an opioid while consuming alcohol receives naloxone (Narcan). After he awakens, what is the most important action for the nurse to perform?
1. Feed the client.
2. Teach the client about the effects of taking pills and alcohol together.
3. Discharge the client from the hospital.
4. Admit the client to a psychiatric facility.

57. 2. This client needs information about the dangers of taking pills and alcohol together. It may not be advisable to feed the client at first in case his level of consciousness decreases again, increasing the possibility of aspiration. Discharge at this point is inappropriate. Unless the client was trying to commit suicide, admission to a psychiatric facility isn't necessary.
CN: Physiological integrity; CNS: Physiological adaptation; CL: Analysis

58. A firefighter is being treated for smoke inhalation. He develops severe hypoxia 48 hours later, requiring intubation and mechanical ventilation. The nurse determines that the client is experiencing:
1. acute respiratory distress syndrome (ARDS).
2. atelectasis.
3. bronchitis.
4. pneumonia.

58. 1. Severe hypoxia after smoke inhalation is typically related to ARDS. The other conditions listed aren't typically associated with smoke inhalation and severe hypoxia.
CN: Physiological integrity; CNS: Physiological adaptation; CL: Application

Crackle, wheeze, or rattle? Each sound is another clue.

59. A client experienced smoke inhalation and developed pulmonary edema. The nurse auscultates the client's breath sounds and anticipates hearing which of the following?
1. Crackles
2. Decreased breath sounds
3. Inspiratory and expiratory wheezing
4. Upper airway rhonchi

59. 1. In pulmonary edema, the most frequently heard sounds are crackles. Decreased breath sounds and inspiratory and expiratory wheezing are associated with asthma, and rhonchi are heard when there's sputum in the airways.
CN: Physiological integrity; CNS: Physiological adaptation; CL: Application

60. A client has developed acute respiratory distress syndrome (ARDS). What is the priority nursing diagnosis for the client?
1. Impaired gas exchange
2. Risk for infection
3. Imbalanced nutrition: Less than body requirements
4. Impaired skin integrity

60. 1. Impaired gas exchange is the priority nursing diagnosis. A client with ARDS usually requires intubation and mechanical ventilation. The other diagnoses are appropriate but not the priority.
CN: Safe, effective care environment; CNS: Management of care; CL: Analysis

61. The nurse is explaining the process of acute respiratory distress syndrome (ARDS) to a client. What is the <u>best</u> explanation for the nurse to tell the client?
1. Alveoli are overexpanded.
2. Alveoli increase perfusion.
3. Alveolar spaces are filled with fluid.
4. Alveoli improve gaseous exchange.

61. 3. In ARDS, the alveolar membranes are more permeable and the spaces are fluid filled. Alveoli collapse, impairing gas exchange. The fluid interferes with gas exchange and reduces perfusion.
CN: Physiological integrity; CNS: Physiological adaptation; CL: Application

62. A 69-year-old client develops acute shortness of breath and progressive hypoxia requiring mechanical ventilation after repair of a fractured right femur. The nurse determines that the hypoxia was probably a result of which condition?
1. Asthma attack
2. Atelectasis
3. Bronchitis
4. Fat embolism

63. A client who developed a fat embolism is receiving 100% F_{IO_2} on a mechanical ventilator and continues to be hypoxic. What is the most important intervention?
1. Add positive end-expiratory pressure (PEEP).
2. Give beta-adrenergic blockers.
3. Give diuretics.
4. Increase the F_{IO_2} on the ventilator.

64. A client with a fat embolism continues to be hypoxic following therapy with positive end-expiratory pressure. What is the priority intervention to reduce oxygen demand?
1. Give diuretics.
2. Give neuromuscular blockers.
3. Put the head of the bed flat.
4. Use bronchodilators.

65. The client is receiving positive end-expiratory pressure (PEEP) therapy. The nurse anticipates that the client will exhibit which of the following?
1. Bradycardia
2. Tachycardia
3. Increased blood pressure
4. Reduced cardiac output

Several answers may seem correct, but *probably* points to the best one.

You're almost there! Keep going!

62. 4. Long bone fractures are correlated with fat emboli, which cause shortness of breath and hypoxia. It's unlikely that the client has developed asthma or bronchitis without a previous history. He could develop atelectasis, but it typically doesn't produce progressive hypoxia.
CN: Physiological integrity; CNS: Physiological adaptation; CL: Analysis

63. 1. PEEP can be added to open up alveoli and keep them open. There's no reason to give the client beta-adrenergic blockers. He may benefit from diuresis, but in the meantime, PEEP should be added to improve oxygenation. The highest amount of oxygen that can be delivered is 100% F_{IO_2}.
CN: Physiological integrity; CNS: Physiological adaptation; CL: Application

64. 2. Neuromuscular blockers cause skeletal muscle paralysis, reducing the amount of oxygen used by the restless skeletal muscles. This should improve oxygenation. Diuretics can be administered to reduce pulmonary congestion, and the head of the bed should be partially elevated to facilitate diaphragm movement. Bronchodilators may be used, but they typically don't have enough of an effect to reduce the amount of hypoxia present. However, diuretics, head elevation, and bronchodilators would improve oxygen delivery, not reduce oxygen demand.
CN: Physiological integrity; CNS: Physiological adaptation; CL: Application

65. 4. PEEP reduces cardiac output by increasing intrathoracic pressure and reducing the amount of blood delivered to the left side of the heart, thereby reducing cardiac output. It doesn't affect heart rate, but a decrease in cardiac output may reduce blood pressure, commonly causing a compensatory tachycardia.
CN: Physiological integrity; CNS: Physiological adaptation; CL: Application

66. The nurse placed a client diagnosed with acute respiratory distress syndrome in the prone position. The nurse determined that this positioning of the client would:
1. improve cardiac output.
2. make the client more comfortable.
3. prevent skin breakdown.
4. recruit more alveoli.

66. 4. A supine position may reduce the ability of posterior alveoli to open and remain open. Turning the client to the prone position may recruit new alveoli in the posterior region of the lung and improve oxygenation status. Cardiac output shouldn't be affected by the prone position. The prone position doesn't make the client more comfortable, and he often requires sedation to tolerate it. Skin breakdown can still occur over the new pressure points.

CN: Physiological integrity; CNS: Physiological adaptation; CL: Application

67. The nurse is aware that which diagnosis is most likely to contribute to the development of acute respiratory distress syndrome (ARDS)?
1. Appendicitis
2. Massive trauma
3. Receiving conscious sedation
4. Right meniscus injury

67. 2. The client with massive trauma will require multiple transfusions. Blood products are preserved with citrate, which causes increased permeability in the lungs, the defect that allows ARDS to develop. Appendicitis, unless it causes overwhelming sepsis, won't lead to ARDS. Conscious sedation and injuries to the meniscus don't lead to ARDS.

CN: Physiological integrity; CNS: Physiological adaptation; CL: Analysis

68. The nurse reviews the assessment of a client with acute respiratory distress syndrome (ARDS). What is the best indicator of improvement in the client?
1. Arterial blood gas (ABG) values
2. Bronchoscopy results
3. Increased blood pressure
4. Sputum culture and sensitivity results

68. 1. Improved ABG results would indicate that the client's oxygenation status is improved. Hypoxia is the problem in ARDS, so bronchoscopy and sputum culture results may have no bearing on the improvement of ARDS. Increased blood pressure isn't relative to the client's respiratory condition.

CN: Physiological integrity; CNS: Physiological adaptation; CL: Analysis

69. A client has been placed on a high level of oxygen. The nurse anticipates that this will cause the client's lungs to do what?
1. Improve oxygen uptake
2. Increase carbon dioxide levels
3. Stabilize carbon dioxide levels
4. Reduce the amount of functional alveolar surface area

In question 70, break kyphoscoliosis down to find its meaning—and a clue.

69. 4. Oxygen toxicity causes direct pulmonary trauma, reducing the amount of alveolar surface area available for gaseous exchange, which results in increased carbon dioxide levels and decreased oxygen uptake.

CN: Physiological integrity; CNS: Physiological adaptation; CL: Application

70. A client has been diagnosed with thoracic kyphoscoliosis. The nurse is aware that this will have what effect on the client's lungs?
1. Improve overall expansion
2. Obstruct deflation
3. Reduce alveolar compression during expiration
4. Restrict expansion

70. 4. Thoracic kyphoscoliosis causes lung compression, restricts lung expansion, and results in more rapid and shallow respiration. It doesn't improve lung expansion because of the compression. It also doesn't cause obstruction or reduce alveolar compression during expiration.

CN: Physiological integrity; CNS: Physiological adaptation; CL: Application

71. A 24-year-old client comes into the clinic complaining of sudden-onset, right-sided chest pain and shortness of breath. The nurse is assessing the client and determines that the most important intervention to implement is:
1. auscultation of breath sounds.
2. chest X-ray.
3. echocardiogram.
4. electrocardiogram (ECG).

72. A client with shortness of breath has decreased-to-absent breath sounds on the right side, from the apex to the base. The nurse interprets this assessment data as indicating which condition?
1. Acute asthma
2. Chronic bronchitis
3. Pneumonia
4. Spontaneous pneumothorax

73. The nurse anticipates that the priority treatment for a client with spontaneous pneumothorax is:
1. antibiotics.
2. bronchodilators.
3. chest tube placement.
4. hyperbaric chamber.

74. A 60-year-old client was in a motor vehicle accident. He is brought to the emergency department by the paramedics. During the assessment, the client complains of difficulty breathing and chest pain. Auscultation of lung fields notes absent breath sounds in the left upper lobe. The nurse interprets this information as indicating which condition?
1. Bronchitis
2. Pneumonia
3. Pneumothorax
4. Tuberculosis (TB)

75. The client is suspected of having a pneumothorax. The nurse anticipates the diagnosis will be confirmed by:
1. auscultating breath sounds.
2. having the client use an incentive spirometer.
3. chest X-ray.
4. thoracic puncture.

Listening to breath sounds sure helps diagnose a lot of conditions, doesn't it?

You're a natural! Keep going!

71. 1. Because the client is short of breath, listening to breath sounds is a good idea. He may need a chest X-ray and an ECG, but a physician must order these tests. Unless a cardiac source for the client's pain is identified, he won't need an echocardiogram.

CN: Physiological integrity; CNS: Physiological adaptation; CL: Application

72. 4. A spontaneous pneumothorax occurs when the client's lung collapses, causing an acute decrease in the amount of functional lung used in oxygenation. The sudden collapse was the cause of his chest pain and shortness of breath. An asthma attack would show wheezing breath sounds, and bronchitis would have rhonchi. Pneumonia would have bronchial breath sounds over the area of consolidation.

CN: Physiological integrity; CNS: Physiological adaptation; CL: Analysis

73. 3. The only way to reexpand the lung is to place a chest tube on the right side so the air in the pleural space can be removed and the lung reexpanded. Antibiotics and bronchodilators would have no effect on lung reexpansion, nor would the hyperbaric chamber.

CN: Physiological integrity; CNS: Physiological adaptation; CL: Application

74. 3. The client may have a left pneumothorax from the trauma he experienced. Auscultation would reveal rhonchi with bronchitis, bronchial breath sounds with pneumonia, and rhonchorous breath sounds with TB.

CN: Physiological integrity; CNS: Physiological adaptation; CL: Application

75. 3. A chest X-ray will show the area of collapsed lung if a pneumothorax is present as well as the volume of air in the pleural space. Listening to breath sounds won't confirm a diagnosis. An incentive spirometer is used to encourage deep breathing. A needle thoracostomy is done only in an emergency and only by someone trained to do it.

CN: Physiological integrity; CNS: Physiological adaptation; CL: Application

76. After a motor vehicle collision, a client has a chest tube inserted in the left upper chest. The tube begins to drain a large amount of dark red fluid. The nurse determines that:
1. the chest tube was inserted improperly.
2. this is an expected result.
3. an artery was nicked when the chest tube was placed.
4. the client is experiencing a hemothorax.

77. A hospitalized client has a central I.V. catheter inserted in the subclavian vein. Shortly after placement, the client develops shortness of breath and appears restless. The priority action by the nurse would be?
1. Administer a sedative.
2. Advise the client to calm down.
3. Auscultate for breath sounds.
4. Check to see if the client can have medication.

78. The nurse is caring for a client who recently had a central venous catheter inserted and now appears short of breath and anxious. The nurse anticipates that the physician will order a:
1. chest X-ray.
2. electrocardiogram.
3. laboratory tests.
4. sedation.

79. The nurse is preparing a client to have a chest tube inserted in the right upper chest. What is the priority role of the nurse?
1. The nurse isn't needed.
2. Preparing the chest tube drainage system
3. Bringing the chest X-ray to the client's room
4. Inserting the chest tube

80. The nurse is auscultating the lungs of a client following chest tube insertion. What assessment finding would indicate to the nurse correct chest tube placement?
1. Bronchial sounds heard at both bases
2. Vesicular sounds heard over upper lung fields
3. Bronchovesicular sounds heard over both lung fields
4. Crackles heard on the affected side

When I'm in distress, what should you do first?

Which breath sounds do I predict hearing after chest tube insertion?

76. 4. Because of the traumatic cause of injury, the client had a hemothorax, in which blood collection causes the collapse of the lung. The placement of the chest tube will drain the blood from the space and reexpand the lung. There's a very slight chance of nicking an intercostal artery during insertion, but it's fairly unlikely if the person placing the chest tube has been trained. The initial chest X-ray would help confirm whether there was blood in the pleural space or just air.

CN: Physiological integrity; CNS: Physiological adaptation; CL: Application

77. 3. Because this is an acute episode, listen to the client's lungs to see if anything has changed. Don't give this client medication, especially sedatives, if he's having difficulty breathing. Give the client emotional support and contact the physician who placed the central venous access.

CN: Physiological integrity; CNS: Physiological adaptation; CL: Analysis

78. 1. Inserting an I.V. catheter in the subclavian vein can result in a pneumothorax, so a chest X-ray should be done. If it's negative, then other tests should be done, but they aren't appropriate as the first intervention. Sedation may depress respirations.

CN: Physiological integrity; CNS: Reduction of risk potential; CL: Application

79. 2. The nurse must anticipate that a drainage system is required and set this up before insertion so the tube can be directly connected to the drainage system. The chest X-ray need not be brought to the client's room. A physician will insert the chest tube.

CN: Physiological integrity; CNS: Physiological adaptation; CL: Application

80. 3. If the chest tube is inserted correctly, normal bronchovesicular breath sounds in that area will be heard and the client's oxygenation status will improve. A chest X-ray should be done to ensure reexpansion. All other sounds noted are abnormal.

CN: Physiological integrity; CNS: Reduction of risk potential; CL: Analysis

81. The nurse is caring for a client who had a chest tube inserted for treatment of a pneumothorax. Which assessment finding best indicates to the nurse that a chest tube is no longer needed?
1. The drainage from the chest tube is minimal.
2. Arterial blood gas (ABG) levels are obtained to ensure proper oxygenation.
3. It's removed and the client is assessed to see if he's breathing adequately.
4. No fluctuation in the water seal chamber occurs when no suction is applied.

Go for the best!

82. A client is scheduled to have a chest tube removed. What is the most important intervention for the nurse to perform prior to the removal?
1. Disconnect the drainage system from the tube.
2. Obtain a chest X-ray to document reexpansion.
3. Obtain an arterial blood gas level to document oxygen status.
4. Sedate the client, and the physician will slip the tube out without warning the client.

I'm number one— and don't you forget it.

83. The nurse is teaching a client about lung cancer. The nurse determines teaching was effective when the client states the primary cause of lung cancer is:
1. genetics.
2. occupational exposures.
3. smoking a pipe.
4. smoking cigarettes.

84. A nurse reinforces the teaching plan for a client who has recently been diagnosed with squamous cell carcinoma of the left lung. The most appropriate information for the nurse to give the client would be?
1. "You have a slow-growing cancer that rarely spreads."
2. "In terms of prognosis, you may have only a few months to live."
3. "Squamous cell cancer is a very rapid-growing cancer."
4. "The cancer has generally metastasized by the time diagnosis is made."

81. 4. One indication of reexpansion is the cessation of fluctuation in the water seal chamber when suction isn't applied. Drainage should be minimal before the chest tube is removed. An ABG analysis may be done to ensure proper oxygenation but isn't necessary if clinical assessment criteria are met. The chest tube isn't removed until it's determined the client's lung has adequately reexpanded and will stay that way. After the lung stays expanded, the chest tube is removed.
CN: Physiological integrity; CNS: Physiological adaptation; CL: Analysis

82. 2. A chest X-ray should be done to ensure and document that the lung is reexpanded and has remained expanded since suction was discontinued. The drainage system shouldn't be disconnected from the tube while still in the client because that could cause a pneumothorax to recur. A pulse oximetry measurement is sufficient to track oxygenation before the tube is removed. Client cooperation is desirable; if the client can hold his breath while the chest tube is removed, there's less chance that air will be drawn back into the pleural space during removal.
CN: Physiological integrity; CNS: Reduction of risk potential; CL: Application

83. 4. As many as 90% of clients with lung cancer smoke cigarettes. Cigarette smoke contains several organ-specific carcinogens. There may be a genetic predisposition for the development of cancer. Occupational hazards such as pollutants can cause cancer. Pipe smokers inhale less often than cigarette smokers and tend to develop cancers of the lip and mouth.
CN: Health promotion and maintenance; CNS: None; CL: Application

84. 1. Squamous cell carcinoma is a slow-growing, rarely metastasizing type of cancer. It has the best prognosis of all lung cancer types.
CN: Physiological integrity; CNS: Physiological adaptation; CL: Analysis

85. The nurse is obtaining assessment data from a client with a suspected diagnosis of lung cancer. The nurse is most concerned if the client exhibits which symptom?
1. Dizziness
2. Generalized weakness
3. Hypotension
4. Recurrent pleural effusions

86. A nurse is admitting a client to the medical unit. The client tells the nurse that the doctor diagnosed him with a <u>centrally located</u> lung tumor. Upon assessment of the client, the nurse anticipates the client to exhibit:
1. coughing.
2. hemoptysis.
3. pleuritic pain.
4. shoulder pain.

Centrally located. That's your clue for question 86.

87. A client with a suspected diagnosis of lung cancer tells the nurse the doctor is scheduling tests to confirm the diagnosis. The nurse understands that the definitive diagnosis will be determined by:
1. bronchoscopy.
2. chest X-ray.
3. computed tomography (CT) scan of the chest.
4. surgical biopsy.

88. Which statements are true about staging lung cancer tumors? Select all that apply.
1. Staging describes the severity of the cancer.
2. Staging helps the physician plan appropriate treatment.
3. Staging systems don't change over time.
4. Surgical biopsy with cytologic cell examination is the only data collection method used to perform staging.
5. Staging helps to determine whether the cancer has spread to distant areas of the body.

89. The nurse is teaching clients about interventions to increase the survival rates of clients with lung cancer. The nurse determines teaching is effective when the client states that which action will increase survival?
1. Early bronchoscopy
2. Early detection
3. High-dose chemotherapy
4. Smoking cessation

85. **4.** Recurring episodes of pleural effusions can be caused by the tumor and should be investigated. Dizziness, generalized weakness, and hypotension aren't typically considered warning signals but may occur in advanced stages of cancer.
CN: Physiological integrity; CNS: Physiological adaptation; CL: Application

86. **1.** Centrally located lung tumors are found in the upper airway and usually produce such symptoms as coughing, wheezing, and stridor. Small cell tumors tend to be located in the lower airways and often cause hemoptysis. Tumors invading the pleural space may cause pleuritic pain. Pancoast tumors that occur in the apices may cause shoulder pain.
CN: Physiological integrity; CNS: Physiological adaptation; CL: Analysis

87. **4.** Only surgical biopsy with cytologic examination of the cells can give a definitive diagnosis of cancer and type. Bronchoscopy gives positive results in only 30% of the cases. Chest X-ray and CT scan can identify location of abnormal tissue but not confirm cancer.
CN: Physiological integrity; CNS: Physiological adaptation; CL: Application

88. **1, 2, and 5.** Staging describes the extent and severity of the cancer and helps the physician determine the most appropriate therapy. Staging systems continue to evolve as cancer is better understood. Multiple data collection methods, such as laboratory results, physical examinations, and imaging results, are used to determine the stage of a cancer.
CN: Physiological integrity; CNS: Physiological adaptation; CL: Analysis

89. **2.** Early detection of cancer when the cells may be premalignant and potentially curable would be most beneficial. However, a tumor must be 1 cm in diameter before it's detectable on a chest X-ray. A bronchoscopy may help early identification but is often not ordered until an abnormal X-ray is seen. High-dose chemotherapy has minimal effect on long-term survival. Smoking cessation won't reverse the process but may prevent further decompensation.
CN: Health promotion and maintenance; CNS: None; CL: Application

90. A client alerts the nurse that his chest tube has accidentally been removed. What is the most appropriate action by the nurse?
1. Position the client on his left side.
2. Position the client on his right side.
3. Apply an occlusive dressing over the site.
4. Reinsert the chest tube that fell out.

91. A client has been diagnosed with lung cancer and requires a wedge resection. The client asks the nurse what a wedge resection is. The most appropriate response by the nurse is that the procedure involves resection of:
1. one entire lung.
2. a lobe of the lung.
3. a small, localized area near the surface of the lung.
4. a segment of the lung, including a bronchiole and its alveoli.

92. The nurse is caring for a client who has just returned to the unit after a lobectomy. During assessment of the client, the nurse is aware that the lobectomy site:
1. remains empty.
2. is filled with a gel by the surgeon.
3. is filled with serous fluid.
4. is filled by overexpansion of the remaining lobe(s).

93. A client who is scheduled for a pneumonectomy asks the nurse how thoracic cavity will be filled. The best response by the nurse would be?
1. The space remains filled with air only.
2. The surgeon fills the space with a gel.
3. Serous fluid fills the space and consolidates the region.
4. The tissue from the other lung grows over to the other side.

You're doing great! Keep up the good work!

What happens when there is only one of me?

90. 3. To prevent the client from sucking air into the pleural space and causing a pneumothorax, an occlusive dressing should be put over the hole where the tube came out. The physician should be called and the client checked for signs of respiratory distress. Positioning the client on either the left or right side won't make a difference. It isn't advisable for the physician to reinsert the old tube because it's no longer sterile.
CN: Physiological integrity; CNS: Reduction of risk potential; CL: Application

91. 3. A small area of tissue close to the surface of the lung is removed in a wedge resection. An entire lung is removed in a pneumonectomy. A lobe is removed in a lobectomy, and a segment of the lung is removed in a segmental resection.
CN: Physiological integrity; CNS: Physiological adaptation; CL: Application

92. 4. The remaining lobe or lobes overexpand slightly to fill the space previously occupied by the removed tissue. The diaphragm is carried higher on the operative side to further reduce the empty space. The space can't remain "empty" because truly empty would imply a vacuum, which would interfere with the intrathoracic pressure changes that allow breathing. The surgeon doesn't use gel to fill the space. Serous fluid overproduction would compress the remaining lobes, diminish their function, and, possibly, cause a mediastinal shift.
CN: Physiological integrity; CNS: Physiological adaptation; CL: Application

93. 3. Serous fluid fills the space and eventually consolidates, preventing extensive mediastinal shift of the heart and remaining lung. Air can't be left in the space. There's no gel that can be placed in the pleural space. The tissue from the other lung can't cross the mediastinum, although a temporary mediastinal shift exists until the space is filled.
CN: Physiological integrity; CNS: Physiological adaptation; CL: Application

94. A client is scheduled to undergo a pneumonectomy. The nurse determines that the client understands the rationale for cutting the phrenic nerve and hemidiaphragm paralysis when the client states the procedure will:
1. paralyze the diaphragm and reduce oxygen demand.
2. reduce postoperative pain.
3. increase the capacity of the remaining lung.
4. reduce the space left by the pneumonectomy.

94. 4. Because the hemidiaphragm is a muscle that doesn't contract when paralyzed, an uncontracted hemidiaphragm remains in an "up" position, which reduces the space left by the pneumonectomy. Serous fluid has less space to fill, thus reducing the extent and duration of mediastinal shift after surgery. Paralyzing the hemidiaphragm doesn't decrease total-body oxygen demand or increase the capacity of the remaining lung. The client will also still experience postoperative pain. Although it's true that the client no longer needs the hemidiaphragm on the operative side to breathe, this alone wouldn't be sufficient justification for cutting the phrenic nerve.
CN: Physiological integrity; CNS: Physiological adaptation; CL: Application

95. A preoperative client is scheduled for surgical resection after being diagnosed with lung cancer. The client correctly states that the procedure will:
1. "remove the tumor and all surrounding tissue."
2. "remove the tumor and as little surrounding tissue as possible."
3. "remove all the tumor and any collapsed alveoli in the same region."
4. "remove as much of the tumor as possible, without removing any alveoli."

95. 2. The goal of surgical resection is to remove the lung tissue that has a tumor in it while saving as much surrounding tissue as possible. It may be necessary to remove alveoli and bronchioles, but care is taken to make sure only what's absolutely necessary is removed.
CN: Physiological integrity; CNS: Physiological adaptation; CL: Application

96. A client with preexisting pulmonary disease has been diagnosed with lung cancer and is being evaluated for surgery. The nurse is aware that the impact of both conditions may:
1. have no effect on the surgery.
2. require the whole lung to be removed.
3. prevent the resection of the entire tumor.
4. prohibit the client from having the surgery done.

96. 4. If the client's preexisting pulmonary disease is restrictive and advanced, it may be impossible to perform surgery, and the client may have to be treated with only chemotherapy and radiation.
CN: Physiological integrity; CNS: Physiological adaptation; CL: Application

97. The nurse is performing preoperative teaching for a client scheduled for surgery. What should be the primary focus of the teaching?
1. Deciding if the client should have the surgery
2. Giving emotional support to the client and his family
3. Giving minute details of the surgery to the client and his family
4. Providing general information to reduce client and family anxiety

The nurse does a lot of teaching but in this case, what would be the main focus?

97. 4. The nurse's role is to provide general information about the surgery and what to expect before and after surgery and to give emotional support during this time. The nurse's role isn't to decide if the client should have surgery or to give minute details of the surgery unless the client or family requests them, in which case the surgeon should answer the questions. Emotional support alone during this time isn't sufficient.
CN: Physiological integrity; CNS: Reduction of risk potential; CL: Application

98. A client has been diagnosed with a benign lung tumor and asks the nurse how it will be treated. What is the best response by the nurse?
1. The tumor is treated with radiation only.
2. The tumor is treated with chemotherapy only.
3. The tumor is left alone unless symptoms are present.
4. The tumor is removed, involving the least possible amount of tissue.

99. The nurse is caring for a client with terminal lung cancer. What is the priority nursing intervention for this client?
1. Provide emotional support.
2. Provide nutritional support.
3. Provide pain control.
4. Prepare the client's will.

Focus!

100. A 165-lb client with a pulmonary embolus is ordered to receive heparin 20 units/kg/hour by I.V. infusion. How many units of heparin should he receive each hour?
1. 1,000
2. 1,200
3. 1,500
4. 1,700

This clue asks you to select the most common, even when all answers are correct.

101. The nurse is conducting a preoperative class for clients scheduled for gastric bypass surgery. One of the clients asks the nurse what the most common source of pulmonary embolism is. The most appropriate response by the nurse is:
1. amniotic fluid.
2. bone marrow.
3. septic thrombi.
4. venous thrombi.

98. 4. The tumor is removed to prevent further compression of lung tissue as the tumor grows, which could lead to respiratory decompensation. If for some reason, it can't be removed, then radiation or chemotherapy may be used to try to shrink the tumor.

CN: Physiological integrity; CNS: Physiological adaptation; CL: Application

99. 3. The client with terminal lung cancer may have extreme pleuritic pain and should be treated to reduce his discomfort. Preparing the client and his family for the impending death and providing emotional support are also important but shouldn't be the primary focus until pain is under control. Nutritional support may be provided, but as the terminal phase advances, the client's nutritional needs greatly decrease. Nursing care doesn't focus on helping the client prepare a will.

CN: Physiological integrity; CNS: Basic care and comfort; CL: Analysis

100. 3. A 165-lb client weighs 75 kg (2.2 lb = 1 kg). 20 units × 75 kg × 1 hour = 1,500 units/hour.

CN: Physiological integrity; CNS: Pharmacological and parenteral therapies; CL: Application

101. 4. Venous thrombi in the thigh and pelvis are the most common sources for pulmonary emboli. Clients who are immobile form clots from this source. When dislodged, the clots are carried through the bloodstream and lodge in the pulmonary vasculature. The other options are also sources but not the most common.

CN: Physiological integrity; CNS: Physiological adaptation; CL: Application

102. Which client is at <u>highest</u> risk for developing a pulmonary embolism?
1. An ambulatory client with an inflammatory joint disease
2. An ambulatory client who has type 1 diabetes
3. A healthy client who's 6 months pregnant
4. A client who has fractures of his pelvis and right femur

103. The nurse is planning care for a client who has undergone a total knee replacement. The <u>most important</u> intervention to prevent the development of a pulmonary embolism would be?
1. Early ambulation
2. Frequent chest X-rays to find a pulmonary embolism
3. Frequent lower extremity scans
4. Intubation of the client

104. Which physiologic effect of a pulmonary embolism would initially affect oxygenation?
1. A blood clot blocks ventilation; perfusion is unaffected.
2. A blood clot blocks ventilation, producing hypoxia despite normal perfusion.
3. A blood clot blocks perfusion and ventilation, producing profound hypoxia.
4. A blood clot blocks perfusion, producing hypoxia despite normal or supernormal ventilation.

105. The nurse is teaching the client about his diagnosis of a pulmonary embolism. The client tells the nurse that the doctor told him that he has a ventilation-perfusion mismatch. Which statement by the client best conveys an understanding of the diagnosis?
1. The area of the lung being ventilated isn't being perfused.
2. The area of the lung being perfused isn't being ventilated.
3. The area of the lung being ventilated is also being perfused.
4. The amount of ventilation occurring doesn't equal perfusion.

Hint! Check out the word *most important!*

Pat yourself on the back and keep going. Good job!

102. 4. Thrombosis formation is caused by abnormalities in blood flow, vein wall integrity, and blood coagulation. The client with pelvic and femur fractures will be immobilized and probably have edema, which leads to venous stasis and predisposes him to the development of deep vein thrombosis. A pulmonary embolus commonly arises from clots in the deep veins of the leg that break off and travel to the pulmonary arteries. The risk of developing venous thrombosis isn't as high with the other conditions.
CN: Physiological integrity; CNS: Physiological adaptation; CL: Application

103. 1. Early ambulation helps reduce pooling of blood, which reduces the tendency of the blood to form a clot that could then dislodge. Frequent chest X-rays or lower extremity scans don't prevent pulmonary embolism. Intubation of the client won't prevent the occurrence of a pulmonary embolism.
CN: Physiological integrity; CNS: Reduction of risk potential; CL: Application

104. 4. The blood clot blocks blood flow to a region of the lung tissue. That area remains ventilated, but because blood flow is blocked, no gas exchange can occur in that region and a ventilation-perfusion mismatch is present. Ventilation isn't initially affected by a blood clot because air can still move normally through the bronchial tree.
CN: Physiological integrity; CNS: Physiological adaptation; CL: Application

105. 1. A pulmonary embolism blocks the flow of blood past a region of the lung tissue, which is still being ventilated because no disorder of the bronchial tree exists. A pulmonary embolism blocks the pulmonary vasculature, not allowing blood to flow to the distal region of the lung and interfering with gas exchange. Blood must flow around each alveolus, or perfuse, for the exchange of carbon dioxide and oxygen to occur across the alveolar-capillary membrane. When an area of lung is ventilated but not perfused, there is a ventilation-perfusion mismatch specific to pulmonary embolism. A mismatch that shows impaired ventilation but normal perfusion indicates a pathological state in the bronchial tree, such as pneumonia or atelectasis.
CN: Physiological integrity; CNS: Physiological adaptation; CL: Application

106. A client has been diagnosed with a pulmonary embolism and begins to experience chest pain. The client asks the nurse what is causing the pain. The most appropriate response by the nurse is:
1. costochondritis.
2. myocardial infarction (MI).
3. inflammatory reaction.
4. referred pain from the pelvis to the chest.

107. A client with a pulmonary embolism tells the nurse that he feels a sense of "impending doom." The nurse recognizes that this manifestation is caused by what?
1. Inflammatory reaction in the lung parenchyma
2. Loss of chest expansion
3. Loss of lung tissue
4. Sudden reduction in adequate oxygenation

Here's a hint for question 107: Think about what causes the condition.

108. A client with pulmonary embolism has developed hemoptysis. The nurse determines that this is most likely related to:
1. alveolar damage in the infarcted area.
2. involvement of major blood vessels where the clot formed.
3. loss of lung parenchyma.
4. loss of lung tissue.

109. A client with a massive pulmonary embolism is scheduled to have arterial blood gas analysis performed. The nurse expects the analysis will identify:
1. metabolic acidosis.
2. metabolic alkalosis.
3. respiratory acidosis.
4. respiratory alkalosis.

110. A client is scheduled to have a ventilation-perfusion ($\dot{V}/\dot{Q}$) scan performed and asks the nurse to explain the tests. The nurse tells the client that the test is frequently done to diagnose a pulmonary embolism and provide information about the:
1. amount of perfusion present in the lung.
2. extent of the occlusion and amount of perfusion lost.
3. location of the pulmonary embolism.
4. location and size of the pulmonary embolism.

106. 3. Pleuritic pain is caused by the inflammatory reaction of the lung parenchyma. The pain isn't associated with costochondritis, MI, or referred pain from the pelvis to the chest.
CN: Physiological integrity; CNS: Physiological adaptation; CL Application

107. 4. The client with a pulmonary embolism has a portion of the lung not involved in oxygenation, causing the client to feel apprehensive. If the area involved is large, the apprehension can be great, giving the client the feeling of "impending doom." The inflammatory reaction in the lung causes chest pain. There's no actual loss of lung tissue, and chest expansion isn't affected.
CN: Physiological integrity; CNS: Physiological adaptation; CL: Application

108. 1. The infarcted area produces alveolar damage that can lead to the production of bloody sputum, sometimes in massive amounts. Clot formation usually occurs in the legs. There's a loss of lung parenchyma and subsequent scar tissue formation, but these don't cause hemoptysis.
CN: Physiological integrity; CNS: Physiological adaptation; CL: Application

109. 4. A client with a massive pulmonary embolism will have a large region of lung tissue unavailable for perfusion. This causes the client to hyperventilate and blow off large amounts of carbon dioxide, which crosses the unaffected alveolar-capillary membrane more readily than does oxygen and results in respiratory alkalosis.
CN: Physiological integrity; CNS: Physiological adaptation; CL: Analysis

110. 2. The $\dot{V}/\dot{Q}$ scan provides information on the extent of occlusion caused by the pulmonary embolism and the amount of lung tissue involved in the area not perfused.
CN: Physiological integrity; CNS: Physiological adaptation; CL: Application

111. A client is suspected of having a pulmonary embolism and asks the nurse how the doctor will <u>definitively</u> determine the diagnosis. The nurse anticipates that the physician will order:
1. arterial blood gas (ABG) analysis.
2. chest X-ray.
3. pulmonary angiogram.
4. ventilation-perfusion (V̇/Q̇) scan.

Watch that word, definitively.

111. 3. A pulmonary angiogram is used to definitively diagnose a pulmonary embolism. A catheter is passed through the circulation to the region of the occlusion; the region can be outlined with an injection of contrast medium and viewed by fluoroscopy. This shows the location of the clot as well as the extent of the perfusion defect. ABG levels can define the amount of hypoxia present. A chest X-ray can't provide a definitive diagnosis of pulmonary embolism. The V̇/Q̇ scan can report whether there's a V̇/Q̇ mismatch present and define the amount of tissue involved.
CN: Physiological integrity; CNS: Reduction of risk potential; CL: Application

112. A definitive diagnosis of pulmonary embolism has been made for a client. The nurse anticipates which medication will be ordered?
1. Warfarin (Coumadin)
2. Heparin
3. Streptokinase (Streptase)
4. Acyclovir (Zovirax)

112. 2. Heparin is started I.V. once a pulmonary embolism is diagnosed to reduce further clot formation. When a therapeutic level of heparin is established, warfarin is started. It can take up to 3 days before a therapeutic level of warfarin is achieved. Streptokinase is a fibrinolytic, and its usefulness in the management of pulmonary embolism is unclear. Acyclovir is an antiviral and is not prescribed after a pulmonary embolism.
CN: Physiological integrity; CNS: Pharmacological and parenteral therapies; CL: Application

Knowing what a treatment should achieve will help you monitor the response.

113. The nurse is teaching a client diagnosed with a pulmonary embolism about the prescribed heparin therapy. The nurse determines that teaching has been effective when the client states heparin is given to:
1. dissolve the clot.
2. break up the pulmonary embolism.
3. slow the development of other clots.
4. prevent clots from breaking off and embolizing to the lung.

113. 3. Heparin slows the development of other clots. It doesn't break up pulmonary embolisms or dissolve clots already formed. Heparin doesn't stop clots from going to the lung.
CN: Physiological integrity; CNS: Pharmacological and parenteral therapies; CL: Application

114. A client who was hospitalized for pulmonary embolism is being discharged on warfarin (Coumadin) therapy. The client asks the nurse to explain how warfarin works. The best response by the nurse is:
1. "It inhibits the formation of blood clots."
2. "It will reduce the size of the pulmonary embolism."
3. "It will reduce blood pressure and prevent venous stasis."
4. "It will dissolve an existing clot."

114. 1. Warfarin inhibits clot formation by interfering with clotting factors that are dependent on vitamin K. Warfarin doesn't dissolve clots and won't reduce the size of the pulmonary embolus. It doesn't reduce blood pressure and won't prevent venous stasis. Coagulation studies will be performed every 2 to 4 weeks while the client is receiving warfarin.
CN: Physiological integrity; CNS: Pharmacological and parenteral therapies; CL: Application

115. A client with a pulmonary embolism has been placed on oxygen therapy. The nurse is reviewing lab work and determines that the therapy is effective when the lab work shows which value?
1. $Paco_2$ greater than 40 mm Hg
2. $Paco_2$ less than 40 mm Hg
3. Pao_2 greater than 60 mm Hg
4. Pao_2 less than 60 mm Hg

Remember, hypo and hyper are opposites.

HYPER HYPO

116. A client hospitalized with a pulmonary embolism develops hypotension. The nurse determines that the hypotension was the result of which of the following?
1. Pressure on the heart and reduced cardiac output
2. Reduced blood flow to the lung, which causes hypotension
3. Reduced blood return to the right side of the heart leading to lower blood pressure
4. Increased pulmonary vascular resistance and reduced blood delivery to the left side of the heart

117. A client with a pulmonary embolism is experiencing chest pain and apprehension. What is the priority intervention by the nurse?
1. Administering analgesics
2. Using guided imagery
3. Positioning the client on his left side
4. Providing emotional support

Always know the whys of a condition, especially the most common ones, like this one.

118. A client with a pulmonary embolism is scheduled to have an umbrella filter placed in the vena cava. The nurse determines that teaching has been effective when the client states:
1. "The filter prevents further clot formation."
2. "The filter collects clots so they don't go to the lung."
3. "The filter breaks up clots into insignificantly small pieces."
4. "The filter contains anticoagulants that are slowly released, dissolving any clots."

115. 3. The goal of oxygen therapy for a client with a pulmonary embolism is to have a Pao_2 greater than 60 mm Hg on an Fio_2 of 40% or less. The normal range of the $Paco_2$ is 35 to 45 mm Hg. In the absence of other pathologic states, it should reach normal levels before the Pao_2 does on room air because carbon dioxide crosses the alveolar-capillary membrane with greater ease.
CN: Physiological integrity; CNS: Reduction of risk potential; CL: Analysis

116. 4. Blood meets resistance and can't perfuse the pulmonary vasculature because of the embolism. Pulmonary vascular resistance is increased, which reduces the amount of blood returned to the left side of the heart, lowers the cardiac output of the heart, and reduces blood pressure, sometimes significantly.
CN: Physiological integrity; CNS: Physiological adaptation; CL Application

117. 1. Once the pulmonary embolism has been diagnosed and the amount of hypoxia determined, chest pain and the accompanying apprehension can be treated with analgesics as long as respiratory status isn't compromised. Using guided imagery and providing emotional support can be used as alternatives. Positioning the client on his left side when a pulmonary embolism is suspected may prevent a clot that has extended through the capillaries and into the pulmonary veins from breaking off and traveling through the heart into the arterial circulation, leading to a massive stroke.
CN: Physiological integrity; CNS: Physiological adaptation; CL: Application

118. 3. The umbrella filter is placed in a client at high risk for the formation of more clots that could potentially become pulmonary emboli. The filter breaks the clots into small pieces that won't significantly occlude the pulmonary vasculature. The filter doesn't prevent further clot formation and doesn't release anticoagulants. The filter doesn't collect the clots, because if it did, it would have to be emptied periodically, causing the client to require surgery in the future.
CN: Physiological integrity; CNS: Physiological adaptation; CL: Application

119. The nurse is providing preoperative teaching for a client with a pulmonary embolism scheduled for an embolectomy. The most appropriate information for the nurse to give the patient is:
1. "It is done to remove an embolism in the lower extremity."
2. "It sucks an embolism out of the lung by bronchoscopy."
3. "It surgically removes the embolism source in the pelvis."
4. "It surgically removes the embolism in the pulmonary vasculature."

120. Nursing management of a client with a pulmonary embolism will primarily focus on which action?
1. Assessing oxygenation status
2. Monitoring the oxygen delivery device
3. Monitoring for other sources of clots
4. Determining whether the client requires another ventilation-perfusion ($\dot{V}/\dot{Q}$) scan

You're doing great! Keep going!

121. The nurse is obtaining a pulse oximetry reading on a client. The nurse is aware that analysis of the results will provide information regarding:
1. amount of carbon dioxide in the blood.
2. amount of oxygen in the blood.
3. percentage of hemoglobin carrying oxygen.
4. respiratory rate.

122. A client is admitted to the hospital with shortness of breath. The physician orders a stat hemoglobin and hematocrit level to be drawn. The client is questioning why he needs to have blood drawn when he is having trouble breathing. What is the best response by the nurse?
1. "Hemoglobin has no effect on oxygenation."
2. "More hemoglobin reduces the client's respiratory rate."
3. "Low hemoglobin levels cause reduced oxygen-carrying capacity."
4. "Low hemoglobin levels cause increased oxygen-carrying capacity."

119. 4. If the pulmonary embolism is large and doesn't respond to treatment, surgical removal may be necessary to restore perfusion to the area of the lung. This is rarely done because of the associated high mortality risk. It's impossible to remove a pulmonary embolism through bronchoscopy because the defect isn't in the bronchial tree. A thrombectomy can be performed at other sources of clot, but when a pulmonary embolism has already occurred, it would have little effect on oxygenation.
CN: Physiological integrity; CNS: Physiological adaptation; CL: Analysis

120. 1. Nursing management of a client with a pulmonary embolism focuses on assessing oxygenation status and ensuring that treatment is adequate. If the client's status begins to deteriorate, it's the nurse's responsibility to contact the physician and attempt to improve oxygenation. Ensuring that the oxygen delivery device is working properly and monitoring for other clot sources are other nursing responsibilities, but they aren't the focus of care. The physician would determine if the client required another $\dot{V}/\dot{Q}$ scan.
CN: Physiological integrity; CNS: Reduction of risk potential; CL: Application

121. 3. Pulse oximetry determines the percentage of hemoglobin carrying oxygen. This doesn't ensure that the oxygen being carried through the bloodstream is actually being taken up by the tissue. Pulse oximetry doesn't provide information about the amount of carbon dioxide or oxygen in the blood or the client's respiratory rate.
CN: Physiological integrity; CNS: Physiological adaptation; CL: Application

122. 3. Hemoglobin carries oxygen to all tissues in the body. If the hemoglobin level is low, the amount of oxygen-carrying capacity is also low. More hemoglobin will increase oxygen-carrying capacity and thus increase the total amount of oxygen available in the blood. If the client has been tachypneic during exertion, or even at rest, because oxygen demand is higher than the available oxygen content, then an increase in hemoglobin may decrease the respiratory rate to normal levels.
CN: Physiological integrity; CNS: Reduction of risk potential; CL: Application

123. A client has been intubated and placed on a ventilator with positive end-expiratory pressure (PEEP). The nurse anticipates that the primary function of PEEP will be to:
1. provide more oxygen to the client.
2. open up bronchioles and allow oxygen to get in the lungs.
3. open up collapsed alveoli and help keep them open.
4. add pressure to the lung tissue, which improves gaseous exchange.

124. The nurse is reviewing a client's chest X-ray report that states that there are bilateral areas of collapsed alveoli in the bases. The nurse initiated coughing and deep breathing exercises, reinforced the use of the incentive spirometer, and encouraged the client to ambulate in the halls at least twice a day. The nurse implemented these interventions into the plan of care based on what knowledge?
1. Alveoli need oxygen to live.
2. Alveoli have no effect on oxygenation.
3. Collapsed alveoli increase oxygen demand.
4. Gaseous exchange occurs in the alveolar membrane.

125. A hospitalized client is experiencing hypoxia. The physician orders continuous positive airway pressure (CPAP) per face mask. The family is concerned and questions the nurse as to why the client needs the mask. What is the most appropriate response by the nurse?
1. "The mask is providing 100% oxygen to the client."
2. "The mask is providing continuous air that the client can breathe."
3. "The mask is providing pressurized oxygen so the client can breathe more easily."
4. "The mask is providing pressurized oxygen at the end of expiration to open collapsed alveoli."

126. A client is being treated with bilevel positive airway pressure (BiPAP). The nurse anticipates that the use of BiPAP will:
1. provide 100% oxygen at both inspiration and expiration.
2. provide pressurized oxygen so the client can breathe more easily.
3. provide pressurized oxygen at the end of expiration to open collapsed alveoli.
4. provide both continuous positive airway pressure (CPAP) and positive end-expiratory pressure (PEEP) to provide optimal oxygenation and ventilation.

Take a deep breath.

123. 3. PEEP delivers positive pressure to the lung at the end of expiration. This helps open collapsed alveoli and helps them stay open so gas exchange can occur in these newly opened alveoli, improving oxygenation. The bronchioles don't participate in gas exchange except to act as a conduit for inspired and expired air. The walls are rigid enough that they generally don't collapse. PEEP doesn't directly add pressure to the lung tissue or provide more oxygen to the client.
CN: Physiological integrity; CNS: Physiological adaptation; CL: Application

124. 4. Gaseous exchange occurs in the alveolar membrane, so if the alveoli collapse, no exchange occurs. Collapsed alveoli receive oxygen, as well as other nutrients, from the bloodstream. Collapsed alveoli have no effect on oxygen demand, although by decreasing the surface area available for gas exchange, they decrease oxygenation of the blood.
CN: Physiological integrity; CNS: Physiological adaptation; CL: Application

125. 3. The mask provides pressurized oxygen continuously through both inspiration and expiration. The mask can be set to deliver any amount of oxygen needed. By providing a client with pressurized oxygen, the client has less resistance to overcome in taking in his next breath, making it easier to breathe. Pressurized oxygen delivered at the end of expiration is positive end-expiratory pressure, not CPAP.
CN: Physiological integrity; CNS: Physiological adaptation; CL: Application

126. 4. BiPAP delivers both CPAP and PEEP. It provides the differing pressures throughout the respiratory cycle, attempting to optimize a client's oxygenation and ventilation. It's used in an effort to avoid intubation for mechanical ventilation. Inspiratory and expiratory pressures are set separately to optimize the client's ventilatory status, and the fraction of inspired oxygen is adjusted to optimize oxygenation. The second choice describes only the CPAP component of BiPAP, and the third choice describes the PEEP component.
CN: Physiological integrity; CNS: Physiological adaptation; CL: Application

127. The nurse is caring for a client with a pleural effusion. The client asks, "What is a pleural effusion?" What is the most appropriate response from the nurse?
1. "It is the collapse of alveoli."
2. "It is the collapse of a bronchiole."
3. "It is the fluid in the alveolar space."
4. "It is the accumulation of fluid between the linings of the pleural space."

Can you see I'm not at my best?

128. The client has developed a pleural effusion. The nurse anticipates that the most appropriate intervention would be?
1. Inserting a chest tube
2. Performing thoracentesis
3. Performing paracentesis
4. Allowing the pleural effusion to drain by itself

I bet you were voted most likely to pick the most likely choice.

129. An 18-year-old client who was involved in a motor vehicle accident is admitted to the hospital with a diagnosis of pneumothorax. A chest tube was inserted and attached to a chest drainage system. The nurse notes bubbling in the water seal chamber and determines further assessment is required. The nurse is aware the bubbling is <u>most likely</u> the result of:
1. air leaks.
2. adequate suction.
3. inadequate suction.
4. kinked chest tubes.

127. 4. Pleural fluid normally seeps continually into the pleural space from the capillaries lining the parietal pleura and is reabsorbed by the visceral pleural capillaries and lymphatics. Any condition that interferes with either the secretion or drainage of this fluid will lead to a pleural effusion. The collapse of alveoli or a bronchiole has no particular name. Fluid within the alveolar space can be caused by heart failure or adult respiratory distress syndrome.
CN: Physiological integrity; CNS: Physiological adaptation; CL: Application

128. 2. Thoracentesis is used to remove excess pleural fluid and restore proper lung status. The fluid is then analyzed to determine if it's transudative or exudative. Transudates are substances that have passed through a membrane and usually occur in low protein states. Exudates are substances that have escaped from blood vessels. They contain an accumulation of cells and have a high specific gravity and a high lactate dehydrogenase level. Exudates usually occur in response to a malignancy, infection, or inflammatory process. A chest tube is rarely necessary because the amount of fluid typically isn't large enough to warrant such a measure. Paracentesis is the removal of fluid from the abdomen. Pleural effusions can't drain by themselves.
CN: Physiological integrity; CNS: Physiological adaptation; CL: Application

129. 1. Bubbling in the water seal chamber of a chest drainage system stems from an air leak. In pneumothorax, an air leak can occur as air is pulled from the pleural space. Bubbling doesn't normally occur with either adequate or inadequate suction. A kinked chest tube can stop the suction and any preexisting bubbling in the water seal chamber.
CN: Physiological integrity; CNS: Reduction of risk potential; CL: Application

130. A comatose client requires a nasopharyngeal airway for suctioning. After the airway is inserted, he gags and coughs. The priority intervention by the nurse would be?
1. Remove the airway and insert a shorter one.
2. Reposition the airway.
3. Leave the airway in place until the client gets used to it.
4. Remove the airway and attempt suctioning without it.

131. The nurse is teaching the family of an older adult client who requires long-term ventilator therapy how to suction the client. The client has a tracheostomy in place and requires frequent suctioning. The nurse determines teaching was effective when the family is observed:
1. using intermittent suction while advancing the catheter.
2. using continuous suction for no longer than 10 seconds while withdrawing the catheter.
3. using continuous suction for no longer than 20 seconds while withdrawing the catheter.
4. using continuous suction while advancing the catheter.

132. A client's arterial blood gas (ABG) analysis reveals a pH of 7.18, $Paco_2$ of 73 mm Hg, Pao_2 of 77 mm Hg, and HCO_3^- of 24 mEq/L. The nurse interprets these values as indicating what?
1. Metabolic acidosis
2. Respiratory alkalosis
3. Metabolic alkalosis
4. Respiratory acidosis

133. A 67-year-old client is in respiratory distress after being admitted with an exacerbation of chronic obstructive pulmonary disease. To promote <u>optimal</u> lung expansion, the nurse should position the client:
1. prone.
2. semi-Fowler's.
3. reverse Trendelenburg's.
4. supine.

It's time to take action with this client. What's first?

What position will promote my expansion?

130. 1. If the client gags or coughs after nasopharyngeal airway placement, the tube may be too long. The nurse should remove it and insert a shorter one. Simply repositioning the airway won't solve the problem. The client won't get used to the tube because it's the wrong size. Suctioning without a nasopharyngeal airway causes trauma to the natural airway.
CN: Physiological integrity; CNS: Reduction of risk potential; CL: Application

131. 2. To prevent hypoxia, continuous suctioning shouldn't last more than 10 seconds at a time during catheter withdrawal. Suction shouldn't be applied while the catheter is being advanced.
CN: Physiological integrity; CNS: Reduction of risk potential; CL: Application

132. 4. Normal ABG values include a pH of 7.35 to 7.45; $Paco_2$ of 35 to 45 mm Hg; Pao_2 of 75 to 100 mm Hg; and HCO_3^- of 22 to 26 mEq/L. This client has a below-normal pH, an elevated $Paco_2$, and normal HCO_3^-, indicating respiratory acidosis. With metabolic acidosis, pH and HCO_3^- are low and $Paco_2$ is normal. In respiratory alkalosis, pH is elevated and $Paco_2$ is low. In metabolic alkalosis, both pH and HCO_3^- are elevated.
CN: Physiological integrity; CNS: Reduction of risk potential; CL: Analysis

133. 2. Semi-Fowler's position (with the head of the bed elevated 30 degrees) promotes optimal lung expansion. A prone position (lying on the abdomen) improves oxygenation in a client with acute respiratory distress syndrome who's receiving mechanical ventilation by recruiting new alveoli in the posterior region of the lung. Reverse Trendelenburg's position (in which the entire bed is raised to a 45-degree angle) may improve lung expansion but is less effective than semi-Fowler's position. Supine positioning (lying flat on the back) doesn't aid lung expansion.
CN: Physiological integrity; CNS: Reduction of risk potential; CL: Application

134. A client is admitted to the hospital with dehydration and pneumonia. Upon admission to the unit, the nurse notes the I.V. has infiltrated. What is the <u>most appropriate</u> action by the nurse?
1. Stop the infusion, remove the I.V. catheter, and restart the infusion in another site.
2. Remove the I.V. catheter and apply a cool compress to the site.
3. Apply moist heat to the site.
4. Gently massage the site.

I've been infiltrated. What's the nurse's most appropriate action?

135. The nurse is preparing to administer an intradermal injection of 5 tuberculin units/0.1 ml of tuberculin purified protein derivative to a client with a suspected case of tuberculosis. What is the most appropriate needle for the nurse to select?
1. ⅝″ to ½″ 25G to 27G needle
2. 1″ to 3″ 20G to 25G needle
3. ½″ to ⅜″ 26G or 27G needle
4. 1″ 20G needle

136. After a right lower lobectomy for lung cancer, a client returns to her room with a chest tube in place. The nurse formulates a care plan with a primary nursing diagnosis of impaired gas exchange related to lung surgery. The nurse determines the outcome has been met when:
1. the client sits upright, leaning slightly forward.
2. the client requests pain medication as needed.
3. the client maintains a pulse oximetry level above 93%.
4. the client is pain free.

What outcome are we headed toward?

134. 1. Immediately after discovering an I.V. infiltration, the nurse should stop the infusion, remove the I.V. catheter, restart the infusion in another site, and apply a warm compress to the infiltrated site. A cool compress doesn't promote fluid absorption. Moist heat shouldn't be applied until the infusion is stopped, the catheter is removed, and another catheter is inserted at a different site. Massaging the site is likely to cause pain and isn't effective in treating an infiltration.

CN: Physiological integrity; CNS: Pharmacological and parenteral therapies; CL: Application

135. 3. Intradermal injections like those used in tuberculin skin tests are administered in small volumes (usually 0.5 ml or less) into the outer skin layers to produce a local effect. A tuberculin syringe with a ½″ to ⅜″ 26G or 27G needle should be inserted about ⅛″ below the epidermis. A ⅝″ to ½″ 25G to 27G needle is appropriate for a subcutaneous injection; a 1″ to 3″ 20G to 25G needle, for an I.M. injection; and a 1″ 20G needle, for an I.V. bolus injection.

CN: Physiological integrity; CNS: Pharmacological and parenteral therapies; CL: Application

136. 3. A pulse oximetry level above 93% and a normal respiratory rate demonstrate probable lung expansion and normal chest tube functioning. Sitting upright and leaning slightly forward suggest that the client has impaired gas exchange because this position increases lung expansion. Requesting pain medication as needed and remaining pain free are expected outcomes associated with a nursing diagnosis of acute pain.

CN: Physiological integrity; CNS: Physiological adaptation; CL: Analysis

137. A client is involved in a motor vehicle accident. Upon admission to the emergency department, he has a heart rate of 130 beats/minute, shallow respirations at a rate of 32 breaths/minute, and a blood pressure of 90/60 mm Hg. Breath sounds are diminished on the right side, and paradoxical chest-wall movement appears on the right side. A chest X-ray reveals a right pneumothorax with multiple rib fractures. The nurse anticipates that this client will have a diagnosis of:
1. tension pneumothorax.
2. flail chest.
3. ruptured diaphragm.
4. massive hemothorax.

138. A healthy client comes to the clinic for a routine examination. When auscultating his lower lung lobes, the nurse should expect to hear which type of breath sounds?
1. Bronchial
2. Tracheal
3. Vesicular
4. Bronchovesicular

I'm listening.

139. A 76-year-old client is admitted for elective knee surgery. Physical examination reveals shallow respirations but no signs of respiratory distress. The nurse determines that this assessment finding indicates:
1. increased elastic recoil of the lungs.
2. increased number of functional capillaries in the alveoli.
3. decreased residual volume.
4. decreased vital capacity.

137. 2. Multiple rib fractures and paradoxical chest-wall movement confirm a diagnosis of flail chest. Tension pneumothorax causes severe respiratory distress, hypotension, diminished breath sounds over the affected area, hyperresonance, distended neck veins, eventual tracheal shift, and, possibly, paradoxical chest-wall movement on the injured side. A ruptured diaphragm leads to hyperresonance on percussion, hypotension, dyspnea, dysphagia, and shifting of heart and bowel sounds in the lower to middle chest. A massive hemothorax produces signs of shock (such as tachycardia and hypotension), dullness on percussion on the injured side, decreased breath sounds on the injured side, respiratory distress, and, possibly, mediastinal shift.

CN: Physiological integrity; CNS: Physiological adaptation; CL: Analysis

138. 3. Vesicular breath sounds are soft, low-pitched sounds normally heard over the lower lobes of the lung. They're prolonged on inhalation and shortened on exhalation. Bronchial breath sounds are loud, high-pitched sounds normally heard next to the trachea; discontinuous, they're loudest during exhalation. Tracheal breath sounds are harsh, discontinuous sounds heard over the trachea during inhalation or exhalation. Bronchovesicular breath sounds are medium-pitched, continuous sounds that occur during inhalation or exhalation and are best heard over the upper third of the sternum and between the scapulae.

CN: Health promotion and maintenance; CNS: None; CL: Application

139. 4. Reduction in vital capacity is a normal physiological change in the older adult. Other normal physiological changes include decreased elastic recoil of the lungs, fewer functional capillaries in the alveoli, and an increase in residual volume.

CN: Health promotion and maintenance; CNS: None; CL: Application

140. A 79-year-old client is admitted with pneumonia. What is the priority nursing diagnosis?
1. Acute pain related to lung expansion secondary to lung infection
2. Risk for imbalanced fluid volume related to increased insensible fluid losses secondary to fever
3. Anxiety related to dyspnea and chest pain
4. Ineffective airway clearance related to retained secretions

What's effective when it comes to exercise and asthma medication?

141. An asthmatic client is being discharged with a prescription for cromolyn (Intal inhaler). The nurse determines teaching was effective when the client makes which statement?
1. "I should use my inhaler no more than 1 hour before I exercise."
2. "I should use my inhaler whenever I feel an asthma attack coming on."
3. "I should stop taking steroids if I need a dose of my inhaler."
4. "I should avoid gargling and rinsing my mouth after using my inhaler."

142. The nurse is preparing to instruct a client on obtaining a sputum analysis. The nurse determines teaching was effective when the client states:
1. "Fluids will be restricted the night before the test."
2. "I will be asked to take several deep abdominal breaths and then to take one more breath, bend forward, and cough into the provided sterile container."
3. "If a bronchoscopy is required for specimen collection, I will have no oral intake for 12 hours before the procedure."
4. "After bronchoscopy, I will receive a drink of water."

140. 4. Pneumonia is an acute infection of the lung parenchyma. The inflammatory reaction may cause an outpouring of exudate into the alveolar spaces, leading to ineffective airway clearance related to retained secretions. Pneumonia also can cause acute pain related to lung expansion and anxiety related to dyspnea and chest pain. However, these diagnoses take lower priority than ineffective airway clearance. Fever associated with pneumonia places the client at risk for imbalanced fluid volume—but this diagnosis also doesn't take priority.
CN: Physiological integrity; CNS: Physiological adaptation; CL: Analysis

141. 1. The client should verbalize the need to use the inhaler no more than 1 hour before exercise when indicated for exercise-induced asthma. Cromolyn is contraindicated during an acute asthma attack. A client who is taking steroids should continue to take them during cromolyn therapy, if appropriate. Gargling and rinsing the mouth after cromolyn administration can reduce mouth dryness.
CN: Physiological integrity; CNS: Pharmacological and parenteral therapies; CL: Analysis

142. 2. If the specimen will be collected by expectoration, the client should be instructed to take several deep abdominal breaths; when he's ready to cough, he should take one more deep abdominal breath, bend forward, and cough into the provided sterile container. He should be instructed to drink plenty of fluids the night before the test. If the specimen will be collected during bronchoscopy, the client should fast for 6 hours before the procedure. After bronchoscopy, he's observed for possible complications. He can have liquids when his gag reflex returns.
CN: Physiological integrity; CNS: Reduction of risk potential; CL: Application

143. A 57-year-old client is admitted with acute bronchitis. During the admission interview, he tells the nurse he's allergic to bananas. The nurse is aware that the client may also be allergic to:
1. iodine-containing drugs.
2. cephalosporins.
3. penicillins.
4. latex.

An allergy to bananas can cause which other allergy?

143. **4.** Clients who are allergic to certain cross-reactive foods—including apricots, avocados, bananas, cherries, chestnuts, grapes, kiwis, passion fruit, peaches, and tomatoes—may also be allergic to latex. When exposed to latex, they may have an allergic response similar to the one these foods produce. Clients with allergies to shellfish may be allergic to iodine-containing drugs. Hypersensitivity reactions to cephalosporins are more common in clients with penicillin allergy. There's no link between food allergies and penicillin.
CN: Physiological integrity; CNS: Reduction of risk potential; CL: Application

144. The care plan for a 42-year-old client with deep vein thrombosis (DVT) includes monitoring the client for complications. The nurse determines that the client is at <u>highest</u> risk to develop:
1. pulmonary embolism.
2. pneumothorax.
3. pulmonary edema.
4. pneumonia.

144. **1.** The most common etiology of pulmonary embolism is thromboembolism from a distant site, particularly from deep veins of the legs and pelvis (90% to 95%). Moreover, the immobilization used to treat DVT is an additional clinical risk factor for pulmonary embolism. Pneumothorax and pulmonary edema aren't complications of DVT. Although immobility also places the client at risk for pneumonia, the risk isn't as great for this client.
CN: Physiological integrity; CNS: Reduction of risk potential; CL: Application

No sweat! You're doing great!

145. A 20-year-old client with cystic fibrosis is being discharged with a high-frequency chest wall oscillating vest. Which statement by the client indicates that the nurse's teaching about the vest has been effective?
1. "I'll wear the vest for 5 minutes each time a treatment is due."
2. "I'll lie down to use the vest."
3. "I'll require help in applying the vest."
4. "I can be in any position to use the vest."

145. **4.** The vest system doesn't require special positioning or breathing to be effective. In most cases, treatments last 15 to 20 minutes and clients can manage therapy without any assistance.
CN: Safe, effective care environment; CNS: Safety and infection control; CL: Analysis

146. The nurse is preparing to obtain an arterial blood gas (ABG) sample on a client. Which action should the nurse take <u>first</u>?
1. Perform Allen's test.
2. Place a rolled towel under the client's wrist.
3. Clean the puncture site with an alcohol or povidone-iodine pad.
4. Palpate the artery with the index and middle fingers of one hand.

> Question 146 asks for the first action.

146. 1. First, perform Allen's test to assess circulation. Next, wash your hands, put on gloves, and place a rolled towel under the client's wrist for support. Then locate the artery and palpate it for a strong pulse. Next, clean the puncture site with an alcohol or povidone-iodine pad. Then palpate the artery with the index and middle fingers of one hand while holding the syringe over the puncture site with the other hand. Holding the needle bevel at a 30- to 45-degree angle, puncture the skin and arterial wall in one smooth motion, watch for blood backflow in the syringe, and fill it to the 5-ml mark. After collecting the sample, press a gauze pad over the puncture site for at least 5 minutes.
CN: Physiological integrity; CNS: Reduction of risk potential; CL: Application

147. A client tells the nurse that he has lost his appetite after receiving radiation treatment for lung cancer. The most appropriate response by the nurse is:
1. "Drink plenty of fluids."
2. "Eat hot meats with spices to improve the taste."
3. "Limit activities immediately before and after meals."
4. "Consume food high in calories."

147. 4. The client should consume high-calorie foods whenever he can eat, to help compensate for the times when he can't eat. Consuming large amounts of fluids creates a feeling of fullness, which can limit food intake. Hot meats tend to cause taste aversions during radiation therapy. Activity increases the appetite.
CN: Physiological integrity; CNS: Physiological adaptation; CL: Application

148. Three days after an abdominal aortic aneurysm repair, a client develops a pulmonary embolus. What is the <u>priority</u> nursing diagnosis?
1. Ineffective peripheral tissue perfusion
2. Impaired physical mobility
3. Ineffective airway clearance
4. Risk for aspiration

148. 1. Pulmonary embolus occurs when a thrombus lodges in a branch of the pulmonary artery, partially or totally occluding it. The lung is adequately ventilated but can't be perfused, resulting in ineffective peripheral tissue perfusion. Although impaired physical mobility is an appropriate nursing diagnosis for this client, it doesn't take priority over ineffective peripheral tissue perfusion. A pulmonary embolus doesn't increase secretions, so ineffective airway clearance isn't an appropriate diagnosis. It also doesn't place the client at risk for aspiration.
CN: Physiological integrity; CNS: Physiological adaptation; CL: Analysis

149. After experiencing an anxiety attack, a client comes to the emergency department complaining of dizziness and light-headedness. Arterial blood gas (ABG) analysis reveals a pH of 7.62, $Paco_2$ of 22 mm Hg, Pao_2 of 96 mm Hg, and HCO_3^- of 24 mEq/L. What is the most appropriate action by the nurse?
1. Do nothing; these ABG values are normal.
2. Encourage the client to breathe into a paper bag.
3. Notify the physician and prepare to give sodium bicarbonate.
4. Notify the physician and prepare to give supplemental oxygen.

150. A nurse teaches a group of police officers about the spread of tuberculosis (TB). Which statement by an officer indicates that the nurse's teaching has been effective?
1. "I could get TB by being in close proximity for a brief time with someone who has the disease."
2. "I could get TB if I inhale infected droplets when an infected individual coughs."
3. "I could get TB if I search the home of someone infected with TB."
4. "I could get TB if I come in contact with blood from an infected person."

151. A client receives midazolam, 2 mg I.V., as sedation before bronchoscopy. Five minutes after he receives the drug, his respiratory rate drops to 4 breaths/minute. What is the most appropriate action by the nurse?
1. Administer naloxone.
2. Administer protamine sulfate.
3. Administer phentolamine (Regitine).
4. Administer flumazenil (Romazicon).

Don't let me in—every breath I take can cause infection.

149. 2. These ABG values reveal respiratory alkalosis (elevated pH, decreased $Paco_2$, and normal Pao_2 and HCO_3^- levels), so the client is most likely hyperventilating from anxiety. Breathing into a paper bag can stop the hyperventilation by increasing carbon dioxide. Doing nothing or giving sodium bicarbonate could worsen respiratory alkalosis. The client has a normal Pao_2 level and doesn't need supplemental oxygen.

CN: Physiological integrity; CNS: Reduction of risk potential; CL: Analysis

150. 2. TB infection typically occurs from inhaling infected droplets after a person with TB coughs. Transmission usually requires close, frequent, prolonged contact. Human immunodeficiency virus—not TB—is spread through contact with an infected person's blood.

CN: Safe, effective care environment; CNS: Safety and infection control; CL: Analysis

151. 4. Flumazenil reverses the effects of benzodiazepines such as midazolam. Naloxone is used to reverse opioids, such as morphine. Protamine sulfate reverses the effects of heparin. Phentolamine is injected into the tissues to reverse the damaging effects of a dopamine infiltration.

CN: Physiological integrity; CNS: Pharmacological and parenteral therapies; CL: Application

152. The nurse notes an order to change the client's chest drainage system from suction to gravity drainage. What is the most appropriate action by the nurse?
1. Detach the tubing from the suction port to provide a vent.
2. Clamp the client's drainage tube.
3. Question the physician's order.
4. Turn off the suction source and leave the tubing connected.

153. A client with cancer develops pleural effusion. During chest auscultation, what would the nurse expect to hear?
1. Crackles
2. Rhonchi
3. Diminished breath sounds
4. Wheezes

What? I can barely hear you.

154. An employee-health nurse who performs annual purified protein derivative (PPD) testing instructs the staff that their results must be read within _____ after administration.
1. 6 to 12 hours
2. 12 to 24 hours
3. 24 to 48 hours
4. 48 to 72 hours

155. A 79-year-old client suddenly develops pulmonary edema. The physician prescribes furosemide (Lasix), 40 mg I.V., and use of a nonrebreather mask. The nurse is aware that the mask will provide the client an oxygen concentration of:
1. 60% to 80%.
2. 80% to 100%.
3. 36%.
4. 44%.

152. 1. When the suction source is turned off, the drainage system should be opened to the atmosphere so intrapleural air can escape from the system. Detaching the tubing from the suction port provides an exit vent for the air and, thus, reduces the risk of tension pneumothorax. Clamping the tube may cause air to accumulate in the pleural space, rapidly leading to tension pneumothorax. There's no need to question the order.

CN: Physiological integrity; CNS: Physiological adaptation; CL: Application

153. 3. In pleural effusion, fluid accumulates in the pleural space, impairing transmission of normal breath sounds. Because of the acoustic mismatch, breath sounds are diminished. Crackles (short explosive or popping sounds) commonly accompany atelectasis, interstitial fibrosis, and left-sided heart failure. Rhonchi (low-pitched sounds with a snoring quality) suggest secretions in the large airways. Wheezes (high-pitched, hissing sounds) result from narrowed airways, as in asthma, chronic obstructive pulmonary disease, or bronchitis.

CN: Physiological integrity; CNS: Physiological adaptation; CL: Application

154. 4. To ensure accurate results, a PPD test must be read 48 to 72 hours after administration.

CN: Health promotion and maintenance; CNS: None; CL: Application

155. 2. The nonrebreather mask delivers oxygen concentrations of 80% to 100%. It's reserved for emergency situations. A partial rebreather mask delivers concentrations of 60% to 80%. A nasal cannula delivers oxygen at flow rates of 1 to 6 L/minute. A flow rate of 4 L/minute delivers an oxygen concentration of 36%; a rate of 6 L/minute delivers an oxygen concentration of 44%.

CN: Physiological integrity; CNS: Physiological adaptation; CL: Application

156. A nurse attending a neighborhood picnic notices an adult at the bottom of the swimming pool. She immediately calls for help and tries to rescue the person. When she pulls him out, he's unresponsive and breathless. What is the most appropriate action by the nurse?
1. Open the airway and begin rescue breathing immediately.
2. Immobilize the cervical spine.
3. Start chest compressions.
4. Perform abdominal thrust.

157. A client with newly diagnosed chronic obstructive pulmonary disease (COPD) presents to the clinic for a routine examination. The nurse teaches him strategies for preventing airway irritation and infection. The nurse determines teaching was successful when the client states:
1. "I should avoid enclosed, crowded areas during the summer."
2. "I'm glad I only need to get the flu vaccine."
3. "I should use products with aerosol sprays."
4. "I should avoid using powders."

158. A client with a suspected pulmonary embolus is brought to the emergency department complaining of shortness of breath and pleuritic chest pain. Select all of the assessment data that would support this diagnosis.
1. Low-grade fever
2. Thick green sputum
3. Bradycardia
4. Frothy sputum
5. Tachycardia
6. Blood-tinged sputum

159. A physician prescribes an I.V. solution to infuse at a rate of 125 ml/hour for a client. How many liters of solution will the client receive during an 8-hour shift? Record your answer using a whole number.

_____ liters

You've done a great job!

156. **1.** The nurse should open the airway and begin rescue breathing immediately—while still in the water, if possible. Immobilizing the cervical spine won't provide the needed oxygenation. Chest compressions should be delivered only if circulation is absent. Performing abdominal thrust in an attempt to remove water from the lungs would delay the start of rescue breathing.
CN: Physiological integrity; CNS: Physiological adaptation; CL: Application

157. **4.** A client with COPD should verbalize the need to avoid exposure to powders, dusts, and smoke from cigarettes, pipes, and cigars. He should stay indoors when the humidity, temperature, and pollen counts are high; avoid enclosed, crowded areas during cold and flu season; and avoid aerosol sprays. He should obtain immunizations against pneumococcal pneumonia as well as influenza.
CN: Health promotion and maintenance; CNS: None; CL: Analysis

158. **1, 5, and 6.** In addition to pleuritic chest pain and dyspnea, a client with a pulmonary embolus may also present with a low-grade fever, tachycardia, and blood-tinged sputum. Thick green sputum would indicate infection, and frothy sputum would indicate pulmonary edema. A client with a pulmonary embolus is tachycardic (to compensate for decreased oxygen supply), not bradycardic.
CN: Physiological integrity; CNS: Physiological adaptation; CL: Application

159. 1. The client is to receive the solution at an infusion rate of 125 ml/hour. 125 ml × 8 hours = 1,000 ml, the total volume in milliliters the client will receive during an 8-hour shift. Convert milliliters to liters by dividing by 1,000. The total volume in liters of normal saline solution that the client will receive in 8 hours is 1 L.
CN: Physiological integrity; CNS: Pharmacological and parenteral therapies; CL: Application

160. A nurse begins the shift by reading the following shift report note on a client.

Miscellaneous reports
H.B. age 78
Hyperventilating, RR 36
bpm. C/O dizziness,
shortness of breath,
tingling in hands and feet,
weakness. Anxious.
ABG: pH 7.48
$Paco_2$: 33 mm Hg

The nurse interprets these results as indicating which of the following?
1. Metabolic acidosis
2. Acute respiratory failure
3. Respiratory alkalosis
4. Anxiety reaction

161. The nurse is assessing a client's respiratory pattern. Which graphic illustrates Cheyne-Stokes respirations?

1.
2.
3.
4.

160. 3. Respiratory alkalosis is defined by a pH greater than 7.45 and $Paco_2$ less than 35 mm Hg, and generally is associated with deep, rapid breathing; light-headedness or dizziness; circumoral and peripheral paresthesia; and carpopedal spasms, twitching, and muscle weakness as it progresses. Metabolic acidosis is defined as a pH less than 7.3, $Paco_2$ less than or equal to 34 mm Hg depending on respiratory compensation, and HCO_3^- less than 22 mEq/L and is caused by an underlying nonrespiratory disorder. Acute respiratory failure is characterized by a pH less than 3, $Paco_2$ greater than 50 mm Hg, and markedly diminished oxygen saturation levels. Although the client may be anxious, the abnormal blood gas levels and corresponding symptoms indicate that treatment of respiratory alkalosis is the primary concern and may greatly reduce the client's anxiety level.

CN: Physiological integrity; CNS: Physiological adaptation; CL: Analysis

161. 2. In Cheyne-Stokes respirations, breaths gradually become faster and deeper than normal and then slower during a 30- to 170-second period with intermittent periods of apnea (option 2). Option 1 shows tachypnea—shallow breathing with an increased respiratory rate. Option 3 shows Kussmaul's breathing—rapid, deep breathing without pauses. Option 4 shows bradypnea—regular breathing at a decreased rate.

CN: Physiological integrity; CNS: Reduction of risk potential; CL: Analysis

Stroke, subdural hematoma, laminectomy—they're all here in this comprehensive chapter on neurosensory disorders in adults. I've got a sixth sense, you're going to do great!

Chapter 6
Neurosensory disorders

1. A nurse is caring for a client with homonymous hemianopia. The most important information for the nurse to teach the client is:
1. scan the environment on the affected side.
2. use memory aids such as pictures.
3. plan for adequate rest.
4. make simple, nonrisky decisions.

A stroke can change my normal views.

2. A client who has recently experienced a thromboembolic stroke is now stable and will begin warfarin. The client asks the nurse why the treatment was ordered. The best response by the nurse would be?
1. It is the standard of care for preventing all types of recurrent ischemic stroke.
2. It is more effective than antithrombotic therapy in the presence of a thrombus.
3. It is cheap and readily available, with few side effects.
4. The stroke was due to atrial fibrillation.

3. A 65-year-old client with a stroke in evolution has been ordered alteplase (t-PA). The order is for 0.9 mg/kg over 1 hour. The client weighs 110 lb. What is the total dose in milligrams (mg) the client will receive?
1. 35 mg
2. 40 mg
3. 45 mg
4. 50 mg

Practice makes calculations easy.

4. A client is admitted to the unit with a thromboembolic stroke. Which medication does the nurse anticipate will be started by day 2?
1. Acetaminophen
2. Aspirin
3. Alteplase (t-PA)
4. Methylprednisolone

1. 1. Scanning the environment can help a client with visual field deficit (also known as a homonymous hemianopia) overcome this loss in visual perception and prevent injury. Clients with other types of perceptual or memory loss may benefit from answers 2 to 4, but these interventions are not specific for a visual field loss.
CN: Physiological integrity; CNS: Physiological adaptation; CL: Application

2. 4. Warfarin is the standard of care for a client with stroke due to atrial fibrillation. Anticoagulation therapy is not routinely indicated in most other types of thromboembolic stroke. Because of increased bleeding risk and required outclient monitoring, careful consideration is needed when ordering warfarin.
CN: Pharmacological and parenteral therapies; CNS: Reduction of risk potential; CL: Application

3. 3. First, convert lbs to kg (2.2 lb = 1 kg) by dividing 110 lb by 2.2 kg to obtain 50 kg. Next, multiply 0.9 mg by 50 kg to obtain a dose of 45 mg. The total dose the client will receive is 45 mg.
CN: Physiological integrity; CNS: Pharmacological and parenteral therapies; CL: Application

4. 2. Aspirin, not acetaminophen, interferes with platelet aggregation and other antiplatelets and is used in the treatment of thromboembolic stroke. Alteplase is only approved by the U.S. Food and Drug Administration (FDA) for treatment within 3 hours of stroke onset. Methylprednisolone is a steroid with mild anticoagulant properties and is not indicated in acute stroke.
CN: Physiological integrity; CNS: Pharmacological and parenteral therapies; CL: Application

CN: Client needs category   CNS: Client needs subcategory   CL: Cognitive level

5. The nurse is caring for a client experiencing a stroke in evolution. What is the priority nursing intervention?
1. Thicken all dietary liquids.
2. Restrict dietary and parenteral fluids.
3. Place the client on oxygen.
4. Have tracheal suction available at all times.

6. The nurse has been caring for a client who experienced a stroke and is now asking for food. What is the most important assessment for the nurse to observe before feeding the client?
1. The gag reflex has returned to normal.
2. Speech has returned to normal.
3. Cranial nerves III, IV, and VI are intact.
4. The client swallows water without coughing.

7. The nurse is caring for a client who had a stroke and now has residual dysphagia. What is the most appropriate diet for this client?
1. Clear liquid
2. Full liquid
3. Mechanical soft
4. Thickened liquid

8. While assessing a 77-year-old client who had a thromboembolic right stroke, the nurse notes the left arm is swollen. The nurse suspects this finding may indicate:
1. elbow contracture secondary to spasticity.
2. loss of muscle contraction decreasing venous return.
3. deep vein thrombosis (DVT) due to immobility of the ipsilateral side.
4. hypoalbuminemia due to protein escaping from an inflamed glomerulus.

9. A client has experienced a brain stem infarction. It is most important for the nurse to assess the client for:
1. aphasia.
2. bradypnea.
3. contralateral hemiplegia.
4. numbness and tingling to the face or arm.

Think: How well can a dysphagic client chew and swallow?

Where is the hemiplegia in a right stroke?

5. 4. Because of a potential loss of the gag reflex and potential altered level of consciousness, tracheal suction should be available at all times. Thickening dietary liquids isn't done until the gag reflex returns or the stroke has evolved and the deficit can be assessed. Unless heart failure is present, restricting fluids isn't indicated. Oxygen is based on saturation results, and oxygen alone will not maintain an airway.
CN: Physiological integrity; CNS: Reduction of risk potential; CL: Application

6. 4. Some stroke clients may have a decreased gag reflex and still be safe to eat. A standardized bedside swallow screen should be performed that includes a water test. Even if the client passes a swallow test, additional precautions may be required. Speech alone is not adequate for assessing the ability to swallow. Cranial nerves III, IV, and VI evaluate eye movement and accommodation.
CN: Physiological integrity; CNS: Reduction of risk potential; CL: Application

7. 4. Thickened liquids are easiest to form into a bolus and swallow. Clear and full liquids are amorphous and can't easily form a bolus. A mechanical soft diet may be too hard to chew and too dry to swallow when dysphagia is present.
CN: Physiological integrity; CNS: Reduction of risk potential; CL: Application

8. 2. In clients with hemiplegia or hemiparesis, loss of muscle contraction decreases venous return and may cause swelling of the affected extremity. Contractures, or bony calcifications, may occur with a stroke but don't appear with swelling. DVT may develop in clients with a stroke but is more likely to occur in the lower extremities. A stroke isn't linked to protein loss.
CN: Physiological integrity; CNS: Physiological adaptation; CL: Analysis

9. 2. The brain stem contains the medulla and the vital cardiac, vasomotor, and respiratory centers. A brain stem infarction leads to vital sign changes such as bradypnea. Contralateral hemiplegia and numbness or tingling in the face or arm may occur, depending on the level of injury. Aphasia is associated with lobar strokes in the cerebral hemispheres.
CN: Physiological integrity; CNS: Physiological adaptation; CL: Application

10. A 40-year-old client asks the nurse what may increase the risk for the development of cataracts. The best response by the nurse is:
1. history of frequent streptococcal throat infections.
2. maternal exposure to rubella during pregnancy.
3. increased intraocular pressure.
4. prolonged use of steroidal anti-inflammatory agents.

11. In caring for a client after cataract surgery, the nurse should notify a physician if the client has which of the following conditions?
1. Blurred vision
2. Eye pain
3. Glare
4. Itching

12. The nurse assesses clear fluid draining from the nose of a client who experienced head trauma 3 hours ago. The nurse suspects this finding may indicate:
1. basilar skull fracture.
2. cerebral concussion.
3. cerebral palsy.
4. sinus infection.

13. A 19-year-old client with a mild concussion is discharged from the emergency department. Before discharge, he complains of a headache. When offered acetaminophen, his mother tells the nurse she would like her son to have something stronger. The most appropriate response by the nurse is:
1. "Your son had a mild concussion; acetaminophen is strong enough."
2. "Aspirin is avoided because of the danger of Reye's syndrome in children or young adults."
3. "Opioids are avoided after a head injury because they may hide a worsening condition."
4. "Stronger medications may lead to vomiting, which increases the intracranial pressure (ICP)."

14. A client is admitted to the hospital with a subarachnoid hemorrhage and is now experiencing severe headache, nuchal rigidity, and projectile vomiting. The nurse is aware that a lumbar puncture (LP) would be contraindicated if:
1. vomiting continues.
2. intracranial pressure (ICP) is increased.
3. the client needs mechanical ventilation.
4. blood is anticipated in the cerebrospinal fluid (CSF).

Which symptom would spell danger?

You're doing a great job!

10. 4. Prolonged use of steroidal anti-inflammatory agents is a risk factor for cataracts. The other risk factors don't contribute to the development of cataracts.
CN: Health promotion and maintenance; CNS: None; CL: Application

11. 2. Pain shouldn't be present after cataract surgery. Pain may be an indication of hyphema, or clouding in the anterior chamber, and infection. The other symptoms might be present.
CN: Physiological integrity; CNS: Physiological adaptation; CL: Application

12. 1. Clear fluid draining from the ear or nose of a client may mean a cerebrospinal fluid leak, which is common in basilar skull fractures. Concussion is associated with a brief loss of consciousness, cerebral palsy is associated with nonprogressive paralysis present since birth, and sinus infection is associated with facial pain and pressure with or without nasal drainage.
CN: Physiological integrity; CNS: Physiological adaptation; CL: Analysis

13. 3. Opioids may mask changes in the level of consciousness (LOC) that indicate increased ICP and shouldn't be given as a first-line drug. Saying acetaminophen is strong enough ignores the mother's question and therefore isn't appropriate. Aspirin is contraindicated in conditions that may have bleeding, such as trauma, and for children or young adults with viral illnesses due to the danger of Reye's syndrome. Stronger medications may not necessarily lead to vomiting but will sedate the client, thereby masking changes in his LOC.
CN: Physiological integrity; CNS: Reduction of risk potential; CL: Application

14. 2. Sudden removal of CSF results in pressures lower in the lumbar area than the brain and favors herniation of the brain; therefore, LP is contraindicated with increased ICP. An LP is performed if brain imaging is negative or inconclusive in the presence of subarachnoid hemorrhage-type symptoms. Vomiting may be caused by reasons other than increased ICP; therefore, LP isn't strictly contraindicated. An LP may be performed on clients requiring mechanical ventilation. Blood in the CSF is diagnostic for subarachnoid hemorrhage.
CN: Physiological integrity; CNS: Physiological adaptation; CL: Application

15. The nurse is assessing a client with head trauma. The nurse notes a urine output of 300 ml/hour, dry skin, dry mucous membranes, and a high serum sodium. The <u>most important</u> intervention for the nurse to implement would be?
1. Evaluate urine specific gravity.
2. Anticipate treatment for renal failure.
3. Provide emollients to the skin to prevent breakdown.
4. Slow the I.V. fluids and notify the physician.

What do you think is the most important intervention?

15. 1. Urine output of 300 ml/hour in the presence of high serum sodium may indicate diabetes insipidus (DI), which is a failure of the pituitary to produce antidiuretic hormone. Sodium disturbances are common in clients with brain injury because of the major role that the central nervous system plays in the regulation of sodium and water homeostasis. Other related conditions include cerebral salt wasting and syndrome of inappropriate antidiuretic hormone. These conditions are respectively differentiated from DI by low serum sodium and low urine output. DI may occur with increased intracranial pressure and head trauma; the nurse evaluates for low urine specific gravity, increased serum osmolarity, and dehydration. There's no evidence that the client is experiencing renal failure. Providing emollients to prevent skin breakdown is important but doesn't need to be performed immediately. Slowing the rate of I.V. fluid would contribute to dehydration when polyuria is present.
CN: Physiological integrity; CNS: Physiological adaptation; CL: Analysis

16. Stool softeners would be given to a client prior to repair of a cerebral aneurysm for which reason?
1. To stimulate the bowel due to loss of nerve innervation
2. To prevent straining, which increases intracranial pressure (ICP)
3. To prevent reflex bradycardia from the Valsalva maneuver
4. To prevent constipation when osmotic diuretics are used

16. 2. Straining when having a bowel movement, sneezing, coughing, and suctioning may lead to increased ICP and should be avoided when potential increased ICP exists. Stool softeners don't stimulate the bowel and aren't used in combination with osmotic diuretics. Although the Valsalva maneuver may lead to an increase in intracranial pressure, the given rationale doesn't apply to this client.
CN: Physiological integrity; CNS: Reduction of risk potential; CL: Application

Knowing why you do something can help prevent errors.

17. A client with a subdural hematoma becomes restless and confused, with dilation of the ipsilateral pupil. The physician orders mannitol for which reason?
1. To reduce intraocular pressure
2. To prevent acute tubular necrosis
3. To promote osmotic diuresis to decrease intracranial pressure (ICP)
4. To draw water into the vascular system to increase blood pressure

17. 3. Mannitol promotes osmotic diuresis by increasing the pressure gradient, drawing fluid from intracellular to intravascular spaces. Although mannitol is used for all the reasons described, the reduction of ICP in this client is of greatest concern.
CN: Physiological integrity; CNS: Pharmacological and parenteral therapies; CL: Application

18. A client with a subdural hematoma was given mannitol to decrease intracranial pressure (ICP). The nurse assesses the client and determines that the mannitol was effective when:
1. urine output increases.
2. pupils are 8 mm and nonreactive.
3. systolic blood pressure remains at 150 mm Hg.
4. blood urea nitrogen (BUN) and creatinine levels return to normal.

19. The nurse is evaluating an arterial blood gas result from a client with a subdural hematoma and notes the $Paco_2$ is 30 mm Hg. How does the nurse interpret this result?
1. Potentially appropriate, as modest lowering of carbon dioxide (CO_2) may reduce intracranial pressure (ICP)
2. Emergent; the client requires aggressive hyperventilation and is poorly oxygenated
3. No response; this is a normal $Paco_2$ value
4. Significant; the client has alveolar hypoventilation

20. The nurse is concerned that a client recovering from a brain injury may be developing foot drop and contractures. What is the best intervention for the nurse to implement?
1. High-topped sneakers or other type of foot-up ankle support
2. Low-dose heparin therapy
3. Physical therapy consultation
4. Sequential compression device

21. The nurse is aware that a client who had a transsphenoidal hypophysectomy should be observed carefully for hemorrhage. The nurse is most concerned when the client displays:
1. bloody drainage from the ears.
2. frequent swallowing.
3. guaiac-positive stools.
4. hematuria.

22. The nurse is preparing to administer vasopressin to a client who has undergone a hypophysectomy. What is the purpose of the medication?
1. To treat growth failure
2. To prevent syndrome of inappropriate antidiuretic hormone (SIADH)
3. To reduce cerebral edema and lower intracranial pressure
4. To replace antidiuretic hormone (ADH) normally secreted from the pituitary

Remember to assess.

Hmmm, does health insurance cover high-topped sneakers?

18. 1. Mannitol promotes osmotic diuresis by increasing the pressure gradient in the renal tubules, thus increasing urine output. Fixed and dilated pupils are symptoms of increased ICP or cranial nerve damage. No information is given about abnormal BUN and creatinine levels or that mannitol is being given for renal dysfunction or blood pressure maintenance.
CN: Physiological integrity; CNS: Physiological adaptation; CL: Application

19. 1. A normal $Paco_2$ value is 35 to 45 mm Hg. CO_2 has vasodilating properties; therefore, slight lowering of $Paco_2$ through hyperventilation in some clients may lower ICP caused by dilated cerebral vessels. Previously, hyperventilation was used routinely to maximally reduce $Paco_2$; however, no studies have shown this to improve outcome in these clients and may actually be harmful. Consequently, hyperventilation should be used only for short periods when immediate control of ICP is necessary Oxygenation is evaluated through Pao_2 and oxygen saturation. Alveolar hypoventilation would be reflected in an increased $Paco_2$.
CN: Physiological integrity; CNS: Physiological adaptation; CL: Analysis

20. 1. High-topped sneakers or other types of foot-up ankle support devices are used to prevent foot drop and contractures in neurological clients. Low-dose heparin therapy and sequential compression boots will prevent deep vein thrombosis. Although a physical therapy consultation is important to initiate other interventions to prevent foot drop, a nurse may use high-topped sneakers independently.
CN: Physiological integrity; CNS: Basic care and comfort; CL: Application

21. 2. Frequent swallowing after brain surgery may indicate fluid or blood leaking from the sinuses into the oropharynx. Blood or fluid draining from the ear may indicate a basilar skull fracture, guaiac-positive stools indicate GI bleeding, and hematuria may result from cystitis or other urological complications.
CN: Physiological integrity; CNS: Physiological adaptation; CL: Analysis

22. 4. After hypophysectomy, or removal of the pituitary gland, the body can't synthesize ADH. Somatropin or growth hormone, not vasopressin, is used to treat growth failure. SIADH results from excessive ADH secretion.
CN: Physiological integrity; CNS: Pharmacological and parenteral therapies; CL: Application

23. A client's intracranial pressure (ICP) is fluctuating between 20 and 25 mm Hg. Which of the following nursing interventions is the <u>most appropriate</u>?
1. Ensure that the mean arterial pressure (MAP) is less than 90 mm Hg.
2. Lower the head of the bed to less than 15 degrees.
3. Encourage visitation.
4. Reassess the client's ABCs (airway, breathing, and circulation).

Be familiar with normal values to recognize an abnormal result.

24. A nurse is planning care for a 33-year-old client who has just undergone a L4–L5 laminectomy. What is the most important intervention for the nurse to include?
1. Encourage the client to be out of bed the first postoperative day.
2. Maximize bracing while in bed.
3. Limit movement in bed and reposition only when necessary.
4. Use a soft mattress.

25. A client who has undergone a lumbar laminectomy is experiencing frequent voiding of small amounts of urine. The nurse suspects the client may have developed which condition?
1. Diabetes insipidus
2. Diabetic ketoacidosis
3. Urine retention
4. Urinary tract infection (UTI)

Assessment is a primary responsibility of the nurse.

26. When assessing a client with a spinal injury at C6, the nurse would expect the highest level of functioning to include which of the following?
1. Significant loss of function at the biceps and shoulders
2. Potential loss of function at the shoulders and biceps and complete loss of function at the wrists and hands
3. Limited wrist control and complete loss of hand function
4. Lack of dexterity in the hands and fingers but allows for limited use of arms

27. A nurse is preparing a client with suspected lumbar herniated nucleus pulposus for magnetic resonance imaging (MRI). The most important action by the nurse would be?
1. Question the client about allergy to iodine.
2. Mark distal pulses on the foot in indelible ink.
3. Teach the client relaxation techniques.
4. Tell the client he may be asked to cough or pant to clear the dye.

23. 4. The nurse should always reassess the client's ABCs when the ICP is elevated (normal is between 0 and 15 mm Hg). MAP should be maintained at or above 90 mm Hg. The head of the bed should be elevated between 15 and 30 degrees to facilitate venous drainage. External stimulation, such as visitors, should be limited as it may increase ICP.
CN: Physiological integrity; CNS: Physiological adaptation; CL: Application

24. 1. In most cases, clients should be out of bed the first postoperative day. Frequent repositioning, use of a chair-like brace for the lower back when out of bed, and a firm mattress will help minimize complications.
CN: Physiological integrity; CNS: Reduction of risk potential; CL: Application

25. 3. Swelling or pressure on the peripheral nerves controlling micturition, anesthesia, or use of an indwelling urinary catheter may lead to urine retention with frequent overflow of small amounts of urine. Diabetes insipidus and diabetic ketoacidosis are shown by polyuria. UTI may be shown by dysuria and frequent voiding of small amounts of urine but would be less likely in this situation.
CN: Physiological integrity; CNS: Basic care and comfort; CL: Analysis

26. 3. A lesion at C6 will result in limited wrist control and complete loss of hand function. Significant loss of function of the biceps and shoulder occurs with C4, with potential loss of function at the shoulder and biceps occurring at C5. An injury at C7 and T1 results in dexterity in the hands and finger but allows for limited use of arms.
CN: Physiological integrity; CNS: Physiological adaptation; CL: Application

27. 3. The MRI scanner is a narrow tube that contains a magnet. The client lies on a platform and is placed in the tube. Some clients may become claustrophobic during the test; teaching relaxation techniques may help to alleviate this. Radiopaque dyes, used in myelography and cardiac catheterization, are usually iodine based and may cause a reaction in those clients who are allergic. No dyes are used in MRI. During cardiac catheterization, a client is asked to cough or pant to clear the dye, and before cardiac catheterization or arteriogram, the nurse marks pedal pulses in ink.
CN: Physiological integrity; CNS: Reduction of risk potential; CL: Application

28. A client is scheduled for chemonucleolysis with chymopapain to relieve the pain of a herniated disk. Which factor should be assessed before the procedure?
1. Allergy to meat tenderizers
2. Allergy to shellfish
3. Ability to lie flat during the procedure
4. Ability to perform full range of motion (ROM) on the affected side

29. When prioritizing care, which client should the nurse assess <u>first</u>?
1. A 17-year-old client 24 hours postappendectomy
2. A 33-year-old client with a recent diagnosis of Guillain-Barré syndrome
3. A 50-year-old client 3 days postmyocardial infarction
4. A 50-year-old client with diverticulitis

Here's a test-taking hint: prioritize.

30. A client is newly diagnosed with myasthenia gravis. The nurse is teaching the client about the cause of this disease. The nurse determines that teaching has been effective when the client states:
1. a postviral illness characterized by ascending paralysis.
2. loss of the myelin sheath surrounding peripheral nerves.
3. inability of basal ganglia to produce sufficient dopamine.
4. destruction of acetylcholine receptors causing muscle weakness.

31. A client has just begun exhibiting signs of myasthenia gravis. The nurse anticipates assessment of the client to include:
1. dysphagia.
2. fatigue improving at the end of the day.
3. ptosis.
4. respiratory distress.

Keep your eyes open for clues.

28. 1. Chymopapain, derived from papaya, is an ingredient in meat tenderizers. Sensitivity to this substance may preclude the use of chymopapain. Allergy to shellfish may be a contraindication to tests using iodine-based dyes. The client may be positioned on the side in a "C" position to allow access to the intervertebral area. Full ROM isn't needed for this procedure.
CN: Physiological integrity; CNS: Pharmacological and parenteral therapies; CL: Application

29. 2. Guillain-Barré syndrome is characterized by ascending paralysis and potential respiratory failure. The order of client assessment should follow client priorities, with disorders of airway, breathing, and then circulation. There's no information to suggest the postmyocardial infarction client has an arrhythmia or other complication. There's no evidence to suggest hemorrhage or perforation for the remaining clients as a priority of care.
CN: Safe, effective care environment; CNS: Management of care; CL: Analysis

30. 4. Myasthenia gravis, an autoimmune disorder, is caused by the destruction of acetylcholine receptors. Guillain-Barré syndrome is a postviral illness characterized by ascending paralysis, multiple sclerosis is caused by loss of the myelin sheath, and Parkinson's disease is caused by the inability of basal ganglia to produce sufficient dopamine.
CN: Health promotion and maintenance; CNS: None; CL: Analysis

31. 3. Ptosis and diplopia are early signs of myasthenia gravis; dysphagia and respiratory distress occur later. Symptoms are typically milder in the morning and may be exacerbated by stress or lack of rest.
CN: Health promotion and maintenance; CNS: None; CL: Application

32. One hour after receiving pyridostigmine bromide (Mestinon), a client reports difficulty swallowing and excessive respiratory secretions. The nurse notifies the physician and prepares to administer which medication?
1. Additional pyridostigmine bromide (Mestinon)
2. Atropine
3. Edrophonium (Tensilon)
4. Acyclovir (Zovirax)

32. 2. These symptoms suggest cholinergic crisis or excessive acetylcholinesterase medication, typically appearing 45 to 60 minutes after the last dose of acetylcholinesterase inhibitor. Atropine, an anticholinergic drug, is used to antagonize acetylcholinesterase inhibitors. The other drugs are acetylcholinesterase inhibitors. Edrophonium is used for the diagnosis and pyridostigmine bromide is used for the treatment of myasthenia gravis and would worsen these symptoms. Acyclovir is an antiviral and would not be used to treat these symptoms.
CN: Physiological integrity; CNS: Pharmacological and parenteral therapies; CL: Analysis

33. A client with suspected myasthenia gravis is to undergo a Tensilon test. The client asks if the Tensilon can be used to treat myasthenia gravis. The best response by the nurse is:
1. "It isn't available in an oral form."
2. "With repeated use, immunosuppression may occur."
3. "Dry mouth and abdominal cramps may be intolerable adverse effects."
4. "The short half-life of Tensilon makes it impractical for long-term use."

33. 4. Although Tensilon is not available in an oral form, the duration of action of Tensilon is 1 to 2 minutes, making it impractical for the long-term management of myasthenia gravis. Immunosuppression with repeated use is an adverse effect of steroid administration, a medication used to treat myasthenia gravis. Dry mouth and abdominal cramps are adverse effects of increased acetylcholine in the parasympathetic nervous system.
CN: Physiological integrity; CNS: Pharmacological and parenteral therapies; CL: Application

34. A 20-year-old client with myasthenia gravis will undergo plasmapheresis. Which action describes the purpose of this procedure?
1. Preventing exacerbations during pregnancy
2. Removing T and B lymphocytes that attack acetylcholine receptors
3. Delivering acetylcholinesterase inhibitor directly into the bloodstream
4. Separating and removing acetylcholine receptor antibodies from the blood

34. 4. The purpose of plasmapheresis in myasthenia gravis is to separate and remove circulating acetylcholine receptor antibodies from the blood of clients refractory to the usual therapies or clients in crisis. Although stress, including pregnancy, may precipitate crisis, this isn't the purpose of the procedure. Plasmapheresis doesn't remove T and B lymphocytes, nor does it deliver acetylcholinesterase inhibitor directly into the bloodstream.
CN: Physiological integrity; CNS: Pharmacological and parenteral therapies; CL: Application

35. When assessing a client with glaucoma, a nurse expects which finding?
1. Complaints of double vision
2. Complaints of halos around lights
3. Intraocular pressure of 15 mm Hg
4. Soft globe on palpation

Way to go!

35. 2. Complaint of halos around lights is a common finding in a client with glaucoma. Symptoms of glaucoma don't include double vision but can include loss of peripheral vision or blind spots, reddened sclera, firm globe, decreased accommodation, halos around lights, and occasional eye pain, but clients may be asymptomatic. Normal intraocular pressure is 10 to 21 mm Hg.
CN: Physiological integrity; CNS: Physiological adaptation; CL: Application

CN: Client needs category   CNS: Client needs subcategory   CL: Cognitive level

36. The nurse is teaching a client newly diagnosed with glaucoma about the importance of medication compliance. The nurse determines that teaching has been effective when the client states that noncompliance may result in:
1. diplopia.
2. permanent vision loss.
3. progressive loss of peripheral vision.
4. pupillary constriction.

37. A nurse is preparing to administer pilocarpine 1%, eyedrops to a client. The order reads: Instill 2 gtt both eyes four times a day. What is the correct administration?
1. Two drops of the drug in both eyes four times daily
2. Two drops on the sclera of both eyes two times daily
3. Two drops over the lacrimal duct of both eyes four times daily
4. Two drops of the drug toward the nasal side of each conjunctival sac three times daily

38. A nurse is evaluating a client to determine the extent of Parkinson's disease. The nurse would observe for which symptom?
1. Bulging eyeballs
2. Diminished distal sensation
3. Increased dopamine levels
4. Muscle rigidity

39. A client is admitted with Parkinson's disease. The client's face is expressionless, and the client's speech is monotone. Which of the following observations by the nurse is <u>most accurate</u>?
1. The client is most likely depressed and should be left alone.
2. These are common symptoms of Parkinson's disease that produce an undesired façade of an alert and responsive individual.
3. The client's antipsychotic medication may need to be adjusted.
4. The client probably has dementia.

Don't get all discombobulated, now. Read with accuracy.

36. 2. Without treatment, glaucoma may progress to irreversible blindness. Treatment won't restore visual damage but will halt disease progression. Blurred or foggy vision, not diplopia, is typical in glaucoma. Central vision loss is typical in glaucoma. Miotics, which constrict the pupil, are used in the treatment of glaucoma to permit outflow of the aqueous humor.
CN: Physiological integrity; CNS: Pharmacological and parenteral therapies; CL: Application

37. 1. Medications placed on the nasal side near the lacrimal duct will enter the nose and be ineffective. Eye drops are generally instilled into the lower conjunctival sac, which is accessed by gently pulling down the lower eyelid to form a pocket into which one drop is instilled.
CN: Physiological integrity; CNS: Pharmacological and parenteral therapies; CL: Application

38. 4. Parkinson's disease is characterized by the slowing of voluntary muscle movement, muscular rigidity, and resting tremor. Bulging eyeballs (exophthalmos) occur in Graves' disease. Diminished distal sensation doesn't occur in Parkinson's disease. Dopamine is deficient in this disorder.
CN: Physiological integrity; CNS: Physiological adaptation; CL: Application

39. 2. The nurse should recognize that these are common symptoms of Parkinson's disease. The symptoms do not indicate depression or dementia, although these are common in Parkinson's disease. Antipsychotic medication will often mimic Parkinson's disease extrapyramidal symptoms and is not indicated. Parkinson's disease is caused by degeneration of the substantia nigra in the basal ganglia of the brain, where dopamine is produced and stored. This degeneration results in motor dysfunction, resulting in symptoms such as an expressionless face and monotone speech.
CN: Physiological integrity; CNS: Physiological adaptation; CL: Application

40. Which client would be most at risk for secondary Parkinson's disease caused by pharmacotherapy?
1. A 30-year-old client with schizophrenia taking chlorpromazine (Thorazine)
2. A 50-year-old client taking nitroglycerin tablets for angina
3. A 60-year-old client taking prednisone for chronic obstructive pulmonary disease
4. A 75-year-old client using naproxen for rheumatoid arthritis

41. Which symptom occurs <u>initially</u> in Parkinson's disease?
1. Akinesia
2. Aspiration of food
3. Dementia
4. Pill rolling movements of the hand

42. To evaluate the effectiveness of levodopa-carbidopa (Sinemet), a nurse should assess the client for:
1. improved visual acuity.
2. decreased dyskinesia.
3. reduction in short-term memory.
4. lessened rigidity and tremor.

43. Two days after starting therapy with trihexyphenidyl, a client complains of a dry mouth. What is the most appropriate nursing intervention?
1. Offer the client ice chips and frequent sips of water.
2. Withhold the drug and notify the physician.
3. Change the client's diet to clear liquid until the symptoms subside.
4. Encourage the use of supplemental puddings and shakes to maintain weight.

44. Which antiparkinsonian drug can cause drug tolerance or toxicity if taken for too long at one time?
1. Amantadine (Symmetrel)
2. Levodopa-carbidopa (Sinemet)
3. Pergolide
4. Selegiline (Eldepryl)

Read question 41 carefully to get the correct answer.

40. 1. Phenothiazines such as chlorpromazine deplete dopamine, which may lead to tremor rigidity (extrapyramidal effects). The other drugs don't place the client at a greater risk for developing Parkinson's disease.

CN: Physiological integrity; CNS: Pharmacological and parenteral therapies; CL: Application

41. 4. Early symptoms of Parkinson's disease include coarse resting tremors of the fingers and thumb. Akinesia and aspiration are late signs of Parkinson's disease. Dementia occurs in only 20% of clients with Parkinson's disease.

CN: Health promotion and maintenance; CNS: None; CL: Application

42. 4. Levodopa-carbidopa increases the amount of dopamine in the central nervous system, allowing for more smooth, purposeful movements. The drug doesn't affect visual acuity and should improve dyskinesia and short-term memory.

CN: Physiological integrity; CNS: Pharmacological and parenteral therapies; CL: Application

43. 1. Trihexyphenidyl is an anticholinergic agent that causes blurred vision, dry mouth, constipation, and urine retention. There's no need to withhold the drug unless hypotension or tachyarrhythmia occurs. A clear liquid diet doesn't provide adequate nutrition and may be more difficult to swallow than thickened liquids if dysphagia is present; it isn't indicated at this time. Weight loss may occur with Parkinson's disease; however, the question relates to effects of trihexyphenidyl.

CN: Physiological integrity; CNS: Pharmacological and parenteral therapies; CL: Analysis

44. 2. Long-term therapy with levodopa-carbidopa can result in drug tolerance or toxicity shown by confusion, hallucinations, or decreased drug effectiveness. The other drugs don't require that the client take a drug holiday.

CN: Physiological integrity; CNS: Pharmacological and parenteral therapies; CL: Application

CN: Client needs category   CNS: Client needs subcategory   CL: Cognitive level

45. A young female client has been recently diagnosed with multiple sclerosis (MS) and wants more information on the disease. In teaching the client, which statement by the nurse is <u>most accurate</u>?
1. MS is an autoimmune disease.
2. MS is more common in men than women.
3. MS is characterized by remyelination.
4. MS is an acute and curable disease.

46. A client with multiple sclerosis (MS) is started on 20 mg of glatiramer (Copaxone) subcutaneously daily. Immediately after the injection, the client experiences flushing and chest pain. What is the <u>most appropriate</u> nursing intervention?
1. Call a code.
2. Call the physician to inform him of the client's adverse reaction.
3. Administer oxygen.
4. Monitor the client to see if the symptoms quickly dissipate.

47. A client is experiencing <u>early</u> symptoms of multiple sclerosis (MS). What would the nurse expect to assess?
1. Diplopia
2. Grief
3. Paralysis
4. Dementia

48. The nurse is <u>teaching</u> a client with multiple sclerosis (MS) about ways to avoid exacerbation of the disease. What is the best information for the nurse to include?
1. Patching the affected eye
2. Sleeping 8 hours each night
3. Taking hot baths for relaxation
4. Drinking 1½ to 2 qt (1.5 to 2 L) of fluid daily

49. A client who was diagnosed with multiple sclerosis (MS) asks the nurse if there are any conditions or activities that may exacerbate MS. What is the best response by the nurse?
1. Pregnancy
2. Range-of-motion (ROM) exercises
3. Swimming
4. Urine retention

Close in on the clues.

Client teaching is very important.

45. 1. MS is a chronic autoimmune disease that is more common in women than in men. It is characterized by multiple areas of demyelination and scarring (sclerosis) of the underlying nerve fibers. There are no known cures for MS, although treatment can help promote remissions and prevent exacerbations.
CN: Physiological integrity; CNS: Physiological adaptation; CL: Application

46. 4. Glatiramer helps to decrease the number of relapses in the MS client. Flushing, chest pain, palpitations, anxiety, shortness of breath, and itching occur in some clients following administration of the medication. They typically are transient and self-limiting and don't need specific treatment.
CN: Physiological integrity; CNS: Pharmacological and parenteral therapies; CL: Analysis

47. 1. Early symptoms of MS include slurred speech and diplopia. Grief isn't a clinical manifestation. Paralysis is a late symptom of MS. Although depression and a short attention span may occur, dementia is rarely associated with MS.
CN: Physiological integrity; CNS: Physiological adaptation; CL: Application

48. 2. MS is exacerbated by exposure to stress, fatigue, and heat. Clients should balance activity with rest. Patching the affected eye may result in improvement in vision and balance but won't prevent exacerbation of the disease. Adequate hydration will help prevent urinary tract infections secondary to a neurogenic bladder.
CN: Physiological integrity; CNS: Reduction of risk potential; CL: Application

49. 1. Pregnancy, stress, fatigue, and heat may exacerbate MS. Exercise to maintain ROM is encouraged; swimming is particularly effective due to weightlessness and the cooling of nerves. Urine retention is common due to neurogenic bladder but doesn't lead to the exacerbation of symptoms.
CN: Physiological integrity; CNS: Reduction of risk potential; CL: Application

50. A client with suspected multiple sclerosis (MS) undergoes a lumbar puncture. The nurse understands that the results of the cerebrospinal fluid (CSF) may show:
1. blood or increased red blood cells.
2. elevated white blood cells (WBCs) or pus.
3. increased glucose concentrations.
4. increased protein levels.

51. A nurse observes a client experiencing involuntary, jerking, rhythmic movements of the eyes. The nurse documents this which condition?
1. Diplopia
2. Exophthalmos
3. Nystagmus
4. Oculogyric crisis

52. What is the <u>most important</u> nursing intervention for a client having a tonic-clonic seizure?
1. Maintaining a patent airway
2. Timing the duration of the seizure
3. Noting the origin of seizure activity
4. Inserting a padded tongue blade to prevent the client from biting his tongue

53. A client recalls smelling an unpleasant odor before his seizure. What would the nurse document this as?
1. Atonic seizure
2. Aura
3. Icterus
4. Postictal experience

54. A client with new-onset seizures of unknown cause is started on phenytoin (Dilantin), 750 mg I.V. now and 100 mg by mouth, three times a day. The nurse understands that the I.V. loading dose was given for which reason?
1. To ensure that the drug reaches the cerebrospinal fluid
2. To prevent the need for surgical excision of the epileptic focus
3. To reduce secretions in case another seizure occurs
4. To more quickly attain therapeutic levels

The question said "loading" dose, not "loaded bases."

50. 4. Elevated gamma globulin fraction in CSF without an elevated level in the blood occurs in MS. WBCs or pus indicates infection. Blood may be found with trauma or subarachnoid hemorrhage. Increased glucose concentration is a nonspecific finding indicating infection or subarachnoid hemorrhage.
CN: Physiological integrity; CNS: Physiological adaptation; CL: Analysis

51. 3. Nystagmus refers to jerking movements of the eye. Diplopia means double vision. Exophthalmos refers to bulging eyeballs, as seen in Graves' disease. Oculogyric crisis involves deviation of the eyes.
CN: Health promotion and maintenance; CNS: None; CL: Application

52. 1. The priority during and after a seizure is to maintain a patent airway. Timing the seizure activity and noting the origin of motor dysfunction are done but not first. Nothing should be placed in the client's mouth during a seizure because teeth may be dislodged or the tongue pushed back, further obstructing the airway.
CN: Safe, effective care environment; CNS: Management of care; CL: Application

53. 2. An aura occurs in some clients as a warning before a seizure. The client may experience a certain smell, a vision such as flashing lights, or a sensation. Atonic seizure or drop attack refers to an abrupt loss of muscle tone. Icterus refers to jaundice. Postictal experience occurs after a seizure, during which the client may be confused, somnolent, and fatigued.
CN: Physiological integrity; CNS: Physiological adaptation; CL: Application

54. 4. A loading dose of phenytoin and other drugs is given to reach therapeutic levels more quickly; maintenance dosing follows. A loading dose of phenytoin can be oral or parenteral. Surgical excision of an epileptic focus is considered when seizures aren't controlled with anticonvulsant therapy. Phenytoin doesn't reduce secretions.
CN: Physiological integrity; CNS: Pharmacological and parenteral therapies; CL: Application

55. A client has just started taking phenytoin (Dilantin) and asks the nurse if there are any adverse effects to be aware of. The best response by the nurse is:
1. dry mouth.
2. furry tongue.
3. somnolence.
4. tachycardia.

56. The laboratory has just notified the nurse that a client on the unit has a phenytoin level of 32 mg/dl. The nurse would expect the client to display which symptom(s)?
1. Ataxia and confusion
2. Sodium depletion
3. Tonic-clonic seizure
4. Urinary incontinence

57. The most important intervention for nurse to implement when giving phenytoin (Dilantin) to a client with a nasogastric (NG) tube for feeding is:
1. check the phenytoin level after giving the drug to check for toxicity.
2. elevate the head of the bed before giving phenytoin through the NG tube.
3. give phenytoin 1 hour before or 2 hours after NG tube feedings to ensure absorption.
4. verify proper placement of the NG tube by placing the end of the tube in a glass of water and observing for bubbles.

58. A client asks the nurse if he can drink alcohol while taking phenytoin. What is the <u>best</u> response by the nurse?
1. Alcohol increases phenytoin activity.
2. Alcohol raises the seizure threshold.
3. Alcohol impairs judgment and coordination.
4. Alcohol decreases the effectiveness of phenytoin.

59. When assessing vital signs in a client with a seizure disorder, which measure is used?
1. Checking for a pulse deficit
2. Checking for pulsus paradoxus
3. Taking axillary instead of oral temperatures
4. Checking the blood pressure for an auscultatory gap

Caution! Can you find the clues here?

So, why doesn't alcohol get along with phenytoin?

55. **3.** Adverse effects of phenytoin include sedation, somnolence, gingival hyperplasia, blood dyscrasia, and toxicity. The other symptoms aren't adverse effects of phenytoin.

CN: Physiological integrity; CNS: Pharmacological and parenteral therapies; CL: Application

56. **1.** A level of 32 mg/dl indicates phenytoin toxicity. Symptoms of toxicity include confusion and ataxia. Phenytoin doesn't cause hyponatremia, seizure, or urinary incontinence. Incontinence may occur during or after a seizure.

CN: Physiological integrity; CNS: Pharmacological and parenteral therapies; CL: Analysis

57. **3.** Nutritional supplements and milk interfere with the absorption of phenytoin, decreasing its effectiveness. Phenytoin levels are checked before giving the drug, and the drug is withheld for elevated levels to avoid compounding toxicity. The head of the bed is elevated when giving all drugs or solutions and isn't specific to phenytoin administration. The nurse verifies NG tube placement by checking for stomach contents before giving drugs and feedings.

CN: Physiological integrity; CNS: Pharmacological and parenteral therapies; CL: Application

58. **4.** Alcohol decreases phenytoin activity, diminishing its effectiveness. Although alcohol also reduces the seizure threshold and impairs judgment and coordination, these effects aren't the primary concern.

CN: Physiological integrity; CNS: Pharmacological and parenteral therapies; CL: Application

59. **3.** To reduce the risk of injury, the nurse should take an axillary temperature or use a non-glass thermometer when taking an oral temperature to prevent injury if a seizure occurs. Pulse deficit occurs in an arrhythmia. Pulsus paradoxus may occur with cardiac tamponade. An auscultatory gap occurs in hypertension.

CN: Physiological integrity; CNS: Reduction of risk potential; CL: Application

60. A client in status epilepticus arrives at the emergency department accompanied by a family member. The nurse asks the client's family member if anything may have predisposed the client to this condition. The nurse is most concerned when the family member states that the client:
1. abruptly stopped anticonvulsant therapy.
2. recently traveled by airplane.
3. had exposure to sunlight.
4. recently suffered an upper respiratory infection.

61. A client comes to the emergency department after hitting his head in a motor vehicle collision. He's alert and oriented. Which nursing intervention should be done <u>first</u>?
1. Assess full range of motion (ROM) to determine the extent of injuries.
2. Call for an immediate chest X-ray.
3. Immobilize the client's head and neck.
4. Open the airway with the head-tilt, chin-lift maneuver.

62. A client is admitted with a C6 spinal injury. The nurse anticipates the client most likely has which condition?
1. Aphasia
2. Hemiparesis
3. Paraplegia
4. Quadriplegia

63. Nursing care of a client with damage to the hippocampus, amygdala, and fornix should focus on which of the following?
1. Frequent monitoring of vital signs
2. Coordination
3. Memory and emotion
4. Pain control

64. A 30-year-old client is admitted to the progressive care unit with a C5 fracture from a motorcycle collision. Which assessment would take <u>priority</u>?
1. Bladder distention
2. Neurological deficit
3. Pulse oximetry readings
4. The client's feelings about the injury

First things first.

Let's see, what do all three of these brain areas have in common?

60. 1. Status epilepticus (seizures not responsive to usual therapies) occurs with the abrupt cessation of anticonvulsant drugs or ethanol intake. The other options don't cause status epilepticus.
CN: Physiological integrity; CNS: Pharmacological and parenteral therapies; CL: Analysis

61. 3. All clients with a head injury are treated as if a cervical spine injury is present until X-rays confirm their absence. ROM would be contraindicated at this time. There is no indication the client needs a chest X-ray. The airway doesn't need to be opened since the client appears alert and not in respiratory distress. The head-tilt, chin-lift maneuver wouldn't be used until cervical spine injury is ruled out.
CN: Safe, effective care environment; CNS: Management of care; CL: Application

62. 4. Quadriplegia occurs as a result of cervical spine injuries. Aphasia refers to difficulty expressing or understanding spoken words and is caused by injury to the Broca and or Wernicke areas of the brain. Hemiparesis describes weakness of one side of the body. Paraplegia occurs as a result of injury to the thoracic cord and below.
CN: Physiological integrity; CNS: Physiological adaptation; CL: Application

63. 1. The hippocampus, amygdala, and fornix make up the limbic system, which regulates emotions. The hippocampus and associated structures are also important for short-term memory. Coordination is a function of the cerebellum. The midbrain, pons, medulla oblongata, and reticular formation regulate vital functions.
CN: Safe, effective care environment; CNS: Management of care; CL: Application

64. 3. After a spinal cord injury, ascending cord edema may cause a higher level of injury. The diaphragm is innervated at the level of C4, so assessment of adequate oxygenation and ventilation is necessary. Although the other options are important, observation for respiratory failure is the priority.
CN: Safe, effective care environment; CNS: Management of care; CL: Application

65. While in the emergency department, a client with C8 quadriplegia develops a blood pressure of 80/44 mm Hg, pulse of 48 beats/minute, and respiratory rate of 18 breaths/minute. The nurse suspects which condition?
1. Autonomic dysreflexia
2. Hemorrhagic shock
3. Neurogenic shock
4. Pulmonary embolism

66. A client is admitted with a newly acquired spinal cord injury at the level of T12. He has limited movement of his upper extremities. The nurse anticipates the physician may prescribe which medication?
1. Acetazolamide (Diamox)
2. Furosemide (Lasix)
3. Methylprednisolone (Solu-Medrol)
4. Sodium bicarbonate

Which nursing intervention comes first?

67. A 22-year-old client with quadriplegia is apprehensive and flushed, with a blood pressure of 210/100 mm Hg and heart rate of 50 beats/minute. Which nursing intervention should be done <u>first</u>?
1. Place the client flat in bed.
2. Assess patency of the indwelling urinary catheter.
3. Give one sublingual nitroglycerin tablet.
4. Raise the head of the bed immediately to 90 degrees.

68. A client with paraplegia from a T10 injury is getting ready to transfer to a rehabilitation hospital. When the nurse offers to assist him, the client throws his suitcase on the floor and says, "You don't want to help me." What is the <u>most appropriate</u> response by the nurse?
1. "You know I want to help you. I offered."
2. "I'll pick these things up for you and come back later."
3. "You seem angry today. Going to rehab may be scary."
4. "When you get to rehab, they won't let you behave like this."

Choose the most therapeutic response.

65. 3. Symptoms of neurogenic shock include hypotension, bradycardia, and warm, dry skin due to loss of adrenergic stimulation below the level of the lesion. Hypertension, bradycardia, flushing, and sweating of the skin are seen with autonomic dysreflexia. Hemorrhagic shock presents with anxiety, tachycardia, and hypotension; this wouldn't be suspected without an injury. Pulmonary embolism presents with chest pain, hypotension, hypoxemia, tachycardia, and hemoptysis; this may be a later complication of spinal cord injury due to immobility.
CN: Physiological integrity; CNS: Physiological adaptation; CL: Analysis

66. 3. Spinal cord injuries below T12 do not affect the upper extremities, unless edema of the spinal cord is present. High doses of methylprednisolone are used within 8 hours of spinal cord injury to reduce cord swelling and limit neurological deficit. The other drugs aren't indicated in this circumstance. Acetazolamide and furosemide are both diuretics.
CN: Physiological integrity; CNS: Pharmacological and parenteral therapies; CL: Application

67. 4. Anxiety, flushing above the level of the lesion, piloerection, hypertension, and bradycardia are symptoms of autonomic dysreflexia, typically caused by such noxious stimuli as a full bladder, fecal impaction, or pressure ulcer. Putting the client flat will cause the blood pressure to increase more. The indwelling urinary catheter should be assessed immediately after the head of the bed is raised. Nitroglycerin is given to relieve chest pain and reduce preload; it isn't used for hypertension or dysreflexia.
CN: Safe, effective care environment; CNS: Management of care; CL: Analysis

68. 3. The nurse should always focus on the feelings underlying a particular action. Options 1 and 4 are confrontational. Offering to pick up the client's belongings doesn't deal with the situation and assumes he can't do it alone.
CN: Psychosocial integrity; CNS: None; CL: Application

69. A client with a cervical spine injury is placed in a Minerva body vest. The client is uncomfortable and would like to try a different device. What is the best response by the nurse?
1. The vest protects the neck against excessive motion.
2. The vest will provide for immobilization of the midcervical segments.
3. The vest will provide significant immobilization including lateral flexion.
4. There are other soft-type collars that can be used.

70. A client with a halo vest is being discharged from the hospital. What is the most important information for the nurse to give the client and family?
1. "Don't use the wheelchair while the halo vest is in place."
2. "Clean the pin sites with peroxide."
3. "Keep the wrench that opens the vest attached to the client at all times."
4. "Perform range-of-motion (ROM) exercises to the neck and shoulders four times daily."

71. A client is admitted with intervertebral disk prolapse and now shows new symptoms of loss of bladder control and paralysis of both legs. Which of the following nursing interventions should be the priority?
1. Obtaining an order for a urinary drainage device
2. Notifying the physician immediately
3. Increasing the frequency of vital signs
4. Administering medication to decrease inflammation

72. Which intervention describes an appropriate bladder program for a client in rehabilitation for a recent spinal cord injury?
1. Insert an indwelling urinary catheter.
2. Schedule intermittent catheterization every 2 to 4 hours.
3. Perform a straight catheterization every 8 hours while the client is awake.
4. Perform Credé's maneuver to the lower abdomen before the client voids.

Teaching is second nature to a nurse.

69. 3. The Minerva vest will provide significant immobilization including lateral flexion. Most soft collars do not limit cervical motion but act as a reminder against excessive motion. More rigid devices such as the Philadelphia collar provide reasonable immobilization of the midcervical segments for flexion and extension but not for lateral flexion.
CN: Physiological integrity; CNS: Physiological adaptation; CL: Application

70. 3. The wrench must be attached at all times to remove the vest in case the client needs cardiopulmonary resuscitation. The vest is designed to improve mobility; the client may use a wheelchair. Peroxide, especially full strength, can disrupt the healing process and normal flora. The purpose of the vest is to immobilize the neck; ROM exercises to the neck are prohibited but should be performed to other areas.
CN: Physiological integrity; CNS: Reduction of risk potential; CL: Application

71. 2. Cauda equina syndrome occurs when there is compression on the nerve roots. It affects areas below the level of these nerve roots. It is an emergency that requires surgical intervention; if not treated, it may lead to permanent loss of bladder and bowel control and paralysis of the legs. Inserting a urinary drainage device, increasing the frequency of vital signs, and administering anti-inflammatory medication may be interventions that are needed; however, they are not the priority.
CN: Safe, effective care environment; CNS: Management of care; CL: Analysis

72. 2. Intermittent catheterization should begin every 2 to 4 hours early in treatment. When residual volume is less than 400 ml, the schedule may advance to every 4 to 6 hours. Indwelling catheters may predispose the client to infection and are removed as soon as possible. Credé's maneuver is applied after voiding to enhance bladder emptying.
CN: Physiological integrity; CNS: Basic care and comfort; CL: Application

73. A 46-year-old client with breast cancer complains of back pain and difficulty moving her legs. Which nursing intervention is the <u>most appropriate</u>?
1. Notify the physician.
2. Position the client on her side, and prop her with a foam wedge.
3. Ask the physician for a physical therapy consultation.
4. Give acetaminophen, and reassure the client that the pain will disappear soon.

74. A client was admitted to the hospital because of a transient ischemic attack secondary to atrial fibrillation. The nurse anticipates the physician will prescribe which medication?
1. Digoxin (Lanoxin)
2. Diltiazem (Cardizem)
3. Warfarin (Coumadin)
4. Quinidine gluconate

75. A client is diagnosed with Ménière's disease. Which nursing diagnosis would take priority for this client?
1. Risk for ineffective cerebral tissue perfusion
2. Imbalanced nutrition: More than body requirements
3. Impaired social interaction
4. Risk for injury

76. A client has just undergone a stapedectomy. How should the nurse position the client?
1. On the affected side
2. On the unaffected side
3. Prone
4. In Sims' position

77. The nurse is assessing a client with Ménière's disease. The nurse anticipates the assessment will identify which symptom?
1. Epistaxis
2. Facial pain
3. Ptosis
4. Tinnitus

78. What is the <u>most important</u> intervention for an occupational nurse to implement when treating a client with a foreign body protruding from the eye?
1. Irrigate the eye with sterile saline.
2. Assess visual acuity with a Snellen chart.
3. Remove the foreign body with sterile forceps.
4. Patch both eyes until seen by the ophthalmologist.

You're doing great! I knew you would!

This question is making my head spin.

73. 1. Symptoms of back pain and neurological deficits may be symptoms of metastasis. The physician should be notified. Repositioning the client, physical therapy, or giving acetaminophen may help the pain but may delay evaluation and treatment.
CN: Health promotion and maintenance; CNS: None; CL: Analysis

74. 3. Atrial fibrillation may lead to the formation of mural thrombi, which may embolize to the brain. Coumadin will prevent further clot formation and prevent clot enlargement. The other drugs are used in the treatment and control of atrial fibrillation but won't affect clot formation.
CN: Physiological integrity; CNS: Pharmacological and parenteral therapies; CL: Application

75. 4. Ménière's disease results in dizziness, so the client should be protected from falling. Ménière's disease doesn't alter cerebral tissue perfusion or directly affect nutrition. Although hearing loss may occur, causing impaired social interaction, this isn't a priority.
CN: Safe, effective care environment; CNS: Management of care; CL: Application

76. 2. The client should be positioned with the operative ear up, on the unaffected side. Although Sims' position is a side-lying position, it doesn't consider which side is best for after ear surgery.
CN: Physiological integrity; CNS: Physiological adaptation; CL: Application

77. 4. Tinnitus, dizziness, and vertigo occur in Ménière's disease. Epistaxis may occur with a variety of blood dyscrasias or local lesions. Facial pain may occur with trigeminal neuralgia. Ptosis occurs with a variety of conditions, including myasthenia gravis.
CN: Physiological integrity; CNS: Physiological adaptation; CL: Application

78. 4. One or both eyes may be patched to prevent pain with extraocular movement or accommodation. Chemicals or small foreign bodies may be irrigated. Assessment of visual acuity isn't a priority, although it may be done after treatment. Protruding objects aren't removed by the nurse because the vitreous body may rupture.
CN: Safe, effective care environment; CNS: Management of care; CL: Application

79. A client with severe eye pain requests a prescription for the topical anesthetic the ophthalmologist instilled. The nurse explains that these drugs should not be used on an ongoing basis for which reason?
1. They are a way for pathogens to enter.
2. They cause dependence and rebound pain.
3. Damage could occur to the cornea due to lack of sensation.
4. The resulting blurred vision from mydriasis makes activity hazardous.

80. An 86-year-old client admitted to the hospital with chest pain is hearing impaired. Which method should be used when assessing the client?
1. Obtain an ear wick.
2. Shout into the better ear.
3. Lower your voice pitch while facing the client.
4. Ask the family to go home and get the client's hearing aid.

81. A client is scheduled for magnetic resonance imaging (MRI) of the head. Which area is essential to assess before the procedure?
1. Food or drink intake within the past 8 hours
2. Prostheses or a pacemaker
3. The presence of carotid artery disease
4. Voiding before the procedure

82. The nurse is providing teaching for a client being discharged with a prescription reading 1 gtt to both ears three times a day. Which of the following statements by the nurse would be most accurate?
1. Place one drop into each ear three times daily.
2. Place one drop into each ear two times daily.
3. Place one drop into each ear four times daily.
4. Place three drops into both ears once daily.

79. 3. Corneal damage may occur with the prolonged use of topical anesthetics. If the bottle isn't touched to the eye or lashes, the entry of pathogens should be limited. Dependence and rebound don't occur from topical anesthetics. Anesthetics don't cause mydriasis.
CN: Physiological integrity; CNS: Reduction of risk potential; CL: Application

80. 3. Hearing loss in an elderly client typically involves the upper ranges; lowering the pitch of your voice and facing the client is essential for the client to use other means of understanding, such as lip reading, mood, and so on. An ear wick is used to allow medications to enter the ear canal. Shouting is typically in the upper ranges and could cause anxiety to an already anxious client. Alternative means of communication such as writing may also be used to assess chest pain while waiting for the family to bring the hearing aid from home.
CN: Physiological integrity; CNS: Basic care and comfort; CL: Application

81. 2. Strong magnetic waves may dislodge metal in the client's body, causing tissue injury. Although the client may be told to restrict food for 8 hours, particularly if contrast is used, metal is an absolute contraindication for this procedure. Voiding beforehand would make the client more comfortable and better able to remain still during the procedure but isn't essential for the test. Having carotid artery disease isn't a contraindication to having an MRI.
CN: Safe, effective care environment; CNS: Safety and infection control; CL: Application

82. 1. The nurse would instruct the client that t.i.d. means three times daily and that gtt means drop.
CN: Physiological integrity; CNS: Pharmacological and parenteral therapies; CL: Application

83. To properly instill eardrops in a 28-year-old client with otitis externa, which method is correct?
1. Pulling the pinna down and back
2. Pulling the pinna up and back
3. Pulling the tragus up and back
4. Separating the palpebral fissures with a clean gauze pad

84. Which instruction given to a client after cataract surgery is incorrect?
1. "Avoid bending and straining."
2. "Avoid high-sodium foods to reduce intraocular pressure."
3. "Don't drive or sleep on the affected side."
4. "Don't use makeup on the affected eye."

85. Which sign or symptom of increased intracranial pressure (ICP) after head trauma would appear first?
1. Bradycardia
2. Large amounts of very dilute urine
3. Restlessness and confusion
4. Widened pulse pressure

86. A client admitted to the emergency department for head trauma is diagnosed with an epidural hematoma. Which of the following would most likely cause this condition?
1. Laceration of the middle meningeal artery
2. Rupture of the carotid artery
3. Trauma to the middle cerebral artery
4. Venous bleeding from the arachnoid space

87. A 23-year-old client has been hit on the head with a baseball bat. The nurse notes clear fluid draining from his ears and nose. Which nursing intervention should be done first?
1. Position the client flat in bed.
2. Notify the physician of potential cerebrospinal fluid leak
3. Suction the nose to maintain airway patency.
4. Insert nasal and ear packing with sterile gauze.

Check out the in before correct.

The words "most likely" help you choose the correct answer.

83. **2.** To straighten the ear canal of an adult, the pinna is pulled up and back. Options 1 and 3 aren't appropriate methods for preparing the ear to receive eardrops. The palpebral fissures are in the eye.
CN: Physiological integrity; CNS: Pharmacological and parenteral therapies; CL: Application

84. **2.** After cataract surgery, there's no need to restrict sodium. Using makeup, bending, straining, lifting, vomiting, and sleeping on the affected side may increase intraocular pressure and put strain on the sutures.
CN: Physiological integrity; CNS: Reduction of risk potential; CL: Application

85. **3.** The earliest symptom of increased ICP is a change in mental status. Bradycardia, widened pulse pressure, and bradypnea occur later. The client may void large amounts of very dilute urine if there's damage to the posterior pituitary.
CN: Physiological integrity; CNS: Physiological adaptation; CL: Analysis

86. **1.** Epidural hematoma or extradural hematoma is usually caused by laceration of the middle meningeal artery. Trauma to the middle cerebral artery would be associated with intracerebral hemorrhage or stroke. Venous bleeding from the arachnoid space is usually observed with subdural hematoma.
CN: Physiological integrity; CNS: Physiological adaptation; CL: Application

87. **2.** Clear or light pink–tinged liquid from the nose (rhinorrhea) or ear (otorrhea) in the presence of a head injury may be leakage of cerebral spinal fluid due to a basilar skull fracture. The physician should be notified and precautions to prevent infection taken. Placing the client flat in bed may increase intracranial pressure and promote pulmonary aspiration. The nose wouldn't be suctioned because of the risk of suctioning brain tissue through the sinuses. Nothing is inserted into the ears or nose of a client with a skull fracture because of the risk of infection.
CN: Physiological integrity; CNS: Physiological adaptation; CL: Analysis

88. A child is admitted to the emergency department with a recent head injury. In educating the client and family, the nurse discusses concerns regarding the lucid period. This is best described as:
1. an interval when the client's speech is garbled.
2. an interval when the client is alert but can't recall recent events.
3. an interval when the client is oriented but then becomes somnolent.
4. an interval when the client has a "warning" symptom, such as an odor or visual disturbance.

89. When teaching the family of a client with C4 quadriplegia how to suction his tracheostomy, the nurse includes which instruction?
1. Suction for 10 to 15 seconds at a time.
2. Regulate the suction machine to −300 cm suction.
3. Apply suction to the catheter during insertion only.
4. Pass the suction catheter into the opening of the tracheostomy tube ¾″ to 1¼″ (2 to 3 cm).

90. Which condition is the leading risk factor for hemorrhagic stroke?
1. Coronary artery disease
2. Diabetes
3. Hypertension
4. Recent viral infection

91. An 86-year-old client with a stroke in evolution and a history of coronary artery disease is brought to the medical-surgical floor. His medications include isosorbide (Isordil). Which condition is a concern?
1. Dehydration
2. Hypocarbia
3. Hypotension
4. Tube feeding

Teaching the family is as important as teaching the client.

You're doing great!

88. 3. A lucid interval is described as a brief period of unconsciousness followed by alertness; after several hours, the client again loses consciousness. This is most common with an epidural hematoma. Therefore, clients should be closely monitored and swift action taken (such as surgical evacuation of the hematoma) if the client deteriorates. Garbled speech is known as dysarthria. An interval in which the client is alert but can't recall recent events is known as amnesia. Warning symptoms or auras typically occur before seizures.
CN: Physiological integrity; CNS: Reduction of risk potential; CL: Application

89. 1. Suction should be applied for 10 to 15 seconds at a time. Suction is regulated to 80 to 120 cm. Suction should be applied only during withdrawal of the catheter. When suctioning the trachea, the catheter is inserted 4″ to 6″ (10 to 15 cm) or until resistance is felt.
CN: Physiological integrity; CNS: Reduction of risk potential; CL: Application

90. 3. Uncontrolled hypertension is the major cause of hemorrhagic stroke. Nurses need to address secondary prevention of stroke by educating clients and their families about blood pressure control. Both diabetes and heart disease increase the probability of stroke by hastening atherosclerosis but are lesser risk factors compared to hypertension. A recent viral infection is not directly linked to this problem.
CN: Physiological integrity; CNS: Reduction of risk potential; CL: Application

91. 3. Isosorbide is a potent vasodilator and can cause hypotension, which reduces brain perfusion and should be avoided in acute stroke. Treatment for an acute stroke and stroke in evolution includes permissive hypertension. Dehydration would be inappropriate in this instance. Hypocarbia is intermittently used in the emergent reduction of intracranial pressure through cerebral vasoconstriction. Nutrition may be delivered by tube when dysphagia exists.
CN: Physiological integrity; CNS: Physiological adaptation; CL: Application

92. Which client on the rehabilitation unit is most likely to develop autonomic dysreflexia?
1. A client with brain injury
2. A client with herniated nucleus pulposus
3. A client with a high cervical spine injury
4. A client with a stroke

92. 3. Autonomic dysreflexia refers to uninhibited sympathetic outflow in clients with spinal cord injuries most commonly above the level of T6. Autonomic dysreflexia is characterized by severe paroxysmal hypertension associated with throbbing headaches, profuse sweating, nasal stuffiness, flushing of the skin above the level of the lesion, bradycardia, apprehension, and anxiety, which is sometimes accompanied by cognitive impairment. The other clients aren't prone to dysreflexia.
CN: Safe, effective care environment; CNS: Management of care; CL: Application

93. Which condition indicates that spinal shock is resolving in a client with C7 quadriplegia?
1. Absence of pain sensation in the chest
2. Return of reflexes below the injury
3. Spontaneous respirations
4. Urinary continence

93. 2. The return of reflexes and spasticity are signs of resolving shock. Spinal or neurogenic shock is characterized by hypotension, bradycardia, dry skin, flaccid paralysis, or the absence of reflexes below the level of injury. The absence of pain sensation in the chest doesn't apply to spinal shock. Spinal shock descends from the injury, and respiratory difficulties occur at C4 and above. Slight muscle contraction at the bulbocavernosus reflex occurs but not enough for urinary continence.
CN: Physiological integrity; CNS: Physiological adaptation; CL: Analysis

94. When discharging a client from the hospital after a laminectomy, the nurse recognizes that the client needs further teaching when he makes which statement?
1. "I'll sleep on a firm mattress."
2. "I won't drive for 2 to 4 weeks."
3. "When I pick things up, I'll bend my knees."
4. "I can't wait to pick up my 1-year-old granddaughter."

94. 4. Lifting more than 10 lb (4.5 kg) for several weeks after surgery is contraindicated. The other responses are appropriate.
CN: Physiological integrity; CNS: Reduction of risk potential; CL: Analysis

95. When assessing a client with herniated nucleus pulposus of L4–L5, the nurse should expect to find which sign or symptom of spinal cord compression?
1. Lower back pain
2. Pain radiating across the buttocks
3. Positive Kernig's sign
4. Urinary incontinence

95. 4. Progressive neurological deficits at L4–L5, including worsening muscle weakness, paresthesia, and loss of bowel and bladder control, are symptoms of spinal cord compression. The other symptoms usually occur in clients with herniated nucleus pulposus without spinal cord compression. Kernig's sign is a symptom of meningitis and is characterized by severe stiffness of the hamstrings causing an inability to straighten the leg when the hip is flexed to 90 degrees.
CN: Physiological integrity; CNS: Physiological adaptation; CL: Analysis

96. A nurse assesses a client who has episodes of autonomic dysreflexia. Which condition can cause autonomic dysreflexia?
1. Headache
2. Lumbar spinal cord injury
3. Neurogenic shock
4. Noxious stimuli

Correct positioning will help relieve your client's symptoms.

97. A client is experiencing an episode of autonomic dysreflexia and becomes hypertensive. The most important intervention by the nurse would be?
1. Elevate the client's legs.
2. Put the client flat in bed.
3. Put the bed in Trendelenburg's position.
4. Put the client in high Fowler's position.

98. A client recovering from a spinal cord injury has a great deal of spasticity. Which medication may be used to control spasticity?
1. Hydralazine
2. Baclofen (Lioresal)
3. Lidocaine (Xylocaine)
4. Methylprednisolone (Medrol)

I know you're feeling fried at this point, but keep going!

99. Client teaching for a client with Gardner-Wells tongs should include which reason for their use?
1. To reduce intracranial pressure (ICP)
2. To reduce dislocations and pain
3. To prevent deep vein thrombosis (DVT)
4. To prevent the need for surgery

100. A client with a T1 spinal cord injury arrives at the emergency department with a blood pressure of 82/40 mm Hg, pulse of 34 beats/minute, dry skin, and flaccid paralysis of the lower extremities. Which condition should be suspected?
1. Autonomic dysreflexia
2. Hypervolemia
3. Neurogenic shock
4. Sepsis

96. 4. Noxious stimuli, such as a full bladder, fecal impaction, or a decubitus ulcer, may cause autonomic dysreflexia. A headache is a symptom of autonomic dysreflexia, not a cause. Autonomic dysreflexia is most commonly seen with injuries at T6 or above. Neurogenic shock isn't a cause of dysreflexia.
CN: Physiological integrity; CNS: Physiological adaptation; CL: Application

97. 4. Putting the client in high Fowler's position can help reduce blood pressure below dangerous levels until other treatment can be started (e.g., removing or treating the stimulus and administration of antihypertensives). Elevating the client's legs, putting the client flat in bed, or putting the bed in Trendelenburg's position places the client in positions that can increase blood pressure.
CN: Physiological integrity; CNS: Reduction of risk potential; CL: Application

98. 2. Baclofen is a skeletal muscle relaxant used to decrease spasms. It may be given orally or intrathecally. Hydralazine is an antihypertensive and afterload-reducing agent. Lidocaine is an antiarrhythmic and a local anesthetic agent. Methylprednisolone, an anti-inflammatory drug, is used to decrease spinal cord edema in the acute phase.
CN: Physiological integrity; CNS: Pharmacological and parenteral therapies; CL: Application

99. 2. Gardner-Wells tongs are used to reduce dislocations, subluxations, pain, and spasm in cervical spinal cord injuries. They may be used to stabilize a neck fracture until a definitive surgical procedure can be performed. Gardner-Wells tongs aren't used to reduce ICP or prevent DVT.
CN: Physiological integrity; CNS: Reduction of risk potential; CL: Application

100. 3. Loss of sympathetic control and unopposed vagal stimulation below the level of the injury typically cause hypotension, bradycardia, pallor, flaccid paralysis, and warm, dry skin in the client in neurogenic shock. Hypervolemia is indicated by a rapid and bounding pulse and edema. Autonomic dysreflexia occurs after neurogenic shock abates. Signs of sepsis would include elevated temperature, increased heart rate, and increased respiratory rate.
CN: Physiological integrity; CNS: Physiological adaptation; CL: Analysis

101. A client has a cervical spine injury at the level of C5. Which condition should the nurse anticipate during the <u>acute</u> phase?
1. Absent corneal reflex
2. Decerebrate posturing
3. Movement of only the right or left half of the body
4. The need for mechanical ventilation

102. When caring for a client with quadriplegia, which nursing intervention takes <u>priority</u>?
1. Forcing fluids to prevent renal calculi
2. Maintaining skin integrity
3. Obtaining adaptive devices for more independence
4. Preventing atelectasis

103. A client with C7 quadriplegia is flushed and anxious and complains of a pounding headache. Which symptom(s) should also be anticipated?
1. Decreased urine output or oliguria
2. Hypertension and bradycardia
3. Respiratory depression
4. Symptoms of shock

104. The nurse is teaching a client who has a diagnosis of a stroke versus a transient ischemic attack (TIA). Which statement by the nurse describing to the client the difference between stroke and TIA would be the <u>most accurate</u>?
1. TIAs resolve in less than 24 hours.
2. TIAs may be hemorrhagic in origin.
3. TIAs may cause a permanent motor deficit.
4. TIAs may predispose the client to a myocardial infarction (MI).

105. A client with a right stroke has a flaccid left side. Which intervention would best prevent shoulder subluxation?
1. Splint the wrist.
2. Use an air splint.
3. Put the affected arm in a sling.
4. Perform range-of-motion exercises on the affected side.

Pay close attention to the word acute.

Keep alert! You've got 44 questions to go!

101. 4. The diaphragm is stimulated by nerves at the level of C4. Initially, this client may need mechanical ventilation due to cord edema. This may resolve in time. Absent corneal reflexes, decerebrate posturing, and hemiplegia occur with brain injuries, not spinal cord injuries.
CN: Physiological integrity; CNS: Physiological adaptation; CL: Application

102. 4. Clients with quadriplegia have paralysis or weakness of the diaphragm, abdominal, or intercostal muscles. Maintenance of airway and breathing take top priority. Although forcing fluids, maintaining skin integrity, and obtaining adaptive devices for more independence are all important interventions, preventing atelectasis has more priority.
CN: Physiological integrity; CNS: Reduction of risk potential; CL: Application

103. 2. Hypertension, bradycardia, anxiety, blurred vision, and flushing above the lesion occur with autonomic dysreflexia due to uninhibited sympathetic nervous system discharge. The other options are incorrect. The most common cause of autonomic dysreflexia is bowel impaction or bladder distension.
CN: Physiological integrity; CNS: Physiological adaptation; CL: Analysis

104. 1. Symptoms of a TIA result from a transient lack of oxygen to the brain and usually resolve within 24 hours, and the average time is less than 30 minutes. Unlike an ischemic stroke, TIAs are not permanent. However, people who have had a TIA are at high risk of having a stroke, and secondary stroke prevention is required. TIAs are due to an ischemic process, not a hemorrhage. The risk factors for stroke, TIA, and MI are similar, but the question asked about the difference between a stroke and TIA.
CN: Physiological integrity; CNS: Physiological adaptation; CL: Analysis

105. 3. Due to the weight of the flaccid extremity, the shoulder may disarticulate. A sling will support the extremity. The other options won't support the shoulder. Air splints are used to support fractured or broken bones.
CN: Physiological integrity; CNS: Basic care and comfort; CL: Application

106. A 40-year-old paraplegic client must perform intermittent catheterization of the bladder. Which instruction should be given?
1. "Clean the meatus from back to front."
2. "Measure the quantity of urine."
3. "Gently rotate the catheter during removal."
4. "Clean the meatus with soap and water."

Which instruction should be given?

107. Which method should be used to assess pupil accommodation?
1. Assessing for peripheral vision
2. Touching the cornea lightly with a wisp of cotton
3. Having the client follow an object upward, downward, obliquely, and horizontally
4. Observing for pupil constriction and convergence while focusing on an object coming toward the client

108. A client at the eye clinic reports difficulty seeing at night. This may result from which nutritional deficiency?
1. Vitamin A
2. Vitamin B$_6$
3. Vitamin C
4. Vitamin K

109. A client with a spinal cord injury has a neurogenic bladder. When planning for discharge, the nurse anticipates the client will need which procedure or program?
1. Intermittent catheterization program
2. Kock pouch
3. Transurethral prostatectomy
4. Ureterostomy

Keep those numbers straight!

110. When using a Snellen alphabet chart, a nurse records a client's vision as 20/40. Which statement best describes 20/40 vision?
1. The client has alterations in near vision and is legally blind.
2. The client can see at 20 feet what the person with normal vision sees at 40 feet.
3. The client can see at 40 feet what the person with normal vision sees at 20 feet.
4. The client has a 20% decrease in acuity in one eye, and 40% decrease in the other eye.

106. 4. Intermittent catheterization may be performed chronically with clean technique, using soap and water to clean the urinary meatus. The meatus is always cleaned from front to back in a woman, or in expanding circles working outward from the meatus in a man. It isn't necessary to measure the urine. The catheter doesn't need to be rotated during removal.

CN: Physiological integrity; CNS: Basic care and comfort; CL: Application

107. 4. Accommodation refers to convergence and constriction of the pupil while following a near object. Assessing for peripheral vision refers to visual fields. Touching the cornea lightly with a wisp of cotton describes assessment of the corneal reflex. Having the client follow an object upward, downward, obliquely, and horizontally refers to cardinal fields of gaze.

CN: Physiological integrity; CNS: Reduction of risk potential; CL: Application

108. 1. Night blindness (nyctalopia) may be caused by a vitamin A deficiency or dysfunctional rod receptors. None of the other deficiencies listed lead to nyctalopia.

CN: Health promotion and maintenance; CNS: None; CL: Application

109. 1. Intermittent catheterization, starting with 2-hour intervals and increasing to 4- to 6-hour intervals, is used to manage neurogenic bladder. A Kock pouch is a type of urinary diversion. Transurethral prostatectomy is indicated for obstruction to urinary outflow by benign prostatic hyperplasia or for the treatment of cancer. An ileostomy or ureterostomy isn't necessary.

CN: Physiological integrity; CNS: Basic care and comfort; CL: Application

110. 2. The numerator refers to the client's vision while comparing the normal vision in the denominator. Legal blindness refers to 20/150 or less. Alterations in near vision may be due to loss of accommodation caused by the aging process (presbyopia) or farsightedness.

CN: Physiological integrity; CNS: Reduction of risk potential; CL: Analysis

111. A nurse would use which of the following instruments in recording intraocular pressure?
1. Goniometer
2. Ophthalmoscope
3. Slit lamp
4. Tonometer

112. After a nurse instills atropine drops into both eyes for a client undergoing an ophthalmic examination, which instruction should be given to the client?
1. "Be careful because the blink reflex is paralyzed."
2. "Avoid wearing your regular glasses when driving."
3. "Be aware that the pupils may be unusually small."
4. "Wear dark glasses in bright light because the pupils are dilated."

113. Which procedure or assessment must a nurse perform when preparing a client for eye surgery?
1. Clipping the client's eyelashes
2. Verifying the affected eye has been patched for 24 hours before surgery
3. Verifying the client has had nothing by mouth since midnight or at least 8 hours before surgery
4. Obtaining informed consent

For eye surgery, which procedure or assessment shall I perform?

114. Which statement indicates that a client needs additional teaching after cataract surgery?
1. "I'll avoid eating until the nausea subsides."
2. "I can't wait to get back to the gym."
3. "I'll avoid bending over to tie my shoelaces."
4. "I'll avoid touching the dropper to my eye when using my eyedrops."

Teaching isn't complete if your client doesn't understand.

115. Cataract surgery results in aphakia. Which statement best describes this term?
1. Absence of the crystalline lens
2. A "keyhole" pupil
3. Loss of accommodation
4. Retinal detachment

111. **4.** A tonometer is a device used in glaucoma screening to record intraocular pressure. A goniometer measures joint movement and angles. An ophthalmoscope examines the interior of the eye, especially the retina. A slit lamp evaluates structures in the anterior chamber of the eye.

CN: Physiological integrity; CNS: Reduction of risk potential; CL: Comprehension

112. **4.** Atropine, an anticholinergic drug, has mydriatic effects causing pupil dilation. This allows more light onto the retina and may cause photophobia and blurred vision. Atropine doesn't paralyze the blink reflex or cause miosis (pupil constriction). Driving may be contraindicated due to blurred vision.

CN: Physiological integrity; CNS: Pharmacological and parenteral therapies; CL: Application

113. **3.** Maintaining nothing-by-mouth status for at least 8 hours before surgical procedures prevents vomiting and aspiration. There's no need to patch an eye before most surgeries unless specifically ordered by the physician or to clip the eyelashes. The physician is responsible for obtaining informed consent; the nurse validates that the consent is obtained.

CN: Physiological integrity; CNS: Reduction of risk potential; CL: Application

114. **2.** Lifting, usually involving the Valsalva maneuver, increases intraocular pressure (IOP) and strain on the surgical site. Preventing nausea and subsequent vomiting will prevent increased IOP, as will avoiding bending or placing the head in a dependent position. Touching the eye dropper to the eye will contaminate the dropper and thus the entire bottle of medication.

CN: Physiological integrity; CNS: Reduction of risk potential; CL: Analysis

115. **1.** Aphakia means without lens. In cataract surgery, the diseased lens is removed and replaced with an artificial lens (called an intraocular lens, or IOL). A keyhole pupil results from iridectomy. Loss of accommodation is a normal response to aging. A retinal detachment is usually associated with retinal holes created by vitreous traction.

CN: Physiological integrity; CNS: Physiological adaptation; CL: Comprehension

116. When developing a teaching session on glaucoma for the community, which statement should the nurse stress?
1. Glaucoma is easily corrected with eyeglasses.
2. White and Asian individuals are at the highest risk for glaucoma.
3. Yearly screening for people ages 20 to 40 years is recommended.
4. Glaucoma can be painless and vision may be lost before the person is aware of a problem.

117. For a client having an episode of acute angle-closure glaucoma, the nurse expects to give which medication?
1. Acetazolamide (Diamox)
2. Atropine
3. Furosemide (Lasix)
4. Urokinase

118. Which symptom would occur in a client with a detached retina?
1. Flashing lights and floaters
2. Homonymous hemianopia
3. Loss of central vision
4. Ptosis

119. A client underwent an enucleation of the right eye for a malignancy. Which intervention will the nurse perform?
1. Instilling miotics as ordered to the affected eye
2. Teaching the client to clean the prosthesis in soap and water
3. Assessing reactivity of the pupils to light and accommodation
4. Teaching the client to prevent straining at stool leading to increased intraocular pressure

120. A nurse should question an order to irrigate the ear canal in which circumstance?
1. Ear pain
2. Hearing loss
3. Otitis externa
4. Perforated tympanic membrane

This question should be painless.

If you're unsure about an order, ask.

116. **4.** Open-angle glaucoma causes a painless increase in intraocular pressure (IOP) with loss of peripheral vision. A variety of miotics and agents to decrease IOP and occasionally surgery are used to treat glaucoma. Blacks have a threefold greater chance of developing glaucoma with an increased chance of blindness than other groups. Individuals older than age 40 years should be screened.
CN: Health promotion and maintenance; CNS: None; CL: Application

117. **1.** Acetazolamide, a carbonic anhydrase inhibitor, decreases intraocular pressure (IOP) by decreasing the secretion of aqueous humor. Atropine dilates the pupil and decreases outflow of aqueous humor, causing a further increase in IOP. Furosemide is a loop diuretic, and urokinase is a thrombolytic agent; they aren't used in the treatment of glaucoma.
CN: Physiological integrity; CNS: Pharmacological and parenteral therapies; CL: Application

118. **1.** Signs and symptoms of retinal detachment include abrupt flashing lights, floaters, loss of peripheral vision, or a sudden shadow or curtain in the vision. Occasionally, vision loss is gradual.
CN: Physiological integrity; CNS: Physiological adaptation; CL: Application

119. **2.** Enucleation of the eye refers to surgical removal of the entire eye; therefore, the client needs instructions about the prosthesis. There are no activity restrictions, and there is no need for miotic eyedrops; however, prophylactic antibiotics may be used in the immediate postoperative period. Miotic eyedrops are used in acute glaucoma to inhibit visual field loss and slow optic nerve damage.
CN: Physiological integrity; CNS: Physiological adaptation; CL: Application

120. **4.** Irrigation of the ear canal is contraindicated with perforation of the tympanic membrane because solution entering the inner ear may cause dizziness, nausea, vomiting, and infection. The other conditions aren't contraindications to irrigation of the ear canal.
CN: Physiological integrity; CNS: Reduction of risk potential; CL: Application

121. Which intervention is essential when instilling Cortisporin suspension, 2 drops in the right ear?
1. Verifying the proper client and route
2. Warming the solution to prevent dizziness
3. Holding an emesis basin under the client's ear
4. Positioning the client in the semi-Fowler's position

121. 1. When giving medications, a nurse follows the five Rs of medication administration: right client, right drug, right dose, right route, and right time. The drops may be warmed to prevent pain or dizziness, but this action isn't essential. An emesis basin would be used for irrigation of the ear. The client should be placed in the lateral position, not semi-Fowler's position, to prevent the drops from draining out for 5 minutes.
CN: Physiological integrity; CNS: Pharmacological and parenteral therapies; CL: Application

122. When teaching the client with Ménière's disease, which instruction should the nurse give about vertigo?
1. "Report dizziness at once."
2. "Drive in daylight hours only."
3. "Get up slowly, turning the entire body."
4. "Change your position using the logroll technique."

122. 3. Turning the entire body, not the head, will prevent vertigo. Dizziness is expected but can be prevented with Ménière's disease. The client shouldn't drive because he may reflexively turn the wheel to correct for vertigo. Turning the client in bed slowly and smoothly will be helpful; logrolling isn't needed.
CN: Physiological integrity; CNS: Reduction of risk potential; CL: Application

Giving I.V. drugs isn't a game. Know the right way to do it.

123. When giving I.V. phenytoin (Dilantin), which method should be used?
1. Administering rapidly
2. Withholding other anticonvulsants
3. Mixing the drug with saline solution only
4. Flushing the I.V. catheter with dextrose solution

123. 3. Phenytoin is compatible only with saline solutions; dextrose causes an insoluble precipitate to form. Phenytoin should be administered slowly (50 mg/minute). There's no need to withhold additional anticonvulsants.
CN: Physiological integrity; CNS: Pharmacological and parenteral therapies; CL: Application

124. An 18-year-old client was hit in the head with a baseball during practice. When discharging him to the care of his mother, the nurse gives which instruction?
1. "Watch him for keyhole pupil for the next 24 hours."
2. "Expect profuse vomiting for 24 hours after the injury."
3. "Wake him every hour and assess his orientation to person, time, and place."
4. "Notify the physician immediately if he has a headache."

124. 3. Changes in level of consciousness (LOC) may indicate expanding lesions such as subdural hematoma; orientation and LOC are assessed frequently for 24 hours. A keyhole pupil is found after iridectomy. Profuse or projectile vomiting is a symptom of increased intracranial pressure and should be reported immediately. A slight headache may last for several days after concussion; severe or worsening headaches should be reported.
CN: Physiological integrity; CNS: Physiological adaptation; CL: Application

Instruct the client's mother about the care for her son's injury.

125. A client is taking carbamazepine (Tegretol). For which of the following potential complications should the nurse be monitoring the client?
1. Acute respiratory distress syndrome (ARDS)
2. Diplopia
3. Elevated levels of phenytoin (Dilantin)
4. Leukocytosis

125. 2. Complications of carbamazepine include diplopia, dizziness, ataxia, and rash. ARDS isn't a complication of carbamazepine. Carbamazepine decreases blood levels of phenytoin and hormonal contraceptives; it also causes agranulocytosis because of the reduction in leukocytes.
CN: Physiological integrity; CNS: Pharmacological and parenteral therapies; CL: Application

126. For a client with damage to the caudate nucleus, putamen, and globus pallidus, which condition should be monitored?
1. Eye movement
2. Modulation of sounds
3. Motor movement
4. Muscle coordination

127. Which of the following should the nurse anticipate in a client with injury to the thalamus, such as in a thalamic stroke?
1. Burning or aching sensation over one half of the body
2. Seizures
3. Problems initiating movement
4. Memory lapses

128. A client is admitted with second-stage Alzheimer's disease. In communicating with the client, which of the following techniques will be the most successful?
1. Listening carefully and deciphering word substitutions
2. Avoiding repeated messages, as this may agitate the client
3. Avoiding yes or no questions
4. Avoiding the subject-verb-object format

129. The family of a client recently admitted to the hospital is describing to the nurse how the client was cooking and was slightly burned because he could not feel the hot temperature of the oven. Which of the following areas of the brain would the nurse suspect to be dysfunctional?
1. Frontal lobe
2. Occipital lobe
3. Parietal lobe
4. Temporal lobe

130. When assessing the ability of a client's pupil to constrict, which cranial nerve (CN) is being tested?
1. II
2. III
3. IV
4. V

Different areas of the brain (Hey, that's me!) regulate different functions.

126. 3. Motor movement is regulated by the basal ganglia, which consists of the caudate nucleus, putamen, and globus pallidus. Eye movement is too vague because there are several cranial nerves responsible for various forms of eye movement. Modulation of sounds occurs from the occipital lobe. The cerebellum regulates muscle coordination.
CN: Safe, effective care environment; CNS: Management of care; CL: Application

127. 1. Damage to the thalamus may result in thalamic syndrome, which is characterized by pain, burning, or an aching sensation over the contralateral side of the body. It is often accompanied by mood swings. Problems initiating movement are associated with the basal ganglia and memory problems with the hippocampus. Seizures are not specific to thalamic injury.
CN: Physiological integrity; CNS: Physiological adaptation; CL: Application

128. 1. Listening and deciphering word substitutions are the most helpful, as the client may have difficulty expressing their thoughts. Sentences should be repeated as often as needed. In questioning the client, yes-no or multiple-choice questions are very helpful. Sentences should be short and literal, following the subject-verb-object format.
CN: Psychosocial integrity; CNS: None; CL: Application

129. 3. The parietal lobe regulates sensory function, which would include the ability to sense hot or cold objects. The frontal lobe regulates thinking, planning, and judgment, and the occipital lobe is primarily responsible for vision function. The temporal lobe regulates memory.
CN: Physiological integrity; CNS: Physiological adaptation; CL: Application

130. 2. CN III, the oculomotor nerve, controls pupil constriction. CN II is the optic nerve, which controls vision. CN IV is the trochlear nerve, which coordinates eye movement. CN V is the trigeminal nerve, which innervates the muscles of chewing.
CN: Physiological integrity; CNS: Physiological adaptation; CL: Application

131. A nurse is discussing the purpose of an EEG with the family of a client with massive cerebral hemorrhage and loss of consciousness. Which of the following responses by the nurse would be the most accurate in describing what the test measures?
1. Extent of intracranial bleeding
2. Sites of brain injury
3. Activity of the brain
4. Percentage of functional brain tissue

What should I be telling the family of a client about an EEG?

132. A nurse is teaching a client and his family about dietary practices related to Parkinson's disease. Which signs and symptoms would be <u>most important</u> for the nurse to address?
1. Fluid overload and drooling
2. Aspiration and anorexia
3. Choking and diarrhea
4. Dysphagia and constipation

133. In assessing a client with a spinal cord injury, the nurse reports that the client can't control his abdominal muscles and is a paraplegic. The spinal cord lesion is most likely at which level?
1. Cervical
2. Lumbar
3. Sacral
4. Thoracic

134. A nurse performs a neurological assessment on a client complaining of headache and dizziness. Which assessment technique helps assess the motor function of cranial nerve VII (facial nerve)?
1. Asking the client to clench his jaw
2. Testing the gag reflex by placing an applicator against the pharynx
3. Asking the client to frown, smile, and raise his eyebrows
4. Asking the client to swallow

Prioritizing hits the mark on this question.

135. An unconscious client is receiving mechanical ventilation. Which nursing diagnosis takes priority?
1. Ineffective airway clearance related to the inability to expectorate
2. Risk for impaired skin integrity related to immobility
3. Imbalanced nutrition: Less than body requirements related to inability to swallow
4. Dressing self-care deficit related to unconsciousness

131. 3. An EEG measures the electrical activity of the brain. Extent of intracranial bleeding and location of the injury site would be determined by computerized tomography or magnetic resonance imaging. Percentage of functional brain tissue would be determined by a series of tests.
CN: Physiological integrity; CNS: Reduction of risk potential; CL: Application

132. 4. The eating problems associated with Parkinson's disease include dysphagia, risk of choking, drooling, aspiration, and constipation. Fluid overload, anorexia, and diarrhea aren't problems specifically related to Parkinson's disease.
CN: Physiological integrity; CNS: Reduction of risk potential; CL: Analysis

133. 4. Complete injuries at or below the thoracic spinal levels (T1–T8) result in paraplegia and the inability to control the abdominal muscles. Accordingly, trunk stability is affected. Functions of the hands, arms, neck, and breathing are associated with cervical injuries. The effects of injuries to the lumbar or sacral regions of the spinal cord are decreased control of the legs and hips, urinary system, and anus.
CN: Physiological integrity; CNS: Physiological adaptation; CL: Application

134. 3. To assess the motor function of cranial nerve VII, the nurse should ask the client to frown, smile, and raise his eyebrows. If these facial expressions are symmetrical, motor function is intact. Jaw clenching is a test for cranial nerve V function. Testing the gag reflex by placing an applicator against the pharynx, and assessing swallowing ability are ways to evaluate cranial nerve IX function. Testing the gag reflex also helps assess cranial nerve X function.
CN: Health promotion and maintenance; CNS: None; CL: Application

135. 1. Ineffective airway clearance related to the inability to expectorate takes priority in an unconscious client. The other nursing diagnoses are appropriate but are less important than airway, breathing, and circulation.
CN: Physiological integrity; CNS: Physiological adaptation; CL: Analysis

136. An 18-year-old client is admitted with a closed head injury sustained in a motor vehicle collision. His intracranial pressure (ICP) shows an upward trend. Which intervention should the nurse perform <u>first</u>?
  1. Reposition the client to avoid neck flexion.
  2. Administer 1 g of mannitol (Osmitrol) I.V. as ordered.
  3. Increase the ventilator's respiratory rate to 20 breaths/minute.
  4. Administer 100 mg of pentobarbital I.V. as ordered.

137. A client arrives at the emergency department after slipping on a patch of ice and hitting his head. A computed tomography scan of the head shows a collection of blood between the skull and dura mater. Which type of head injury does this finding suggest?
  1. Subdural hematoma
  2. Subarachnoid hemorrhage
  3. Epidural hematoma
  4. Contusion

138. After falling 208 feet (6 m), a 36-year-old construction worker sustains a C6 fracture with spinal cord transection. Which other findings should the nurse expect?
  1. Quadriplegia with gross arm movement and diaphragmatic breathing
  2. Quadriplegia and loss of respiratory function
  3. Paraplegia with intercostal muscle loss
  4. Loss of bowel and bladder control

139. A client with a subarachnoid hemorrhage is prescribed a 1,000-mg loading dose of phenytoin (Dilantin) I.V. Which consideration is <u>most important</u> when administering this dose?
  1. Therapeutic drug levels should be maintained between 20 and 30 mg/ml.
  2. Rapid phenytoin administration can cause cardiac arrhythmias.
  3. Phenytoin should be mixed in dextrose in water before administration.
  4. Phenytoin should be administered through an I.V. catheter in the client's hand.

In this case, save the best for first.

136. 1. The nurse should first attempt a nursing intervention, such as repositioning the client to avoid neck flexion, which increases venous return and lowers ICP. If nursing measures prove ineffective, notify the physician.
CN: Safe, effective care environment; CNS: Management of care; CL: Application

137. 3. An epidural hematoma occurs when blood collects between the skull and dura mater. In a subdural hematoma, venous blood collects between the dura mater and arachnoid mater. In a subarachnoid hemorrhage, blood collects between the pia mater and arachnoid membrane. A contusion is a bruise on the brain's surface.
CN: Physiological integrity; CNS: Physiological adaptation; CL: Application

138. 1. A client with a spinal cord injury at levels C5–C6 has quadriplegia with gross arm movement and diaphragmatic breathing. Injuries at levels C1–C4 lead to quadriplegia with total loss of respiratory function. Paraplegia with intercostal muscle loss occurs with injuries at T1–L2. Injuries below L2 cause paraplegia and loss of bowel and bladder control.
CN: Physiological integrity; CNS: Physiological adaptation; CL: Application

Hint! Hint! It's most important to consider what?

Caution

139. 2. Phenytoin I.V. should not exceed 50 mg/minute, as rapid administration can depress the myocardium, causing lethal dysrhythmias. Therapeutic drug levels range from 10 to 20 mg/ml. Phenytoin is only compatible with normal saline, not dextrose in water. It is very irritating to the blood vessels and may cause purple glove syndrome when administered I.V. in a hand.
CN: Physiological integrity; CNS: Pharmacological and parenteral therapies; CL: Application

140. A nurse is developing a discharge teaching plan for a client who has been prescribed phenytoin (Dilantin). Which instruction should the plan include?

1. "Take the drug on an empty stomach."
2. "You can consume alcoholic beverages in moderation."
3. "You can take any phenytoin brand because all brands are the same."
4. "Don't stop taking the drug except with medical supervision."

141. A 20-year-old client who fell approximately 31 feet (9 m) is unresponsive and breathless. A cervical spine injury is suspected. How should the first responder open the client's airway for rescue breathing?

1. By inserting a nasopharyngeal airway
2. By inserting an oropharyngeal airway
3. By performing the jaw-thrust maneuver
4. By performing the head-tilt, chin-lift maneuver

142. An 87-year-old client is admitted with a stroke. During the admission interview and assessment, his speech is slow, nonfluent, and labored. How should the nurse document this finding?

1. Receptive aphasia
2. Wernicke's aphasia
3. Expressive aphasia
4. Global aphasia

Which instruction shall I include in the teaching plan?

Documentation is key. Remember to always write it down!

140. 4. Abrupt phenytoin withdrawal may trigger status epilepticus, so the client should be warned not to stop taking the drug unless the physician approves. Taking phenytoin with food minimizes GI distress. Alcoholic beverages can decrease the drug's effectiveness. Changing phenytoin brands may alter the therapeutic effect.

CN: Physiological integrity; CNS: Pharmacological and parenteral therapies; CL: Application

141. 3. If the client has a suspected cervical spine injury, the jaw-thrust maneuver should be used to open the airway. If the tongue or relaxed throat muscles are obstructing the airway, a nasopharyngeal or oropharyngeal airway can be inserted; however, the client must have spontaneous respirations when the airway is open. The head-tilt, chin-lift maneuver requires neck hyperextension, which can worsen a cervical spine injury.

CN: Physiological integrity; CNS: Physiological adaptation; CL: Analysis

142. 3. Expressive (Broca's) aphasia results from damage to Broca's area, located in the frontal lobe of the brain's dominant hemisphere. Typically, the client with expressive aphasia has difficulty expressing himself and his speech is slow, nonfluent, and labored; however, comprehension of written and verbal communication is intact. With receptive (Wernicke's) aphasia (which results from injury to Wernicke's area, located in the temporal lobe of the dominant hemisphere), the client can't comprehend written or verbal communication; his speech is normal, but he conveys information poorly. With global aphasia—a combination of receptive and expressive aphasia—most of the brain's communication system is damaged. Global aphasia results from extensive damage to Broca's and Wernicke's areas.

CN: Physiological integrity; CNS: Physiological adaptation; CL: Application

143. A nurse is developing a teaching plan for a client who will undergo a stapedectomy for treatment of otosclerosis. Which point should the plan include?
1. Ringing in the ears is common after surgery.
2. Vertigo and dizziness are common after surgery.
3. Hearing should return immediately after surgery.
4. Excessive drainage is common after surgery.

144. A client has just been diagnosed with primary open-angle glaucoma and requires teaching about the disease. Which nursing diagnosis takes priority?
1. Risk for injury related to peripheral vision loss
2. Chronic pain related to increased intraocular pressure
3. Ineffective health maintenance related to medication adverse effects
4. Deficient knowledge related to new diagnosis of glaucoma

145. When teaching a client how to administer mydriatic agents, which instruction should the nurse provide?
1. "Your pupils will be small and your night vision will be diminished."
2. "Blurred vision is an adverse effect and you should report it to the physician immediately."
3. "Eye pain is common after administration."
4. "Compress the lacrimal sac for 1 minute after instillation."

143. 2. Vertigo is the most frequent complication of stapedectomy. The client should move slowly to avoid triggering or worsening vertigo and should ask for assistance with ambulation. Ringing in the ears (tinnitus) rarely follows this surgery and should be reported to the physician. Hearing typically decreases after surgery because of ear packing and tissue swelling, but commonly returns over the next 2 to 6 weeks. Usually, postoperative drainage and pain are minimal; excessive drainage should be reported.
CN: Physiological integrity; CNS: Reduction of risk potential; CL: Application

144. 1. Risk for injury related to peripheral vision loss takes priority because open-angle glaucoma limits peripheral vision; the client risks injury from stumbling over peripheral objects that he can't see. Angle-closure glaucoma—not open-angle glaucoma—commonly causes acute pain. Primary open-angle glaucoma is an incurable disease that requires lifelong treatment; adverse effects of medications are common. Although ineffective health maintenance is an appropriate diagnosis for this client, safety takes priority. Deficient knowledge is appropriate for any client with a new diagnosis, but it takes lower priority than safety.
CN: Physiological integrity; CNS: Reduction of risk potential; CL: Analysis

145. 4. To prevent systemic absorption, the client should compress the lacrimal sac for 1 minute after instilling a mydriatic agent. The drug makes the pupils large and causes light sensitivity. Blurred vision is an expected effect of mydriatics and need not be reported immediately. The client should discontinue the drug if eye pain occurs.
CN: Physiological integrity; CNS: Pharmacological and parenteral therapies; CL: Application

146. A nurse is performing a neurological assessment on a client during a routine physical examination. To assess the Babinski reflex, indicate the point where the nurse should place the tongue blade to begin the stroke of the foot.

146. To test for the Babinski reflex, use a tongue blade to slowly stroke the lateral side of the underside of the foot. Start at the heel and move toward the great toe. The normal response in an adult is plantar flexion of the toes. Upward movement of the great toe and fanning of the little toes, called the Babinski reflex, is abnormal.

CN: Health promotion and maintenance; CNS: None; CL: Application

147. The nurse is assessing a client's deep tendon reflexes. Which graphic shows assessing the biceps reflex?

1.

2.

3.

4.

147. 3. To test the biceps reflex, the client's elbow is flexed at a 45-degree angle. The nurse places her thumb or index finger over the biceps tendon and strikes the digit with the pointed end of the reflex hammer, watching and feeling for the contraction of the biceps muscle and flexion of the forearm. Option 1 shows assessment of the patellar reflex. Option 2 shows assessment of the brachioradialis reflex. Option 4 shows assessment of the triceps reflex.

CN: Physiological integrity; CNS: Reduction of risk potential; CL: Analysis

Here's a test that covers nursing care for clients with a disorder of the musculoskeletal system. So get moving! (Get it? Moving? Hmmm. I must be losing my touch.)

Chapter 7
Musculoskeletal disorders

1. A 70-year-old female client complains of lower back pain and is diagnosed with osteoporosis. The nurse is aware that this client is most at risk for which condition?
1. Pain
2. Fracture
3. Hardening of the bones
4. Increased bone matrix and remineralization

2. A 76-year-old woman with a history of osteoporosis experienced a right hip fracture and is admitted to the hospital. The client had a total hip replacement. The most important nursing diagnosis for this client would be?
1. Acute pain
2. Self-care deficit
3. Risk for impaired skin integrity
4. Imbalanced nutrition: Less than body requirements

3. The nurse is teaching a client about the risk factors of osteoporosis. It is most important for the nurse to include which factors? Select all that apply.
1. Inadequate dietary intake of calcium
2. Blood pressure medications
3. Family history
4. Smoking
5. Oral hypoglycemics

4. The nurse is teaching the client about the primary cause of osteoporosis. What is the most important information for the nurse to provide?
1. "Alcoholism is the primary cause of osteoporosis."
2. "Malnutrition is the primary cause of osteoporosis."
3. "Hormonal imbalance is the primary cause of osteoporosis."
4. "Osteogenesis imperfecta is the primary cause of osteoporosis."

1. 2. The primary complication of osteoporosis is fractures. With osteoporosis, bones soften, and there's a decrease in bone matrix and remineralization. Pain may occur, but fractures can be life threatening.
CN: Physiological integrity; CNS: Physiological adaptation; CL: Application

2. 1. Relieving pain and making the client comfortable are the highest priorities. All of the other nursing diagnoses would be lower priorities.
CN: Physiological and safety integrity; CNS: Physiological adaptation; CL: Analysis

A client may have different postoperative risk factors.

3. 1, 3, and 4. Inadequate dietary intake of calcium, family history, and smoking are risk factors of osteoporosis. There is no evidence that blood pressure medications or oral hypoglycemics are risk factors.
CN: Physiological integrity; CNS: Physiological adaptation; CL: Application

4. 3. Hormonal imbalance, faulty metabolism, and poor dietary intake of calcium cause primary osteoporosis. Alcoholism, malnutrition, osteogenesis imperfecta, rheumatoid arthritis, liver disease, scurvy, lactose intolerance, hyperthyroidism, and trauma cause secondary osteoporosis.
CN: Physiological integrity; CNS: Physiological adaptation; CL: Application

5. A 42-year-old client recently had a total hysterectomy and bilateral oophorectomy. Which of the following responses by the client indicates that the nurse's teaching about osteoporosis has been effective?
 1. "Osteoporosis affects only women over 65 years."
 2. "My risk for osteoporosis is low because I still have my thyroid gland."
 3. "I'm still producing hormones, so I don't have to worry about osteoporosis."
 4. "I need to take precautions to protect myself from osteoporosis because I have had surgically induced menopause."

6. The nurse is teaching a class on primary prevention of osteoporosis. What is the most important information for the nurse to provide?
 1. Maintain the optimal calcium intake.
 2. Place items within reach of the client.
 3. Install bars in the bathroom to prevent falls.
 4. Use a professional alert system in the home in case a fall occurs when the client is alone.

7. The nurse is providing discharge teaching for a client who was hospitalized with gout. The nurse determines that teaching was effective when the client states the need to reduce the intake of:
 1. tofu.
 2. liver.
 3. tomatoes.
 4. blackberries.

8. The nurse is planning interventions for a client with an acute gout attack. What would the priority intervention for this client be?
 1. Instruct the client on relaxation techniques and promote bed rest.
 2. Instruct the client about relaxation techniques.
 3. Administer prescribed analgesics.
 4. Force fluids.

9. A nurse is interviewing a client who has a pattern of nonchronic gout. Which statement by the client best describes the pattern of nonchronic gout?
 1. Frequent painful attacks
 2. Generally painful joints at all times
 3. Painful attacks with pain-free periods
 4. Painful attacks with less painful periods, but pain never subsides

I'm a primary means of prevention.

5. 4. Menopause at any age puts women at risk for osteoporosis because of the associated hormonal imbalance. This client's thyroid gland won't protect her from osteoporosis. With her ovaries removed, she's no longer producing hormones.
CN: Physiological integrity; CNS: Physiological adaptation; CL: Analysis

6. 1. Primary prevention of osteoporosis includes maintaining optimal calcium intake. Placing items within reach of the client, using a professional alert system in the home, and installing bars in bathrooms are all secondary and tertiary prevention methods to prevent falls.
CN: Health promotion and maintenance; CNS: None; CL: Application

7. 2. A client with gout should reduce his or her intake of purine-rich food, such as liver. Blackberries, tofu, and tomatoes are not rich in purine.
CN: Physiological integrity; CNS: Basic care and comfort; CL: Application

8. 3. Administering prescribed analgesics to relieve pain should be the priority. Pain control is a priority. The other actions are appropriate measures to institute but aren't the priority.
CN: Physiological integrity; CNS: Physiological adaptation; CL: Analysis

9. 3. The usual pattern of gout involves painful attacks with pain-free periods. Chronic gout may lead to frequent attacks with persistently painful joints.
CN: Physiological integrity; CNS: Physiological adaptation; CL: Application

10. The health care provider has prescribed a diet that limits purine-rich foods. Which of the following foods would the nurse teach the client to avoid eating? Select all that apply.
1. Bananas, wine, and cheese
2. Milk, ice cream, vegetables, and yogurt
3. Anchovies, sardines, and kidneys
4. Sweetbreads and lentils
5. Meat and dried fruits

11. The nurse has provided teaching to a client who has been newly diagnosed with gout. The nurse evaluates that teaching has been effective when the client makes which statement?
1. "Weight loss will decrease purine levels."
2. "Weight loss will decrease inflammation."
3. "Weight loss will increase uric acid levels and decrease stress on joints."
4. "Weight loss will decrease uric acid levels and decrease stress on joints."

12. The health care provider informs the client diagnosed with gout that his X-rays are normal. Which of the following statements by the health care provider would be <u>most appropriate</u> when the client asks if he still has gout?
1. "No, you're cured."
2. "Yes, X-rays are unreliable."
3. "Yes, X-rays are normal in the early stages of gout."
4. "Yes, X-ray changes are only seen with acute attacks."

13. The nurse is evaluating the effectiveness of colchicine (Colcrys) that was prescribed for a client who has recently been diagnosed with gout. The nurse determines the drug has been effective when? Select all that apply.
1. The client has decreased inflammation.
2. The client has decreased infections.
3. The client has fewer gout attacks.
4. The client says that pain is manageable.
5. The client is able to accomplish desired daily living activities.

14. Which of the following statements by a client diagnosed with gout indicates that the client understands the discharge instructions?
1. "I'll increase my fluids so that the inflammation will be reduced."
2. "Increasing fluid intake will increase the calcium my body absorbs."
3. "Increasing fluid intake will cause my body to excrete more uric acid."
4. "Increasing fluids will help provide a cushion for my bones."

You'll answer these questions in no time!

Question 12 asks you to choose the most appropriate answer. That means more than one may be suitable.

I'm just a little guy, but I'm ready to take action.

10. **3 and 4.** Anchovies, sardines, kidneys, sweetbreads, and lentils are high in purines. Bananas and dried fruits are high in potassium. Milk, ice cream, and yogurt are rich in calcium. Wine, cheese, preserved fruits, meats, and vegetables contain tyramine.
CN: Physiological integrity; CNS: Basic care and comfort; CL: Application

11. **4.** Weight loss will decrease uric acid levels and decrease stress on joints. Weight loss will not decrease purine levels, increase uric acid levels, or decrease inflammation.
CN: Health promotion and maintenance; CNS: None; CL: Application

12. **3.** X-rays are normal in the early stages of gout and can be very valuable in the diagnosis of gout. Telling the client that he's cured would be incorrect, because he may be in the early stages of gout when X-rays appear normal. With chronic gout, X-rays show damage to cartilage and bone. When X-ray changes occur, they're present during attacks and remissions.
CN: Physiological integrity; CNS: Physiological adaptation; CL: Application

13. **1, 3, 4, and 5.** The action of colchicine is to decrease inflammation by reducing the migration of leukocytes to synovial fluid, which will decrease pain and the number of gout attacks. Colchicine doesn't decrease infection.
CN: Physiological integrity; CNS: Pharmacological and parenteral therapies; CL: Application

14. **3.** Fluids promote the excretion of uric acid. Fluids do not decrease inflammation, increase calcium absorption, or provide a cushion for weakened bones.
CN: Physiological integrity; CNS: Physiological adaptation; CL: Application

15. The nurse is performing an admission assessment on a client with osteoarthritis. Which of the following clinical manifestations would the nurse expect to find?
1. Joint pain after exercise relieved by rest
2. Symmetrical swelling of the joints of both hands
3. Morning stiffness lasting longer than 30 minutes
4. Fever

16. The health care provider has prescribed indomethacin (Indocin) for a client with gout. What is the most important information for the nurse to give the client about nonsteroidal anti-inflammatory drugs (NSAIDs)?
1. "Bleeding is not a problem with NSAIDs."
2. "Take NSAIDs with food to avoid an upset stomach."
3. "Take NSAIDs on an empty stomach to increase absorption."
4. "Don't take NSAIDs at bedtime because they may cause excitement."

17. The nurse is obtaining a health history from a client who has been taking ibuprofen (Motrin). What is (are) the most important question(s) for the nurse to ask the client? Select all that apply.
1. "How often do you take this medication?"
2. "Have you had any difficulty with breathing?"
3. "Do you monitor your blood pressure regularly?"
4. "Have you ever had tarry, black stools?"
5. "Have you ever vomited blood?"

Your client depends on you for information.

18. A client asks the nurse for information about osteoarthritis. What is the most appropriate information for the nurse to include?
1. Osteoarthritis is rarely debilitating.
2. Osteoarthritis is a rare form of arthritis.
3. Osteoarthritis afflicts people over age 60.
4. Osteoarthritis is the most common form of arthritis.

19. The health care provider orders 2 g of ampicillin (Omnipen) in 50 ml of D5W to infuse I.V. piggyback (IVPB) over 30 minutes for a client who had a right total knee replacement secondary to osteoarthritis. The nurse will set the I.V. infusion pump at what rate in milliliters per hour?
_____ ml/hour

---

15. 1. The most common symptom of osteoarthritis is joint pain after exercise or weight-bearing, usually relieved by rest. The other options are all symptoms of rheumatoid arthritis.
CN: Physiological integrity; CNS: Physiological adaptation; CL: Application

16. 2. Indomethacin, like other NSAIDs, should be taken with food because it can be irritating to the gastrointestinal (GI) mucosa and lead to GI bleeding. It can cause drowsiness, not excitement, and potential bleeding complications.
CN: Physiological integrity; CNS: Pharmacological and parenteral therapies; CL: Application

17. 1, 2, 4, and 5. Questions 4 and 5 are appropriate for the client who is taking ibuprofen because the medication can lead to irritation of the gastrointestinal (GI) mucosa, which can increase the risk of a GI bleed and vomiting. Knowing how often the client takes the medication is important because the client should not exceed 3,600 mg/day. If the client exceeds the medication amount, this can lead to renal failure, which will cause the blood pressure to increase. If the client has a history of respiratory problems, ibuprofen can increase the risk for developing hypersensitivity reactions.
CN: Physiological integrity; CNS: Pharmacological therapies; CL: Application

18. 3. Osteoarthritis is the most common form of arthritis and can be extremely debilitating. It can afflict people of any age, although most are elderly.
CN: Physiological integrity; CNS: Physiological adaptation; CL: Application

19. 100. 60/30 = 2 × 50 ml/hour = 100 ml/hour
CN: Physiological integrity; CNS: Pharmacological and parenteral therapies; CL: Application

20. The health care provider orders heparin 7,500 units subcutaneous for a client who had a left total hip replacement secondary to osteoarthritis. The pharmacy sent heparin 5,000 units/0.5 ml to the unit. How many milliliters would the nurse administer to the client?

21. Which of the following are causes of <u>primary</u> osteoarthritis?
1. Overuse of joints, aging, and obesity
2. Obesity, aging, and diabetes mellitus
3. Congenital abnormality, aging, overuse of joints
4. Diabetes mellitus, congenital abnormality, aging

22. The nurse is caring for a client with osteoarthritis of the knee. The nurse determines that discharge teaching has been effective when the client makes which statement?
1. "I'll take my ibuprofen (Motrin) on an empty stomach."
2. "I'll try taking a warm shower in the morning."
3. "I'll wear my knee splint every night."
4. "I'll jog at least a mile every morning."

23. The health care provider prescribed salicylates for a client with osteoarthritis. The nurse assesses the client and determines further intervention is necessary when the client exhibits which of the following?
1. Hearing loss
2. Increased pain in joints
3. Decreased calcium absorption
4. Increased bone demineralization

24. A 69-year-old client is admitted to the medical-surgical unit for osteoarthritis. During the health history, the nurse learns that the client has been on prolonged bed rest. What is the most appropriate nursing intervention for this client?
1. Encourage and educate coughing and deep breathing and limit fluid intake.
2. Turn the client every 2 hours and encourage coughing and deep breathing.
3. Provide only passive range of motion (ROM) and decrease stimulation.
4. Have the client lie as still as possible and give adequate pain medicine.

Don't be fooled. What does primary mean in this question?

What did you say?

20.
$$\frac{5{,}000 \text{ units} = 0.5 \text{ ml}}{7{,}500 \text{ units} = \text{X ml}}$$
$$\frac{\cancel{5{,}000}\text{X}}{\cancel{5{,}000}} = \frac{3{,}750 \text{ ml}}{5{,}000} = 0.75 \text{ ml}$$

CN: Physiological integrity; CNS: Pharmacological and parenteral therapies; CL: Application

21. 1. Primary osteoarthritis may be caused by the overuse of joints, aging, or obesity. Congenital abnormalities and diabetes mellitus can cause secondary osteoarthritis.

CN: Physiological integrity; CNS: Physiological adaptation; CL: Application

22. 2. A client with osteoarthritis has joint stiffness that may be partially relieved with a warm shower on arising in the morning. Ibuprofen should be taken with food, as should all nonsteroidal anti-inflammatory medications. Splints are usually used by clients with rheumatoid arthritis. Because the problem is continued stress on the joint, the client may want to try to an exercise that puts less strain on the joint, such as swimming.

CN: Physiological integrity; CNS: Basic care and comfort; CL: Application

23. 1. Many elderly people already have diminished hearing, and salicylate use can lead to further or total hearing loss. Salicylates do not increase pain in joints, decrease calcium absorption, or increase bone demineralization.

CN: Physiological integrity; CNS: Pharmacological and parenteral therapies; CL: Application

24. 2. A bedridden client needs to be turned every 2 hours, have adequate nutrition, and cough and deep breathe. Hydration, active and passive ROM, and adequate pain medication are also appropriate nursing measures. To prevent contractures, the client shouldn't limit his fluid intake or lie as still as possible.

CN: Physiological integrity; CNS: Basic care and comfort; CL: Application

25. A client asks the nurse, "What is the difference between rheumatoid arthritis and osteo-arthritis?" What is the most appropriate response by the nurse?
1. Osteoarthritis is gender specific; rheumatoid arthritis is not.
2. Osteoarthritis is a systemic disease; rheumatoid arthritis is localized.
3. Osteoarthritis is a localized disease; rheumatoid arthritis is systemic.
4. Osteoarthritis has dislocations and subluxations; rheumatoid arthritis does not.

26. The nurse is performing an assessment on a client with a diagnosis of osteoarthritis. Which of the following clinical manifestations would the nurse expect to find?
1. Elevated sedimentation rate
2. Multiple subcutaneous nodules
3. Asymmetrical joint involvement
4. Signs and symptoms of inflammation, such as heat, fever, and malaise

27. When assessing a client with osteoarthritis, which of the following instructions would be considered <u>primary</u> prevention of injury from osteoarthritis? Select all that apply.
1. The client should avoid repetitive tasks.
2. The client should avoid physical activity.
3. The client should warm up before exercising.
4. The client should perform only repetitive tasks.

28. The client asks the nurse for information about osteoarthritis. What is the most appropriate information for the nurse to include about the disease?
1. It is a systemic inflammatory joint disease.
2. It is a disease involving fusion of the joints in the hands.
3. It is an inflammatory joint disease, with degeneration and loss of articular cartilage in synovial joints.
4. It is a noninflammatory joint disease, with degeneration and loss of articular cartilage in synovial joints.

29. The most appropriate clothing for a client with osteoarthritis would be?
1. Zippered clothing
2. Tied shoes to promote stability
3. Velcro clothing, slip-on shoes, and rubber grippers
4. Buttoned clothing, slip-on shoes, and rubber grippers

It's important to know the difference between these two common diseases.

You've finished 29 questions already!

25. 3. Osteoarthritis is a localized disease, whereas rheumatoid arthritis is systemic. Osteoarthritis is not gender specific, but rheumatoid arthritis is gender specific. Clients have dislocations and subluxations in both disorders.
CN: Physiological integrity; CNS: Physiological adaptation; CL: Application

26. 3. Asymmetrical joint involvement is present in osteoarthritis. Elevated sedimentation rate, multiple subcutaneous nodules, and such signs and symptoms of inflammation as heat, fever, and malaise are all present in rheumatoid arthritis.
CN: Physiological integrity; CNS: Physiological adaptation; CL: Analysis

27. 1 and 3. Primary prevention of injury from osteoarthritis includes warming up before exercise and avoiding repetitive tasks. Bed rest would contribute to many other systemic complications. Physical activity is important to remain fit and healthy and to maintain joint function.
CN: Health promotion and maintenance; CNS: None; CL: Application

28. 4. Osteoarthritis is a noninflammatory joint disease, with degeneration and loss of articular cartilage in synovial joints. Rheumatoid arthritis is a systemic inflammatory joint disease. Arthrodesis is fusion of the joints.
CN: Physiological integrity; CNS: Physiological adaptation; CL: Application

29. 3. Velcro clothing, slip-on shoes, and rubber grippers make it easier for the client to dress and grip objects. Zippers, ties, and buttons may be difficult for the client to use.
CN: Physiological integrity; CNS: Basic care and comfort; CL: Application

30. The nurse is caring for a client with osteoarthritis who is refusing to perform independent care. What is the <u>most important</u> nursing intervention for this client?
1. Perform the care for the client.
2. Explain to the client the purpose to maintain complete independence.
3. Encourage and support the client to perform as much self-care that the pain will allow.
4. Inform the client that once the care has been completed independently, she will receive pain medication.

31. The nurse asks a client in the late stages of osteoarthritis to describe the joint pain the client is currently experiencing. The nurse anticipates that the client will describe the pain as:
1. grating.
2. a dull ache.
3. a dull and deep aching pain.
4. deep aching relieved only with rest.

32. A client is admitted to the medical-surgical unit for osteoarthritis and weakness in the left lower extremity. The client uses a walker at home. The health care provider ordered a cane and physical therapy for the client. The client asks the nurse about the difference between the cane and walker. What is the best response by the nurse?
1. A walker is a better choice than a cane.
2. The cane should be used on the affected side.
3. The cane should be used on the unaffected side.
4. A client with osteoarthritis should be encouraged to ambulate without the cane.

33. The nurse is providing discharge teaching for a client with osteoarthritis. What is the most important information for the nurse to include?
1. Learn to pace activity.
2. Remain as sedentary as possible.
3. Return to a normal level of activity.
4. Include vigorous exercise in your daily routine.

What would be the best way to help the client?

If your client describes his pain, maybe I can help.

30. 3. A client with osteoarthritis should be encouraged or supported to perform as much of his or her care. The nurse's goal should be to allow the client to maintain his or her self-care abilities with help as needed but not to perform the care for the client. It is never appropriate to use pain medication as a bargaining tool.
CN: Psychosocial integrity; CNS: None; CL: Analysis

31. 1. In the late stages of osteoarthritis, the client often describes joint pain as grating. As the disease progresses, the cartilage covering the ends of bones is destroyed and bones rub against each other. Osteophytes, or bone spurs, may also form on the ends of bones. A dull ache and deep aching pain with or without relief with rest is often seen in the earlier stages of osteoarthritis.
CN: Physiological integrity; CNS: Physiological adaptation; CL: Application

32. 3. A cane should be used on the unaffected side. A client with osteoarthritis should be encouraged and educated to ambulate with a cane, walker, or other assistive device as needed; the assistive devices take the weight and stress off of joints.
CN: Physiological integrity; CNS: Basic care and comfort; CL: Application

33. 1. A client with osteoarthritis should pace his or her activities and avoid overexertion. Overexertion can increase degeneration and cause pain. The client should not become sedentary because he or she will have a high risk of pneumonia and contractures.
CN: Physiological integrity; CNS: Basic care and comfort; CL: Application

CN: Client needs category   CNS: Client needs subcategory   CL: Cognitive level

Case Study: Clinical Reasoning
Questions: 34–36

Mr. Smith is a 79-year-old client who is admitted to the Armstrong Community Memorial Hospital. The client is diagnosed with a left hip fracture secondary to a fall. The client is scheduled for a left total hip replacement (LTHR). The client's comorbidities are hypertension and diabetes. The client is a full code with no known allergies (NKA).

34. Which of the following nursing diagnoses would the nurse select as a priority for this client?
1. Disturbed sleep pattern
2. Ineffective coping
3. Risk for infection
4. Acute pain

34. 4. Acute pain is a priority nursing diagnosis for the nurse to select. Keeping the pain at an acceptable level will allow the client to participate in the plan of care. With a hip fracture, the priority is to control the pain. Relieving the pain and making the client restful are the highest the priority. All of the other nursing diagnoses would be lower priorities.
CN: Physiological integrity; CNS: Physiological adaptation; CL: Application

35. The client asks the nurse if anything affects how long it takes for the hip to heal. What is (are) the best response(s) by the nurse? Select all that apply.
1. The age of the client
2. The height of the client
3. The weight of the client
4. The client's comorbidities
5. The client's marital status

35. 1 and 4. The age and comorbidities of the client are important because they can affect the blood supply to the fracture, which can decrease the healing process. An older client and one with comorbidities such as hypertension and diabetes will have slowed bone healing due to a decrease in blood supply. The weight and the height of the client do not directly delay bone healing unless the client is malnourished. The client's marital status has no effect on healing. If help is needed, services for help with activities can be contracted.
CN: Physiological integrity; CNS: Physiological adaptation; CL: Application

36. A nurse is caring for the client who is 2 days postoperative and complaining of severe pain in the left leg. The nurse administers the prescribed morphine sulfate, 2 mg I.V. The client continues to complain of severe pain. The nurse assesses the client's left leg and finds the extremity cool to touch with absent pulses and a capillary refill greater than 3 seconds. What is the priority action of the nurse?
1. Notify the health care provider.
2. Document the clinical findings.
3. Readminister the prescribed morphine sulfate.
4. Reassess the left lower extremities within 1 hour.

36. 1. Skin cool to touch, no pulse, and capillary refill greater than 3 seconds are indications that the client's circulation is impaired. There are several complications that can impede circulation such as compartment syndrome or deep vein thrombosis (DVT), which requires immediately action to prevent damage to the nerves and tissues and necrosis. These complications can lead to loss of the leg. The nurse needs to collaborate with the health care provider for additional plans of care. Pain that is caused by tissue ischemia will not be relieved by morphine sulfate. Reassessing the left leg within 1 hour is delay in care and can cause more complications, which can lead to an irreversible outcome for the client.
CN: Physiological integrity; CNS: Physiological adaptation; CL: Application

37. A client was prescribed an anti-inflammatory drug for osteoarthritis 5 days ago. The client says the pain has decreased a little but not completely. Which of the following nursing interventions would be the <u>most appropriate</u>?
1. Notify the health care provider and suggest increasing the dose.
2. Notify the health care provider and suggest stopping the medication.
3. Notify the health care provider and suggest adding another medication.
4. Continue the present dose and offer other pain relief measures.

38. A client is diagnosed with a herniated nucleus pulposus (herniated disk). Which of the following statements should the nurse include in teaching the client about a herniated disk?
1. The disk slips out of alignment.
2. The disk shatters, and fragments place pressure on nerve roots.
3. The nucleus tissue itself remains centralized, and the surrounding tissue is displaced.
4. The nucleus of the disk puts pressure on the annulus, causing pressure on the nerve root.

39. The nurse is caring for a client who is admitted for a herniated nucleus pulposus. The client's pain level is a 10 out of 10. The health care provider ordered a morphine sulfate (Duramorph) patient-controlled analgesic (PCA), which is implemented for the client. What is the priority nursing assessment for this client?
1. Neurological system
2. Respiratory system
3. Gastrointestinal system
4. Cardiovascular system

40. A client complains of low back pain that radiates down the right leg, with numbness and weakness of the right leg. Based on the subjective data, the nurse recognizes these complaints as related to which disorder?
1. Herniated nucleus pulposus
2. Muscular dystrophy
3. Parkinson's disease
4. Osteoarthritis

41. A client has decided on <u>conservative</u> treatment for a herniated nucleus pulposus. The nurse anticipates that the treatment will include which of the following?
1. Surgery
2. Bone fusion
3. Bed rest, pain medication, physiotherapy
4. Strenuous exercise, pain medication, physiotherapy

You might have to stick with me for a while so I can do my job.

Why am I feeling so much pressure?

The word conservative is a clue to the right answer.

37. 4. Anti-inflammatory medications may take 2 to 3 weeks to provide full benefits. If the client can tolerate the pain, continue on the medication and offer other pain measures, such as rest, massage, heat, or cold. Increasing, stopping, or adding another medication is not appropriate because the medication hasn't been taken long enough to provide full benefit.
CN: Physiological integrity; CNS: Pharmacological and parenteral therapies; CL: Application

38. 4. With a herniated nucleus pulposus, or herniated disk, the nucleus of the disk puts pressure on the annulus, causing pressure on the nerve root. The disk itself does not slip, rupture, or shatter. The nucleus tissue usually moves from the center of the disk.
CN: Physiological integrity; CNS: Physiological adaptation; CL: Application

39. 2. The respiratory system is the highest priority nursing assessment because morphine sulfate can lead to respiratory depression, which can cause death for the client. The other systems are priorities, but they are low priorities.
CN: Physiological integrity; CNS: Physiological adaptation; CL: Analysis

40. 1. Compression of nerves by the herniated nucleus pulposus causes back pain that radiates into the leg, with numbness and weakness of the leg. Muscular dystrophy causes wasting of skeletal muscles. Parkinson's disease is characterized by progressive muscle rigidity and tremors. Osteoarthritis causes deep, aching joint pain.
CN: Physiological integrity; CNS: Physiological adaptation; CL: Analysis

41. 3. Conservative treatment of a herniated nucleus pulposus may include bed rest, pain medication, and physiotherapy. Aggressive treatment may include surgery such as a bone fusion.
CN: Physiological integrity; CNS: Reduction of risk potential; CL: Application

CN: Client needs category   CNS: Client needs subcategory   CL: Cognitive level

42. Which of the following instructions should the nurse include in the preoperative teaching for a client scheduled for closed spine surgery?
1. An endoscope is used to perform the surgery.
2. Intense physical therapy is needed after the procedure.
3. There is a greater associated risk with closed spine surgery.
4. Recovery time is twice as long as with open spine surgery.

43. The nurse provided teaching to the client with a herniated lumbar disk. The nurse determines further teaching is necessary when the client makes which statement?
1. "I can strengthen my back muscles by doing pelvic tilt exercises."
2. "I need to maintain a healthy weight to limit back strain."
3. "I should bend at the waist when picking up objects."
4. "I should increase my fiber and fluid intake."

44. The nurse is caring for a client with low back pain. Which action may the nurse delegate to the nursing assistant?
1. Assess pain level.
2. Palpate the abdomen for distension.
3. Reposition the client from side-lying to back.
4. Assess the client's skin for skin breakdown.

45. A client asks the nurse what is the purpose of applying a cold pack to a sprained ankle. What is the best response by the nurse?
1. "It decreases pain and increases circulation."
2. "It numbs the nerves and dilates the blood vessels."
3. "It promotes circulation and reduces muscle spasm."
4. "It constricts local blood vessels and decreases swelling."

46. The nurse is teaching a community class about back injuries. Which of the following statements by the nurse would be the most accurate concerning the area that is common for vertebral herniation?
1. It is the L1–L2, L4–L5 vertebra.
2. It is the L1–L2, L5–S1 vertebra.
3. It is the L4–L5, L5–S1 vertebra.
4. It is the L5–S1, S2–S3 vertebra.

I think I need further instruction.

42. 1. Closed spine surgery uses endoscopy to fix a herniated disk. It is less risky than open surgery and has a shorter recovery time; it is commonly done as a same-day surgical procedure. Physical therapy may be less intensive or not needed at all.

CN: Physiological integrity; CNS: Reduction of risk potential; CL: Application

43. 3. The client should bend at the knees, not the waist, to maintain proper body mechanics. Pelvic tilt exercises are recommended to strengthen back muscles. Increasing fiber and fluid intake helps soften stool, thereby preventing straining, which increases intraspinal pressure. Any extra weight carried by the client increases back strain.

CN: Physiological integrity; CNS: Physiological adaptation; CL: Application

44. 3. The nursing assistant is able to perform routine tasks. The registered is responsible for assessment, teaching, and evaluation of clients.

CN: Safe, effective care environment; CNS: Management of care; CL: Application

45. 4. Application of a cold pack causes the blood vessels to constrict, which reduces the leakage of fluid into the tissues and prevents swelling. It may have an effect on muscle spasms. Cold therapy may reduce pain by numbing the nerves and tissues. Cold therapy doesn't promote circulation or dilate the blood vessels.

CN: Physiological integrity; CNS: Basic care and comfort; CL: Application

46. 3. The most common areas of herniation are L4–L5, L5–S1.

CN: Health promotion and maintenance; CNS: None; CL: Application

47. A 50-year-old client is admitted to the emergency department with severe lower back pain, weakness, and atrophy of the leg muscles. Based on the clinical manifestations, which diagnostic tests would the nurse expect the physician to order?
1. Chest X-ray, magnetic resonance imaging (MRI), and computed tomography (CT) scan
2. Lumbar puncture, chest X-ray, MRI, and CT scan
3. Lumbar puncture, chest X-ray, and myelography
4. Myelography, MRI, and CT scan

48. The nurse is preparing a client for discharge. Which one of the following discharge instructions should be included when teaching the client how to prevent back injury?
1. Sleep on your side and carry objects at arm's length.
2. Sleep on your back and carry objects at arm's length.
3. Sleep on your side and carry objects close to your body.
4. Sleep on your back and carry objects close to your body.

49. A client is being discharged home with a prescription for skeletal muscle relaxants. What is the most important information for the nurse to tell the client?
1. Change your position quickly to avoid dizziness.
2. Double a missed dose to ensure proper muscle relaxation.
3. Cough and cold medications are appropriate to take, if needed.
4. Avoid activities that require alertness; muscle relaxants can cause drowsiness.

50. The nurse suspects that a client with a recent fracture has developed compartment syndrome. The assessment of the client may find which symptom?
1. Body-wide decrease in bone mass
2. A growth in and around the bone tissue
3. Inability to perform active movement; pain with passive movement
4. Inability to perform passive movement; pain with active movement

51. The nurse is caring for a client who has returned to the unit following the application of a cast for a fracture of the right ulna. The client is now complaining of severe pain, numbness, and tingling of the right arm. What is the most important action of the nurse?
1. Administer acetaminophen (Tylenol) as prescribed.
2. Lower the arm below the level of the heart.
3. Immediately report the client's symptoms.
4. Apply a heating pad.

Teach! Teach! Teach!

Now I know why they call them relaxants.

47. 4. Tests used to diagnose a herniated nucleus pulposus include myelography, MRI, and CT scan. Chest X-ray and lumbar puncture are not conclusive for a herniated disk.
CN: Physiological integrity; CNS: Physiological adaptation; CL: Application

48. 3. By sleeping on the side and carrying objects close to the body, there is less strain on the back. Sleeping on the back and carrying objects at arm's length adds pressure to the back.
CN: Health promotion and maintenance; CNS: None; CL: Application

49. 4. Client teaching should include avoiding activities that require alertness; muscle relaxants can cause drowsiness. Tell the client to change position slowly to avoid dizziness. The client shouldn't double a missed dose or take cough and cold medications because this will increase the likelihood of adverse effects.
CN: Physiological integrity; CNS: Pharmacological and parenteral therapies; CL: Application

50. 3. With compartment syndrome, the client cannot perform active movement, and pain occurs with passive movement. Osteoporosis brings a body-wide decrease in bone mass. A bone tumor shows growth in and around the bone tissue.
CN: Physiological integrity; CNS: Physiological adaptation; CL: Application

51. 3. Severe pain, numbness, and tingling are symptoms of impaired circulation due to compartment syndrome, which is a medical emergency. Don't give analgesics until the client has been assessed and treated. Lowering the arm below the level of the heart and applying heat will decrease venous outflow and impair the circulation even more.
CN: Physiological integrity; CNS: Physiological adaptation; CL: Application

52. The nurse is assessing a client with a hemorrhage from compartment syndrome. Which of the following symptoms would the nurse expect to find? Select all that apply.
1. Edema
2. Increased venous pressure
3. Decreased venous circulation
4. Increased arterial circulation

53. A client has developed compartment syndrome following application of a cast from a fractured tibia. The nurse is aware that the <u>priority</u> goal of intervention is to:
1. prevent tissue death, which can occur within 2 to 4 hours.
2. decrease the swelling in the extremity.
3. prevent further complications.
4. decrease the level of pain.

You'll have this answer in no time.

54. The nurse is caring for a client with compartment syndrome. The nurse anticipates that the client may require which measure?
1. Casting
2. Amputation
3. Fasciotomy
4. Observation; no treatment necessary

55. A client is admitted to the emergency department with a foot fracture, and a brace is applied. The nurse determines that teaching about the brace has been effective when the client makes which statement?
1. "The brace will act as a splint."
2. "The brace will allow for movement."
3. "The brace will help to prevent infection."
4. "The brace will encourage direct contact."

56. A nurse is assessing a client who is experiencing new-onset signs and symptoms of paresthesia. What is the most appropriate question for the nurse to ask the client?
1. "Have you had any changes in range of motion (ROM)?"
2. "Do you have any numbness and tingling?"
3. "Do you have any pain and blanching?"
4. "How long have you had fever and chills?"

52. 1, 2, and 3. The hemorrhage in compartment syndrome causes edema, increased venous pressure, and decreased venous and arterial circulation.
CN: Physiological integrity; CNS: Physiological adaptation; CL: Application

53. 1. Following development of compartment syndrome, there is an increase in pressure within the affected compartment that compromises circulation to the muscle tissue and to nerves. This may lead to death of these tissues and can occur within 2 to 4 hours. Decreasing pain levels, preventing further complication, and decreasing the swelling in the affected extremity are important goals of treatment, but they are not the priority of treatment.
CN: Physiological integrity; CNS: Physiological adaptation; CL: Application

54. 3. Treatment of compartment syndrome includes fasciotomy, which involves cutting the fascia over the affected area to permit muscle expansion. Amputation and casting are not treatments for compartment syndrome.
CN: Physiological integrity; CNS: Physiological adaptation; CL: Application

55. 1. The purpose of the brace is to act as a splint, maintain immobility, and prevent direct contact. A brace does not prevent infection.
CN: Physiological integrity; CNS: Reduction of risk potential; CL: Application

56. 2. Paresthesia is described as numbness and tingling. It is not associated with fever and chills or changes in ROM, nor is it described as pain or blanching.
CN: Physiological integrity; CNS: Physiological adaptation; CL: Analysis

57. A client has been treated for compartment syndrome by undergoing a fasciotomy. Which nursing diagnosis has the <u>highest priority</u> for this client?
1. Chronic pain
2. Risk for infection
3. Impaired gas exchange
4. Decreased cardiac output

58. The community health nurse found an elderly female client lying in the snow. The client was unable to move the right leg because of a fracture. What action should the nurse take <u>first</u>?
1. Immobilize the fracture in its present position.
2. Elevate the leg on whatever is available.
3. Realign the fracture ends.
4. Reduce the fracture.

59. A client is receiving discharge teaching on early signs and symptoms of compartment syndrome to report to the health care provider. The nurse recognizes that teaching has been effective when the client makes which statement?
1. "I will contact my health care provider when I notice redness."
2. "I will contact my health care provider when I notice swelling."
3. "I will contact my health care provider when I have numbness and tingling."
4. "I will contact my health care provider when I notice a change in my skin color."

60. Which of the following symptoms are considered signs of a fracture?
1. Tingling, coolness, and loss of pulses
2. Loss of sensation, redness, and coolness
3. Coolness, redness, and new site of pain
4. Redness, warmth, and pain at the site of injury

61. A nurse is performing a neurovascular assessment. It is most important for the nurse to include which of the following in the assessment?
1. Orientation, movement, pulses, and warmth
2. Capillary refills, movement, pulses, and warmth
3. Orientation, pupillary response, temperature, and pulses
4. Respiratory pattern, orientation, pulses, and temperature

57. 2. Risk for infection is the most appropriate diagnosis following a fasciotomy. A fasciotomy involves the excision of the fascia and leaving the wound unsutured. The wound is covered with dressings that are moistened with sterile saline. The client may develop infection in this open wound. Although there is pain involved, the pain should decrease due to the surgical decompression of the fascia. Gas exchange and cardiac output should not be affected by the fasciotomy.
CN: Physiological integrity; CNS: Physiological adaptation; CL: Analysis

58. 1. Initial treatment of obvious and suspected fractures includes immobilizing and splinting the limb. Any attempt to realign or reset the fracture at the stem may cause further injury and complications. The leg may be elevated only after immobilization.
CN: Safe, effective care environment; CNS: Management of care; CL: Analysis

59. 3. Numbness and tingling is known as paresthesia, which is the earliest sign of compartment syndrome. Pain, heat, and swelling are also signs and symptoms of compartment syndrome, but they occur after paresthesia, making them late signs and symptoms. Skin pallor isn't a sign of compartment syndrome.
CN: Physiological integrity; CNS: Physiological adaptation; CL: Analysis

Knowing normal signs will alert you to what is wrong.

60. 4. Signs of a fracture may include redness, warmth, numbness or loss of sensation, and new site of pain. Coolness, tingling, and loss of pulses are signs of a vascular problem.
CN: Physiological integrity; CNS: Physiological adaptation; CL: Application

61. 2. A correct neurovascular assessment should include capillary refill, movement, pulses, and warmth. Neurovascular assessment involves nerve and blood supply to an area. Respiratory pattern, orientation, temperature, and pupillary response aren't part of a neurovascular examination.
CN: Physiological integrity; CNS: Reduction of risk potential; CL: Application

62. A nurse has instructed a client to accurately measure the circumference of both calves each morning and to report any increase in size. The nurse determines that teaching has been effective when the client makes which statement?
1. "I'll use a measuring tape to check circumference."
2. "I'll use the standardized chart for limb circumference."
3. "I only have to call if one leg is significantly larger than the other."
4. "I can measure my calves either near the knee or closer to the ankle."

Question 62 will help determine how you measure up.

63. The nurse is performing a neurovascular assessment on a client who was admitted with a right fractured femur. The nurse noticed that the pulses are not palpable. What is the <u>most important</u> action of the nurse?
1. Alert the charge nurse immediately.
2. Reassesses the pulses again in 1 hour.
3. Notify the health care provider immediately.
4. Verify the clinical findings with a Doppler ultrasonography.

64. A client with a left arm cast complains of a foul odor. What is the appropriate action by the nurse?
1. Assess further because this may be a sign of an infection.
2. Teach the client proper cast care, including hygiene measures.
3. This is normal, especially when a cast is in place for a few weeks.
4. Assess further because this may be a sign of neurovascular compromise.

65. The nurse is collaborating with the orthopaedic technician regarding interventions to reduce the roughness of a cast. What is the best intervention?
1. Petal the edges.
2. Elevate the limb.
3. Break off the rough area.
4. Distribute pressure evenly.

66. The nurse is aware that elevating a limb with a cast will prevent swelling. Which of the following actions best describes how this should be done?
1. Place the limb with the cast close to the body.
2. Place the limb with the cast at the level of the heart.
3. Place the limb with the cast below the level of the heart.
4. Place the limb with the cast above the level of the heart.

62. 1. The correct method for measuring calf circumference is to use a measuring tape: place the tape at the level where the calf circumference is largest and measure at the same place each time. The client was instructed to report any increase in circumference. A significant increase in calf circumference size might be unilateral or bilateral. There's no standardized chart for limb circumference.

CN: Health promotion and maintenance; CNS: None; CL: Application

63. 4. If pulses are not palpable, verify the assessment with Doppler ultrasonography. If pulses cannot be found with Doppler ultrasonography, immediately notify the physician.

CN: Safe, effective care environment; CNS: Management of care; CL: Application

64. 1. A foul odor from a cast may be a sign of an infection. The nurse needs to assess for fever, malaise, and, possibly, an elevation in white blood cells. Odor from a cast is never normal, and it is not a sign of neurovascular compromise, which would include decreased pulses, coolness, and paresthesia.

CN: Physiological integrity; CNS: Reduction of risk potential; CL: Analysis

65. 1. Petaling the edges will reduce the roughness of the cast. Elevating the limb will prevent swelling. Never break a rough area off the cast. Distributing pressure evenly will prevent pressure ulcers.

CN: Physiological integrity; CNS: Basic care and comfort; CL: Application

66. 4. To reduce swelling, place the limb with the cast above the level of the heart. To elevate a cast, the limb may need to be extended from the body. Placing it below or at the level of the heart will not reduce swelling.

CN: Physiological integrity; CNS: Basic care and comfort; CL: Application

67. A client asks the nurse to explain the reason why a plaster cast cannot get wet. What would be the nurse's <u>best</u> response?
1. A wet cast can cause a foul odor.
2. A wet cast will weaken or be destroyed.
3. A wet cast is heavy and difficult to maneuver.
4. It is okay to get the cast wet, just use a hair dryer to dry it off.

68. A client comes to the emergency department complaining of dull, deep bone pain unrelated to movement. The client asks the nurse if this could be a fracture. The best response by the nurse is:
1. "These are classic symptoms of a fracture."
2. "Fracture pain is sharp and related to movement."
3. "Fracture pain is sharp and unrelated to movement."
4. "Fracture pain is dull and deep and related to movement."

69. The nurse is caring for a client with skeletal traction to the right leg. The client complains of severe right leg pain. Which action should the nurse perform <u>first</u>?
1. Perform pin care.
2. Notify the health care provider.
3. Check the client's alignment in bed.
4. Remove the weights from the traction.

70. A 70-year-old male client is admitted to the medical-surgical unit with a fractured femur. The client is placed in Russell's traction. The client asks the nurse to help him with back care. The <u>most appropriate</u> intervention by the nurse is:
1. telling the client that he can't have back care while he's in traction.
2. telling the client to use the trapeze to lift his back off the bed.
3. supporting the weight to give the client more slack to move.
4. removing the weight to give the client more slack to move.

71. The trauma nurse is caring for a client who was involved in an automobile accident. The trauma nurse would assess the client for which of the following <u>classic</u> fractures?
1. Brachial and clavicle
2. Brachial and humerus
3. Humerus and clavicle
4. Occipital and humerus

Your client depends on you to know the answers.

You're doing great! Keep going!

It's important to understand the different types of fractures.

67. **2.** A wet cast will weaken or be destroyed. A foul odor is a sign of infection. It's never okay to get a cast wet. Fiberglass casts do not lose integrity or strength when wet or damp.

CN: Physiological integrity; CNS: Reduction of risk potential; CL: Application

68. **2.** Fracture pain is sharp and related to movement. Pain that is dull and deep and unrelated to movement is not typical of a fracture.

CN: Health promotion and maintenance; CNS: None; CL: Analysis

69. **3.** A client who complains of severe leg pain may need realignment to ease some pressure on the fracture site. If this is ineffective, then the physician may need to be notified. The weights ordered may be too heavy, but the nurse can't remove them without a physician's order. Performing pin care isn't appropriate at this time.

CN: Safe, effective care environment; CNS: Management of care; CL: Application

70. **2.** The traction must not be disturbed to maintain correct alignment. Therefore, the client should use the trapeze to lift his back off of the bed. The client can have back care as long as he uses the trapeze and does not disturb the alignment. The weight should not be moved without a health care provider's order; it should hang freely without touching anything.

CN: Physiological integrity; CNS: Basic care and comfort; CL: Application

71. **3.** Classic fractures that occur with trauma are those of the humerus and clavicle. There are no brachial bones, and occipital bones are not involved in a traumatic injury.

CN: Physiological integrity; CNS: Physiological adaptation; CL: Analysis

CN: Client needs category   CNS: Client needs subcategory   CL: Cognitive level

72. The nurse is caring for a client who has been placed in traction prior to surgery. The client asks the nurse what is the purpose of the traction. What is the best response by the nurse?
  1. "Traction allows for more activity."
  2. "Traction will help prevent skin breakdown."
  3. "Traction helps with repositioning while in bed."
  4. "Traction helps to prevent trauma and overcome muscle spasms."

73. A 75-year-old client with Paget's disease is undergoing diagnostic exams for a suspected fracture. The nurse should expect to observe which of the following types of fracture?
  1. Linear
  2. Oblique
  3. Transverse
  4. Longitudinal

74. The nurse is caring for a client who has been admitted to the hospital with a diagnosis of Paget's disease and hypertension. Which of the following nursing diagnoses would be a priority plan of care for the client?
  1. Social isolation
  2. Ineffective coping
  3. Impaired physical mobility
  4. Ineffective health maintenance

75. The emergency room nurse is caring for a 20-year-old female client who is complaining of severe pain to the right upper arm. The nurse suspects domestic abuse. Which of the following X-ray findings would indicate the need for additional investigation?
  1. Longitudinal fracture
  2. Transverse fracture
  3. Oblique fracture
  4. Spiral fracture

76. A 25-year-old male client has just had a plaster cast applied to the right forearm following the reduction of a closed radius fracture due to an in-line skating accident. What is the priority assessment for the nurse to perform?
  1. Sensation and movement of the fingers
  2. Whether the client is having any pain
  3. Whether the cast is completely dry
  4. Whether the cast needs petaling

72. 4. Traction prevents trauma and overcomes muscle spasms. Traction doesn't help in preventing skin breakdown, repositioning the client, or allowing the client to become active.
CN: Physiological integrity; CNS: Basic care and comfort; CL: Application

73. 3. A transverse fracture commonly occurs with such bone diseases as osteomalacia and Paget's disease. Linear, longitudinal, and oblique fractures generally occur with trauma.
CN: Physiological integrity; CNS: Physiological adaptation; CL: Application

74. 3. Impaired physical mobility is the priority nursing diagnosis to implement in a plan of care for a client with Paget's disease. A client with Paget's disease needs to remain active to prevent complications from developing. The other nursing diagnoses are appropriate; however, they are not priorities.
CN: Physiological integrity; CNS: Physiological adaptation; CL: Application

75. 4. Spiral fractures are commonly seen in the upper extremities and are related to physical abuse. Longitudinal and oblique fractures generally occur with trauma. A transverse fracture commonly occurs with such bone diseases as osteomalacia and Paget's disease.
CN: Physiological integrity; CNS: Physiological adaptation; CL: Application

76. 1. Neurovascular checks are most important because they are used to determine if any impairment exists after cast application and reduction of the fracture. Checking to see if the cast is completely dry isn't the nurse's highest priority. Petaling to smooth the cast edge is done when the cast is completely dry.
CN: Physiological integrity; CNS: Reduction of risk potential; CL: Application

77. A nurse is caring for a client with a femoral shaft fracture. Which of the following assessment findings is serious and warrants immediate intervention by nurse?
1. Decreased urine output
2. Constipation
3. Hemorrhage
4. Pain

78. The nurse is assessing a client who is admitting for a long bone fracture. Which assessment finding would be noted as a life-threatening complication?
1. Fat emboli
2. Bone emboli
3. Serous emboli
4. Platelet emboli

79. A client is diagnosed with fat emboli. Which signs and symptoms would the nurse expect to find during assessment?
1. Tachypnea, tachycardia, shortness of breath, and paresthesia
2. Paresthesia, bradypnea, bradycardia, and petechial rash on chest and neck
3. Bradypnea, bradycardia, shortness of breath, and petechial rash on chest and neck
4. Tachypnea, tachycardia, shortness of breath, and petechial rash on chest and neck

80. A client has developed a fat embolus. The nurse is aware that the treatment of choice would be which of the following?
1. Antibiotics, I.V. fluids, steroids, and oxygen
2. Theophylline (Theo-24), morphine, oxygen, and I.V. fluids
3. Morphine (Duramorph), oxygen, I.V. fluids, and antibiotics
4. Albuterol (AccuNeb), oxygen, I.V. fluids, and steroids

81. The nurse is caring for a client diagnosed with a fracture. The health care provider ordered a high-protein diet. The nurse explains to the client that the high-protein diet is ordered for which of the following reasons?
1. Protein promotes gluconeogenesis.
2. Protein has anti-inflammatory properties.
3. Protein promotes cell growth and bone union.
4. Protein decreases pain medication requirements.

Wow! This is a serious complication.

Assessment is a key skill for nurses in every field.

77. 3. Femoral shaft fractures may cause hemorrhage, with as much as 1,000 to 1,500 ml of blood loss. Constipation and decreased urine output aren't direct complications of a fracture. Pain may occur, but it can be controlled with analgesia.
CN: Physiological integrity; CNS: Physiological adaptation; CL: Analysis

78. 1. A life-threatening complication of long bone fractures is the development of fat emboli. Bone or platelet emboli are rare occurrences and infrequently associated with long bone fractures. There are no emboli known as serous emboli.
CN: Physiological integrity; CNS: Physiological adaptation; CL: Analysis

79. 4. Signs and symptoms of fat emboli include tachypnea, tachycardia, shortness of breath, and a petechial rash on the chest and neck. The fat molecules enter the venous circulation and travel to the lung, obstructing pulmonary circulation. Bradycardia, bradypnea, and paresthesia are not usual symptoms.
CN: Health promotion and maintenance; CNS: None; CL: Analysis

80. 1. Treatment of a fat embolus may include oxygen, I.V. fluids, steroids to counteract inflammation in the lungs and correct cerebral edema, and antibiotics to prevent infection. Albuterol, morphine, and theophylline aren't commonly used to treat fat emboli.
CN: Physiological integrity; CNS: Physiological adaptation; CL: Analysis

81. 3. High-protein intake promotes cell growth and bone union. Protein does not promote gluconeogenesis, exert anti-inflammatory properties, or decrease pain medication requirements.
CN: Physiological integrity; CNS: Basic care and comfort; CL: Application

82. The nurse is instructing a nursing assistant on the proper care of a client in Buck's extension traction following a fracture of the left fibula. Which of the following observations would indicates that teaching has been effective?
1. The leg in traction is kept externally rotated.
2. The weights are allowed to hang freely over the end of the bed.
3. The nursing assistant instructs the client to perform ankle rotation exercises.
4. The nursing assistant lifts the weights when assisting the client to move up in bed.

83. The nurse is caring for a 70-year-old client who has undergone a right total hip replacement. The nurse is aware that the client should be repositioned:
1. every 1 to 2 hours, from the unaffected side to the back.
2. every 4 to 6 hours, from the unaffected side to the back.
3. every 1 to 2 hours, from the affected side to the back.
4. every 4 to 6 hours, from the affected side to the back.

84. A client is receiving nutritional counseling following an application of a plaster cast for a fracture. The client asks the nurse why vitamin D intake is important. What is the best response by the nurse?
1. Absorption and use of potassium and phosphorus
2. Absorption and use of calcium and phosphorus
3. Excretion of calcium and phosphorus
4. Excretion of potassium and calcium

85. After surgical repair of the client's hip, which of the following positions would be <u>best</u> for this client?
1. Prone
2. Adduction
3. Abduction
4. Subluxated

86. While caring for a client after a left hip replacement, the nurse determines that discharge teaching has been effective when the client states:
1. "I must remain on bed rest."
2. "I have no activity restrictions."
3. "I am allowed limited weight bearing."
4. "I cannot bear any weight for 2 months."

87. Which of the following interventions would help prevent deep vein thrombosis (DVT) after hip surgery?
1. Bed rest
2. Egg crate mattress
3. Vigorous pulmonary care
4. Subcutaneous heparin and pneumatic compression boots

Placing the client in the correct position after hip surgery is critical.

82. 2. In Buck's traction, the weights should hang freely without touching the bed or floor. Lifting the weights would break the traction. The client should be moved up in bed, allowing the weight to move freely along with the client. The leg should be kept in straight alignment. Performing ankle rotation exercises could cause the leg to go out of alignment.
CN: Physiological integrity; CNS: Basic care and comfort; CL: Application

83. 1. The client should be turned at least every 2 hours and always from the unaffected side to the back. The client should never be placed on the affected side. Turning the client every 4 to 6 hours places her at greater risk for skin breakdown.
CN: Physiological integrity; CNS: Reduction of risk potential; CL: Application

84. 2. Vitamin D increases the absorption and use of calcium and phosphorus. Vitamin D does not affect potassium, nor does it reduce the absorption or affect the excretion of calcium and phosphorus.
CN: Physiological integrity; CNS: Pharmacological and parenteral therapies; CL: Application

85. 3. After surgical repair of the hip, the desired position of the legs and hips is abduction. Adduction, prone, or subluxated positions do not keep the prosthesis within the acetabulum.
CN: Physiological integrity; CNS: Reduction of risk potential; CL: Application

86. 3. After a hip replacement, the client's activity is usually ordered as limited weight bearing. The client is allowed to move with restrictions for approximately 2 to 3 months. The hip should not be flexed more than 90 degrees. Abduction past the midline of the body is prohibited. Progressive weight bearing reduces the complications of immobility.
CN: Physiological integrity; CNS: Basic care and comfort; CL: Application

87. 4. To prevent DVT after hip surgery, subcutaneous heparin and pneumatic compression boots are used. Bed rest can cause DVT. Egg crate mattresses and pulmonary care do not prevent DVT.
CN: Physiological integrity; CNS: Reduction of risk potential; CL: Application

88. The nurse is preparing the client for discharge. Which of the following discharge instructions should the nurse provide to the client after hip surgery?
1. "Do not flex the hip more than 30 degrees, do not cross your legs, and get help putting on your shoes."
2. "Do not flex the hip more than 60 degrees, do not cross your legs, and get help putting on your shoes."
3. "Do not flex the hip more than 90 degrees, do not cross your legs, and get help putting on your shoes."
4. "Do not flex the hip more than 120 degrees, do not cross your legs, and get help putting on your shoes."

89. A nurse witnessed an accident. Which of the following interventions would apply to a client with a suspected fracture at the scene of the accident? Select all that apply.
1. Do not move the client.
2. Immobilize the extremity.
3. Move the client to safety immediately.
4. Sit the client up to facilitate the airway.

90. The nurse is evaluating a client on crutches using a three-point gait. Which assessment made by the nurse would indicate that the client is using the crutches appropriately?
1. The client is placing weight on the feet.
2. The client is placing weight on the axillary areas.
3. The client is placing weight on the palms of the hands.
4. The client is placing weight on the palms and axillary areas.

91. A client with a right hip fracture is complaining of left-sided leg pain and edema and has a positive Homans' sign. Based on the clinical findings, which of the following potential complications is a priority for the nurse to address?
1. Deep vein thrombosis (DVT)
2. Pulmonary embolism
3. Fat emboli
4. Infection

92. Which nursing intervention would be appropriate for a client in traction?
1. Add and remove weights as the client wants.
2. Assess the pin sites every shift and as needed.
3. Make sure the knots in the rope catch on the pulley.
4. Give range of motion (ROM) to all joints, including those immediately proximal and distal to the fracture, every shift.

Make sure your initial intervention is the correct one.

88. 3. Discharge instructions should include not flexing the hip more than 90 degrees, not crossing the legs, and getting help to put on shoes. These restrictions prevent dislocation of the new prosthesis.
CN: Physiological integrity; CNS: Reduction of risk potential; CL: Application

89. 2 and 3. At the scene of an accident, a client with a suspected fracture should have the extremity immobilized and be moved to safety. If the client is in a safe place, do not try to move him. Never try to sit the client up; this could make the fracture worse.
CN: Safe, effective care environment; CNS: Safety and infection control; CL: Application

90. 3. To avoid damage to the brachial plexus nerves in the axilla, the palms of the hands should bear the client's weight. Minimal weight should be placed on the affected leg.
CN: Physiological integrity; CNS: Basic care and comfort; CL: Application

91. 1. Unilateral leg pain and edema with a positive Homans' sign (not always present) might be symptoms of DVT. Symptoms of fat emboli include restlessness, tachypnea, and tachycardia and are more common in long bone injuries. It is unlikely an infection would occur on the opposite side of the fracture without cause. Tachycardia, chest pain, and shortness of breath may be symptoms of a pulmonary embolism.
CN: Physiological integrity; CNS: Reduction of risk potential; CL: Application

92. 2. Nursing care for a client in traction may include assessing pin sites every shift and as needed and making sure the knots in the rope do not catch on the pulley. Add and remove weights as the health care provider orders, and give ROM to all joints, except those immediately proximal and distal to the fracture, every shift.
CN: Physiological integrity; CNS: Basic care and comfort; CL: Application

CN: Client needs category   CNS: Client needs subcategory   CL: Cognitive level

93. The nurse is assisting the health care provider with the application of a cast. Which of the following nursing interventions would be included in the immediate cast care?
1. Rest the cast on the bedside table.
2. Dispose of the plaster water in the sink.
3. Support the cast with the palms of the hands.
4. Wait until the cast dries before cleaning the surrounding skin.

94. The health care provider has just removed the cast from a 20-year-old client's lower leg. During the removal, a small superficial abrasion occurred over the ankle. Which statement by the client indicates the need for additional client teaching?
1. "The dry, peeling skin will go away by itself."
2. "I must use a moisturizing lotion on the dry areas."
3. "I can wash the abrasion on my ankle with soap and water."
4. "I will wait until the abrasion is healed before I go swimming."

95. Which statement by the client who recently had a cast applied indicates that the nurse's teaching has been effective?
1. "Heat is a normal sensation as a cast dries."
2. "I'll call my health care provider if I feel any heat."
3. "The cast will need to be removed if I feel any heat."
4. "The heat I feel is most likely caused by an infection."

96. A nurse is providing care for a client with a leg cast. To help prevent foot drop, which action by the nurse would be the <u>most</u> appropriate?
1. Encouraging bed rest
2. Supporting the foot with 45 degrees of flexion
3. Supporting the foot with 90 degrees of flexion
4. Placing a stocking on the foot to provide warmth

97. The nurse is caring for a client with a hip-spica cast. The nurse is teaching the client caregivers about the need to avoid gas-forming foods. Which of the following statements indicates that the nurse's teaching has been effective?
1. "Gas-forming foods should be avoided to prevent flatus."
2. "Gas-forming foods should be avoided to prevent diarrhea."
3. "Gas-forming foods should be avoided to prevent constipation."
4. "Gas-forming foods should be avoided to prevent abdominal distension."

So, when can I sign your cast?

The word *prevent* is a hint. Look for a preventive measure, not a treatment.

93. 3. After helping the health care provider to apply a cast, support it with the palms of the hands; do not rest the cast on a hard or sharp surface. Dispose of the plaster water in a sink with a plaster trap or in a garbage bag. Clean the surrounding skin before the cast dries.

CN: Safe, effective care environment; CNS: Management of care; CL: Application

94. 2. The dry, peeling skin will heal in a few days with normal cleaning; therefore, lotions are unnecessary. Vigorous scrubbing isn't necessary. Washing the abrasion and delaying swimming until healing are correct procedures to follow after removal of a cast.

CN: Physiological integrity; CNS: Reduction of risk potential; CL: Application

95. 1. Normally, as the cast dries, a client may complain of heat from the cast. Offer reassurance. The cast will not need to be removed, and the heath care provider does not need to be notified. Heat from the cast is not a sign of infection.

CN: Physiological integrity; CNS: Reduction of risk potential; CL: Application

96. 3. To prevent foot drop in a leg with a cast, the foot should be supported with 90 degrees of flexion. Bed rest can cause foot drop. Keeping the extremity warm will not prevent foot drop.

CN: Health promotion and maintenance; CNS: None; CL: Application

97. 4. A client with a hip-spica cast should avoid gas-forming foods to prevent abdominal distension. Gas-forming foods may cause flatus, but that is not a reason to avoid them. Gas-forming foods generally do not cause diarrhea or constipation.

CN: Physiological integrity; CNS: Reduction of risk potential; CL: Application

98. A client is demonstrating to the nurse the understanding of touchdown weight bearing prior to discharge. Which of the following outcomes demonstrates that the nurse's teaching is successful?
1. Full weight bearing on the affected extremity
2. 30% to 50% weight bearing on the affected extremity
3. No weight on the extremity but may touch the floor with it
4. No weight on the extremity and keep it elevated at all times

99. A client has attended the sports medicine clinic to learn ways to prevent the risk of experiencing a sports-related injury. Which activity indicates that the client understands how to prevent sports-related injury?
1. Warming up
2. Building strength
3. Pacing the activity
4. Working with moderate intensity

100. A client has just returned from the postanesthesia care unit after undergoing internal fixation of a left femoral neck fracture. The nurse should place the client in which position?
1. The client should be positioned on his back with two pillows between his legs.
2. The client should be positioned on the left side with his right knee bent.
3. The client should be positioned on the right side with his left knee bent.
4. The client should be sitting at a 90-degree angle.

101. Which of the following clinical manifestations would lead the nurse to suspect a fat embolus in a client who has a left femur fracture?
1. Dyspnea
2. Sudden headache
3. Numbness in the left leg
4. Muscle spasm in the left thigh

102. Which statement best explains an open reduction of a fractured femur?
1. Traction will be used.
2. A cast will be applied.
3. Crutches will be used after surgery.
4. Some form of screw, plate, nail, or wire is usually used to maintain alignment.

"Screws, nails, wires—who knew open reduction was so much like home repair?"

98. 3. Touchdown weight bearing involves no weight on the extremity, but the client may touch the floor with the affected extremity. Full weight bearing allows for full weight to be put on the affected extremity. Partial weight bearing allows for 30% to 50% weight bearing on the affected extremity. Non–weight bearing is no weight on the extremity.
CN: Physiological integrity; CNS: Basic care and comfort; CL: Application

99. 1. The best way to prevent sports-related injuries is to warm up. Pacing the activity, building strength, and using moderate intensity are also prevention measures, but warming up is the most effective.
CN: Physiological integrity; CNS: Reduction of risk potential; CL: Application

100. 1. The operative leg must be kept abducted to prevent dislocation of the hip. Placing the client on the left or right side with knee bent does not promote abduction. Acute flexion of the operated hip may cause dislocation. The head of the bed may be raised 35 to 49 degrees.
CN: Physiological integrity; CNS: Reduction of risk potential; CL: Application

101. 1. A fat embolism usually presents as an acute respiratory distress. Symptoms include chest pain, cyanosis, dyspnea, tachypnea, and apprehension. A sudden headache is not a symptom of a fat embolism. Muscle spasms in the left thigh are a neuromuscular response of the local muscle around the femoral fracture. Numbness would be a neurovascular response.
CN: Physiological integrity; CNS: Physiological adaptation; CL: Application

102. 4. Open reduction means that the tissue must be surgically opened and the fractured bones realigned. To maintain proper alignment, a screw, plate, nail, or wire is inserted to prevent the bones from separating. Although traction may have been used before surgery, it won't be needed any longer once the fracture is reduced. A cast or crutches may be used after surgery, but the question asks specifically about the surgical procedure.
CN: Physiological integrity; CNS: Physiological adaptation; CL: Application

CN: Client needs category   CNS: Client needs subcategory   CL: Cognitive level

103. Which of the following clinical manifestations would lead the nurse to suspect that the client has a dislocation of the left hip?
1. Pain relieved with pressure
2. Pain in the inguinal area, abnormal gait
3. Internal rotation of the knee, abduction of the leg
4. Pain in the hip, the thigh appears longer than the unaffected leg

103. 2. A dislocated hip will create problems with walking, and pain is often due to a pinched nerve in the joint. Pressure should not be applied to a painful joint or fracture unless there's hemorrhage. The leg is usually adducted and shortened.
CN: Physiological integrity; CNS: Physiological adaptation; CL: Analysis

104. A 20-year-old client developed osteomyelitis 2 weeks after a fishhook was removed from the client's foot. Which rationale best explains the expected long-term antibiotic therapy needed?
1. Bone has poor circulation.
2. Tissue trauma requires antibiotics.
3. Feet are normally more difficult to treat.
4. Fishhook injuries are highly contaminated.

Why am I so difficult to treat?

104. 1. Bone has very poor blood circulation, making it difficult to treat an infection in the bone. This requires the long-term use of intravenous (I.V.) antibiotics to make sure the infection is cleared. Tissue trauma does not always require antibiotics, at least not long term. Feet are not more difficult to treat than other parts of the body unless the client has a circulatory problem or diabetes mellitus. Fishhooks may not be any more contaminated than another instrument that caused an injury.
CN: Physiological integrity; CNS: Pharmacological and parenteral therapies; CL: Application

105. The nurse is teaching a client diagnosed with degenerative joint disease about the condition. The nurse recognizes teaching has been effective when the client makes which statement?
1. "It is a noninflammatory joint disease."
2. "It is an immune-mediated joint disease."
3. "It is a joint inflammation after a viral infection."
4. "It is a joint inflammation related to systemic infections."

105. 1. Degenerative joint disease is joint disease due to the noninflammatory wear and tear on joints and is often seen in athletes. It is not immune-mediated, inflammatory, or caused by systemic infections.
CN: Physiological integrity; CNS: Physiological adaptation; CL: Application

106. Client education about gout includes which information?
1. Good foot care will reduce complications.
2. Increased dietary intake of purine is needed.
3. Production of uric acid in the kidney affects joints.
4. Uric acid crystals cause inflammatory destruction of the joint.

The words "most appropriate" in question 107 are a clue to the answer.

106. 4. The client needs to know that uric acid crystals collect in the joint of the great toe and cause inflammation. The kidney excretes uric acid, an end product of metabolism. A diet low in purines would be indicated. Good foot care does not affect the development of complications, but increasing water intake may help prevent urinary stone formation.
CN: Physiological integrity; CNS: Reduction of risk potential; CL: Application

107. A client has been treated with I.V. antibiotics for osteomyelitis. The treatment has not been effective. Which intervention would be the <u>most appropriate</u> for this client?
1. Bone grafts
2. Hyperbaric oxygen therapy
3. Amputation of the extremity
4. Debridement of necrotic tissue

107. 4. The tissues may need to be debrided to eliminate necrotic tissue and allow new tissue to form. A bone graft would be done after debridement. Hyperbaric oxygen therapy is a new treatment modality that has been used in the successful treatment of osteomyelitis, but it is not universally available. Amputation is not indicated in the treatment of acute osteomyelitis.
CN: Physiological integrity; CNS: Physiological adaptation; CL: Application

108. A high-protein diet is ordered for a client recovering from a fracture. The nurse explains to the client that which of the following is the reason for this diet?
1. Protein promotes gluconeogenesis.
2. Protein has anti-inflammatory properties.
3. Protein promotes cell growth and bone union.
4. Protein decreases pain medication requirements.

109. The nurse is caring a client who has been admitted to the hospital with a musculoskeletal injury. Cold therapy is ordered for which of the following reasons?
1. It promotes analgesia and circulation.
2. It numbs the nerves and dilates the vessels.
3. It promotes circulation and reduces muscle spasms.
4. It causes local vasoconstriction and prevents edema or muscle spasm.

110. What discharge information should be given to a client with a cast?
1. Use powder under the cast as needed.
2. Itching under the cast indicates infection.
3. Keep the extremity in a dependent position.
4. Report fever and foul odors around the cast.

111. The nurse is assessing a client and determines that which of the following is a risk factor for traction-related complications?
1. Coronary artery disease
2. Diabetes mellitus
3. Hypertension
4. Hip fracture

112. A client tells the nurse that she experiences pain and numbness in the fingers when typing on a computer keyboard. Which action will help the nurse assess for Phalen's sign?
1. Having the client hold both wrists in acute flexion with the dorsal surfaces touching for 60 seconds
2. Having the client hold both hands above her head with her arms straight for 30 seconds
3. Having the client extend her wrists while the nurse provides resistance
4. Tapping gently over the median nerve in the wrist

Which action will help the nurse assess for Phalen's sign?

108. 3. High-protein intake promotes cell growth and bone union. Protein does not decrease pain medication requirements, have anti-inflammatory properties, or promote gluconeogenesis.
CN: Physiological integrity; CNS: Basic care and comfort; CL: Application

109. 4. Cold causes the blood vessels to constrict, which reduces the leakage of fluid into the tissues and prevents swelling and muscle spasms. Cold therapy may reduce pain by numbing the nerves and tissues. Heat therapy promotes circulation, enhances flexibility, reduces muscle spasms, and also provides analgesia.
CN: Physiological integrity; CNS: Basic care and comfort; CL: Application

110. 4. Fever, foul odor, and warmth over a specific area of the cast after it is dry may be signs of infection. Itchy skin results from dry skin, and powder should not be used. The extremity should be elevated for 24 to 48 hours.
CN: Health promotion and maintenance; CNS: None; CL: Application

111. 2. Because people with diabetes commonly have microvascular compromise and delayed wound healing, they need careful monitoring for early signs of skin breakdown. The other conditions do not increase the risk of traction-related complications.
CN: Physiological integrity; CNS: Reduction of risk potential; CL: Analysis

112. 1. Acute wrist flexion places pressure on the inflamed median nerve, causing the pain and numbness of carpal tunnel syndrome (Phalen's sign). Holding the hands above the head with arms straight for 30 seconds is not an assessment technique. Tapping gently over the median nerve tests for Tinel's sign, which is another sign of carpal tunnel syndrome. Placing the wrists in extension against resistance tests the strength.
CN: Physiological integrity; CNS: Physiological adaptation; CL: Application

113. A client has a knee-high cast removed 6 weeks after suffering an ankle fracture. Palpation reveals a hard, nontender lump at the fracture site. How should the nurse interpret this finding?
1. Abnormal; the bone may have healed in misalignment, possibly from the short leg cast
2. Abnormal; remodeling should have occurred by now, so the findings suggest malunion
3. Normal; callus formation normally occurs at this stage and may feel like a lump on the bone
4. Normal; swelling and bruising may persist after a traumatic fracture

114. A client is being discharged from the emergency department after cast application for a tibial fracture. The nurse is aware that the client is at risk for ineffective breathing pattern related to long bone fracture secondary to fat embolus. Based on this diagnosis, which instruction should the nurse provide for this client?
1. Cough and deep breathe at least every 2 hours.
2. Restrict your fluid intake to 1 L per day.
3. Keep the leg elevated and apply ice for the first 24 to 48 hours.
4. Call the physician at once if you experience apprehensiveness, shortness of breath, fever, or palpitations.

115. A client who is receiving acetaminophen (Tylenol) for osteoarthritis complains of continuing pain. The health care provider prescribes celecoxib (Celebrex). Which medication instruction should the nurse provide to this client?
1. Report black and tarry stools to the health care provider.
2. Use a stool softener or fiber laxative daily to prevent constipation.
3. If you miss a dose, take a double dose the next day.
4. Don't take the medication with dairy products.

116. A client has an above-the-knee amputation 4 days after a <u>traumatic injury</u>. Which nursing diagnosis is <u>most</u> appropriate?
1. Risk for impaired skin integrity related to decreased peripheral circulation
2. Decreased cardiac output related to shock caused by decreased fluid volume
3. Impaired gas exchange related to fat embolism caused by surgical removal of bone and tissue
4. Acute pain related to phantom limb pain caused by surgical removal of leg after traumatic injury

Which instruction should the nurse provide?

This question is a double-hinter.

113. 3. Callus formation is a normal stage of bone repair. It is characterized by an overgrowth of bone that is reabsorbed gradually during the remodeling stage. This deformity is painless, whereas misalignment and malunion typically cause pain. Swelling and bruising should have disappeared by this time.

CN: Physiological integrity; CNS: Physiological adaptation; CL: Analysis

114. 4. Fat embolism is a complication of a long bone fracture. Signs and symptoms include apprehension; altered mental status; respiratory distress; tachycardia; tachypnea; fever; and petechiae over the neck, upper arms, and chest. Coughing and deep-breathing exercises as well as leg elevations with ice applications can help prevent other complications of a long bone fracture but have no effect on fat emboli. The client should also be instructed that drinking plenty of fluids to stay well hydrated will help him avoid embolic complications.

CN: Physiological integrity; CNS: Reduction of risk potential; CL: Application

115. 1. Black and tarry stools are a sign of gastrointestinal (GI) bleeding and may necessitate a medication change. Dairy products help reduce GI irritation. The celecoxib dose should never be doubled. Constipation isn't an adverse effect of this drug.

CN: Physiological integrity; CNS: Pharmacological and parenteral therapies; CL: Application

116. 4. Phantom limb pain is common after limb amputation and may be more severe with traumatic injury. Because the limb was severed traumatically rather than removed because of poor circulation, peripheral circulation should be adequate. Fat embolism is more typical with long bone fractures. The risk of shock is relatively low on the fourth postoperative day.

CN: Psychosocial integrity; CNS: None; CL: Analysis

117. A nurse is assigned to care for a 70-year-old client with <u>acute</u> rheumatoid arthritis. Which assessment finding should the nurse expect to find during the physical examination?
1. Radial deviation of the distal phalanges
2. Tender, painful, and stiff joints
3. Heberden's nodes
4. Bouchard's nodes

118. A client with lactose intolerance requires dietary teaching. Which foods should the nurse advise the client to eat to ensure adequate calcium intake?
1. Cheese and yogurt
2. Beef liver and broccoli
3. Bananas and avocados
4. Collard greens and spinach

119. An elderly client in a nursing home is particularly susceptible to bone loss. The nurse is aware that bone loss may be caused by which of the following?
1. Chronic use of stool softeners
2. Calcium channel blockers
3. Lack of sunlight exposure
4. Decreased mobility

120. A client with a torn meniscus caused by a football injury arrives at the outpatient surgery clinic for an arthroscopic meniscectomy. What is the most important information for the nurse to give the client?
1. Exactly how the procedure will be performed
2. Avoidance of weight bearing for 2 weeks after the surgery
3. Postoperative exercises, such as straight-leg raising and quadriceps setting
4. The possibility of severe postoperative pain for 24 to 48 hours after surgery

121. A client is ready to be discharged after arthroscopic knee surgery. Which instruction should the nurse expect the health care provider to provide?
1. Ice and elevate the extremity for 12 hours after discharge.
2. Infection isn't a potential problem because of the small incision size.
3. Swelling and coolness of the joint and limb are normal right after surgery.
4. Take acetaminophen with codeine every 4 hours as necessary for pain relief.

I need my rays!

Exercise your knowledge by teaching your client.

117. **2.** Tender, painful, and stiff joints characterize acute rheumatoid arthritis. The other assessment findings characterize osteoarthritis, including nodules on the dorsolateral aspects of the distal interphalangeal joints (Heberden's nodules), flexion and deviation deformities, like radial deviation of the distal phalanges, and nodules on the proximal interphalangeal joints (Bouchard's nodes).
CN: Physiological integrity; CNS: Physiological adaptation; CL: Application

118. **4.** Dark green, leafy vegetables are the best nondairy sources of calcium. Bananas and avocados are good sources of vitamin K. Beef liver and broccoli supply iron. Cheese and yogurt are dairy products, which this client should avoid because of the lactose intolerance.
CN: Physiological integrity; CNS: Basic care and comfort; CL: Application

119. **3.** Lack of sunlight exposure decreases absorption of vitamin D, which must be present for calcium to be absorbed from the small intestine. Calcium channel blockers do not affect serum calcium levels. Stool softeners do not increase peristalsis, so they do not impair calcium absorption. Decreased mobility is a result, not a cause, of bone loss. Immobility results in a loss of bone density.
CN: Health promotion and maintenance; CNS: None; CL: Analysis

120. **3.** The best time to teach about postoperative care is preoperatively. Straight-leg raising and quadriceps setting exercises help maintain the strength of the affected extremity. The health care provider, not the nurse, should explain the surgical procedure. Weight bearing may begin as soon as the day of surgery. Usually, pain is mild to moderate after arthroscopic surgery.
CN: Physiological integrity; CNS: Basic care and comfort; CL: Application

121. **4.** Mild to moderate pain is normal after this type of surgery and can be relieved by oral narcotic analgesics. To minimize swelling, the client should ice and elevate the extremity for at least 24 hours after surgery. Infection is a potential problem after an invasive procedure. Swelling and coolness of the joint and limb may indicate complications from tourniquet use during surgery.
CN: Physiological integrity; CNS: Basic care and comfort; CL: Application

122. A perimenopausal client is at high risk for osteoporosis because of family history, lactose intolerance, and small body frame. The client asks the nurse how to prevent osteoporosis. What is the most important information for the nurse to provide for this client?
1. Increase the amount of calcium and vitamin D in your diet.
2. Hormone replacement therapy (HRT) is recommended.
3. Have a bone density test yearly.
4. It is not necessary to stop smoking.

Counsel your client about health history risk factors.

122. 1. Adequate calcium and vitamin D intake are an important part of an overall prevention program. Bone density tests can evaluate the risk for osteoporosis but do not need to be done yearly. Smoking is a risk factor for developing osteoporosis. Studies show that estrogen in HRT may influence the development of breast and uterine cancers.

CN: Physiological integrity; CNS: Pharmacological and parenteral therapies; CL: Analysis

123. A client is diagnosed with Ewing's sarcoma. The nurse anticipates that which test would be most appropriate in determining the extent of metastasis?
1. Bone scan
2. Computed tomography (CT) scan
3. Magnetic resonance imaging (MRI)
4. Positron emission tomography (PET)

123. 1. A bone scan views the entire skeletal structure, indicating areas of possible metastases. CT scan, MRI, and PET scan visualize only one body area at a time.

CN: Physiological integrity; CNS: Reduction of risk potential; CL: Application

124. An 80-year-old client with pneumonia is admitted to the hospital. The client has a past medical history that includes chronic rheumatoid arthritis. Which assessment finding should the nurse expect during the physical examination?
1. Thickened plaque overlying the flexor tendon of the ring finger
2. Cystic swelling on the dorsum of the wrist
3. Flattened thenar eminence
4. Swan-neck deformity

Pay close attention to the word chronic and what it implies.

124. 4. In chronic rheumatoid arthritis, the fingers may show hyperextension of the proximal interphalangeal joints with fixed flexion of the distal interphalangeal joints, referred to as swan-neck deformities. Flattened thenar eminence characterizes thenar atrophy, a condition that suggests an ulnar nerve disorder. The first sign of a Dupuytren's contracture is a thickened plaque overlying the flexor tendon of the ring finger and possibly the little finger at the level of the distal palmar crease. Ganglia are cystic, round, usually nontender swellings located along tendon sheaths or joint capsules; ganglia frequently involve the dorsum of the wrist.

CN: Physiological integrity; CNS: Physiological adaptation; CL: Application

125. A 64-year-old client with complications related to metastatic cancer and complaints of back pain is admitted to the hospital. Which assessment finding should the nurse expect during the physical examination?
1. A gibbous
2. A rounded thoracic convexity
3. An accentuation of the normal lumbar curve
4. Gentle concavities in the cervical and lumbar regions and a convexity in the thorax

125. 1. A gibbous is an angular deformity of collapsed vertebra and is frequently caused by metastatic cancer or tuberculosis of the spine. A rounded thoracic convexity, kyphosis, is common in aging, especially in women. Gentle curves of the normal spine include concavities in the cervical and lumbar regions and a convexity of the thorax. An accentuation of the normal lumbar curve, called lordosis, frequently develops to compensate for the protuberant abdomen of pregnancy or marked obesity.

CN: Physiological integrity; CNS: Physiological adaptation; CL: Application

126. An elderly client with rheumatoid arthritis is being treated with prednisone (Deltasone). The nurse is aware that complications occurring with long-term therapy include which of the following?
1. Breast and uterine cancer
2. Osteoporosis and diabetes mellitus
3. Weight loss and lactose intolerance
4. Deep vein thrombosis (DVT), pulmonary embolus, and stroke

127. A client with a femoral fracture is in skeletal traction. During the initial shift assessment, the nurse finds that the weight used in traction is heavier than specified by the nursing care plan. Which action should the nurse take <u>first</u>?
1. Ask the health care provider during rounds if the order for the weight was changed.
2. Check the health care provider's orders to see if the orders included a weight change.
3. Assume that if the weight was changed, the health care provider ordered it.
4. Remove the weight and replace it with the weight specified in the plan.

128. The nurse is assessing a client's response to skeletal traction applied to the lower extremity. Which finding would be considered to be <u>normal</u>?
1. Coolness and pallor below the fracture level
2. Moderate to severe muscle spasms around the fracture area
3. Serous drainage and crust formation at the pin insertion site
4. Erythema and swelling immediately around the pin insertion site

129. Which nursing diagnosis is appropriate for a client with diabetes who is placed in skeletal traction after a motor vehicle collision?
1. Imbalanced nutrition: Less than body requirements related to malabsorption of nutrients
2. Risk for injury related to subluxation of the joint above the pin insertion site
3. Risk for autonomic dysreflexia related to bed rest
4. Risk for infection related to the skeletal pin

130. A client in skeletal traction complains of pain and received a dose of an analgesic 1 hour ago. The nurse educates and offers the client an alternative pain-management measure. Which of the following actions should be implemented based on the nurse's scope of practice?
1. Acupressure and shiatsu
2. Relaxation and imagery
3. Hypnosis and therapeutic touch
4. Swedish massage and the Feldenkrais method

I can see the finish line! Keep going!

What's the first thing you would do?

Which nursing diagnosis is appropriate?

126. 2. Long-term prednisone therapy can increase the loss of calcium from bones, slow down the formation of new bone tissue (resulting in osteoporosis), and alter glucose metabolism (resulting in diabetes mellitus). Breast and uterine cancer, DVT, pulmonary embolus, stroke, weight loss, and lactose intolerance are not common adverse effects of prednisone.

CN: Physiological integrity; CNS: Pharmacological and parenteral therapies; CL: Analysis

127. 2. First, the nurse should check the physician's orders to see if a weight change was ordered. If it was, the nurse responsible for ensuring implementation of the care plan should investigate why the change was not incorporated in the plan.

CN: Safe, effective care environment; CNS: Management of care; CL: Analysis

128. 3. Serous drainage around the pin insertion site is a normal finding; some institutions do not recommend crust removal because of its protective nature. A pale extremity may indicate arterial compromise. Erythema and swelling signal infection. Severe muscle spasms may indicate improper alignment of the body or traction.

CN: Physiological integrity; CNS: Reduction of risk potential; CL: Analysis

129. 4. This client has a significant risk of osteomyelitis secondary to the skeletal pin. A dangerous bone infection that's hard to eradicate, osteomyelitis should be prevented at all costs—especially in a client with diabetes, who is already prone to infection. Based on the information provided, the other nursing diagnoses aren't appropriate.

CN: Physiological integrity; CNS: Reduction of risk potential; CL: Analysis

130. 2. Relaxation and imagery are effective adjuncts to pharmacological pain management that the nurse can implement without a physician's order. Although the other therapies may promote pain management, they require special training or certification.

CN: Physiological integrity; CNS: Basic care and comfort; CL: Application

131. The nurse is examining the hands of a client with osteoarthritis and notes Heberden's nodes on the second (pointer) finger. Briefly write an answer to identify the area on the finger where the nurse observed the nodes.

_____

_____

_____

132. A client is diagnosed with gout. Which foods should the nurse instruct the client to eat in moderation? Select all that apply.
  1. Green, leafy vegetables
  2. Chocolate
  3. Sardines
  4. Liver
  5. Cod
  6. Eggs

133. A client is in the emergency department with a suspected fracture of the right hip. Which assessment(s) should the nurse expect to find? Select all that apply.
  1. The right leg is longer than the left leg.
  2. The right leg is shorter than the left leg.
  3. The right leg is externally rotated.
  4. The right leg is internally rotated.
  5. The right leg is abducted.
  6. The right leg is adducted.

No bones about it. You did it!

131. Heberden's nodes appear on the distal interphalangeal joints. These bony and cartilaginous enlargements are usually hard and painless and typically occur in middle-aged and elderly clients with osteoarthritis.

CN: Physiological integrity; CNS: Physiological adaptation: CL: Application

132. 3, 4, and 5. Clients with gout should avoid foods that are high in purines, such as liver, cod, and sardines. They should also avoid anchovies, sweetbreads, lentils, and alcoholic beverages, especially beer and wine. Green, leafy vegetables, chocolate, and eggs are not high in purines.

CN: Physiological integrity; CNS: Basic care and comfort; CL: Application

133. 2, 3, and 6. In a hip fracture, the affected leg is shorter, adducted, and externally rotated.

CN: Physiological integrity; CNS: Physiological adaptation; CL: Application

Chapter 8
Gastrointestinal disorders

1. A client asks the nurse what caused the development of a hiatal hernia? What is the best response by the nurse?
1. Increased intrathoracic pressure
2. Weakness of the esophageal muscle
3. Increased esophageal muscle pressure
4. Weakness of the diaphragmatic muscle

2. Risk factors for the development of hiatal hernias are those that lead to increased abdominal pressure. The nurse understands that which of the following complications is most likely to result in a hiatal hernia?
1. Obesity
2. Volvulus
3. Constipation
4. Intestinal obstruction

3. A client is admitted with a hiatal hernia. The nurse should assess the client for which symptom?
1. Left arm pain
2. Lower back pain
3. Esophageal reflux
4. Abdominal cramping

4. A nurse is preparing to teach a client with a hiatal hernia. The nurse should provide instruction on which diagnostic test?
1. Colonoscopy
2. Lower GI series
3. Barium swallow
4. Abdominal X-ray series

You know what they say, "You are what you eat."

crackle crackle

Which test allows the radiologist to see the stomach in relation to the diaphragm?

1. 4. A hiatal hernia is caused by weakness of the diaphragmatic muscle and increased intra-abdominal—not intrathoracic—pressure. This weakness allows the stomach to slide into the esophagus. The esophageal supports weaken, but esophageal muscle weakness or increased esophageal muscle pressure isn't a factor in hiatal hernia.
CN: Physiological integrity; CNS: Physiological adaptation; CL: Application

2. 1. Obesity may cause increased abdominal pressure that pushes the lower portion of the stomach into the thorax. A volvulus is a type of intestinal obstruction. Constipation has no effect on a hiatal hernia. Obstructions may complicate a rolling hiatal hernia, but they don't cause the hernia.
CN: Physiological integrity; CNS: Physiological adaptation; CL: Analysis

3. 3. Esophageal reflux is a common symptom of hiatal hernia. This seems to be associated with chronic exposure of the lower esophageal sphincter to the lower pressure of the thorax, making it less effective. Left arm pain is a common symptom of heart attack. Lower back pain can be caused by lumbar strain. Abdominal cramping can be caused by intestinal infection.
CN: Physiological integrity; CNS: Physiological adaptation; CL: Application

4. 3. A barium swallow with fluoroscopy shows the position of the stomach in relation to the diaphragm. A colonoscopy and a lower GI series show disorders of the intestine. An abdominal X-ray series will show structural defects but not necessarily a hiatal hernia, unless it's sliding or rolling at the time of the X-ray.
CN: Health promotion and maintenance; CNS: None; CL: Application

CN: Client needs category   CNS: Client needs subcategory   CL: Cognitive level

5. A client is admitted with right lower quadrant pain, anorexia, nausea, low-grade fever, and elevated white blood cell count. Based on these assessments, which of the following complications is the client most likely experiencing?
1. A fecalith
2. Bowel kinking
3. Internal bowel occlusion
4. Abdominal wall swelling

6. The nurse is assessing a client with suspected appendicitis. The nurse would expect the client to use which of the following terms to describe their pain?
1. Aching
2. Fleeting
3. Intermittent
4. Steady

7. Which of the following positions would the nurse assist a client to assume for the relief of pain experienced with appendicitis?
1. Prone
2. Sitting
3. Supine, stretched out
4. Lying with legs drawn up

8. Which nursing intervention should be the <u>priority</u> when caring for a client with appendicitis?
1. Assessing for pain
2. Encouraging oral intake of clear fluids
3. Providing discharge teaching
4. Assessing for symptoms of peritonitis

9. The nurse is teaching the client about gastritis. Which of the following statements by the nurse would be the most accurate in describing gastritis?
1. Erosion of the gastric mucosa
2. Inflammation of a diverticulum
3. Inflammation of the gastric mucosa
4. Reflux of stomach acid into the esophagus

Evaluate each position to determine which one will ease your client's pain.

Does anyone know what's causing me all this pain?

5. 1. The client is experiencing appendicitis. A fecalith is a fecal calculus, or stone, that occludes the lumen of the appendix and is the most common cause of appendicitis. Bowel wall swelling, kinking of the appendix, and external occlusion, not internal occlusion, of the bowel by adhesions can also be causes of appendicitis.
CN: Physiological integrity; CNS: Physiological adaptation; CL: Analysis

6. 4. The pain begins in the epigastrium or periumbilical region and then shifts to the right lower quadrant and becomes steady. The pain may be moderate to severe.
CN: Physiological integrity; CNS: Physiological adaptation; CL: Application

7. 4. Lying still with the legs drawn up toward the chest helps relieve tension on the abdominal muscles, which helps to reduce the amount of discomfort felt. Lying flat or sitting may increase the amount of pain experienced.
CN: Physiological integrity; CNS: Physiological adaptation; CL: Application

8. 4. The focus of care is to assess for peritonitis, or inflammation of the peritoneal cavity. Peritonitis is most commonly caused by appendix rupture and invasion of bacteria, which could be lethal. The client with appendicitis will have pain that should be controlled with analgesia. The nurse should discourage oral intake in preparation for surgery. Discharge teaching is important; however, in the acute phase, management should focus on minimizing preoperative complications and recognizing when such may be occurring.
CN: Safe, effective care environment; CNS: Management of care; CL: Application

9. 3. Gastritis is an inflammation of the gastric mucosa that may be acute (often resulting from exposure to local irritants) or chronic (associated with autoimmune infections or atrophic disorders of the stomach). Erosion of the mucosa results in ulceration. Inflammation of a diverticulum is called diverticulitis; reflux of stomach acid is known as gastroesophageal reflux disease.
CN: Physiological integrity; CNS: Physiological adaptation; CL: Analysis

10.   A 30-year-old client is complaining of reflux in his esophagus 1 to 2 hours after eating or when lying down for the last 2 weeks. The nurse recognizes that this symptom is related to which of the following disorders?
1. Myocardial infarction (MI)
2. Lumbar strain
3. Hiatal hernia
4. Intestinal infection

11.   Which nursing intervention should be included in the <u>immediate</u> postoperative management of a client who has undergone gastric resection?
1. Monitoring gastric pH to detect complications
2. Assessing for bowel sounds
3. Providing nutritional support
4. Monitoring for symptoms of hemorrhage

12.   A client is being admitted with acute gastritis. The nurse knows the immediate collaborative treatment plan will include which of the following?
1. Reducing work stress
2. Completing a gastric resection
3. Treating the underlying cause
4. Administering enteral tube feedings

13.   Upon reviewing the history of a client with chronic gastritis, which of the following may be a risk factor for the development of this condition?
1. Adolescent client
2. Antibiotic usage
3. Gallbladder disease
4. *Helicobacter pylori* infection

You'll most likely know this answer if you just give it some thought.

I can cause a stomach to writhe in pain!

10. **3.** Esophageal reflux is a common symptom of hiatal hernia. This condition seems to be associated with chronic exposure of the lower esophageal sphincter to the lower pressure of the thorax, making it less effective. MI may present with indigestion but not reflux. This symptom isn't associated with the other conditions.

CN: Physiological integrity; CNS: physiological adaptation; CL: Analysis

11. **4.** The client should be monitored closely for signs and symptoms of hemorrhage, such as bright red blood in the nasogastric tube suction, tachycardia, or a drop in blood pressure. Gastric pH may be monitored to evaluate the need for histamine-2 receptor antagonists. Bowel sounds may not return for up to 72 hours postoperatively. Nutritional needs should be addressed soon after surgery.

CN: Physiological integrity; CNS: Reduction of risk potential; CL: Analysis

12. **3.** Discovering and treating the cause of gastritis is the most beneficial approach. Reducing the amount of stress and reducing or eliminating oral intake until the symptoms are gone are important in the recovery phase. A gastric resection is only an option when serious erosion has occurred.

CN: Safe, effective care environment; CNS: Safety and infection control; CL: Analysis

13. **4.** *H. pylori* infection can lead to chronic atrophic gastritis. Chronic gastritis can occur at any age but is more common in older adults. It may be caused by conditions that allow reflux of bile acids into the stomach. Drugs such as nonsteroidal antiinflammatory agents, not antibiotics, may cause gastritis. Chronic gastritis isn't related to gallbladder disease.

CN: Health promotion and maintenance; CNS: None; CL: Analysis

14. A client with chronic gastritis asks why they need to have injections of vitamin B$_{12}$. Which response by the nurse is most appropriate?
1. "Your white blood cell count is low."
2. "It will give you more energy."
3. "Your condition does not allow vitamin B$_{12}$ to be absorbed."
4. "It is necessary for people with this disorder."

Hmmm. I should be absorbable under normal conditions.

14. 3. With gastritis, the stomach lining becomes thin and atrophic, decreasing the stomach acid secretion (the source of intrinsic factor). This causes a reduction in the absorption of vitamin B$_{12}$, which can lead to pernicious anemia. Chronic gastritis does not cause a decrease in the white blood count. While vitamin B$_{12}$ injections may increase a client's energy, this is not the most appropriate answer to the client's question.

CN: Physiological integrity; CNS: Physiological adaptation; CL: Analysis

15. In which developmental stage would the nurse note that a client is at risk of developing diverticulosis?
1. Infant
2. School age
3. Young adult
4. Older adult

15. 4. As clients age, the incidence of diverticulosis increases. Almost two-thirds of the population is diagnosed with diverticulosis by age 85.

CN: Health promotion and maintenance; CNS: None; CL: Application

16. A client newly diagnosed with diverticulosis is being discharged. The client asks the nurse what type of diet may have contributed to the diagnosis. What is the best response by the nurse?
1. Low-fiber diet
2. High-fiber diet
3. High-protein diet
4. Low-carbohydrate diet

Looks like the door is wide open for my entrance!

16. 1. Low-fiber diets have been implicated in the development of diverticula because these diets decrease the bulk in the stool and predispose the person to the development of constipation. A high-fiber diet is recommended to help prevent diverticulosis. A high-protein or low-carbohydrate diet has no effect on the development of diverticulosis.

CN: Physiological integrity; CNS: Basic care and comfort; CL: Analysis

17. Which mechanism can facilitate the development of diverticulosis into diverticulitis?
1. Treating constipation with chronic laxative use, leading to dependence on the laxatives
2. Chronic constipation causing an obstruction, reducing forward flow of intestinal contents
3. Herniation of the intestinal mucosa, rupturing the wall of the intestine
4. Undigested food blocking the diverticulum, predisposing the area to bacterial invasion

17. 4. Undigested food can block the diverticulum, decreasing blood supply to the area and predisposing the area to the invasion of bacteria. Chronic laxative use is a common problem in elderly clients, but it doesn't cause diverticulitis. Chronic constipation can cause an obstruction—not diverticulitis. Herniation of the intestinal mucosa causes an intestinal perforation.

CN: Physiological integrity; CNS: Physiological adaptation; CL: Analysis

Sometimes you have to read between the lines.

18. While reviewing the clinical presentation of clients with diverticular disease, the nurse understands that which of the following symptoms indicates diverticulosis?
1. No symptoms exist
2. Change in bowel habits
3. Anorexia and low-grade fever
4. Episodic, dull or steady midabdominal pain

18. 1. Diverticulosis is an asymptomatic condition. The other choices are signs and symptoms of diverticulitis.

CN: Physiological integrity; CNS: Physiological adaptation; CL: Analysis

19. Which test should the nurse expect to be ordered for a client suspected of having diverticulosis?
1. Abdominal ultrasound
2. Barium enema
3. Barium swallow
4. Gastroscopy

20. The nurse has provided discharge teaching for a client who was hospitalized and treated for acute diverticulitis. Which statement by the client indicates understanding of the discharge instructions?
1. "I'll reduce my fluid intake."
2. "I'll decrease the fiber in my diet."
3. "I'll take all of my antibiotics."
4. "I'll exercise to increase my intra-abdominal pressure."

It's time for us to get to work.

21. Crohn's disease can be described as a chronic relapsing disease. Which area of the GI system may be involved with this disease?
1. The entire length of the large colon
2. Only the sigmoid area
3. The entire large colon through the layers of mucosa and submucosa
4. The small intestine and colon, affecting the entire thickness of the bowel

22. A client presents with a recurrence of Crohn's disease. Which area of the alimentary canal does the nurse suspect is involved?
1. Ascending colon
2. Descending colon
3. Sigmoid colon
4. Terminal ileum

Sometimes you just have to blame it on your jeans—I mean genes.

23. A nurse is preparing the teaching plan for a client with Crohn's disease. Which factor should the nurse include as a possible link to the development of this disease?
1. Constipation
2. Diet
3. Heredity
4. Lack of exercise

19. **2.** A barium enema will cause diverticula to fill with barium and be easily seen on an X-ray. An abdominal ultrasound can tell more about structures, such as the gallbladder, liver, and spleen, than the intestine. A barium swallow and gastroscopy view upper GI structures.
CN: Health promotion and maintenance; CNS: None; CL: Application

20. **3.** Antibiotics are used to reduce the inflammation and potential infectious process. The client typically isn't allowed anything orally until the acute episode subsides. Parenteral fluids are given until the client feels better; then it's recommended that the client drink eight 8-oz glasses of water per day and gradually increase fiber in the diet to improve intestinal motility. During the acute phase, activities that increase intra-abdominal pressure should be avoided to decrease pain and the chance of intestinal obstruction.
CN: Physiological integrity; CNS: Physiological adaptation; CL: Analysis

21. **4.** Crohn's disease more commonly involves any segment of the small intestine, the colon, or both, affecting the entire thickness of the bowel. However, it can also affect the digestive system anywhere from the mouth to the anus. Options 1 and 3 describe ulcerative colitis. Option 2 is too specific and, therefore, not likely.
CN: Physiological integrity; CNS: Physiological adaptation; CL: Application

22. **4.** Studies have shown that the terminal ileum is the most common site for recurrence in clients with Crohn's disease. The other areas may be involved but aren't as common.
CN: Physiological integrity; CNS: Physiological adaptation; CL: Application

23. **3.** Although the definitive cause of Crohn's disease is unknown, it's thought to be associated with infectious, immune, or psychological factors. Because it has a higher incidence in siblings, it may have a genetic cause.
CN: Health promotion and maintenance; CNS: None; CL: Analysis

24. A nurse is reviewing the causes of ulcerative colitis with a client. Which factor is believed to cause ulcerative colitis?
1. Acidic diet
2. Altered immunity
3. Chronic constipation
4. Emotional stress

25. A client is admitted with an anorectal fistula. The nurse is aware that the client most likely has which condition?
1. Crohn's disease
2. Diverticulitis
3. Diverticulosis
4. Ulcerative colitis

NCLEX questions sure can be a fistula full of trouble!

26. A client with Crohn's disease experiences 20 watery stools per day. When assessing the client, the nurse would anticipate which finding?
1. Tenting skin turgor
2. Decreased heart rate
3. Dilute urine
4. Elevated blood pressure

27. Which associated disorder might a client with ulcerative colitis exhibit?
1. Gallstones
2. Hydronephrosis
3. Nephrolithiasis
4. Toxic megacolon

Many GI disorders have similar symptoms. Pay attention to which one the question is asking about.

28. Which associated disorder might a client with Crohn's disease exhibit most often?
1. Ankylosing spondylitis
2. Colon cancer
3. Malabsorption
4. Lactase deficiency

24. 2. Several theories exist regarding the cause of ulcerative colitis. One suggests altered immunity as the cause based on the extraintestinal characteristics of the disease, such as peripheral arthritis and cholangitis. Diet and constipation have no effect on the development of ulcerative colitis. Emotional stress may exacerbate the attacks but isn't believed to be the primary cause.
CN: Health promotion and maintenance; CNS: None; CL: Analysis

25. 1. As the disease progresses, the lesions of Crohn's disease become transmural; that is, they involve all thicknesses of the bowel. These lesions may perforate the bowel wall, forming fistulas with adjacent structures. Fistulas don't develop in diverticulitis or diverticulosis. The ulcers that occur in the submucosal and mucosal layers of the intestine in ulcerative colitis usually don't progress to fistula formation as in Crohn's disease.
CN: Physiological integrity; CNS: Physiological adaptation; CL: Analysis

26. 1. Signs and symptoms of dehydration include poor (tenting) skin turgor, increased heart rate, concentrated urine, and decreased blood pressure. Other signs are dry skin and mouth, sunken eyes, and lethargy.
CN: Physiological integrity; CNS: Physiological adaptation; CL: Analysis

27. 4. Toxic megacolon is extreme dilation of a segment of the diseased colon caused by paralysis of the colon, resulting in complete obstruction. This disorder is associated with both Crohn's disease and ulcerative colitis. The other disorders are more commonly associated with Crohn's disease.
CN: Physiological integrity; CNS: Physiological adaptation; CL: Analysis

28. 3. Because of the transmural nature of Crohn's disease lesions, malabsorption may occur with Crohn's disease. Although ankylosing spondylitis and colon cancer are more commonly associated with ulcerative colitis, they may be seen in clients with Crohn's disease. Lactase deficiency is caused by a congenital defect in which an enzyme isn't present.
CN: Physiological integrity; CNS: Physiological adaptation; CL: Analysis

29. A client with Crohn's disease is admitted with fever, weight loss, leg cramping, diarrhea, frequent premature ventricular contractions, and abdominal pain. The nurse reviews the client's lab data and determines immediate intervention is required when the results identify which of the following?
1. Hypoalbuminemia
2. Leukocytosis
3. Increased erythrocyte sedimentation rate
4. Hypokalemia

30. The nurse determines that which diet would be most appropriate for a client with ulcerative colitis?
1. Low fat, low protein
2. Low residue, high protein
3. High calorie, low fiber
4. High residue, high fiber

31. If a client had irritable bowel syndrome, which diagnostic test would determine if the diagnosis is Crohn's disease or ulcerative colitis?
1. Abdominal computed tomography (CT) scan
2. Abdominal X-ray
3. Barium swallow
4. Colonoscopy with biopsy

32. Which intervention should be included in the collaborative management of a client with Crohn's disease?
1. Increasing oral intake of fiber
2. Administering laxatives as ordered
3. Using long-term steroid therapy as prescribed
4. Increasing physical activity

33. A client with Crohn's disease is experiencing an exacerbation. Which instruction would be a <u>priority</u> in planning his care?
1. Increasing current weight
2. Encouraging ambulation
3. Promoting bowel rest
4. Controlling rectal bleeding

One of these tests can help you distinguish between two GI disorders.

29. 4. A low potassium level can lead to cardiac arrest. The client is already having leg cramps and arrhythmias, so this finding is the priority.
CN: Physiological integrity; CNS: Physiological adaptation; CL: Analysis

30. 2. Clients with ulcerative colitis should follow a low-residue, high-protein diet. More protein is needed for tissue healing. High-residue food, such as grains and nuts, should be avoided. There is no need for clients with ulcerative colitis to follow a low-fat diet.
CN: Physiological integrity; CNS: Basic care and comfort; CL: Application

31. 4. A colonoscopy with biopsy can be performed to determine the state of the colon's mucosal layers, presence of ulcerations, and level of cytologic involvement. An abdominal X-ray or a CT scan wouldn't provide the cytologic information necessary to diagnose which disease it is. A barium swallow doesn't involve the intestine.
CN: Physiological integrity; CNS: Physiological adaptation; CL: Analysis

32. 3. Management of Crohn's disease may include long-term steroid therapy to reduce the extensive inflammation associated with the deeper layers of the bowel wall. Other management focuses on bowel rest (not increasing oral intake) and reducing diarrhea with medications (not giving laxatives). The pain associated with Crohn's disease may require bed rest, not an increase in physical activity.
CN: Physiological integrity; CNS: Basic care and comfort; CL: Application

33. 3. Promoting bowel rest is the priority during an acute exacerbation. This is accomplished by decreasing activity and initially putting the client on nothing-by-mouth status. Weight loss may occur, but the priority is bowel rest. Rectal bleeding usually isn't expected in Crohn's disease.
CN: Safe, effective care environment; CNS: Management of care; CL: Analysis

CN: Client needs category   CNS: Client needs subcategory   CL: Cognitive level

34. A nurse would expect to prepare a client with ulcerative colitis for surgery if the client develops which condition?
1. Gastritis
2. Bowel herniation
3. Bowel outpouching
4. Bowel perforation

Certain complications may require surgery.

35. Which medication would the nurse expect to find on the electronic medication administration record (E-MAR) for treating the pain associated with irritable bowel disease?
1. Acetaminophen
2. Opiates
3. Steroids
4. Stool softeners

36. The nurse is prioritizing care for a client 2 days after surgery for a stoma creation that resulted from ulcerative colitis. What is the most important issue for the nurse to address?
1. Body image
2. Ostomy care
3. Sexual concerns
4. Skin care

Question 36 is asking you to prioritize.

37. The nursing assessment of a client with colon cancer may also include a past medical history of which condition?
1. Appendicitis
2. Hemorrhoids
3. Hiatal hernia
4. Ulcerative colitis

38. A nurse is providing nutritional teaching for a client with a family history of colon cancer. Which dietary choice by the client demonstrates understanding of the appropriate diet to follow?
1. Vegetarian chili
2. Hot dogs and sauerkraut
3. Egg salad on rye bread
4. Spaghetti and meat sauce

39. Which diagnostic test should be performed annually after age 50 years to screen for colon cancer?
1. Abdominal computed tomography (CT) scan
2. Abdominal X-ray
3. Colonoscopy
4. Fecal occult blood test

Screening for colon cancer should be on the "to do" list of anyone over age 50 years.

40. A client with colon cancer is scheduled to receive radiation therapy prior to surgery. What should the nurse include in her teaching about the use of radiation therapy?
1. It helps reduce the size of the tumor.
2. It eliminates the malignant cells.
3. It may cure the cancer.
4. It helps heal the bowel after surgery.

34. 4. Bowel perforation, obstruction, hemorrhage, and toxic megacolon are common complications of ulcerative colitis that may require surgery. Gastritis and herniation aren't associated with irritable bowel diseases, and outpouching of the bowel wall is diverticulosis.
CN: Physiological integrity; CNS: Physiological adaptation; CL: Application

35. 3. The pain of irritable bowel disease is caused by inflammation, which steroids can reduce. Acetaminophen has little effect on the pain, and opiates won't treat its underlying cause. Stool softeners aren't necessary.
CN: Physiological integrity; CNS: Pharmacological and parenteral therapies; CL: Analysis

36. 2. Although all of these are concerns the nurse should address, being able to safely manage the ostomy is crucial for the client before discharge.
CN: Safe, effective care environment; CNS: Management of care; CL: Analysis

37. 4. Chronic ulcerative colitis, granulomas, and familial polyposis seem to increase a person's chance of developing colon cancer. The other conditions listed have no known effect on colon cancer risk.
CN: Health promotion and maintenance; CNS: None; CL: Application

38. 1. A high-fiber, low-fat food, such as vegetarian chili, increases motility and decreases the chance of constipation and is recommended to help avoid colon cancer. The other choices don't represent a high-fiber, low-fat diet.
CN: Physiological integrity; CNS: Basic care and comfort; CL: Application

39. 4. Surface blood vessels of polyps and cancers are fragile and often bleed with the passage of stools, so a fecal occult blood test should be performed annually. Abdominal X-ray and CT scan can help establish tumor size and metastasis. A colonoscopy can help to locate a tumor as well as polyps but is only recommended every 10 years.
CN: Health promotion and maintenance; CNS: None; CL: Application

40. 1. Radiation therapy is used before surgery to reduce the size of the tumor, making it easier to be resected. Radiation therapy isn't curative, can't eliminate the malignant cells (although it helps to define tumor margins), and could slow postoperative healing.
CN: Physiological integrity; CNS: Physiological adaptation; CL: Application

41. The nurse anticipates that a client with colon cancer will most likely exhibit which symptom?
1. A change in appetite
2. A change in bowel habits
3. An increase in body weight
4. An increase in body temperature

42. A client has just had surgery for colon cancer. The nurse is aware that the client is most at risk for developing which condition?
1. Peritonitis
2. Diverticulosis
3. Partial bowel obstruction
4. Complete bowel obstruction

43. Which symptom, if reported by a client, would lead the nurse to suspect gastric cancer?
1. Abdominal cramping
2. Constant hunger
3. Feeling of fullness
4. Weight gain

44. A client is seen in the outpatient surgical clinic for a suspected diagnosis of gastric cancer. The nurse anticipates the diagnostic testing of the client will include which test?
1. Barium enema
2. Colonoscopy
3. Endoscopy
4. Serum chemistry levels

45. A client with gastric cancer anticipates having surgery for a gastric resection. What is the <u>most important</u> nursing intervention during the preoperative period?
1. Discharge planning
2. Correction of nutritional deficits
3. Prevention of deep vein thrombosis (DVT)
4. Instruction regarding radiation treatment

It's important to ask the client about his symptoms.

Read the question carefully and know what disorder is being addressed.

You're really pumping up now!

41. 2. The most common complaint of the client with colon cancer is a change in bowel habits. The client may have anorexia, secondary abdominal distention, or weight loss. Fever isn't related to colon cancer.
CN: Physiological integrity; CNS: Physiological adaptation; CL: Application

42. 1. Bowel spillage could occur during surgery, resulting in peritonitis. Diverticulosis doesn't result from surgery for colon cancer. Complete or partial intestinal obstruction may occur *before* bowel resection.
CN: Physiological integrity; CNS: Physiological adaptation; CL: Application

43. 3. The client with gastric cancer may report a feeling of fullness in the stomach but not enough to cause him to seek medical care. Abdominal cramping isn't associated with gastric cancer. Anorexia and weight loss (not increased hunger or weight gain) are common symptoms of gastric cancer.
CN: Physiological integrity; CNS: Physiological adaptation; CL: Application

44. 3. An endoscopy will allow direct visualization of the tumor. A colonoscopy or a barium enema would help to diagnose colon cancer, not gastric cancer. Serum chemistry levels don't contribute data useful to the assessment of gastric cancer.
CN: Health promotion and maintenance; CNS: None; CL: Application

45. 2. Clients with gastric cancer commonly have nutritional deficits and may be cachectic. Discharge planning before surgery is important, but correcting the nutritional deficit is a higher priority. Prevention of DVT also isn't a high priority prior to surgery, although it assumes greater importance after surgery. At present, radiation therapy hasn't been proven effective for gastric cancer, and teaching about it preoperatively wouldn't be appropriate.
CN: Safe, effective care environment; CNS: Management of care; CL: Application

CN: Client needs category   CNS: Client needs subcategory   CL: Cognitive level

46. Which factor is the <u>priority</u> postoperative care need of the client after gastric resection?
1. Body image
2. Nutritional needs
3. Skin care
4. Spiritual needs

Do you know the key to the treatment of GI disorders in general?

46. 2. After gastric resection, a client may require total parenteral nutrition or jejunostomy tube feedings to maintain adequate nutritional status, which promotes healing. Body image isn't much of a problem for this client at this point because clothing can cover the incision site. Wound care of the incision site is necessary to prevent infection; otherwise, the skin shouldn't be affected. Spiritual needs may be a concern, depending on the client, and should be addressed as the client demonstrates readiness to share concerns.

CN: Safe, effective care environment; CNS: Management of care; CL: Analysis

47. The nurse is providing discharge instructions for a client who has undergone a gastric resection. The nurse is aware that the client is at risk for:
1. constipation.
2. dumping syndrome.
3. gastric spasm.
4. intestinal spasms.

47. 2. Dumping syndrome is a problem that occurs postprandially after gastric resection because ingested food rapidly enters the jejunum without proper mixing and without the normal duodenal digestive processing. Diarrhea, not constipation, may also be a symptom. Gastric or intestinal spasms don't occur, but antispasmodics may be given to slow gastric emptying.

CN: Physiological integrity; CNS: Reduction of risk potential; CL: Application

48. A client reports having several episodes of rectal bleeding, ribbon-shaped stools, and abdominal cramping. The nurse recognizes these signs and symptoms as related to which disorder?
1. Hemorrhoids
2. Irritable bowel syndrome (IBS)
3. Colorectal cancer
4. Liver cancer

Knowing what to teach your clients can help avoid problems down the road.

48. 3. Rectal bleeding, ribbon-shaped stool, and abdominal cramping are all associated with colorectal cancer, but these signs and symptoms aren't all associated with the other conditions. IBS can produce abdominal cramping but not rectal bleeding. Hemorrhoids can cause rectal bleeding. Liver cancer isn't related to these symptoms.

CN: Physiological integrity; CNS: Physiological adaptation; CL: Analysis

49. A client with which condition may be at risk for the development of rectal cancer?
1. Adenomatous polyps
2. Diverticulitis
3. Hemorrhoids
4. Peptic ulcer disease

49. 1. A client with adenomatous polyps has a higher risk for developing rectal cancer than others do. Clients with diverticulitis are more likely to develop colon cancer. Hemorrhoids don't increase the chance of any type of cancer. Clients with peptic ulcer disease have a higher incidence of gastric cancer.

CN: Health promotion and maintenance; CNS: None; CL: Analysis

50. A client recently diagnosed with colon cancer tells the nurse that he's been having trouble sleeping and is preoccupied with thoughts of how his life will change after surgery. Which is the most appropriate nursing diagnosis?
1. Anxiety related to upcoming surgery
2. Powerlessness related to illness
3. Disturbed sleep pattern related to fear of the unknown
4. Ineffective coping related to the diagnosis of colon cancer

You made it to question 50!

50. 3. The client is having trouble sleeping because of his concerns about life changes. Although he may be experiencing anxiety and powerlessness, the information supports a diagnosis of insomnia. There is no evidence of ineffective coping.

CN: Safe, Physiological integrity; CNS: Basic care and comfort; CL: Analysis

51. Which condition may lead to hemorrhoids?
1. Diarrhea
2. Diverticulosis
3. Portal hypertension
4. Rectal bleeding

51. 3. Portal hypertension and other conditions associated with persistently high intra-abdominal pressure such as pregnancy can lead to hemorrhoids. The passing of hard stool, not diarrhea, can aggravate hemorrhoids. Diverticulosis has no relationship to hemorrhoids. Rectal bleeding can be a symptom of hemorrhoids.
CN: Physiological integrity; CNS: Physiological adaptation; CL: Analysis

52. Which assessment is most relevant with the diagnosis of hemorrhoids?
1. Abdominal assessment
2. Diet history
3. Digital rectal examination
4. Sexual history

Now let me think. Which treatment would be appropriate?

52. 3. Digital rectal examination is important to assess for internal hemorrhoids and to determine if other causes of the pain and bleeding are present. Abdominal assessment isn't necessary for hemorrhoids. Diet history is relevant because constipation can worsen hemorrhoids, but it isn't as important to diagnosis as a digital rectal examination. Sexual history may also be relevant, but again, the history isn't as important as a digital rectal examination.
CN: Physiological integrity; CNS: Physiological adaptation; CL: Analysis

53. Which of the following should be part of the teaching plan for a client with hemorrhoids?
1. Recommending a high-fiber diet
2. Applying cold to reduce swelling
3. Using astringent lotions to reduce swelling
4. Elevating the buttocks to reduce engorgement

53. 1. A high-fiber diet will add bulk to the stool and ease its passage through the rectum. Application of cold isn't recommended because it can cause injury to the tissue. Astringent lotions can be used to reduce pain, but they aren't a treatment. The buttocks should be elevated only when prolapsed hemorrhoids are present.
CN: Physiological integrity; CNS: Physiological adaptation; CL: Application

54. Which response should a nurse offer to a client who asks why he's having a vagotomy to treat his ulcer?
1. To repair a hole in the stomach
2. To reduce the ability of the stomach to produce acid
3. To prevent the stomach from sliding into the chest
4. To remove a potentially malignant lesion in the stomach

Client education is an important tool for obtaining compliance.

54. 2. A vagotomy is performed to eliminate the acid-secreting stimulus to gastric cells. A perforation would be repaired with a gastric resection. Repair of hiatal hernia (fundoplication) prevents the stomach from sliding through the diaphragm. Removal of a potentially malignant tumor wouldn't reduce the entire acid-producing mechanism.
CN: Physiological integrity; CNS: Reduction of risk potential; CL: Application

55. The nurse should be aware that which condition is most likely to <u>directly</u> cause peritonitis?
1. Cholelithiasis
2. Gastritis
3. Perforated ulcer
4. Incarcerated hernia

55. 3. The most common cause of peritonitis is a perforated ulcer, which can pour contaminants into the peritoneal cavity, causing inflammation and infection within the cavity. The other conditions—cholelithiasis, gastritis, and incarcerated hernia—don't by themselves cause peritonitis. However, if cholelithiasis leads to rupture of the gallbladder, gastritis leads to erosion of the stomach wall, or an incarcerated hernia leads to rupture of the intestines, peritonitis may develop.
CN: Physiological integrity; CNS: Physiological adaptation; CL: Analysis

56. Which assessment finding would a client in the early stages of peritonitis exhibit?
1. Abdominal distention
2. Abdominal pain and rigidity
3. Hyperactive bowel sounds
4. Right upper quadrant pain

57. Which laboratory result would the nurse anticipate in a client with peritonitis?
1. Partial thromboplastin time above 100 seconds
2. Hemoglobin level below 10 mg/dl
3. Potassium level above 5.5 mEq/L
4. White blood cell (WBC) count above 15,000/µl

In my case, more is not necessarily better.

58. A recently admitted client is suspected of having peritonitis. He's requesting a glass of water to drink. Which would be the nurse's best response to the client?
1. "I can give you small amounts of water frequently."
2. "You're getting your fluids intravenously."
3. "I'll check with the physician."
4. "Until your diagnosis is confirmed and bowel function returns, it wouldn't be safe to give you anything to drink."

59. Which of the following would be the <u>priority</u> focus of nursing care for a client with peritonitis?
1. Fluid and electrolyte balance
2. Gastric irrigation
3. Pain management
4. Psychosocial issues

What is the priority focus with this client?

56. 2. Abdominal pain causing rigidity of the abdominal muscles is characteristic of peritonitis. Abdominal distention may occur as a late sign but not early on. Bowel sounds may be normal or decreased but not increased. Right upper quadrant pain is characteristic of cholecystitis or hepatitis.
CN: Health promotion and maintenance; CNS: None; CL: Application

57. 4. Because of infection, the client's WBC count will be elevated. A partial thromboplastin time longer than 100 seconds may suggest disseminated intravascular coagulation, a serious complication of septic shock. A hemoglobin level below 10 mg/dl may occur from hemorrhage. A potassium level above 5.5 mEq/L may suggest renal failure.
CN: Physiological integrity; CNS: Reduction of risk potential; CL: Application

58. 4. The client with peritonitis commonly isn't allowed anything orally until the source of the peritonitis is confirmed and treated. I.V. fluids are given to maintain hydration and hemodynamic stability and to replace electrolytes. However, saying to a client that, "You're getting your fluids intravenously," doesn't explain to the client why he can't have fluids orally. Checking with the physician isn't necessary.
CN: Physiological integrity; CNS: Physiological adaptation; CL: Application

59. 1. Peritonitis can advance to shock and circulatory failure, so fluid and electrolyte balance is the priority focus of nursing management. Gastric irrigation may be needed periodically to ensure patency of the nasogastric tube. Although pain management is important for comfort and psychosocial care will address concerns such as anxiety, focusing on fluid and electrolyte balance will maintain hemodynamic stability.
CN: Safe, effective care environment; CNS: Management of care; CL: Analysis

60. Which factor is most commonly associated with the development of pancreatitis?
1. Alcohol abuse
2. Hypercalcemia
3. Hyperlipidemia
4. Pancreatic duct obstruction

61. Which action of pancreatic enzymes can cause pancreatic damage?
1. Utilization by the intestine
2. Autodigestion of the pancreas
3. Reflux into the pancreas
4. Clogging of the pancreatic duct

Read question 61 carefully before you answer. Make sure you know what it's asking.

62. Which laboratory test would the nurse expect to be ordered to diagnose pancreatitis?
1. Amylase level
2. Hemoglobin level
3. Blood glucose level
4. White blood cell (WBC) count

What sign are you looking for?

63. A client with pancreatitis may exhibit Cullen's sign on physical examination. Which assessment finding best describes Cullen's sign?
1. Jaundiced sclera
2. Pain that occurs with movement
3. Bluish discoloration of the left flank area
4. Bluish discoloration of the periumbilical area

64. Which factor should be the initial focus of nursing management in a client with acute pancreatitis?
1. Dietary management
2. Prevention of skin breakdown
3. Management of hypoglycemia
4. Pain control

60. **1.** Alcohol abuse is the major cause of acute pancreatitis in males, although gallbladder disease is more commonly implicated in women. Hypercalcemia, hyperlipidemia, and pancreatic duct obstruction are also causes of pancreatitis but occur less frequently.
CN: Physiological integrity; CNS: Reduction of risk potential; CL: Application

61. **2.** In pancreatitis, pancreatic enzymes become activated and begin to autodigest the pancreas. The enzymes are activated but aren't used properly by the intestine. Reflux of bile into the pancreatic duct and clogging of the pancreatic duct may occur before autodigestion of the pancreas occurs.
CN: Physiological integrity; CNS: Physiological adaptation; CL: Analysis

62. **1.** Amylase is an enzyme secreted by the pancreas; when elevated, it's useful in diagnosing pancreatitis. Hemoglobin level can be low in pancreatitis, but there are other causes for this. The blood glucose level may be elevated with pancreatitis, but this factor isn't diagnostic. The WBC count may also be elevated in pancreatitis, but this symptom can be due to infection.
CN: Health promotion and maintenance; CNS: None; CL: Analysis

63. **4.** Cullen's sign is bluish discoloration of the periumbilical area from subcutaneous intraperitoneal hemorrhagic pancreatitis. Jaundiced sclera occurs with hepatitis. Pain with movement is a common finding with peritonitis. Turner's sign is the bluish discoloration of the left flank area, which can be present in peritonitis.
CN: Health promotion and maintenance; CNS: None; CL: Analysis

64. **4.** The priority is to provide adequate pain control. This is essential to minimize discomfort and restlessness, which may stimulate pancreatic secretion further. Initially, the client with acute pancreatitis isn't permitted food and oral intake. Although prevention of skin breakdown is important, it isn't the initial focus. Clients are at risk for hyperglycemia, not hypoglycemia.
CN: Physiological integrity; CNS: Physiological adaptation; CL: Analysis

CN: Client needs category   CNS: Client needs subcategory   CL: Cognitive level

65. When admitting a client to the hospital with suspected acute pancreatitis, which electrolyte disorder would be expected?
1. Hypoglycemia
2. Hypernatremia
3. Hypocalcemia
4. Hyperkalemia

66. If a gastric ulcer perforates, which action should be included in the management of the client?
1. Removal of the nasogastric (NG) tube
2. Antacid administration
3. H₂-receptor antagonist administration
4. Fluid and electrolyte replacement

67. A client presents to the emergency department with abdominal pain, weight loss, steatorrhea, and a random glucose of 417 mg/dl. The nurse should expect which diagnostic test to be ordered?
1. Upper GI series
2. Lower GI series
3. Ultrasound of the abdomen
4. Colonoscopy

68. In alcohol-related pancreatitis, which intervention is the best way to reduce the exacerbation of pain?
1. Lying in a supine position
2. Taking aspirin
3. Eating a low-fat diet
4. Abstaining from alcohol

69. A client with cirrhosis complains that his skin always feels itchy. The nurse recognizes that the itching is a result of which abnormality associated with cirrhosis?
1. Prolonged prothrombin time
2. Decreased protein level
3. Increased bilirubin level
4. Increased aspartate aminotransferase level

Give yourself a pat on the back: You're doing great!

I'm really feeling under the influence.

I'm itching to be done with this question.

65. 3. The client with acute pancreatitis may exhibit hypocalcemia due to the deposit of calcium in areas of fat necrosis. Hyperglycemia, not hypoglycemia, may occur due to reduced insulin production caused by islet of Langerhans involvement. Hypokalemia and hyponatremia may occur because potassium is lost in emesis, but hypernatremia is unlikely.
CN: Physiological integrity; CNS: Physiological adaptation; CL: Analysis

66. 4. The client should be treated with antibiotics as well as fluid, electrolyte, and blood replacement. NG tube suction should also be performed to prevent further spillage of stomach contents into the perineal cavity. Antacids and H₂-receptor antagonists aren't helpful in this situation.
CN: Physiological integrity; CNS: Physiological adaptation; CL: Application

67. 3. The symptoms described correlate with chronic pancreatitis. An abdominal ultrasound could reveal pancreatic changes. The other tests are of no value in evaluating the pancreas.
CN: Physiological integrity; CNS: Physiological adaptation; CL: Analysis

68. 4. Abstaining from alcohol is imperative to reduce the injury to the pancreas; in fact, it may be enough to completely control pain. Lying in a supine position usually aggravates the pain because it stretches the abdominal muscles. Taking aspirin can cause bleeding in hemorrhagic pancreatitis. During an attack of acute pancreatitis, the client usually isn't allowed to ingest anything orally.
CN: Physiological integrity; CNS: Reduction of risk potential; CL: Application

69. 3. High bilirubin levels irritate peripheral nerves, causing an intense itching sensation. Itching isn't a symptom of prolonged prothrombin time, decreased protein levels, or increased aspartate aminotransferase levels.
CN: Physiological integrity; CNS: Physiological adaptation; CL: Analysis

70. A client presents with dark urine, fatigue, and generalized pruritus. Lab results reveal elevated serum bilirubin and increased bile salts. The diagnosis is made of biliary cirrhosis. The client asks what is happening in his body. What is the nurse's best response?
1. "There is an obstruction of the bile ducts causing biliary inflammation."
2. "Your liver is releasing toxins, which are poisonous to your circulation."
3. "The alcohol you have consumed has caused small nodules to form in your liver."
4. "The weakened heart muscle has limited blood flow to the liver."

71. Which assessment finding would <u>strongly</u> indicate the possibility of cirrhosis?
1. Dry skin
2. Hepatomegaly
3. Peripheral edema
4. Pruritus

72. For a definitive diagnosis of cirrhosis, the nurse will assist with which diagnostic test?
1. Albumin level
2. Bromsulphthalein dye excretion
3. Liver biopsy
4. Liver enzyme levels

73. Which of the following assessment findings would be consistent with a client's diagnosis of cirrhosis?
1. Increased carbon dioxide level
2. Increased pH level
3. Increased prothrombin time
4. Increased white blood cell (WBC) count

74. The nurse is aware that the most important intervention when caring for a client with esophageal varices is which of the following?
1. Recognizing hemorrhage
2. Controlling blood pressure
3. Encouraging nutritional intake
4. Teaching the client about varices

One of these findings is a red flag for cirrhosis.

70. 1. Biliary cirrhosis is caused by decreased bile flow from obstruction of the bile ducts outside of the liver. This obstruction leads to inflammation and possible necrosis of the liver cells and ducts. The other responses do not occur with biliary cirrhosis.
CN: Physiological integrity; CNS: Physiological adaptation; CL: Analysis

71. 2. The client with cirrhosis has a liver that is enlarged (hepatomegaly), fibrotic, and nodular, which makes it palpable. The client may develop dry skin, pruritus, and peripheral edema, but these symptoms may have other causes.
CN: Physiological integrity; CNS: Physiological adaptation; CL: Analysis

72. 3. A liver biopsy can reveal the exact cause of the hepatomegaly. The albumin level will be low, but that can be caused by poor nutritional states. Bromsulphthalein dye excretion may be reduced, but other hepatocirculatory disorders could also cause this. Liver enzymes may be elevated, but other liver conditions may cause these elevations.
CN: Physiological integrity; CNS: Physiological adaptation; CL: Application

73. 3. Clotting factors may not be produced normally when a client has cirrhosis, increasing the potential for bleeding. There's no associated change in carbon dioxide level or pH unless the client is developing other comorbidities, such as metabolic alkalosis. The WBC count can be elevated in acute cirrhosis but isn't always altered.
CN: Physiological integrity; CNS: Physiological adaptation; CL: Application

74. 1. Recognizing the rupture of esophageal varices, or hemorrhage, is the focus of nursing care because the client could succumb to this quickly. Controlling blood pressure is also important because it helps reduce the risk of variceal rupture. It's also important to teach the client what foods he should avoid, such as spicy foods, and what varices are.
CN: Physiological integrity; CNS: Physiological adaptation; CL: Application

75. Several children at a day care center have been infected with hepatitis A virus. What is the most important information the nurse can provide to reduce the risk of hepatitis A transmission?
1. Hand washing after diaper changes
2. Isolation of the sick children
3. Use of masks during contact with the children
4. Sterilization of all eating utensils

76. A client is being evaluated for hepatitis A. Which activity places him at the highest risk for contracting hepatitis A?
1. Helping his roommate with an epistaxis episode
2. Receiving an elective blood transfusion after surgery
3. Eating a shrimp platter at a local restaurant
4. Having sexual intercourse with his fiancée

77. The nurse is teaching a client with a peptic ulcer about discharge instructions. The client asks the nurse which type of analgesic he may take. Which of the following responses by the nurse would be the most accurate?
1. Aspirin
2. Acetaminophen
3. Naproxen
4. Ibuprofen

78. The nurse is performing an assessment on a client being evaluated for viral hepatitis. Which symptom will the nurse most likely assess on this client?
1. Arthralgia
2. Excitability
3. Headache
4. Polyphagia

Remember, hepatitis A is highly contagious.

75. 1. Children in day care centers are at risk of hepatitis A infection, which is transmitted via fecal-oral route due to poor hand hygiene practices and poor sanitation. Isolation of sick children, use of mask during contact, and sterilization of all eating utensils would not be useful in breaking the chain of infection.
CN: Safe, effective care environment; CNS: Safety and infection control; CL: Application

76. 3. Hepatitis A can be caused by contact with contaminated feces and may be transmitted through infected water, milk, or food, especially shellfish from contaminated waters. Hepatitis B is caused by blood contact and sexual contact. Hepatitis C is usually caused by contact with infected blood, including blood transfusions.
CN: Health promotion and maintenance; CNS: None; CL: Application

77. 2. Acetaminophen is recommended for pain relief because it does not promote irritation of the mucosa. Aspirin and nonsteroidal anti-inflammatory drugs such as naproxen and ibuprofen may cause irritation of the mucosa and subsequent bleeding.
CN: Physiological integrity; CNS: Pharmacological and parenteral therapies; CL: Application

78. 1. Arthralgia is common in clients with viral hepatitis. Other symptoms of viral hepatitis include lethargy, flulike symptoms, anorexia, nausea and vomiting, abdominal pain, diarrhea, constipation, and fever. Excitability, headache, and polyphagia are not symptoms of viral hepatitis.
CN: Physiological integrity; CNS: Physiological adaptation; CL: Application

79. A client is admitted with a diagnosis of hepatic encephalopathy. The nurse's assessment documentation will include which of the following?
1. Asterixis
2. Proficient concentration
3. Increased energy
4. Talkativeness

80. Which dietary instructions should the nurse give to a client with toxic hepatitis?
1. No foods or drinks allowed.
2. Eat low-calorie foods.
3. Consume only low-residue foods.
4. Eat high-calorie foods.

81. Which diagnostic test is the most accurate for diagnosing liver cancer?
1. Abdominal ultrasound
2. Abdominal flat plate X-ray
3. Cholangiogram
4. Computed tomography (CT) scan

82. Immediately after a liver biopsy, which complication should a client be closely monitored for?
1. Abdominal cramping
2. Hemorrhage
3. Nausea and vomiting
4. Potential infection

83. A client with a diagnosed liver disorder is scheduled to have an invasive procedure. The nurse will monitor which test result to ensure the safety of the client?
1. Coagulation studies
2. Liver enzyme levels
3. Serum chemistries
4. White blood cell count

You're almost there!

Closely monitor a client for complications following surgery.

Caution

79. 1. Asterixis, also known as liver flap, is commonly present in clients with hepatic encephalopathy. It can be easily elicited by applying a blood pressure cuff and noting if the flapping is present when the cuff is released. Lack of concentration, fatigue, and introversion are also symptoms of encephalopathy.
CN: Physiological integrity; CNS: Physiological adaptation; CL: Application

80. 4. Instructions to a client with toxic hepatitis should include consuming a high-calorie diet. The client is allowed to eat and drink and does not need to consume low-calorie or low-residue foods.
CN: Physiological integrity; CNS: Basic care and comfort; CL: Application

81. 4. A client with suspected liver cancer will likely undergo CT imaging to identify tumors. The results of a CT scan are much more definitive than the findings of an ultrasound or X-ray. A cholangiogram evaluates the gallbladder, not the liver.
CN: Health promotion and maintenance; CNS: None; CL: Analysis

82. 2. The liver is very vascular, and taking a biopsy could cause the client to hemorrhage. The client may experience some discomfort but, typically, not cramping. Nausea and vomiting may be present, and infection may occur but not immediately after the procedure.
CN: Physiological integrity; CNS: Reduction of risk potential; CL: Application

83. 1. The liver produces coagulation factors. If the liver is affected negatively, production of these factors may be altered, placing the client at risk for hemorrhage. The other laboratory tests should also be monitored, but the results may not necessarily relate to the safety of the procedure.
CN: Physiological integrity; CNS: Reduction of risk potential; CL: Analysis

84. A nurse is providing instructions to a client who will undergo a liver biopsy the next morning. The client asks the nurse about what potential problems could occur. It is <u>most important</u> for the nurse to provide information for which condition?
1. Paralytic ileus
2. Hemorrhage
3. Renal shutdown
4. Constipation

85. Which procedure is <u>most likely necessary</u> for a client with a small tumor confined to one liver segment or lobe?
1. Chemotherapy only
2. Cryoablation or liver resection
3. Liver transplant
4. Radiation therapy only

86. The nurse is counseling a client on how to prevent cholecystitis. What is the <u>most important</u> guideline for the nurse to include?
1. Eat a low-protein diet.
2. Eat a low-fat, low-cholesterol diet.
3. Limit exercise to 10 minutes a day.
4. Keep weight proportional to height.

What to do, what to do. I hope someone knows what to do.

The correct answer carries a lot of weight towards preventing cholecystitis.

84. 2. Because the most common adverse effect of a liver biopsy is bleeding, the nurse should provide relevant information regarding the potential for hemorrhage. There's no reason to provide the client with information about paralytic ileus. Renal shutdown isn't an expected complication after a liver biopsy. The nurse would have no reason to suspect that the client will have a problem with constipation after a liver biopsy.
CN: Physiological integrity; CNS: Reduction of risk potential; CL: Application

85. 2. If the tumor is confined and small, the best treatment would be cryoablation of the tumor or liver resection, removing the segment involved. Chemotherapy and radiation therapy may also be used to reduce the chance of cancerous hepatocytes from regrowing. Liver transplantation usually isn't indicated for liver cancer.
CN: Physiological integrity; CNS: Physiological adaptation; CL: Application

86. 4. Obesity is a known cause of cholecystitis, and maintaining a recommended weight will help to protect against cholecystitis. Excessive dietary intake of cholesterol is associated with the development of gallstones in many people. Dietary protein isn't implicated in cholecystitis. Liquid protein and low-calorie diets (with rapid weight loss of more than 5 lb [2.3 kg] per week) are implicated as the cause of some cases of cholecystitis. Regular exercise (30 minutes/three times a week) may help to reduce weight and improve fat metabolism. Reducing stress may reduce bile production, which may also indirectly decrease the chances of developing cholecystitis.
CN: Health promotion and maintenance; CNS: None; CL: Application

87. Which assessment finding best describes Murphy's sign?
1. Periumbilical ecchymosis is observed.
2. On deep palpation and release, pain is elicited.
3. On palpation and deep inspiration, pain is elicited and the client stops breathing in.
4. Abdominal muscles are tightened in anticipation of palpation.

88. A client is suspected of having cholecystitis. The nurse will prepare the client for which of the following diagnostic tests?
1. Abdominal computed tomography (CT) scan
2. Abdominal ultrasound
3. Barium swallow
4. Endoscopy

Question 89 is asking you to prioritize again.

89. Which intervention should be the priority of nursing management for a client hospitalized for acute cholecystitis?
1. Administration of antibiotics
2. Assessment for complications
3. Preparation for lithotripsy
4. Preparation for surgery

90. A nurse has given discharge instructions to a client with chronic cholecystitis. Which response by the client indicates the teaching has been effective?
1. "I need to rest more."
2. "I should avoid taking antacids."
3. "I should increase the fat in my diet."
4. "I will take my anticholinergic medications as prescribed."

87. 3. Murphy's sign is elicited when the client reacts to pain and stops breathing in. It's a common finding in clients with cholecystitis. Periumbilical ecchymosis (Cullen's sign) is present in peritonitis. Pain on deep palpation and release is rebound tenderness. Tightening up abdominal muscles in anticipation of palpation is guarding, not Murphy's sign.
CN: Physiological integrity; CNS: Physiological adaptation; CL: Application

88. 2. An abdominal ultrasound can show if the gallbladder is enlarged, if gallstones are present, if the gallbladder wall is thickened, or if distention of the gallbladder lumen is present. An abdominal CT scan can be used to diagnose cholecystitis, but it usually isn't necessary. A barium swallow looks at the stomach and the duodenum. Endoscopy looks at the esophagus, stomach, and duodenum.
CN: Health promotion and maintenance; CNS: None; CL: Application

89. 2. The client with acute cholecystitis should first be monitored for such complications as perforation, fever, abscess, fistula, and sepsis. After assessment, antibiotics will be administered to reduce the infection. Lithotripsy is used for only a small percentage of clients. Surgery is usually done after the acute infection has subsided.
CN: Safe, effective care environment; CNS: Management of care; CL: Application

90. 4. Conservative therapy for chronic cholecystitis includes weight reduction by increasing physical activity, a low-fat (not low-protein) diet, antacid use to treat dyspepsia, and anticholinergic use to relax smooth muscles and reduce ductal tone and spasm, thereby reducing pain.
CN: Physiological integrity; CNS: Reduction of risk potential; CL: Application

91. Documentation of an assessment by the nurse for a client diagnosed with a duodenal ulcer will most likely reveal which of the following findings?
1. Hematemesis
2. Malnourishment
3. Melena
4. Pain with eating

92. To reduce occurrences of the dumping syndrome, the nurse should instruct a client to do which of the following?
1. Sip fluids with meals.
2. Eat three meals daily.
3. Rest after meals for 30 minutes.
4. Eat a high-carbohydrate, low-fat, and low-protein diet.

93. Assessment of a client with a duodenal ulcer will reveal which of the following characteristics?
1. Early satiety
2. Pain on eating
3. Dull upper epigastric pain
4. Pain on an empty stomach

94. The nurse has just admitted a client to the unit with a diagnosis of suspected peptic ulcer. The nurse anticipates that the doctor will order which test?
1. Abdominal X-ray
2. Barium swallow
3. Computed tomography (CT) scan of the abdomen
4. Esophagogastroduodenoscopy (EGD)

95. The nurse is preparing to administer ranitidine (Zantac) to a client diagnosed with peptic ulcer disease. The client asks the nurse what the purpose of the medication is. What is the most appropriate response by the nurse?
1. Neutralize acid
2. Reduce acid secretions
3. Stimulate gastrin release
4. Protect the mucosal barrier

I know some food will relieve this pain.

91. 3. The client with a duodenal ulcer may have bleeding at the ulcer site, which shows up as melena. The other findings are consistent with a gastric ulcer.
CN: Physiological integrity; CNS: Physiological adaptation; CL: Application

92. 3. To reduce the occurrences of the dumping syndrome, clients should be taught to lie down after eating for 30 minutes; take fluids only between meals, none with meals; eat smaller amounts more frequently in a semirecumbent position; and eat a low-carbohydrate diet, with high-protein and moderate-fat foods, and avoid sweets.
CN: Physiological integrity; CNS: Reduction of risk potential; CL: Application

93. 4. Pain of a duodenal ulcer on an empty stomach is relieved by taking food or antacids. The other symptoms are those of a gastric ulcer.
CN: Physiological integrity; CNS: Physiological adaptation; CL: Application

94. 4. The EGD can visualize the entire upper GI tract as well as allow for tissue specimens and electrocautery as needed. The barium swallow could locate a gastric ulcer and may be an initial test performed. A CT scan and an abdominal X-ray aren't useful in the diagnosis of an ulcer.
CN: Health promotion and maintenance; CNS: None; CL: Application

95. 2. Ranitidine is a histamine-2 receptor antagonist that reduces acid secretion by inhibiting gastrin secretion. Antacids neutralize acid, and mucosal barrier fortifiers protect the mucosal barrier.
CN: Physiological integrity; CNS: Pharmacological and parenteral therapies; CL: Application

96. The nurse is reviewing the computerized laboratory results of a client with suspected pancreatitis. Which lab results would confirm the client's diagnosis of pancreatitis?
1. Elevated amylase, elevated lipase, elevated serum glucose, and decreased serum calcium levels
2. Elevated amylase, elevated lipase, decreased serum glucose, and decreased serum calcium levels
3. Decreased amylase, decreased lipase, elevated serum glucose, and increased serum calcium levels
4. Decreased amylase, decreased lipase, decreased serum glucose, and increased serum calcium levels

97. Which instruction should a nurse give a client with pancreatitis during discharge teaching?
1. Consume high-fat meals.
2. Consume low-calorie meals.
3. Limit daily intake of alcohol.
4. Avoid beverages that contain caffeine.

98. After a liver biopsy, a nurse should place a client in which position?
1. Left side-lying position, with the bed flat
2. Right side-lying position, with the bed flat
3. Left side-lying position, with the bed in semi-Fowler's position
4. Right side-lying position, with the bed in semi-Fowler's position

99. A client with irritable bowel syndrome is being prepared for discharge. Which dietary instructions should be included in the teaching?
1. Low fiber, low fat
2. High fiber, low fat
3. Low fiber, high fat
4. High fiber, high fat

It's irritating to give up my cup of joe.

96. 1. Inflammation of the pancreas causes it to excrete pancreatic enzymes. The inflammation also causes a blockage of the ducts from the pancreas to the GI tract; therefore, the pancreatic enzymes are released into the blood, resulting in an elevation of amylase and lipase levels. Carbohydrate metabolism is impaired secondary to damage to pancreatic beta cells. This impairment causes the client to become hyperglycemic. As in many other disease processes, serum calcium level decreases because of the saponification of calcium by fatty acids in the area of the inflamed pancreas.

CN: Physiological integrity; CNS: Physiological adaptation; CL: Analysis

97. 4. A client with pancreatitis must avoid foods or beverages that can cause a relapse of the disease. Caffeine must be avoided because it's a stimulant that will further irritate the pancreas. The client with pancreatitis must avoid all alcohol because chronic alcohol use is one of the causes of pancreatitis. The diet should be low in fats and high in calories, especially carbohydrates.

CN: Physiological integrity; CNS: Reduction of risk potential; CL: Application

98. 2. Lying the client on his right side with the bed flat will splint the biopsy site and minimize bleeding. The other positions won't do this and may cause increased bleeding at the site or internally.

CN: Physiological integrity; CNS: Reduction of risk potential; CL: Application

99. 2. The client with irritable bowel syndrome needs to be on a diet that contains at least 25 g of fiber per day. Fatty foods are to be avoided because they may precipitate symptoms.

CN: Physiological integrity; CNS: Basic care and comfort; CL: Application

100. A client presents to the emergency department, reporting that he has been vomiting every 30 to 40 minutes for the past 8 hours. The nurse is aware that the client is at risk for which of the following?
1. Metabolic acidosis and hyperkalemia
2. Metabolic acidosis and hypokalemia
3. Metabolic alkalosis and hyperkalemia
4. Metabolic alkalosis and hypokalemia

101. Five days after undergoing surgery, a client develops a small-bowel obstruction. A Miller-Abbott tube is inserted for bowel decompression. Which nursing diagnosis takes <u>priority</u>?
1. Imbalanced nutrition: Less than body requirements
2. Acute pain
3. Deficient fluid volume
4. Excess fluid volume

102. A client presents to the clinic for a follow-up appointment after diagnostic tests show he has gastroesophageal reflux disease. Which instruction should the nurse provide?
1. "Lie down and rest after each meal."
2. "Avoid alcohol and caffeine."
3. "Drink 16 oz of water with each meal."
4. "Eat three well-balanced meals every day."

Closely examine the answers to question 100; it's easy to confuse them.

100. 4. Gastric acid contains large amounts of potassium, chloride, and hydrogen ions. Excessive loss of these substances, such as from vomiting, can lead to metabolic alkalosis and hypokalemia. It doesn't cause metabolic acidosis or hyperkalemia.
CN: Physiological integrity; CNS: Reduction of risk potential; CL analysis

101. 3. Fluid shifts to the site of the bowel obstruction, causing a fluid deficit in the intravascular spaces. If the obstruction isn't resolved immediately, the client may experience imbalanced nutrition: less than body requirements; however, deficient fluid volume takes priority. The client also may experience pain, but that nursing diagnosis is also of lower priority than deficient fluid volume.
CN: Safe, effective care environment; CNS: Management of care; CL: Analysis

102. 2. A client with gastroesophageal reflux disease should avoid alcohol, caffeine, and foods that increase acidity, all of which can cause epigastric pain. To further prevent reflux, the client should remain upright for 2 to 3 hours after eating; avoid eating for 2 to 3 hours before bedtime; avoid bending and wearing tight clothing; avoid drinking large fluid volumes with meals; and eat small, frequent meals to help reduce gastric acid secretion.
CN: Physiological integrity; CNS: Reduction of risk potential; CL: Application

103. When teaching an elderly client how to prevent constipation, which instruction should the nurse include?
1. "Drink six glasses of fluid each day."
2. "Avoid grain products and nuts."
3. "Add at least 4 g of bran to your cereal each morning."
4. "Be sure to get regular exercise."

104. In a client with diarrhea, which outcome indicates that fluid resuscitation is successful?
1. The client passes formed stools at regular intervals.
2. The client reports a decrease in stool frequency and liquidity.
3. The client exhibits firm skin turgor.
4. The client no longer experiences perianal burning.

105. When teaching a community group about measures to prevent colon cancer, which instruction should a nurse include?
1. "Limit fat intake to 20% to 25% of your total daily calories."
2. "Include 15 to 20 g of fiber in your daily diet."
3. "Get an annual rectal examination after age 35."
4. "Undergo sigmoidoscopy annually after age 50."

106. A 30-year-old client experiences weight loss, abdominal distention, crampy abdominal pain, and intermittent diarrhea after the birth of her second child. Diagnostic tests reveal gluten-induced enteropathy. Which foods must she eliminate from her diet permanently?
1. Milk and dairy products
2. Protein-containing foods
3. Cereal grains (except rice and corn)
4. Carbohydrates

If you keep moving, you'll keep moving.

Eliminating the wrong answers can be as important as selecting the right one.

103. 4. Exercise helps prevent constipation. Fluids and dietary fiber promote normal bowel function. The client should drink 8 to 10 glasses of fluid per day. Although adding bran to cereal helps prevent constipation by increasing dietary fiber, the client should start with a small amount of bran and gradually increase the amount as tolerated to a maximum of 2 g daily.

CN: Health promotion and maintenance; CNS: None; CL: Application

104. 3. Firm skin turgor would be one indication of successful fluid resuscitation. Other indications would include moist mucous membranes and urine output of at least 30 ml/hour. Passage of formed stools at regular intervals and a decrease in stool frequency and liquidity indicate successful resolution of diarrhea. The absence of perianal burning indicates that the irritation from the diarrhea is gone.

CN: Physiological integrity; CNS: Basic care and comfort; CL: Analysis

105. 1. To help prevent colon cancer, fats should account for no more than 20% to 25% of total daily calories and the diet should include 25 to 30 g of fiber per day. A digital rectal examination isn't recommended as a stand-alone test for colorectal cancer. For colorectal cancer screening, the American Cancer Society advises clients over age 50 to have a flexible sigmoidoscopy every 5 years, yearly fecal occult blood tests, a double-contrast barium enema every 5 years, or a colonoscopy every 10 years.

CN: Health promotion and maintenance; CNS: None; CL: Application

106. 3. To manage gluten-induced enteropathy, the client must eliminate gluten, which means avoiding all cereal grains except rice and corn. In initial disease management, clients eat a high-calorie, high-protein diet with mineral and vitamin supplements to help normalize the nutritional status. Lactose intolerance is sometimes an associated problem, so milk and dairy products are limited until improvement occurs. Cereal grains are the only carbohydrates this client must eliminate.

CN: Physiological integrity; CNS: Basic care and comfort; CL: Application

107. After a right hemicolectomy for treatment of colon cancer, a 57-year-old client is reluctant to turn while on bed rest. What is the most appropriate intervention by the nurse?
1. Asking a coworker to help turn the client
2. Explaining to the client why turning is important
3. Allowing the client to turn when he's ready to do so
4. Telling the client that the physician's order states he must turn every 2 hours

108. A nurse assists a physician during paracentesis. When documenting the procedure, which information should the nurse include?
1. The nurse's role during the procedure
2. The reason for the procedure
3. The physician's name and the client's response to the procedure
4. Diagnostic tests performed before obtaining the specimen

109. A client has a percutaneous endoscopic gastrostomy tube inserted for continuous tube feedings. What is the best position for the nurse to place the client in before starting the feeding?
1. Semi-Fowler's
2. Supine
3. Reverse Trendelenburg
4. High Fowler's

110. An enema is prescribed for a client with suspected appendicitis. What is the most appropriate action by the nurse?
1. Prepare 750 ml of irrigating solution warmed to 100° F (37.8° C).
2. Question the physician about the order.
3. Provide privacy and explain the procedure to the client.
4. Assist the client to left lateral Sims' position.

Good record keeping is a key factor in client care.

When in doubt ... always ask!

107. 2. The appropriate action is to explain the importance of turning to avoid postoperative complications. Asking a coworker to help turn the client against his will would infringe on his rights. Allowing him to turn when he's ready would increase his risk for postoperative complications. Telling him he must turn because of the physician's orders would put him on the defensive and exclude him from participating in care decisions.
CN: Physiological integrity; CNS: Reduction of risk potential; CL: Application

108. 3. The nurse should document the date and time of the procedure, the physician's name, pertinent information about the procedure (including tests done on the specimen obtained), the client's response, and client teaching. Documentation should include response to her interventions during the procedure. The reason for the procedure doesn't need to be documented.
CN: Physiological integrity; CNS: Reduction of risk potential; CL: Analysis

109. 1. To prevent aspiration of stomach contents, the nurse should place the client in semi-Fowler's position. The supine and reverse Trendelenburg positions may cause aspiration. High Fowler's position isn't necessary and may not be tolerated as well as semi-Fowler's.
CN: Physiological integrity; CNS: Reduction of risk potential; CL: Application

110. 2. Enemas are contraindicated in an acute abdominal condition of unknown origin (such as suspected appendicitis) as well as after recent colon or rectal surgery or myocardial infarction, so questioning the physician about the order would be the correct thing to do. The other answers are correct only when enema administration is appropriate.
CN: Safe, effective care environment; CNS: Safety and infection control; CL: Application

111. A 75-year-old client is admitted to the hospital with lower GI bleeding. His hemoglobin on admission to the emergency department is 7.3 g/dl. The physician prescribes 2 units of packed red blood cells (RBCs) to infuse over 1 hour each. Each unit of packed RBCs contains 250 ml. The blood administration set has a drip factor of 10 gtt/ml. What is the flow rate in drops per minute? Record your answer using a whole number.

_____ gtt/minute

112. A nurse is assessing a client's abdomen. Identify the area where the nurse's hand should be placed to palpate the liver.

113. A nurse is caring for a client who has had extensive abdominal surgery and is in critical condition. Dextrose 5% in half-normal saline solution is infusing through a triple-lumen central catheter at 125 ml/hour. The physician's orders include gentamicin 80 mg I.V. piggyback in 50 ml D5W over 30 minutes; ranitidine (Zantac) 50 mg I.V. in 50 ml D5W over 30 minutes; one unit of 250 ml of packed red blood cells (RBCs) over 3 hours; and a nasogastric tube flush with 30 ml normal saline solution every 2 hours. How many milliliters should the nurse document as the intake for the 8-hour shift? Record your answer using a whole number.

_____ milliliters

111. 42. Each unit of packed RBCs contains 250 ml. Each unit is to infuse over 1 hour (60 minutes). Use the following equation: 250 ml/60 minutes = 4.16 ml. Multiply by the drip factor: 4.16 ml × 10 gtt = 41.6 gtt/minute (42 gtt/minute).

CN: Physiological integrity; CNS: Pharmacological and parenteral therapies; CL: Analysis

112. The nurse can palpate the liver by standing at the client's right side and placing her right hand on the client's abdomen to the right of midline. The nurse should point the fingers of her right hand toward the client's head, just under the right rib margin.

CN: Health promotion and maintenance; CNS: None; CL: Application

113. 1,470. The regular I.V. at 125 ml × 8 hours = 1,000 ml; gentamicin piggyback = 50 ml; ranitidine (Zantac) piggyback = 50 ml; packed RBCs = 250 ml; and nasogastric flushes of 30 ml × 4 = 120 ml. Totaled together, this equals 1,470 ml.

CN: Physiological integrity; CNS: Pharmacological and parenteral therapies; CL: Application

This chapter covers diabetes mellitus and other endocrine disorders, typically a difficult area for nursing students. Don't worry, though, I'll help you through all the tough spots.

Chapter 9
Endocrine disorders

Make sure you don't confuse hyper and hypo!

1. The nurse is admitting a client who is diagnosed with a new onset of type 1 diabetes mellitus. While performing the initial physical assessment and nursing history, the nurse expects to find which of the following signs/symptoms?
   1. Polydipsia, polyuria, and weight loss
   2. Weight gain, tiredness, and bradycardia
   3. Irritability, diaphoresis, and tachycardia
   4. Diarrhea, abdominal pain, and weight loss

2. A client presents with diaphoresis, palpitations, jitters, and tachycardia approximately 1.5 hours after taking his regular morning insulin. What is the most appropriate intervention by the nurse?
   1. Check blood glucose level and administer carbohydrates.
   2. Give nitroglycerin and perform an electrocardiogram (ECG).
   3. Call the physician for additional insulin order.
   4. Restrict salt, administer diuretics, and perform a paracentesis.

3. The nurse is caring for a preoperative client with insulin-dependent diabetes. On the morning of surgery, the nurse should carry out which of the following nursing actions?
   1. Clarify the insulin dose with the physician.
   2. Administer an oral antidiabetic agent.
   3. Administer an I.V. insulin infusion.
   4. Administer the full daily insulin dose.

1. 1. Symptoms of diabetes mellitus (uncontrolled) include polydipsia, polyuria, and weight loss. Weight gain, tiredness, and bradycardia are symptoms of hypothyroidism. Irritability, diaphoresis, and tachycardia are symptoms of hypoglycemia. Symptoms of Crohn's disease include diarrhea, abdominal pain, and weight loss.
CN: Physiological integrity; CNS: Reduction of risk potential; CL: Analysis

2. 1. The client is experiencing symptoms of hypoglycemia. Checking the blood glucose level and administering carbohydrates will elevate blood glucose. ECG and nitroglycerin are treatments for myocardial infarction. This client has a low blood glucose; additional insulin will lower blood glucose further. Restricting salt, administering diuretics, and performing a paracentesis are treatments for ascites.
CN: Physiological integrity; CNS: Physiological adaptation; CL: Application

3. 1. Because of the many treatment approaches to diabetes, clarify the drug orders with the physician. If the client takes his full daily dose of intermediate-acting insulin when he isn't allowed anything orally before surgery, he'll become hypoglycemic. Clients with type 1 diabetes don't take oral antidiabetic agents. I.V. insulin infusions may be ordered, along with a dextrose infusion, but must be ordered and clarified by the physician.
CN: Physiological integrity; CNS: Physiological adaptation; CL: Application

4. The nurse is teaching a health promotion class in the community. Which of the following would the nurse encourage in order to prevent type 2 diabetes mellitus?
1. A fat-free diet and nonimpact exercise three times weekly
2. Maintenance of ideal weight and participation in regular exercise
3. A very low–carbohydrate diet with moderate amounts of fat
4. Smoking cessation and a diet high in protein and fat

Health promotion can be prevention.

5. The nurse is caring for a client with type 2 diabetes. One hour after taking an oral diabetic drug, the client becomes nauseated and vomits. Which nursing intervention should be taken?
1. Give the oral diabetic drug again.
2. Give subcutaneous insulin and monitor blood glucose.
3. Monitor blood glucose closely and look for signs of hypoglycemia.
4. Monitor blood glucose and assess for symptoms of hyperglycemia.

Teach your client about the link between diet and diabetes.

6. When teaching a newly diagnosed diabetic client about diet and exercise, what is the most important information for the nurse to provide?
1. Exercise will increase blood glucose.
2. Management of fluid, protein, and electrolytes
3. Reduction of calorie intake before exercising
4. Dietary goals, food consistency, and physical activity

7. A nurse is teaching a client with diabetes mellitus about chronic complications associated with the disease. Which information should be included in the teaching?
1. Buy shoes that are a half size larger.
2. Annual eye examinations are recommended.
3. Excessive exercise increases insulin resistance.
4. Podiatry visits are necessary every 5 years.

4. 2. Everyone should be encouraged to prevent type 2 diabetes by achieving and maintaining ideal body weight and participating in regular exercise. A low-fat diet can be encouraged, but some fat is required in all diets. Carbohydrates should make up the majority of a healthy diet. Diets high in fat are never encouraged.

CN: Health promotion and maintenance; CNS: None; CL: Application

5. 3. When a client who has taken an oral anti-diabetic agent vomits, the nurse should monitor glucose and assess him frequently for signs of hypoglycemia. Most of the medication has probably been absorbed, and any food taken in may be lost. Therefore, repeating the dose would further lower glucose levels later in the day. Giving insulin also will lower glucose levels, causing hypoglycemia. The client wouldn't have hyperglycemia if most of the oral diabetic drug was absorbed.

CN: Physiological integrity; CNS: Pharmacological and parenteral therapies; CL: Analysis

6. 4. Diabetic clients must be taught the relationship among dietary goals, consistency of food composition, and regular physical activity. Exercise will usually decrease blood glucose. Management of fluids, proteins, and electrolytes is important for a client with acute renal failure. The diabetic client may need to intake additional calories before exercising.

CN: Health promotion and maintenance; CNS: None; CL: Application

7. 2. Retinopathy is a chronic complication of diabetes mellitus. Therefore, yearly eye examinations are recommended. Because of the risk of serious foot injuries, shoes should fit properly and be the correct size. Exercise decreases insulin resistance. A podiatrist should be seen on a yearly basis or more often, as needed.

CN: Physiological integrity; CNS: Reduction of risk potential; CL: Application

8. The nurse is teaching a client with newly diagnosed diabetes mellitus about rotation of insulin injection sites. Which of the following is the correct information to give the client?
1. Rotation within one anatomic site is preferred.
2. Rotation from one anatomic site to another is best.
3. Rotation of sites does not affect speed of absorption.
4. Rotation of sites does not prevent lipohypertrophy.

It's all about location, location, location.

8. 1. Rotation within one anatomic site is preferred to rotation from one site to another to prevent day-to-day changes in absorption. Speed of absorption is affected by choice of site. Lipohypertrophy can be prevented by rotation of sites.

CN: Physiological integrity; CNS: Pharmacological and parenteral therapies; CL: Application

9. The nurse is providing diabetic education to a group of clients with newly diagnosed diabetes. One of the clients asks why the glycosylated hemoglobin blood test (A$_{1C}$) is done in addition to the daily capillary blood glucose tests. What is the best response by the nurse?
1. It provides hemoglobin level in addition to blood glucose level.
2. It is used to assess long-term glycemic control.
3. It provides information about a red blood cell's life span.
4. It provides information about serum protein and albumin.

9. 2. The glycosylated hemoglobin is a good indicator of the average blood glucose level during the previous 120 days, which is the life span of red blood cells. It is used to assess long-term glycemic control. It does not provide a hemoglobin or serum blood glucose level. It does not provide information about serum protein or albumin.

CN: Physiological integrity; CNS: Reduction of risk potential; CL: Application

10. The nurse is providing diabetic education to a group of clients with previously diagnosed diabetes. One of the clients asks what the advantage is in using a continuous subcutaneous pump. What is the best response by the nurse?
1. It is easy to use and requires very little education.
2. It eliminates the potential for ketoacidosis.
3. It is cheaper to use than traditional insulin injections.
4. It allows flexibility in meal timing.

10. 4. Continuous subcutaneous insulin infusion (CSII) provides a basal dose of insulin with increases in insulin at mealtimes and is more effective in controlling blood glucose levels than a multiple-injection schedule. CSII allows flexibility in meal timing because if a meal is skipped or taken later than planned, the mealtime dose of insulin is not given. Use of this pump requires intensive education for the client. The potential for more frequent and severe ketoacidosis may increase because of inexperience in pump use, infection, or accidental cessation/obstruction of the infusion. CSII is more costly than traditional insulin injections, and not all costs are covered by insurance.

CN: Physiological integrity; CNS: Pharmacological and parenteral therapies; CL: Application

11. The nurse is admitting a new client with a diagnosis of myxedema. During the initial assessment, the nurse is most concerned when the client presents with which findings?
1. Hypertension and weight loss
2. Heat intolerance and emotional lability
3. Corneal ulcerations and increased appetite
4. Bradycardia and decreased intellectual function

11. 4. Myxedema is caused by hypothyroidism. Signs and symptoms of hypothyroidism include slowing of the heart rate and decreased intellectual functions, such as slurring speech, impaired memory, and inattentiveness. Hypertension, weight loss, heat intolerance, emotional lability, and increased appetite are all signs and symptoms of hyperthyroidism. Corneal ulcerations may be seen in hyperthyroidism due to exophthalmos because edema behind the eye may prevent eyelids from closing completely.

CN: Physiological integrity; CNS: Physiological adaptation; CL: Analysis

12. The nurse is caring for a client who is 1 day postoperative from a total thyroidectomy. The nurse determines it is necessary to call the rapid response team (RRT) when the client displays which of the following?
1. Blood pressure of 150/92 mm Hg
2. Harsh, high-pitched respiratory sounds
3. Weak voice and/or hoarseness
4. Decreased deep tendon reflexes

13. The nurse is assessing a newly admitted client who is diagnosed with hypocalcemia. In order to assess the thyroid gland properly, which of the following techniques would the nurse use?
1. Have the client flex his neck onto his chest and cough while the nurse palpates the anterior neck with her fingertips.
2. Place hands around the client's neck, with the thumbs in the front of the neck, and gently massage the anterior neck.
3. Ask the client to slightly flex his neck forward and toward the side being examined and then to swallow.
4. Have the client hyperextend his neck and take slow, deep inhalations while the nurse palpates the neck with her fingertips.

14. The nurse is educating a client who is diagnosed with hypothyroidism. The nurse explains the importance of medication adherence and the potential effects of trauma, emergency surgery, or severe infection, which would place the client at risk for which condition?
1. Laryngeal spasms
2. Malignant hyperthermia
3. Myxedema coma
4. Thyroid storm

15. When the nurse is assessing a client who is being treated for hypothyroidism, which of these findings would indicate a potentially serious complication?
1. Chills, fever, and hypotension
2. Palpitations and chest pain
3. Decreased visual acuity
4. Low platelet counts

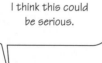

I think this could be serious.

12. 2. Stridor, or harsh, high-pitched respiratory sounds, indicates respiratory obstruction, which may be caused by laryngeal spasms or swelling. A blood pressure of 150/92 mm Hg is high but not enough to call the RRT. A weak voice and/or hoarseness may be expected if the laryngeal nerve is affected. Decreased deep tendon reflexes are not a concern. Hyperactive deep tendon reflexes would indicate a low calcium level, which may occur with damage to the parathyroid glands.
CN: Physiological integrity; CNS: Reduction of risk potential; CL: Application

13. 3. This approach is the correct method for palpating the thyroid gland. This allows relaxation of the sternocleidomastoid muscle. Having the client flex his neck onto his chest wouldn't allow for palpation. Massaging the area or checking during inhalation doesn't allow for the movement of tissue that swallowing provides.
CN: Physiological integrity; CNS: Reduction of risk potential; CL: Analysis

14. 3. Myxedema coma can be precipitated by opioids, stress (such as surgery), trauma, and infections. It represents the most severe form of hypothyroidism. Laryngeal spasms are caused by low calcium, which would be related to the parathyroid gland. The client would be hypothermic, not hyperthermic. Thyroid storm is a complication of hyperthyroidism.
CN: Physiological integrity; CNS: Pharmacological and parenteral therapies; CL: Application

15. 2. Palpitations and chest pain are cardiac symptoms, which can be precipitated with thyroid replacement therapy, especially in clients with pre-existing heart disease. Chills, fever, and hypotension could indicate several complications, such as sepsis related to infection, or transfusion reactions, which are not related to hypothyroid therapy. Decreased visual acuity and low platelet count are not related to hypothyroidism.
CN: Physiological integrity; CNS: Physiological adaptation; CL: Application

16. A client presents with weight gain, intolerance to cold, constipation, and lethargy. Which test should the nurse expect to be ordered?
1. Liver function tests
2. Hemoglobin A_{1C}
3. T_4 and thyroid-stimulating hormone
4. 24-hour urine free cortisol measurement

Know which test to order to ensure a proper diagnosis.

16. **3.** The client's symptoms suggest hypothyroidism. Levels of thyroid-stimulating hormone and T_4 should be measured if hypothyroidism is suspected. Liver function tests are used to determine liver disease. Hemoglobin A_{1C} measurement is used to assess hyperglycemia. As part of the screening process for Cushing's syndrome, a 24-hour urine free cortisol measurement is completed.

CN: Physiological integrity; CNS: Physiological adaptation; CL: Application

17. The nurse is admitting a client with hypothyroidism. During the initial assessment, which of the following symptoms should the nurse be alert for?
1. Polyuria, polydipsia, and weight loss
2. Heat intolerance, nervousness, weight loss, and hair loss
3. Coarsening of facial features and extremity enlargement
4. Tiredness, cold intolerance, weight gain, and constipation

17. **4.** Tiredness, cold intolerance, weight gain, and constipation are symptoms of hypothyroidism, secondary to a decrease in cellular metabolism. Polyuria, polydipsia, and weight loss are symptoms of type 1 diabetes mellitus. Hyperthyroidism has symptoms of heat intolerance, nervousness, weight loss, and hair loss. Coarsening of facial features and extremity enlargement are symptoms of acromegaly.

CN: Physiological integrity; CNS: Physiological adaptation; CL: Application

18. A client is admitted with an adrenal malfunction. The nurse demonstrates an understanding of the function of the adrenal gland by identifying which hormones as being released by the adrenal medulla?
1. Epinephrine and norepinephrine
2. Glucocorticoids, mineralocorticoids, and androgens
3. Thyroxine, triiodothyronine, and calcitonin
4. Insulin, glucagon, and somatostatin

18. **1.** The medulla of the adrenal gland causes the release of epinephrine and norepinephrine. Glucocorticoids, mineralocorticoids, and androgens are released from the adrenal cortex. Thyroxine, triiodothyronine, and calcitonin are secreted by the thyroid gland. The islet cells of the pancreas secrete insulin, glucagon, and somatostatin.

CN: Physiological integrity; CNS: Physiological adaptation; CL: Analysis

19. A client is scheduled for several tests. Which test should be performed <u>after</u> the thyroid function tests?
1. Ultrasound of the carotid arteries
2. EEG
3. Chest X-ray
4. Computed tomography scan of the head with contrast

Sometimes the order of the tests performed is as important as the results.

19. **4.** Contrast media contains iodine and can alter thyroid function test results. The other studies don't require contrast media and don't need to be performed after the thyroid function tests.

CN: Physiological integrity; CNS: Reduction of risk potential; CL: Application

20. The nurse is caring for a client who has experienced a cerebral vascular accident. The client is displaying oliguria and hyponatremia. The nurse suspects which of the following disorders?
1. Thyrotoxic crisis
2. Diabetes insipidus
3. Primary adrenocortical insufficiency
4. Syndrome of inappropriate antidiuretic hormone (SIADH)

21. The nurse admits a client with a diagnosis of chronic adrenal insufficiency. The nurse is aware that adrenal insufficiency develops secondary to inadequate secretion of which pituitary hormone?
1. Adrenocorticotropic hormone (ACTH)
2. Antidiuretic hormone (ADH)
3. Follicle-stimulating hormone (FSH)
4. Thyroid-stimulating hormone (TSH)

22. A nurse is caring for a client with diabetes insipidus. Which laboratory value is most important for the nurse to monitor?
1. Glucose
2. Hemoglobin
3. Creatinine
4. Sodium

23. A 37-year-old client complains of muscle weakness, anorexia, and darkening of his skin. The nurse reviews his laboratory data and notes findings of low serum sodium and high serum potassium levels. The nurse recognizes that these signs and symptoms are associated with which condition?
1. Addison's disease
2. Cushing's disease
3. Diabetes insipidus
4. Thyrotoxic crisis

You've already made big strides. Keep at it!

20. 4. SIADH is a condition in which the client has excessive levels of antidiuretic hormone (ADH) and can't excrete the dilute urine. Therefore, the client retains fluids. This disorder causes a dilutional hyponatremia. Thyrotoxic crisis occurs with severe hyperthyroidism. Diabetes insipidus creates an ADH deficiency, causing dilute urine and hypernatremia. Primary adrenocortical insufficiency (Addison's disease) is caused by deficiency of a cortical hormone.

CN: Physiological integrity; CNS: Reduction of risk potential; CL: Application

21. 1. Inadequate secretion of ACTH from the pituitary gland results in adrenal insufficiency. ADH is secreted by the pituitary gland but doesn't affect the adrenal gland. FSH is also secreted by the pituitary gland but doesn't affect the adrenal gland; it stimulates the gonads. TSH is also secreted by the pituitary gland and stimulates the thyroid gland.

CN: Physiological integrity; CNS: Reduction of risk potential; CL: Application

22. 4. Diabetes insipidus occurs as a result of decreased release of antidiuretic hormone, which disturbs fluid and electrolyte balance, especially sodium. Clients need to be closely monitored for hypernatremia.

CN: Physiological integrity; CNS: Reduction of risk potential; CL: Analysis

23. 1. The clinical picture of Addison's disease includes muscle weakness, anorexia, darkening of the skin's pigmentation, low sodium level, and high potassium level. Cushing's syndrome presents with obesity, "buffalo hump," "moon face," and thin extremities. Symptoms of diabetes insipidus include excretion of large volumes of dilute urine, leading to hypernatremia and dehydration. Thyrotoxic crisis can occur with severe hyperthyroidism.

CN: Physiological integrity; CNS: Physiological adaptation; CL: Application

24. The nurse is caring for a postoperative client who has undergone removal of the pituitary gland and tumor (hypophysectomy). The nurse is aware that the client may be at risk for:
1. hypernatremia and concentrated urine.
2. dilute urine with a low specific gravity.
3. hyponatremia and concentrated urine.
4. dilute urine with a high specific gravity.

25. The nurse is caring for a postoperative client who has had a surgical removal of the pituitary gland (hypophysectomy) and has developed diabetes insipidus (DI). The nurse is aware that if fluids are restricted, the client is at risk for which of the following?
1. Hypertension and bradycardia
2. Glucosuria and weight gain
3. Fluid overload and hyponatremia
4. Severe dehydration and hypernatremia

26. When caring for a client with a diagnosis of diabetes insipidus, which nursing intervention should be the priority?
1. Watching for signs and symptoms of septic shock
2. Maintaining adequate fluid intake
3. Checking weight every 3 days
4. Monitoring urine for specific gravity greater than 1.030

27. The nurse has just completed an assessment of a client who has suffered a head injury. During the assessment, the client consumed three glasses of water. Additionally, the nurse noted the client's output of a large amount of dilute urine with a specific gravity of less than 1.005. The nurse is aware that the client is at risk for which condition?
1. Diabetes mellitus
2. Diabetes insipidus
3. Diabetic ketoacidosis
4. Syndrome of inappropriate antidiuretic hormone (SIADH)

Knowing how much water a client should have can be a real juggling act.

24. **2.** DI results from a lack of antidiuretic hormone (ADH). This causes the kidneys to excrete very dilute urine with a low specific gravity. Sodium is high in clients with DI due to hemoconcentration. Very concentrated urine is a sign of syndrome of inappropriate antidiuretic hormone (SIADH).
CN: Physiological integrity; CNS: Physiological adaptation; CL: Application

25. **4.** A client with DI excretes high volumes of urine, even without fluid replacement. Therefore, limiting fluid intake will cause severe dehydration and hypernatremia. A client undergoing a fluid deprivation test may experience tachycardia and hypotension. A client with DI will usually experience weight loss, and his urine doesn't contain glucose. Fluid overload and hypernatremia are signs of syndrome of inappropriate antidiuretic hormone (SIADH).
CN: Physiological integrity; CNS: Physiological adaptation; CL: Analysis

26. **2.** In a client with diabetes insipidus, maintaining fluid intake is essential to prevent severe dehydration. The client is at risk for developing hypovolemic shock because of increased urine output. Weight should be measured on a daily basis to check for adequate fluid balance. Urine specific gravity should be monitored for low osmolality, generally less than 1.005, due to the body's inability to concentrate urine.
CN: Safe, effective care environment; CNS: Management of care; CL: Application

27. **2.** Diabetes insipidus (DI) results from lack of antidiuretic hormone (ADH), which can occur if the pituitary gland is involved in a head injury. DI is characterized by a great thirst (polydipsia) and large amounts of water-like urine, which has a specific gravity of 1.001 to 1.005. Diabetes mellitus presents with polydipsia, polyuria, and polyphagia, but the client also has hyperglycemia. Diabetic ketoacidosis presents with weight loss, polyuria, and polydipsia, and the client has a severe acidosis. A client with SIADH can't excrete dilute urine; the client retains fluid and develops a sodium deficiency.
CN: Physiological integrity; CNS: Physiological adaptation; CL: Analysis

28. A client with diabetes insipidus is receiving desmopressin (DDAVP). Immediate intervention is necessary if the client develops which adverse effect?
1. Rash and difficulty breathing
2. Abdominal cramping
3. Burning at the injection site
4. Headache

29. The nurse is caring for a client who is diagnosed with diabetes insipidus. The nurse assesses the client carefully based on the understanding that which of the following complications must be prevented?
1. Decreased hemoglobin and hyponatremia
2. Hypertension and bradycardia
3. Hypotension and increased urine output
4. High urine specific gravity and hypertension

30. The nurse is caring for a client who has been admitted with a suspected diagnosis of diabetes insipidus (DI). The nurse can expect which of the following tests to confirm the diagnosis?
1. Capillary blood glucose test
2. Fluid deprivation test
3. Serum ketone test
4. Urine glucose test

You're doing great!

31. The nurse is admitting a client who is suspected of having adrenal insufficiency, or Addison's disease. An initial serum chemistry test is done. The nurse expects to see which of the following abnormalities?
1. Hyponatremia and hyperkalemia
2. Hypernatremia and hypokalemia
3. Hyperglycemia and hypernatremia
4. Hypercalcemia and hyperglycemia

28. 1. Rash and difficulty breathing may indicate an allergic reaction to the medication, which requires immediate intervention. The other symptoms may occur but aren't life threatening.
CN: Physiological integrity; CNS: Pharmacological and parenteral therapies; CL: Application

29. 3. A lack of antidiuretic hormone (ADH) causes diabetes insipidus (DI). This causes the kidneys to excrete large amounts of very dilute urine with a low specific gravity. This can cause hypovolemic hypotension and tachycardia. It also causes hemodilution, which results in increased hemoglobin and hypernatremia.
CN: Physiological integrity; CNS: Physiological adaptation; CL: Application

30. 2. The fluid deprivation test involves withholding water for 4 to 18 hours and checking urine output for amount and specific gravity, weight, postural blood pressure, and urine osmolarity periodically. Plasma osmolarity is also checked. A client with diabetes insipidus will have an increased serum osmolarity (of less than 300 mOsm/kg). Urine osmolarity won't increase. The capillary blood glucose test allows a rapid measurement of glucose in whole blood. The serum ketone test documents diabetic ketoacidosis. The urine glucose test monitors glucose levels in urine, but diabetes insipidus doesn't affect urine glucose levels.
CN: Physiological integrity; CNS: Reduction of risk potential; CL: Analysis

31. 1. Addison's disease is characterized by low serum sodium (hyponatremia) and high serum potassium (hyperkalemia). Serum glucose is low due to decreased glyconeogenesis and depletion of muscle and liver glycogen. Serum calcium is not usually affected to a significant degree.
CN: Physiological integrity; CNS: Physiological adaptation; CL: Application

CN: Client needs category   CNS: Client needs subcategory   CL: Cognitive level

32. The nurse is caring for a client who is diagnosed with Addison's disease. While completing the initial assessment and reviewing serum laboratory test results, the nurse expects to find which of the following signs and symptoms?
1. Weight gain and loss of skin pigment
2. Fatigue and muscle weakness
3. Hypertension and hypernatremia
4. Increased appetite and hypokalemia

33. The nurse is caring for a client with Addison's disease. Which of the following serum laboratory values indicates that the treatment being given is effective?
1. Sodium of 147 mEq/L
2. Potassium of 2.9 mEq/L
3. Sodium of 142 mEq/L
4. Potassium of 6.0 mEq/L

34. The nurse is caring for a client who has been admitted with a diagnosis of addisonian crisis. In planning care for this client, which outcome should be <u>priority</u>?
1. Preventing irreversible shock
2. Preventing infection
3. Relieving anxiety
4. Lowering blood pressure

35. The nurse is caring for a client who is admitted with untreated hypothyroidism. Which of the following laboratory serum values will the nurse expect to see?
1. High T_3 and T_4 and low thyroid-stimulating hormone (TSH)
2. High T_3 and T_4 and normal TSH
3. Low T_3 and T_4 and low TSH
4. Low T_3 and T_4 and high TSH

How low can I go?

32. 2. Manifestations of adrenal insufficiency or Addison's disease include fatigue, muscle weakness, weight loss, hyperpigmentation, hypotension, hyponatremia, decreased appetite, and hyperkalemia.

CN: Physiological integrity; CNS: Physiological adaptation; CL: Application

33. 3. Adrenal insufficiency causes a low sodium level and a high potassium level. A sodium value of 142 mEq/L is within the normal range and indicates the therapy is effective. All of the other lab values are outside of the normal range.

CN: Physiological integrity; CNS: Physiological adaptation; CL: Application

34. 1. In addisonian crisis, there's an uncontrolled loss of sodium in the urine and impaired mineralocorticoid function, resulting in loss of extracellular fluid and low blood volume and possible irreversible shock. Preventing infection isn't an appropriate goal in this life-threatening situation. Relieving anxiety is appropriate after the client is stabilized. The client in addisonian crisis is hypotensive, so blood pressure should be raised not lowered.

CN: Safe, effective care environment; CNS: Management of care; CL: Analysis

35. 4. Thyroid cells may fail to produce sufficient levels of thyroid hormones. This causes low serum levels, and the client has a decreased metabolic rate. This signals the hypothalamus and anterior pituitary gland to make more TSH in an attempt to trigger more production of thyroid hormones from the thyroid gland; thus, we see low serum thyroid hormone levels and a high serum TSH level.

CN: Physiological integrity; CNS: Physiological adaptation; CL: Application

36. The nurse is planning care for a client with Addison's disease. What is the most appropriate nursing diagnosis?
1. Fatigue
2. Excess fluid volume
3. Ineffective thermoregulation
4. Impaired gas exchange

I can relax my way right through this question.

37. The nurse is planning care for a client with Addison's disease. What is the most appropriate outcome for this client?
1. Taking in less than 1,000 ml of fluid a day
2. Participating in relaxation techniques
3. Ambulating in the hall five to six times per day
4. Knowing which high-sodium foods to avoid

38. The nurse is providing education to a client with Addison's disease about managing the disease process. What is the most important information for the nurse to include?
1. Eat a low-sodium diet.
2. Restrict fluids to 1,000 ml/day.
3. Wear Medic-Alert bracelet.
4. Take daily cortisone on an empty stomach.

39. The nurse is admitting a client who is diagnosed with untreated Cushing's syndrome. While performing the initial assessment, the nurse can expect to see which of the following signs and symptoms?
1. Moon face and truncal obesity
2. Weight loss and heat intolerance
3. Changes in skin texture and low body temperature
4. Polyuria and dehydration

36. 1. Clients with Addison's disease experience fatigue related to decreased metabolic energy production and altered body chemistry. Clients with Addison's disease experience fluid volume deficit, secondary to decreased mineralocorticoid secretion. Heat intolerance is a symptom of hyperthyroidism. The respiratory system isn't directly affected, and gas exchange shouldn't be affected.
CN: Health promotion and maintenance; CNS: None; CL: Analysis

37. 2. Stress can precipitate a hypotensive crisis in clients with Addison's disease. These clients need to learn ways to identify and cope with stressors. Fluids shouldn't be restricted; fluid intake should be 3 qt (3 L) or more per day. Activity should be monitored closely for fatigue and weakness. Sodium shouldn't be restricted.
CN: Physiological integrity; CNS: Physiological adaptation; CL: Analysis

38. 3. Clients with Addison's disease should wear a Medic-Alert bracelet. Replacement therapy must not be discontinued; abruptly stopping the medication is very dangerous. These clients must take in extra sodium and fluids. Cortisone medication should be taken with food or milk to prevent gastric distress.
CN: Physiological integrity; CNS: Physiological adaptation; CL: Application

39. 1. Overproduction of adrenocortical hormone results in redistribution of fat, which manifests as a moon face, truncal obesity, and a buffalo hump. Weight loss and heat intolerance indicate thyroid hormone overproduction. Changes in skin texture and low body temperature indicate thyroid hormone underproduction. Polyuria and dehydration indicate diabetic ketoacidosis.
CN: Physiological integrity; CNS: Physiological adaptation; CL: Application

40. The nurse is planning care for a client who is diagnosed with Cushing's syndrome. Which of the following nursing diagnoses would be appropriate for this client?
1. Risk for fluid volume deficit
2. Risk for infection
3. Impaired gas exchange
4. Acute pain

Here's to you! You've finished 40 questions already! That's excellent!

41. The nurse is reviewing the diagnoses of her assigned clients and notes that one of the clients has Cushing's syndrome. The nurse is aware that this client is at risk for which of the following?
1. Hypoglycemia and dehydration
2. Hypotension and hyperglycemia
3. Hyponatremia and dehydration
4. Hypertension and heart failure

42. The nurse is admitting a client with newly diagnosed Cushing's syndrome. Which of the following serum laboratory results might be expected for this client?
1. Decreased sodium and decreased glucose
2. Decreased cortisol and increased glucose
3. Increased cortisol and decreased sodium
4. Increased cortisol and increased sodium

43. The nurse is caring for a client who is diagnosed with Cushing's disease. It is most important for the nurse to assess the client for which condition?
1. Diabetes insipidus
2. Syndrome of inappropriate antidiuretic hormone (SIADH)
3. Addison's disease
4. Diabetes mellitus

40. 2. High levels of corticosteroids cause reduced inflammatory and immune responses, putting the client with Cushing's syndrome at increased risk for infection. Sodium and water are retained, causing fluid overload. Problems with gas exchange are not associated with Cushing's syndrome, nor is acute pain.
CN: Physiological integrity; CNS: Physiological adaptation; CL: Application

41. 4. Increased mineralocorticoid activity resulting in sodium and water retention in a client with Cushing's syndrome commonly contributes to hypertension and heart failure. Hypoglycemia and dehydration are uncommon in a client with Cushing's syndrome. Diabetes mellitus and hyperglycemia may develop, but hypotension is not part of the disease process. Dehydration also is not a complication of Cushing's syndrome.
CN: Physiological integrity; CNS: Physiological adaptation; CL: Analysis

42. 4. Increased cortisol, glucose, and sodium are found in clients with Cushing's syndrome.
CN: Physiological integrity; CNS: Physiological adaptation; CL: Application

43. 4. Glucose metabolism is profoundly affected by hypercortisolism. The liver is stimulated to convert more glycogen to glucose, and the insulin receptors are less sensitive so that blood glucose does not move as easily into the cells. Addison's disease is caused by low levels of cortisol. Diabetes insipidus and SIADH are not related to Cushing's disease.
CN: Physiological integrity; CNS: Physiological adaptation; CL: Application

44. Treatment for Cushing's syndrome may involve removal of one of the adrenal glands, which could cause a <u>temporary</u> state of which condition?
1. Hyperkalemia
2. Adrenal insufficiency
3. Excessive adrenal hormone
4. Syndrome of inappropriate antidiuretic hormone (SIADH)

44. 2. Removing a major source of adrenal hormones may cause a state of temporary adrenal insufficiency, requiring short-term replacement therapy. When both adrenal glands are removed, the client requires lifelong hormone replacement. A client with Cushing's syndrome would have a low—not high—potassium level. The client wouldn't have excessive adrenal hormone if all or part of the adrenal glands were removed. SIADH doesn't involve the adrenal gland; it involves the pituitary gland.
CN: Physiological integrity; CNS: Physiological adaptation; CL: Analysis

45. The nurse is caring for a client with newly diagnosed Cushing's disease. Which of the following signs and/or symptoms would the nurse expect to find on initial assessment?
1. Bruising and hypotension
2. Truncal obesity and petechiae
3. Hypertension and emaciation
4. Weight loss and moon face

45. 2. Cushing's disease causes truncal obesity due to fat redistribution and petechiae due to capillary fragility. Other manifestations include hypertension and weight gain.
CN: Physiological integrity; CNS: Physiological adaptation; CL: Application

46. The nurse is providing education for a client with Cushing's disease. Which of the following information would be important to include?
1. Avoid a low-sodium diet.
2. Physical changes are disease related.
3. High fluid intake is important.
4. Restrict protein intake.

> Explaining physical changes that may result from corticosteroid use can help ease your client's mind.

46. 2. The client may have a disturbed body image related to fat redistribution, moon face, buffalo hump, striae, acne, and facial hair (in women). Explaining that these are disease related is a start to addressing client feelings. The clients should take in minimal amounts of sodium. Fluids are often restricted, and a high-protein diet is encouraged.
CN: Physiological integrity; CNS: Physiological adaptation; CL: Application

47. The nurse is providing community education about prevention of diabetes mellitus to a group of clients. The nurse realizes that which of the following clients in the group is most at risk for developing type 2 diabetes mellitus?
1. A young adult who regularly plays basketball
2. An elderly sedentary woman
3. A middle-age woman who is a postal worker
4. A middle-age man with a normal weight

47. 2. The risk for developing type 2 diabetes is increased in clients over 65 years of age. The risk is increased with lack of exercise. The risk is decreased with exercise and maintenance of normal weight.
CN: Physiological integrity; CNS: Reduction of risk potential; CL: Application

48. The nurse is providing education for a client who is insulin dependent and often skips the ordered dose of insulin at home. The nurse teaches the client that omitting the insulin can result in which of the following?
1. Diabetic ketoacidosis
2. Hypoglycemia
3. Pancreatitis
4. Diabetes insipidus

49. A client with diabetes presents with polyphagia, polydipsia, and oliguria; he also complains of headache, malaise, and some visual changes. Assessment shows signs of dehydration. The nurse determines the client may be experiencing which condition?
1. Diabetes insipidus
2. Diabetic ketoacidosis
3. Hypoglycemia
4. Syndrome of inappropriate antidiuretic hormone (SIADH)

50. The nurse is admitting a client who is scheduled for a thyroidectomy. The initial serum laboratory tests indicate high levels of T_3 and T_4. The nurse expects to see which of the following related to levels of thyroid-stimulating hormone (TSH) for this client?
1. High
2. Low
3. Normal
4. Not important

51. A client exhibiting exophthalmos, weight loss, and tachycardia would be evaluated by checking the levels of which hormones?
1. Amylase, lipase, and trypsin
2. Triiodothyronine (T_3), thyroxine (T_4), and thyroid-stimulating hormone (TSH)
3. Glucocorticoids, mineralocorticoids, and androgens
4. Vasopressin and oxytocin

I'm a real shot in the arm towards your client's good health.

Do you know which glands produce which hormones? Here's a chance to test your knowledge.

48. 1. A client who fails to regularly take his insulin is at risk for hyperglycemia, which could lead to diabetic ketoacidosis. Hypoglycemia wouldn't occur because the lack of insulin would lead to increased levels of sugar in the blood. A client with chronic pancreatitis may develop diabetes (secondary to the pancreatitis), but insulin-dependent diabetes mellitus doesn't lead to pancreatitis. Diabetes insipidus isn't related to insulin levels.
CN: Physiological integrity; CNS: Physiological adaptation; CL: Application

49. 2. Early manifestations of diabetic ketoacidosis include polydipsia, polyphagia, and polyuria. As the client dehydrates and loses electrolytes, this condition often leads to oliguria, malaise, and visual changes. Diabetes insipidus may result in dehydration but not polyphagia and polydipsia. Symptoms of hypoglycemia include diaphoresis, tachycardia, and nervousness. A client with SIADH is unable to excrete a dilute urine, causing hyponatremia.
CN: Physiological integrity; CNS: Physiological adaptation; CL: Application

50. 2. The best indicator of primary hyperthyroidism (such as Graves' disease) is suppression of TSH below 0.1 µg/ml. This occurs when circulating levels of thyroid hormones are high. High levels of thyroid hormones signal the pituitary gland to stop producing TSH. This is important to differentiate between thyroid and pituitary dysfunction.
CN: Physiological integrity; CNS: Reduction of risk potential; CL: Analysis

51. 2. The symptoms reflect a potential dysfunction of the thyroid gland. T_3, T_4, and TSH are all secreted by the thyroid gland. Amylase, lipase, and trypsin are enzymes produced by the pancreas that aid in digestion. Glucocorticoids, mineralocorticoids, and androgens are produced by the adrenal gland. The pituitary gland secretes vasopressin and oxytocin.
CN: Health promotion and maintenance; CNS: None; CL: Analysis

52. The nurse is teaching a client with hypothyroidism about the thyroid gland. Which of the following statements by the nurse would be the most accurate about which gland controls the secretion of thyroid hormone?
1. Adrenal gland
2. Parathyroid gland
3. Pituitary gland
4. Thyroid gland

53. The nurse is admitting a client who is diagnosed with hyperthyroidism. The client asks what can be done for this disorder. What is the best response by the nurse?
1. Oral thyroid hormones
2. Lithotripsy
3. Radioactive iodine therapy
4. Laryngectomy

54. The nurse is providing education about the thyroid gland and aging to a group of nursing students. Which of the following would be appropriate to include in this discussion?
1. The thyroid gland increases in size with increasing age.
2. Older adults require higher doses of replacement therapy.
3. Thyroid hormone secretion increases with age.
4. The basal metabolic rate decreases with age.

55. A client with hyperthyroidism develops a high fever, extreme tachycardia, and systolic hypertension. The nurse suspects which of the following?
1. Hepatic coma
2. Thyroid storm
3. Myxedema
4. Laryngeal spasm

52. 3. By secretion of thyroid-stimulating hormone, the pituitary gland controls the rate of thyroid hormone released. The adrenal gland isn't involved with the thyroid gland. The parathyroid gland secretes parathyroid hormones, depending on the levels of calcium and phosphorus in the blood. The thyroid gland secretes thyroid hormone but doesn't control how much is released.
CN: Physiological integrity; CNS: Physiological adaptation; CL: Application

53. 3. The client (if not pregnant) can receive radioactive iodine (RAI) in the form of oral ^{131}I. The thyroid gland picks up the RAI, and some of the thyroid-producing cells are destroyed by the local radiation. Lithotripsy is a procedure to break up stones, such as found in the renal system. Oral thyroid hormones are contraindicated because the client already has too much of them. A laryngectomy involves removal of the larynx.
CN: Physiological integrity; CNS: Reduction of risk potential; CL: Application

54. 4. The basal metabolic rate decreases with age because the thyroid gland decreases in size and output of hormones as the client ages. Older adults require lower doses of replacement thyroid hormone; too large a dose may adversely affect the heart muscle.
CN: Physiological integrity; CNS: Reduction of risk potential; CL: Application

I think there's a storm on the way.

55. 2. Thyroid storm is a form of severe hyperthyroidism that can be precipitated by stress, injury, or infection. Hepatic coma occurs in clients with profound liver failure. Myxedema is related to hypothyroidism. Laryngeal spasms are a possible complication that can occur after thyroid surgery and do not involve fever or hypertension.
CN: Physiological integrity; CNS: Physiological adaptation; CL: Analysis

56. The nurse is providing health maintenance education to a group of clients. As the nurse talks about thyroid disorders, one of the clients asks about risk factors for Graves' disease. Which of the following would be most at risk for developing this disease?
1. A 40-year-old male
2. A 30-year-old female
3. A 15-year-old female
4. A 35-year-old male

56. 2. Graves' disease is diagnosed most often in women between 20 and 40 years of age, affecting women about 5 to 10 times more often than men.
CN: Physiological integrity; CNS: Reduction of risk potential; CL: Application

57. A client is admitted with a diagnosis of hyperparathyroidism. The nurse anticipates the client to present with which of the following?
1. Exophthalmos
2. Renal calculi
3. Weight gain
4. Weight loss

57. 2. Hyperparathyroidism is overproduction of parathyroid hormone, characterized by elevated serum calcium, bone calcification, or renal calculi. Exophthalmos and weight loss are signs of hyperthyroidism, and weight gain is a sign of hypothyroidism.
CN: Physiological integrity; CNS: Physiological adaptation; CL: Application

58. A client presents with flushed skin, exophthalmos, and perspiration and states that he has been "irritable" and having palpitations. The nurse interprets these symptoms as indicating which disorder?
1. Hyperthyroidism
2. Hyperparathyroidism
3. Hypothyroidism
4. Type 1 diabetes mellitus

> The words most important are a clue to how to answer question 59.

58. 1. Signs and symptoms of hyperthyroidism include nervousness, palpitations, irritability, exophthalmos, heat intolerance, weight loss, and weakness. Hyperparathyroidism is characterized by weakness and anorexia. Signs and symptoms of hypothyroidism include fatigue, cool skin, and sensitivity to cold. Type 1 diabetes mellitus presents with polyuria, polydipsia, and weight loss.
CN: Physiological integrity; CNS: Physiological adaptation; CL: Analysis

59. Which of the following would be <u>most important</u> for the nurse to assess in a client with anterior pituitary hypofunction?
1. Date of least menstrual period
2. Weight gain
3. Changes in urinary output
4. Chest pain

59. 1. Amenorrhea is a sign of decreased follicle-stimulating hormone, which is one of the anterior pituitary hormones. Weight gain is associated with Cushing's syndrome, which is associated with the adrenal cortex. Urinary output is related to posterior pituitary function, and chest pain is not related to hormone levels.
CN: Health promotion and maintenance; CNS: None; CL: Application

60. A client is brought into the emergency department with a brain stem contusion. Two days after admission, the client has a large amount of urine and a serum sodium level of 155 mEq/dl. Which condition may be developing?
1. Myxedema coma
2. Diabetes insipidus
3. Type 1 diabetes mellitus
4. Syndrome of inappropriate antidiuretic hormone (SIADH)

61. A client is exhibiting Kussmaul's respirations, abdominal discomfort, and lethargy. If random serum glucose is 325 mg/dl, which additional test should be conducted?
1. Complete blood count (CBC)
2. Serum ketones
3. Blood urea nitrogen (BUN)/creatinine
4. Liver enzymes

62. The nurse is admitting a client with the diagnosis of <u>diabetic ketoacidosis</u> (DKA). The nurse should anticipate administration of which of the following treatments?
1. Glucagon and I.V. fluids
2. Blood products
3. Glucocorticoids
4. Insulin and I.V. fluids

63. The nurse is caring for a client who was admitted with a diagnosis of diabetic ketoacidosis (DKA). The nurse is aware of possible complications related to fluid and electrolyte imbalances. Which of the following laboratory tests would be the priority to monitor as the client receives initial treatment of insulin and I.V. fluids?
1. Serum potassium
2. A_{1C}
3. Serum calcium
4. Serum nitrogen

Make sure you know which disorder the question is asking you to treat.

This question calls for a concentrated effort.

60. 2. Two leading causes of diabetes insipidus are hypothalamic or pituitary tumors and closed head injuries. Myxedema coma is a form of hypothyroidism. Type 1 diabetes mellitus isn't caused by a brain injury. A client with SIADH would have hyponatremia and oliguria; this client's sodium level was 155 mEq/dl, which is above normal levels of 135 to 145 mEq/dl.
CN: Physiological integrity; CNS: Reduction of risk potential; CL: Application

61. 2. Clients with Kussmaul's respirations, abdominal discomfort, lethargy, and serum glucose levels above 300 mg/dl could be diagnosed with diabetic ketoacidosis. Serum ketones would aid in confirming the diagnosis. CBC, BUN/creatinine, and liver enzymes are not indicated in a diabetic ketoacidosis workup.
CN: Physiological integrity; CNS: Reduction of risk potential; CL: Application

62. 4. A client with DKA would receive insulin to lower glucose and I.V. fluids to correct hypotension. Glucagon is given to treat hypoglycemia; DKA involves hyperglycemia. Blood products aren't needed to correct DKA. Glucocorticoids aren't needed because the adrenal glands aren't involved.
CN: Physiological integrity; CNS: Pharmacological and parenteral therapies; CL: Application

63. 1. Regardless of the initial high potassium value, there is a large total-body potassium deficit with DKA. With insulin therapy, serum potassium levels fall rapidly as insulin allows potassium to enter cells. Hypokalemia will cause cardiac complications and is a common cause of death in the treatment of DKA. A_{1C} values indicate overall glucose control over the past 3 to 4 months. Serum calcium and nitrogen are not priorities in managing DKA.
CN: Physiological integrity; CNS: Reduction of risk potential; CL: Application

64. The home health nurse is visiting a new type 1 diabetic client and finds the client lethargic with very deep, rapid respirations. The client reports nausea and abdominal pain. The nurse observes dehydration, dry skin, and weight loss. The nurse suspects which of the following diabetic complications?
1. Hypoglycemia
2. Diabetes insipidus
3. Myxedema
4. Ketoacidosis

65. The nurse is preparing to administer I.V. insulin to a client diagnosed with diabetic ketoacidosis. The client is at risk for which conditions?
1. Hypokalemia and hypoglycemia
2. Hypocalcemia and hyperkalemia
3. Hyperkalemia and hyperglycemia
4. Hypernatremia and hypercalcemia

Keep your eyes open for the highs and lows.

66. Which nursing diagnosis would have the highest priority for a client with hyperosmolar hyperglycemic nonketotic syndrome (HHNS)?
1. Risk for infection
2. Risk for acute confusion
3. Deficient fluid volume
4. Impaired skin integrity

67. The nurse and a nursing student are caring for a client who is diagnosed with hyperglycemic hyperosmolar state (HHS). The student asks the nurse how HHS differs from diabetic ketoacidosis (DKA). Which is the correct reply by the nurse?
1. HHS displays little or no ketones.
2. HHS has no potential for hypokalemia.
3. HHS presents with lower blood glucose than DKA.
4. HHS presents with normal hydration.

It is important to know what you are looking for.

68. The nurse is preparing an insulin infusion for a client in diabetic ketoacidosis (DKA). Which of the following would be the appropriate type of insulin to use for I.V. infusion?
1. Lantus
2. NPH
3. Humalog
4. Regular

64. 4. Classic symptoms of diabetic ketoacidosis include polyuria, weight loss, nausea and vomiting, altered mental status, abdominal pain, and Kussmaul's respirations (deep, rapid respirations meant to correct acidosis). Hypoglycemia and diabetes insipidus do not cause Kussmaul's respirations. Myxedema is caused by low thyroid function.
CN: Physiological integrity; CNS: Reduction of risk potential; CL: Application

65. 1. Blood glucose needs to be monitored because there's a chance for hyperglycemia or hypoglycemia. Hypoglycemia might occur if too much insulin is administered. Hypokalemia might occur because I.V. insulin forces potassium into cells, thereby lowering the plasma levels of potassium. The client may have hyperkalemia prior to starting the insulin therapy, but hypokalemia will occur with insulin administration. Calcium and sodium levels aren't affected.
CN: Physiological integrity; CNS: Pharmacological and parenteral therapies; CL: Application

66. 3. A client with HHNS has severe dehydration, which requires immediate intervention. The other nursing diagnoses are all appropriate but aren't the priority.
CN: Physiological integrity; CNS: Physiological adaptation; CL: Analysis

67. 1. Both HHS and DKA are caused by hyperglycemia and dehydration. HHS differs from DKA in that ketone levels are low or absent and blood glucose levels are much higher. In HHS as well as DKA, the serum potassium level may drop quickly when insulin therapy allows potassium to enter cells.
CN: Physiological integrity; CNS: Reduction of risk potential; CL: Application

68. 4. Regular insulin can be given intravenously. The other types listed can only be given by the subcutaneous route.
CN: Physiological integrity; CNS: Pharmacological and parenteral therapies; CL: Application

69. The nurse is caring for a client admitted to the emergency department with weakness, thirst, and an inability to concentrate. Laboratory results show a serum glucose of 712 mg/dl, urine negative for ketones, and minimal electrolyte imbalance. For which diabetic complication should the client be evaluated?
1. Hypoglycemia
2. Diabetes insipidus
3. Diabetic ketoacidosis (DKA)
4. Hyperglycemic hyperosmolar state (HHS)

70. The nurse is providing education about sick-day rules to a group of clients with type 1 diabetes mellitus. Which of the following information is appropriate to include?
1. Monitor blood glucose at least once a day.
2. Do not take insulin until you feel well.
3. Drink 8 to 12 oz of fluid each waking hour.
4. If nauseated, cease all oral intakes.

71. The nurse is caring for a client with type 1 diabetes mellitus. At 3:00 a.m., the nurse finds the client manifesting mild confusion and diaphoresis and complaining of palpitations. Which of the following should the nurse do first?
1. Give 10 to 15 g of carbohydrate orally.
2. Call the physician for additional insulin order.
3. Administer 1 mg of glucagon subcutaneously.
4. Check blood glucose level.

72. The nurse checks on a diabetic client and finds the client lethargic, difficult to arouse, and profusely diaphoretic. The nurse immediately checks the client's blood glucose and finds it to be 40 mg/dl. Which of the following interventions is the priority?
1. Obtain a urine sample and assess for ketones.
2. Give 10 to 15 g of carbohydrate orally.
3. Give 1 mg of glucagon subcutaneously.
4. Call the physician for addition insulin order.

I'm taking a sick day.

69. 4. A serum glucose level over 600 mg/dl and no ketones in the urine suggest HHS. Hypoglycemia is usually due to excessive insulin administration. Dysfunctions in antidiuretic hormone secretion from the pituitary gland lead to diabetes insipidus. DKA manifests with urine and serum ketones.

CN: Physiological integrity; CNS: Physiological adaptation; CL: Application

70. 3. To prevent dehydration, sick clients should drink 8 to 12 oz of sugar-free liquids every waking hour. Clients who are ill should monitor their blood glucose at least every 4 hours and continue to take insulin or oral agents. If nauseated, clients should consume more easily tolerated foods or liquids equal to the carbohydrate content of usual meals.

CN: Physiological integrity; CNS: Pharmacological and parenteral therapies; CL: Analysis

71. 4. Check the blood glucose first when symptoms arise and then proceed with treatment according to results. If the client is hypoglycemic, administration of carbohydrate is appropriate. If fully conscious, carbohydrate may be given orally. If unconscious, subcutaneous or intramuscular glucagon is appropriate. This client is showing signs/symptoms of hypoglycemia, so additional insulin would lower the blood glucose further.

CN: Physiological integrity; CNS: Reduction of risk potential; CL: Application

72. 3. The client has hypoglycemia. Since the client is lethargic and difficult to arouse, giving oral glucose is not advised due to the potential for aspiration. The priority is to administer glucagon subcutaneously or intramuscularly to treat the hypoglycemia and avoid the potential for aspiration. Ketones are produced with hyperglycemia. Additional insulin would lower the blood glucose further.

CN: Physiological integrity; CNS: Reduction of risk potential; CL: Application

73. The nurse is caring for a middle-aged athletic client with hyperparathyroidism. The client has been further diagnosed with kidney stones. The client is currently showing signs of apathy and depression, and despite the client's athleticism, the nurse's assessment finds flabby musculature. Based on the diagnosis and signs and symptoms, the nurse suspects which of the following conditions?
1. Hypercalcemia
2. Hypocalcemia
3. Hypernatremia
4. Hyponatremia

74. The nurse is providing education to a client who has been diagnosed with hyperparathyroidism. The nurse determines further teaching is necessary when the client states that they will continue to take:
1. acetaminophen.
2. aspirin.
3. potassium-wasting diuretics.
4. thiazide diuretics.

Oh so many contraindications to know!

75. The serum calcium level of a client with hyperparathyroidism is 14.6 mg/dl. Which treatment should the nurse anticipate?
1. Withholding fluids
2. Starting oral calcium supplements
3. Giving vitamin D supplements
4. Administering I.V. fluids at 200 ml/hour

76. The nurse admits a client whose initial laboratory tests reveal hyperphosphatemia and hypocalcemia. The nurse suspects which of the following disorders?
1. Cushing's syndrome
2. Graves' disease
3. Hypoparathyroidism
4. Hypothyroidism

77. A 55-year-old client is admitted with hyperthyroidism. What is the most important nursing intervention?
1. Keeping the client warm
2. Encouraging the client to increase activity
3. Providing a calm, restful environment
4. Placing the client in high Fowler's position

73. 1. An overactive parathyroid gland (hyperparathyroidism) produces an increased amount of parathyroid hormone, which promotes the release of calcium from the bone and increases serum calcium (which may cause kidney stones). The client is demonstrating signs/symptoms of hypercalcemia. Hypocalcemia would cause muscle cramps and possible tetany. Hyperparathyroidism does not directly affect sodium levels.
CN: Physiological integrity; CNS: Reduction of risk potential; CL: Analysis

74. 4. Thiazide diuretics shouldn't be used because they decrease renal excretion of calcium, thereby raising serum calcium levels even higher. There are no contraindications to acetaminophen or aspirin for clients with hyperparathyroidism. Potassium loss isn't an issue for clients with hyperparathyroidism.
CN: Physiological integrity; CNS: Pharmacological and parenteral therapies; CL: Application

75. 4. Normal calcium levels are 8.5 to 10.5 mg/dl, so a level of 14.6 mg/dl is dangerously high. To decrease the calcium level, intake of calcium should be reduced, and calcium excretion should be promoted by administering I.V. and oral fluids and diuretics. Vitamin D increases the calcium level.
CN: Physiological integrity; CNS: Physiological adaptation; CL: Analysis

76. 3. The parathyroid gland works to balance calcium by decreasing bone calcium and increasing serum calcium. Calcium and phosphorus levels are inversely related. Therefore, a low-functioning parathyroid gland would manifest as hyperphosphatemia and hypocalcemia. Excessive adrenocortical activity indicates Cushing's syndrome. Excessive thyroid hormone levels indicate Graves' disease (hyperthyroidism). Low thyroid hormone levels indicate hypothyroidism.
CN: Physiological integrity; CNS: Physiological adaptation; CL: Analysis

77. 3. Clients with hyperthyroidism are typically anxious, diaphoretic, nervous, and fatigued; they need a calm, restful environment in which to relax and get adequate rest. Clients with hyperthyroidism are usually warm and diaphoretic and need a cool environment. Activity shouldn't be increased. A high Fowler's position would benefit a client who is dyspneic, but this is not usually the case for hyperthyroidism.
CN: Safe, effective care environment; CNS: Management of care; CL: Application

78. A nurse is providing teaching to a client with hypoparathyroidism. Which vitamin therapy should she include in her teaching?
1. Vitamin A
2. Vitamin C
3. Vitamin D
4. Vitamin E

79. The nurse is caring for a 47-year-old client admitted with joint pain and weakness. The client describes a gradual coarsening of facial features and enlargement of hands and feet over the past year. The nurse is aware that these are early clinical manifestations of which condition?
1. Acromegaly
2. Cushing's syndrome
3. Graves' disease
4. Pheochromocytoma

One of us needs to get involved.

80. A nurse is teaching a client about mixing insulin. The physician has ordered, "Regular insulin 6 units mixed with NPH insulin 10 units." Put the following steps related to mixing insulin in the correct order.

1. Withdraw 6 units of regular insulin.

2. Inject 10 units of air into the NPH vial.

3. Inject 6 units of air into the regular insulin.

4. Withdraw 10 units of NPH insulin.

5. Roll bottle of NPH gently to mix.

81. A client is diagnosed with a somatotrophin-secreting tumor that could lead to development of acromegaly, Cushing's syndrome, and hypopituitarism. Which gland is related to this tumor?
1. Adrenal gland
2. Hypothalamus
3. Pituitary gland
4. Thyroid gland

Here's a case for knowing your hormones cold.

78. 3. A client with hypoparathyroidism has a decreased serum calcium level. Variable doses of vitamin D preparations enhance the absorption of calcium from the GI tract. Vitamins A, C, and E aren't involved with this process.
CN: Physiological integrity; CNS: Pharmacological and parenteral therapies; CL: Analysis

79. 1. Acromegaly is marked by coarsening of facial features and soft tissue swelling of the hands and feet. Cushing's syndrome causes thin extremities, truncal obesity, and a "moon face." Graves' disease causes bulging of the eyes, weight loss, and heat intolerance. Pheochromocytoma is a tumor of the adrenal gland that causes hypertension.
CN: Physiological integrity; CNS: Physiological adaptation; CL: Application

80. The correct order is as follows:

5. Roll bottle of NPH gently to mix.
2. Inject 10 units of air into the NPH vial.
3. Inject 6 units of air into the regular insulin.
1. Withdraw 6 units of regular insulin.
4. Withdraw 10 units of NPH insulin.

Always withdraw the clear or shorter acting (regular) insulin before the cloudy or longer acting (NPH) insulin. This prevents contamination of the shorter acting insulin vial with the longer acting insulin. Make sure the total adds up after drawing up the NPH.
CN: Physiological integrity; CNS: Pharmacological and parenteral therapies; CL: Analysis

81. 3. Tumors that affect the pituitary gland would lead to acromegaly, Cushing's syndrome, and hypopituitarism. Tumors of the adrenal gland would cause symptoms such as hypertension. The hypothalamus secretes corticotropin-releasing factor, which stimulates the anterior pituitary to secrete corticotropin. Tumors affecting the thyroid gland would involve thyroid hormones.
CN: Physiological integrity; CNS: Physiological adaptation; CL: Application

82. The nurse is reviewing a client's chart and notes a low serum calcium level. The nurse assesses the client and notes development of a carpopedal spasm when blood flow in the arm is occluded for a few minutes with a blood pressure cuff. The nurse interprets this as which sign?
1. Negative Chvostek's sign
2. Positive Chvostek's sign
3. Negative Trousseau's sign
4. Positive Trousseau's sign

83. After undergoing a thyroidectomy, a client develops hypocalcemia and tetany caused by inadvertent damage to the parathyroid glands. Which medication should the nurse anticipate administering?
1. Calcium gluconate
2. Potassium chloride
3. Sodium bicarbonate
4. Sodium phosphorus

84. After undergoing a thyroidectomy, a client develops a positive Trousseau's sign and muscle hyperexcitability, which can lead to tetany. These signs are caused by which of the following?
1. Hyperkalemia
2. Hypercalcemia
3. Hypokalemia
4. Hypocalcemia

85. Which test should a nurse expect to be ordered for a client with severe abdominal pain in the midepigastric region, back tenderness, nausea, and vomiting?
1. Amylase
2. C-peptide
3. Stool culture
4. Colonoscopy

86. A 48-year-old client has been admitted with complaints of acute abdominal pain in the midepigastric region, back tenderness, nausea, and vomiting. The nurse recognizes these findings to be associated with which condition?
1. Acute pancreatitis
2. Crohn's disease
3. Hypophysectomy
4. Pheochromocytoma

82. 4. A Trousseau's sign is positive when a carpopedal spasm is induced by occluding the blood flow of an arm for 1 to 4 minutes using a blood pressure cuff. Chvostek's sign is positive when a sharp tapping over the facial nerve, in front of the parotid gland and anterior to the ear, causes the mouth, nose, and eye to twitch. When positive, these signs indicate a low calcium level and muscle hyperexcitability.
CN: Physiological integrity; CNS: Reduction of risk potential; CL: Application

83. 1. Immediate treatment for a client who develops hypocalcemia and tetany after thyroidectomy is calcium gluconate. Potassium chloride and sodium bicarbonate aren't indicated. Sodium phosphorus wouldn't be given because phosphorus levels are already elevated.
CN: Physiological integrity; CNS: Pharmacological and parenteral therapies; CL: Analysis

84. 4. Damage to the parathyroid glands can occur inadvertently during a thyroidectomy. This causes a decrease in serum calcium, which causes muscle hyperexcitability and can lead to tetany. Immediate treatment for a client who develops hypocalcemia and tetany after thyroidectomy is calcium gluconate. Potassium is not affected by damage to the parathyroids.
CN: Physiological integrity; CNS: Reduction of risk potential; CL: Analysis

85. 1. Severe abdominal pain in the midepigastric region, back tenderness, nausea, and vomiting may be due to irritation of the pancreas. Therefore, an amylase level test should be ordered. C-peptide, a stool culture, and a colonoscopy wouldn't be ordered for the presenting symptoms.
CN: Physiological integrity; CNS: Physiological adaptation; CL: Analysis

86. 1. Signs and symptoms of acute pancreatitis include midepigastric abdominal pain, back pain, nausea, and vomiting. Crohn's disease is associated with right lower quadrant abdominal pain (in acute disease) and cramping abdominal pain (in chronic disease). Hypophysectomy is the surgical removal of the pituitary gland. Pheochromocytoma is a tumor of the adrenal gland and doesn't cause abdominal or back symptoms.
CN: Physiological integrity; CNS: Physiological adaptation; CL: Application

87. The nurse is modifying the plan of care for a client who is recovering from acute pancreatitis. Which of these measures would be the most appropriate to include in the care plan?
1. Eat small, frequent meals that are bland, high carbohydrate, high protein, and low fat.
2. Consume no more than one alcoholic drink per day and limit coffee to three cups per day.
3. Include fruits and vegetables that are high in vitamin C and K and increase fiber.
4. Maintain a diet that is low residue, low protein, and high in calcium.

88. An attack of pancreatitis has been brought on by gallstones and gallbladder disease. The client will require reinforcement about the need to follow which type of diet?
1. High-calorie, high-protein diet
2. High-fiber diet, encouraging fluid intake
3. Low-fat diet, avoiding heavy meals
4. Diet high in protein, calcium, and vitamin D

89. The nurse is teaching a group of nursing students about the incidence and risk for diabetes mellitus. To assist in growth of cultural awareness, the nurse explains that which of the following populations are at higher risk for diabetes mellitus than the rest of the populations? Select all that apply.
1. Caucasians
2. African Americans
3. Canadians
4. American Indians
5. Mexican Americans

90. A client is in diabetic ketoacidosis, secondary to infection. As the condition progresses, which symptoms might the nurse see?
1. Kussmaul's respirations and a fruity odor on the breath
2. Shallow respirations and severe abdominal pain
3. Decreased respirations and increased urine output
4. Cheyne-Stokes respirations and foul-smelling urine

Teach your client the importance of making healthy food choices.

Keep your eyes— and nose—alert to symptoms.

87. **1.** In order to restore energy and nutrients, small, frequent meals that are high carbohydrate, high protein, and low fat are advised. Spicy foods, caffeine, and alcohol should be avoided. The other instructions do not relate to pancreatitis.
CN: Physiological integrity; CNS: Basic care and comfort; CL: Application

88. **3.** A client who survives an acute pancreatitis attack caused by gallstones or gallbladder disease requires reinforcement to maintain a low-fat diet and to avoid heavy meals. A high-calorie, high-protein diet is appropriate for clients with hyperthyroidism. A diet high in fiber, encouraging fluid intake, is recommended for constipation. A client with Cushing's syndrome should follow a diet high in protein, calcium, and vitamin D.
CN: Physiological integrity; CNS: Reduction of risk potential; CL: Application

89. **2, 4, and 5.** African Americans, American Indians, and Mexican Americans are all at higher risk for diabetes mellitus.
CN: Physiological integrity; CNS: Reduction of risk potential; CL: Application

90. **1.** Coma and severe acidosis are ushered in with Kussmaul's respirations (rapid and deep but not labored respirations) and a fruity odor on the breath (acidemia). Shallow respirations and severe abdominal pain may be symptoms of pancreatitis. Decreased respirations and increased urine output aren't symptoms related to acidemia. Cheyne-Stokes respirations and foul-smelling urine do not result from diabetic ketoacidosis.
CN: Physiological integrity; CNS: Physiological adaptation; CL: Application

91. A nurse is preparing to administer "Regular insulin 4 units subcutaneously" to a client with type 1 diabetes mellitus. Which equipment does the nurse need to perform the injection?
1. 27-gauge, ½" needle
2. 22-gauge, ½" needle
3. 27-gauge, 1" needle
4. 22-gauge, 1" needle

91. 1. To administer medication, the nurse will be using a subcutaneous injection, which should be administered with a 25-gauge to 27-gauge, ⅝" to ½" needle. A 22-gauge needle is too large for a subcutaneous injection. A 1" needle will deliver the medication into the muscle of most clients, rather than subcutaneous tissue.
CN: Physiological integrity; CNS: Pharmacological and parenteral therapies; CL: Application

Don't give up now. You're doing great!

92. Clients with insulin-dependent diabetes mellitus may require which change to their daily routine during periods of infection?
1. No changes
2. Less insulin
3. More insulin
4. Oral antidiabetic agents

92. 3. During periods of infection or illness, insulin-dependent clients may need even more insulin to compensate for increased blood glucose levels. Since the client has insulin-dependent diabetes, oral antidiabetic agents wouldn't be indicated.
CN: Physiological integrity; CNS: Pharmacological and parenteral therapies; CL: Application

93. A physician prescribes an oral antidiabetic medication and weekly glucose monitoring for a 42-year-old male client recently diagnosed with type 2 diabetes. The client is moderately overweight and has a poor diet and a stressful job. He asks how his diagnosis will affect his life. What is the best response by the nurse?
1. "The medication will help maintain a steady glucose level, but you need to cut back on snacking."
2. "Type 2 diabetes is common and easily treated. You don't have to make changes."
3. "I'll refer you to a diabetes nurse educator. She'll help you develop a plan."
4. "You may want to change careers because your job is so stressful."

93. 3. A referral to a diabetic nurse educator who can develop an ongoing relationship and spend time assessing the client's personal needs and developing a workable plan with him would be the most appropriate. Although the medication does help to maintain steady glucose levels, this response ignores the other factors contributing to the client's poor health habits. Telling the client that he won't have to make any lifestyle changes is inappropriate, as is suggesting he change careers.
CN: Health promotion and maintenance; CNS: None; CL: Application

Make sure you know the standard guidelines of common disorders.

94. A nonpregnant client tells the nurse that two recent fasting blood glucose results were 132 mg/dl and 146 mg/dl. The nurse should expect which of the following actions to occur?
1. These are normal results; no further action is needed.
2. These results indicate diabetes mellitus; further follow-up is needed.
3. The fasting blood glucose tests should be repeated two more times.
4. The client should be scheduled for an HbA$_{1C}$ test.

94. 2. Based on the American Diabetes Association guidelines, fasting blood glucose of 126 mg/dl or more, on at least two occasions, is indicative of diabetes mellitus. These are not normal results. Further tests to make a definitive diagnosis of diabetes mellitus should be random blood glucose or glucose tolerance tests, not a fasting blood glucose or HbA$_{1C}$ test.
CN: Physiological integrity; CNS: Reduction of risk potential; CL: Analysis

95. The nurse is caring for a client who is diagnosed with a unilateral pheochromocytoma and is scheduled for surgery to remove the left adrenal gland. The nurse is aware that the main manifestation of this disease process is which of the following?
1. Hypertension
2. Renal failure
3. Hyponatremia
4. Heart failure

95. 1. A pheochromocytoma is usually a benign tumor of the adrenal medulla that secretes epinephrine and norepinephrine, resulting in hypertension and paroxysmal tachycardia. The other conditions are not directly associated with pheochromocytoma.
CN: Physiological integrity; CNS: Reduction of risk potential; CL: Analysis

96. The nurse is caring for a client with an adrenal medulla tumor. Which of the following symptoms would the nurse expect to assess?
1. Carpopedal spasm
2. Hyperglycemia
3. Hypertension
4. "Moon face"

97. The nurse is administering corticosteroid therapy to a client. The nurse should be alert for which of the following adverse effects of this therapy?
1. Hyponatremia
2. Hypoglycemia
3. Change in metabolism
4. Heart failure

98. The nurse is caring for a client who is diagnosed with hyperparathyroidism. The client asks what conditions may contribute to the development of hyperparathyroidism. What is the most appropriate response by the nurse?
1. Chronic renal failure
2. Thyroidectomy
3. Elevated serum calcium level
4. Steroid use

99. A previously healthy 70-year-old male client has a serum glucose level of 1,200 mg/dl, a normal serum bicarbonate level, and urine free from acetone. The nurse should suspect which condition?
1. Diabetic ketoacidosis (DKA)
2. Diabetes insipidus
3. Hyperglycemic hyperosmolar state (HHS)
4. Syndrome of inappropriate antidiuretic hormone (SIADH)

100. The nurse is providing education for a client newly diagnosed with Addison's disease who is receiving a maintenance dose of steroids. What is the most important information for the nurse to include?
1. Importance of restricting fluids
2. Watching for signs of hypoglycemia
3. Taking steroids exactly as prescribed
4. Adjusting steroid doses based on dietary intake and exercise

You should feel on top of the world! You're almost finished.

Always note the stated age. It can influence the answer.

96. 3. Tumors of the adrenal medulla usually produce hypertension because they release excessive amounts of epinephrine and norepinephrine. Carpopedal spasm occurs as a result of hypocalcemia. Hyperglycemia is a result of low insulin levels. Clients with Cushing's syndrome usually have a "moon face."

CN: Physiological integrity; CNS: Physiological adaptation; CL: Application

97. 3. A major adverse effect of corticosteroid therapy is a slowing of metabolism. This therapy also produces hyperglycemia and hypernatremia. Heart failure is not usually directly related to corticosteroid therapy.

CN: Physiological integrity; CNS: Pharmacological and parenteral therapies; CL: Analysis

98. 1. Because failing kidneys can't convert vitamin D, the serum calcium level declines, causing hyperparathyroidism from increased release of parathyroid hormones. Thyroidectomy may lead to hypoparathyroidism if the parathyroid is also removed during surgery. Hyperparathyroidism may cause serum calcium levels to rise. Steroid use induces calcium to leave bone, suppressing parathyroid hormone.

CN: Physiological integrity; CNS: Physiological adaptation; CL: Analysis

99. 3. Elderly clients are at risk for developing a hyperosmolar state as their taste preferences shift to softer, higher carbohydrate foods. The urine free from acetone indicates that the client isn't experiencing breakdown of fats and proteins, so the nurse shouldn't suspect DKA. The client's laboratory values don't indicate a disturbance in the production, secretion, or use of antidiuretic hormone, which would result in diabetes insipidus or SIADH.

CN: Physiological integrity; CNS: Physiological adaptation; CL: Analysis

100. 3. A client with Addison's disease needs more steroids than the body produces. Taking a lower dose may trigger an addisonian crisis; taking a higher dose increases the effects of potassium depletion, hyperglycemia, and fluid retention, leading to a life-threatening situation. Fluid restriction isn't desirable and could cause dehydration. Steroids tend to increase, not decrease, blood sugar. Steroid doses aren't adjusted for diet and exercise, although the client may need to administer insulin and adjust insulin doses.

CN: Physiological integrity; CNS: Pharmacological and parenteral therapies; CL: Application

CN: Client needs category CNS: Client needs subcategory CL: Cognitive level

101. A client is being treated for adrenal crisis (addisonian crisis). Which laboratory values are <u>most</u> important for the nurse to monitor?
1. Serum bicarbonate and sodium
2. Serum glucose and ketones
3. Serum sodium and potassium
4. Serum calcium and magnesium

Be careful! Combo answers can be tricky!

102. A client newly diagnosed with diabetic ketoacidosis has a serum glucose level of 485 mg/dl. After treatment, the serum glucose level drops to 185 mg/dl, and the cardiac monitor starts to show ventricular ectopic beats. Which factor is the <u>most probable</u> cause of the arrhythmia?
1. Decreased serum chloride level
2. Decreased serum potassium level
3. Elevated serum glucose level
4. Elevated serum sodium level

103. When teaching a diabetic client about nutritional planning, which food selection would be considered one healthy serving of carbohydrate?
1. One small orange
2. ½ cup of vanilla ice cream
3. 2 slices of white bread
4. 2 cups of whole-grain rice

Teaching is crucial for clients with diabetes.

104. An unemployed client with no health insurance hasn't filled his prescriptions for some time. According to his roommate, the client has been "getting sicker by the day." Which problem suggests the client isn't taking his prescribed levothyroxine (Synthroid)?
1. Diarrhea and vomiting
2. Rapid heart rate
3. Warm, dry, flushed skin
4. Temperature of 94° F (34.4° C)

105. A client with newly diagnosed diabetes mellitus is ready for discharge. What is the most important information for the nurse to include?
1. Foot care and the need for a high-calorie diet
2. How to balance diet, exercise, and medication
3. Fasting before health care maintenance visits
4. Avoiding all carbohydrates and drinking 2 qt (2 L) of water daily

101. 3. If steroid replacement therapy is inadequate, sodium loss and potassium retention persist. If the steroid dose is too high, sodium and water are retained, and large amounts of potassium are excreted. Steroid replacement can affect glucose, but the replacement doesn't have as great an impact on ketones, bicarbonate, calcium, or magnesium as it does on sodium and potassium.
CN: Physiological integrity; CNS: Reduction of risk potential; CL: Analysis

102. 2. Correction of an elevated serum glucose level may alter the serum potassium level, predisposing the client to arrhythmias. Serum chloride and sodium changes are more likely to contribute to an altered level of consciousness, whereas elevated serum glucose contributes to long-term effects of diabetes mellitus, such as coronary artery disease, hypertension, and peripheral vascular disease.
CN: Physiological integrity; CNS: Physiological adaptation; CL: Analysis

103. 1. One small orange is one serving of a healthy carbohydrate. Besides providing vitamins and water content, an orange contains fiber. Vanilla ice cream contains both carbohydrate and saturated fat. Two slices of white bread are two servings of carbohydrate. Two cups of whole-grain rice are approximately three to four servings of a carbohydrate.
CN: Physiological integrity; CNS: Basic care and comfort; CL: Application

104. 4. Levothyroxine is prescribed for hypothyroidism, which causes a hypodynamic state; failure to maintain levothyroxine therapy can lead to a low body temperature. The other problems indicate a hypermetabolic state; although the client may also experience these symptoms, they stem from infection and dehydration.
CN: Physiological integrity; CNS: Physiological adaptation; CL: Application

105. 2. With type 1, type 2, or gestational diabetes mellitus, balancing diet, exercise, and medication is essential to diabetes control. High-calorie and noncarbohydrate diets are contraindicated in diabetes. While fasting may reduce the serum glucose level temporarily, glycosylated hemoglobin tests show the effectiveness of long-term diabetes control.
CN: Physiological integrity; CNS: Physiological adaptation; CL: Application

106. Which statement indicates to the nurse that a client with diabetes understands proper foot care?
1. "I'll call for a physician's appointment if my feet start to ache."
2. "I'll rotate insulin injection sites from my left foot to my right foot."
3. "I'll go barefoot around the house to avoid pressure areas on my feet."
4. "I'll wear cotton socks with well-fitting shoes."

107. A 17-year-old client with diabetes has a decreased level of consciousness, with a fingerstick glucose level of 45. Her family reports that she has been skipping meals in an effort to lose weight. Which nursing intervention is <u>most</u> appropriate?
1. Placing a Salem sump tube and providing tube feedings
2. Administering a 500-ml bolus of normal saline solution
3. Administering 1 mg of glucagon intramuscularly or subcutaneously
4. Calling the physician for orders

108. A client is admitted to the medical floor with a diagnosis of pancreatitis. Which of the following nursing interventions is the <u>priority</u>?
1. Maintain oral intake and avoid analgesics.
2. Control pain and maintain NPO status.
3. Allow client to dictate food and alcohol servings.
4. Support surgical management interventions.

109. The nurse is providing education for a client diagnosed with Cushing's disease. Which statement indicates that he understands his disease?
1. "My blood sugar is low, so I don't need to watch my diet."
2. "I should increase my fluid intake to 3 L a day."
3. "I will weigh myself daily and report any gain."
4. "With this disease process, it is okay to increase my sodium intake."

110. The nurse is admitting a client who has been diagnosed with untreated hypothyroidism. What manifestations can the nurse expect to find during the initial assessment? Select all that apply.
1. Cold intolerance
2. Tachycardia
3. Hypotension
4. Weight gain
5. Mental sluggishness

Focus on proper care to get this one right!

Lookin' good. Only 5 questions to go!

Read series answers carefully to be certain all are correct.

Caution

106. 4. Cotton socks wick moisture away from the skin, helping to prevent fungal infections; proper shoe fit helps avoid pressure areas. Aching isn't a common sign of foot problems; however, a tingling sensation in the feet indicates neurovascular changes. Injecting insulin into the foot is not recommended. Going barefoot can cause injury.
CN: Physiological integrity; CNS: Reduction of risk potential; CL: Analysis

107. 3. Administering 1 mg of glucagon intramuscularly or subcutaneously helps restore the client's physiological integrity. Providing a feeding tube is appropriate only in a less urgent situation; during the time it takes to insert a nasogastric tube, administer a feeding, and wait for digestion to occur, the client may suffer permanent brain damage and seizures from severe hypoglycemia. A blood pressure drop wasn't mentioned; a bolus of normal saline solution would correct only the client fluid status, not her glucose level. Calling the physician would delay treatment at a time when rapid intervention is crucial.
CN: Physiological integrity; CNS: Physiological adaptation; CL: Application

108. 2. The priority for patient care is to provide pain control and decrease gastrointestinal activity. Alcohol and caffeine are contraindicated in pancreatitis because they provoke exacerbations and make signs/symptoms worse. Surgery is not a primary intervention for treatment of pancreatitis.
CN: Physiological integrity; CNS: Physiological adaptation; CL: Application

109. 3. Excess fluid volume can be a complication of Cushing's disease due to sodium and water retention. This can lead to fluid overload, heart failure, and pulmonary edema quickly. Weight gain is an indicator of fluid retention and should be reported. Sodium intake should be kept to a minimum, and fluid restriction may be needed to maintain balance. Hyperglycemia occurs instead of hypoglycemia.
CN: Health promotion and maintenance; CNS: None; CL: Application

110. 1, 3, 4, and 5. Cardiac functions are decreased resulting in bradycardia and hypotension. Weight gain is common due to decreased metabolism. Intolerance to cold often occurs due to lowered body temperature and slowed metabolism. Neurological manifestations include slurring/slowness of speech, impaired memory, and inattentiveness, all of which result is mental sluggishness.
CN: Physiological integrity; CNS: Physiological adaptation; CL: Analysis

CN: Client needs category   CNS: Client needs subcategory   CL: Cognitive level

111. A client is admitted with a diagnosis of diabetic ketoacidosis. An insulin drip is initiated with 50 units of insulin in 100 ml of normal saline solution. The I.V. is being infused via an infusion pump, and the pump is currently set at 10 ml/hour. The nurse determines that the client is receiving how many units of insulin each hour? Record your answer using a whole number.

_____ units

112. A client with Addison's disease is scheduled for discharge after being hospitalized for an adrenal crisis. Which statements by the client would indicate that the nurse's teaching has been effective? Select all that apply:
1. "I have to take my steroids for 10 days."
2. "I need to weigh myself daily to be sure I don't eat too many calories."
3. "I need to call my physician to discuss my steroid needs before I have dental work."
4. "I will call the physician if I start to feel fatigued, weak, or dizzy."
5. "If I feel like I have the flu, I'll carry on as usual because this is an expected response."
6. "I need to obtain and wear a medical alert bracelet."

113. A client who suffered a brain injury after falling off a ladder has recently developed syndrome of inappropriate antidiuretic hormone (SIADH). What findings indicate that the treatment being received for SIADH is effective? Select all that apply.
1. Decrease in body weight
2. Rise in blood pressure; drop in heart rate
3. Absence of wheezes in the lungs
4. Increase in urine output
5. Decrease in urine osmolarity

111. 5. To determine the number of insulin units the client is receiving per hour, the nurse must first calculate the number of units in each milliliter of fluid (50 units/100 ml = 0.5 units/ml). Next, she should multiply the units/ml by the rate of ml/hour (0.5 units × 10 ml/hour = 5 units/hour).
CN: Physiological integrity; CNS: Pharmacological and parenteral therapies; CL: Application

112. 3, 4, and 6. Dental work can be a cause of physical stress; therefore, the client's physician needs to be informed and may need to adjust the steroid dosage. Fatigue, weakness, and dizziness are symptoms of inadequate dosing; the physician should be notified if these symptoms occur. A medical alert bracelet allows health care providers to access the client's history of Addison's disease if it can't be communicated by the client. For this client, routine administration of steroids is a lifetime treatment. Daily weight is monitored for changes in fluid balance, not caloric intake. Influenza is an added physical stressor; the client shouldn't "carry on as usual."
CN: Physiological integrity; CNS: Reduction of risk potential; CL: Analysis

113. 1, 4, and 5. SIADH is an abnormality involving an excessive release of antidiuretic hormone. The predominant feature is water retention with oliguria, edema, and weight gain. Successful treatment should result in a reduction of weight, increased urine output, and a decrease in urine concentration (osmolarity).
CN: Physiological integrity; CNS: Physiological adaptation; CL: Analysis

Congratulations! You finished! You're a class act!

For more information about genitourinary system disorders, visit the Web site of the National Institute of Diabetes and Digestive and Kidney Diseases at **www2.niddk.nih.gov.**

Chapter 10
Genitourinary disorders

1. Which statement by the nurse best explains why it's important to empty the bowel before treatment with intracavitary radiation for cancer of the cervix?
1. "Feces in the bowel increase the risk for ileus."
2. "An empty bowel allows the applicator to be positioned with little or no discomfort."
3. "Bowel movements increase the risk of inadvertent contamination of the vagina and urethra."
4. "Pressure changes in the pelvis associated with bowel movements can alter the position of the applicator and the radiation source."

2. A physician tells a client to return 1 week after treatment to have a repeat culture done to verify the cure. This order would be appropriate for a woman with which condition?
1. Genital warts
2. Genital herpes
3. Gonorrhea
4. Syphilis

3. The nurse is reviewing clients' lab results. Which client is at <u>greatest</u> risk for having a false-positive Venereal Disease Research Laboratory (VDRL) result?
1. An alcoholic
2. A narcotics addict
3. A transfusion recipient
4. A breast-feeding mother

You're the greatest at choosing the correct answer.

1. 4. A position change of the radioactive implant could deliver more radiation to healthy tissue and less to the malignant lesion. This increases the risk of injury to healthy tissue and decreases the effectiveness of treatment on the cancer. Feces in the bowel increase the likelihood of a bowel movement, which can change the position of the applicator and radiation source. Feces in the bowel don't increase the risk of ileus or inadvertent contamination of the vagina and urethra from a bowel movement. Applicators are usually inserted under anesthesia in the operating room.
CN: Physiological integrity; CNS: Reduction of risk potential; CL: Analysis

2. 3. Gonococcal infections can be completely eliminated by drug therapy. This is documented by a negative culture 4 to 7 days after therapy is finished. Genital warts aren't curable and are identified by appearance, not culture. Genital herpes isn't curable and is identified by the appearance of the lesions or by cytologic studies. The diagnosis of syphilis is by darkfield microscopy or serological tests.
CN: Physiological integrity; CNS: Physiological adaptation; CL: Application

3. 2. The VDRL test is a nontreponemal test used to check for the presence of reagins in the client's serum. It isn't specific for syphilis, so false-positive results occur for a variety of reasons, most commonly in clients with chronic infection, autoimmune disease, and narcotics addiction. History of alcoholism, transfusion, or breast-feeding alone doesn't constitute a risk of a false-positive VDRL result.
CN: Physiological integrity; CNS: Physiological adaptation; CL: Analysis

CN: Client needs category   CNS: Client needs subcategory   CL: Cognitive level

4. Which statement made by a client with a chlamydial infection indicates an understanding of the potential complications?
1. "I'm glad I'm not pregnant; I'd hate to have a malformed baby from this disease."
2. "I hope this medicine works before this disease gets into my urine and destroys my kidneys."
3. "If I had known a diaphragm would put me at risk for this, I would've taken birth control pills."
4. "I need to treat this infection so it doesn't spread into my pelvis because I want to have children someday."

Your client relies on you for accurate instruction.

5. A client with genital herpes asks the nurse what comfort measure can be recommended. What is the best response by the nurse?
1. Wear loose cotton underwear.
2. Apply a water-based lubricant to the lesions.
3. Rub rather than scratch in response to an itch.
4. Pour hydrogen peroxide and water over the lesions.

6. Giving instructions for breast self-examination is particularly important for clients with which medical problem?
1. Cervical dysplasia
2. A dermoid cyst
3. Endometrial polyps
4. Ovarian cancer

7. A 32-year-old client has an elevated temperature and decreased hematocrit when she returns for a follow-up visit after having a vaginal hysterectomy. The nurse is aware that the client may be experiencing which of the following?
1. Hematoma
2. Hypovolemia
3. Infection
4. Thromboembolism

4. 4. Chlamydia is a common cause of pelvic inflammatory disease and infertility. It doesn't cause birth defects or affect the kidneys. It can cause conjunctivitis and respiratory infection in neonates exposed to infected cervicovaginal secretions during delivery. Use of a diaphragm isn't a risk factor.

CN: Physiological integrity; CNS: Reduction of risk potential; CL: Application

5. 1. Wearing loose cotton underwear promotes drying and helps avoid irritation of the lesions. The use of lubricants is contraindicated because they can prolong healing time and increase the risk of secondary infection. Lesions shouldn't be rubbed or scratched because of the risk of tissue damage and additional infection. Cool, wet compresses can be used to soothe the itch. The use of hydrogen peroxide and water on lesions isn't recommended.

CN: Physiological integrity; CNS: Basic care and comfort; CL: Application

6. 4. Clients with ovarian cancer are at increased risk for breast cancer. Breast self-examination supports early detection and treatment and is very important. There isn't a known relationship between breast cancer and cervical dysplasia, or endometrial polyps, or dermoid cysts, so breast self-examination is no more or less important for these clients.

CN: Health promotion and maintenance; CNS: None; CL: Application

7. 1. An elevated temperature and decreased hematocrit are signs of hematoma, a delayed complication of abdominal and vaginal hysterectomy. Symptoms of hypovolemia include increased hematocrit and hemoglobin values. Temperature is a classic sign of infection, but a decreased hematocrit isn't. Abrupt onset of fever is a symptom of thromboembolism, but other symptoms include dyspnea, chest pain, cough, hemoptysis, restlessness, and signs of shock.

CN: Physiological integrity; CNS: Reduction of risk potential; CL: Application

8. Which client is at <u>greatest</u> risk for dehydration?
1. A 48-year-old having intracavitary radiation for cancer of the cervix
2. A 59-year-old 1 week after a radical vulvectomy
3. A 67-year-old receiving adjuvant tamoxifen therapy for breast cancer
4. A 72-year-old with a vesicovaginal fistula

Dehydration is risky business.

9. In which group is it <u>most important</u> for a client to understand the importance of an annual Papanicolaou test?
1. Clients with a history of recurrent candidiasis
2. Clients with a pregnancy before age 20
3. Clients infected with the human papillomavirus (HPV)
4. Clients with a long history of oral contraceptive use

10. The nurse reviews a client's history and determines that which factor indicates a risk for candidiasis?
1. Nulliparity
2. Menopause
3. Use of corticosteroids
4. Use of spermicidal jelly

The symptoms are the clue.

11. A 22-year-old female visiting the clinic describes her chief complaint as "frothy greenish vaginal discharge." The nurse anticipates setting up for a wet mount procedure to diagnose which of the following?
1. Candidiasis
2. *Gardnerella vaginalis* vaginitis
3. Gonorrhea
4. Trichomoniasis

8. 1. Regardless of age, dehydration is a risk caused by fluid loss secondary to tissue destruction at the site of irradiation. After radical vulvectomy, wound drains are generally removed by postoperative day 4 or 5 and don't create a significant risk of dehydration. Tamoxifen therapy is unrelated to dehydration. Although urine may escape through the vagina as a result of a vesicovaginal fistula, it doesn't cause an unusual amount of urine or other fluid to be lost.
CN: Physiological integrity; CNS: Physiological adaptation; CL: Analysis

9. 3. HPV causes genital warts, which are associated with an increased incidence of cervical cancer. Recurrent candidiasis, pregnancy before age 20, and use of oral contraceptives don't increase the risk of cervical cancer.
CN: Health promotion and maintenance; CNS: None; CL: Analysis

10. 3. Small numbers of the fungus *Candida albicans* commonly are found in the vagina. Because corticosteroids decrease host defense, they increase the risk of candidiasis. Pregnancy, not nulliparity, increases the risk of candidiasis. Candidiasis is rare before menarche and after menopause. The use of oral contraceptives, not spermicidal jelly, increases the risk of candidiasis.
CN: Health promotion and maintenance; CNS: None; CL: Application

11. 4. The discharge associated with infection caused by *Trichomonas* organisms is homogenous, greenish gray, watery, and frothy or purulent. The discharge associated with candidiasis is thick and white and resembles cottage cheese in appearance, while that associated with infection due to *Gardnerella vaginalis* is thin and grayish white, with a marked fishy odor. With gonorrhea, vaginal discharge is purulent when present, but in many women, gonorrhea is asymptomatic.
CN: Physiological integrity; CNS: Physiological adaptation; CL: Application

12. A 19-year-old woman reports an intermittent milky vaginal discharge. She is not sexually active and denies itching or burning. Which factor is the most likely cause of the milky-appearing discharge?
1. Inadequate cleaning of the perineal area
2. Sensitivity to a feminine hygiene product
3. Normal fluctuation in estrogen and progesterone levels
4. Reaction to heat and moisture from wearing tight clothing

13. Which nursing intervention is appropriate for a client who had breast reconstruction surgery?
1. Prevent hypothermia.
2. Maintain even pressure on the wound.
3. Position the client on the operative side.
4. Raise the client's arms over her head four times daily.

Postoperative care depends on the type of surgery.

14. A client who had intracavitary radiation treatment for cancer of the cervix 1 month earlier reports small amounts of vaginal bleeding. The nurse interprets this as which of the following?
1. Recurrence of the carcinoma
2. Development of a rectovaginal fistula
3. Expected effect of the radiation therapy
4. Infection secondary to a change in vaginal flora

It's equally important to teach your client what and what *not* to do.

15. A nurse enters the room of a client who had a left modified mastectomy 8 hours earlier. Which assessment indicates that the nursing assistant assigned to the client needs <u>further instruction</u> and guidance?
1. The client is squeezing a ball in her left hand.
2. The client is wearing a robe with elastic cuffs.
3. The client's affected arm is elevated on a pillow.
4. A blood pressure cuff is on the client's right arm.

12. 3. Vaginal fluid is clear, milky, or cloudy, depending on the fluctuating levels of estrogen and progesterone. A milky-appearing vaginal discharge is normal and isn't associated with inadequate cleaning, sensitivity, or reaction to heat or moisture.
CN: Health promotion and maintenance; CNS: None; CL: Application

13. 1. Hypothermia causes a decrease in surface circulation. This can lead to ischemia of the skin or muscle graft and ultimately to tissue necrosis in clients who had breast reconstruction surgery. Because of the importance of maintaining good circulation, pressure on the breast wound must be avoided, so the client is positioned on the back or nonoperative side. Arms shouldn't be lifted above shoulder level for 4 to 6 weeks.
CN: Physiological integrity; CNS: Reduction of risk potential; CL: Application

14. 3. After intracavitary radiation, some vaginal bleeding occurs for 1 to 3 months. Intermittent painless vaginal bleeding is a classic symptom of cervical cancer, but given the client's history, bleeding is more likely a result of the radiation than recurrent cancer. The passage of feces through the vagina, not vaginal bleeding, is a sign of rectovaginal fistula. Vaginal infections show various types of vaginal discharge but not vaginal bleeding.
CN: Physiological integrity; CNS: Physiological adaptation; CL: Application

15. 2. Elastic cuffs can contribute to the development of lymphedema and should be avoided. Simple exercises, such as squeezing a ball, help promote circulation and should be started as soon as possible after surgery. Elevation of the affected arm promotes venous and lymphatic return from the extremity. Blood pressure measurements in the affected arm also should be avoided.
CN: Safe, effective care environment; CNS: Management of care; CL: Analysis

16. A postoperative client who is at risk for evisceration has returned to the unit after an abdominal hysterectomy. The nurse would assess the client for which of the following?
1. Tachycardia accompanied by a weak, thready pulse
2. Hypotension with a decreased level of consciousness (LOC)
3. Shallow, rapid respirations and increasing vaginal drainage
4. Low-grade fever with increasing serosanguineous incisional drainage

17. Which finding indicates that oxycodone (OxyContin) given to a client with breast cancer metastasized to the bone is exerting the desired effect?
1. Bone density is increased.
2. Pain is 0 to 2 on a 10-point scale.
3. Alpha-fetoprotein level is decreased.
4. Serum calcium level is within normal range.

18. Which instruction should the nurse give to a client with prostatitis who's receiving co-trimoxazole double strength (Bactrim DS)?
1. Don't expect improvement of symptoms for 7 to 10 days.
2. Drink six to eight glasses of fluid daily while taking this medication.
3. If a sore mouth or throat develops, take the medication with milk or an antacid.
4. Use a sunscreen of at least SPF-15 with para-aminobenzoic acid (PABA) to protect against drug-induced photosensitivity.

19. The nurse administers tamsulosin (Flomax) to a client with benign prostatic hyperplasia (BPH)? The nurse is aware that which of the following is a priority assessment?
1. Voiding pattern
2. Size of the prostate
3. Creatinine clearance
4. Serum testosterone level

16. **4.** Signs of impending evisceration are low-grade fever and increasing serosanguineous drainage. Tachycardia; weak, thready pulse; hypotension; decreased LOC; shallow, rapid respirations; and vaginal drainage after abdominal hysterectomy are all unrelated to impending evisceration, although they may be associated with other serious problems such as shock.
CN: Physiological integrity; CNS: Reduction of risk potential; CL: Application

17. **2.** Oxycodone is an opioid analgesic used for alleviating severe pain, especially in terminal illness. If a client's pain has decreased to 0 to 2 on a 10-point scale (0 is no pain and 10 is the worst pain), the medication is working as desired. The drug doesn't directly affect bone density, alpha-fetoprotein level, or serum calcium level.
CN: Physiological integrity; CNS: Pharmacological and parenteral therapies; CL: Analysis

18. **2.** Six to eight glasses of fluid daily are needed to prevent renal problems, such as crystalluria and stone formation. The symptoms should improve in a few days if the drug is effective. Sore throat and sore mouth are adverse effects that should be reported right away. The drug causes photosensitivity, but a PABA-free sunscreen should be used because PABA can interfere with the drug's action.
CN: Physiological integrity; CNS: Pharmacological and parenteral therapies; CL: Application

19. **1.** The alpha-adrenergic blocker tamsulosin (Flomax) relaxes the smooth muscle of the bladder neck and prostate, so the urinary voiding symptoms (frequency, urgency, hesitancy) of BPH are reduced in many clients. These drugs don't affect the size of the prostate, renal function, or production or metabolism of testosterone.
CN: Physiological integrity; CNS: Pharmacological and parenteral therapies; CL: Application

20. A nursing diagnosis addressing risk for impaired tissue integrity would be <u>most appropriate</u> for which client?
1. A client with endometriosis
2. A client taking oral contraceptives
3. A client with a vaginal packing in place
4. A client having reconstructive breast surgery

The appropriate nursing diagnosis helps everyone work toward the same goal.

21. A 27-year-old man arrives at the clinic with priapism. The nurse is aware that the client is at risk for which condition?
1. Disseminated intravascular coagulation (DIC)
2. Hydronephrosis
3. Penile gangrene
4. Testicular atrophy

22. What is the <u>most important</u> information for the nurse to give a client to decrease the risk of toxic shock syndrome?
1. Avoid douching.
2. Wear loose cotton underwear.
3. Use pads, not tampons, overnight.
4. Avoid sexual intercourse during menses.

23. The nurse is reviewing discharge instructions for a client who had a dilation and curettage procedure. Which statement should the nurse include in the discharge instructions?
1. Tampons may be used during exercise.
2. Avoid strenuous work and sexual intercourse for at least 2 weeks.
3. Stay on bed rest for 3 days; then gradually resume normal activity.
4. Take a soaking tub bath each day to promote relaxation.

I really shouldn't have worked so hard.

20. 4. Reconstructive breast surgery places the client at risk for insufficient blood supply to the muscle graft and skin, which can lead to tissue necrosis. Endometriosis and oral contraceptives aren't generally associated with altered tissue perfusion. Pressure from vaginal packing can sometimes put pressure on the bladder neck and interfere with voiding.
CN: Physiological integrity; CNS: Reduction of risk potential; CL: Analysis

21. 3. Priapism is a condition in which the penis is persistently erect and painful. It's a urological emergency because gangrene secondary to ischemia can result if venous drainage of the corpora cavernosa doesn't occur. Priapism doesn't cause DIC, hydronephrosis, or testicular atrophy.
CN: Physiological integrity; CNS: Reduction of risk potential; CL: Application

22. 3. The cause of toxic shock syndrome is a toxin produced by *Staphylococcus aureus* bacteria. It occurs most commonly in menstruating women using tampons. Tampons, particularly when left in place for more than 8 hours (such as overnight), are believed to provide a good environment for growth of the bacteria, which then enter the bloodstream through breaks in the vaginal mucosa. Douching, use of loose cotton underwear, and sexual intercourse during menstruation have no direct association with toxic shock syndrome.
CN: Health promotion and maintenance; CNS: None; CL: Analysis

23. 2. Strenuous work, which can result in increased bleeding, should be avoided for 2 weeks to allow time for healing. Sexual intercourse should also be avoided for 2 weeks to allow healing and thus decrease the risk of infection. Tampons and tub baths should be avoided for 1 week. Overall activity should be gradually resumed, reaching preoperative levels in the 2-week period, but bed rest isn't necessary. No other restrictions are routinely necessary.
CN: Physiological integrity; CNS: Reduction of risk potential; CL: Application

24. Which assessment finding is expected in a client receiving bicalutamide (Casodex) and leuprolide (Lupron) for advanced prostate cancer?
1. Abdominal distention
2. Acromegaly
3. Colicky pain
4. Hot flashes

25. Which assessment finding is <u>abnormal</u> in a 72-year-old male client?
1. Decreased sperm count
2. Small, firm testes on palpation
3. History of slowed sexual response
4. Decreased plasma testosterone level

26. Which comment made by a client being treated for chronic prostatitis indicates to the nurse that further teaching is necessary?
1. "I miss not being able to have sex."
2. "I enjoy frequent soaking in a hot tub of water."
3. "Cutting down on coffee hasn't been as hard as I expected."
4. "I'm used to getting up and moving, not just sitting for long periods."

27. The nurse is aware that perineal pain in the absence of any observable cause is suggestive of which condition?
1. Endometriosis
2. Internal hemorrhoids
3. Prostatitis
4. Renal calculus

What is abnormal about this client's findings?

Client teaching includes making sure your client understands your instructions.

24. 4. Bicalutamide, a nonsteroidal antiandrogen, and leuprolide, a gonadotropin-releasing hormone agonist, decrease the production of testosterone. This helps to decrease the production of cancer cells involved in the prostate cancer. Because androgens are responsible for the development of the male genitalia and secondary male sex characteristics, low androgen levels can cause genital atrophy, breast enlargement, and hot flashes. Abdominal distention, acromegaly, and colicky pain aren't caused by bicalutamide and leuprolide therapy.

CN: Physiological integrity; CNS: Pharmacological and parenteral therapies; CL: Analysis

25. 1. Sperm continues to be produced despite the age-related degenerative changes that occur in the male reproductive system. Among the normal age-related changes are decreased size and increased firmness of the testes, a decrease in sexual potency, and decreased production of testosterone and progesterone.

CN: Physiological integrity; CNS: Physiological adaptation; CL: Application

26. 1. Ejaculation can aid in the treatment of chronic prostatitis by decreasing the retention of prostatic fluid. Coffee should be eliminated from the diet because it can increase prostate secretion. Warm sitz baths and not sitting for too long at a time promote comfort.

CN: Physiological integrity; CNS: Physiological adaptation; CL: Application

27. 3. Prostatitis can cause prostate pain, which is felt as perineal discomfort. Endometriosis can cause pain low in the abdomen, deep in the pelvis, or in the rectal or sacrococcygeal area, depending on the location of the ectopic tissue. Hemorrhoids cause rectal pain and pressure. Renal calculi typically produce flank pain.

CN: Health promotion and maintenance; CNS: None; CL: Analysis

28. Which assessment finding would be a cause for alarm in a client taking finasteride (Proscar)?
1. Azotemia
2. Breast enlargement
3. Decreased prostate size
4. Flushing

Which assessment finding is cause for alarm? Here's a hint: I think it's a waste.

28. **1.** Azotemia, a buildup of nitrogenous waste products in the blood, indicates impaired renal function. Finasteride, an antiandrogenic agent, is prescribed for chronic urinary retention with large residual volumes secondary to benign prostatic hypertrophy. Azotemia in a client on finasteride therapy can indicate the drug isn't effective in relieving the urinary symptoms associated with benign prostatic hypertrophy or that an unrelated renal problem has occurred. Breast enlargement, decrease in prostate size, and flushing are expected effects of finasteride.
CN: Physiological integrity; CNS: Pharmacological and parenteral therapies; CL: Application

29. Which treatment is appropriate for a client with cervical polyps who has been treated with cryosurgery?
1. Daily douche
2. Oral antibiotics
3. Intravaginal antibiotic cream
4. Use of tampons for 72 hours

29. **3.** Intravaginal antibiotic cream is commonly used to aid healing and prevent infection. Oral antibiotics are used for clients with acute cervicitis or perimetritis. Douching is generally avoided for 2 weeks, as is the use of tampons.
CN: Physiological integrity; CNS: Reduction of risk potential; CL: Application

30. Which nursing intervention would be correct for a woman having intracavitary radiation for cancer of the cervix?
1. High-residue diet
2. Fowler's position when in bed
3. Intermittent urinary catheterization
4. Bed rest

30. **4.** Clients having intracavitary radiation therapy are on strict bed rest, with the head of the bed elevated no more than 10 to 15 degrees to avoid displacing the radiation source. A low-residue diet is used to prevent diarrhea during treatment. An order for Fowler's position when in bed is incorrect. An indwelling urinary catheter, not intermittent urinary catheterization, is used to prevent urine from distending the bladder and changing the position of tissues relative to the radiation source.
CN: Physiological integrity; CNS: Physiological adaptation; CL: Analysis

31. Which condition of the female reproductive system generally requires the identification and treatment of sexual partners?
1. Bartholinitis
2. Candidiasis
3. Chlamydia
4. Endometriosis

31. **3.** Chlamydia is a common sexually transmitted disease requiring the treatment of all current sexual partners to prevent reinfection. Bartholinitis results from obstruction of a duct. Sexual partners may become infected, although men can usually be treated with over-the-counter products. Candidiasis is a yeast infection that typically occurs as a result of antibiotic use. Endometriosis occurs when endometrial cells are seeded throughout the pelvis and isn't a sexually transmitted disease.
CN: Health promotion and maintenance; CNS: None; CL: Application

32. The nurse is providing information to a client taking metronidazole (Flagyl). What is the most important information for the nurse to include?
1. Breathlessness and cough are common adverse effects.
2. Urine may develop a greenish tinge while the client is taking this drug.
3. Mixing this drug with alcohol causes severe nausea and vomiting.
4. Heart palpitations may occur and should be immediately reported.

33. Hydrocodone with acetaminophen has been prescribed for a client with metastatic prostate cancer. Which of the following is an adverse effect of the medication that the nurse should instruct the client to report?
1. Blurred vision
2. Diarrhea
3. Unusual dreams
4. Vomiting

34. The nurse is planning care for a client having hysterosalpingography. What is the most important nursing intervention for the nurse to provide?
1. Give the client a perineal pad to wear after the procedure.
2. Give the client nothing by mouth after midnight the night before the procedure.
3. Position the client in the knee-chest position during the procedure.
4. Keep the client in a dorsal recumbent position for 4 hours after the procedure.

35. The nurse is instructing a client with vulvovaginal candidiasis on the use of the prescribed Nystatin vaginal tablets. Which of the following statements indicates that the client needs additional teaching?
1. "I will need to refrigerate the Nystatin tablets."
2. "I can get up to do other activities after inserting the medicine."
3. "I will finish all the tablets even if I am feeling better."
4. "I should report any increased skin irritation to my doctor."

Drugs and alcohol typically don't mix.

You've got it all under control. Keep going!

32. 3. When mixed with alcohol, metronidazole causes a disulfiram-like effect involving nausea, vomiting, and other unpleasant symptoms. Urine may turn reddish brown, not greenish, from the drug. Cardiovascular or respiratory effects aren't associated with use of this drug.
CN: Physiological integrity; CNS: Pharmacological and parenteral therapies; CL: Application

33. 4. Vomiting is an adverse reaction to the drug that should be reported because it impairs the client's quality of life and places the client at risk for dehydration. Taking the medication with food may prevent vomiting. If not, other opiate analgesics may be better tolerated. Blurred vision and diarrhea aren't associated with the use of hydrocodone with acetaminophen. Unusual dreams are a common adverse effect but don't need to be reported unless they're bothersome to the client.
CN: Physiological integrity; CNS: Pharmacological and parenteral therapies; CL: Application

34. 1. A perineal pad is needed after hysterosalpingography because the contrast medium may leak from the vagina for several hours and stain the clothing. The bowel needs to be cleaned before the procedure, but the client doesn't have to refrain from having anything by mouth after midnight. The procedure is performed with the client in the lithotomy position, and no special positioning is required after the procedure.
CN: Physiological integrity; CNS: Basic care and comfort; CL: Application

35. 2. The client needs to continue lying down for at least 30 minutes after insertion of the vaginal tablets. Refrigerating Nystatin tablets, finishing all the tablets, and reporting any increased skin irritation to the doctor are all important interventions concerning this medication.
CN: Physiological integrity; CNS: Pharmacological and parenteral therapies; CL: Application

36. A 36-year-old client who has never had mumps or a measles, mumps, and rubella (MMR) immunization reports that he was just notified that an 8-year-old child of a family with whom he stayed recently has been diagnosed with mumps. Which treatment should the client receive?
1. I.V. antibiotics
2. Ice packs to the scrotum
3. Application of a scrotal support
4. Administration of gamma globulin

37. Which statement by a client scheduled for a vasectomy indicates he needs further teaching about the procedure?
1. "I'm glad I won't have to worry about contraception as soon as this procedure is done."
2. "I'll need to place an ice pack over the incision several times a day when I first go home."
3. "I know this procedure can be reversed, but the success rate is low."
4. "I'll have to limit my usual activities for about 1 week."

38. Which area of client teaching should be stressed when the goal is preventing the development of phimosis in a 20-year-old uncircumcised client?
1. Proper cleaning of the prepuce
2. Importance of regular ejaculation
3. Technique of testicular self-examination
4. Proper hand washing before touching the genitals

39. Which statement should be included when teaching a client newly diagnosed with testicular cancer?
1. Testicular cancer isn't responsive to chemotherapy, but it's highly curative with surgery.
2. Radiation therapy is never used, so the unaffected testicle remains healthy.
3. Testicular self-examination is still important because there's increased risk for a second tumor.
4. Taking testosterone after orchiectomy prevents changes in appearance and sexual function.

Look for signs that your client doesn't understand the information.

You can ease your client's worries through effective teaching efforts.

36. 4. Gamma globulin provides passive immunity to mumps. Antibiotic therapy is used in the treatment of bacterial orchitis. Ice and the use of a scrotal support are used as comfort measures in the treatment of orchitis.
CN: Health promotion and maintenance; CNS: None; CL: Application

37. 1. After vasectomy, the client remains fertile for several weeks until sperm stored distal to the severed vas are evacuated. After this occurs, sperm are still produced, but they don't enter the ejaculate and are absorbed by the body. The other statements are accurate.
CN: Physiological integrity; CNS: Physiological adaptation; CL: Analysis

38. 1. Proper cleaning of the preputial area to remove secretions is critical to the prevention of noncongenital phimosis. Regular ejaculation can decrease the symptoms of chronic prostatitis, but it has no effect on the development of phimosis. Testicular self-examination is important in the early detection and treatment of testicular cancer. Hand washing is important in preventing the spread of infection.
CN: Health promotion and maintenance; CNS: None; CL: Application

39. 3. A history of a testicular malignancy puts the client at increased risk for a second tumor. Testicular self-examination allows for early detection and treatment and is critical. Chemotherapy is added for clients who have evidence of metastasis after irradiation. Radiation therapy is used on the retroperitoneal lymph nodes. Testosterone usually isn't needed because the unaffected testis usually produces sufficient hormone.
CN: Physiological integrity; CNS: Reduction of risk potential; CL: Application

40. The nurse is teaching a client about penile hygiene. What is the most important information for the nurse to include?
1. Use warm water without soap.
2. Dry all areas of the penis thoroughly.
3. Wash from the base of the shaft to the tip.
4. Avoid retracting the foreskin if not circumcised.

You've made it through 40 questions in no time!

40. 2. Careful drying is essential to avoid maceration of the penis. To decrease the risk of genitourinary infection, wash the penis from the tip to the base to reduce the risk for introducing pathogens into the urethral meatus. Effective cleaning requires soap and thorough rinsing. It's also essential to remove secretions that accumulate under the foreskin because they can lead to inflammation and are associated with the development of penile cancer. The foreskin in uncircumcised men must be retracted for cleaning and then replaced to prevent paraphimosis.

CN: Health promotion and maintenance; CNS: None; CL: Application

41. The physician tells a client who underwent an orchiectomy for testicular cancer that a persistent elevation in alpha-fetoprotein level remains. The nurse is aware that this finding is consistent with which statement?
1. Fertility is maintained.
2. The cancer has recurred.
3. There's metastatic disease.
4. Testosterone levels are low.

41. 3. Alpha-fetoprotein is a tumor marker elevated in nonseminomatous malignancies of the testicle. After the tumor is removed, the level should decrease. A persistent elevation after orchiectomy indicates a tumor is present someplace outside the testicle that was removed. The level of alpha-fetoprotein isn't related to fertility or testosterone level. A recurrence of the cancer is indicated by a postsurgical decrease in alpha-fetoprotein level followed by an elevation as a new tumor starts to grow.

CN: Physiological integrity; CNS: Physiological adaptation; CL: Analysis

42. Which discharge instruction should be given to a client after a prostatectomy?
1. Avoid straining at stool.
2. Report clots in the urine right away.
3. Soak in a warm tub daily for comfort.
4. Return to your usual activities in 3 weeks.

This test has been a real strain on my brain.

42. 1. Straining at stool after prostatectomy can cause bleeding. Small blood clots or pieces of tissue commonly are passed in the urine for up to 2 weeks postoperatively. Tub baths are prohibited because they cause dilation of pelvic blood vessels. Other activities are resumed based on the guidance of the physician. Sexual intercourse and driving are usually prohibited for about 3 weeks. Exercising and returning to work are usually prohibited for about 6 weeks.

CN: Physiological integrity; CNS: Reduction of risk potential; CL: Application

43. After a biopsy of the prostate, which symptom should a nurse instruct a client to report?
1. Pain on the following day
2. Discolored semen
3. Difficulty urinating
4. Temperature greater than 99° F (37.2° C)

43. 3. Difficulty urinating suggests urethral obstruction. Mild pain is expected for 1 to 3 days after the biopsy. Semen may be discolored for up to a month after the biopsy. Temperature higher than 101° F (38.3° C) should be reported because it suggests infection.

CN: Physiological integrity; CNS: Reduction of risk potential; CL: Analysis

44. Two days after a transrectal biopsy of the prostate, a client calls the clinic to report that his stool is streaked with blood. Which response by the nurse is appropriate?
1. Tell the client to take a laxative.
2. Tell the client to come in for examination.
3. Reassure the client that this is an expected occurrence.
4. Ask the client to collect a stool specimen for testing.

45. A nurse is caring for clients who have a history of genital herpes infection. Which client is <u>most</u> at risk for an outbreak of genital herpes?
1. A client who complains of a headache and fever
2. A client who complains of vaginal and urethral discharge
3. A client who complains of dysuria and lymphadenopathy
4. A client who complains of genital pruritus and paresthesia

Teach your client the prodromal symptoms of an outbreak of genital herpes.

46. Which instruction should be given to a female client newly diagnosed with genital herpes?
1. Obtain a Papanicolaou (Pap) test every year.
2. Have your partner use a condom when lesions are present.
3. Use a water-soluble lubricant for relief of pruritus.
4. Limit stress and emotional upset as much as possible.

47. A client newly diagnosed with genital herpes is crying and wringing her hands as the nurse approaches her. Which nursing diagnosis is the most appropriate to this situation?
1. Acute pain
2. Impaired tissue integrity
3. Anxiety
4. Deficient knowledge

44. 3. After a transrectal prostatic biopsy, blood in the stool is expected for a number of days. Because blood in the stool is expected, testing the stool or examining the client isn't necessary. Stool softeners are prescribed if the client complains of constipation; straining at stool can precipitate bleeding, but laxatives generally aren't necessary.
CN: Physiological integrity; CNS: Reduction of risk potential; CL: Application

45. 4. Pruritus and paresthesia as well as redness of the genital area are prodromal symptoms of recurrent herpes infection. These symptoms occur 30 minutes to 48 hours before the lesions appear. Headache and fever are symptoms of viremia associated with the primary infection. Vaginal and urethral discharge is also a local sign of primary infection. Dysuria and lymphadenopathy are local symptoms of primary infection that may also occur with recurrent infection.
CN: Physiological integrity; CNS: Physiological adaptation; CL: Analysis

46. 4. Stress, anxiety, and emotional upset seem to predispose to recurrent outbreaks of genital herpes. Because a relationship has been found between genital herpes and cervical cancer, a Pap test is recommended every 6 months. Sexual intercourse should be avoided during outbreaks, and a condom should be used between outbreaks; it isn't known if the virus can be transmitted at this time. During an outbreak, creams and lubricants should be avoided because they may prolong healing.
CN: Physiological integrity; CNS: Physiological adaptation; CL: Application

47. 3. The client is demonstrating anxiety; this problem needs to be incorporated into the plan of care. Acute pain and impaired tissue integrity are not nursing diagnoses for the client. The client may have deficient knowledge concerning the new diagnosis; however, that is not being demonstrated at this time.
CN: Psychosocial integrity; CNS: None; CL: Application

48. A client is describing how she palpates her breasts for breast self-examination. Which statement indicates the need for further teaching?
1. "I put lotion on my breasts before I begin to palpate them."
2. "I palpate both breasts standing up and then lying on my back."
3. "I'm careful to palpate under each arm and up to 2 in. below my collarbone."
4. "I start at the outer edge of the breast and work in to the nipple in smaller and smaller circles."

Make sure your client understands the proper technique for breast self-examination.

49. During a routine physical examination, a firm mass is palpated in the right breast of a 35-year-old female client. Which finding or client history would suggest cancer of the breast as opposed to fibrocystic disease?
1. Mass located in upper, outer quadrant
2. Cyclic change in mass size
3. History of anovulatory cycles
4. Increased vascularity of the breast

50. The nurse is aware that the highest risk for developing a postoperative wound infection exists with a client who has experienced which of the following?
1. Radical prostatectomy
2. Perineal prostatectomy
3. Suprapubic prostatectomy
4. Transurethral resection of the prostate (TURP)

Read this question carefully.

51. A client with pneumonia is transferred to the intensive care unit for mechanical ventilation. His blood pressure is 70/40 mm Hg, his heart rate is 115 beats/minute, and his respiratory rate is 32 breaths/minute with accessory muscle use. I.V.s are infusing at 150 ml/hour. Urine output is 50 ml for the past 4 hours. This client is most at risk for which of the following?
1. Postrenal failure
2. Prerenal failure
3. Intrarenal failure
4. Chronic renal failure

48. 3. Breast self-examination requires palpation of all breast tissue. This includes checking the area above the breast up to the collarbone and all the way over to the shoulder as well as the area between the breast and the underarm, including the underarm itself. Lotion or powder helps the fingers glide over the skin and facilitates palpation. Breasts need to be palpated in both erect and lying positions. Any pattern of palpation may be used in performing breast self-examination as long as each quadrant of the breast, tail, and axilla are examined.
CN: Health promotion and maintenance; CNS: None; CL: Application

49. 4. Increase in breast size or vascularity is consistent with cancer of the breast. Masses associated with fibrocystic disease of the breast are firm, most commonly located in the upper outer quadrant of the breast, and increase in size prior to menstruation. They may be bilateral in a mirror image and are typically well demarcated and freely moveable.
CN: Health promotion and maintenance; CNS: None; CL: Application

50. 2. The incision in a perineal prostatectomy is close to the rectum, which normally contains gram-negative organisms that can cause infection if introduced into other areas of the body. Therefore, a perineal incision will become contaminated more often than either no external incision, as with TURP, or abdominal incisions, as with radical or suprapubic prostatectomy.
CN: Physiological integrity; CNS: Reduction of risk potential; CL: Analysis

51. 2. Prerenal refers to renal failure due to an interference with renal perfusion. Decreased cardiac output causes a decrease in renal perfusion, which leads to a lower glomerular filtration rate. The other answers don't apply to this scenario.
CN: Physiological integrity; CNS: Physiological adaptation; CL: Analysis

52. A client admitted for acute pyelonephritis is about to start antibiotic therapy. Which symptom would the nurse expect this client to present?
1. Hypertension
2. Flank pain on the affected side
3. Pain that radiates toward the unaffected side
4. No tenderness with deep palpation over the costovertebral angle

53. The nurse is providing discharge instructions for a client treated for acute pyelonephritis. What is the most important information for the nurse to include?
1. Avoid taking any dairy products.
2. Return for follow-up urine cultures.
3. Stop taking the prescribed antibiotics when the symptoms subside.
4. Recurrence is unlikely because you've been treated with antibiotics.

54. A client is complaining of severe flank and abdominal pain. A flat plate of the abdomen shows urolithiasis. Which intervention is important?
1. Strain all urine.
2. Limit fluid intake.
3. Enforce strict bed rest.
4. Encourage a high-calcium diet.

55. A client is receiving a radiation implant for the treatment of bladder cancer. Which intervention is appropriate?
1. Flush all urine down the toilet.
2. Restrict the client's fluid intake.
3. Place the client in a semiprivate room.
4. Monitor the client for signs and symptoms of cystitis.

Here's another question about client teaching, an essential topic on NCLEX examinations.

52. 2. The client may complain of pain on the affected side because the kidney is enlarged and might have formed an abscess. Hypertension is associated with chronic pyelonephritis. Pain may radiate down the ureters or to the epigastrium. The client would have tenderness with deep palpation over the costovertebral angle.
CN: Physiological integrity; CNS: Physiological adaptation; CL: Application

53. 2. The client needs to return for follow-up urine cultures because bacteriuria may be present but asymptomatic. Intake of dairy products won't contribute to pyelonephritis. Antibiotics need to be taken for the full course of therapy regardless of symptoms. Pyelonephritis typically recurs as a relapse or new infection and frequently recurs within 2 weeks of completing therapy.
CN: Health promotion and maintenance; CNS: None; CL: Application

54. 1. Urine should be strained for calculi and sent to the laboratory for analysis. Fluid intake of 3 to 4 qt (3 to 4 L) per day is encouraged to flush the urinary tract and prevent further calculi formation. Ambulation is encouraged to help pass the calculi through gravity. A low-calcium diet is recommended to help prevent the formation of calcium calculi.
CN: Physiological integrity; CNS: Reduction of risk potential; CL: Application

55. 4. Cystitis is the most common adverse reaction of clients undergoing radiation therapy; symptoms include dysuria, frequency, urgency, and nocturia. Urine of clients with radiation implants for bladder cancer should be sent to the radioisotopes laboratory for monitoring. It's recommended that fluid intake be increased. Clients with radiation implants require a private room.
CN: Physiological integrity; CNS: Physiological adaptation; CL: Application

56. The nurse is assessing a client who has undergone a radical cystectomy and ileal conduit for the treatment of bladder cancer. The nurse is aware that <u>immediate</u> intervention is necessary when the client presents with which finding?
1. A red, moist stoma
2. A dusky colored stoma
3. Urine output more than 30 ml/hour
4. Slight bleeding from the stoma when changing the appliance

57. The nurse is providing instruction about skin care at the stoma site for a client with an ileal conduit. What is the most important information for the nurse to provide?
1. Change the appliance at bedtime.
2. Leave the stoma open to air while changing the appliance.
3. Clean the skin around the stoma with mild soap and water and dry it thoroughly.
4. Cut the faceplate or wafer of the appliance no more than 4 mm larger than the stoma.

58. A client is diagnosed with cystitis. The nurse provides teaching aimed at preventing a recurrence. Which instruction does the nurse provide to the client?
1. Bathe in a tub.
2. Wear cotton underwear.
3. Use a feminine hygiene spray.
4. Limit your intake of cranberry juice.

59. When performing a physical assessment, the nurse discovers a client's urinary drainage bag lying next to him. Based on this finding, the nurse identifies which <u>priority</u> nursing diagnosis?
1. Risk for infection
2. Reflex urinary incontinence
3. Impaired comfort
4. Risk for compromised human dignity

Question 56 asks you to prioritize responses according to which is most urgent.

EMERGENCY

56. 2. The stoma should be red and moist, indicating adequate blood flow. A dusky or cyanotic stoma indicates insufficient blood supply and is an emergency needing prompt intervention. Urine output less than 30 ml/hour or no urine output for more than 15 minutes should be reported. Slight bleeding from the stoma when changing the appliance may occur because the intestinal mucosa is fragile.
CN: Physiological integrity; CNS: Reduction of risk potential; CL: Application

57. 3. Cleaning the skin around the stoma with mild soap and water and drying it thoroughly helps keep the area clean from urine, which can irritate the skin. Change the appliance in the early morning when urine output is less to decrease the amount of urine in contact with the skin. The stoma should be covered with a gauze pad when changing the appliance to prevent seepage of urine onto the skin. The faceplate or wafer of the appliance shouldn't be more than 3 mm larger than the stoma to reduce the skin area in contact with urine.
CN: Physiological integrity; CNS: Basic care and comfort; CL: Application

58. 2. Cotton underwear prevents infection because it allows for air to flow to the perineum. Women should shower instead of taking a tub bath to prevent infection. Feminine hygiene spray can act as an irritant. Cranberry juice helps prevent cystitis because it increases urine acidity; alkaline urine supports bacterial growth, so cranberry juice intake should be increased, not limited.
CN: Health promotion and maintenance; CNS: None; CL: Application

59. 1. The drainage bag shouldn't be placed alongside the client or on the floor because of the increased risk of infection caused by microorganisms. It should hang on the bed in a dependent position. The other nursing diagnoses are not appropriate for this assessment finding.
CN: Safe, effective care environment; CNS: Management of care; CL: Application

60. A urine culture has been ordered for a male client. The nurse instructs the client to:
1. void in a clean container.
2. clean the foreskin of the penis if uncircumcised before specimen collection.
3. void into a urinal and then pour the urine into the specimen container.
4. begin the stream of urine in the toilet and catch the urine in a sterile container midstream.

If I can't do my job properly, I get a little hyper.

61. A client with a history of chronic renal failure is admitted to the unit with pulmonary edema after missing his dialysis treatment yesterday. His laboratory result levels are serum potassium 6.0 mEq/L, serum sodium 130 mEq/L, and serum bicarbonate 18 mEq/L. The nurse interprets that the client has which of the following conditions?
1. Alkalemia
2. Hyperkalemia
3. Hypernatremia
4. Hypokalemia

62. A client with acute renal failure has a serum potassium level of 7.0 mEq/L. The nurse's priority for this client is to assess which of the following?
1. Urine specific gravity
2. Electrocardiogram (ECG) results
3. Mental status
4. Blood pressure

63. A client has just received a renal transplant and has started cyclosporine therapy to prevent graft rejection. What is the most important information for the nurse to tell the client?
1. Report any signs of depression or a decreased appetite.
2. Report any dizziness and bleeding from the incision.
3. Report any fever, a flushed feeling, or lethargy.
4. Report any stomach discomfort or dyspepsia.

60. 4. Catching urine midstream reduces the amount of contamination by microorganisms at the meatus. Voiding in a clean container is done for a random specimen, not a clean-catch specimen for urine culture. When cleaning an uncircumcised male, the foreskin should be retracted and the glans penis should be cleaned to prevent specimen contamination. Voiding in a urinal doesn't allow for an uncontaminated specimen because the urinal isn't sterile.
CN: Physiological integrity; CNS: Reduction of risk potential; CL: Application

61. 2. The kidneys are responsible for excreting potassium. In renal failure, the kidneys are no longer able to excrete potassium, resulting in hyperkalemia. The kidneys are responsible for regulating the acid–base balance; in renal failure, acidemia would be seen. Generally, hyponatremia would be seen because of the dilutional effect of water retention. Hypokalemia is generally seen in clients undergoing diuresis.
CN: Physiological integrity; CNS: Physiological adaptation; CL: Analysis

62. 2. Acute renal failure can result in hyperkalemia, which can manifest in widening of the PR and QRS intervals on the ECG. Urine specific gravity, mental status, and blood pressure are not a priority with this client.
CN: Safe, effective care environment; CNS: Management of care; CL: Application

63. 3. Fever, a flushed feeling, or lethargy suggests infection, which is the major complication to watch for in clients on cyclosporine therapy because it's an immunosuppressive drug. The other symptoms aren't indicative of cyclosporine therapy.
CN: Physiological integrity; CNS: Pharmacological and parental therapies; CL: Application

64. A client received a kidney transplant 2 months ago. He's admitted to the hospital with the diagnosis of acute rejection. Which assessment finding should the nurse anticipate?
 1. Hypotension
 2. Normal body temperature
 3. Decreased white blood cell (WBC) counts
 4. Elevated blood urea nitrogen (BUN) and creatinine levels

65. A client is diagnosed with chronic renal failure and is told he must start hemodialysis. What is the most important client teaching for the nurse to provide?
 1. Follow a high-potassium diet.
 2. Strictly follow the hemodialysis schedule.
 3. There will be few changes in your lifestyle.
 4. Use alcohol on the skin to clean it because of integumentary changes.

66. A client is to undergo a kidney transplantation with a living donor. What is the most important preoperative assessment by the nurse?
 1. Urine output
 2. Signs of graft rejection
 3. Signs and symptoms of infection
 4. Client's support system and understanding of lifestyle changes

67. A client is undergoing peritoneal dialysis. The dialysate dwell time is completed, and the clamp is opened to allow the dialysate to drain. The nurse notes that drainage has stopped and that only 500 ml has drained; the amount of dialysate instilled was 1,500 ml. Which intervention should be done <u>first</u>?
 1. Change the client's position.
 2. Call the physician.
 3. Check the catheter for kinks or obstruction.
 4. Clamp the catheter and instill more dialysate at the next exchange time.

It's important that your client follow scheduled treatment.

This question is asking for the first thing you should do.

64. 4. In a client with acute renal graft rejection, evidence of deteriorating renal function (elevated BUN and creatinine levels) is expected. The client would most likely have acute hypertension. The nurse would see fever and elevated WBC counts because the body is recognizing the graft as foreign and is attempting to fight it.
CN: Physiological integrity; CNS: Reduction of risk potential; CL: Analysis

65. 2. To prevent life-threatening complications, the client must follow the dialysis schedule. The client should follow a low-potassium diet because potassium levels increase in chronic renal failure. The client should know that hemodialysis is time-consuming and will definitely cause a change in current lifestyle. Alcohol would further dry the client's skin more than it already is.
CN: Physiological integrity; CNS: Reduction of risk potential; CL: Application

66. 4. The client undergoing a renal transplantation will need vigilant follow-up care and must adhere to the medical regimen. The client is most likely anuric or oliguric preoperatively but postoperatively will require close monitoring of urine output to make sure the transplanted kidney is functioning optimally. Rejection can occur postoperatively. Although the client will always need to be monitored for signs and symptoms of infection, it's most important postoperatively because of the initiation of immunosuppressive therapy.
CN: Psychosocial integrity; CNS: None; CL: Application

67. 3. The first intervention should be to check for kinks and obstructions because that could be preventing drainage. After checking for kinks, have the client change position to promote drainage. Don't give the next scheduled exchange until the dialysate is drained because abdominal distention will occur, unless the output is within the parameters set by the physician. If unable to get more output despite checking for kinks and changing the client's position, the nurse should then call the physician to determine the proper intervention.
CN: Physiological integrity; CNS: Reduction of risk potential; CL: Analysis

68. A client receiving hemodialysis treatments arrives at the hospital with a blood pressure of 200/100 mm Hg, a heart rate of 110 beats/minute, and a respiratory rate of 36 breaths/minute. Oxygen saturation on room air is 89%. He complains of shortness of breath, and plus 2 pedal edema is noted. His last hemodialysis treatment was yesterday. Which intervention should be done first?
1. Administer oxygen.
2. Elevate the foot of the bed.
3. Restrict the client's fluids.
4. Prepare the client for hemodialysis.

69. A client with renal insufficiency is admitted with a diagnosis of pneumonia. He's being treated with I.V. antibiotics, which can be nephrotoxic. Which laboratory value(s) should be monitored closely?
1. Blood urea nitrogen (BUN) and creatinine levels
2. Arterial blood gas (ABG) levels
3. Platelet count
4. Potassium level

70. A client had a transurethral prostatectomy for benign prostatic hypertrophy and is currently being treated with a continuous bladder irrigation. He's complaining of an increase in severity of bladder spasms. Which intervention should the nurse do <u>first</u>?
1. Administer an oral analgesic.
2. Stop the irrigation and call the physician.
3. Administer a belladonna and opium suppository as ordered by the physician.
4. Check for the presence of clots and make sure the catheter is draining properly.

71. A client has returned from surgery with continuous bladder irrigation. The nurse is aware that proper maintenance of a continuous bladder irrigation system includes:
1. regulating irrigant flow to maintain red urine.
2. regulating irrigant flow to maintain pink urine.
3. maintaining a slow flow rate of irrigant to prevent bladder distention.
4. stopping the irrigation if there's leakage of large amounts of urine around the catheter.

Lots to do, but what's the most important?

I guess I better learn to go with the flow.

68. 1. Airway and oxygenation are always the first priority. Because the client is complaining of shortness of breath and his oxygen saturation is only 89%, the nurse needs to try to increase the partial pressure of arterial oxygen by administering oxygen. The foot of the bed may be elevated to reduce edema, but this isn't a priority. The client is in pulmonary edema from fluid overload and will need to be dialyzed and have his fluids restricted, but the first intervention should be aimed at the immediate treatment of hypoxia.
CN: Physiological integrity; CNS: Physiological adaptation; CL: Analysis

69. 1. BUN and creatinine levels should be monitored closely to detect elevations due to nephrotoxicity. ABG determinations are inappropriate for this situation. Platelets and potassium levels should be monitored according to routine.
CN: Physiological integrity; CNS: Reduction of risk potential; CL: Analysis

70. 4. Blood clots and blocked outflow of the urine can increase spasms. The irrigation shouldn't be stopped as long as the catheter is draining because clots will form. A belladonna and opium suppository should be given to relieve spasms but only after assessment of the drainage. Oral analgesics should be given if the spasms are unrelieved by the belladonna and opium suppository.
CN: Physiological integrity; CNS: Physiological adaptation; CL: Analysis

71. 2. The irrigant should be infused at a rate fast enough to maintain pink urine. Red urine indicates inadequate irrigation and possible clot formation. Bladder distention shouldn't occur as long as the system is draining properly and no clots are obstructing the outflow of urine. Leakage of urine around the catheter indicates clot formation on the catheter tip, needing manual irrigation. The irrigation shouldn't be stopped because of the potential for clot formation.
CN: Physiological integrity; CNS: Physiological adaptation; CL: Application

72. A client has an indwelling urinary catheter, and urine is leaking from a hole in the collection bag. Which nursing intervention would be <u>most appropriate</u>?
1. Cover the hole with tape.
2. Remove the catheter and insert a new one using sterile technique.
3. Disconnect the drainage bag from the catheter and replace it with a new bag.
4. Place a towel under the bag to prevent spillage of urine on the floor, which could cause the client to slip and fall.

73. A client is admitted with a diagnosis of hydronephrosis secondary to calculi. The calculi have been removed, and postobstructive diuresis is occurring. What is the most important intervention by the nurse?
1. Take vital signs every 8 hours.
2. Weigh the client every other day.
3. Assess the urine output every shift.
4. Monitor the client's electrolyte levels.

74. A client is admitted with severe nausea, vomiting, and diarrhea. He is hypotensive and is noted to have severe oliguria with elevated blood urea nitrogen (BUN) and creatinine levels. The nurse anticipates the physician will most likely write an order for which treatment?
1. Force oral fluids.
2. Give furosemide 20 mg I.V.
3. Start hemodialysis after a temporary access is obtained.
4. Start I.V. fluid of normal saline solution bolus followed by a maintenance dose.

75. A client has a history of chronic renal failure and receives hemodialysis treatments three times a week through an arteriovenous (AV) fistula in the left arm. What is the most important intervention for the nurse to provide?
1. Keep the AV fistula site dry.
2. Keep the AV fistula wrapped in gauze.
3. Take the blood pressure in the left arm.
4. Assess the AV fistula for a bruit and thrill.

Which answer is most likely to be correct?

72. 2. The system is no longer a closed system, and bacteria might have been introduced into the system, so a new sterile catheter should be inserted. Taping up the hole and placing a towel under the bag leave the system open, which increases the risk of infection. Replacing the drainage bag by disconnecting the old one from the catheter opens up the entire system and isn't recommended because of the increased risk of infection.

CN: Safe, effective care environment; CNS: Safety and infection control; CL: Analysis

73. 4. Postobstructive diuresis seen in hydronephrosis can cause electrolyte imbalances; laboratory values must be checked so electrolytes can be replaced as needed. Vital signs should initially be taken every 30 minutes for the first 4 hours and then every 2 hours. Urine output needs to be assessed hourly. The client's weight should be taken daily to assess fluid status more closely.

CN: Physiological integrity; CNS: Reduction of risk potential; CL: Analysis

74. 4. The client is prerenal secondary to hypovolemia. I.V. fluids should be given to rehydrate the client, urine output should increase, and the BUN and creatinine levels will normalize. The client wouldn't be able to tolerate oral fluids because of the nausea, vomiting, and diarrhea. The client isn't fluid overloaded, and his urine output won't increase with furosemide. The client won't need dialysis because the oliguria and increased BUN and creatinine levels are due to dehydration.

CN: Physiological integrity; CNS: Physiological adaptation; CL: Analysis

75. 4. Assessment of the AV fistula for a bruit and thrill is important because, if not present, it indicates a nonfunctioning fistula. When not being dialyzed, the AV fistula site may get wet. Immediately after a dialysis treatment, the access site is covered with adhesive bandages. No blood pressures or venipunctures should be taken in the arm with the AV fistula.

CN: Physiological integrity; CNS: Physiological adaptation; CL: Application

76. The nurse is obtaining a health history on a client. Which statement made by the client indicates a risk of renal calculi?
1. "I've been drinking a lot of cola soft drinks lately."
2. "I've been jogging more than usual."
3. "I've had more stress since we adopted a child last year."
4. "I'm a vegetarian and eat cheese two or three times each day."

77. The nurse is assessing a client who reports painful urination during and after voiding. The nurse suspects the client may have a problem with which area of the client's urinary system?
1. Bladder
2. Kidneys
3. Ureters
4. Urethra

78. A client is ordered diuretics. Which of the following would be the best time of day for the nurse to schedule this medication?
1. Anytime
2. Nighttime
3. Morning
4. Noon

79. Which nursing intervention would be the <u>most appropriate</u> for a client with postoperative urinary retention?
1. Give a diuretic.
2. Pour warm water over the perineum.
3. Consider inserting a bladder catheter.
4. Lay the client flat in bed.

80. A client has not voided 10 hours following an inguinal hernia repair. The nurse determines that the nursing diagnosis for this client would be urinary retention related to which of the following?
1. Dehydration
2. History of smoking
3. Duration of surgery
4. Preoperative atropine

This is the best time of day.

I never meant to put anyone at risk.

76. 4. Renal calculi are commonly composed of calcium. Diets high in calcium may predispose a person to renal calculi. Milk and milk products are high in calcium. Cola soft drinks don't contain ingredients that would increase the risk of renal calculi. Jogging and increased stress aren't considered risk factors for renal calculi formation.
CN: Health promotion and maintenance; CNS: None; CL: Analysis

77. 1. Pain during or after voiding indicates a bladder problem, usually infection. Kidney and ureter pain would be in the flank area, and problems of the urethra would cause pain at the external orifice that's commonly felt at the start of voiding.
CN: Health promotion and maintenance; CNS: None; CL: Application

78. 3. A diuretic given in the morning has time to work throughout the day. Diuretics given at nighttime will cause the client to get up to go to the bathroom frequently, interrupting sleep.
CN: Physiological integrity; CNS: Pharmacological and parenteral therapies; CL: Application

79. 2. Urinary retention reflects bladder distention from urine. Sitting the client upright and pouring warm water over the perineum may help the client void. A diuretic isn't necessary. If these measures aren't successful, the nurse should consider inserting a bladder catheter to drain the bladder. This procedure needs an order from the primary health care provider.
CN: Physiological integrity; CNS: Basic care and comfort; CL: Application

80. 4. Anticholinergic medications, such as atropine, may cause urinary retention, particularly for the client who has surgery in the pelvic area (inguinal hernia, hysterectomy). Dehydration, smoking, and duration of surgery aren't risk factors for retention, although opiate analgesics are risk factors.
CN: Physiological integrity; CNS: Reduction of risk potential; CL: Application

81. The nurse is caring for a client with urine retention. The physician has ordered the client to be catheterized. Which of the following catheters would be the most appropriate for the nurse to select to perform the procedure?
1. Coudé
2. Indwelling urinary
3. Straight
4. Three way

All catheters are not created equal.

82. An 80-year-old male client reports urine retention. Which factor may contribute to this client's problem?
1. Benign prostatic hyperplasia (BPH)
2. Diabetes
3. Diet
4. Hypertension

83. A 75-year-old client is admitted with dehydration. The client's laboratory results are serum sodium 145 mg/dl, serum potassium 5.0 mEq/L, blood urea nitrogen 29 mg/dl, and serum creatinine 1.3 mg/dl. Based on these results, the nurse determines that the client is at risk for developing which of the following conditions?
1. Acute confusion
2. Urinary retention
3. Acute renal failure
4. Cardiac arrhythmias

84. A client with an overactive neurogenic bladder is complaining of a dry mouth from his medication oxybutynin (Ditropan). The nurse is aware that this adverse effect is commonly found with which of the flowing drug classifications?
1. Anti-infective
2. Corticosteroid
3. Urinary antiseptic
4. Spasmolytic

A nurse needs to be able to prioritize.

85. A client is injected with radiographic contrast medium and immediately shows signs of dyspnea, flushing, and pruritus. Which intervention should take priority?
1. Check vital signs.
2. Make sure the airway is patent.
3. Apply a cold pack to the I.V. site.
4. Call the physician.

81. 3. Urine retention is usually a temporary problem that requires insertion of a straight catheter. An indwelling urinary catheter is used for longer term bladder problems. A catheter coudé is used only when it's difficult to insert a standard catheter, usually because of an enlarged prostate. A three-way catheter is used for clients who need bladder irrigation such as after a prostate resection.
CN: Physiological integrity; CNS: Basic care and comfort; CL: Application

82. 1. BPH is common among elderly men and typically results in urine retention, frequency, dribbling, and difficulty starting the urine stream. Diabetes, diet, and hypertension usually don't affect urine retention.
CN: Physiological integrity; CNS: Reduction of risk potential; CL: Application

83. 3. The laboratory results indicate an elevated serum blood urea nitrogen (normal ranges are from 5 to 25 mg/dl), which is reflective of dehydration. Volume depletion or dehydration is a risk factor for developing acute renal failure due to decreased perfusion of the kidneys. The serum potassium, sodium, and creatinine levels are within high-normal range.
CN: Physiological integrity; CNS: Reduction of risk potential; CL: Application

84. 4. Oxybutynin belongs to the spasmolytic drug classification. A common side effect is dry mouth. The other drug classifications do not commonly have an adverse effect of dry mouth.
CN: Physiological integrity; CNS: Pharmacological and parenteral therapies; CL: Application

85. 2. The client is showing symptoms of an allergy to the iodine in the contrast medium. The first action is to make sure the client's airway is patent. If compromised, call a cardiac arrest code. Checking vital signs and calling for the physician are important nursing actions but should follow making sure the airway is patent. A cold pack isn't indicated.
CN: Physiological integrity; CNS: Physiological adaptation; CL: Analysis

86. An 80-year-old man is admitted for a cystoscopy with biopsy of the bladder. After obtaining a history, surgery is postponed. Which reason would be the cause to postpone this client's surgery?
  1. The client stopped taking his anticoagulant 3 days ago.
  2. The client has a urinary tract infection.
  3. The client has previously been treated for carcinoma of the bladder.
  4. The client took an antibiotic prior to the procedure.

87. A client who underwent a cystoscopy is scheduled to be discharged to home within 24 hours. What is the most important information for the nurse to give the client?
  1. Expect bloody urine for about a week.
  2. Drink 8 to 10 glasses of water every 8 hours.
  3. Try to urinate frequently and measure your output.
  4. Check the color, consistency, and amount of urine in the indwelling urinary catheter bag every 4 to 8 hours.

It's important to share vital client information.

88. Before a renal biopsy, which information is most important to tell the physician?
  1. The client signed a consent form.
  2. The client understands the procedure.
  3. The client has normal urinary elimination.
  4. The client regularly takes aspirin or nonsteroidal anti-inflammatory drugs (NSAIDs).

89. Kegel exercises are used to gain control of bladder function in women with stress incontinence and in some men after prostate surgery. Which instruction would help the client perform these exercises?
  1. Completely empty the bladder.
  2. Do the exercise 200 times per day.
  3. Sit or stand with your legs together.
  4. Drink small amounts of fluid frequently.

Kegel exercises can help the client gain bladder control.

86. 2. Bladder biopsies shouldn't be done when an active urinary tract infection is present because sepsis may result. Anticoagulants should be discontinued for 3 to 5 days before the procedure. The client who has been treated for bladder cancer may still require the procedure to check effectiveness of treatment. Antibiotics are sometimes given prophylactically prior to the procedure.
CN: Physiological integrity; CNS: Reduction of risk potential; CL: Analysis

87. 3. The bladder needs to be emptied frequently, and output should be measured to make sure the bladder is emptying. Blood in the urine isn't normal except for small amounts during the first 24 hours after the procedure. Large amounts of fluids help flush microorganisms out of the body, but 8 to 10 glasses every 8 hours may not be reasonable. Also, clients don't tend to think in time periods, so instructions should be given per day. The client may not have an indwelling urinary catheter.
CN: Physiological integrity; CNS: Reduction of risk potential; CL: Application

88. 4. Aspirin and NSAIDs cause increased bleeding times and commonly result in hemorrhaging when biopsies are performed. It's the physician's responsibility to make sure the client understands the procedure, which is needed for informed consent. It isn't necessary to report that the client has normal urinary elimination.
CN: Physiological integrity; CNS: Reduction of risk potential; CL: Application

89. 2. Exercises begin with tightening and relaxing the vagina, rectum, and urethra four or five times during each session and gradually increasing to 25 times for each session. The client stops the flow of urine during urination to practice holding the flow. Standing or sitting with the legs apart facilitates the exercise. Clients should drink plenty of fluids to prevent urinary problems.
CN: Physiological integrity; CNS: Physiological adaptation; CL: Application

90. A client with chronic pyelonephritis is preparing to be discharged from the hospital. What is the most important information for the nurse to tell the client?
1. Stay on bed rest for up to 2 weeks.
2. Use analgesia on a regular basis for up to 6 months.
3. Have a urine culture every 2 weeks for up to 6 months.
4. Antibiotic treatment may be needed for several weeks or months.

91. A client had transurethral prostatectomy for benign prostatic hypertrophy. He's currently being treated with continuous bladder irrigation and is complaining of an increase in severity of bladder spasms. What should the nurse do first for this client?
1. Administer an oral analgesic.
2. Stop the irrigation and call the physician.
3. Administer a belladonna and opium suppository as ordered by the physician.
4. Check for the presence of clots and make sure that the catheter is draining properly.

92. Which client is at greatest risk for developing acute renal failure?
1. A dialysis client who gets influenza
2. A teenager who has an appendectomy
3. A pregnant woman who has a fractured femur
4. A client with diabetes who has a heart catheterization

93. Which nursing intervention should be done for a client with urinary calculus?
1. Save any calculi larger than 0.25 cm.
2. Strain the urine, limit oral fluids, and give pain medications.
3. Encourage fluid intake, strain the urine, and give pain medications.
4. Insert an indwelling urinary catheter, check intake and output, and give pain medications.

Remember, it's what you should do first that's important.

I never did understand calculus.

90. 4. Chronic pyelonephritis can be a long-term condition requiring antibiotic treatment for several weeks or months as well as close monitoring to prevent permanent damage to the kidneys. Bed rest and analgesia may be used during the acute stage but usually aren't required long-term. A urine culture is done 2 weeks after stopping antibiotics to make sure the infection has been eradicated.
CN: Physiological integrity; CNS: Reduction of risk control; CL: Application

91. 4. Blood clots and blocked outflow of urine can increase spasms. The irrigation shouldn't be stopped as long as the catheter is draining because clots will form. A belladonna and opium suppository should be given to relieve spasm only after assessment of the drainage. Oral analgesics should be given if the spasms are unrelieved by the belladonna and opium suppository.
CN: Physiological integrity; CNS: Reduction of risk potential; CL: Analysis

92. 4. Clients with diabetes are prone to renal insufficiency and renal failure. The contrast used for heart catheterization must be eliminated by the kidneys, which further stresses them and may produce acute renal failure. A dialysis client already has end-stage renal disease and wouldn't develop acute renal failure. A teenager who has an appendectomy and a pregnant woman who fractures a femur aren't at increased risk for renal failure.
CN: Health promotion and maintenance; CNS: None; CL: Analysis

93. 3. Encourage fluid intake and strain all urine, saving all calculi, including "flecks." Give pain medications because renal calculi are painful. Indwelling urinary catheters aren't usually needed.
CN: Physiological integrity; CNS: Physiological adaptation; CL: Application

94. The nurse is caring for a client who is receiving hemodialysis treatments. Which of the following interventions would be the most appropriate for this client?
1. Palpate for a thrill on the arm with the fistula.
2. Palpate for a thrill on the arm without the fistula.
3. Document the absence of a bruit as a normal finding.
4. Take the blood pressure on the arm with the fistula.

95. A client has passed a renal calculus. The nurse sends the specimen to the laboratory so it can be analyzed for:
1. antibodies.
2. type of infection.
3. composition of calculus.
4. size and number of calculi.

96. Which symptom may indicate <u>acute</u> rejection of a transplanted kidney?
1. Increased urine output
2. Hypotension
3. Pain at the graft site
4. Decreased white blood cell (WBC) count

97. A client has been placed on prednisone therapy. The client asks the nurse if any adverse reactions can occur when taking the medication. What is the most appropriate response by the nurse?
1. Acne and bleeding gums
2. Sodium retention and constipation
3. Mood swings and increased temperature
4. Increased blood glucose levels and decreased wound healing

98. Steroids, such as prednisone and methylprednisolone, are used to suppress the inflammatory immune response following a kidney transplant. Which information should be given to a client with a transplant?
1. Alopecia may occur.
2. Weight loss is common.
3. Cholesterol levels may become elevated.
4. Hypokalemia may result.

Don't give up now. You're doing great!

Yes, I know I am kind of a-cute!

94. **1.** The nurse would palpate for a thrill and auscultate for a bruit on the arm with a fistula, but no procedures (blood pressure, I.V. access, or blood draw) should be done on the arm with a fistula because it could damage the fistula. The absence of a thrill or bruit should be reported promptly to the physician because it indicates an occlusion and is not a normal finding.
CN: Physiological integrity; CNS: Reduction of risk potential; CL: Application

95. **3.** The calculus should be analyzed for composition to determine appropriate interventions such as dietary restrictions. Calculi don't result from infections. The size and number of calculi aren't relevant, and they don't contain antibodies.
CN: Physiological integrity; CNS: Reduction of risk potential; CL: Application

96. **3.** Signs and symptoms of acute rejection of a transplanted kidney include pain at the graft site, decreased (not increased) urine output, hypertension (not hypotension), elevated (not decreased) WBC count, fever, and elevated creatinine level.
CN: Physiological integrity; CNS: Physiological adaptation; CL: Analysis

97. **4.** Steroid use tends to increase blood glucose levels, particularly in clients with diabetes and borderline diabetes. Steroids also contribute to poor wound healing and may cause acne, mood swings, and sodium and water retention. Steroids don't affect bleeding tendencies, constipation, or thermoregulation.
CN: Physiological integrity; CNS: Pharmacological and parenteral therapies; CL: Analysis

98. **4.** Steroids may decrease serum potassium levels but don't increase cholesterol levels. Hirsutism may occur but not alopecia. Weight gain is commonly reported, not weight loss.
CN: Physiological integrity; CNS: Pharmacological and parenteral therapies; CL: Analysis

99. A nurse suspects that a client with polyuria is experiencing water diuresis. The nurse assesses the laboratory values for which of the following?
1. High urine specific gravity
2. High urine osmolarity
3. Normal to low urine specific gravity
4. Elevated urine pH

100. A client with bladder cancer has had his bladder removed and an ileal conduit created for urine diversion. While changing this client's pouch, the nurse observes that the area around the stoma is red, weeping, and painful. What should the nurse conclude?
1. The skin wasn't lubricated before the pouch was applied.
2. The pouch faceplate doesn't fit the stoma.
3. A skin barrier was applied properly.
4. Stoma dilation wasn't performed.

101. A client is diagnosed with prostate cancer. The physician is most likely to order which test to monitor the client's progress?
1. Serum creatinine
2. Complete blood count (CBC)
3. Prostate-specific antigen (PSA)
4. Serum potassium

102. When teaching a client about cystitis, a nurse explains that females are more prone to the disorder than males. Which factor explains a female's increased susceptibility?
1. Higher estrogen levels
2. Inadequate fluid intake
3. Urethral proximity to the rectum
4. Continuous nature of the mucosa

103. A client presents with a possible urinary tract infection. Which urine characteristic should the nurse assess <u>first</u>?
1. Urine clarity
2. Urine specific gravity
3. Urine acetone
4. Urine protein

You've finished 100 questions. Way to go!

Location. It's a hint to help you answer question 102.

99. 3. Water diuresis causes low urine specific gravity, low urine osmolarity, and a normal to elevated serum sodium level. High urine specific gravity indicates dehydration. Elevated urine pH can result from potassium deficiency, a high-protein diet, or uncontrolled diabetes.
CN: Physiological integrity; CNS: Physiological adaptation; CL: Application

100. 2. If the pouch faceplate doesn't fit the stoma properly, the skin around the stoma will be exposed to continuous urine flow from the stoma, causing excoriation and red, weeping, painful skin. A lubricant shouldn't be used because it would prevent the pouch from adhering to the skin. When properly applied, a skin barrier prevents skin excoriation. Stoma dilation isn't performed with an ileal conduit, although it may be done with a colostomy, if ordered.
CN: Physiological integrity; CNS: Basic care and comfort; CL: Analysis

101. 3. The PSA test is used to monitor prostate cancer progression; higher PSA levels indicate a greater tumor burden. Serum creatinine levels may suggest blockage from an enlarged prostate. CBC is used to diagnose anemia and polycythemia. Serum potassium levels identify hypokalemia and hyperkalemia.
CN: Physiological integrity; CNS: Physiological adaptation; CL: Application

102. 3. In females, the urethra and rectum are in close proximity, posing a greater risk for urethral contamination with feces after a bowel movement. Decreased estrogen levels may reduce vaginal and urethral lubrication, increasing the chance of irritation during coitus. Males and females can have equivalent fluid intake. The mucosa is continuous in both males and females.
CN: Physiological integrity; CNS Physiological adaptation; CL: Application

103. 1. First, the nurse should assess urine clarity; cloudy urine usually indicates drainage, which may reflect infection. Urine specific gravity yields information about fluid balance. Neither urine acetone nor urine protein indicates infection.
CN: Health promotion and maintenance; CNS: None; CL: Analysis

104. A 70-year-old male client is diagnosed with syphilis in the secondary stage. Which finding should the nurse expect during assessment?
1. Chronic bone and joint irritation
2. Tender lymphadenopathy
3. Generalized rash on the palms and soles
4. Personality changes and mental confusion

104. 3. In secondary syphilis, a maculopapular nonpruritic rash appears on the palms and soles. Chronic bone and joint irritation aren't related to secondary syphilis. During the second stage of syphilis, nontender lymphadenopathy occurs. Personality changes occur during the late stage of syphilis.

CN: Physiological integrity; CNS: Basic care and comfort; CL: Application

105. Which medication is <u>most likely</u> to be prescribed for a client with gonorrhea?
1. Penicillin G benzathine (Bicillin)
2. Azithromycin (Zithromax)
3. Ceftriaxone (Rocephin)
4. Trichloroacetic acid (TCA)

105. 3. According to the Centers for Disease Control guidelines, ceftriaxone (Rocephin) or cefixime (Suprax) is the drug of choice for treating gonorrhea. Penicillin is used to treat syphilis. Azithromycin is used for chlamydial infection. Topical trichloroacetic acid is used for human papillomavirus.

CN: Physiological integrity; CNS: Pharmacological and parenteral therapies; CL: Application

The question is, which one of us can help?

106. In a client with renal failure, which assessment finding may indicate hypocalcemia?
1. Headache
2. Serum calcium level of 10 mg/dl
3. Increased blood coagulation
4. Diarrhea

106. 4. In renal failure, calcium absorption from the intestine declines, leading to increased smooth-muscle contractions, causing diarrhea. Central nervous system changes in renal failure rarely cause headache. A serum calcium level of 9 to 10.5 mg/dl is a normal calcium level. As renal failure progresses, bleeding tendencies increase.

CN: Health promotion and maintenance; CNS: None; CL: Application

107. A 27-year-old client, who became paraplegic after a swimming accident, is experiencing autonomic dysreflexia. Which condition is the <u>most common</u> cause of autonomic dysreflexia?
1. Upper respiratory infection
2. Incontinence
3. Bladder distention
4. Diarrhea

There may be many causes, but which is *most* common?

107. 3. Autonomic dysreflexia is a potentially life-threatening complication of spinal cord injury, occurring from obstruction of the urinary system or bowel. An upper respiratory infection could obstruct the respiratory system but not the urinary or bowel system. Incontinence and diarrhea don't result in obstruction of the urinary system or bowel, respectively.

CN: Physiological integrity; CNS: Physiological adaptation; CL: Analysis

108. When teaching a client how to prevent recurrences of acute glomerulonephritis, which instruction should the nurse include?
1. "Avoid physical activity."
2. "Strain all urine."
3. "Seek early treatment for respiratory infection."
4. "Monitor urine specific gravity every day."

109. After radical prostatectomy for prostate cancer, a client has an indwelling catheter removed. He then begins to have periods of incontinence. During the postoperative period, which intervention should be implemented first?
1. Kegel exercises
2. Fluid restriction
3. Artificial sphincter use
4. Self-catheterization

110. When providing discharge teaching for a client with uric acid calculi, the nurse should include an instruction to <u>avoid</u> which type of food?
1. Cottage cheese
2. Beets
3. Spinach
4. Organ meats

111. When a client with nephrotic syndrome manifests anasarca, the nurse relates this assessment finding to which abnormally low laboratory value?
1. Cholesterol
2. Prothrombin time
3. Albumin
4. Calcium

108. 3. Hemolytic streptococci are common in throat infections and can cause an immune reaction that causes glomerular damage. Therefore, the client should seek early treatment for respiratory infection. Avoiding physical activity may promote urination but doesn't prevent recurrence of glomerulonephritis. Straining all urine helps identify renal calculi that have passed through the urine. Daily monitoring of urine specific gravity helps assess hydration status but doesn't aid in glomerulonephritis prevention.

CN: Physiological integrity; CNS: Reduction of risk potential; CL: Analysis

109. 1. Kegel exercises are noninvasive and are recommended as the initial intervention for incontinence. Fluid restriction is useful for a client with increased detrusor contraction related to acidic urine. Artificial sphincter use isn't a primary intervention for postprostatectomy incontinence. Self-catheterization may be used as a temporary measure but isn't a primary intervention.

CN: Physiological integrity; CNS: Physiological adaptation; CL: Application

110. 4. To control uric acid calculi, the client should avoid high-purine foods such as organ meats. Beets and spinach are high in oxalate. Cottage cheese is high in calcium.

CN: Physiological integrity; CNS: Reduction of risk potential; CL: Application

111. 3. When the glomeruli are damaged, as in nephrotic syndrome, the kidneys are excessively permeable to plasma protein, causing proteinuria and hypoalbuminemia. This leads to a decreased oncotic pressure, which results in anasarca (massive generalized edema).

CN: Physiological integrity; CNS: Physiological adaptation; CL: Application

112. After a retropubic prostatectomy, a client requires continuous bladder irrigation. The client has an I.V. of dextrose 5% in water infusing at 40 ml/hour and a triple-lumen urinary catheter with normal saline solution infusing at 200 ml/hour. The nurse empties the urinary catheter drainage bag three times during an 8-hour period for a total of 2,780 ml. How many milliliters does the nurse calculate as urine? Record your answer using a whole number.

_____ milliliters

113. A nurse is caring for a client with chronic renal failure. The laboratory results indicate hypocalcemia and hyperphosphatemia. When assessing the client, the nurse should be alert for which symptom(s)? Select all that apply.
1. Trousseau's sign
2. Cardiac arrhythmias
3. Constipation
4. Decreased clotting time
5. Drowsiness and lethargy
6. Fractures

114. A 26-year-old client with chronic renal failure plans to receive a kidney transplant. Recently, the physician told the client that he's a poor candidate for transplant because of chronic uncontrolled hypertension and diabetes mellitus. Now the client tells the nurse, "I want to go off dialysis. I'd rather not live than be on this treatment for the rest of my life." Which response is appropriate? Select all that apply.
1. Take a seat next to the client and sit quietly.
2. Say to the client, "We all have days when we don't feel like going on."
3. Leave the room to allow the client to collect his thoughts.
4. Say to the client, "You're feeling upset about the news you got about the transplant."
5. Say to the client, "The treatments are only 3 days a week. You can live with that."

112. 1,180. During 8 hours, 1,600 ml of bladder irrigation has been infused (200 ml × 8 hours = 1,600 ml/8 hours). The nurse then subtracts this amount of infused bladder irrigation from the total volume in the drainage bag (2,780 ml − 1,600 ml = 1,180 ml) to determine urine output.

CN: Physiological integrity; CNS: Basic care and comfort; CL: Analysis

113. **1, 2, and 6.** Hypocalcemia is a calcium deficit that causes nerve fiber irritability and repetitive muscle spasms. Signs and symptoms of hypocalcemia include Trousseau's sign, cardiac arrhythmias, diarrhea, increased clotting, anxiety, and irritability. The calcium–phosphorus imbalance leads to brittle bones and pathological fractures.

CN: Physiological integrity; CNS: Reduction of risk potential; CL: Application

114. **1 and 4.** Silence is a therapeutic communication technique that allows the nurse and client to reflect on what has taken place or been said. By waiting quietly and attentively, the nurse encourages the client to initiate and maintain conversation. By reflecting the client's implied feelings, the nurse also promotes communication. Using such platitudes as "We all have days when we don't feel like going on" fails to address the client's needs. The nurse shouldn't leave the client alone because he may harm himself. Reminding the client of the treatment frequency doesn't address his feelings.

CN: Psychosocial integrity; CNS: None; CL: Analysis

115. The radiology nurse is reviewing a list of home medications of a 53-year-old client who is scheduled for an outpatient I.V. pyelogram (IVP) at 10:00 a.m. The client took the following medications at home with sips of water at 8:00 a.m. Which of the medications would prompt the nurse to contact the physician?
1. Metoprolol (Lopressor) 25 mg by mouth
2. Sitagliptin (Januvia) 100 mg by mouth
3. Metformin (Glucophage) 500 mg by mouth
4. Lorazepam (Ativan) 0.5 mg by mouth

116. The nurse is caring for a 22-year-old client with acute glomerulonephritis. The nurse would anticipate to expect which manifestations? Select all that apply.
1. Fatigue
2. Periorbital edema
3. Thromboemboli
4. Cola-colored urine
5. Hypertension
6. Proteinuria
7. Hyperlipidemia

117. The nurse is reviewing admission orders for a 78-year-old client with a pneumonia diagnosis. The client has no known drug allergies, and the client's serum labs are as follows: white blood cells (WBC) 15.2 K/ml, hemoglobin 11.2 g/dl, blood urea nitrogen (BUN) 29 mg/dl, and creatinine 2.8 mg/dl. The nurse should contact the physician to question which of the following orders?
1. Gentamicin 150 mg I.V. piggyback (IVPB) every 24 hours
2. Doxycycline 100 mg IVPB every 12 hours
3. Rocephin 1 g IVPB every 24 hours
4. Zithromax 500 mg IVPB every 24 hours

118. The spouse of a client diagnosed with acute glomerulonephritis asked the nurse to clarify foods that are a complete source of protein. Which examples of complete protein foods should the nurse discuss with the spouse? Select all that apply.
1. Nuts
2. Eggs
3. Fish
4. Legumes
5. Soy

119. A client diagnosed with acute renal failure voided 260 ml of urine on Tuesday. What is the maximum amount of fluid the client may consume orally on Wednesday?
1. 360 ml
2. 500 ml
3. 740 ml
4. 760 ml

115. 3. Metformin, a biguanide oral hypoglycemic agent, should be held 24 hours before and 48 hours after IVP to reduce potential of lactic acidosis and renal failure. Sitagliptin, metoprolol, and lorazepam do not produce harmful effects when IV contrast is administered.
CN: Physiological integrity; CNS: Pharmacological and parenteral therapies; CL: Application

116. 1, 2, 4, 5, and 6. Fatigue, periorbital edema, hematuria (cola-colored urine), hypertension, and proteinuria are common manifestations of acute glomerulonephritis. Thromboemboli and hyperlipidemia are common manifestations of nephrotic syndrome.
CN: Physiological integrity; CNS: Physiological adaptation; CL: Application

117. 1. The aminoglycoside gentamicin may be nephrotoxic when administered to a client with altered renal function. This client's BUN and creatinine are elevated. The client is elderly, placing the client at increased risk for nephrotoxic effects of medications.
CN: Physiological integrity; CNS: Pharmacological and parenteral therapies; CL: Analysis

118. 2, 3, and 5. Eggs, fish, and soy (as well as milk, cheese, meat, and poultry) contain all essential amino acids and are considered a source of complete protein. When renal function is impaired, urea accumulates in the body as a result of impaired protein metabolism. Complete proteins are efficiently metabolized by the body, reducing urea accumulation.
CN: Physiological integrity; CNS: Basic care and comfort; CL: Application

119. 4. The nurse adds the client's urine output for the previous 24 hours (260 ml) to 500 ml, which is the standard amount for insensible losses. 260 ml + 500 ml = 760 ml
CN: Physiological integrity; CNS: Basic care and comfort; CL: Application

120. The intensive care unit nurse is explaining the procedure for continuous renal replacement therapy (CRRT) to a client with acute renal failure. Which statement best describes how the nurse should tell the client how CRRT will be initiated?
1. "I will attach the machine to the central venous catheter the physician placed in your upper chest."
2. "I will attach the machine to the catheter the physician placed in your abdomen."
3. "I will attach the machine to the fistula the physician placed in your arm."
4. "I will attach the machine to the shunt the physician placed in your arm."

You've reached question 120. Only 5 more to go.

121. The nurse is reviewing the urinalysis results on four different adult clients. Which client would the nurse anticipate to receive an I.V. fluid bolus?
1. Mr. Compton: specific gravity 1.005
2. Mr. Bailey: specific gravity 1.022
3. Mr. Sanchez: specific gravity 1.030
4. Mrs. Wu: specific gravity 1.045

122. A 72-year-old male tells the nurse he has been taking saw palmetto by mouth twice a day for the past 3 years as treatment for urinary hesitancy due to an enlarged prostate. What should the nurse assesses the client for?
1. Hypertension
2. Jaundice
3. Joint pain
4. Dry mouth

123. A 23-year-old female is at the clinic for her yearly gynecological assessment. She expresses concern about a family friend who recently had a hysterectomy due to cancer and asks the nurse how she can prevent getting this type of cancer. Which of the following statements should the nurse tell the client? Select all that apply.
1. "Not smoking reduces risk for cervical cancer."
2. "A high-fat diet decreases risk for ovarian cancer."
3. "Using condoms reduces risk for cervical cancer."
4. "Limiting your number of sexual partners reduces risk for cervical cancer."
5. "A vaccine called Gardasil, given as an injection two times over a 6-month period, can reduce risk for cervical cancer."

120. 1. Through CRRT, blood from a double-lumen central venous line is slowly filtered and returned to the client. The slow filtration promotes hemodynamic stability and minimizes complications related to changes in extracellular fluid composition. The peritoneal catheter is used for peritoneal dialysis. The fistula and shunt are used for hemodialysis.

CN: Physiological integrity; CNS: Physiological adaptation; CL: Application

121. 4. Specific gravity measures the ratio of the density of urine as compared to the density of an equal volume of water and is a reflection of the client's hydration status. Normal specific gravity in adults ranges between 1.016 and 1.030. An elevated specific gravity indicates the client is in need of hydration.

CN: Physiological integrity; CNS: Reduction of risk potential; CL: Analysis

122. 2. Saw Palmetto is used by more than 2 million men to treat benign prostatic hypertrophy and may cause damage to the liver and pancreas. Assessment for signs of jaundice relates to identification of saw palmetto's potential adverse effects on the liver.

CN: Physiological integrity; CNS: Pharmacological and parenteral therapies; CL: Application

123. 1, 3, and 4. Not smoking, using condoms, and limiting the number of sexual partners reduce risk for cervical cancer. A high-fat diet increases risk for ovarian cancer. Gardasil is given as three intramuscular injections over a 6-month period.

CN: Physiological integrity; CNS: Reduction of risk potential; CL: Application

124. The nurse is to prepare a client diagnosed with acute kidney injury (AKI) for a renal radiological study. The physician orders the client to have the bowel evacuated before the study. Which of the following orders for method of bowel evacuation would the nurse question? Select all that apply.
1. Soap suds cleansing enema until clear
2. Fleet enema until clear
3. Bisacodyl (Dulcolax) 15 mg orally
4. Magnesium citrate 240 ml orally
5. Castor oil (Emulsoil) 30 ml orally

125. A 78-year-old African-American male who is alert and oriented has been receiving hemodialysis three times per week for the last 5 years. The client's condition has gradually declined and he tells the dialysis nurse, "I do not want to do this anymore. I am tired and ready to let my body shut down. I know I will die, but I am ready." What is the most appropriate response by the nurse?
1. "I understand. My grandmother decided to give up too."
2. "You are just having a really bad day. You will feel better tomorrow."
3. "Have you thought about how your children will react?"
4. "Are you saying you no longer want to receive dialysis treatments?"

124. 2 and 4. Fleet enema and magnesium citrate are hyperosmolar solutions, which are contraindicated for those with renal problems. The salt content in these solutions can cause toxicity. Soap suds enema, bisacodyl, and castor oil may be used.

CN: Physiological integrity; CNS: Pharmacological and parental therapies; CL: Application

125. 4. Clarification is a therapeutic communication technique that is helpful in validating the intended meaning of the client's statement. Insinuating that the client decided to "give up" is judgmental. Telling the client he is having a "bad day" invalidates his feelings. Asking how his children will react places guilt on the client.

CN: Psychosocial integrity; CNS: None; CL: Application

You were right on target with chapter 10. Now aim to do as well on chapter 11.

So, you think the care of the client with a skin disorder isn't your strong suit, eh? Maybe you'd like to check out this Web site before taking on this chapter: **www.aad.org**. Enjoy!

Chapter 11
Integumentary disorders

1. The nurse is providing care for a client admitted to the burn unit. Select the most appropriate statement that identifies the nutritional needs of the client.
1. The client needs 100 cal/kg throughout hospitalization.
2. The hypermetabolic state after a burn injury contributes to poor healing.
3. A cool environment decreases caloric demand.
4. Maintaining a hypermetabolic rate decreases the client's risk of infection.

Don't let this chapter get under your skin.

2. The nurse is assessing a 30-year-old client admitted to the emergency department with a deep partial-thickness burn on his arm after a fire in the workplace. The nurse documents the assessment findings as:
1. pain and redness.
2. minimal damage to the epidermis.
3. necrotic tissue through all layers of skin.
4. necrotic tissue through most of the dermis.

3. The nurse is assessing a client in the emergency room who was bitten by a brown recluse spider. Documentation of the assessment is correct when which of the following assessments has been recorded in the client's record?
1. Bull's-eye rash
2. Painful rash around a necrotic lesion
3. Herald patch of oval lesions
4. Line of papules and vesicles that appear 1 to 3 days after exposure

1. 2. A burn injury causes a hypermetabolic state resulting in protein and lipid catabolism that affects wound healing. Calories need to be 1.5 to 2 times the basal metabolic rate, with at least 1.5 to 2 g/kg of body weight of protein daily. An environmental temperature within normal range lets the body function efficiently and devote caloric expenditure to healing and normal physiological processes. If the temperature is too warm or too cold, the body gives energy to warming or cooling, which takes away from energy used for tissue repair. High metabolic rates increase the risk of infection.

CN: Physiological integrity; CNS: Basic care and comfort; CL: Application

2. 4. A deep partial-thickness burn causes necrosis of the epidermal and dermal layers. Redness and pain are characteristics of a superficial injury. Superficial burns cause slight epidermal damage. Necrosis through all skin layers is seen with full-thickness injuries.

CN: Physiological integrity; CNS: Physiological adaptation; CL: Application

3. 2. Necrotic, painful rashes are associated with the bite of a brown recluse spider. A bull's-eye rash located primarily at the site of the bite is a classic sign of Lyme disease. A herald patch—a slightly raised, oval lesion about 2 to 6 cm in diameter and appearing anywhere on the body—is indicative of pityriasis rosea. A linear, papular, vesicular rash is characteristic of exposure to poison ivy.

CN: Physiological integrity; CNS: Physiological adaptation; CL: Application

4. A potential exposure to tuberculosis has occurred at a large, rural high school. The school nurse provides instruction to a group of community nurses who have volunteered to assist in the administration of the Mantoux test for the students. The school nurse determines that further instructions are not required when a volunteer nurse makes which statement?
1. "Use the deltoid muscle."
2. "Rub the site to help absorption."
3. "Read the results within 72 hours."
4. "Read the results by checking for a rash."

5. A woman walks into the health clinic and frantically tells the nurse she is worried she might have lice. The nurse performs an assessment and determines that the client has lice when she observes which of the following?
1. Diffuse pruritic wheals
2. Oval, white dots stuck to the hair shafts
3. Pain, redness, and edema with an embedded stinger
4. Pruritic papules, pustules, and linear burrows of the finger and toe webs

6. The client has experienced a bite from a dog. The nurse documents this in the client's record as which type of injury?
1. Abrasion
2. Crush injury
3. Fracture
4. Puncture wound

7. A 19-year-old client comes to the clinic with dark red lesions on her hands, wrist, and waistline. She has scratched several of the lesions, and they are open and bleeding. The nurse instructs the client to try pressing on the itchy lesions. The nurse explains that pressing on the skin:
1. spreads the beneficial microorganisms.
2. is suggested before scratching.
3. promotes breaks in the skin.
4. stimulates nerve endings.

8. A client arrives at the office of his physician complaining of a rash. The nurse assesses the client and notes several palpable, elevated masses, each about 0.5 cm. The nurse documents these assessment findings using which term?
1. Erosions
2. Macules
3. Papules
4. Vesicles

Sometimes timing is everything.

Your most important skill is assessment.

4. 3. The test results should be read 48 to 72 hours after placement by measuring the diameter of the induration that develops at the site. The Mantoux test is injected intradermally on the volar surface of the forearm, not I.M. Rubbing the site could cause leakage from the injection site. An induration develops, not a rash.

CN: Physiological integrity; CNS: Reduction of risk potential; CL: Application

5. 2. Nits, the eggs of lice, are seen as white oval dots. Diffuse pruritic wheals are associated with an allergic reaction. Bites from honeybees are associated with a stinger, pain, and redness. Pruritic papules, vesicles, and linear burrows are diagnostic for scabies.

CN: Physiological integrity; CNS: Physiological adaptation; CL: Application

6. 2. The bite of a large dog can exert between 150 to 400 psi of pressure, causing a crush injury, not a fracture. An abrasion is caused by friction. A bite from a small animal such as a cat will cause puncture wounds.

CN: Physiological integrity; CNS: Physiological adaptation; CL: Application

7. 4. Pressing the skin stimulates nerve endings and can reduce the sensation of itching. Scratching (not pressing) the skin spreads microorganisms and opens portals of entry for bacteria. Scratching isn't recommended at all. Pressing the skin doesn't promote breaks in the skin.

CN: Physiological integrity; CNS: Physiological adaptation; CL: Application

8. 3. Papules are masses elevated up to 0.5 cm, and nodules and tumors are masses elevated more than 0.5 cm. Erosions are characterized as loss of the epidermis layer. Macules and patches are nonpalpable, flat changes in skin color. Fluid-filled lesions are vesicles and pustules.

CN: Health promotion and maintenance; CNS: None; CL: Application

9. A nurse is teaching a female client about the use of isotretinoin (Accutane). The nurse determines that teaching was effective when the client states the need to take:
1. contraceptive precautions.
2. antiemetics.
3. analgesics.
4. antidiarrheals.

10. A client complains of small, red, pruritic dots between his fingers and toes. Based on the assessment data, the nurse recognizes that the client most likely has which condition?
1. Contusion
2. Herpes zoster
3. Scabies
4. Varicella

11. The home health care nurse is assessing a client. During the assessment, the client tells the nurse that the doctor has recently prescribed nystatin (Mycostatin). The nurse determines that further teaching is not necessary when the client states:
1. "I need to take the drug right after meals."
2. "I need to take the drug right before meals."
3. "I need to mix the drug with small amounts of food"
4. "I need to take half the dose before and half after meals."

12. A client is examined and found to have pinpoint, pink-to-purple, nonblanching macular lesions 1 to 3 mm in diameter. The nurse documents this assessment as:
1. ecchymosis.
2. hematoma.
3. petechiae.
4. purpura.

13. A client has a rash consisting of scattered lesions on various parts of the body. Based on the assessment, the nurse recognizes these lesions as being:
1. annular.
2. confluent.
3. diffuse.
4. linear.

What type of rash is this lesion suggesting?

9. **1.** Even small amounts of isotretinoin are associated with severe birth defects. Most female clients are also prescribed oral contraceptives. The other medications aren't necessary for a client on isotretinoin.

CN: Physiological integrity; CNS: Pharmacological and parenteral therapies; CL: Application

10. **3.** Scabies are seen as linear burrows between the fingers and toes caused by a mite. Contusions don't have small pruritic dots. The varicella zoster virus causes herpes zoster, characterized by papulovesicular lesions that erupt along a dermatome, usually with hyperesthesia, pain, and tenderness. The papulovesicular lesions of varicella are distributed over the trunk, face, and scalp and don't follow a dermatome.

CN: Physiological integrity; CNS: Physiological adaptation; CL: Application

11. **1.** Nystatin oral solution should be swished around the mouth after eating for the best contact with mucous membranes. Taking the drug before or with meals doesn't allow for the best contact with the mucous membranes.

CN: Physiological integrity; CNS: Pharmacological and parenteral therapies; CL: Application

12. **3.** Petechiae are small macular lesions 1 to 3 mm in diameter. Ecchymosis is a purple-to-brown bruise, macular or papular, and varied in size. A hematoma is a collection of blood from ruptured blood vessels more than 1 cm in diameter. Purpura is seen as purple macular lesions larger than 1 cm.

CN: Physiological integrity; CNS: Physiological adaptation; CL: Application

13. **3.** A diffuse rash usually has widely distributed scattered lesions. An annular rash is ring shaped. Confluent lesions are touching or adjacent to each other. Linear rashes are lesions arranged in a line.

CN: Physiological integrity; CNS: Physiological adaptation; CL: Application

14. A nurse is assessing a client recently admitted to the hospital and observes hair loss in small round circles on the client's scalp. The nurse documents this assessment finding as:
1. alopecia.
2. amblyopia.
3. exotropia.
4. seborrhea.

15. A client is diagnosed with atopic dermatitis. He is upset and asks how to avoid another outbreak. The nurse determines that the client needs information regarding:
1. avoiding bacterial infections.
2. avoiding fungal infections.
3. hereditary factors.
4. avoiding viral infections.

16. A client has rough papules on the soles of his feet that are sometimes painful when he walks. The nurse suspects that the client has:
1. filiform warts.
2. flat warts.
3. plantar warts.
4. venereal warts.

17. A client has recently been diagnosed with tinea corporis. The nurse would document this assessment finding as:
1. a fungal infection of the skin.
2. a group of small, red, papular lesions.
3. a flat, scaling papular lesion with raised borders.
4. itching and sweating of the feet accompanied by a foul odor.

18. The nurse is caring for a client who has thick, discolored nails that have "ice pick" pits and ridges and splintered hemorrhages and that easily separate from the nail bed. The nurse explains to the client that these findings are associated with which condition?
1. Paronychia
2. Psoriasis
3. Seborrhea
4. Scabies

14. 1. Alopecia is the correct term for thinning hair loss. Exotropia and amblyopia are eye disorders. Seborrhea is a chronic inflammatory dermatitis.

CN: Physiological integrity; CNS: Physiological adaptation; CL: Application

15. 3. Atopic dermatitis is a hereditary disorder associated with a family history of asthma, allergic rhinitis, or atopic dermatitis. Atopic dermatitis isn't a bacterial, fungal, or viral infection.

CN: Physiological integrity; CNS: Physiological adaptation; CL: Application

16. 3. Plantar warts are rough papules commonly found on the soles of the feet. Filiform warts are long, spiny projections from the skin surface. Flat warts are flat-topped, smooth-surfaced lesions. Venereal warts appear on the genital mucosa and are confluent papules with rough surfaces.

CN: Physiological integrity; CNS: Physiological adaptation; CL: Application

17. 3. Tinea corporis, or ringworm, is a flat, scaling papular lesion with raised borders. Candidiasis is a fungal infection of the skin or mucous membranes commonly found in the oral, vaginal, and intestinal mucosal tissue. Molluscum contagiosum is a viral skin infection with small, red, papular lesions. Tinea pedis is a superficial fungal infection on the feet, commonly called athletes' foot, that causes itching and sweating and a foul odor.

CN: Physiological integrity; CNS: Physiological adaptation; CL: Application

18. 2. Psoriasis, a chronic skin disorder with an unknown cause, shows these characteristic skin changes. A paronychia is a bacterial infection of the nail bed. Seborrhea is a chronic inflammatory dermatitis known as cradle cap. Scabies are mites that burrow under the skin, generally between the webbing of the fingers and toes.

CN: Physiological integrity; CNS: Physiological adaptation; CL: Application

19. A client found unconscious at home is brought to the emergency department. Physical examination shows cherry-red mucous membranes, nail beds, and skin. The nurse interprets these findings as indicating which of the following?
1. Spider bite
2. Aspirin ingestion
3. Hydrocarbon ingestion
4. Carbon monoxide poisoning

20. A client is diagnosed with a fungal infection of the scalp. The nurse would document this as:
1. tinea capitis.
2. tinea corporis.
3. tinea cruris.
4. tinea pedis.

21. The client has been diagnosed with secondary syphilis. Which is an appropriate assessment for the nurse to enter into the client's record?
1. Chancre ulcers
2. No significant symptoms
3. Nodular, pustular, annular lesions
4. Destructive lesions involving many organs and tissues

22. An intubated client with full-thickness, circumferential burns to the chest is experiencing pressure from edema that is inhibiting chest wall expansion. The nurse anticipates that which of the following is the priority intervention for the client?
1. Cricothyrotomy
2. Escharotomy
3. Needle thoracentesis
4. Insertion of a chest tube

23. A client has just arrived at the emergency department after sustaining a major burn injury. During the first 8 hours after the injury, the nurse will assess the client for which of the following?
1. Hyponatremia and hypokalemia
2. Hyponatremia and hyperkalemia
3. Hypernatremia and hypokalemia
4. Hypernatremia and hyperkalemia

Color can be a classic sign of some conditions.

19. 4. Cherry-red skin indicates exposure to high levels of carbon monoxide. Spider bite reactions are usually localized to the area of the bite. Nausea and vomiting and pale skin are symptoms of aspirin ingestion. Hydrocarbon or petroleum ingestion usually causes respiratory symptoms and tachycardia.
CN: Physiological integrity; CNS: Physiological adaptation; CL: Analysis

20. 1. Tinea capitis is a fungal infection of the scalp. Tinea corporis describes fungal infections of the body. Tinea cruris describes fungal infections of the inner thigh and inguinal creases, and tinea pedis is the term for fungal infections of the foot.
CN: Physiological integrity; CNS: Physiological adaptation; CL: Application

21. 3. Nodular, pustular, annular lesions and generalized lymphadenopathy occur in secondary syphilis. The chancre, a painless, shallow ulcer, develops in primary syphilis and appears 3 weeks after exposure. The latent phase occurs between the secondary and tertiary stages. Tertiary syphilis has destructive lesions involving many organs and tissues.
CN: Physiological integrity; CNS: Physiological adaptation; CL: Application

22. 2. Escharotomy is a surgical incision used to relieve pressure from edema. It's needed with circumferential burns that prevent chest expansion or circulatory compromise. Cricothyrotomy is an emergency procedure that involves puncturing the trachea through the cricothyroid membrane to create an airway. This client is already intubated. Needle thoracentesis and insertion of a chest tube are performed to relieve a pneumothorax.
CN: Physiological integrity; CNS: Physiological adaptation; CL: Analysis

23. 2. During the first 48 hours after a burn, capillary permeability increases, allowing fluids to shift from the plasma to the interstitial spaces. This fluid is high in sodium, causing a decrease in serum sodium levels. Potassium also leaks from the cells into the plasma, causing hyperkalemia.
CN: Physiological integrity; CNS: Physiological adaptation; CL: Analysis

24. A client has just been admitted to the hospital after sustaining partial-thickness burns to both lower extremities and portions of the trunk. The nurse is aware that the most important I.V. fluid to administer is:
1. albumin.
2. dextrose 5% in water.
3. lactated Ringer's solution.
4. normal saline solution with 2 mEq of potassium per 100 ml.

25. The nurse is preparing a plan of care for a client requiring a dressing change. What is the most important nursing intervention?
1. Write the order in the client's care plan.
2. Put a sign above the head of the client's bed.
3. Tell the nurse about the treatment in the report.
4. Document the dressing change in the narrative note.

26. What is the most appropriate nursing diagnosis for a client with a reddened sacrum unrelieved by position change?
1. Sedentary lifestyle
2. Risk for impaired skin integrity
3. Noncompliance
4. Impaired skin integrity

27. The client has sustained the initial phase of a burn injury. The nurse anticipates that the primary focus of the client's care is:
1. enhancing self-esteem.
2. promoting hygiene.
3. reducing anxiety.
4. preventing infection.

28. The home health nurse assesses four clients. The nurse determines that which client is at highest risk for <u>impaired</u> wound healing after surgery?
1. A 65-year-old client with hypertension
2. A 60-year-old client who's slightly overweight
3. A 78-year-old client in general good health
4. A 75-year-old client with poorly controlled diabetes mellitus

You're doing great!

Preventing infection is always a priority.

24. **3.** Lactated Ringer's solution replaces lost sodium and corrects metabolic acidosis, both of which commonly occur following a burn. Albumin is used as adjunct therapy, not primary fluid replacement. Dextrose isn't given to burn clients during the first 24 hours because it can cause pseudodiabetes. The client is hyperkalemic from the potassium shift from the intracellular space to the plasma, so potassium would be detrimental.
CN: Physiological integrity; CNS: Pharmacological and parenteral therapies; CL: Application

25. **1.** Writing the order in the client's care plan notifies everyone of the treatment. Posting a sign above the head of the bed is a good reminder but doesn't ensure that the treatment will be performed. Verbally reporting to the nurse on the upcoming shift doesn't ensure the dressing change will be done. Although the intervention should be documented in the narrative note, this doesn't guarantee that the next nurse will do the treatment.
CN: Safe, effective care environment; CNS: Management of care; CL: Application

26. **4.** This client has an actual—not potential—skin impairment. There isn't enough information to indicate a sedentary lifestyle or noncompliance.
CN: Physiological integrity; CNS: Basic care and comfort; CL: Application

27. **4.** Because the body's protective barrier is damaged and the immune system is compromised, preventing infection is the primary goal. Enhancing self-esteem, promoting hygiene, and reducing anxiety are important but aren't the primary focus.
CN: Physiological integrity; CNS: Physiological adaptation; CL: Application

28. **4.** Poorly controlled diabetes is a serious risk factor for impaired wound healing. Other factors that delay wound healing include advanced age, inadequate blood supply, nutritional deficiencies, and obesity.
CN: Physiological integrity; CNS: Physiological adaptation; CL: Analysis

29. The charge nurse is instructing a new graduate nurse on the procedure of obtaining a wound culture for a client with a suspected infection. The nurse determines that teaching has been effective when the graduate nurse states:
1. "Thoroughly irrigate the wound before collecting the culture."
2. "Use a sterile swab to wipe the crusty area around the outside of the wound."
3. "Gently roll a sterile swab from the center of the wound outward to collect drainage."
4. "Use one sterile swab to collect drainage from several possible infected sites along the incision."

30. The nurse is assessing a client with an abdominal incision and suspects there is a potential for <u>delayed</u> wound healing. Which assessment data that would validate this suspicion?
1. Sutures dry and intact
2. Wound edges in close approximation
3. Purulent drainage on soiled wound dressing
4. Sanguineous drainage in wound collection drainage bag

31. A nurse is instructing a nursing assistant on the procedure of changing bed linens. The nursing assistant asks the nurse what to do if the linens are soiled with drainage from a pressure ulcer. What is the most appropriate response by the nurse?
1. "You will need to use a mask."
2. "You will need to use clean gloves."
3. "You will need to use sterile gloves."
4. "You will need to use shoe protectors."

32. The nurse is caring for a bedridden older adult. What is the most important nursing intervention?
1. Slide instead of lift the client when turning.
2. Turn and reposition the client at least every 8 hours.
3. Apply lotion after bathing the client and vigorously massage the skin.
4. Post a turning schedule at the client's bedside and adapt position changes to the client's situation.

33. A client has recently had a skin graft. What is the <u>most important</u> instruction for the nurse to give the client?
1. Continue physical therapy.
2. Protect the graft from direct sunlight.
3. Use cosmetic camouflage techniques.
4. Apply lubricating lotion to the graft site.

Always take the necessary protective measures.

29. 3. Rolling a swab from the center outward is the right way to culture a wound. Irrigating the wound washes away drainage, debris, and many of the microorganisms colonizing or infecting the wound. The outside of the wound may be colonized with microorganisms from this wound or another wound or with the normal microorganisms on the client's skin. These may grow in culture and confuse the interpretation of results. All sources of drainage in an incision or surgical wound may not be infected or may be infected with different microorganisms, so each swab should be used on only one site.

CN: Safe, effective care environment; CNS: Safety and infection control; CL: Application

30. 3. Purulent drainage contains white blood cells, which fight infection, and indicates possible delay in wound healing. The sutures from a wound draining purulent secretions would pull away with an infection. Wound edges can't approximate with an infection in the wound. Sanguineous drainage indicates bleeding, not infection.

CN: Physiological integrity; CNS: Physiological adaptation; CL: Analysis

31. 2. Clean gloves protect the hands and wrists from microorganisms in the linens. Sterile gloves allow one to touch a sterile object or area without contaminating it. A mask protects the wearer and client from droplet nuclei and large-particle aerosols. Shoe protectors prevent static and microorganism transmission from the floor of one room to another.

CN: Safe, effective care environment; CNS: Safety and infection control; CL: Analysis

32. 4. A turning schedule with a signing sheet will make sure the client gets turned. When moving a client, lift, rather than slide, the client to avoid shearing. A client in bed for prolonged periods should be turned every 1 to 2 hours. Apply lotion to keep the skin moist, but avoid vigorous massage to avoid damaging capillaries.

CN: Physiological integrity; CNS: Basic care and comfort; CL: Analysis

33. 2. To avoid burning and sloughing, the client must protect the graft from direct sunlight. The other three interventions are all helpful to the client and his recovery.

CN: Physiological integrity; CNS: Physiological adaptation; CL: Analysis

34. The nurse is teaching the client how to prevent development of basal cell epithelioma. What is the priority instruction for the nurse to give the client?
1. Avoid burns.
2. Avoid exposure to the sun.
3. Avoid immunosuppression.
4. Avoid exposure to radiation.

35. The nurse is assessing an older client's skin turgor and finds inelasticity present. The nurse interprets this assessment as indicating:
1. overhydration.
2. normal skin turgor.
3. a normal part of the aging process.
4. dehydration.

36. A client has a stage II sacral pressure ulcer that is being treated with a transparent film dressing. The nurse is aware that:
1. the dressing maintains a moist environment for the wound.
2. the dressing is allowed to dry out before removal.
3. a gauze dressing covers the transparent film dressing.
4. the transparent film dressing should be tightly packed into the wound.

37. A 19-year-old client presents with second-degree sunburn on her face and both arms. What is the initial intervention by the nurse?
1. Administer analgesic medication as ordered.
2. Apply cold, moist towels to the burns.
3. Apply sterile, dry towels to the burns.
4. Apply vitamin A, D, and E ointment to the burns.

38. A client received burns to his entire back and left arm. The nurse uses the Rule of Nines to calculate that he has sustained burns to what percentage of his body?
1. 9%
2. 18%
3. 27%
4. 36%

39. The nurse is performing a sterile dressing change. What is the most important intervention by the nurse?
1. Change the sterile field after sterile water is spilled on it.
2. Put on sterile gloves; then open a container of sterile saline.
3. Place a sterile dressing ½″ (1.3 cm) from the edge of the sterile field.
4. Clean the wound with a circular motion, moving from outer circles toward the center.

34. 2. The sun is the best-known and most common cause of basal cell epithelioma. Burns, immunosuppression, and radiation are less common causes.
CN: Physiological integrity; CNS: Reduction of risk potential; CL: Application

35. 3. Inelastic skin turgor is a normal part of aging. Overhydration causes the skin to appear edematous and spongy. Normal skin turgor is dry and firm. Dehydration causes inelastic skin with tenting.
CN: Health promotion and maintenance; CNS: None; CL: Application

36. 1. A transparent film dressing keeps the wound moist and enhances autolysis of necrotic tissue. There's no need to cover the transparent film dressing with a gauze dressing. The dressing should never be allowed to dry or be packed into the wound.
CN: Physiological integrity; CNS: Physiological adaptation; CL: Analysis

37. 2. Cold, moist towels help stop the burning process. Analgesics should be administered as ordered after the burning process has been controlled. Dry towels would retain the heat and aren't used. Ointments are applied during the healing phase but not initially.
CN: Physiological integrity; CNS: Basic care and comfort; CL: Application

38. 3. According to the Rule of Nines, the posterior trunk, anterior trunk, and legs are each 18% of the total body surface. The head, neck, and arms are each 9% of total body surface, and the perineum is 1%. In this case, the client received burns to his back (18%) and one arm (9%), totaling 27% of his body.
CN: Physiological integrity; CNS: Reduction of risk potential; CL: Application

39. 1. A sterile field is considered contaminated when it becomes wet. Moisture can act as a wick, allowing microorganisms to contaminate the field. The outside of containers such as sterile saline bottles aren't sterile. The containers should be opened before sterile gloves are put on, and the solution poured over the sterile dressings placed in a sterile basin. The outer inch of a sterile field isn't considered sterile. Wounds should be cleaned from the most contaminated area to the least contaminated area, for example, from the center outward.
CN: Safe, effective care environment; CNS: Safety and infection control; CL: Application

40. The client has sustained a burn wound. What is the most important intervention by the nurse to decrease hypertrophied scarring during later stages of healing?
1. Remove all tissue in the wound area.
2. Apply continuous pressure using elastic wraps.
3. Wear clothing to protect the burn from the sun.
4. Maintain wound dressing changes.

41. The nurse is providing instructions to a family who will be caring for a bed-bound client who is going home. The nurse determines that teaching was effective when the family members state the need to avoid the use of a:
1. waterbed.
2. ring or donut.
3. gel flotation pad.
4. polyurethane foam mattress.

42. A postoperative client signals the nurse and states, "I felt something pop." The nurse enters the room and notes a wound evisceration. What is the most important action by the nurse?
1. Give prophylactic antibiotics as ordered.
2. Place the client on nothing-by-mouth (NPO) status.
3. Explain to the client what's happening and give support.
4. Cover the protruding internal organs with sterile gauze moistened with sterile saline.

43. The nurse is teaching a client's family the procedure for a dressing change they will do when the client is discharged. What is the most important action for the nurse to tell the client's family that they should do <u>first</u>?
1. Put on gloves.
2. Wash hands thoroughly.
3. Slowly remove the soiled dressing.
4. Observe the dressing for the amount, type, and odor of drainage.

44. The nurse is teaching a class of unlicensed assistive personnel (UAP) about the importance of mobility and turning clients. A UAP ask the nurse how often a client who is confined to bed should be turned. What is the best response by the nurse?
1. "Turn every half hour."
2. "Turn every 1 to 2 hours."
3. "Turn once every 8 hours."
4. "Keep the client on his back as much as possible."

You're doing very well. The remaining questions should be a snap.

I should know better than to indulge.

Prioritize!

40. 2. Using elastic wraps and bandages to apply continuous pressure during the early stages of wound healing can help prevent keloid scar formation. Removing tissue, especially eschar, promotes wound healing as do dressing changes, but neither directly decreases scar formation. Wearing clothing prevents sunburn but doesn't decrease scar formation.
CN: Physiological integrity; CNS: Physiological adaptation; CL: Application

41. 2. Rings or donuts shouldn't be used because they restrict circulation. The waterbed distributes pressure over the entire surface. Gel pads give with weight. Foam mattresses distribute pressure evenly.
CN: Physiological integrity; CNS: Reduction of risk potential; CL: Application

42. 4. Covering the wound with moistened gauze is the priority to prevent the organs from drying. Both the gauze and the saline must be sterile to reduce the risk of infection. Because evisceration usually requires emergency surgery, the nurse should place the client on NPO status. Evisceration is a frightening situation for any client. While the nurse works quickly to get the client treated, she can provide support to reduce the client's anxiety. Antibiotics will usually be ordered and should be started as soon as possible.
CN: Physiological integrity; CNS: Physiological adaptation; CL: Analysis

43. 2. The first thing that someone who is changing a dressing must do is wash their hands. Putting on gloves, removing the dressing, and observing the drainage are all parts of the procedure for a dressing change.
CN: Safe, effective care environment; CNS: Management of care; CL: Application

44. 2. Turning the client every 1 to 2 hours will prevent pressure areas from developing and help prevent atelectasis and other pulmonary complications. Turning every half hour is too frequent, and turning every 8 hours would make the client vulnerable to the development of complications. The client should spend time on his back according to the turning schedule. During that period, the head of the bed should be raised to prevent the client from aspirating.
CN: Physiological integrity; CNS: Basic care and comfort; CL: Application

45. What is the <u>most important</u> information for the nurse to teach a client about hypersensitivity skin test results?
1. Wash the sites daily with a mild soap.
2. Have the sites read on the correct date.
3. Keep the skin test areas moist with a mild lotion.
4. Stay out of direct sunlight until the tests are read.

46. The nurse is reviewing lab results of a client diagnosed with disseminated herpes zoster who is receiving hydrocortisone (Solu-Cortef). Which laboratory value does the nurse anticipate will be elevated?
1. Calcium
2. Glucose
3. Magnesium
4. Potassium

47. A client has been admitted to the burn unit with extensive full-thickness burns. What is the nurse's <u>priority</u> in implementing the treatment plan for the client?
1. Fluid status
2. Body image
3. Level of pain
4. Risk of infection

48. A nurse is performing a skin assessment on a recently admitted client. The nurse analyzes the assessment findings and determines that which is the most important risk factor?
1. Family history of pressure ulcers
2. Presence of existing pressure ulcers
3. Overall risk of developing pressure ulcers
4. Potential areas of pressure ulcer development

49. A client with extensive burns has a new donor site. What is the most important intervention by the nurse?
1. Make the site dependent.
2. Avoid pressure on the site.
3. Keep the site fully covered.
4. Allow ventilation of the site.

50. A client has been diagnosed with late-stage Lyme disease. The nurse anticipates that the client may exhibit which of the following?
1. Arthritis
2. Lung abscess
3. Renal failure
4. Sterility

It's most important that you read this question carefully.

You're almost at question 50, and you're doing OK. Does that take some of the pressure off?

45. 2. An important facet of evaluating skin tests is to read the skin test results at the proper time. Evaluating the skin test too late or too early will give inaccurate and unreliable results. Both the gauze and the saline must be sterile to reduce the risk of infection. There's no need to wash the sites with soap. The sites should be kept dry. Direct sunlight isn't prohibited.
CN: Health promotion and maintenance; CNS: None; CL: Application

46. 2. Corticosteroids increase blood sugar and tend to lower serum potassium and calcium levels. Their effect on magnesium isn't substantial.
CN: Physiological integrity; CNS: Pharmacological and parenteral therapies; CL: Analysis

47. 1. In early burn care, the client's greatest need is fluid resuscitation because of large-volume fluid loss through the damaged skin. Body image, pain, and infection are important concerns in the nursing care of a burn client but don't take precedence over fluid management in the early phase of burn care.
CN: Safe, effective care environment; CNS: Management of care; CL: Analysis

48. 2. Areas of existing pressure ulcers need immediate treatment and therefore are the most important. Family history of pressure ulcers isn't a risk factor for the development of pressure ulcers. Overall risk and potential areas of pressure development are important in planning care but don't take priority.
CN: Safe, effective care environment; CNS: Management of care; CL: Analysis

49. 2. A universal concern in the care of donor sites for burn care is to keep the site away from sources of pressure. Placing the site in a position of dependence isn't a justified aspect of donor site care. Ventilation of the site and keeping the site fully covered are practices in some institutions but aren't hallmarks of donor site care.
CN: Physiological integrity; CNS: Physiological adaptation; CL: Application

50. 1. If Lyme disease goes untreated, arthritis, neurological problems, and cardiac abnormalities may arise as late complications. Lung abscess, renal failure, and sterility aren't complications of Lyme disease.
CN: Physiological integrity; CNS: Physiological adaptation; CL: Application

51. A client is admitted with suspected malignant melanoma on his left shoulder. During the physical assessment, the nurse would anticipate observing:
1. a brown birthmark that has lightened in color.
2. a brown or black mole with red, white, or blue areas.
3. petechiae.
4. a red birthmark that has recently become darker.

52. A nurse educator is teaching a group of clients about hygiene. Which statement by a client indicates the need for further teaching?
1. "The skin absorbs fluids."
2. "The skin serves as the body's first line of defense."
3. "The skin excretes waste products."
4. "The skin changes vitamin D to a form the body can use."

53. The nurse is teaching a client how to care for his skin. The nurse determines that the client understands teaching about sebum when the client makes which statement?
1. "It is the most superficial layer of the skin."
2. "It is the oil secreted by the skin."
3. "It is a pouch-like depression from which a hair grows."
4. "It is the deepest layer of the skin."

54. The nurse is planning care for a client with a late-stage burn wound to promote healing. What is the most important intervention for the nurse to include?
1. Removing eschar from the skin
2. Applying continuous-compression wraps
3. Wearing clothing to protect the burn from the sun
4. Maintaining wound care irrigation

55. A client has an inflamed area on the right forearm that's causing considerable discomfort. The nurse would anticipate the physician to prescribe which measure?
1. Warm, moist compresses
2. An elastic bandage
3. Hydrocortisone cream
4. Nonadherent dressing

56. An elderly client has a sore on the inside of his ankle that he says won't heal. After noting varicosities and coarse discoloration around the sore, the nurse should suspect which condition?
1. Acute venous insufficiency
2. Chronic venous insufficiency
3. Acute arterial occlusive disease
4. Chronic arterial occlusive disease

Why is everyone always trying to change me?

With your knowledge of burns, this question should take minimal effort.

You've answered 55 questions! Hang in there!

51. **2.** Melanomas have an irregular shape and lack uniformity in color. They may appear brown or black with red, white, or blue areas. Melanoma lesions don't appear as petechiae or as birthmarks that have changed color.
CN: Health promotion and maintenance; CNS: None; CL: Application

52. **4.** The skin doesn't change vitamin D to a form the body can use. (The sun helps to convert vitamin D.) The skin absorbs fluids, serves as the body's first line of defense, and excretes waste products.
CN: Physiological integrity; CNS: Physiological adaptation; CL: Analysis

53. **2.** Sebum is the oil secreted by the skin. The epidermis and dermis are skin layers. A follicle is a pouch-like depression from which a hair grows.
CN: Physiological integrity; CNS: Physiological adaptation; CL: Application

54. **2.** Applying continuous-compression wraps aids skin healing and prevents hypertrophied tissue from forming. The other interventions are appropriate for the client with a burn wound but don't necessarily help minimize scarring.
CN: Physiological integrity; CNS: Reduction of risk potential; CL: Application

55. **1.** Warm, moist compresses increase circulation to the area, reducing discomfort and redness. An elastic bandage decompresses the area but doesn't ease inflammation. Hydrocortisone cream is useful on an inflamed area that itches. A nonadherent dressing doesn't relieve inflammation or pain.
CN: Physiological integrity; CNS: Basic care and comfort; CL: Application

56. **2.** Classic signs of chronic venous insufficiency include skin discoloration (from blood extravasation in subcutaneous tissue) and stasis ulcers, usually found on the ankle's medial aspect. Asymmetric moderate edema, normal pulses, and deep muscle pain relieved by elevation are signs of acute venous insufficiency. Acute or chronic arterial occlusive disease usually causes intermittent claudication and severe burning pain.
CN: Physiological integrity; CNS: Physiological adaptation; CL: Application

57. A nurse prepares a client for a shave biopsy of a skin lesion. What is the priority information for the nurse to include in the teaching plan?
1. How to care for the suture line
2. The need for a skin graft
3. The need for sedation
4. How to care for the dressing

58. The physician orders a wet-to-dry dressing for a client who has a pressure ulcer with infected, necrotic tissue. The nurse understands that the purpose of this dressing is:
1. to prevent extension of the infection.
2. to debride the wound.
3. to keep the wound moist.
4. to reduce pain.

59. A client has been receiving moist saline dressings to an open ulcer of the foot for 10 days. The nurse is assessing the current status of the wound and determines that treatment has been effective when the area appears as which of the following?
1. Red, swollen tissue
2. Dry, crusted scab
3. Deep, wide keloid
4. Warm, painful tissue

60. When changing a dressing on a pressure ulcer, a nurse notes necrotic wound tissue. Based on this assessment finding, the nurse anticipates that the physician will order which procedure?
1. Wound incision and drainage
2. Wound culturing
3. Wound debridement
4. Wound irrigation with an antiseptic

61. After a traumatic injury, a client's wound heals and a smooth, pink, thickened, rubbery lesion forms over the wound. The nurse interprets this assessment as indicating a(n):
1. erosion.
2. fissure.
3. keloid.
4. abscess.

62. A client is diagnosed with urticaria. How would the nurse describe this manifestation?
1. Elevated, firm circumscribed lesion in the dermis, 1 to 2 cm in diameter
2. Flat, nonpalpable, irregularly shaped lesion, more than 1 cm in diameter
3. Transient, elevated, solid, firm, irregularly shaped area of cutaneous edema, with a variable diameter
4. Elevated, circumscribed lesion in the dermis or subcutaneous layer, filled with liquid or semisolid material

Observe the time in a question of this type.

These questions aren't easy, but you've got a good handle on it.

57. 4. Dressing care should be included in the teaching plan. A shave biopsy removes only the first or second layer of skin, causing a superficial wound with no suture line and minimal scarring. There's no need for a skin graft or sedation with a shave biopsy.
CN: Physiological integrity; CNS: Physiological adaptation; CL: Application

58. 2. A wet-to-dry dressing placed over a necrotic area adheres to dead tissue and is debrided as the dressing is removed. Antibiotics, not dressings, help prevent extension of the infection. Keeping the wound moist would prevent the necessary debridement. The dressing has no analgesic effect.
CN: Physiological integrity; CNS: Physiological adaptation; CL: Application

59. 2. Ten days into healing, an ulcer should be at the end of the lag phase of healing, as indicated by a dry, crusted scab. Tissue is red, swollen, warm, or painful during the inflammatory phase, which occurs 2 to 7 days after the ulcer develops. A deep, wide keloid may appear 3 weeks to 2 years after ulcer development.
CN: Physiological integrity; CN: Physiological adaptation; CL: Application

60. 3. For healing to occur, necrotic (dead) tissue must be removed from the wound; usually, this is done by debridement. Wound incision and drainage and wound culturing are done when infection is present or suspected. Wound irrigation with an antiseptic may damage sensitive tissue and prevent healing.
CN: Physiological integrity; CNS: Physiological adaptation; CL: Application

61. 3. A keloid results from a defect in the healing process in which excess collagen develops at the healing site. Erosion refers to loss of part or all of the skin surface, usually from infection or pressure. A fissure is a slit in the wound. Abscess, which results from accumulation of purulent drainage, causes the wound to appear red, swollen, and tender.
CN: Physiological integrity; CNS: Physiological adaptation; CL: Analysis

62. 3. A wheal is a transient, elevated, firm lesion of irregular shape and size. A nodule is an elevated lesion in the dermis with a diameter of 1 to 2 cm. A patch is a flat lesion with a diameter exceeding 1 cm. A cyst is an elevated, circumscribed lesion filled with liquid or semisolid material.
CN: Physiological integrity; CNS: Physiological adaptation; CL: Application

63. A 70-year-old client who spilled hot coffee on his lap 3 days ago has multiple blisters. While the nurse is providing care for the client, two of the blisters break. What is the most appropriate action by the nurse?
1. Remove the raised skin because the blister has been compromised.
2. Wash the area vigorously with soap and water.
3. Apply alcohol to the area.
4. Clean the area with normal saline solution and cover it with a dressing.

64. A client undergoes cryosurgery to remove a cancerous skin lesion. The nurse determines that the treatment was effective when assessment of the client includes:
1. dry, itchy patches.
2. oozing and pain.
3. dryness, tenderness, and sutures.
4. swelling, blistering, and tenderness.

65. A client with facial lacerations requires hospitalization for 1 week. During assessment, the nurse notes scabs on the wounds. These assessment findings would be indicative of which phase of wound healing?
1. Contraction phase
2. Inflammatory phase
3. Proliferative phase
4. Remodeling phase

Know your assessment facts; they're critical in nursing and on the NCLEX.

66. An 85-year-old female client who has spent a great deal of time outdoors tells the home health nurse that her skin is dry and itchy. What is the most important information for the nurse to give the client?
1. "Soak in a bubble bath once per day."
2. "Bathe with antimicrobial soap once per day."
3. "Bathe with mild soap and water or with water only."
4. "Scrub the skin vigorously to remove dead skin cells."

Only four more questions to go. Whew!

67. The nurse is assessing a client who has a maculopapular rash on his trunk, which follows skin cleavage lines in a Christmas tree pattern. The client reports that the rash started as a small lesion 4 days ago. The nurse would document the findings as:
1. tinea corporis.
2. pityriasis rosea.
3. allergic reaction to a drug.
4. eczema.

63. 4. To maintain asepsis, the nurse should clean the area with normal saline solution and cover it with a dressing. Removing the raised skin would cause further skin damage. Washing the area vigorously with soap and water would damage the tissue and cause drying. Alcohol would dry out the tissue.
CN: Safe, effective care environment; CNS: Safety and infection control; CL: Application

64. 4. Cryosurgery leaves a wound resembling a burn, with swelling, blistering, and tenderness. Oozing and pain suggest an infection. The wound wouldn't be dry or itchy and wouldn't have sutures.
CN: Physiological integrity; CNS: Physiological adaptation; CL: Analysis

65. 3. During the proliferative phase of wound healing, which lasts from the 4th to 21st day after injury, granulation tissue appears (scabs form) and the wound edges start to pull together. Contraction, the third phase of wound healing, may begin around the 7th day and involves a significant decrease in the wound surface. The inflammatory phase, the first healing phase, immediately follows the injury and lasts 4 to 6 days; it involves control of bleeding and release of chemicals needed for healing. The remodeling phase, the final phase, may lead to scar flattening and correction of any deformities that occurred during the third phase.
CN: Physiological integrity; CNS: Basic care and comfort; CL: Analysis

66. 3. Bathing with mild soap and water or with water only can relieve skin itching and dryness. Bubble baths and antimicrobial soap can be very drying to an elderly person's sensitive skin. Scrubbing vigorously may worsen skin dryness.
CN: Physiological integrity; CNS: Basic care and comfort; CL: Application

67. 2. Pityriasis rosea starts with a "herald patch" and then erupts in a Christmas tree pattern on the trunk. Tinea corporis is a skin infestation, usually seen as fine lines under the skin. Allergic reactions to drugs typically affect the entire body. Eczema is an erythematous papular rash typically affecting the antecubital and popliteal fossae.
CN: Physiological integrity; CNS: Physiological adaptation; CL: Analysis

68. At an outpatient clinic, a medical assistant interviews a client and documents her findings as follows:

Progress notes	
12/13/10 0900	Client very anxious because new black mole with shades of brown noted on upper outer right thigh. Asymmetrical in shape with an irregular border. ——— *M. Rosenfeld, MA*

After reading the chart note, a nurse begins planning the client's care based on which nursing diagnosis?

1. Deficient knowledge related to potential diagnosis of basal cell carcinoma
2. Fear related to potential diagnosis of malignant melanoma
3. Risk for impaired skin integrity related to potential squamous cell carcinoma
4. Readiness for enhanced knowledge: Skin care precautions related to benign mole

69. The nurse is examining the back of a client and notes a rash with a discrete lesion configuration. Which graphic shows a discrete lesion configuration?

Hooray! You've finished Part II. I see your future success in Part III.

68. 2. Documentation reveals that the client is anxious about her symptoms. These symptoms (asymmetry, variable color, and border irregularity) most closely resemble malignant melanoma. The nursing note contains no indication that the client currently has deficient knowledge. The characteristics of the lesion aren't consistent with basal or squamous cell carcinoma or a benign nevus (mole).

CN: Physiological integrity; CNS: Physiological adaptation; CL: Analysis

69. 1. In a discrete pattern, individual lesions are separate and distinct. Option 2 shows a grouped pattern, in which lesions are clustered together. Option 3 is a confluent pattern. In this configuration, lesions merge so that individual lesions aren't visible or palpable. Option 4 is a linear pattern, in which lesions form a line.

CN: Physiological integrity; CNS: Physiological adaptation; CL: Analysis

Part III

Care of the psychiatric client

Before you take the tests relating to psychiatric care, take this test relating to tests (and treatments, too) in psychiatric care.

Chapter 12
Essentials of psychiatric care

1. The preceptor is teaching a graduate nurse about electroconvulsive therapy (ECT). The preceptor determines that further teaching is not needed when the graduate nurse makes which statement?
1. ECT is used to treat clients with major depression.
2. ECT is used to treat antisocial personality disorder.
3. ECT is used to treat clients diagnosed with schizophrenia.
4. ECT is used to treat clients diagnosed with somatoform disorders.

2. A client diagnosed with bipolar disorder becomes verbally aggressive during group therapy. The client states "I hate all of you." What is the <u>most appropriate</u> response by the nurse?
1. "You're behaving in an unacceptable manner."
2. "If you continue to talk like that, I will dismiss you from the group."
3. "Other people are not comfortable with your statement, please stop it."
4. "You're frightening the group; let's walk down the hall to release some energy."

3. A client is demonstrating hostility toward the nursing staff he just met. The nurse interprets the behavior as:
1. intellectualization.
2. transference.
3. triangulation.
4. splitting.

All of these options might be acceptable, but which is *most* appropriate?

1. 1. ECT is most commonly used for the treatment of major depression in clients who haven't responded to antidepressants or who have medical problems that contraindicate the use of antidepressants. ECT isn't commonly used for treatment of personality disorders. ECT doesn't appear to be of value to individuals with chronic schizophrenia and isn't the treatment of choice for clients with somatoform disorders.
CN: Psychosocial integrity; CNS: None; CL: Application

2. 4. This response informs the client that, although the behavior is unacceptable, the client is still worthy of help. The other responses are nontherapeutic and blaming.
CN: Safe, effective care environment; CNS: Management of care; CL: Application

3. 2. Transference is the unconscious assignment of negative or positive feelings evoked by a significant person in the client's past to another person. Intellectualization is a defense mechanism in which the client avoids dealing with emotions by focusing on facts. Triangulation refers to conflicts involving three family members. Splitting is a defense mechanism commonly seen in clients with personality disorders in which the world is perceived as all good or all bad.
CN: Psychosocial integrity; CNS: None; CL: Analysis

4. The nurse is aware that cognitive-behavioral therapy is most appropriate for a client who is experiencing low self-esteem. What is the best intervention for the nurse to use for facilitation of this therapy?
1. Conditional positive regard
2. Analysis of free association
3. Classical conditioning
4. Examination of negative thought patterns

5. A client in group therapy states, "I didn't think anyone else felt like I did as a child." The nurse interprets this statement as:
1. altruism.
2. universality.
3. catharsis.
4. existential factor.

The 11 curative factors of who??

6. The nurse is teaching a group of students about the benefits of using group psychotherapy. Which statement best describes the rationale for group psychotherapy?
1. It decreases the focus on the individual.
2. It fosters the physician–client relationship.
3. It confronts the individuals with their shortcomings.
4. It fosters a new learning environment.

Sometimes it helps to know you aren't alone.

7. A client whose wife recently died in an automobile accident is now being treated at the outpatient psychiatric clinic. The nurse anticipates that the most effective treatment would be?
1. Electroconvulsive therapy
2. Group therapy
3. Hypnotherapy
4. Individual therapy

4. 4. Popular cognitive-behavioral approaches examine the validity of habitual patterns of thinking and belief systems that influence feelings and behaviors. "Unconditional positive regard" is a phrase from Carl Rogers's client-centered therapy and describes a supportive, nonjudgmental, neutral approach by a therapist. Analysis of free associations is characteristic of Freudian psychoanalysis. Classical conditioning is characteristic of a pure behavioral intervention.
CN: Psychosocial integrity; CNS: None; CL: Application

5. 2. One of the 11 curative factors of group therapy identified by Yalom is universality, which assists group participants in recognizing common experiences and responses. This action helps reduce anxiety and allows other group members to provide support and understanding. Altruism, catharsis, and existential factors are other curative factors Yalom described, but they don't describe this particular incident. Altruism refers to finding meaning through helping others; catharsis is an open expression of previously suppressed feelings; and existential factors describe the recognition that one has control over the quality of one's life.
CN: Psychosocial integrity; CNS: None; CL: Application

6. 4. In a group, the individual has the opportunity to learn that others have the same problems and needs. The group can also provide an arena where new methods of relating to others can be tried. Decreasing focus on the individual isn't a key advantage (and sometimes isn't an advantage at all). Groups don't, by themselves, foster the physician–client relationship, and they aren't always used to confront individuals.
CN: Psychosocial integrity; CNS: None; CL: Analysis

7. 2. The client history suggests he is experiencing complicated mourning. Group therapy has been shown to be effective with this condition.
CN: Psychosocial integrity; CNS: None; CL: Application

8. An adolescent client verbalizes to the nurse about being fat and ugly and states, "Everybody makes fun of me." The nurse interprets this statement as:
1. anxiety of the unknown.
2. anxiety related to loss of respect.
3. anxiety related to separation anxiety.
4. anxiety related to change in body image.

9. The nurse is assessing a client who recently lost his spouse. The nurse determines that the client is experiencing the normal grief response when the:
1. client uses chemicals.
2. client becomes an overachiever.
3. client demonstrates hyperactivity.
4. client demonstrates lack of warmth toward others.

10. The nurse observes two clients playing basketball during exercise activity. The clients are engaged in aggressive communication and begin to fight. What is the most appropriate nursing intervention?
1. Remove the clients to separate areas and set limits.
2. Remind the clients that fighting is not allowed.
3. Show the clients how they should play basketball.
4. Obtain an order to place both clients in seclusion.

11. A client is prescribed sertraline (Zoloft). It is most important for the nurse to provide information to the client about which adverse effects? Select all that apply.
1. Agitation
2. Agranulocytosis
3. Sleep disturbance
4. Intermittent tachycardia
5. Dry mouth
6. Seizures

In psychiatric care, the nurse needs to recognize clues.

8. 4. Anxiety about body image and changes in physical appearance is a common fear of adolescents. Fear of the unknown is associated with toddlerhood. Fear of loss of respect, love, and emerging self-esteem is associated with the school-age developmental phase. Anxiety related to guilt is also associated with the school-age developmental phase.
CN: Psychosocial integrity; CNS: None; CL: Application

9. 4. Hostile reactions, such as loss of warmth when interacting with others, occur during normal grieving. Chemical use, overachieving, and hyperactivity commonly correlate with complicated grieving.
CN: Psychosocial integrity; CNS: None; CL: Application

10. 1. Setting limits and removing the clients from the situation is the best way to handle aggression. Reminders of appropriate behavior aren't likely to be effective at this time, and seclusion and restraints are reserved for more serious situations. It is inappropriate behavior for the nurse to participate in the game at this time.
CN: Psychosocial integrity; CNS: None; CL: Application

11. 1, 3, and 5. Common adverse effects of sertraline include agitation, sleep disturbance, and dry mouth. Agranulocytosis, intermittent tachycardia, and seizures are adverse effects of clozapine (Clozaril).
CN: Physiological integrity; CNS: Pharmacological and parenteral therapies; CL: Application

12. The nurse is preparing discharge instructions for a client who will be taking lithium that has been prescribed for bipolar disorder. What is the most important information for the nurse to give the client? Select all that apply.
1. The potential for addiction
2. Signs and symptoms of drug toxicity
3. The potential for tardive dyskinesia
4. A low-tyramine diet
5. The need to consistently monitor blood levels
6. The expected time frame for noticing improvements in mood

12. 2, 5, and 6. Client education should cover the signs and symptoms of drug toxicity as well as the need to report them to the physician. The client should be instructed to monitor his lithium levels on a regular basis to avoid toxicity. The nurse should explain that 7 to 21 days may pass before the client notes a change in his mood. Lithium doesn't have addictive properties. Tardive dyskinesia isn't associated with lithium. Tyramine is a potential concern for clients taking monoamine oxidase inhibitors.

CN: Physiological integrity; CNS: Pharmacological and parenteral therapies; CL: Application

13. A nurse is administering haloperidol (Haldol) to a client experiencing psychosis. What are the most appropriate nursing interventions? Select all that apply.
1. Review subcutaneous objectives.
2. Closely monitor vital signs, especially temperature.
3. Provide the client the opportunity to pace.
4. Monitor blood glucose levels.
5. Provide the client with hard candy.
6. Monitor for signs and symptoms of urticaria.

13. 2, 3, and 5. Neuroleptic malignant syndrome is a life-threatening adverse effect of antipsychotic medications such as haloperidol. It's associated with a rapid increase in temperature. The most common extrapyramidal adverse effect, akathisia, is a form of psychomotor restlessness that can typically be relieved by pacing. Haloperidol and the anticholinergic medications that are provided to alleviate its extrapyramidal effects can result in a dry mouth. Providing the client with hard candy to suck on can help with this problem. Haloperidol isn't given subcutaneously and doesn't affect blood glucose levels. Urticaria isn't usually associated with haloperidol administration.

CN: Physiological integrity; CNS: Pharmacological and parenteral therapies; CL: Analysis

14. A nurse is caring for an adolescent who lost her best friend in a car accident. The driver was under the influence of alcohol. The adolescent says, "It can't be possible. It is not true." The nurse interprets that the adolescent is in what stage of the Kübler-Ross grieving process?
1. Denial
2. Anger
3. Bargaining
4. Acceptance

14. 1. Denial is when the individual has difficulty believing the loss occurred. The client's statements do not reflect anger, bargaining, or acceptance of the loss.

CN: Psychosocial integrity; CNS: None; CL: Application

Here's to you! You've just zipped through another important NCLEX topic.

Can't remember much about a particular somatoform disorder? Type this address into your Web browser: **www.emedicine.com**. Then search for the disorder.

Chapter 13
Somatoform & sleep disorders

I hope I stay awake long enough to finish these questions.

1. The nurse is teaching a student nurse about somatoform disorders. Which of the following statements by the nurse would be the most accurate in describing somatoform disorders?
1. Individuals experience physical symptoms without an organic cause.
2. Individuals attend psychotherapy sessions.
3. Individuals are considered to be hypochondriacs.
4. Individuals are frustrated about the inability to find the source of their symptoms.

2. The nurse is preparing a teaching plan for a family who has a member diagnosed with a somatoform disorder. The most important information for the nurse to provide would be that these disorders:
1. are limited to one organ system.
2. occur with a recent physical illness.
3. are physical conditions with organic pathological causes.
4. occur in the absence of organic findings.

3. A nurse and senior nursing student are caring for a client with somatoform disorders. The student tells the nurse that associated physical symptoms occur because the client is delusional. What is the best response by the nurse?
1. "Physical symptoms are associated with psychological symptoms."
2. "Tell me more about your rationale."
3. "Let's review the symptoms of delusion."
4. "Tell me more about the symptoms of somatoform disorder."

1. 1. A client with a somatization disorder has a history of multiple physiological complaints without associated demonstrable organic pathological causes. The etiology of the disease takes priority.
CN: Health promotion and maintenance; CNS: None; CL: Application

2. 4. The essential feature of somatoform disorders is the complaint of physical symptoms with no organic etiology. The complaint is not limited to one organ. There is no relationship to other physical illnesses.
CN: Psychosocial integrity; CNS: None; CL: Application

3. 3. The nurse should respond using therapeutic communication. The response includes the rationale, which will help the nurse understand the student's line of reasoning. Reviewing the symptoms is too vague and does not help the nurse narrow down faulty thinking.
CN: Psychosocial integrity; CNS: None; CL: Analysis

CN: Client needs category   CNS: Client needs subcategory   CL: Cognitive level

4. A nurse is caring for a client who's demonstrating an ego defense mechanism. Which finding supports the nurse's observations?
1. Repression of anger
2. Suppression of grief
3. Denial of depression
4. Preoccupation with pain

Remember, you're looking for a *defense mechanism.*

5. The nurse is caring for an 86-year-old client in an extended care facility who is anxious most of the time and frequently complains of a number of vague symptoms that interfere with his ability to eat. The nurse determines these symptoms are associated with which disorder?
1. Conversion disorder
2. Hypochondriasis
3. Severe anxiety
4. Sublimation

6. The nurse is preparing a care plan for a client experiencing hypochondriasis. What is the <u>most</u> <u>appropriate</u> nursing diagnosis for this client?
1. Risk for injury related to constant fear of illness
2. Grieving related to unresolved issues with loss
3. Risk for situational low self-esteem related to feelings of worthlessness
4. Deficient diversional activity related to unknown etiology

Accurate nursing diagnoses make sure all staff are working toward the same goal!

7. A college student frequently visited the health center during the past year with multiple vague complaints of GI symptoms before course examinations. Although physical causes have been eliminated, the student continues to express her belief that she has a serious illness. The nurse interprets this as:
1. conversion disorder.
2. depersonalization.
3. hypochondriasis.
4. anxiety disorder.

4. 1. One psychodynamic theory states that somatization is the transformation of aggressive and hostile wishes toward others into physical complaints. Repressed anger originating from past disappointments and unfilled needs for nurturing and caring are expressed by soliciting other people's concern and rejecting them as ineffective. Denial, suppression, and preoccupation aren't the defense mechanisms underlying the dynamics of somatization disorders.
CN: Psychosocial integrity; CNS: None; CL: Application

5. 2. Complaints of vague physical symptoms that have no apparent medical causes are characteristic of clients with hypochondriasis. In many cases, the GI system is affected. Conversion disorders are characterized by one or more neurological symptoms. The client's symptoms don't suggest severe anxiety. A client experiencing sublimation channels maladaptive feelings or impulses into socially acceptable behavior.
CN: Psychosocial integrity; CNS: None; CL: Analysis

6. 3. Hypochondriasis is a disorder manifested by fear, risk for situational low self-esteem, and feelings of worthlessness. Risk for injury, grieving, and deficient diversional activity have no correlation to the disorder.
CN: Safe, effective care environment; CNS: Management of care; CL: Application

7. 3. Hypochondriasis in this case is shown by the client's belief that she has a serious illness, although pathological causes have been eliminated. The disturbance usually lasts at least 6 months, and the GI system is commonly affected. Exacerbations are usually associated with identifiable life stressors such as, in this case, course examinations. Conversion disorders are characterized by one or more neurological symptoms. Depersonalization refers to persistent, recurrent episodes of feeling detached from one's self or body. Anxiety disorders generally have stages that may not be associated with hypochondriasis.
CN: Psychosocial integrity; CNS: None; CL: Analysis

8. What is a priority nursing goal for a client diagnosed with hypochondriasis?
1. Determining the cause of the sleep disturbance
2. Relieving the fear of serious illness
3. Recovering the lost or altered function
4. Giving positive reinforcement for accomplishments related to physical appearance

Nursing goals target emotional outcomes as well as physical ones.

9. A client with a diagnosis of hypochondriasis is being seen in the outpatient clinic. Which of the following interventions would the nurse implement? Select all that apply.
1. Teach the client adaptive coping strategies.
2. Help the client eliminate the stress in her life.
3. Confront the client with the statement, "It's all in your head."
4. Encourage the client to focus on identification of physical symptoms.
5. Assess the client's prior coping strategies.

10. After repeated office visits and diagnostic tests for assorted complaints, a client is referred to a psychiatrist. The client states, "I can't imagine why I should see a psychiatrist." What is the <u>most likely</u> explanation for the client's statement?
1. The client probably believes psychiatrists are only for "mentally ill" people.
2. The client probably doesn't understand the correlation between symptoms and stress.
3. The client probably believes his physician has made an error in diagnosis.
4. The client probably believes his physician wants to get rid of him as a client.

Meditating is so therapeutic.

11. The nurse anticipates that which therapeutic modality will be used to treat an individual diagnosed with hypochondriasis?
1. Suicide precautions
2. Relaxation exercises
3. Electroconvulsive therapy (ECT)
4. Aversion therapy

8. 2. The nursing goal for hypochondriasis is relief of fear. For insomnia, the goal is focused on determining the cause of the sleep disturbance. The nursing goal for a conversion disorder focuses on the recovery of the lost or altered function. An appropriate goal for body dysmorphic disorder focuses on positive reinforcement for accomplishments related to physical appearance.
CN: Psychosocial integrity; CNS: None; CL: Application

9. 1. Because of weak ego strength, a client with hypochondriasis is unable to use coping mechanisms effectively. The nursing focus is to teach adaptive coping mechanisms. It isn't realistic to eliminate all stress. A client should never be confronted with the statement, "It's all in your head," because this wouldn't facilitate a long-term therapeutic relationship, which is necessary to offer reassurance that no physical disease is present. Calling attention to physical symptoms is counterproductive to treatment. Assessing prior coping strategies is essential prior to teaching new adaptive skills.
CN: Psychosocial integrity; CNS: None; CL: Application

10. 3. The preoccupation in hypochondriasis is related to bodily functions or physical sensations. Repeated physical examinations, diagnostic tests, and reassurance from the physician don't allay the concerns about bodily disease. There's a belief that a health care professional has poor insight if he sees the concern about having a serious illness as excessive or unreasonable. The other responses aren't valid.
CN: Psychosocial integrity; CNS: None; CL: Analysis

11. 2. Relaxation exercises help to decrease anxiety in a client with hypochondriasis. In a hypochondriasis disorder, no threat of suicide exists. ECT and aversion therapy aren't therapeutic strategies for hypochondriasis.
CN: Psychosocial integrity; CNS: None; CL: Application

12. A client is given triazolam (Halcion) for a sleep disorder. The nurse is reinforcing some teaching precautions concerning the medication. The nurse determines that the client understands the precautions when the client makes which statement?
1. "I take the medication with citrus juice."
2. "I shouldn't confuse this medication with Haldol."
3. "It's okay to take a short drive after taking the medication."
4. "It's okay to smoke while I take this medication."

13. A nurse is developing a teaching plan for sleep hygiene. Which of the following interventions should the nurse include? Select all that apply.
1. Keep the room warm.
2. Eat a large meal before bedtime.
3. Schedule bedtime when you feel tired.
4. Avoid caffeine, excessive fluid intake, alcohol, and stimulating drugs before bedtime.
5. Prepare the room for sleep and turn off distracting noise.
6. Participate in a prayer routine.

14. A nurse is interviewing a client newly admitted to the unit. While stating a list of medications, the client falls asleep. The nurse understands that the client is most likely exhibiting which disorder?
1. Hypersomnia
2. Insomnia
3. Narcolepsy
4. Parasomnia

15. Treatments for sleep disorders include which method?
1. Behavior therapy
2. Biofeedback
3. Group therapy
4. Insight-oriented psychotherapy

Who needs help to sleep?

12. 2. Haldol is an antipsychotic that has a spelling similar to Halcion and is used for clients with psychoses, Tourette's syndrome, severe behavioral problems in children, and emergency sedation of severely agitated psychotic clients. Halcion is one of a group of sedative-hypnotic medications that can be used only for a limited time because of the risk of dependence. Grapefruit and grapefruit juices can alter the absorption of Halcion. The client should avoid driving and other tasks that require alertness or motor skills because the medication may cause drowsiness. Smoking reduces drug effectiveness.
CN: Physiological integrity; CNS: Pharmacological and parenteral therapies; CL: Analysis

13. 4, 5, and 6. Caffeine, excessive fluid intake, alcohol, and stimulating drugs act as stimulants; avoiding them should promote sleep. Maintaining a cool temperature in the room will better facilitate sleeping. Excessive fullness or hunger may interfere with sleep. Setting a regular bedtime and wake-up time facilitates physiological patterns. The room should be conducive to sleep, eliminating any distractions such as television and radio. Participation in a prayer or meditation routine can help the client prepare for a restful night.
CN: Health promotion and maintenance; CNS: None; CL: Application

14. 3. Narcolepsy is also known as sleep attacks. Hypersomnia, or somnolence, refers to excessive sleepiness or seeking excessive amounts of sleep. Insomnia is a sleep disorder in which an individual has difficulty initiating or maintaining sleep. Parasomnia refers to unusual or undesired behavior that occurs during sleep, such as nightmares and sleepwalking.
CN: Physiological integrity; CNS: Physiological adaptation; CL: Analysis

15. 2. Biofeedback, relaxation therapy, and psychopharmacology are appropriate treatments for sleep disorders. Behavior therapy, group therapy, and insight-oriented psychotherapy are treatments related to somatoform disorders.
CN: Physiological integrity; CNS: Basic care and comfort; CL: Application

16. What is the nursing intervention <u>most appropriate</u> for an individual experiencing symptoms of depression?
1. Consult the physician about prescribing a bedtime sleep medication.
2. Allow the client to sit at the nurses' station for comfort.
3. Allow the client to watch television until he's sleepy.
4. Encourage the client to take a warm bath before retiring.

17. The nurse is observing an individual who is sleeping. The nurse determined the client is in REM sleep. Which characteristics represent REM sleep?
1. Disorientation and dozing off
2. Jerky limb movements and position changes
3. Decreased physiological activity levels, pulse rate slowed
4. Increased physiological activity levels, rapid eye movements

18. A client with sleep terror disorder might have autonomic signs of intense anxiety. It is most important for the nurse to assess the client for which of the following?
1. Tachycardia
2. Pupil constriction
3. Cool, clammy skin
4. Decreased muscle tone

19. Which considerations are important in planning care for individuals experiencing sleep deprivation? Select all that apply.
1. Sleep is influenced by biological rhythms.
2. The natural body clock follows a 24-hour cycle.
3. Long sleepers have more rapid eye movement periods.
4. Periods of sleep deprivation result in alterations in mental status.

I'm being terrorized again!

16. **4.** Sleep-inducing activities, such as a warm bath, help promote relaxation and sleep. Although consulting a physician about prescribing a bedtime sleep medication is possible, it wouldn't be the best nursing intervention for this client. Encouraging the client to watch television or sit at the nurses' station wouldn't necessarily promote sleep. In fact, these activities may provide too much stimulation, further preventing sleep.

CN: Physiological integrity; CNS: Basic care and comfort; CL: Application

17. **4.** Highly active brain and physiological activity levels characterize the rapid eye movement (REM) stage of sleep. Delta rhythm and theta rhythm sleep are characterized by disorientation and disorganization. During REM sleep, body movement ceases except for the eyes. The pulse rate slows by 5 or 10 beats/minute during non-REM sleep, not REM sleep.

CN: Physiological integrity; CNS: Physiological adaptation; CL: Analysis

18. **1.** Autonomic arousal includes tachycardia, which should be closely monitored by the nurse to prevent the occurrence of further complications such as arrhythmia. Sweating, increased muscle tone, and pupillary dilation are responses that may also occur but aren't considered life threatening.

CN: Physiological integrity; CNS: Physiological adaptation; CL: Application

19. **4.** Sleep deprivation can lead to hallucinations and delusions. Uninterrupted sleep is an important nursing consideration in planning care. All other data are expected and shouldn't cause sleep deprivation. Genetics play a role in sleep deprivation.

CN: Physiological integrity; CNS: Physiological adaptation; CL: Application

20. A nurse is instructing a 38-year-old male client undergoing treatment for anxiety and insomnia. The practitioner has prescribed lorazepam (Ativan) 1 mg by mouth three times per day. The nurse determines that the teaching regarding the client's medication has been effective when the client makes which statement?
1. "I'll avoid coffee."
2. "I'll avoid aged cheese."
3. "I'll avoid sunlight."
4. "I'll maintain adequate salt intake."

21. A client diagnosed with a sleep disorder awakens with a piercing scream. The nurse understands this behavior is associated with which condition?
1. Hypersomnia
2. Nightmare disorder
3. Sleep terror disorder
4. Sleepwalking

22. What is the most appropriate nursing diagnosis for a client with a sleep disorder?
1. Sleep pattern disturbance
2. Risk for injury
3. Risk for situational low self-esteem
4. Disturbed sensory perception (auditory)

23. An individual is experiencing a conversion disorder "paralysis" of the legs. What is the best response by the nurse?
1. "Tell me how this paralysis as hindered your lifestyle."
2. "Tell me whether you understand that the diagnostic tests are normal."
3. "Can you show me how much you can move your legs?"
4. "Tell me what you plan to do when you return home."
5. "Let's talk about your plans for the future."

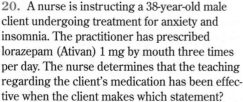
In question 20, you're looking for what could exacerbate the client's symptoms.

Nursing diagnoses are the professional language of nursing.

20. 1. Lorazepam is a benzodiazepine used to treat various forms of anxiety and insomnia. Caffeine is contraindicated because it's a stimulant and increases anxiety. A client on a monoamine oxidase inhibitor should avoid aged cheeses. Clients taking certain antipsychotic medications should avoid sunlight. Salt intake has no effect on lorazepam.
CN: Physiological integrity CNS: Pharmacological and parenteral therapies; CL: Analysis

21. 3. Sleep terror disorder refers to an abrupt arousal from sleep with a piercing scream or cry. Hypersomnia is excessive sleepiness or seeking excessive amounts of sleep. Nightmares are frightening dreams that lead to awakenings from sleep and are severe enough to interfere with social or occupational functioning. Sleepwalking refers to motor activity initiated during sleep in which the individual may leave the bed and walk around.
CN: Psychosocial integrity; CNS: None; CL: Analysis

22. 2. A client with a sleep disorder may be at risk for injury due to drowsiness and decreased concentration. Risk for situational low self-esteem may be related to an alteration in self-concept or self-esteem. No evidence of a disturbed sensory perception (auditory) problem exists. The client cannot participate with family functions due to disorganized thinking because of interruptive sleep patterns. The diagnoses should focus on those areas that will promote safety.
CN: Safe, effective care environment; CNS: Management of care; CL: Analysis

23. 4. The paralysis is used as an unhealthy way of expressing unmet psychological needs. The nurse should avoid speaking about the paralysis to shift the client's attention to the mental aspect of the disorder. The other options focus too much on the paralysis, which doesn't allow for recognition of the underlying psychological motivations.
CN: Psychological integrity; CNS: None; CL: Application

24. Which statement is correct regarding conversion disorders?
1. The symptoms can be controlled.
2. The psychological conflict is repressed.
3. The client is aware of the psychological conflict.
4. The client shouldn't be made aware of the conflicts underlying the symptoms.

25. A client is admitted for abrupt onset of paralysis in his left arm. Although no physiological cause has been found, the symptoms are exacerbated when he speaks of losing custody of his children in a recent divorce. These assessment findings are characteristic of which of the following disorders?
1. Body dysmorphic disorder
2. Conversion disorder
3. Delusional disorder
4. Malingering

26. A client has been hospitalized with a diagnosis of conversion-disorder blindness. Which statement best explains this manifestation?
1. The client is suppressing her true feelings.
2. The client's anxiety has been relieved through her physical symptoms.
3. The client is acting indifferent because she doesn't want to show her actual fear.
4. The client's needs are being met, so she doesn't need to be anxious.

27. A client with hypochondriasis complains of pain in his right side that he hasn't had before. Which response by the nurse is best?
1. "It's time for group therapy now."
2. "Tell me about this new pain you're having. You'll miss group therapy today."
3. "I'll report this pain to your physician. In the meantime, group therapy starts in 5 minutes. You must leave now to be on time."
4. "I'll call your physician and see whether he'll order a new pain medication. Why don't you get some rest for now?"

You've run through 24 questions. You're almost there.

You deserve a pat on the back for answering these questions.

24. 2. In conversion disorder, physical symptoms are manifestations of a repressed psychological conflict. The client isn't able to control or produce symptoms and is unaware of the psychological conflict. Understanding the principles and conflicts behind the symptoms can prove helpful during a client's therapy.
CN: Psychosocial integrity; CNS: None; CL: Analysis

25. 2. Conversion disorders are characterized by one or more neurological symptoms associated with psychological conflict. Body dysmorphic disorder is an imagined belief that there's a defect in the appearance of all or part of the body. The client doesn't have a delusion; this is the sole manifestation of a delusional disorder. Malingering is the intentional production of symptoms to avoid obligations or obtain rewards.
CN: Psychosocial integrity; CNS: None; CL: Analysis

26. 2. Conversion accomplishes anxiety reduction through the production of a physical symptom symbolically linked to an underlying conflict. The client isn't aware of the internal conflict. Hospitalization doesn't remove the source of the conflict.
CN: Psychosocial integrity; CNS: None; CL: Analysis

27. 3. The amount of time focused on discussing physical symptoms should be decreased. Lack of positive reinforcement may help stop the maladaptive behavior. However, avoiding the statement altogether demeans the client and doesn't address the underlying problem. Asking the client to further explain the pain emphasizes physical symptoms and prevents the client from attending group therapy. All physical complaints need to be evaluated for physiological causes by the physician.
CN: Psychosocial integrity; CNS: None; CL: Application

28. What is the best nursing intervention to help a client with conversion-disorder blindness to eat?
1. Direct the client to independently locate items on the tray and feed himself.
2. See to the needs of the other clients in the dining room and then feed this client last.
3. Establish a "buddy" system with other clients who can feed the client at each meal.
4. Expect the client to feed himself after explaining the location of food on the tray.

29. A client diagnosed with conversion disorder is experiencing left-sided paralysis. The client tells the nurse he has received a lot of attention in the hospital and it's unfortunate others outside the hospital don't find him interesting. Which nursing diagnosis is appropriate for this client?
1. Interrupted family processes
2. Ineffective health maintenance
3. Ineffective coping
4. Social isolation

30. What is the most appropriate nursing intervention to increase the self-esteem of a client with conversion disorder?
1. Focus attention on the client as a person rather than on the symptom.
2. Discuss the client's childhood to link present behaviors with past traumas.
3. Encourage the client to use avoidant-interactional patterns rather than assertive patterns.
4. Assist the client in developing short-term goals.

31. A nurse is teaching family members about signs and symptoms of conversion disorder to observe for in the client. It is most important for the nurse to include which sign or symptom?
1. Delusions
2. Feelings of depression or euphoria
3. A feeling of dread accompanied by somatic signs
4. One or more neurological symptoms associated with psychological conflict or need

A client with a disorder of psychologic origin may need the same interventions as one with a disorder of physical origin.

It's nice to feel special.

28. 4. The client is expected to maintain some level of independence by feeding himself while, at the same time, the nurse provides some direction and is supportive in a matter-of-fact way. Feeding the client leads to dependence.
CN: Psychosocial integrity; CNS: None; CL: Application

29. 3. The client can't express his internal conflicts in appropriate ways. There are no defining characteristics to support the other nursing diagnoses.
CN: Psychosocial integrity; CNS: None; CL: Application

30. 1. Focusing on the client directs attention away from the symptom. This approach eventually reduces the client's need to gain attention through physical symptoms. Small goals ensure success and reinforce self-esteem. Discussion of childhood has no correlation with self-esteem. Avoiding interactional situations doesn't foster self-esteem.
CN: Psychosocial integrity; CNS: None; CL: Application

31. 4. Symptoms of conversion disorders are neurological in nature (paralysis, blindness). Delusional disorders are characterized by delusions. Mood disorders are characterized by abnormal feelings of depression or euphoria. Anxiety is characterized by a feeling of dread.
CN: Health promotion and maintenance; CNS: None; CL: Application

32. Which nursing diagnosis is appropriate for a client with conversion disorder who has little energy to expend on activities or interactions with friends?
1. Powerlessness
2. Hopelessness
3. Impaired social interaction
4. Compromised family coping

33. A client diagnosed with conversion disorder has a nursing diagnosis of interrupted family processes related to the client's disability. Which goal is appropriate for this client?
1. The client will resume former roles and tasks.
2. The client will take over roles of other family members.
3. The client will rely on family members to meet all client needs.
4. The client will focus energy on problems occurring in the family.

34. A new client admitted to a psychiatric unit is diagnosed with conversion disorder. The client shows a lack of concern for his sudden paralysis, although his athletic abilities have always been a source of pride to him. The nurse understands that the client is demonstrating:
1. acute dystonia.
2. la belle indifference.
3. malingering.
4. secondary gain.

35. Which nursing intervention is the <u>most appropriate</u> for a client who had pseudoseizures and is diagnosed with conversion disorder?
1. Explain that the pseudoseizures are imaginary.
2. Promote dependence so that unfilled dependency needs are met.
3. Encourage the client to discuss his feelings about the pseudoseizures.
4. Promote independence and withdraw attention from the pseudoseizures.

Mingle, mingle, mingle!

32. 3. When clients focus their mental and physical energy on somatic symptoms, they have little energy to expend on social or diversional activities. Such a client needs nursing assistance to become involved in social interactions. Although the other diagnoses are common for a client with conversion disorder, the information given in the question doesn't support them.
CN: Psychosocial integrity; CNS: None; CL: Application

33. 1. The client who uses somatization has typically adopted a sick role in the family, characterized by dependence. Increasing independence and resumption of former roles are necessary to change this pattern. The client shouldn't be expected to take on the roles or responsibilities of other family members. Focusing energy on problems occurring in the family doesn't address the nursing diagnosis and related factors.
CN: Psychosocial integrity; CNS: None; CL: Application

34. 2. La belle indifference is a lack of concern about the present illness. Acute dystonia refers to muscle spasms. Malingering is voluntary production of symptoms. Secondary gain refers to the benefits of illness.
CN: Psychosocial integrity; CNS: None; CL: Application

35. 4. Successful performance of independent activities enhances self-esteem. Telling the client that the symptoms are imaginary may jeopardize the nurse–client relationship. Positive reinforcement encourages the use of maladaptive responses. The focus shouldn't be on the disability because it may provide positive gains for the client.
CN: Psychosocial integrity; CNS: None; CL: Application

36. Which therapeutic approach would enable a client to cope effectively with life stress without using conversion?
1. Focus on the symptoms.
2. Ask for clarification of the symptoms.
3. Listen to the client's symptoms in a matter-of-fact manner.
4. Point out that the client's symptoms are an escape from dealing with conflict.

37. Which statement made by a client with a pain disorder shows the nurse that the goal of stress management was attained?
1. "My arm hurts."
2. "I enjoy being dependent on others."
3. "I don't really understand why I'm here."
4. "My muscles feel relaxed after that progressive relaxation exercise."

38. What is the priority nursing diagnosis for a client with hypochondriasis disorder?
1. Disturbed sensory perception (visual)
2. Hopelessness
3. Imbalanced nutrition: Less than body requirements
4. Risk for other-directed violence

39. A nurse is teaching the family of a client diagnosed with a somatoform pain disorder. Which of the following statements by the nurse most accurately describes this disorder?
1. A preoccupation with pain in the absence of physical disease
2. A physical or somatic complaint without any demonstrable organic findings
3. A morbid fear or belief that one has a serious disease where none exists
4. One or more neurological symptoms associated with psychological conflict or need

Focus on what the client is saying.

36. **3.** Listening in a matter-of-fact manner doesn't focus on the client's symptoms. All other interventions focus on the client's symptoms, which draw attention to the physical symptoms, not the underlying cause.

CN: Health promotion and maintenance; CNS: None; CL: Application

37. **4.** The client is experiencing positive results from the relaxation exercise. All other responses alert the nurse that the client needs further interventions.

CN: Physiological integrity; CNS: Basic care and comfort; CL: Analysis

38. **3.** A client with hypochondriasis has a preoccupying fear of having a serious disease and is at risk for not getting adequate nutrition. Delusions are not a symptom of hypochondriasis. Although hopelessness may be present, it is not the primary focus. Clients with hypochondriasis are not prone to violence toward themselves or others.

CN: Safe, effective care environment; CNS: Management of care; CL: Application

39. **1.** Somatoform pain disorder is a preoccupation with pain in the absence of physical disease. A physical or somatic complaint refers to somatoform disorders in general. A morbid fear of serious illness is hypochondriasis. Neurological symptoms are associated with conversion disorders.

CN: Psychosocial integrity; CNS: None; CL: Application

40. The nurse is caring for a client who conceals the true motivations for his thoughts, actions, or feelings. The nurse interprets this as:
1. displacement.
2. rationalization.
3. regression.
4. substitution.

What a relief!

41. Which nursing goal is most appropriate for a client with a pain disorder?
1. The client will express less fear.
2. The client will increase independence.
3. The client will express relief from pain.
4. The client will adapt coping strategies to deal with stress.

42. Which conditions or situations are most likely to result in difficulty sleeping? Select all that apply.
1. Shift work
2. Sleep apnea
3. Reduction of external stimuli
4. Caffeine intake in the evening
5. Consistent bedtime routine
6. Excessive worry or anxiety

43. Based on a nursing diagnosis of ineffective coping for a client with somatoform pain disorder, which nursing goal is most realistic?
1. The client will be free from injury.
2. The client will recognize sensory impairment.
3. The client will discuss beliefs about spiritual issues.
4. The client will verbalize reduction of physical symptoms.

40. 2. Rationalization is a process by which an individual deals with emotional conflict or internal or external stressors by concealing the true motivations for his thoughts, actions, and feelings through the elaboration of reassuring or self-serving but incorrect explanations. This process isn't a defense mechanism related to pain disorders. Displacement, substitution, and regression are defense mechanisms that would be expected from a client with a pain disorder.
CN: Psychosocial integrity; CNS: None; CL: Application

41. 3. Relief of pain should be a priority for clients experiencing pain. Expression of less fear applies to a client with hypochondriasis. A focus on independence is appropriate for a client diagnosed with conversion disorder. The development of coping strategies would be beneficial for a client with a somatization disorder.
CN: Physiological integrity; CNS: Physiological adaptation; CL: Application

42. 1, 2, 4, and 6. Shift work can disrupt the circadian rhythm. Sleep apnea can cause a reduction in oxygen to the brain, which can reduce the quality of rest. Caffeine is a stimulant and, if taken too close to bedtime, can interfere with falling asleep. Excessive worry or anxiety causes an increase in adrenaline, which enhances alertness and reduces sleepiness. A consistent bedtime routine and reduction of external stimuli promote good sleep.
CN: Health promotion and maintenance; CNS: None; CL: Analysis

43. 4. Expression of feelings enables the client to ventilate emotions, which decreases anxiety and draws attention away from the physical symptoms. The client isn't experiencing a safety issue. There's no apparent correlation with any sensory-perceptual alterations. Spiritual issues are related to spiritual distress, and no evidence exists to support that the client is having spiritual distress.
CN: Physiological integrity; CNS: Basic care and comfort; CL: Analysis

44. Which statement made by a client best meets the diagnostic criteria for pain disorder?
1. "I can't move my right leg."
2. "I'm having severe stomach and leg pain."
3. "I'm so afraid I might have human immuno-deficiency virus."
4. "I'm having chest pain and pain radiating down my left arm that began more than 1 hour ago."

45. Which nursing diagnosis is most appropriate for a client with somatoform pain disorder?
1. Interrupted family processes
2. Disturbed body image
3. Ineffective denial
4. Ineffective coping

46. Which statement made by a nurse promotes independence in self-care in a client diagnosed with somatoform pain disorder?
1. "I'll call you for all the group activities."
2. "I'll help you on a daily basis with your care."
3. "The staff will help you with your basic needs for today."
4. "We'll wait until you have no more pain before you participate in activities."

47. Which <u>initial</u> therapeutic intervention is the most appropriate for a client diagnosed with ineffective coping related to a pain disorder?
1. Make an accurate assessment.
2. Promote expression of feelings.
3. Promote insight into the disorder.
4. Help the client develop alternative coping strategies.

48. A client with a somatoform pain disorder may obtain primary and secondary gain. Which statement best describes secondary gain?
1. It brings some stability to the family.
2. It decreases the preoccupation with the physical illness.
3. It enables the client to avoid some unpleasant activity.
4. It promotes emotional support or attention for the client.

Remember, diagnostic criteria for psychologic problems come from the latest edition of the *Diagnostic and Statistical Manual of Mental Disorders*, currently known as DSM-IV-TR.

What is the *initial* intervention?

44. 2. The diagnostic criteria for pain disorders state that pain in one or more anatomic sites is the predominant focus of the clinical presentation and is of sufficient severity to warrant clinical attention. A client with a conversion disorder can experience a motor neurological symptom such as paralysis. Hypochondriasis is a morbid fear or belief that one has a serious disease where none exists. Unremitting chest pain with radiation of pain down the left arm is symptomatic of a myocardial infarction.
CN: Psychosocial integrity; CNS: None; CL: Application

45. 4. A somatoform pain disorder is closely associated with the client's inability to handle stress and conflict. Although interrupted family processes and ineffective denial may be present, they aren't the primary focus. Disturbed body image isn't directly correlated with this disorder.
CN: Safe, effective care environment; CNS: Management of care; CL: Application

46. 3. Limited time in assisting a client will help the client develop independence. All other options would promote dependence on the staff.
CN: Safe, effective care environment; CNS: Management of care; CL: Application

47. 1. It's essential to accurately assess the client first before any interventions. Promoting expression of feelings and insight and helping the client develop coping strategies are appropriate interventions that can be implemented after the initial assessment.
CN: Psychosocial integrity; CNS: None; CL: Application

48. 4. Secondary gain refers to the benefits of the illness that allow the client to receive emotional support or attention. A dysfunctional family may disregard the real issue, although some conflict is relieved. Somatoform pain disorder is a preoccupation with pain in the absence of physical disease. Primary gain enables the client to avoid some unpleasant activity.
CN: Psychosocial integrity; CNS: None; CL: Analysis

49. Which nursing intervention is appropriate for a client diagnosed with a somatoform pain disorder?
1. Reinforce the client's behavior when it isn't focused on pain.
2. Allow the client to verbalize anxieties related to body image.
3. Allow the client to verbalize relief of fear related to the illness.
4. Assist the client in recovery of the lost or altered function of a body part.

50. A client has primary insomnia and requires pharmaceutical assistance to sleep. The physician orders secobarbital sodium (Seconal) 75 mg by mouth at bedtime. The nurse has secobarbital sodium 25-mg tablets on hand. How many tablets should the nurse administer to the client? Record your answer using a whole number.

_____ tablets

51. A home health nurse is caring for a client diagnosed with a conversion disorder manifested by paralysis in the left arm. An organic cause for the deficit has been ruled out. Which nursing intervention is <u>most appropriate</u> for this client?
1. Perform all physical tasks for the client to foster dependence.
2. Allot an hour each day to discuss the paralysis and its cause.
3. Identify primary or secondary gains that the physical symptom provides.
4. Allow the client to withdraw from all physical activities.

52. A client with somatoform disorder states that her frequent headaches result from a brain tumor. However, a tumor hasn't shown up on diagnostic tests. The nurse interprets the client's form of somatization as which disorder?
1. Conversion disorder
2. Pain disorder
3. Hypochondriasis
4. Body dysmorphic disorder

Remember to use the correct formula when calculating the appropriate drug dose.

Have you sorted out the various forms of somatization? Don't try to rush. You can do it!

49. 1. Help the client get attention and see himself as valuable without using pain. Verbalization of anxieties related to body image may be beneficial in a client with body dysmorphic disorder. Fear of illness is related to hypochondriasis. The recovery of a lost or altered function of a body part is related to conversion disorders.
CN: Psychosocial integrity; CNS: None; CL: Application

50. 3. Each tablet contains 25 mg of the medication. The correct formula to calculate this drug dose is:
Dose of each tablet × X = Prescribed dose
25 mg × X (# of tablets) = 75 mg
25X = 75
X = 75/25
X = 3
CN: Physiological integrity; CNS: Pharmacological and parenteral therapies; CL: Analysis

51. 3. Primary or secondary gains should be identified because they're etiological factors that can be used in problem resolution. The nurse should encourage the client to be as independent as possible and should intervene only when the client requires assistance. The nurse shouldn't focus on the disability. The nurse should encourage the client to perform physical activities to the greatest extent possible.
CN: Psychosocial integrity; CNS: None; CL: Application

52. 3. In hypochondriasis, a physical symptom is interpreted as severe or life threatening and causes exaggerated worry. In conversion disorder, the client loses a motor or sensory function but lacks appropriate concern about the loss. In pain disorder, pain is the dominant feature. In body dysmorphic disorder, the client is preoccupied with a perceived defect in appearance.
CN: Psychosocial integrity; CNS: None; CL: Application

53. A college student frequently visited the health center before course examinations. Physical causes for these visits have been eliminated. Based on the following progress note entry in the client's chart, the nurse suspects which disorder?

Progress notes

9/9/10	19-year-old client states "I'm having
2130	abdominal discomfort. It happens on
	and off, especially the last week while
	I'm trying to study for midterm
	exams. I know that there's something
	really wrong." Client denies that these
	symptoms are related to eating.
	Normal bowel sounds auscultated.
	Abdomen soft and nontender to
	palpation. Vital signs: Temp, 98.20° F;
	BP, 114/72 mm Hg; heart rate,
	76 beats/minute; respiratory rate,
	20 breaths/minute. Client denies
	nausea, vomiting, diarrhea or loss of
	appetite. ——— *Natalie Jones, RN*

1. Conversion disorder
2. Depersonalization
3. Hypochondriasis
4. Somatoform disorder

54. A 26-year-old client is diagnosed with somatoform disorder. What is the most important information for the nurse to provide when discussing the care plan with the client's wife?
1. "Tell your husband that his symptoms are all in his head to force him to deal with reality."
2. "Tell your husband that his symptoms are an attempt to get attention and that you'll be more attentive."
3. "Accept the reality of the symptoms as your husband presents them and don't dispute them."
4. "Realize that your husband is creating the symptoms on purpose."

55. A client with a diagnosis of somatoform disorder has been admitted to the psychiatric unit and has difficulty breathing, numbness, and loss of movement in his left arm. He seems unusually calm and unconcerned about his loss. The nurse recognizes these symptoms as which disorder?
1. Conversion disorder
2. Hypochondriasis
3. Body dysmorphic disorder
4. Pain disorder

Hooray for you! You're the best!

53. 3. Hypochondriasis in this case is shown by the client's belief that she has a serious illness, although pathological causes have been eliminated. The disturbance usually lasts at least 6 months, and the GI system is commonly affected. Exacerbations are usually associated with identifiable life stressors that, in this case, can be related to the client's examinations. Conversion disorders are characterized by one or more neurological symptoms. Depersonalization refers to persistent, recurrent episodes of feeling detached from one's self or body. Somatoform disorders generally have a chronic course with few remissions.
CN: Psychosocial integrity; CNS: None; CL: Analysis

54. 3. For a client with somatoform disorder, caregivers should accept the symptoms and avoid disputing them. The symptoms aren't contrived or all in the client's head. They're neither an attempt to get attention nor created "on purpose."
CN: Psychosocial integrity; CNS: None; CL: Application

55. 1. Conversion disorder is characterized by loss of motor, sensory, or visceral functioning accompanied by the client's indifference to the loss. In hypochondriasis, the client interprets a physical symptom as severe or life threatening and worries over it excessively. Body dysmorphic disorder is a preoccupation with a perceived defect in appearance. In pain disorder, pain is the dominant physical symptom.
CN: Psychosocial integrity; CNS: None; CL: Application

Chapter 14
Anxiety & mood disorders

1. Select the statement most <u>typical</u> of a client experiencing periodic panic attacks.
1. "Yesterday, I sat up in bed and just felt so scared."
2. "I have difficulty sleeping because I'm so anxious."
3. "Sometimes, I have the most wild and vivid dreams."
4. "When I drink beer, I fall asleep without any problems."

2. A client with generalized anxiety disorder states, "I'm afraid I'm going to die from cancer. My mother had cancer." What is the most appropriate response by the nurse?
1. "We all live in fear of dying from cancer."
2. "Did your father also have cancer?"
3. "I wouldn't worry about it just yet. You seem to be in good health."
4. "Has something happened that is causing you to worry?"

3. A client with a history of panic attacks tells the nurse, "I feel so trapped," right after an attack. The nurse determines that the client is <u>most likely</u> expressing which fear?
1. Loss of control
2. Loss of identity
3. Loss of memory
4. Loss of maturity

Question 1 is typical of what you'll be asked throughout the test.

Remember: You're in control, so read the question carefully and choose the most likely response.

1. 1. A person who suffers a panic attack while sleeping experiences an abrupt awakening and feelings of fear. People with severe anxiety commonly have symptoms related to a sleep disorder; they wouldn't typically experience a sleep panic attack. A panic attack while sleeping often causes an inability to remember dreams. Intake of alcohol initially produces a drowsy feeling, but after a short period of time, alcohol causes restless, fragmented sleep and strange dreams.
CN: Psychosocial integrity; CNS: None; CL: Analysis

2. 4. By asking the client about what is making him/her worry, the nurse assists the client in determining the cause of the anxiety. The other responses deflect and minimize the client's concerns.
CN: Psychosocial integrity; CNS: None; CL: Analysis

3. 1. People who fear loss of control during a panic attack commonly make statements about feeling trapped, getting hurt, or having little or no personal control over their situations. People who experience panic attacks don't tend to have loss of identity or memory impairment. People who have panic attacks also don't regress or become immature.
CN: Psychosocial integrity; CNS: None; CL: Application

4. A nurse who is caring for a client with panic disorder receives an order for alprazolam (Xanax) from the physician. The nurse reviews the clients chart and determines further intervention is needed when the medical history includes:
1. intermittent insomnia.
2. acute-angle glaucoma.
3. seizure disorder.
4. tartrazine hypersensitivity.

5. What is the <u>most important</u> nursing intervention to include in the plan of care for a client experiencing an acute panic attack?
1. Tell the client to take deep breaths.
2. Have the client talk about the anxiety.
3. Encourage the client to verbalize feelings.
4. Ask the client about the cause of the attack.

Don't panic! Stay calm and remember to prioritize.

6. The nurse is teaching a client and family about the management of panic attacks. What is the most important information for the nurse to include?
1. Identifying when anxiety is escalating
2. Determining how to stop a panic attack
3. Addressing strategies to reduce physical pain
4. Preventing the client from depending on others

7. What is the most important question for a nurse to ask a client with <u>agoraphobia</u>?
1. How realistic are your goals?
2. Are you able to go shopping?
3. Do you struggle with impulse control?
4. Who else in your family has panic disorder?

For the NCLEX, you should memorize the definitions of common fears such as agoraphobia.

4. 2. Acute-angle glaucoma is a medical problem that contraindicates the use of alprazolam. Alprazolam causes drowsiness and sedation, so sleep shouldn't be interrupted. Seizure disorder isn't a contraindication for the use of alprazolam. Tartrazine hypersensitivity is associated with yellow dye used in some convenience foods and isn't a contraindication for the use of alprazolam.
CN: Physiological integrity; CNS: Pharmacological and parenteral therapies; CL: Application

5. 1. During a panic attack, the nurse should remain with the client and direct what's said toward changing the physiological response, such as taking deep breaths. During an attack, the client is unable to talk about anxious situations and isn't able to address feelings, especially uncomfortable feelings and frustrations. While having a panic attack, the client is also unable to focus on anything other than the symptoms, so the client won't be able to discuss the cause of the attack.
CN: Safe, effective care environment; CNS: Management of care; CL: Analysis

6. 1. By identifying the presence of anxiety, it's possible to take steps to prevent its escalation. A panic attack can't be stopped. The nurse can take steps to assist the client safely through the attack. Later, the nurse can assist the client to alleviate the precipitating stressors. Clients who experience panic disorder don't tend to be in physical pain. The client experiencing a panic disorder may need to periodically depend on other people when having a panic attack.
CN: Psychosocial integrity; CNS: None; CL: Application

7. 2. The client with agoraphobia typically restricts himself to home and can't carry out normal socializing and life-sustaining activities. Clients with panic disorder are able to set realistic goals and tend to be cautious and reclusive rather than impulsive. Although there's a familial tendency toward panic disorder, information about client needs must be obtained to determine how agoraphobia affects the client's life.
CN: Psychosocial integrity; CNS: None; CL: Application

8. The nurse has been working with a female client who is interested in lifestyle changes as behavior modification to treat her panic attacks. What is the most important information for the nurse to tell the client?
1. Cigarettes can trigger panic episodes.
2. Fermented foods can cause panic attacks.
3. Hormonal therapy can induce panic attacks.
4. Tryptophan can predispose a person to panic attacks.

9. What is the <u>priority</u> nursing intervention when caring for a client with a panic disorder?
1. Make the client role-play the panic attack.
2. Assist the client to develop an exercise program.
3. Teach the client to identify cognitive distortions.
4. Teach the client to identify sources of anxiety.

10. The nurse is planning care for a client with panic disorder. What is the most appropriate nursing intervention?
1. Identify childhood trauma.
2. Monitor nutritional intake.
3. Institute suicide precautions.
4. Monitor episodes of disorientation.

11. Which statement indicates a positive response about treatment progress from the client diagnosed with panic disorder with agoraphobia?
1. "I went to the mall with my friend last Saturday."
2. "I'm hyperventilating only when I have a panic attack."
3. "Today, I decided that I can stop taking my medication."
4. "Last night, I decided to eat more than a bowl of cereal."

I'm too anxious to look. Have you finished 10 questions yet?

8. 1. Cigarettes contain nicotine, which can be a stimulant, a depressant, or a tranquilizer, and can trigger panic attacks. None of the other options causes panic attacks.
CN: Psychosocial integrity; CNS: None; CL: Application

9. 4. The client must be aware of the connection between sources of anxiety and the symptoms of a panic attack. Role-playing a panic attack isn't useful. Role-playing coping strategies would be useful for the client. Later in treatment, the client can develop an exercise program as part of the overall plan to handle stress. Learning to identify cognitive distortions is a useful strategy to teach the client after he's begun to work on identifying sources of anxiety.
CN: Psychosocial integrity; CNS: None; CL: Analysis

10. 3. Clients with panic disorder are at risk for suicide because they can be impulsive. Childhood trauma is associated with posttraumatic stress disorder, not panic disorder. Nutritional problems don't typically accompany panic disorder. Clients aren't typically disoriented; they may have a temporary altered sense of reality, but that lasts only for the duration of the attack.
CN: Psychosocial integrity; CNS: None; CL: Application

11. 1. Clients with panic disorder tend to be socially withdrawn. Going to the mall is a sign of working on avoidance behaviors. Hyperventilation is a key symptom of panic disorder. Teaching breathing control is a major intervention for clients with panic disorder. The client taking medications for panic disorder, such as antidepressants and benzodiazepines, must be weaned off these drugs. Most clients with panic disorder with agoraphobia don't have nutritional problems.
CN: Psychosocial integrity; CNS: None; CL: Analysis

12. Which group therapy intervention is of <u>primary</u> importance to a client with panic disorder?
1. Explore how secondary gains are derived from the disorder.
2. Discuss new ways of thinking and feeling about panic attacks.
3. Work to eliminate manipulative behavior used for meeting needs.
4. Learn the risk factors and other demographics associated with panic disorder.

13. The nursing team members planning care for a client with social phobia would primarily address which symptom?
1. Self-harm
2. Poor self-esteem
3. Compulsive behavior
4. Avoidance of social situations

14. A client with social phobia is most likely to make which statement?
1. "Without people around, I just feel so lost."
2. "There's nothing wrong with my behavior."
3. "I like to be the center of attention."
4. "I know I can't accept that award for my brother."

15. The nurse is aware that socially phobic clients typically fear which event?
1. Dental procedures
2. Meeting strangers
3. Being bitten by a dog
4. Having a car collision

12. 2. Restructuring an anxiety-producing event allows the client to gain control over the situation. Discussing new ways of thinking and feeling about panic attacks can enable others to learn and benefit from a variety of intervention strategies. There are usually no secondary gains obtained from having a panic disorder. People with panic disorder aren't using the disorder as a way to manipulate others. Learning the risk factors could be accomplished in another format such as a psychoeducational program.
CN: Psychosocial integrity; CNS: None; CL: Analysis

13. 4. Clients with social phobia avoid social situations for fear of being humiliated or embarrassed. They generally don't tend to be at risk for self-harm and usually don't demonstrate compulsive behavior. Not all individuals with social anxiety have low self-esteem.
CN: Psychosocial integrity; CNS: None; CL: Application

14. 4. People who have a social phobia usually undervalue themselves and their talents. They don't like to be in feared social situations or around many people. They tend to stay away from situations in which they may feel humiliated and embarrassed. They fear social gatherings and dislike being the center of attention. They're very critical of themselves and believe that others also will be critical.
CN: Psychosocial integrity; CNS: None; CL: Application

15. 2. Fear of meeting strangers is a common example of social phobia. Fears of having a dental procedure, being bitten by a dog, or having a collision are not social phobias.
CN: Psychosocial integrity; CNS: None; CL: Application

CN: Client needs category   CNS: Client needs subcategory   CL: Cognitive level

16. The nurse is assessing a client for blood-injection-injury phobia. The most predictive finding would be?
1. Episodes of fainting
2. Gregarious personality
3. Difficulty managing anger
4. Dramatic, overreactive personality

Why would anyone be afraid of us?

17. A client with a phobic disorder would benefit most from which individual counseling approach?
1. Have the client keep a daily journal.
2. Help the client identify the source of the anxiety.
3. Teach the client effective ways to problem solve.
4. Develop strategies to prevent the client from using substances.

18. The nurse is aware that the behaviors of clients with phobias can best be modified using:
1. aversion therapy.
2. imitation or modeling.
3. positive reinforcement.
4. systematic desensitization.

Along with assessment, you also need to familiarize yourself with common treatments.

19. Which statement best describes the need for a strong support system when teaching the client and family about phobias?
1. The use of a family support system is only temporary.
2. The need to be assertive can be reinforced by the family.
3. The family needs to set limits on inappropriate behaviors.
4. The family plays a role in promoting client independence.

16. 1. Many people with a history of blood-injection-injury phobia report frequently fainting when exposed to this type of situation. All personality styles can develop phobias, so personality type doesn't provide information for assessing phobias. Information about a client's difficulty managing anger isn't related to a specific phobic disorder. Individuals with blood-injection-injury phobias aren't being dramatic or overreactive.
CN: Psychosocial integrity; CNS: None; CL: Analysis

17. 2. By understanding the source of the anxiety, the client will understand how this anxiety has been displaced as a phobic response. Keeping a journal is an effective method in many situations; however, its use is limited in the treatment of phobias. Problem solving is a more useful technique for clients with obsessive-compulsive disorder than for clients with phobias. People with phobias don't tend to self-medicate like clients with other psychiatric disorders.
CN: Psychosocial integrity; CNS: None; CL: Application

18. 4. Systematic desensitization is a common behavior modification technique successfully used to help treat phobias. Aversion therapy and positive reinforcement are not behavior modification techniques used with treatment of phobias. Imitation and modeling are social learning techniques, not behavior modification techniques.
CN: Psychosocial integrity; CNS: None; CL: Application

19. 4. The family plays a vital role in supporting the client in treatment and preventing the client from using the phobia to obtain secondary gains. Family support must be ongoing, not temporary. The family can be more helpful by focusing on effective handling of anxiety, rather than focusing on developing assertiveness skills. People with phobias are already restrictive in their behavior; more restrictions aren't necessary.
CN: Psychosocial integrity; CNS: None; CL: Analysis

20. What is the nursing intervention of primary importance during the administration of paroxetine (Paxil) to the depressed client with a phobic disorder?
1. Monitor renal function.
2. Determine electrocardiogram (ECG) changes.
3. Assess for sleeping difficulties.
4. Observe for extrapyramidal symptoms.

21. The nurse suspects a client may have posttraumatic stress disorder. It would be most important for the nurse to assess the client for which of the following?
1. Eating disorder
2. Schizophrenia
3. Suicide
4. "Sundown" syndrome

22. The nurse explains that the therapeutic action of tricyclic antidepressants (TCAs) for clients experiencing posttraumatic stress disorder is to:
1. prevent hyperactivity and purposeless movements.
2. increase the client's ability to concentrate.
3. help prevent experiencing the trauma again.
4. facilitate the grieving process.

23. The nurse is planning care for a client with posttraumatic stress disorder who states that the experience was "bad luck." What is the most important intervention for the nurse to include?
1. Encourage the client to verbalize the experience.
2. Assist the client in defining the experience as a trauma.
3. Work with the client to take steps to move on with life.
4. Help the client accept positive and negative feelings.

How do I know you aren't going to hurt me?

Don't deny it. You're doing great!

20. 1. Clients with impaired renal function shouldn't take paroxetine. ECG changes aren't adverse effects of paroxetine. Other than a transient period of drowsiness occurring when the client begins to take the drug, sleep difficulties don't tend to be a problem. Extrapyramidal symptoms aren't seen with paroxetine.
CN: Physiological integrity; CNS: Pharmacological and parenteral therapies; CL: Analysis

21. 3. Clients who experience posttraumatic stress disorder are at high risk for suicide and other forms of violent behaviors. Eating disorders are possible but aren't a common complication of posttraumatic stress disorder. Clients with posttraumatic stress disorder don't usually have their extreme anxiety manifest itself as schizophrenia. "Sundown" syndrome is an increase in agitation accompanied by confusion. It's commonly seen in clients with dementia, not clients with posttraumatic stress disorder.
CN: Psychosocial integrity; CNS: None; CL: Application

22. 3. Tricyclic antidepressant medication will decrease the frequency of reenactment of the trauma for the client. It will help memory problems and sleeping difficulties and will decrease numbing. The medication won't prevent hyperactivity and purposeless movements or increase the client's concentration. No medication will facilitate the grieving process.
CN: Physiological integrity; CNS: Pharmacological and parenteral therapies; CL: Application

23. 2. The client must define the experience as traumatic to realize the situation wasn't under his personal control. Encouraging the client to verbalize the experience without first addressing the denial isn't a useful strategy. The client can move on with life only after acknowledging the trauma and processing the experience. Acknowledgment of the actual trauma and verbalization of the event should come before the acceptance of feelings.
CN: Psychosocial integrity; CNS: None; CL: Analysis

24. The nurse is teaching a client with posttraumatic stress about relationships. What is the most important information for the nurse to provide?
1. Encourage the client to resume former roles as soon as possible.
2. Assess the client's discomfort when talking about feelings to family members.
3. Explain that avoiding emotional attachment protects against anxiety.
4. Warn the client that he'll have a tendency to be overdependent in relationships.

25. The nurse is caring for a client diagnosed with posttraumatic stress disorder. The client tells the nurse, "My family doesn't believe anything about posttraumatic stress disorder." What is the most appropriate intervention by the nurse?
1. Provide the family with information.
2. Teach the family about problem solving.
3. Discuss the family's view of the problem.
4. Assess for the presence of family violence.

Caring for clients commonly means working with their families—a skill you can expect the exam to test.

26. While caring for a client with posttraumatic stress disorder, the family notices that loud noises cause a serious anxiety response. What is the best explanation for the nurse to give the family?
1. Environmental triggers can cause the client to become hyperaroused and have exaggerated startle reactions.
2. Clients commonly experience extreme fear about normal environmental stimuli.
3. After a trauma, the client can't respond to stimuli in an appropriate manner.
4. The response indicates that another emotional problem needs investigation.

27. What is the primary psychological symptom a nurse should expect to find in a hospitalized client who is the lone survivor of a train collision?
1. Denial
2. Indifference
3. Perfectionism
4. Trust

24. **3.** The client may tend to avoid interpersonal relationships to protect himself against unrelieved anxiety. Because relationships tend to be avoided, the client won't express feelings to family members at this time and won't resume roles and responsibilities for a while. Clients with posttraumatic stress disorder don't tend to become overdependent in relationships but do tend to withdraw from them.
CN: Psychosocial integrity; CNS: None; CL: Application

25. **1.** If the family can understand posttraumatic stress disorder, they can more readily participate in the client's care and be supportive. Learning problem-solving skills doesn't help clarify posttraumatic stress disorder. After being given information about posttraumatic stress disorder, the family can then ask questions and present its views. The family must first have information about posttraumatic stress disorder; then the discussion about violence to self or others can be addressed.
CN: Safe, effective care environment; CNS: Management of care; CL: Application

26. **1.** Repeated exposure to environmental triggers can cause the client to experience a hyperarousal state because there's a loss of physiological control of incoming stimuli. After experiencing a trauma, the client may have strong reactions to stimuli similar to those that occurred during the traumatic event. However, not all stimuli will cause an anxiety response. The client's anxiety response is typically seen after a traumatic experience and doesn't indicate the presence of another problem.
CN: Psychosocial integrity; CNS: None; CL: Application

27. **1.** Denial can act as a protective response. The client tends to be overwhelmed and disorganized by the trauma, not indifferent to it. Perfectionism is more commonly seen in clients with eating disorders, not in clients with posttraumatic stress disorder. Clients who have had a severe trauma commonly experience an inability to trust others.
CN: Psychosocial integrity; CNS: None; CL: Analysis

28. A client is suffering from posttraumatic stress disorder and says, "I've decided to just avoid everything and everyone." The nurse suspects the client is at <u>greatest risk</u> for which of the following?
1. Becoming homeless
2. Exhausting finances
3. Terminating employment
4. Using substances

29. What is the best therapeutic technique to use when speaking with a client with posttraumatic stress disorder about the trauma?
1. Obtain validation of what the client says from another party.
2. Request that the client write down what's being said.
3. Ask questions to convey an interest in the details.
4. Listen attentively and remain with the client.

30. A client's survivor guilt is best indicated by which statement?
1. "I think I can see the purpose of my survival."
2. "I can't help but feel that everything is their fault."
3. "I now understand why I'm not able to forgive myself."
4. "I wish I could stop sabotaging my family relationships."

31. What is the best nursing action to assist a client with posttraumatic stress disorder and his family to handle interpersonal conflict at home?
1. Have the family teach the client to identify defensive behaviors.
2. Have the family discuss how to change dysfunctional family patterns.
3. Have the family agree not to tell the client what to do about problems.
4. Have the family arrange for the client to participate in social activities.

Mirror, mirror, on the wall, what's the greatest risk of all?

Thirty questions! Your survival skills are kicking in!

28. 4. The use of substances is a way for the client to deny problems and self-medicate distress. There are few homeless people with posttraumatic stress disorder as the cause of their homelessness. Most clients with posttraumatic stress disorder can manage money and maintain employment.
CN: Psychosocial integrity; CNS: None; CL: Application

29. 4. An effective communication strategy for a nurse to use with a posttraumatic stress disorder client is listening attentively and staying with the client. There's no need to obtain validation about what the client says by asking for information from another party, to ask the client to write what's being said, or to distract him by asking questions.
CN: Psychosocial integrity; CNS: None; CL: Application

30. 3. Survivor guilt occurs when the person has almost constant thoughts about the other people who perished in the event. The survivor doesn't understand why he survived when a friend or loved one didn't. Blaming self, not others, is a component of survivor guilt. Survivor guilt and impaired interpersonal relationships are two different categories of responses to trauma.
CN: Psychosocial integrity; CNS: None; CL: Analysis

31. 2. Discussion of dysfunctional family patterns allows the family to determine why and how these patterns are maintained. Having family members point out the defensive behaviors of the client may inadvertently produce more defensive behavior. Families can be a source of support and assistance; therefore, inflexible rules aren't useful to either the client or the family. The family shouldn't be encouraged to arrange social activities for the client. Social activities outside of the home don't help the family handle conflict within the home.
CN: Psychosocial integrity; CNS: None; CL: Application

CN: Client needs category   CNS: Client needs subcategory   CL: Cognitive level

32. Family members of a client diagnosed with posttraumatic stress disorder tell the nurse they cannot understand why the client has this disorder, especially because the client did not directly experience a personal trauma. What is the most appropriate intervention by the nurse?
1. Advise them to obtain a second psychiatric evaluation.
2. Ask them what they perceive the client's problem to be.
3. Explain the effect of learning about another's experience.
4. Identify the time period the client manifested symptoms.

32. 3. Posttraumatic stress disorder can occur if a person has experienced the traumatic event, witnessed the event happening to another person, or learned that trauma has happened to a family member or close friend. After educating the family about posttraumatic stress disorder, a second evaluation may not be necessary. Encouraging family members to discuss the situation and share their perceptions can be helpful, but it isn't their responsibility or within their abilities to diagnose the health problem. Symptoms of posttraumatic stress disorder usually appear 6 or more months after the event has occurred for at least a 1-month duration. This information isn't as important as an explanation of what constitutes a traumatic event.
CN: Psychosocial integrity; CNS: None; CL: Analysis

33. The effectiveness of monoamine oxidase inhibitor (MAOI) drug therapy in a client with posttraumatic stress disorder can be demonstrated by which client self-report?
1. "I'm sleeping better and don't have nightmares."
2. "I'm not losing my temper as much."
3. "I've lost my craving for alcohol."
4. "I've lost my phobia for water."

33. 1. MAOIs are used to treat sleep problems, nightmares, and intrusive daytime thoughts in individuals with posttraumatic stress disorder. MAOIs aren't used to help control flashbacks or phobias or to decrease the craving for alcohol.
CN: Physiological integrity; CNS: Pharmacological and parenteral therapies; CL: Analysis

34. What is the <u>major purpose</u> of group therapy for adolescents who witnessed the violent death of a peer?
1. To learn violence prevention strategies
2. To talk about appropriate expression of anger
3. To discuss the effect of the trauma on their lives
4. To develop trusting relationships among their peers

> The term *major purpose* indicates that there may be more than one right answer. You need to choose the best answer.

34. 3. By discussing the effect of the trauma on their lives, the adolescents can grieve and develop effective coping strategies. Learning violence prevention strategies isn't the most immediate concern after a trauma occurs nor is working on developing healthy relationships. It's appropriate to talk about how to express anger constructively after the trauma is addressed.
CN: Psychosocial integrity; CNS: None; CL: Application

35. Which symptom of posttraumatic stress disorder can be treated with hypnosis?
1. Addiction
2. Confabulation
3. Dissociation
4. Hallucinations

35. 3. Hypnosis is one of the main therapies for clients who dissociate. Hypnosis isn't a treatment of choice for clients with addictive disorders or hallucinations. Confabulation isn't a symptom of posttraumatic stress disorder.
CN: Psychosocial integrity; CNS: None; CL: Application

36. A nurse is assigned a client with anxiety disorder. What is the most appropriate intervention by the nurse to demonstrate caring?
1. Verbalize concern about the client.
2. Arrange group activities for the client.
3. Have the client sign the treatment plan.
4. Hold psychoeducational groups on medications.

It's important for the client to know you care.

37. The nurse is talking to a child with generalized anxiety disorder about school. The nurse anticipates that:
1. the child has been fighting with peers for the past month.
2. the child can't stop lying to parents and teachers.
3. the child has gained 15 lb (6.8 kg) in the past month.
4. the child expresses concerns about grades.

38. The nurse is aware that a client who has generalized anxiety disorder may also have which disorder?
1. Bipolar disorder
2. Gender identity disorder
3. Panic disorder
4. Schizoaffective disorder

What do you know about the relationship between anxiety and caffeine?

39. The nurse determines that nutritional teaching for a client with generalized anxiety disorder was successful when the client makes which statement?
1. "I've stopped drinking so much diet cola."
2. "I've reduced my intake of carbohydrates."
3. "I now eat less at dinner and before bedtime."
4. "I've cut back on my use of dairy products."

36. 1. The nurse who verbally expresses concern about a client's well-being is acting in a caring and supportive manner. Arranging for group activities may be an action where the nurse has no direct client contact and is therefore unable to have interpersonal contact with clients. Having a client sign the treatment plan may not be viewed as a sign of caring. Having a psychoeducational group on medications may be viewed by clients as a teaching experience and not interpersonal contact because the nurse may have limited interactions with them.
CN: Psychosocial integrity; CNS: None; CL: Application

37. 4. Children with generalized anxiety disorder will worry about how well they're performing in school. Children with generalized anxiety disorder don't tend to be involved in conflict. They're more oriented toward good behavior. Children with generalized anxiety disorder don't tend to lie to others. They would want to do their best and try to please others. A weight gain of 15 lb isn't a typical characteristic of a child with anxiety disorder.
CN: Psychosocial integrity; CNS: None; CL: Analysis

38. 3. Approximately 75% of clients with generalized anxiety disorder also may have a diagnosis of phobia, panic disorder, or substance abuse. Clients with generalized anxiety disorder don't tend to have a coexisting diagnosis of gender identity disorder, bipolar disorder, or schizoaffective disorder.
CN: Psychosocial integrity; CNS: None; CL: Application

39. 1. Clients with generalized anxiety disorder can decrease anxiety by eliminating caffeine from their diets. It isn't necessary for clients with generalized anxiety to decrease their carbohydrate intake, eat less at dinner or before bedtime (unless there are other compelling health reasons), or cut back on their use of dairy products.
CN: Physiological integrity; CNS: Basic care and comfort; CL: Application

40. A client with generalized anxiety disorder is refusing the prescribed benzodiazepine medication. What is the most likely explanation by the client for his response?
1. "I don't think the psychiatrist likes me."
2. "I want to solve my problems on my own."
3. "The voices tell me that I don't have to take the medication."
4. "I think my family gains by keeping me medicated."

40. 2. It's common for a client with generalized anxiety disorder to refuse to take medication because he believes that using a medication is a sign of personal weakness and that he can't solve problems by himself. Fear that the psychiatrist dislikes him reflects paranoid thinking that isn't usually seen in a client with generalized anxiety disorder. Auditory hallucinations and paranoia about the motives of friends and family members aren't characteristic of clients with generalized anxiety disorder.
CN: Psychosocial integrity; CNS: None; CL: Analysis

40 down, 54 to go!

41. The nurse is assisting a client with generalized anxiety disorder in verbalizing feelings. What is important for the nurse to consider?
1. The client may intellectualize the anxiety.
2. The client may regard the problem as genetic.
3. The client may decide that verbalizing feelings isn't beneficial.
4. The client may believe only medications are useful.

41. 1. Clients who experience generalized anxiety disorder commonly need assistance acknowledging anxiety instead of denying or intellectualizing it. Although scientists believe that there may be a tendency for anxiety to be familial, the problem isn't regarded as genetic. A client who's unwilling to express feelings may not view therapy as helpful. The most effective treatment of generalized anxiety disorder combines psychotherapy and pharmacotherapy.
CN: Psychosocial integrity; CNS: None; CL: Analysis

42. The nurse anticipates that an adult client with a long-standing history of generalized anxiety disorder would most likely make which statement?
1. "I was, and still am, an impulsive person."
2. "I've always been hyperactive but not in useful ways."
3. "When I was in college, I never thought I would finish."
4. "All my life I've had intrusive dreams and scary nightmares."

Certain psychological disorders tend to appear at particular ages—that's information to know for the NCLEX.

42. 3. For many people who have a generalized anxiety disorder, the age of onset is during young adulthood. The symptoms of impulsiveness and hyperactivity aren't commonly associated with a diagnosis of generalized anxiety disorder. Intrusive dreams and nightmares are associated with posttraumatic stress disorder rather than generalized anxiety disorder.
CN: Psychosocial integrity; CNS: None; CL: Analysis

43. The nurse is assessing a client with generalized anxiety disorder for muscle tension. The nurse anticipates that the client will display which symptom?
1. Difficulty sleeping
2. Restlessness
3. Strong startle response
4. Tachycardia

43. 2. Restlessness is a symptom associated with muscle tension. Difficulty sleeping and a strong startle response are considered symptoms of vigilance and scanning of the environment, not muscle tension. Tachycardia is classified as a symptom of autonomic hyperactivity, not muscle tension.
CN: Physiological integrity; CNS: Physiological adaptation; CL: Application

44. What is the <u>priority</u> nursing action for a client with generalized anxiety disorder who is working to develop coping skills?
   1. Determine whether the client has fears or obsessive thinking.
   2. Monitor the client for overt and covert signs of anxiety.
   3. Teach the client how to use effective communications skills.
   4. Assist the client to identify coping mechanisms used in the past.

45. The nurse is caring for a client who is experiencing escalating anxiety. What is the most appropriate intervention by the nurse?
   1. Explore the client's feelings about current life stressors.
   2. Have the client discuss the need to flee from painful situations.
   3. Encourage the client to develop a realistic view of self.
   4. Provide appropriate phone numbers for hotlines and clinics.

46. The nurse is teaching the family of an adult client about generalized anxiety disorder. It is most important for the nurse to do which of the following?
   1. Explain how the family can handle the confusion related to memory loss.
   2. Teach the family to assist the client with coping strategies as needed.
   3. Teach the family how to cope with the client's sudden and unexpected travel behavior.
   4. Have the family determine when and for what reasons the client should take medication.

47. A client with generalized anxiety disorder tells the nurse that he wants to stop taking his lorazepam (Ativan). What is the most appropriate response by the nurse?
   1. "Stopping the drug may cause depression."
   2. "Stopping the drug increases cognitive abilities."
   3. "Stopping the drug decreases sleeping difficulties."
   4. "Stopping the drug can cause withdrawal symptoms."

Thorough teaching plans typically include ways to contact support organizations.

You should be familiar with the symptoms that discontinuing key medications may cause.

44. 4. To help a client develop effective coping skills, the nurse must know the client's baseline functioning. Determining whether the client has fears or obsessive thinking, monitoring for signs of anxiety, and teaching about effective communications skills are later priorities, not initial ones.
CN: Safe, effective care environment; CNS: Management of care; CL: Application

45. 4. By having information on hotlines and clinics, the client can pursue help when the anxiety is escalating. Discussion about current life stressors isn't useful when focusing on how best to handle the client's escalating anxiety. Fleeing from painful situations and discussing views of oneself aren't the best strategies, neither allows for problem solving.
CN: Psychosocial integrity; CNS: None; CL: Application

46. 2. The family can be there for support, but they negate the client's ability to function if they take control of the situation and don't allow the client to use his own coping skills. A client who has confusion related to memory loss is commonly struggling with dissociative amnesia, not a generalized anxiety disorder. Sudden and unexpected travel behavior is a problem for families who have members with dissociative identity disorder, not generalized anxiety disorder. The client must handle and use medication as prescribed.
CN: Psychosocial integrity; CNS: None; CL: Application

47. 4. Stopping antianxiety drugs such as benzodiazepines can cause the client to have withdrawal symptoms. Stopping a benzodiazepine doesn't tend to cause depression, increase cognitive abilities, or decrease sleeping difficulties.
CN: Physiological integrity; CNS: Pharmacological and parenteral therapies; CL: Application

48. Five days after running out of medication, a client taking clonazepam (Klonopin) says to the nurse, "I know I shouldn't have just stopped the drug like that, but I'm OK." What is the most appropriate response by the nurse?
1. "Let's monitor you for problems, in case something else happens."
2. "You could go through withdrawal symptoms for up to 2 weeks."
3. "You have handled your anxiety, and you now know how to cope with stress."
4. "If you're fine now, chances are you won't experience withdrawal symptoms."

They'll notice I'm gone in a few weeks.

49. A client taking alprazolam (Xanax) reports light-headedness and nausea every day while getting out of bed. What is the most important action by the nurse?
1. Take the client's blood pressure.
2. Monitor body temperature.
3. Teach the Valsalva maneuver.
4. Obtain a blood chemical profile.

50. A client with generalized anxiety disorder complains of a headache and upset stomach to the nurse. The nurse assesses the client and is aware that the client may:
1. have a variety of somatic complaints.
2. experience an alteration in self-care skills.
3. undergo unhealthy binge eating episodes.
4. experience secondary gains from mental illness.

Stay focused on the topic at hand.

51. The nurse needs to communicate with a client experiencing mania. It is most important for the nurse to do which of the following?
1. Address the client in a light and joking manner.
2. Focus and redirect the conversation as necessary.
3. Allow the client to talk about several different topics.
4. Ask only open-ended questions to facilitate conversation.

48. 2. Withdrawal syndrome symptoms can appear after 1 or 2 weeks because the benzodiazepine has a long half-life. Looking for another problem unrelated to withdrawal isn't the nurse's best strategy. The act of discontinuing an antianxiety medication doesn't indicate that a client has learned to cope with stress. Every client taking medication needs to be monitored for withdrawal symptoms when the medication is stopped abruptly.
CN: Physiological integrity; CNS: Pharmacological and parenteral therapies; CL: Analysis

49. 1. The nurse should take a blood pressure reading to validate orthostatic hypotension. A body temperature reading or chemistry profile won't yield useful information about hypotension. The Valsalva maneuver is performed to lower the heart rate and isn't an appropriate intervention.
CN: Physiological integrity; CNS: Reduction of risk potential; CL: Application

50. 1. Clients with anxiety disorders commonly experience somatic symptoms. They don't usually experience problems with self-care. Eating problems aren't a typical part of the diagnostic criteria for anxiety disorders. Not all clients obtain secondary gains from mental illness.
CN: Psychosocial integrity; CNS: None; CL: Application

51. 2. To decrease stimulation, the nurse should attempt to redirect and focus the client's communication, not allow the client to talk about different topics. By addressing the client in a light and joking manner, the conversation may contribute to the client's feeling out of control. For a manic client, it's best to ask closed questions because open-ended questions may enable the client to talk endlessly, again possibly contributing to the client's feeling out of control.
CN: Psychosocial integrity; CNS: None; CL: Application

52. A nurse is providing teaching for a client with bipolar disorder who is scheduled for electroconvulsive therapy (ECT). The client asks the nurse if there are any adverse effects from the therapy. What is the best response by the nurse?
1. Cholestatic jaundice
2. Hypertensive crisis
3. Mouth ulcers
4. Respiratory distress

53. A client who has just had electroconvulsive therapy (ECT) asks the nurse for a drink of water. What is the <u>most important</u> intervention by the nurse?
1. Take the client's blood pressure.
2. Monitor the gag reflex.
3. Obtain a body temperature.
4. Determine the level of consciousness.

54. The nurse is assessing the behavior of a client with hypomania. The nurse would expect the client to be:
1. on the verge of depression and crisis.
2. indecisive and vacillating, with a diminished ability to think.
3. irritable, with an elevated mood and symptoms of mania.
4. disorganized, tending to exhibit impaired judgment.

55. A client with bipolar disorder is complaining of headache, agitation, and indigestion. The nurse understands that this client is <u>most likely</u> experiencing which of the following?
1. Depression
2. Cyclothymia
3. Hypomania
4. Mania

What harm could result from a glass of water?

The words most likely *can help you focus on the answer.*

52. 4. Respiratory distress or even arrest may occur as a complication of the anesthesia used with ECT. Cholestatic jaundice, hypertensive crisis, and mouth ulcers don't occur during or as a result of ECT.
CN: Physiological integrity; CNS: Physiological adaptation; CL: Application

53. 2. The nurse must check the client's gag reflex before allowing the client to have a drink after an ECT procedure. Blood pressure and body temperature don't influence whether the client may have a drink after the procedure. The client would obviously be conscious if he's requesting a glass of water.
CN: Physiological integrity; CNS: Physiological adaptation; CL: Analysis

54. 3. When a client is hypomanic, there's evidence of an elevated and irritable mood, along with mild or beginning symptoms of mania. A hypomanic client is experiencing a period of mild elation, not a depression or crisis. Indecision and vacillation with a diminished ability to think are symptoms more likely seen in a major depressive episode than in a hypomanic episode. A client with hypomania tends to be creative and more productive than usual, rather than disorganized with impaired judgment.
CN: Psychosocial integrity; CNS: None; CL: Analysis

55. 4. Headache, agitation, and indigestion are symptoms suggestive of mania in a client with a history of bipolar disorder. These symptoms are not suggestive of depression, cyclothymia, or hypomania.
CN: Physiological integrity; CNS: Physiological adaptation; CL: Application

56. A client with bipolar disorder tells the nurse that he has suddenly stopped taking his medication. The nurse assesses the client and is aware that which behavior would indicate the client is experiencing a manic episode?
1. Binge eating
2. Relationship avoidance
3. Sudden relocation
4. Thoughtless spending

Know the behaviors associated with each disorder.

57. A client who is experiencing a manic episode has been admitted to the unit. What is the most important intervention by the nurse to provide adequate nutrition for the client?
1. Determine the client's metabolic rate.
2. Make the client sit down for each meal and snack.
3. Give the client foods to be eaten while he's active.
4. Have the client interact with a dietician twice a week.

58. The nurse is providing discharge teaching for a client who will be taking lithium. The nurse determines that teaching was effective when the client states the need to notify the health care provider if he experiences:
1. black tongue.
2. increased lacrimation.
3. periods of excitability.
4. persistent GI upset.

Lithium has adverse effects specifically associated with pregnancy.

59. A client with bipolar disorder tells the nurse she just found out she is pregnant and is concerned because she takes lithium. What is the most important information for the nurse to provide the client?
1. Use of lithium usually results in serious congenital problems.
2. Thyroid problems can occur in the first trimester of the pregnancy.
3. Lithium causes severe urine retention and increased risk of toxicity.
4. Women who take lithium are very likely to have a spontaneous abortion.

56. 4. Thoughtless or reckless spending is a common symptom of a manic episode. Binge eating isn't a behavior that's characteristic of a client during a manic episode. Relationship avoidance doesn't occur in a client experiencing a manic episode; during episodes of mania, a client may in fact interact with many people and participate in unsafe sexual behavior. Sudden relocation isn't a characteristic of impulsive behavior demonstrated by a client with bipolar disorder.
CN: Psychosocial integrity; CNS: None; CL: Application

57. 3. By giving the client high-calorie foods that can be eaten while he's active, the nurse facilitates the client's nutritional intake. Determining the client's metabolic rate isn't useful information when the client is experiencing mania. During a manic episode, the client can't be still or focused long enough to interact with a dietitian or sit still long enough to eat.
CN: Physiological integrity; CNS: Basic care and comfort; CL: Application

58. 4. Persistent GI upset indicates a mild-to-moderate toxic reaction. Black tongue is an adverse reaction of mirtazapine (Remeron), not lithium. Increased lacrimation and periods of excitability aren't adverse effects of lithium.
CN: Physiological integrity; CNS: Pharmacological and parenteral therapies; CL: Application

59. 1. Use of lithium during pregnancy results in congenital defects, especially cardiac defects. Thyroid problems don't occur in the first trimester of the pregnancy. In lithium toxicity, a condition called nontoxic goiter may occur. An adverse effect of lithium is polyuria, not urine retention. The rate of spontaneous abortion for women taking lithium is no greater than for nonusers.
CN: Physiological integrity; CNS: Pharmacological and parenteral therapies; CL: Application

60. A nurse is teaching a client with bipolar disorder about the drug carbamazepine (Tegretol). The nurse determines teaching was effective when the client makes which statement?
1. "My hair will fall out if I take this drug."
2. "I will drink plenty of water so I don't develop kidney problems."
3. "I need to have my blood counts checked periodically."
4. "I can't take any other drugs with this one."

61. The nurse is developing a plan of care for a client with bipolar disorder. It would be most important for the nurse to include which suggestion?
1. Obtain medication for sleep.
2. Work on solving a problem.
3. Exercise before bedtime.
4. Develop a sleep ritual.

62. Family members of a client with bipolar disorder tell the nurse that they are distressed about the client's episodes of manic behavior and are unsure of what to do. What is the most important information for the nurse to give the family?
1. Ways to protect oneself from the client's behavior
2. How to proceed with an involuntary commitment
3. How to confront the client about the reckless behavior
4. When to safely increase medication during manic periods

63. A client who is taking lithium asks the nurse why it is necessary to have his blood drawn for a lithium level. What is the <u>most appropriate</u> response by the nurse?
1. Lithium levels are obtained to determine liver and renal damage.
2. Lithium levels demonstrate whether the client is taking a therapeutic dose range of the drug.
3. Lithium levels indicate whether the drug has passed through the blood-brain barrier.
4. Lithium levels are unnecessary if the client takes the drug as ordered.

My immediate sleep goal is a 10-minute nap.

Monitoring blood levels helps ensure that adequate doses of lithium are being administered.

60. 3. The most dangerous adverse effect of carbamazepine is bone marrow depression. Other medications may be taken with carbamazepine. Hair loss doesn't occur in clients taking carbamazepine. Clients who take lithium, not carbamazepine, must be closely monitored for nephrogenic diabetes insipidus. The interactions of all drugs being taken must be monitored because some drugs can either increase or decrease the blood level of carbamazepine.
CN: Physiological integrity; CNS: Pharmacological and parenteral therapies; CL: Analysis

61. 4. A sleep ritual or nighttime routine helps the client to relax and prepare for sleep. Obtaining sleep medication is a temporary solution. Working on problem solving may excite the client rather than tire him. Exercise before retiring is inappropriate.
CN: Physiological integrity; CNS: Reduction of risk potential; CL: Application

62. 1. Family members need to assess their needs and develop ways to protect themselves. Clients who have symptoms of impulsive or reckless behavior might not be candidates for hospitalization. Confronting the client during a manic episode may escalate the behavior. The family must never increase the dosage of prescribed medication without first consulting the primary health care provider.
CN: Safe, effective care environment; CNS: Safety and infection control; CL: Application

63. 2. Lithium levels determine whether an effective dose of lithium is being given to maintain a therapeutic level of the drug. The drug is contraindicated for clients with renal, cardiac, or liver disease. Lithium levels aren't drawn for the purpose of determining whether the drug passes through the blood-brain barrier. Taking the drug as ordered doesn't eliminate the need for blood work.
CN: Physiological integrity; CNS: Pharmacological and parenteral therapies; CL: Application

64. What is the most important information for the nurse to include when providing <u>nutritional counseling</u> for family members of a client with bipolar disorder?
1. If sufficient roughage isn't eaten while taking lithium, bowel problems will occur.
2. If the intake of carbohydrates increases, the lithium level will increase.
3. If the intake of calories is reduced, the lithium level will increase.
4. If the intake of sodium increases, the lithium level will decrease.

65. The nurse teaches a client with bipolar disorder effective coping strategies. The nurse determines that teaching was successful when the client makes which statement?
1. "I can decide what to do to prevent family conflict."
2. "I can handle problems without asking for any help."
3. "I can stay away from my friends when I feel distressed."
4. "I can ignore things that go wrong instead of getting upset."

66. The nurse is developing a plan of care for a client with depression who has been admitted to the inpatient unit because of an attempted suicide. What is the <u>priority</u> goal for this client?
1. The client will seek out the nurse when feeling self-destructive.
2. The client will identify and discuss actual and perceived losses.
3. The client will learn strategies to promote relaxation and self-care.
4. The client will establish healthy and mutually caring relationships.

67. A nurse is caring for a client who reports that he thinks about suicide every day. The nurse anticipates that the client's care will include which of the following?
1. A no-suicide contract
2. Weekly outpatient therapy
3. A second psychiatric opinion
4. Intensive inpatient treatment

It's important to know how medications interact with foods.

You shouldn't have to ask what short-term goal is most appropriate!

64. **4.** Any time the level of sodium increases, such as with a change in dietary intake, the level of lithium will decrease. The intake of roughage and carbohydrates in the diet isn't related to the metabolism of lithium. Reducing the number of calories the client eats doesn't affect the lithium level in the body.

CN: Physiological integrity; CNS: Reduction of risk potential; CL: Analysis

65. **1.** The client should be focusing on his strengths and abilities to prevent family conflict. Not being able to ask for help is problematic and not a good coping strategy. Avoiding problems also isn't a good coping strategy. It's better to identify and handle problems as they arise. Ignoring situations that cause discomfort won't facilitate solutions or allow the client to demonstrate effective coping skills.

CN: Psychosocial integrity; CNS: None; CL: Analysis

66. **1.** By seeking out the nurse when feeling self-destructive, the client can feel safe and begin to see that there are coping skills to assist in dealing with self-destructive tendencies. Discussion of losses also is important when dealing with feelings of depression, but the priority intervention is still to promote immediate client safety. Although relationship building and learning strategies to promote relaxation and self-care are important goals, safety is the priority intervention.

CN: Safe, effective care environment; CNS: Management of care; CL: Analysis

67. **4.** For a client thinking about suicide on a daily basis, inpatient care would be the best intervention. Although a no-suicide contract is an important strategy, this client needs additional care. The client needs a more intensive level of care than weekly outpatient therapy. Immediate intervention is paramount, not a second psychiatric opinion.

CN: Safe, effective care environment; CNS: Management of care; CL: Application

68. The nurse is developing short-term goals for a client who repeatedly makes statements about not deserving things. The nurse determines that which of the following is an appropriate <u>short-term goal</u>?
1. Identify distorted thoughts.
2. Describe self-care patterns.
3. Discuss family relationships.
4. Explore communication skills.

69. The nurse is caring for a client who is manifesting negative expectations. The nurse determines that which of the following is an appropriate intervention for this client?
1. Encourage the client to discuss spiritual matters.
2. Assist the client to learn how to problem solve.
3. Help the client explore issues related to loss.
4. Have the client identify positive aspects of self.

70. The nurse is concerned that a client admitted with depression may be suicidal. What is the <u>most appropriate</u> action by the nurse?
1. Speak to family members to ascertain whether the client is suicidal.
2. Talk to the client to determine whether the client is an attention seeker.
3. Arrange for the client to be placed on immediate suicidal precautions.
4. Ask a direct question such as, "Do you ever think about killing yourself?"

71. A client diagnosed with <u>major depression</u> has been admitted to an inpatient unit. The client's family members are upset and tell the nurse they do not understand what is wrong. What is the best response by the nurse?
1. Address how depression is a lifelong illness.
2. Explain that depression is an illness and can be treated.
3. Describe how depression masks a person's true feelings.
4. Teach how depression causes frequent disorganized thinking.

You're doing great in the short term, and your long-term goal is in sight.

Depression affects the entire family.

68. **1.** It's important to identify distorted thinking because self-deprecating thoughts lead to depression. Self-care patterns don't necessarily reflect distorted thinking. Family relationships might not influence distorted thinking patterns. A form of communication called negative self-talk would be explored only after distorted thinking patterns were identified.
CN: Psychosocial integrity; CNS: None; CL: Application

69. **4.** An important intervention used to counter negative expectations is to focus on the positive and have the client explore positive aspects of himself. Discussion of spiritual matters doesn't address the need to change negative expectations. Learning how to problem solve won't modify the client's negative expectations. If the client dwells on the negative and focuses on loss, it will be natural to have negative expectations.
CN: Psychosocial integrity; CNS: None; CL: Application

70. **4.** The best approach to determining whether a client is suicidal is to ask about thoughts of suicide in a direct and caring manner. Assessing for attention-seeking behaviors doesn't deal directly with the problem. The client should be assessed directly, not through family members. Assessment must be performed before determining whether suicide precautions are necessary.
CN: Psychosocial integrity; CNS: None; CL: Application

71. **2.** The nurse must help the family understand depression, its impact on the family, and recommended treatments. Depression doesn't need to be a lifelong illness. It's important to help families understand that depression can be successfully treated and that, in some situations, depression can reoccur during the life cycle. The feelings expressed by the client are genuine; they reflect cognitive distortions and disillusionment. Disorganized thinking is more commonly associated with schizophrenia rather than with depression.
CN: Psychosocial integrity; CNS: None; CL: Application

72. A client diagnosed with major depression asks the nurse why he is taking mirtazapine (Remeron) instead of imipramine hydrochloride (Tofranil). What is the best response by the nurse?
1. The newer serotonin reuptake inhibitor drugs are better tested drugs.
2. The serotonin reuptake inhibitors have few adverse effects.
3. The serotonin reuptake inhibitors require a low dose of antidepressant drug.
4. The serotonin reuptake inhibitors are as good as other antidepressant drugs.

73. A nurse is selecting interventions to enhance the self-esteem of a client with depression. What is the most appropriate intervention for this client?
1. Playing cards
2. Praying daily
3. Taking medication
4. Writing poetry

74. An adolescent who is depressed and reportedly having difficulty in school is brought to the community mental health center by his parents for evaluation. The nurse performs an assessment and suspects the client may also be experiencing which of the following?
1. Anxiety disorder
2. Behavioral difficulties
3. Cognitive impairment
4. Labile moods

75. The nurse is developing a plan of care for a client with a risk of suicide. What is the most important nursing intervention for the nurse to include?
1. Using a caring approach
2. Developing a strong relationship with the client
3. Establishing a suicide contract to ensure his safety
4. Encouraging avoidance of overstimulating activities

You've completed 75 questions. The rest should be smooth sailing.

72. 2. The serotonin reuptake inhibitors are drugs with few adverse effects and are unlikely to be toxic in an overdose. All drugs must be tested through a government-specified protocol. Comparison of two different types of antidepressant medications isn't useful. The final statement doesn't give the client helpful information.
CN: Physiological integrity; CNS: Pharmacological and parenteral therapies; CL: Analysis

73. 4. Writing poetry or engaging in some other creative outlet will enhance self-esteem. Playing cards and praying don't necessarily promote self-esteem. Taking medication will decrease symptoms of depression after a blood level is established, but it won't, by itself, promote self-esteem.
CN: Psychosocial integrity; CNS: None; CL: Application

74. 2. Adolescents tend to demonstrate severe irritability and behavioral problems rather than simply a depressed mood. Anxiety disorder is more commonly associated with small children rather than with adolescents. Cognitive impairment is typically associated with delirium or dementia. Labile mood is more characteristic of a client with cognitive impairment or bipolar disorder.
CN: Psychosocial integrity; CNS: None; CL: Analysis

75. 3. Establishing a suicide contract with the client demonstrates that the nurse's concern for his safety is a priority and that his life is of value. When a client agrees to a suicide contract, it decreases his risk of a successful attempt. Caring alone ignores the underlying mechanism of the client's wish to commit suicide. Merely developing a strong relationship with the client isn't addressing the potential the client has for harming himself. Encouraging the client to stay away from activities could cause isolation, which would be detrimental to the client's well-being.
CN: Psychosocial integrity; CNS: None; CL: Application

76. Which nursing diagnosis is most likely to be on the care plan of a client with a phobia about elevators?
1. Social isolation related to a lack of social skills
2. Disturbed sleep pattern related to a fear of elevators
3. Ineffective coping related to poor coping skills
4. Anxiety related to fear of elevators

77. Which behavior modification technique is most beneficial in the treatment of phobias?
1. Aversion therapy
2. Imitation or modeling
3. Positive reinforcement
4. Systematic desensitization

No need to fear this question—focus on which technique would be useful.

78. What is the best statement for the nurse to make when teaching the client and family about phobias and the need for a strong family support system?
1. The use of a family support system is only temporary.
2. The need to be assertive can be reinforced by the family.
3. The family must set limits on inappropriate behaviors.
4. The family plays a role in promoting client independence.

79. The nurse has provided medication teaching for a client who will be taking alprazolam (Xanax) upon discharge from the hospital. The nurse determines that teaching was effective when the client states the need to avoid which of the following?
1. Shellfish
2. Alcohol
3. Coffee
4. Cheese

76. 3. Poor coping skills can cause ineffective coping. Such a client isn't relegated to social isolation, and lack of social skills has nothing to do with phobia. Fear of elevators is a manifestation, not the cause, of altered thoughts and anxiety.
CN: Psychosocial integrity; CNS: None; CL: Analysis

77. 4. Systematic desensitization is a common behavior modification technique that has been successfully used to help treat phobia. Aversion therapy and positive reinforcement aren't behavior modification techniques used with the treatment of phobias. The techniques of imitation or modeling are social learning techniques, not behavior modification techniques.
CN: Psychosocial integrity; CNS: None; CL: Application

78. 4. The family plays a vital role in supporting a client in treatment and in preventing the client from using the phobia to obtain secondary gains. Family support must be ongoing, not temporary. The family can be more helpful by focusing on effective handling of anxiety, rather than focusing energy on developing assertiveness skills. People with phobias are already restrictive in their behavior; more restrictions aren't necessary.
CN: Psychosocial integrity; CNS: None; CL: Analysis

79. 2. Alcohol should be avoided because of additive depressive effects. Ingestion of shellfish, coffee, and cheese isn't problematic.
CN: Physiological integrity; CNS: Pharmacological and parenteral therapies; CL: Application

80. A female client describes her unpredictable episodes of acute anxiety as "just awful." She says that she feels like she's about to die and can hardly breathe. The nurse interprets these symptoms as indicating which condition?
1. Agoraphobia
2. Dissociative disorder
3. Posttraumatic stress disorder (PTSD)
4. Panic disorder

81. A client who was diagnosed with major depression 3 weeks ago tells the nurse that he is feeling better since he started taking the prescribed antidepressant medication. The nurse is aware that it is most important to assess the client for which of the following?
1. Manic depression
2. Potential for violence
3. Substance abuse
4. Suicidal ideation

82. The nurse is performing an initial admission assessment on a 40-year-old client with a diagnosis of major depression. The client was brought to the hospital by her husband who states that the client refused to get out of bed for 2 days, has not eaten, is tired all the time, and has neglected her household responsibilities. What is the most important question for the nurse to ask the client at this time?
1. "What has been troubling you?"
2. "Why do you dislike yourself?"
3. "How do you feel about your life?"
4. "What can we do to help?"

83. A client with bipolar disorder has been receiving lithium (Eskalith) for 2 weeks. He also takes chemotherapeutic drugs that cause him to feel nauseated and anorexic. It is most important for the nurse to assess the client for which of the following?
1. Hyperpyrexia
2. Marked arthritis
3. Hypotonic reflexes with muscle weakness
4. Oliguria

Don't panic if the answer isn't immediately clear—read through the question carefully and eliminate the obvious incorrect options first.

Timing is critical here. Read the question again if you have any doubts about what's being asked.

80. 4. This client is describing the characteristics of someone with panic disorder. Agoraphobia is characterized by fear of public places; dissociative disorder, by lost periods of time; and PTSD, by hypervigilance and sleep disturbance.
CN: Psychosocial integrity; CNS: None; CL: Application

81. 4. After a client has been on antidepressants and is feeling better, he commonly then has the energy to harm himself. Manic depression isn't treated with antidepressants. Nothing in the client's history suggests a potential for violence. There are no signs or symptoms suggesting substance abuse.
CN: Safe, effective care environment; CNS: Safety and infection control; CL: Analysis

82. 3. The nurse must develop nursing interventions based on the client's perceived problems and feelings. Asking the client to draw a conclusion may be difficult for her at this time. *Why* questions can place the client in a defensive position. Requiring the client to find possible solutions is beyond the scope of her present abilities.
CN: Psychosocial integrity; CNS: None; CL: Analysis

83. 3. Lithium alters sodium transport in nerve and muscle cells, slowing the speed of impulse transmission, so look for hypotonic reflexes and muscle weakness. Lithium has no known effect on body temperature or on the transmission of pain impulses. The drug doesn't cause arthritis. Oliguria and other signs of renal failure occur late in severe lithium toxicity.
CN: Physiologic integrity; CNS: Pharmacological and parenteral therapies; CL: Application

84. A client with a history of bipolar disorder was admitted to the psychiatric unit 2 days ago. The client stopped taking lithium (Eskalith) 2 weeks ago and is now in a manic phase. The nurse would anticipate the client's assessment to include which finding?
1. Flight of ideas
2. Echolalia
3. Clang associations
4. Neologism

85. An acutely manic client kisses a nurse on the lips and asks her to marry him. The nurse is taken by surprise. What is the most appropriate response by the nurse?
1. Seclude the client for his inappropriate behavior.
2. Ask the client what he's trying to prove by his behavior.
3. Ask the client to fold some laundry.
4. Tell the client his behavior is offensive.

86. The nurse is preparing discharge instructions for a client taking lithium (Eskalith). What is the most important information for the nurse to give the client?
1. Limit fluids to 1,500 ml daily.
2. Maintain a high fluid intake.
3. Take advantage of the warm weather by exercising outside whenever possible.
4. When feeling a cold coming, it's OK to take over-the-counter (OTC) remedies.

87. A nurse is teaching a client who was recently diagnosed with dysthymic disorder about the condition. What is the most appropriate information for the nurse to include?
1. It involves a mood range from moderate depression to hypomania.
2. It involves a single manic episode.
3. It's a form of depression that occurs in the fall and winter.
4. It's a mood disorder similar to major depression but of mild to moderate severity.

84. 1. Flight of ideas is a speech pattern characterized by rapid transition from topic to topic, typically without finishing one idea. It's common in mania. Echolalia (repetition of words heard), clang associations (use of rhyming), and neologism (inverted words) aren't seen in mania states.
CN: Psychosocial integrity; CNS: None; CL: Application

85. 3. Having the client help with laundry rechannels his energy in a positive activity. The client needs direction and structure, not seclusion. Asking the client what he's trying to prove ignores his impaired judgment and poor impulse control. Telling the client that his behavior is offensive doesn't assist him in controlling his behavior.
CN: Psychosocial integrity; CNS: None; CL: Application

86. 2. Clients taking lithium need to maintain a high fluid intake. Exercising outside may not be safe; photosensitivity occurs with lithium use, and activity in warm weather could increase sodium loss, predisposing the client to lithium toxicity. The client shouldn't take OTC drugs without the physician's approval.
CN: Physiological integrity; CNS: Pharmacological and parenteral therapies; CL: Application

87. 4. Dysthymic disorder is a mood disorder similar to major depression, but it remains mild to moderate in severity. Cyclothymic disorder is a mood disorder characterized by a mood range from moderate depression to hypomania. Bipolar I disorder is characterized by a single manic episode with no past major depressive episodes. Seasonal affective disorder is a form of depression occurring in the fall and winter.
CN: Psychosocial integrity; CNS: None; CL: Application

I'd better read this question carefully to determine which statement is true.

88. A depressed client who is taking a prescribed tricyclic antidepressant tells the nurse he is sleepy all the time and does not feel like doing anything. What is the best response by the nurse?
1. Tell the client to stop taking the drug until he sees his physician.
2. Advise the client to continue taking the drug to see whether these effects wear off.
3. Ask the physician whether the medication can be given in one dose at bedtime.
4. Advise the client to get another opinion.

89. A depressed client is now taking trazodone (Desyrel). The client asks the nurse when the medication should be taken. What is the best response by the nurse?
1. In the morning
2. At bedtime
3. At any time during the day
4. When the client has an urge for a cigarette

90. A nurse is teaching a client about tricyclic antidepressants. The nurse determines that teaching has been effective when the client makes which statement?
1. "This drug causes photosensitivity."
2. "I should avoid milk and dairy products."
3. "I should notify my physician if my mood doesn't improve within 7 days."
4. "Mood improvement takes up to 28 days."

91. The nurse is developing interventions for a client newly diagnosed with type 1 diabetes who has a blood-injection-injury phobia. What is the most appropriate intervention for this client?
1. Teach the client to avoid fainting by tensing the muscles of the legs and abdomen.
2. Quickly expose the client to feared situations.
3. Have the client avoid as much medical care as possible.
4. Focus on treating the symptoms with an antianxiety medication.

I just don't feel like doing anything.

All I'm asking for is a little patience.

88. 3. Many tricyclic antidepressants can be given safely in one dose; when an antidepressant is taken at bedtime, the adverse effect of drowsiness can help the client sleep. It's inappropriate for the nurse to tell the client to stop taking the drug, to continue taking it until the undesired effects wear off, or to seek a second opinion.
CN: Physiological integrity; CNS: Pharmacological and parenteral therapies; CL: Application

89. 2. Trazodone has a strong sedative effect and is commonly prescribed as a sleep aid to be taken at bedtime. Wellbutrin is used for smoking cessation.
CN: Physiological integrity; CNS: Pharmacological and parenteral therapies; CL: Application

90. 4. The client's mood may not improve until the third or fourth week of tricyclic antidepressant therapy. The client needs to be reassured that the drug works slowly. The drug doesn't cause photosensitivity or interact with milk and dairy products.
CN: Physiological integrity; CNS: Pharmacological and parenteral therapies; CL: Application

91. 1. The client may be able to avoid fainting and relieve hypotension by tensing the larger muscle groups. Desensitization by slowly, not quickly, exposing the client to blood injection is indicated to reduce fear. Clients with blood-injection-injury phobia may avoid all medical care, which is dangerous to their health. Antianxiety medications may help on a short-term basis only.
CN: Psychosocial integrity; CNS: None; CL: Application

92. A socially phobic client has a nursing diagnosis of fear related to being embarrassed in the presence of others. What should the goals be for this client? Select all that apply.
1. Manage his fear in group situations.
2. Develop a plan to avoid situations that may cause stress.
3. Verbalize feelings that occur in stressful situations.
4. Develop a plan for responding to stressful situations.
5. Deny feelings that may contribute to irrational fears.
6. Use suppression to deal with underlying fears.

93. The nurse recognizes improvement in a client with the nursing diagnosis of ineffective role performance related to the need to perform rituals. The nurse identifies which behaviors as indicating improvement? Select all that apply.
1. The client refrains from performing rituals during stress.
2. The client verbalizes that he uses "thought stopping" when obsessive thoughts occur.
3. The client verbalizes the relationship between stress and ritualistic behaviors.
4. The client avoids stressful situations.
5. The client rationalizes ritualistic behavior.
6. The client performs ritualistic behaviors in private.

94. After interviewing a client diagnosed with recurrent depression, the nurse determines the client's potential to commit suicide. What factors should the nurse consider as contributing to the client's suicide potential? Select all that apply.
1. Psychomotor retardation
2. Impulsive behaviors
3. Overwhelming feelings of guilt
4. Chronic, debilitating illness
5. Decreased physical activity
6. Repression of anger

92. 1, 3, and 4. Improving stress-management skills, verbalizing feelings, and anticipating and planning for stressful situations are adaptive responses to stress. Avoidance, denial, and suppression are maladaptive defense mechanisms.
CN: Psychosocial integrity; CNS: None; CL: Application

93. 1, 2, and 3. Refraining from rituals demonstrates that the client manages stress appropriately. Using "thought stopping" demonstrates the client's ability to employ appropriate interventions for obsessive thoughts. Verbalizing the relationship between stress and behaviors indicates that the client understands the disease process. Avoiding, rationalizing, and hiding behaviors demonstrate maladaptive methods for managing stress and anxiety.
CN: Psychosocial integrity; CNS: None; CL: Analysis

Congratulations! Good job!

94. 2, 3, 4, and 6. Impulsive behavior, overwhelming guilt, chronic illness, and anger repression are factors that contribute to suicide potential. Psychomotor retardation and decreased activity are symptoms of depression but don't typically lead to suicide because the client doesn't have the energy to harm himself.
CN: Psychosocial integrity; CNS: None; CL: Analysis

CN: Client needs category   CNS: Client needs subcategory   CL: Cognitive level

This chapter covers a host of cognitive disorders. Are your own cognitive powers ready? OK, let's go!

Chapter 15
Cognitive disorders

1. The nurse is asking a client in the psychiatric crisis unit specific questions about recent substance use. Which assessment finding could indicate to the nurse that the client is experiencing mild to moderate delirium?
1. Time and place disorientation
2. Impaired abstract thinking
3. Persistent memory disturbance
4. Changes in personality

2. The nurse is explaining the symptoms of dementia to a military family member who has not seen his mother in 15 months. Which characteristics of dementia of the Alzheimer's type would the nurse address in her teaching session? Select all that apply.
1. Experiences an impending sense of doom
2. Forgets that food is cooking on the stove
3. Becomes lost walking on her own street
4. Unable to write and to sign her name
5. Begins to fear using public transportation
6. Unable to understand new information

3. During an interaction with the spouse of a client with Alzheimer's disease, the nurse is asked the following question: "What exactly is Alzheimer's disease?" Which is the correct explanation for the nurse to tell the spouse?
1. "Often, Alzheimer's disease is a combination of several common autoimmune diseases that attack and shrink brain tissue."
2. "It is a brain disease that results from the development of abnormal structures called neurofibrillary tangles found in the person's brain."
3. "The disease is a genetic disease that changes a person's brain tissue, causing it to deteriorate due to an accumulation of excessive fluid."
4. "A biological and psychosocial component of undiagnosed moderate depression is causing a steady decline in daily performance."

What is the best response???

1. 1. Clients with delirium experience disorientation to time, then place, and then person. Impaired abstract thinking and noted changes in personality are characteristics of dementia. Persistent memory disturbance is associated with an amnestic disorder.
CN: Physiological integrity; CNS: Physiological adaptation; CL: Analysis

2. 2, 3, 4, and 6. Common symptoms of dementia of the Alzheimer's type include forgetting things such as cooking food and where specific items were placed, becoming lost in one's own neighborhood, being unable to write or even sign one's name to a document, and being unable to understand new information. A client experiencing an impending sense of doom and fearing public transportation is most likely dealing with a panic attack with agoraphobia.
CN: Health promotion and maintenance; CNS: None; CL: Application

3. 2. People with Alzheimer's disease have a disease of the brain where abnormal structures composed of twisted protein fibers (neurofibrillary tangles) are found within the nerve cells. These neurofibrillary tangles attack the inside of the neurons. The possible link of autoimmune diseases to Alzheimer's disease as well as the genetic errors identified on chromosomes 14, 19, and 21 along with biological and neurochemical problems are currently being investigated.
CN: Physiological integrity; CNS: Physiological adaptation; CL: Analysis

4. The home health nurse notices that the elderly, diabetic client she sees every week is starting to demonstrate some difficulty answering questions about her chronic disease strategies and self-management activities. Which action would the nurse take to validate her suspicion of the client having cognitive changes and possibly the beginning stages of dementia?
1. Speak to the doctor about ordering cardiac diagnostic studies.
2. Petition the insurance company for a weekly home health aide.
3. Request that another nurse visit and perform a mental status exam.
4. Arrange to speak to a family caregiver as soon as possible.

The answer is on the tip of my tongue, but I just can't remember.

5. A nurse is caring for a client with delirium. Which nursing intervention has the <u>highest priority</u>?
1. Providing a safe environment
2. Offering recreational activities
3. Providing a structured environment
4. Instituting measures to promote sleep

6. The nurse notices that a client with dementia about to eat his dinner picks up his spoon, looks at it, puts it down, and then picks up his fork, looks at it, and puts it back on the table. He sits staring at the utensils and his dinner. How does the nurse interpret this behavior?
1. A risk for altered nutrition
2. A disruption in metabolic functioning
3. A disturbance in executive functioning
4. A potential sensory-motor deficit

7. The family of a client with increasing dementia asks the nurse how to convince one sibling who refuses to acknowledge their elderly mother's personality change. Which information would the nurse address in teaching the family about personality change in dementia? Select all that apply.
1. Loss of interest in surroundings
2. Lack of consideration for others
3. Difficulty learning new things
4. Disregard for the concept of time
5. Inability to do things in sequence
6. Decreased performance of daily activities

4. 4. By speaking to the consistent family caregiver, that person may be able to validate for the nurse the presence of the slow and progressive changes that occur in the early stages of dementia. In the early stages of dementia, the client will have recurrent memory impairment and will attempt to hide these cognitive losses. Communication with the physician would be for the purpose of sharing the nurse's assessment findings, not to request a cardiac workup. The need for a possible home health aide can be addressed when speaking to the caregiver, rather than acting without family consultation. There is no need to request that a different home health nurse perform the mental status assessment.

CN: Safe, effective care environment; CNS: Management of care; CL: Application

5. 1. The nurse's highest priority when caring for a client with delirium is to ensure client safety. Offering recreational activities, providing a structured environment, and promoting sleep are all appropriate interventions after safety measures are in place.

CN: Safe, effective care environment; CNS: Management of care; CL: Analysis

6. 3. The client's inability to initiate activities or perform routine tasks are examples of the loss of the ability to think and reason abstractly; hence, a disturbance or interference in the client's executive functioning has occurred. This behavior does not indicate a problem with nutrition or with metabolic or sensory-motor functioning.

CN: Physiological integrity; CNS: Physiological adaptation; CL: Analysis

7. 1 and 2. Clients with dementia often manifest a loss of interest in their surroundings, a lack of consideration for others, and a tendency to be self-absorbed as manifestations of a personality change. Having difficulty learning new things and the loss or disregard for the concept of time are cognitive changes that occur in dementia. The inability to do things in an orderly sequence and the decreased performance of daily activities indicate the functional changes seen in clients with dementia.

CN: Physiological integrity; CNS: Physiological adaptation; CL: Application

8. Which intervention should help a client diagnosed with Alzheimer's disease perform activities of daily living?
 1. Have the client perform all basic care without help.
 2. Tell the client morning care must be done by 9 a.m.
 3. Give the client a written list of activities he's expected to do.
 4. Encourage the client and give ample time to complete basic tasks.

9. The nurse has taught a family about the medication donepezil (Aricept). The nurse determines that teaching was successful when the family makes which statement?
 1. "We will need to figure out a schedule to get dad's weekly blood work done."
 2. "When dad's Alzheimer's disease worsens, he will need to stop taking this drug."
 3. "This drug may slow down dad's pulse, since he has preexisting heart disease."
 4. "Aricept acts like a diuretic medication, so dad should take it in the morning."

10. The home health nurse is speaking to the spouse caregiver of a client with Alzheimer's disease. The client has been taking donepezil (Aricept). The nurse is most concerned when the caregiver makes which statement?
 1. "In the last few days, the main thing that my husband wants to eat is bread."
 2. "Yesterday, I managed to weigh my husband, and he lost 8 lb this month."
 3. "Somehow, this medication has been making him sleep in longer in the morning."
 4. "My husband no longer has any interest in listening to the radio with me."

11. Which nursing intervention will help a client with progressive memory deficit function in his environment?
 1. Help the client do simple tasks by giving step-by-step directions.
 2. Avoid frustrating the client by performing basic care routines for the client.
 3. Stimulate the client's intellectual functioning by discussing new topics daily.
 4. Promote the client's sense of humor by telling jokes and discussing cartoons.

12. Which intervention is a priority action of the nurse providing care to a client diagnosed with Alzheimer's disease?
 1. Avoid physical contact with the client.
 2. Confine the client to his room after 8:00 p.m.
 3. Provide a high level of sensory stimulation.
 4. Monitor the client's activities carefully.

A gentle, calm approach is comforting and nonthreatening.

Mmmmm? Let me think about what you said.

Look for the answer that makes the most safety sense.

8. **4.** Clients with Alzheimer's disease respond to the effect of those around them. A gentle, calm approach is comforting and nonthreatening, and a tense, hurried approach may agitate the client. The client has problems performing independently. The inherent expectations of deadlines and activity lists may lead to frustration.
CN: Physiological integrity; CNS: Basic care and comfort; CL: Application

9. **3.** Donepezil has the potential to cause bradycardia in clients with cardiac disease. Weekly blood work is not necessary for clients on donepezil. Donepezil can be used for mild, moderate, or severe Alzheimer's disease. Donepezil does not act like a diuretic; it can cause urinary retention, and the client may have difficulty passing his urine.
CN: Physiological integrity; CNS: Pharmacological and parenteral therapies; CL: Application

10. **2.** A side effect of Aricept is weight loss, and it would be important to discuss the weight loss with the primary care provider. The desire to eat bread (carbohydrates), the ability to sleep longer, and the lack of interest in listening to the radio are not changes related to the use of donepezil (Aricept).
CN: Physiological integrity; CNS: Pharmacological and parenteral therapies; CL: Application

11. **1.** Clients with cognitive impairment should do the tasks that they are capable of performing. By receiving simple directions in a step-by-step fashion, the client can better process information and perform tasks. Stimulation of intellect can be accomplished by discussing familiar topics to the client. The discussion of new topics may add to the client's confusion. Clients with cognitive impairment may not be able to understand jokes, and cartoons may add to their confusion.
CN: Psychosocial integrity; CNS: None; CL: Application

12. **4.** Whenever a client's safety is at risk, careful observation and supervision are of ultimate importance in avoiding injury. Physical contact is implemented during basic care. Confining the client may cause agitation and combativeness. A high level of sensory stimulation may be too stimulating and distracting.
CN: Safe, effective care environment; CNS: Management of care; CL: Application

13. Which nursing intervention is the <u>most important</u> in caring for a client diagnosed with Alzheimer's disease?
1. Provide the client with a safe and comfortable environment.
2. Supervise food selections for client health and enjoyment of meals.
3. Initiate the client meeting other clients for social interactions.
4. Encourage the client to independently perform her daily physical care.

14. The nurse administered haloperidol (Haldol) to a client with dementia who was experiencing severe agitation. It is most important for the nurse to assess the client for which adverse effects? Select all that apply.
1. Photosensitivity
2. Bradycardia, apnea, and hypotension
3. Urinary output
4. Skin irritations
5. Insomnia, nightmares, and early morning awakenings
6. Dizziness

Let me take a good look at you!

15. A client diagnosed with Alzheimer's disease tells the nurse that today she has a luncheon date with her daughter, who is not visiting that day. Which response by the nurse would be <u>most appropriate</u>?
1. "Where are you planning on having your lunch?"
2. "You're confused and don't know what you're saying."
3. "I think you need some more medication and I'll bring it to you."
4. "Today is Monday, March 8, and we'll be eating lunch in the dining room."

You're already at question 15 and doing great. Keep going!

16. During a visit to the outpatient clinic, a spouse asks the nurse if she needs to be concerned about her 80-year-old husband consistently referring to items as "whatchamacallits." What is the best response by the nurse?
1. "Sometimes, a change in cognitive functioning is occurring when a person has difficulty finding the right word to say."
2. "You need to write down the word you think your husband wanted to say when he says whatchamacallit."
3. "Tell me if he also has periods of dizziness, balance problems, and walks leaning forward with an unsteady gait."
4. "I don't think you need to worry about this, as it is an unpleasant but normal behavior associated with aging."

13. 1. Providing client safety is the number one priority when caring for any client, particularly when a client is already compromised and at greater risk for injury. The other options may be part of caring for a client with Alzheimer's disease, but they are not the priority.
CN: Safe, effective care environment; CNS: Safety and infection control; CL: Application

14. 1, 3, and 6. A client on haloperidol (Haldol) must be monitored for photosensitivity reactions to sunlight, urinary retention, dizziness, and drowsiness. Haloperidol (Haldol) does not cause bradycardia, apnea, hypotension, dermatological problems, or disturbances in sleep.
CN: Physiological integrity; CNS: Physiological adaptation; CL: Application

15. 4. The best nursing response is to reorient the client to the date and environment. Humoring the client isn't therapeutic. Medication won't provide immediate relief for memory impairment. Confrontation can provoke an outburst.
CN: Psychosocial integrity; CNS: None; CL: Application

16. 1. Many people with dementia experience changes in cognitive functioning, such as increasing and persistent forgetfulness, difficulty finding the right word to say, and trouble with abstract thinking. Writing down forgotten words, asking about other physical problems, and minimizing the caregiver's concern do not answer the caregiver's question.
CN: Physiological integrity; CNS: Physiological adaptation; CL: Application

17. A 65-year-old man recovering from a mild stroke questions the nurse about his risk for vascular dementia. What is the best response by the nurse?
  1. "It is hard to predict the risk factors for vascular dementia, since anything that affects your heart and your circulation increases your risk."
  2. "The factors that increase your risk of stroke, such as hypertension, high cholesterol, and smoking, will also increase your risk for vascular disease."
  3. "Usually, only the people who suffer from traumatic brain injuries are the ones who will develop vascular dementia as they age."
  4. "I suggest that if you are worried, you ask your primary care provider to order a diagnostic workup and a brain magnetic resonance imaging study."

What places you at risk???

17. 2. Controlling hypertension and high cholesterol and not smoking will decrease a person's risk for vascular dementia. The other options present incorrect information. Risk factors are known. Other people, in addition to brain-injured persons, can develop vascular dementia. Talking about a diagnostic workup does not address one's lifestyle risks.
CN: Physiological integrity; CNS: Physiological adaptation; CL: Application

18. A nurse is teaching the family of a client with dementia. Which of the following explanations of dementia by the nurse would be most appropriate?
  1. Personal neglect in hygiene and other types of self-care
  2. Poor judgment and inability to be reasonable, especially in social situations
  3. Memory loss for familiar people occurring as a natural consequence of aging
  4. Loss of intellectual abilities sufficient to impair the ability to perform basic care

18. 4. The ability to perform self-care is an important measure of the progression of dementia. Memory loss reflects underlying physical, metabolic, and pathological processes. Personal neglect and poor judgment typically occur in dementia but aren't considered defining characteristics.
CN: Physiological integrity; CNS: Physiological adaptation; CL: Application

19. While interacting with a client who is suspected of having a dementia disorder, the nurse asks the client what was on his tray for breakfast. This question allows the nurse to assess which area?
  1. Food preferences
  2. Recent memory
  3. Remote memory
  4. Speech clarity

19. 2. Persons with dementia have difficulty with recent memory or learning, which may be a key to early detection. Assessing food preferences may be helpful in determining what the client likes to eat, but this assessment has no direct correlation in assessing dementia. Speech difficulties, such as rambling, irrelevance, and incoherence, may be related to delirium.
CN: Health promotion and maintenance; CNS: None; CL: Application

20. The client states, "Just because I get a little confused at times, my doctor told my wife that I have the beginnings of Alzheimer's disease!" Which response by the nurse would be most appropriate?
  1. "Anyone who has struggled with your health problems can easily have periods of confusion, but it may be premature to be diagnosed with Alzheimer's disease."
  2. "The symptoms of Alzheimer's disease occur over time and in stages, and in the beginning, forgetfulness and confusion are often experienced."
  3. "A diagnosis of Alzheimer's disease is a serious health concern, and I suggest that you and your wife meet and discuss this with the doctor."
  4. "I think that you should be worried about this, and your doctor should not have had this discussion with only your wife."

20. 2. Loss of short-term memory, forgetfulness, and increasing levels of confusion are the characteristics of the beginning phases of Alzheimer's disease. As the symptoms progress, they become more obvious, and the person can become more defensive and depressed. The other options do not give the client information about Alzheimer's disease or help to explain the disease process.
CN: Health promotion and maintenance; CNS: None; CL: Analysis

21. The nurse is teaching the client and his family about cognitive vascular impairment that occurs when a person has vascular dementia. Which comment by a family member would indicate the need for additional teaching?
1. "The vision and speaking problems dad has are part of his vascular dementia."
2. "Now I know that inadequate blood flow to the brain affects the ability to think."
3. "It is good to know that vascular dementia is not anything like Alzheimer's disease."
4. "I understand how regular strokes and small strokes can cause changes in the brain."

22. The family of a client recently admitted with vascular dementia asks the nurse about the cause of the client's condition. Which of the following would be the most accurate response by the nurse?
1. "It is caused by high blood pressure."
2. "It is caused by low oxygen levels."
3. "It is caused by an infection."
4. "It is caused by toxins."

23. During the admission assessment, the nurse focuses on the client's reflexes, muscle strength, coordination, eye movements, and mental status. What symptoms does the nurse identify that are suggestive of vascular dementia? Select all that apply.
1. Swinging leg
2. Losing bladder control
3. Laughing inappropriately
4. Shuffling gait
5. Hyperextending the head
6. Aching joint deformities

24. The spouse of a client diagnosed with vascular dementia asks the nurse how this disorder differs from Alzheimer's disease. Which response from the nurse is most appropriate?
1. "Vascular dementia can be either an insidious onset or a more abrupt onset, depending on the change in blood flow to the brain."
2. "Vascular dementia can be treated with medications to improve the prognosis and prevent further circulatory decline."
3. "Personality change is a common characteristic seen in vascular dementia, and it tends to occur in the final stages of the disease."
4. "The inability to perform motor activities and language difficulties happen in the severe stage of vascular dementia."

This question is asking specifically about vascular dementia.

Let's see! What is the cause?

21. 3. Vascular dementia and Alzheimer's disease are both types of dementias, with vascular dementia ranked as the second most common cause of dementia after Alzheimer's disease. The other statements are all true about vascular dementia.
CN: Physiological integrity; CNS: Physiological adaptation; CL: Analysis

22. 1. Vascular dementia is a result of small strokes that can either destroy or damage cerebral tissue. Strokes may be caused by high blood pressure, high cholesterol levels, heart disease, or diabetes. Hypoxia, infection, and toxins aren't causes of dementia.
CN: Physiological integrity; CNS: Physiological adaptation; CL: Application

23. 2, 3, and 4. The typical symptoms of vascular dementia are confusion, memory deficits, wandering, shuffling gait, loss of bladder and bowel control, and inappropriate laughter. Leg swinging, head hyperextension, and joint deformities are not symptoms associated with vascular dementia.
CN: Physiological integrity; CNS: Physiological adaptation; CL: Analysis

24. 1. Vascular dementia differs from Alzheimer's disease in that it can have either an abrupt or insidious onset depending on the disruption of blood flow to the brain. Vascular dementia has a poor prognosis with a shortened lifespan. Personality change is common in Alzheimer's disease. The inability to carry out motor activities and language difficulties are common in Alzheimer's disease.
CN: Health promotion and maintenance; CNS: None; CL: Analysis

25. A progression of symptoms that occurs in steps rather than a gradual deterioration indicates which type of dementia?
1. Alzheimer's dementia
2. Parkinson's dementia
3. Substance-induced dementia
4. Vascular dementia

26. The client's grandson, a biology major in college, asks the nurse what pathological change occurs in the brain and causes Alzheimer's disease. What is the best response by the nurse?
1. Impairment in glucose metabolism
2. Atrophy of the frontal lobe of the brain
3. Degeneration of the cholinergic system
4. Intracranial bleeding in the limbic system

27. An elderly client has experienced memory and attention deficits that developed over a 3-day period. The nurse is aware that these symptoms are characteristic of which disorder?
1. Alzheimer's disease
2. Amnesia syndrome
3. Delirium
4. Dementia

28. A home care nurse visits a married couple's extended family, composed of children in elementary school and high school, grandparents, and an unmarried adult brother. Which age group is at high risk for developing a state of delirium?
1. Adolescent
2. Elderly
3. Middle-aged
4. School-aged

29. Which nursing diagnosis is most appropriate for an elderly client experiencing visual and auditory hallucinations?
1. Interrupted family processes
2. Ineffective role performance
3. Impaired verbal communication
4. Disturbed sensory perception

You've taken the first steps towards understanding the many types of dementia.

Which one of these changes is a cause of Alzheimer's symptoms?

Age is an important factor when assessing a client.

25. 4. Vascular dementia differs from Alzheimer's disease in that vascular dementia has a more abrupt onset and progresses in steps. At times, the dementia seems to clear up, and the individual shows fairly lucid thinking. Dementia of the Alzheimer's type has a slow onset with a progressive and deteriorating course. Dementia of Parkinson's sometimes resembles the dementia of Alzheimer's disease. Substance-induced dementia is related to the persisting effects of use of a substance.
CN: Physiological integrity; CNS: Physiological adaptation; CL: Analysis

26. 3. Research related to Alzheimer's disease indicates that the enzyme needed to produce acetylcholine is dramatically reduced. The other pathophysiological changes don't cause the symptoms of Alzheimer's disease
CN: Physiological integrity; CNS: Physiological adaptation; CL: Analysis

27. 3. Delirium is characterized by an abrupt onset of fluctuating levels of awareness, clouded consciousness, perceptual disturbances, and disturbed memory and orientation. Alzheimer's disease is a progressive dementia. Amnesia refers to recent short-term and long-term memory loss. Dementia is characterized by general impairment in intellectual functioning and occurs in a progressive, irreversible course.
CN: Physiological integrity; CNS: Physiological adaptation; CL: Application

28. 2. The elderly population, because of normal physiological changes, is highly susceptible to delirium. All the other options are incorrect.
CN: Health promotion and maintenance; CNS: None; CL: Application

29. 4. The client is experiencing visual and auditory hallucinations related to a sensory alteration. The other options don't address the hallucinations the client is experiencing.
CN: Safe, effective care environment; CNS: Management of care; CL: Analysis

30. The nurse is teaching a group of caregivers who live with family members that have mild to moderate changes in their cognitive functioning. Which goal will the nurse identify as a <u>priority</u> of care for the clients?
1. Promote frequent socialization.
2. Maintain optimal physical health.
3. Provide frequent changes in caregivers.
4. Provide an overstimulating environment.

31. A newly admitted client diagnosed with delirium has a history of hypertension and anxiety. The client had been taking digoxin, furosemide (Lasix), and diazepam (Valium) for anxiety. The nurse suspects that this client's impairment may be the result of which of the following?
1. Opportunistic infection
2. Metabolic acidosis
3. Drug intoxication
4. Hepatic encephalopathy

32. A client who has experienced cerebral hypoxia demonstrates sensory-perceptual alterations. Which environment would the nurse create for this client?
1. A softly lit room around the clock with the curtains kept open
2. A brightly lit room around the clock with the curtains closed
3. A low-lit room situated near the nurses' station with soft background music
4. A well-lit room without glare during the day and a darkened room for sleeping

33. As a nurse enters a client's room, the client says, "They're crawling on my sheets! Get them off my bed!" The nurse interprets this assessment finding as:
1. aphasia.
2. dysarthria.
3. illusions.
4. hallucinations.

Sometimes we're not a good combination.

Your clients depend on you for meeting their environmental needs as well as their physical ones.

30. 2. A client's cognitive impairment may hinder self-care abilities. More socialization, frequent changes in caregivers, and an overstimulating environment would only increase anxiety and confusion.
CN: Health promotion and maintenance; CNS: None; CL: Application

31. 3. This client was taking several medications that have a propensity for producing delirium: digoxin (a cardiac glycoside), furosemide (a thiazide diuretic), and diazepam (a benzodiazepine). Sufficient supporting data do not exist to view the other options as causes.
CN: Physiological integrity; CNS: Physiological adaptation; CL: Analysis

32. 4. A quiet, shadow-free environment produces the fewest sensory-perceptual distortions for a client with cognitive impairment associated with delirium.
CN: Psychosocial integrity; CNS: None; CL: Application

33. 4. The presence of a sensory stimulus correlates with the definition of a hallucination, which is a false sensory perception. Aphasia refers to a communications problem. Dysarthria is difficulty in speech production. Illusions are incorrectly perceived sensory stimuli.
CN: Psychosocial integrity; CNS: None; CL: Application

CN: Client needs category   CNS: Client needs subcategory   CL: Cognitive level

34. A delirious client is shouting for someone to get the bugs off her. Which response by the nurse is the most appropriate?
1. "Don't worry. I'll stay here and talk to you while I brush the bugs away for you."
2. "You need to try and relax. The crawling sensation will go away sooner if you can relax."
3. "There are no bugs on your legs or in the bed. It's just your imagination playing tricks on you."
4. "I see that you are frightened, and I will stay with you. I don't see any bugs crawling on you."

This question is really starting to bug me.

34. 4. Never argue about hallucinations with a client. Instead, promote an environment of trust and safety by acknowledging the client's perceptions.

CN: Physiological integrity; CNS: Basic care and comfort; CL: Application

35. The nurse is giving a report to the nurse on the next shift. Which description of a client's experience and behavior can be shared as an example of the client experiencing an illusion?
1. "The client tried to push me away, hit me, and cursed at me every time I went into the room to take vital signs."
2. "Repeatedly the client yelled, 'I keep hearing my mother's voice telling me to get dressed and run away.'"
3. "Whenever I went to leave the room, the client became anxious and grabbed my hand and begged me to stay."
4. "Every time the client looked at the shadows on a wall she said, 'There are frightening faces on that wall.'"

35. 4. An illusion is an inaccurate perception or false response to a sensory stimulus. Auditory hallucinations are associated with sound and are more common in schizophrenia. Anxiety and agitation can be secondary to illusions.

CN: Physiological integrity; CNS: Physiological adaptation; CL: Analysis

36. The nurse explains to the client and his family that the changes occurring in Alzheimer's disease are irreversible. The nurse is aware that which of the following is an <u>expected</u> neurological change of aging?
1. Widening of the central sulci
2. Depletion of neurotransmitters
3. Neurofibrillary tangles and plaques
4. Degeneration of the temporal lobes

I feel like I'm tied up in knots.

36. 3. Aging isn't necessarily associated with significant decline, but neurofibrillary tangles and plaques are expected changes. These normal occurrences are sometimes referred to as benign senescent forgetfulness of age-associated memory impairment.

CN: Physiological integrity; CNS: Physiological adaptation; CL: Analysis

37. The nurse is teaching a caregiver how to effectively interact with her elderly parent who suffers from impaired memory and impaired judgment. What is the most important information for the nurse to provide? Select all that apply.
1. Perform all the client's care and activities of daily living.
2. Speak slowly and use understandable words and phrases.
3. Keep music playing to promote environmental stimulation.
4. Allow ample time for the client to respond to a question.
5. Orient and reorient the client as needed throughout the day.
6. Approach the client from the front when beginning a conversation.

37. 2, 4, 5, and 6. When interacting with a client with cognitive impairment, a person should speak slowly and use simple, understandable language, allow ample time to answer a question, orient and reorient at each interaction as needed, and approach the client from the front where the speaker can be seen. The caregiver must not do care and activities that the client can perform. The caregiver wants to provide a low-stimulus environment, so continuous music would cause agitation.

CN: Physiological integrity; CNS: Physiological adaptation; CL: Application

38. During morning care, a nurse asks a client with dementia, "How was your night?" The client replies, "My husband and I went out to dinner and a movie and had a wonderful evening!" The nurse interprets the client's statement as which of the following?
1. Interpretation
2. Perseveration
3. Confabulation
4. Disorientation

38. 3. Confabulation is the process in which an individual makes up stories to answer questions. It's considered a defensive tactic to protect the individual's self-esteem and prevent others from noticing the memory loss. Interpretation is assigning meaning and understanding to a question in order to reply appropriately. Perseveration is persistent repetition of the same word or idea in response to different questions. Disorientation is a state of mental confusion characterized by incorrect perceptions of time, place, or person.
CN: Psychosocial integrity; CNS: None; CL: Application

39. A nursing assistant tells a nurse, "The client with amnesia looks fine but responds to questions in a vague, distant manner. What should I be doing to take care of her?" Which response is the <u>most appropriate</u>?
1. "Give her ample time and plenty of space to test her independence."
2. "Keep her busy and make sure she doesn't take naps during the day."
3. "Whenever you think she needs direction, use short, simple sentences."
4. "Spend as much time talking as you can with her and ask her questions."

Teaching nursing assistants helps to improve the quality of care they provide.

39. 3. Confusion, anxiety, and disruptions in the ability to perform basic care are often apparent in clients with amnesia. Offering simple directions to promote daily functions and reduce confusion helps increase feelings of safety and security. Giving this client ample time and plenty of space may make her feel insecure. Excessive talking and asking her questions that she won't be able to answer will intensify her anxiety level. There is no significant rationale for keeping her busy all day with no rest periods. This action will make the client tired and less functional at performing other basic tasks.
CN: Safe, effective care environment; CNS: Management of care; CL: Application

40. The nurse is assessing an elderly client diagnosed with amnestic disorder related to traumatic head trauma. What assessment finding can be expected during the interaction between the nurse and client?
1. Speech patterns are altered and difficult to understand.
2. The inability to concentrate occurs since diagnosis.
3. There is a noted disruption in intellectual functioning.
4. Recent recall of life events is severely impaired.

40. 4. The primary area affected in an amnestic disorder is memory. The client cannot recall previously learned information or learn new information; all other areas of cognition are normal.
CN: Physiological integrity; CNS: Physiological adaptation; CL: Analysis

41. A client with mild Alzheimer's disease desires to remain at home living with his extended family. What is the <u>most appropriate</u> nursing intervention?
1. Provide mandated written directions for all activities of daily living.
2. Obtain a physician's order for either a mild anxiolytic or sleeping pill.
3. Advise the client to attend occupational therapy three times a week.
4. Maintain a stable, predictable environment and daily routine.

Question 41 is asking which action is *most appropriate.*

41. 4. Clients in the early stages of Alzheimer's disease remain fairly functional with familiar surroundings and a predictable routine. They become easily disoriented with surprises and social overstimulation. Requiring that a client in the early stages of Alzheimer's disease follow mandated written directions for daily activities is unnecessary and disempowering. Anxiolytics or sleeping medication can impair memory and worsen the problem. Advising the client to attend occupational therapy is nonproductive and will only serve to frustrate and fatigue the client.
CN: Psychosocial integrity; CNS: None; CL: Application

42. The nurse is providing care to a client with Alzheimer's type dementia. Which nursing intervention is most important?
1. Establish a routine that reinforces memories and supports former habits.
2. Maintain an environment with cheerful and pleasant surroundings.
3. Structure a daily and precise routine that can be used after discharge.
4. Control the environment by providing structure and consistent boundaries.

43. The wife of a 78-year-old client with Alzheimer's disease reported to the nurse that she often finds her husband wandering in the backyard in the middle of the night. The client is dressed only in his underwear, and he says to his wife, "I'm just taking out the trash before I go to work." What is the priority nursing diagnosis for the wife of this client?
1. Knowledge deficit
2. Sleep deprivation
3. Risk for loneliness
4. Self-neglect

44. Which nursing diagnosis is appropriate for a client diagnosed with an amnestic disorder?
1. Complicated grieving
2. Ineffective denial
3. Defensive coping
4. Risk for injury

45. The nurse is planning care for a client living with his family who has been diagnosed with Alzheimer's disease. The family reports that the client is disoriented, doesn't recognize objects to be used for care, and finds and eats uncooked food. Which nursing diagnosis is <u>most important</u>?
1. Disturbed sleep pattern
2. Risk for powerlessness
3. Impaired home maintenance
4. Risk for poisoning

46. The nurse is reviewing the chart of a man admitted with amnestic disorder. Which medical condition may be associated with an amnestic disorder?
1. Drug overdose
2. Cerebral anoxia
3. Anticonvulsant medication
4. Environmental toxins

You need to determine what is most important!

You've reached question 45. Now's the time to kick it into high gear!

42. 4. By controlling the environment and providing structure and consistent boundaries, the nurse is helping to keep the client safe and secure, which is a top priority nursing measure. Establishing a routine that reinforces memories, supports former habits, maintains pleasant surroundings, and structures a daily routine fosters a supportive environment; however, keeping the client safe and secure takes priority.
CN: Safe, effective care environment; CNS: Management of care; CL: Application

43. 1. The priority nursing diagnosis is knowledge deficit related to her distress about her husband's behavior and her lack of understanding about Alzheimer's disease. The other nursing diagnoses are appropriate but do not reflect the priority needs of this caregiver.
CN: Safe, effective care environment; CNS: Management of care; CL: Analysis

44. 4. Changes in cognitive ability place a client at high risk for injury. The client isn't aware of a loss and therefore doesn't recognize the extent of the diagnosis amnestic disorder. The client isn't in denial but has an impaired ability to learn new information or to remember past information. The client isn't aware of a need to cope with the consequences of his diagnosis.
CN: Safe, effective care environment; CNS: Management of care; CL: Analysis

45. 3. Impaired home maintenance is occurring due to the client's progressive decline in cognitive functioning. The nurse's priority is to assist the client and family meet their need for information, supervision, and assistance in providing safe care. Disturbed sleep pattern, risk for powerlessness, and risk for poisoning are important diagnoses for the nurse's consideration, but they are not the top priority.
CN: Safe, effective care environment; CNS: Management of care; CL: Analysis

46. 2. A variety of medical conditions are related to amnestic disorders, such as head trauma, stroke, cerebral neoplastic disease, herpes simplex, encephalitis, poorly controlled insulin-dependent diabetes, and cerebral anoxia. The other three options are substance induced.
CN: Physiological integrity; CNS: Physiological adaptation; CL: Application

47. The nurse is preparing to teach a group of caregivers about medication management for family members with Alzheimer's disease. What is the most important information for the nurse to include? Select all that apply.
1. Evaluate whether the client is able to safely self-medicate.
2. Perform a visual mouth inspection after giving a pill.
3. Use only one pharmacy for all of the client's prescriptions.
4. Check to be certain that the client can swallow the pill.
5. Consult with the pharmacy about altering the dosage.
6. Know what to do if the client refuses to take the medication.

47. 1, 2, 3, 4, and 6. A teaching plan would include evaluating whether the client is able to safely self-medicate, performing a visual mouth inspection after giving a pill, using only one pharmacy for all of the client's prescriptions, checking to ascertain that the client can swallow the pill, and knowing what to do if the client refuses to take the medication. The caregiver should consult with the pharmacist about obtaining an alternative form of the drug if the client can no longer swallow a pill or capsule. The health care prescriber would be consulted to change or alter the medication dose.
CN: Health promotion and maintenance; CNS: None; CL: Analysis

> Use the hints to your advantage.

48. The home health nurse is consulting with a family about making changes in their home in order to create a safe environment for a person who has Alzheimer's disease. What is the <u>most important</u> information for the nurse to provide? Select all that apply.
1. Keep all household cleaning products in a locked cabinet.
2. Supervise the client when cooking or fixing a snack.
3. Place all matches and cigarette lighters in a safe place.
4. Install locks on places where garden equipment is kept.
5. Monitor the use of stoves, ovens, and heating appliances.
6. Mount heat sensors or smoke detectors in each room.

48. 1, 2, 3, 4, and 5. To create a safe home environment, the nurse would discuss keeping all household cleaning products in a locked cabinet, supervising the client when cooking or fixing a snack, placing all matches and cigarette lighters in a safe place, installing locks on places where garden equipment is kept, and monitoring the use of stoves, ovens, and heating appliances. Some people place heat sensors beside a stove or oven, but they are not needed in every room. Extra smoke detectors are not required. Smoke detectors are typically placed on each floor of the house, not in each room.
CN: Safe, effective care environment; CNS: Management of care; CL: Application

49. The client's daughter tells the nurse, "I do not understand what the doctor said about my father having transient global amnesia." What is the most appropriate response by the nurse? Select all that apply.
1. "Your father will draw a blank when asked about things that happened a day, a month, or a year ago."
2. "Transient global amnesia is usually harmless, and it is unlikely that it will be experienced again."
3. "After this type of amnesia, your father will undergo a period of depression and feelings of hopelessness."
4. "It remains to be determined whether your dad will have a lack of insight and permanent memory problems."
5. "The stroke was the cause of the transient global amnesia and the sudden, temporary memory loss."
6. "Even though there is memory loss, your dad does remember you and recognizes the people he knows well."

49. 1, 2, 5, and 6. Transient global amnesia is a sudden, temporary episode of memory loss that can be attributed to a more common neurological condition, such as a stroke. During an episode of transient global amnesia, a person's recall of recent events vanishes. The person also draws a blank when asked to remember things that happened a day, a month, or even a year ago. However, the person does recognize familiar people. Transient global amnesia is rare, usually harmless, and unlikely to happen again. Episodes are usually short lived, and afterward, one's memory returns. After an episode of transient global amnesia, a person does not have a lack of insight, does not experience feelings of depression and hopelessness, and does not have permanent memory problems.
CN: Physiological integrity; CNS: Physiological adaptation; CL: Analysis

CN: Client needs category   CNS: Client needs subcategory   CL: Cognitive level

50. During conversation with a client, the nurse observes that he shifts from one topic to the next on a regular basis. Which disorder is the client most likely to have?
1. Flight of ideas
2 Concrete thinking
3 Ideas of reference
4. Loose associations

Hey! You've answered 50 questions. Awesome!

51. A daughter reports to the nurse that she thinks her mother's dementia is becoming worse. Which assessment finding would indicate to the nurse that the client's dementia is worsening?
1. The client resists logical explanations.
2. The client stops redirecting negative energy.
3. The client maintains a nondefensive position.
4. The client becomes increasingly agitated.

52. For the family of a client with Alzheimer's disease, one goal is effective communication. Which outcome is successful for this goal?
1. Family members don't use humor with the client.
2. Family members speak to the client in a loud voice.
3. Family members give the client one-step commands.
4. Family members don't touch the client while speaking.

For effective communications, think clear and concise.

53. Immediately after visiting hours, a nurse monitors for wandering behavior in a client with Alzheimer's disease. The nurse anticipates the client may:
1. need to walk after eating a complete meal.
2. feel tense due to an uncomfortable situation.
3. be demonstrating eccentric behavior.
4. have difficulty following directions.

As a nurse, you will often need to prioritize!

54. For a client with dementia who lives in a long-term care facility, which outcome takes the highest nursing care priority?
1. Maintaining the client's optimal level of functioning
2. Identifying coping methods the client can use to handle stress
3. Facilitating client conversation with five people each day
4. Having the client use physical activity to work off aggressive energy

50. 4. Loose associations are conversations that constantly shift in topic. Loose associations don't necessarily start in a disorganized way; the conversations can begin cogently and then become loose. Flight of ideas is characterized by conversation that's disorganized from the onset. Concrete thinking implies highly definitive thought processes. Ideas of reference are characterized by a delusional belief that things irrelevant to the client, such as newspaper headlines, are referring to the client directly.
CN: Psychosocial integrity; CNS: None; CL: Application

51. 4. A client with dementia who becomes increasingly agitated may be unable to perform expected tasks. Communication must be clear and concise; giving logical explanations is inappropriate. This client may revert to old ways of coping, and trying to change the client rarely proves successful; the nurse should try to decrease the source of negativity. The client with dementia is rarely defensive.
CN: Psychosocial integrity; CNS: None; CL: Analysis

52. 3. Giving one-step commands keeps communication simple, clear, concise, and pleasant. Humor must be used judiciously so as not to confuse the client. Speaking in a loud voice may be interpreted as shouting and cause agitation. Depending on the situation, the use of touch may be appropriate, helping to reassure and soothe the client.
CN: Psychosocial integrity; CNS: None; CL: Application

53. 2. Tension and stress may cause a client with Alzheimer's disease to want to get away from an uncomfortable situation. Exercise is an important health promotion activity, but it doesn't help explain wandering behavior. Eccentric behavior is rarely related to wandering. Many clients with dementia have difficulty following directions; however, wandering typically results from disorientation.
CN: Psychosocial integrity; CNS: None; CL: Application

54. 1. The highest nursing care priority is to maintain the client's optimal level of functioning. Reducing the client's stress is the nurse's responsibility. Having a conversation with five people each day is unrealistic for this client. Expecting a client with dementia to use physical activity to decrease aggressive energy is also unrealistic.
CN: Safe, effective care environment; CNS: Management of care; CL: Application

55. A nurse is assessing a client for dementia. What history would the nurse expect to find in a client with dementia? Select all that apply.
1. There's a slow progression of symptoms.
2. The client admits to feelings of sadness.
3. The client acts apathetic and pessimistic.
4. The family can't determine when the symptoms first appeared.
5. There are changes in the client's basic personality.
6. The client has great difficulty paying attention to others.

56. A delusional client approaches a nurse, states, "I am the Easter Bunny," and insists that the nurse refer to him as such. Which nursing interventions should the nurse implement when working with this client? Select all that apply.
1. Consistently use the client's name in interaction.
2. Smile at the humor of the situation.
3. Agree that the client is the Easter Bunny.
4. Logically point out why the client could not be the Easter Bunny.
5. Provide as-needed medication.
6. Provide the client with structured activities.

55. **1, 4, 5, and 6.** Common characteristics of dementia are a slow onset of symptoms, which makes it difficult to determine when they first occurred. It progresses to noticeable changes in the client's personality and impaired ability to pay attention to other people. Feelings of sadness, apathy, and pessimism are symptoms of depression.

CN: Health promotion and maintenance; CNS: None; CL: Analysis

56. **1 and 6.** Continued reality-based orientation is necessary, so it is appropriate to use the client's name in any interaction. Structured activities can help the client refocus and resolve his delusion. The nurse shouldn't contribute to the delusion by going along with the situation. Logical arguments and as-needed medication aren't likely to change the client's beliefs.

CN: Psychosocial integrity; CNS: None; CL: Analysis

> Wow! You completed this chapter in record time. There's nothing wrong with your cognitive skills!

No, this chapter doesn't cover quirks of the rich and famous. It's all about mental disorders affecting the personality. Have a blast!

Chapter 16
Personality disorders

1. A client tells the nurse that his coworkers are sabotaging the computer. When the nurse asks questions, the client becomes argumentative. What is the most appropriate intervention for the nurse to implement?
   1. Encourage the client to vent his anger about his coworkers.
   2. Tell the client that his coworkers haven't touched his computer.
   3. Use clear and consistent speech when talking to the client.
   4. Tell the client to go to his room and stay there until he calms down.

2. A nurse is distinguishing characteristics of schizotypal personality disorder from schizoid personality disorder. What is the most appropriate statement by the nurse?
   1. Schizotypals are characterized by emotional detachment.
   2. Schizotypals are characterized by disinterest in close relationships.
   3. Schizotypals are indifferent to praise or criticism.
   4. Schizotypals have magical thinking or perceptual distortions.

3. The nurse is assessing a new client who was just admitted to the psychiatric unit. Which of the following assessment questions by the nurse would determine if the client has a schizotypal personality disorder? Select all that apply.
   1. "Do you feel that people often want to reject you or that they find you odd?"
   2. "Does anxiety make you want to self-mutilate?"
   3. "Do people of the opposite sex frequently find you attractive?"
   4. "Do you feel that other people take advantage of you?"
   5. "Have you ever felt like you had some special powers like ESP or some sort of magical influence over other?"
   6. "Do you tend to stay by yourself, even though you would like to be with others?"
   7. "Have you ever been arrested or pulled over by the police?"

1. **3.** Using clear and consistent speech when talking with the client helps him focus on reality and fosters a therapeutic relationship. Encouraging the client to vent his anger at his coworkers validates his suspicious thoughts and may make him more argumentative. Trying to convince him that his coworkers haven't touched his computer or telling him to go to his room may make him more defensive.
CN: Psychosocial integrity; CNS: None; CL: Analysis

2. **4.** Emotional detachment, disinterest in close relationships, and indifference to praise or criticism are features of schizoid personality disorder.
CN: Psychosocial integrity; CNS: None; CL: Analysis

Understanding a client's traits will help you deal with him effectively.

3. **1, 5, and 6.** Self-mutilation describes borderline personality disorders. Attractiveness to the opposite sex describes histrionic personality disorders. Feelings that others are taking advantage describe paranoid personality disorder. Being arrested or in trouble with the law describes antisocial personality disorder behaviors.
CN: Psychosocial integrity; CNS: None; CL: Analysis

4. Which of the following nursing diagnoses would be most appropriate for a client with a schizotypal personality disorder?
1. Ineffective coping related to repetitive behaviors such as hand washing
2. Risk for self-mutilation related to social anxiety
3. Risk for violence toward others related to lack of remorse for behaviors
4. Impaired thought processes related to ideas of reference and magical thinking

5. A nurse is caring for a client with schizotypal personality disorder. What is the most appropriate response by the nurse?
1. "You are to participate in all of the classes offered here on the unit."
2. "You may work on your assigned work sheets in your room."
3. "You are to conduct the community meeting this morning."
4. "You will help teach our medication class today to the entire group."

6. Which of the following behaviors can a nurse expect to see in a client with a personality disorder? Select all that apply.
1. Compliance with the rules of the unit
2. Tendency to provoke interpersonal conflict
3. Inflexibility
4. Maladaptive responses to stress
5. Trouble in social and professional relationships
6. Personal boundaries are blurred

7. Which of the following responses from the nurse would enhance a therapeutic relationship with a client with a personality disorder?
1. "What would you like to do today?"
2. "After you attend the morning community meeting, you may work on your homework."
3. "You remind me of a friend of mine."
4. "We will have you get comfortable on the unit first before we have you work on any homework."

What should we expect to see?

4. 4. People with a schizotypal personality disorder have ideas of reference and magical thinking. Repetitive behaviors describe obsessive-compulsive personality disorder, self-mutilation describes borderline personality disorders, and violence toward others with lack of remorse describes antisocial personality disorder.

CN: Safe, effective care environment; CNS: Management of care; CL: Application

5. 2. Clients with schizotypal personality disorders tend to isolate; this should be respected by the nurse. Answer choices 1, 3, and 4 are approaches that cause clients with schizoid personality disorders to be with the rest of the unit (attending, teaching, and conducting groups on the unit). The nurse may receive quite a bit of resistance from the client when there is a tone of control from the nurse.

CN: Safe, effective care environment; CNS: Management of care; CL: Application

6. 2, 3, 4, 5, and 6. These behaviors are evident regardless of the type of personality disorder. You will not see compliance with the unit rules with any personality disorder.

CN: Psychosocial integrity; CNS: None; CL: Analysis

7. 2. This response reflects a firm yet supportive approach. Responses 1 and 4 leave the nurse open for manipulation by the client. The client could suggest any activity that might not be therapeutic. The client could also never become comfortable on the unit. That is not the reason for their admission—to become comfortable. Response 3 is an example of countertransference. It is important for the nurse to discuss countertransference with other staff, not with the client with a personality disorder.

CN: Safe, effective care environment; CNS: Management of care; CL: Analysis

CN: Client needs category   CNS: Client needs subcategory   CL: Cognitive level

8. A client with paranoid personality disorder is discussing current problems with a nurse. What is the <u>most important</u> intervention for the nurse to implement?
1. Have the client look at sources of frustration.
2. Have the client focus on ways to interact with others.
3. Have the client discuss the use of defense mechanisms.
4. Have the client clarify thoughts and beliefs about an event.

Remember to prioritize!

9. A client with a paranoid personality disorder makes an inappropriate and unreasonable report to a nurse. What is the most appropriate intervention by the nurse?
1. Use logic to address the client's concern.
2. Confront the client about the stated misperception.
3. Use nonverbal communication to address the issue.
4. Tell the client matter-of-factly that you don't share his interpretation.

10. What is the <u>most appropriate</u> short-term goal for a client with paranoid personality disorder and impaired social skills?
1. Obtain feedback from other people.
2. Discuss anxiety-provoking situations.
3. Address positive and negative feelings about self.
4. Identify personal feelings that hinder social interaction.

11. A nurse is caring for a client with schizotypal personality disorder. The nurse would expect to observe which of the following?
1. Exhibitionism
2. Impulsiveness
3. Bodily illusions
4. Repetitive behaviors

8. **4.** Clarifying thoughts and beliefs helps the client avoid misinterpretations. Clients with a paranoid personality disorder tend to mistrust people and don't see interacting with others as a way to handle problems. They tend to be aggressive and argumentative rather than frustrated. The client's priority must be to interpret his thoughts and beliefs realistically, rather than discuss defensive mechanisms. A paranoid client will focus on defending self rather than acknowledging the use of defense mechanisms.
CN: Safe, effective care environment; CNS: Management of care; CL: Analysis

9. **4.** Telling the client you don't share his interpretation helps the client differentiate between realistic and emotional thoughts and conclusions. When the nurse uses logic to respond to a client's inappropriate statement, the nurse risks creating a power struggle with the client. The use of nonverbal communication will probably be misinterpreted and arouse the client's suspicion. It's unwise to confront a client with a paranoid personality disorder as the client will immediately become defensive.
CN: Psychosocial integrity; CNS: None; CL: Analysis

10. **4.** The client must address the feelings that impede social interactions before developing ways to address impaired social skills. Feedback can only be obtained after action is taken to improve or change the situation. Discussion of anxiety-provoking situations is important but doesn't help the client with impaired social skills. Addressing the client's positive and negative feelings about self won't directly influence impaired social skills.
CN: Psychosocial integrity; CNS: None; CL: Application

11. **3.** Clients with schizotypal personality disorders tend to have bodily illusions. Clients with histrionic personality disorder tend to be exhibitionists, borderlines are impulsive, and obsessive-compulsive individuals engage in repetitive behaviors.
CN: Psychosocial integrity; CNS: None; CL: Application

12. A nurse is assessing a client to determine if the client has an avoidant personality disorder. What are the most appropriate questions for the nurse to ask the client? Select all that apply.
1. Have you found yourself being worried that people won't like you?
2. Do you tend to drive yourself pretty hard, frequently feeling like you need to do just a little more?
3. Do you tend toward being a perfectionist?
4. Do you think that you would find it pretty easy to lie?
5. Have you often felt hurt by others, so that you are pretty wary of opening yourself to other people?
6. Do you tend to be very careful about selecting friends, perhaps only having one or two close friends in your whole life?
7. Is it hard for you to argue with your spouse because you are worried that he or she will really get mad at you and start to dislike you?

12. 1, 5, and 6. Questions 2 and 3 describe obsessive-compulsive personality disorder, question 4 describes antisocial personality disorder, and question 7 describes dependent personality disorder.
CN: Psychosocial integrity; CNS: None; CL: Application

13. A client with paranoid personality disorder responds aggressively during a psychoeducational group therapy session to something another client said about him. The nurse interprets this behavior as indicating which of the following?
1. The client doesn't want to participate in the group.
2. The client took the statement as a personal criticism.
3. The client is impulsive and was acting out of frustration.
4. The client was attempting to handle emotional distress.

Cheers to you—you're doing great!

13. 2. Clients with paranoid personality disorder tend to be hypersensitive and take what other people say as a personal attack on their character. The client is driven by the suspicion that others will inflict harm. Group participation would be minimal because the client is directing energy toward emotional self-protection. Clients with a paranoid personality tend to be rigid and guarded rather than expressive and acting out. The client with a paranoid personality disorder is acting to defend himself, not handle emotional distress.
CN: Psychosocial integrity; CNS: None; CL: Analysis

14. Which of the following nursing diagnoses would be appropriate for a client with an avoidant personality disorder?
1. Risk for self-mutilation related to a desperate need for attention
2. Ineffective coping related to negative attitudes toward health behavior
3. Anxiety related to fear of criticism, disapproval, and rejection
4. Risk for injury related to uncontrolled anger and hostility toward others

14. 3. Clients with avoidant personality disorder fear criticism, disapproval, and rejection. Self-mutilation describes borderline personality disorder. Negative attitudes toward health behaviors and uncontrolled anger and hostility describe antisocial personality disorder.
CN: Safe, effective care environment; CNS: Management of care; CL: Application

15. Which of the following outcomes would be appropriate for the nurse to expect from a client with an avoidant personality disorder?
1. Demonstrates an ability to use constructive criticism
2. Participates in impulse control training
3. Demonstrates a reduction in clinging, splitting, and manipulation behaviors
4. Demonstrates a decrease in attention-seeking behaviors

Let me think about this.

15. 1. Avoidant personality disorder clients experience fear of rejection and/or criticism and are very reluctant to participate in social situations because of this fear. Selections 2, 3, and 4 describe a cluster B personality disorder: borderline, antisocial, histrionic, or narcissistic.
CN: Safe, effective care environment; CNS: Management of care; CL: Application

CN: Client needs category   CNS: Client needs subcategory   CL: Cognitive level

16. The nurse is caring for a client with an avoidant personality disorder. The nurse anticipates assessment of the client's behavior to include which characteristics? Select all that apply.
1. Vigilant and suspiciousness
2. Distant personal relationships
3. Stealing, lying, and vandalism
4. Unstable relationships
5. View themselves as inferior to others
6. Inflexible, rigid, and needs to be in control
7. Social phobias

17. A nurse caring for a client with an avoidant personality disorder has established an outcome of demonstration of newly acquired social skills in social situations. Which of the following interventions would address this outcome?
1. Discuss with counselor factors that interfere with social interaction.
2. Identify social skills that the client already performs well.
3. Go to hospital cafeteria, purchase desired item, and eat in cafeteria.
4. Complete a work sheet on social skills.

18. Which statement made by a client with paranoid personality disorder shows that teaching about social relationships is effective?
1. "As long as I live, I won't abide by social rules."
2. "Sometimes, I can see what causes relationship problems."
3. "I'll find out what problems others have so I won't repeat them."
4. "I don't have problems in social relationships; I never really did."

19. The nurse is developing <u>long-term</u> goals for a client with paranoid personality disorder who is trying to improve peer relationships. What is the most appropriate goal?
1. The client will verbalize a realistic view of self.
2. The client will take steps to address disorganized thinking.
3. The client will become appropriately interdependent on others.
4. The client will become involved in activities that foster social relationships.

The word long-term is a clue to the correct choice.

16. 5 and 7. Suspiciousness is characteristic of paranoid personality disorder. Distant personal relationships are characteristic of schizoid personality disorder. Stealing, lying, and vandalism are characteristic of antisocial disorder. Unstable relationships are characteristic of borderline personality disorder. Inflexible, rigid, and the need to be in control are characteristic of obsessive-compulsive disorder.
CN: Psychosocial integrity; CNS: None; CL: Application

17. 3. This describes actually performing the skill in a social situation. The other selections address social skills, but there is no performance associated with them.
CN: Psychosocial integrity; CNS: None; CL: Application

18. 2. Progress is shown when the client addresses behaviors that negatively impact relationships. Clients with paranoid personality disorder tend to have impaired social relationships and are very uncomfortable in social settings. Clients with paranoid personality disorder struggle to understand and express their feelings about social rules. Knowing other people's problems isn't useful; the client must focus on his own issues. Not recognizing the problem indicates the client is in denial.
CN: Psychosocial integrity; CNS: None; CL: Application

19. 4. An appropriate long-term goal is for the client to increase interactions and social skills and make the commitment to become involved with others on a long-term basis. To verbalize a realistic view of self is a short-term goal. The client with a paranoid personality disorder doesn't tend to have disorganized thinking. A client with paranoid personality disorder won't allow himself to be interdependent on others.
CN: Psychosocial integrity; CNS: None; CL: Analysis

20. A client is admitted exhibiting the following: pervasive pattern of social inhibition, agoraphobia, fear of criticism, feelings of inferiority to others, and feelings of being totally unattractive to others. The nurse interprets this behavior as characteristic of which disorder?
1. Dependent personality disorder
2. Histrionic personality disorder
3. Narcissistic personality disorder
4. Avoidant personality disorder

21. A client with antisocial personality disorder is trying to convince a nurse that he deserves special privileges and that an exception to the rules should be made for him. What is the <u>best</u> response by the nurse?
1. "I believe we need to sit down and talk about this."
2. "Don't you know better than to try to bend the rules?"
3. "What you're asking me to do for you is unacceptable."
4. "Why don't you bring this request to the community meeting?"

22. Which two words describe cluster C personality disorders?
1. Odd and eccentric
2. Dramatic and emotional
3. Anxious and fearful
4. Erratic and eccentric

23. Which of the following assessment questions by the nurse would determine if the client has a histrionic personality disorder? Select all that apply.
1. "Do you frequently feel let down by people?"
2. "If a friend hurts you, do you sometimes feel like hurting yourself, perhaps by cutting or burning yourself?"
3. "Do you find that most people aren't quite up to your standards?"
4. "Do you think that you would make a good actor or actress?"
5. "Do you think that compared to other people, you are a very special person?"
6. "Do people of the opposite sex frequently find you attractive?"

Therapeutic interventions must be appropriate for the client.

What is the most important question to ask?

20. 4. The description is characteristic of avoidant personality disorder. Histrionic and narcissistic are cluster B and are quite emotionally labile in their demonstration of symptoms. Clients with dependent personality disorders generally cling to others in their personal relationships.
CN: Psychosocial integrity; CNS: None; CL: Application

21. 3. These clients often try to manipulate the nurse to get special privileges or make exceptions to the rules on their behalf. By informing the client directly when actions are inappropriate, the nurse helps the client learn to control unacceptable behaviors by setting limits. By sitting down to talk about the request, the nurse is telling the client there's room for negotiation when there is none. The second option humiliates the client. The client's behavior is unacceptable and shouldn't be brought to a community meeting.
CN: Psychosocial integrity; CNS: None; CL: Application

22. 3. Anxious and fearful describes cluster C personality disorders. Odd and eccentric describe cluster A personality disorders. Dramatic and emotional describe cluster B personality disorders. Erratic describes cluster B and eccentric describes cluster A personality disorders.
CN: Psychosocial integrity; CNS: None; CL: Application

23. 4 and 6. Questions 1 and 2 assess borderline personality disorders. Questions 3 and 5 assess narcissistic personality disorder.
CN: Psychosocial integrity; CNS: None; CL: Application

24. When reviewing a client's chart, the nurse notes the progress note below. Which statement about the client's condition is <u>most</u> accurate?

Progress notes	
9/15/10 1130	Client, age 28, admitted to unit with diagnosis of antisocial perso- nality disorder and suicide attempt after cutting his right wrist. Right wrist dressing appears dry and intact. Client states, "I don't want to be here and I'm not following your treatment plan or any of your rules. I'm going to tell everyone here not to follow your rules." ——— Barbara Jones, RN

1. The client requires psychotropic drugs to treat his condition, which he refuses.
2. The client manipulates other clients but not his family.
3. The client may not be motivated to change his behavior or his lifestyle.
4. The client could quickly make behavior changes if motivated.

25. The nurse would expect to observe which of the following behaviors in a client who has a histrionic personality disorder?
1. Exploitation of others to meet their own needs and desires
2. Portray a demeanor of grandiosity
3. Portray excessive provocative behaviors
4. Expression of feelings of emptiness and boredom

26. Which of the following behavioral patterns is characteristic of individuals with histrionic personality disorders?
1. Berating themselves and their abilities
2. Overreacting to minor stimuli
3. Suspicious and mistrustful of others
4. Social withdrawal and distant relationships

What am I looking for?

24. 3. Clients with antisocial personality disorder feel nothing is wrong with their behavior and have no desire to change. These clients don't benefit from psychotropic drug therapy. They attempt to manipulate all people with whom they come in contact. A quick behavior change isn't realistic expectation for clients with this disorder.
CN: Psychosocial integrity; CNS: None; CL: Application

25. 3. Histrionic personality disorders exhibit provocative behaviors. Exploitation of others and grandiosity are descriptions of narcissistic personality disorder. Feelings of emptiness and boredom are descriptions of borderline personality disorder.
CN: Psychosocial integrity; CNS: None; CL: Application

26. 2. Clients with a histrionic personality disorder are emotional and overreact to stimuli. Berating themselves describes an avoidant personality disorder. Suspiciousness describes a paranoid personality disorder. Socially withdrawn and distant relationships describe schizotypal personality disorder.
CN: Psychosocial integrity; CNS: None; CL: Application

27. A nurse notices other clients on the unit avoiding a client diagnosed with antisocial personality disorder. When discussing appropriate behavior in group therapy, which comment is <u>expected</u> about this client by his peers?
1. Lack of honesty
2. Belief in superstitions
3. Show of temper tantrums
4. Constant need for attention

28. Which of the following nursing diagnoses would be appropriate for a client with a histrionic personality disorder?
1. Impaired social interaction related to seductive and self-dramatizing behaviors
2. Risk for other-directed violence related to pacing and threatening stances
3. Chronic low self-esteem related to overt aggressiveness
4. Defensive coping related to absence of guilt and superior attitude toward others

29. What is the <u>most appropriate</u> goal for a client with antisocial personality disorder with a high risk for violence directed at others?
1. The client will discuss the desire to hurt others rather than act.
2. The client will be given something to destroy to displace the anger.
3. The client will develop a list of resources to use when anger escalates.
4. The client will understand the difference between anger and physical symptoms.

30. A client with antisocial personality disorder says, "I always want to blow things off." Which response by the nurse is most appropriate?
1. "Try to focus on what needs to be done and just do it."
2. "Let's work on considering some options and strategies."
3. "Procrastinating is a part of your illness that we'll work on."
4. "The best thing to do is decide on some useful goals to accomplish."

Read this question carefully. It seems to be asking you for a positive response, but it isn't.

Time to prioritize.

27. 1. Clients with antisocial personality disorder tend to engage in acts of dishonesty, shown by lying. Clients with schizotypal personality disorder tend to be superstitious. Clients with histrionic personality disorders tend to overreact to frustrations and disappointments, have temper tantrums, and seek attention.
CN: Psychosocial integrity; CNS: None; CL: Application

28. 1. Clients with histrionic personality disorders consistently draw attention to themselves. Risk for other-directed violence, chronic low self-esteem, and defensive coping would be appropriate for a client with an antisocial personality disorder.
CN: Safe, effective care environment; CNS: Management of care; CL: Application

29. 1. By discussing the desire to be violent toward others, the nurse can help the client get in touch with the pain associated with the angry feelings. It isn't helpful to have the client destroy something. The client needs to talk about strong feelings in a nonviolent manner, not refer to a list of crisis references. Helping the client understand the relationship between feelings and physical symptoms can be done after discussing the desire to hurt others.
CN: Psychosocial integrity; CNS: None; CL: Analysis

30. 2. By considering options or strategies, the client gains skills to overcome ineffective behaviors. The client tends to be irresponsible and needs guidance on what specifically to focus on to change behavior. Clients with an antisocial personality disorder don't tend to struggle with procrastination; instead, they show reckless and irresponsible behaviors. It's premature to decide on goals when the client needs to address the mental mind-set and work to change the irresponsible behavior.
CN: Psychosocial integrity; CNS: None; CL: Application

31. The nurse is developing outcomes for a client with a histrionic personality disorder. What is the most appropriate outcome for this client?
1. Contracts for safety and is free of self-inflicted injury
2. Participates in impulse control training
3. Participates in anger management classes
4. Participates in group without being the center of attention

32. Which nursing intervention has priority in the plan of care for a client with antisocial personality disorder who shows defensive behaviors?
1. Help the client accept responsibility for his own decisions and behaviors.
2. Work with the client to feel better about himself by taking care of basic needs.
3. Teach the client to identify the defense mechanisms used to cope with distress.
4. Confront the client about the disregard of social rules and the feelings of others.

33. A client with antisocial personality disorder is trying to manipulate the health care team. What is the best strategy for the staff to implement?
1. Focus on how to teach the client more effective behaviors for meeting basic needs.
2. Help the client verbalize underlying feelings of hopelessness and learn coping skills.
3. Remain calm and don't emotionally respond to the client's manipulative actions.
4. Help the client eliminate the intense desire to have everything in life turn out perfectly.

34. A client with dependent personality disorder is working to increase self-esteem. Which statement by the client shows teaching was successful?
1. "I'm not going to look just at the negative things about myself."
2. "I'm most concerned about my level of competence and progress."
3. "I'm not as envious of the things other people have as I used to be."
4. "I find I can't stop myself from taking over things others should be doing."

Teach the client skills to overcome ineffective behaviors.

The staff must work together as a team.

31. **4.** A client with histrionic personality disorder thrives on being the center of attention. Contracting for safety and impulse control training would be appropriate for a client with borderline personality disorder. Anger management class would be appropriate for antisocial personality disorder.
CN: Safe, effective care environment; CNS: Management of care; CL: Application

32. **1.** Clients with antisocial personality disorder tend to blame other people for their behaviors and need to be taught how to take responsibility for their actions. Clients with antisocial personality disorder don't tend to have problems with self-care habits or meeting their basic needs. Clients with antisocial personality disorder will deny they're defensive or distressed. Most often, these clients feel justified with retaliatory behavior. To confront the client would only cause him to become even more defensive.
CN: Psychosocial integrity; CNS: None; CL: Analysis

33. **3.** The best strategy to use with a client trying to manipulate staff is to stay calm and refrain from responding emotionally. Negative reinforcement of inappropriate behavior increases the chance it will be repeated. Later, it may be possible to address how to meet the client's basic needs. Clients with antisocial personality disorder don't tend to experience feelings of hopelessness or to desire life events to turn out perfectly. In most cases, these clients negate responsibility for their behavior.
CN: Psychosocial integrity; CNS: None; CL: Analysis

34. **1.** As the client makes progress on improving self-esteem, self-blame and negative self-evaluations will decrease. Clients with dependent personality disorder tend to feel fragile and inadequate and would be extremely unlikely to discuss their level of competence and progress. These clients focus on self and aren't envious or jealous. Individuals with dependent personality disorders don't take over situations because they see themselves as inept and inadequate.
CN: Psychosocial integrity; CNS: None; CL: Application

35. The nurse is reviewing the behaviors of a client with a histrionic personality disorder. The nurse determines that a change in behavior may be occurring when the client does what?
1. Draws attention and dresses provocatively
2. Is easily influenced by others or circumstances
3. Shows concern about hurting someone else's feelings
4. Describes intimate relationships with casual acquaintances

36. A client with antisocial personality disorder talks about personal life changes that need to occur. Which client statement shows group therapy is having a <u>positive</u> therapeutic effect?
1. "I'm not doing as bad as I thought I was."
2. "I wish I could believe I can change, but it's probably too late."
3. "I see all the problems, but I'm not sure there are good solutions."
4. "I'm finally learning how to live my life without living on the edge."

37. A nurse tells a client with a personality disorder that he must clean his room before he can go to the dayroom. The client asks if he can play one game of pool first. What is the most appropriate response by the nurse?
1. "You can play one quick game. Then you have to clean your room."
2. "No, you may not."
3. "No, you may not play pool first. The rules were explained to you."
4. "Yes, you may play a quick game. But don't tell the other clients about this."

38. Which of the following describes relationships of a client with a histrionic personality disorder?
1. Cold and distant
2. Shallow and smothering
3. Close and clingy
4. Distrustful and jealous

35. 3. A client with a histrionic personality disorder typically is insensitive to anyone else's experience. Exhibiting concern for another's feelings would indicate a change in the histrionic personality disorder client's behavior. Selections 1, 2, and 4 describe typical behaviors of a client with a histrionic personality disorder.
CN: Psychosocial integrity; CNS: None; CL: Application

36. 4. The client is becoming aware of risky behaviors and how problematic these behaviors are. The first option indicates denial, and the client is somewhat defensive about making a change. The second option indicates defeat, and the client seems to feel stuck. The third option indicates problem identification but also uncertainty and ambivalence about the client's ability to change.
CN: Psychosocial integrity; CNS: None; CL: Analysis

37. 3. This response is firm and reinforces the rules. Allowing the client to play one game before cleaning his room and telling him not to tell anyone else encourages manipulative behavior. Saying no to the client without an explanation doesn't outline or reinforce the rules.
CN: Psychosocial integrity; CNS: None; CL: Analysis

38. 2. A client with histrionic personality disorder has shallow and smothering relationships. Cold and distant relationships describe a client with schizoid personality disorder. Close and clingy relationships characterize dependent personality disorders. Distrustful and jealous characterize paranoid personality disorder relationships.
CN: Psychosocial integrity; CNS: None; CL: Application

39. The nurse is assessing a client who was just admitted to the psychiatric unit. What are the most appropriate questions by the nurse to determine if the client has an obsessive-compulsive personality disorder? Select all that apply.
1. "Do you tend to drive yourself pretty hard, frequently feeling like you need to do just a little more?"
2. "Is it hard for you to argue with your spouse, because you are worried that he or she will get really mad at you and start to dislike you?"
3. "Does anxiety make you want to self-mutilate?"
4. "Do you keep things to yourself just to make sure the wrong people don't get the right information?"
5. "Do you keep lists or sometimes feel a need to keep checking things such as whether the door is locked?"
6. "Do you tend to be a perfectionist?"
7. "Have you found yourself being worried that people won't like you?"

Questions, questions. I want to ask the correct ones!

40. Which of the following behavior patterns would a nurse expect to observe in a client with an obsessive-compulsive personality disorder?
1. Inflexible and lack of spontaneity
2. Submissive and clinging
3. Impulsive and unstable emotionally
4. Cheerful and carefree

41. A nurse admits a client who has an obsessive-compulsive personality disorder to the unit. The nurse expects this client to be preoccupied with which of the following?
1. Their own attractiveness
2. Their own needs and desires being met
3. Rules and regulations of the unit
4. Isolating from all the other clients on the unit

42. Which of the following nursing diagnoses would be appropriate for a client with an obsessive-compulsive disorder?
1. Disturbed sensory perception related to body illusions experienced
2. Risk for self-directed violence related to evidence of recent self-mutilation
3. Risk for injury related to uncontrolled angry outbursts, hitting the wall
4. Ineffective coping related to indecisiveness and preoccupation with details

39. 1, 5, and 6. These questions describe the obsessive-compulsive personality disorder. Question 2 describes a dependent personality disorder. Self-mutilation describes borderline personality disorders. Keeping things to oneself so the wrong people don't get the right information describes the paranoid personality disorder. Being worried about people not liking you describes an avoidant personality disorder.
CN: Psychosocial integrity; CNS: None; CL: Application

40. 1. Inflexibility and lack of spontaneity describe the obsessive-compulsive personality disorder. Submissive and clinging describe the dependent personality disorder. Impulsivity and unstable emotions describe borderline personality disorder, and cheerful and carefree describe the narcissistic personality disorder.
CN: Psychosocial integrity; CNS: None; CL: Application

41. 3. The client with an obsessive-compulsive disorder is preoccupied with rules and regulations of the unit. The histrionic personality disorder client will be concerned about their own attractiveness. The narcissistic personality disorder client will be looking to see how their own needs and desires will be met. Clients with schizotypal personality disorder will socially isolate from others on the unit.
CN: Psychosocial integrity; CNS: None; CL: Application

42. 4. Because clients with an obsessive-compulsive personality disorder are so preoccupied with details, they become indecisive. Body illusions are experienced by schizotypal personality disorder clients. Self-mutilation is a characteristic of borderline clients. Uncontrolled angry outbursts and hitting the wall would be seen in an antisocial personality disorder client.
CN: Psychosocial integrity; CNS: None; CL: Application

43. The nurse recently admitted a client with an obsessive-compulsive personality disorder. What is the most appropriate outcome for this client?
1. Participates in impulse control training
2. Demonstrates a reduction in clinging, splitting, manipulation, and other distancing behaviors
3. Demonstrates a decreased suspicion and increased security
4. Participates in recreational therapy on the unit

44. A nurse is providing care for a client who has obsessive-compulsive disorder. It is important for the nurse to do which of the following?
1. Use a friendly, gentle, reassuring approach because it is the best way to treat clients with an obsessive-compulsive disorder.
2. Guard against engaging in power struggles with these clients. Their need for control is very high.
3. Be aware that clients with this personality disorder can instill guilt when they are not getting what they want.
4. Teach and role model assertiveness.

45. What behaviors would a nurse expect to see in a client who has a schizoid personality disorder?
1. Fearful and anxious
2. Erratic and emotional
3. Odd and eccentric
4. Emotional and dramatic

46. The nurse is assessing a new client who was just admitted to the psychiatric unit. Which of the following assessment questions by the nurse would determine if the client has a schizoid personality disorder? Select all that apply.
1. "Do you tend to be a perfectionist?"
2. "Have you found yourself being worried that people won't like you?"
3. "Do you enjoy making most decisions in your house, or would you prefer that others make the most important decisions?"
4. "During the course of your life, have you had only about one or two friends?"
5. "Over the years, have you been able to take care of yourself in a physical fight?"
6. "Do you prefer to be alone?"

Is this behavior expected?

43. 4. The obsessive-compulsive personality overemphasizes work to the exclusion of participating in pleasurable leisure activities. For the client to be able to participate in recreational therapy on the unit is a good first step. Impulse control training, splitting and manipulation, and distancing behaviors describe the borderline personality disorder. Decrease in suspicion and increased security would be outcomes for a client with a paranoid personality disorder.
CN: Psychosocial integrity; CNS: None; CL: Application

44. 2. Guarding against engaging in power struggles describes how a nurse should approach a client with obsessive-compulsive personality disorder. A friendly, gentle, reassuring approach is the best way to treat clients with an avoidant personality disorder. Antisocial personality disorder clients instill guilt in staff when they don't get what they want. Teaching and role modeling assertiveness are strategies for dependent and histrionic personality disorders.
CN: Safe, effective care environment; CNS: Management of care; CL: Application

45. 3. Odd and eccentric behaviors are seen in clients with a cluster A personality disorder: paranoid, schizotypal, and schizoid disorders. Fearful and anxious describe clients with a cluster C personality disorder: avoidant, dependent, and obsessive-compulsive disorders. Erratic, emotional, and dramatic describe clients with a cluster B personality disorder: borderline, antisocial, histrionic, and narcissistic disorders.
CN: Psychosocial integrity; CNS: None; CL: Application

46. 4 and 6. Clients with schizoid personality disorders will only have about one or two friends and prefer to be alone. Clients with obsessive-compulsive personality disorders are perfectionists. Clients with avoidant personality disorders are worried that people won't like them. Clients with dependent personality disorders would prefer that others make important decisions. Clients with antisocial personality disorders can take care of themselves in a physical fight.
CN: Psychosocial integrity; CNS: None; CL: Application

47. Which of the following behavior patterns would a nurse expect to observe in a client with a schizoid personality disorder?
1. Emotional coldness and flattened affect
2. Submissive and clinging
3. Impulsive and unstable emotionally
4. Cheerful and carefree

48. What would be an important guideline for nurses working with clients with borderline personality disorder?
1. When behavioral problems emerge, calmly review the therapeutic goals and boundaries of treatment.
2. Try to prevent or reduce untoward effects of manipulation.
3. Remain neutral and avoid engaging in power struggles.
4. Respect a client's need for social isolation.

49. Which nursing intervention has <u>priority</u> for a client with borderline personality disorder?
1. Maintain consistent, realistic limits.
2. Give instructions for meeting basic self-care needs.
3. Engage in daytime activities to stimulate wakefulness.
4. Have the client attend group therapy on a daily basis.

Prioritizing is a crucial part of nursing!

50. Which of the following nursing diagnoses would be appropriate for a client with a schizoid personality disorder?
1. Impaired social interaction related to seductive and self-dramatizing behaviors
2. Risk for other-directed violence related to pacing and threatening stances
3. Ineffective coping related to difficulty in developing close relationships
4. Defensive coping related to absence of guilt and superior attitude toward others

51. The nurse is identifying nursing outcomes for a client with a schizoid personality disorder. What is the most appropriate outcome?
1. Demonstrates an ability to use constructive criticism
2. Participates in two of the four scheduled groups on the unit
3. Demonstrates a reduction in clinging, splitting, and manipulation behaviors
4. Demonstrates a decrease in attention-seeking behaviors

47. 1. Clients with schizoid personality disorder are emotionally cold and have a flattened affect. Submissive and clinging behaviors describe the dependent personality disorder. Impulsivity and unstable emotions describe borderline personality disorder, and cheerful and carefree describe the narcissistic personality disorder.

CN: Psychosocial integrity; CNS: None; CL: Application

48. 1. Reminding the borderline client of the goals and boundaries of treatment helps the client to focus on therapy. Manipulation is an issue with antisocial personality clients. Power struggles are an issue for the narcissistic client, and respecting the client's need for social isolation describes a client with schizotypal personality disorder.

CN: Safe, effective care environment; CNS: Safety and infection control; CL: Application

49. 1. Clients with borderline personality disorder who are needy, dependent, and manipulative will benefit greatly from maintaining consistent, realistic limits. They don't tend to have difficulty meeting their self-care needs and don't tend to have sleeping difficulties. They enjoy attending group therapy because they typically attempt to use the opportunity to become the center of attention.

CN: Safe, effective care environment; CNS: Management of care; CL: Application

50. 3. Clients with schizoid personality disorders consistently have difficulty in cultivating close relationships, even within their own family. Clients with histrionic personality disorders consistently draw attention to themselves. Risk for other-directed violence, chronic low self-esteem, and defensive coping would be appropriate for a client with an antisocial personality disorder.

CN: Safe, effective care environment; CNS: Management of care; CL: Application

51. 2. Clients with a schizoid personality disorder prefer solitary activities and do not enjoy close relationships. However, for this client to attend two out of four unit groups would be a step toward gaining some comfort in being around people. Avoidant personality disorder clients experience fear of rejection and/or criticism and are very reluctant to participate in social situations because of this fear. Selections 3 and 4 describe a cluster B personality disorders: borderline, antisocial, histrionic, or narcissistic.

CN: Safe, effective care environment; CNS: Management of care; CL: Application

52. What might be an effective intervention for a client with a schizoid personality disorder?
1. Participates in impulse control training
2. Participates in anger management classes
3. Participates in group without being the center of attention
4. Participates in social skills training

What is the best thing to do?

53. The nurse is assessing a client for narcissistic personality disorder. What are the best questions for the nurse to ask the client? Select all that apply.
1. "Do you frequently feel let down by people?"
2. "Do you find that most people aren't quite up to your standards?"
3. "Do you feel that other people take advantage of you?"
4. "Do you find that people often have a tendency to be disloyal or dishonest?"
5. "If people give you a hard time, do you tend to put them in their place quickly?"
6. "Are you a very special person?"
7. "Would you say it is fairly easy for you to get jealous?"

54. A nurse is assessing a client with a narcissistic personality disorder. The nurse anticipates the client's behavior to be characterized as which of the following?
1. Grandiose and entitled
2. Submissive and clinging
3. Impulsive and unstable emotionally
4. Provocative and seductive

You've finished 54 questions. That should motivate you to keep going.

55. A client with dependent personality disorder is working on goals for self-care. Which short-term goal is <u>most important</u> to the client's everyday activities of daily living?
1. Do all self-care activities independently.
2. Write a daily schedule for each day of the week.
3. Do self-care activities in a minimal amount of time.
4. Determine activities that can be performed without help.

It's most important that I answer this question correctly.

52. 4. Clients with schizoid personality disorder could benefit from social skills training because they are detached from others and loners. A client with histrionic personality disorder thrives on being the center of attention. Impulse control training would be appropriate for a client with borderline personality disorder. Anger management class would be appropriate for a client with antisocial personality disorder.
CN: Safe, effective care environment; CNS: Management of care; CL: Application

53. 2, 5, and 6. Clients with narcissistic personality disorders feel others are not up to their standards, they put people in their place quickly, and they feel that they are very special people. Clients with borderline personality disorders feel let down by people. Clients with paranoid personality disorders feel that others take advantage of them, feel that people tend to be disloyal or dishonest, and get jealous easily.
CN: Psychosocial integrity; CNS: None; CL: Application

54. 1. Grandiosity and a sense of entitlement describe the behavior pattern of a client with a narcissistic personality disorder. Submissive and clinging describe the dependent personality disorder. Impulsivity and unstable emotions describe borderline personality disorder, and provocative and seductive behaviors describe the histrionic personality disorder.
CN: Psychosocial integrity; CNS: None; CL: Application

55. 4. By determining activities that can be performed without assistance, the client can then begin to practice them independently. If the nurse only encourages a client to perform self-care activities independently, nothing may change. Writing a daily schedule doesn't help the client focus on what needs to be done to promote self-care. The amount of time needed to perform self-care activities isn't important. If time pressure is put on the client, there may be more reluctance to perform self-care activities.
CN: Psychosocial integrity; CNS: None; CL: Application

CN: Client needs category   CNS: Client needs subcategory   CL: Cognitive level

56. Which of the following nursing diagnoses would be appropriate for a client with a narcissistic personality disorder?
1. Risk for self-mutilation related to a desperate need for attention
2. Ineffective coping related to negative attitudes toward health behavior
3. Impaired social interaction related to use of control strategies and disruption of close relationships
4. Risk for injury related to uncontrolled anger and hostility toward others

57. Which of the following nursing outcomes would be appropriate for a client with a narcissistic personality disorder?
1. Identifies factors that interfere with social interaction
2. Demonstrates a reduction in clinging and splitting behaviors
3. Demonstrates ability to reframe negative self-thoughts into more realistic appraisals
4. Seeks help when experiencing self-destructive impulses

58. Which of the following responses would a nurse expect from a client with a narcissistic personality disorder?
1. "You owe me 5 more minutes on my smoke break since you let us out late from group."
2. "You are the only nurse that understands me; I don't like the other nurses at all. They are mean."
3. "I don't know what I should wear today or what groups I should go to."
4. "I can't go to group today because one of the clients hurt my feelings yesterday in group."

59. A client with dependent personality disorder is having trouble performing activities of daily living. Which nursing intervention should help facilitate the client's daily activities?
1. Have the client eat three meals a day.
2. Work with the client to establish a budget.
3. Make a chart to document hygiene practices.
4. Discuss how the client can obtain a driver's license.

Think carefully. You know the answer to this one.

56. 3. Clients with narcissistic personality disorder have relationships that are characterized by disruption (frequently provoke arguments) or control (consistently in power struggles). Risk for self-mutilation describes clients with borderline personality disorder. Negative attitudes toward health behavior and risk for injury related to uncontrolled anger and hostility toward others describe antisocial personality disorder.

CN: Safe, effective care environment; CNS: Management of care; CL: Application

57. 1. A client with narcissistic personality disorder portrays a demeanor of grandiosity and a lack of empathy for others with relationships that are characterized by disruption (frequently provoke arguments) or control (consistently in power struggles). To be able to identify factors that interfere with social interaction would be most appropriate for a client with narcissistic personality disorder. Reduction in clinging, splitting, and seeking help when self-destructive behaviors are experienced and would be appropriate for a client with borderline personality disorder. Reframing negative self-thoughts would be appropriate for a client with a dependent personality disorder.

CN: Safe, effective care environment; CNS: Management of care; CL: Application

58. 1. Clients with narcissistic personality disorder have a sense of entitlement. Splitting staff is a typical response from a client who has a borderline personality disorder. Indecisiveness is a characteristic of a client with a dependent personality disorder. Holding grudges is a characteristic of a client with a paranoid personality disorder.

CN: Psychosocial integrity; CNS: None; CL: Application

59. 2. Clients with dependent personality disorder tend to withdraw from adult responsibilities. Managing money through the use of a budget is a first step toward assuming adult responsibilities. These clients don't tend to have problems with nutritional intake. Hygiene issues usually aren't a problem for clients with dependent personality disorder. Clients with a dependent personality disorder don't have any special reasons for not obtaining a driver's license.

CN: Psychosocial integrity; CNS: None; CL: Application

60. A client with a dependent personality disorder is taking fluoxetine (Prozac) for depression. Which instruction is included in client teaching?
1. Drink only wine and beer when taking this drug.
2. Add as-needed doses if depression becomes worse.
3. Expect 3 to 4 weeks to go by before effects are seen.
4. Be aware that alterations in usual sleep patterns, especially nightmares, may occur.

61. The nurse has the following clients:

A dependent personality disorder client who is seeking care from another client after experiencing a recent divorce

A borderline personality disorder client who is cutting her wrists and arms since admission to the unit

An avoidant personality disorder client who refuses to go to groups on the unit

A paranoid personality disorder client who is suspicious of the male clients in the unit and refuses to attend the community morning meeting

Which client is the nurse's first priority to see at the beginning of the shift?
1. Dependent personality disorder client
2. Borderline personality disorder client
3. Avoidant personality disorder client
4. Paranoid personality disorder client

62. Which of the following tasks could be delegated to a psychiatric technician on the unit? Select all that apply.
1. Assist a client with personal daily living activities.
2. Conduct educational sessions.
3. Administer medications to clients.
4. Develop recreational activities.
5. Teach clients about their medications.
6. Write medical orders from the physician.
7. Contribute to the planning and implementing of individual treatment plans.
8. Assist in the admission process by interviewing patients and record keeping.
9. Take vitals on clients.

63. Of all of the cluster groupings of personality disorders, which group is apt to be most challenging to the management of the milieu of the unit for the nurse?
1. Cluster A
2. Cluster B
3. Cluster C
4. Cluster D

It takes me a while, but I'll get the job done.

60. 3. The client must take the drug for 3 to 4 weeks before therapeutic effects are seen. The nurse must caution the client against the use of alcohol, including wine and beer, when taking fluoxetine. The client is to take the drug as prescribed. Additional doses must not be self-administered. Fluoxetine treats disruptions in sleep and doesn't cause nightmares.
CN: Physiological integrity; CNS: Pharmacological and parenteral therapies; CL: Application

61. 2. The nurse has to attend to the physical safety of the borderline personality disorder client first. The behaviors of the other three clients with personality disorders affect the milieu of the unit and can be addressed later.
CN: Safe, effective care environment; CNS: Management of care; CL: Application

62. 1, 2, 4, 5, 7, 8, and 9. All of these tasks could be delegated to a psychiatric technician or unlicensed personnel except administering medications and writing medical orders from the physician. The certified medication aide could dispense medications, but writing medical orders from the physician requires a nurse's license to perform.
CN: Safe, effective care environment; CNS: Management of care; CL: Application

63. 2. Cluster B will be the most challenging to maintain a positive milieu for all clients. Cluster B personality disorder clients are very labile emotionally and are quite dramatic. Clusters A and C avoid close relationships and are apt to isolate in their rooms. There is no such cluster D nomenclature for personality disorders.
CN: Safe, effective care environment; CNS: Management of care; CL: Application

CN: Client needs category   CNS: Client needs subcategory   CL: Cognitive level

64. Which of the following clients needs to be assigned as a 1:1 with a psychiatric technician?
1. A client with histrionic personality disorder who frequently faints when a male individual is near
2. A client with antisocial personality disorder who steals food from other clients' meal trays
3. A client with an obsessive-compulsive personality disorder who insists all the rules of the unit be followed
4. A client with borderline personality disorder who has acted on stated suicidal thoughts and has cut herself

65. A nurse is evaluating the effectiveness of an assertiveness group that a client with dependent personality disorder attended. Which client statement indicates the group had therapeutic value?
1. "I can't seem to do the things other people do."
2. "I wish I could be more organized like other people."
3. "I want to talk about something that's bothering me."
4. "I just don't want people in my family to fight anymore."

66. What contributes to the difficulty in creating a therapeutic alliance with clients with personality disorders? Select all that apply.
1. Client's suspiciousness
2. Aloofness from clients
3. Secretive style and hostility of clients
4. Transference from the nurse
5. Setting limits

67. The nurse is expecting the psychiatrist to order an antidepressant for a client with borderline personality disorder. Which of the following would be best for this client?
1. Monoamine oxidase inhibitors (MAOIs) work best for those with a borderline personality disorder because the effects are felt very quickly.
2. Selective serotonin reuptake inhibitors (SSRIs) in addition to an atypical antipsychotic treat dysphoria, mood instability, and impulsivity in clients with borderline personality disorder.
3. Antipsychotics treat illusions, ideas of reference, paranoid thinking, anxiety, and hostility in clients.
4. Anxiolytics will reduce the anxiety seen in borderline personality disorder clients.

You're doing great!

How do I know which is the best?

64. 4. Because of the labile emotion and impulsivity characteristics of a client with borderline personality disorder, it is necessary to implement 1:1 staffing for this borderline client to ensure safety of the client. The other client behaviors do need to be addressed but do not require 1:1 staffing.
CN: Safe, effective care environment; CNS: Management of care; CL: Application

65. 3. By asking to talk about a bothersome situation, the client has taken the first step toward assertive behavior. To smooth over or minimize troubling events isn't an assertive position. The first option reflects a lack of self-confidence; it's not an assertive statement. Statements that express the client's wishes aren't assertive statements.
CN: Psychosocial integrity; CNS: None; CL: Analysis

66. 1, 2, and 3. Client behaviors of suspicion, aloofness, secretive style, and hostility contribute to the difficulty in obtaining a therapeutic alliance with clients with a personality disorder. It is countertransference that the nurse experiences that could possibly affect the therapeutic alliance with personality-disordered clients. Setting limits is a crucial component of the therapeutic alliance with clients with personality disorders. These limits will need to be repeated to instill responsibility to clients for their behaviors.
CN: Psychosocial integrity; CNS: None; CL: Analysis

67. 2. SSRIs and atypical antipsychotics do treat dysphoria, mood instability, and impulsivity in clients with borderline personality disorder. This is the best selection of medications for a client with borderline personality disorder. MAOI medications have food restrictions, and clients with borderline personality disorder would not comply with such restrictions. Antipsychotics are prescribed for psychotic behaviors: illusions, ideas of reference, and paranoid thinking. Anxiolytics may be prescribed for clients with borderline personality disorder, but these medications are limited in addressing only the anxiety these clients would have. Borderline personality disorder clients experience more symptoms than just anxiety.
CN: Safe, effective care environment; CNS: Management of care; CL: Analysis

68. A nurse notices that a client with dependent personality disorder is depressed. Which factor is assessed as contributing to depression?
1. Unmet needs
2. Sense of smothering
3. Messy, unkempt appearance
4. Difficulty delaying gratification

I wonder what caused the change?

69. A client with dependent personality disorder makes the following statement: "I'll never be able to take care of myself." Which response by the nurse is best?
1. "How can you say that? You can function."
2. "Let's talk about what's making you feel so fearful."
3. "I think we need to work on identifying your strengths."
4. "Can we talk about this tomorrow at the family meeting?"

Keep in mind the type of personality this client has.

70. A client on your unit says the Mafia has a contract out on him. He refuses to leave his semi-private room and insists on frisking his roommate before allowing him to enter. Which action should the nurse take first?
1. Transfer the client to a private room.
2. Acknowledge the client's fear when he refuses to leave his room or wants to frisk his roommate.
3. Transfer the roommate to another room.
4. Lock the client out of his room for a while each day so he can see he's safe.

First things first!

68. **1.** Having many unmet needs is a precursor to depression. Clients with dependent personality disorder don't experience a sense of smothering, a problem seen in clients with panic disorder. Poor hygiene is often a manifestation, not a cause, of depression. Clients with problems delaying gratification tend to have anxiety problems, not problems with depression.
CN: Psychosocial integrity; CNS: None; CL: Analysis

69. **2.** The client with dependent personality disorder is afraid of abandonment and being unable to care for himself. Talking about his fears is a useful strategy. The first option is inappropriate because the nurse doesn't recognize the client's feelings. When the client makes a desperate statement, the nurse must respond to the client's feelings, rather than insert her opinion. Working on identifying a client's strengths will add to his feelings of not being strong enough to care for himself. Waiting to talk about his concern until the family meeting minimizes its importance.
CN: Psychosocial integrity; CNS: None; CL: Analysis

70. **2.** Acknowledging underlying feelings may help defuse the client's anxiety without promoting his delusional thinking. This, in turn, may help the client distinguish between his emotional state and external reality. Transferring either client to another room would validate the client's delusional thinking. Locking the client out of his room may further escalate the client's anxiety and stimulate aggressive acting-out behavior.
CN: Psychosocial integrity; CNS: None; CL: Application

71. A client with schizotypal personality disorder is sitting in a puddle of urine. He's playing in it, smiling, and softly singing a child's song. Which action would be best?
1. Admonish the client for not using the bathroom.
2. Firmly tell the client that his behavior is unacceptable.
3. Ask the client whether he's ready to get cleaned up now.
4. Help the client to the shower and change the bedclothes.

72. A client with avoidant personality disorder says occupational therapy (OT) is boring and he doesn't want to go. Which action by the nurse is most appropriate?
1. State firmly that you'll escort him to OT.
2. Arrange with OT for the client to do a project on the unit.
3. Ask the client to talk about why OT is boring.
4. Arrange for the client not to attend OT until he feels better.

73. A client with paranoid personality disorder works toward the goal of increasing social interaction. Which behavior indicates that the client is meeting this goal?
1. The client develops and follows a schedule of group activities.
2. The client verbalizes aggressive feelings to the nurse.
3. The client visits the consumer center to use the Internet.
4. The client explores somatic complaints with the staff.

You've passed the 71 mark. Not too much more to go!

Which answer will help the client increase his social interaction?

71. 4. A client with a schizotypal personality disorder can experience high levels of anxiety and regress to childlike behaviors. This client may require help meeting self-care needs. The client may not respond to the other options or those options may generate more anxiety.

CN: Psychosocial integrity; CNS: None; CL: Application

72. 1. If given the chance, a client with avoidant personality disorder typically elects to remain immobilized. The nurse should insist that the client participate in OT. Arranging for the client to do a project on the unit validates and reinforces the client's desire to avoid going to OT. Addressing an invalid issue such as the client's perceived boredom avoids the real issue: the client's need for therapy. There's no indication that the client is incapable of participating in OT.

CN: Psychosocial integrity; CNS: None; CL: Application

73. 1. By developing and following a schedule of group activities, the client increases opportunities to use social skills and increase interactions with others. Verbalizing aggressive feelings doesn't give the client opportunities to increase social interaction. Using a computer at the consumer center is a solitary activity. Talking to the staff about somatic complaints doesn't provide opportunities for social interaction.

CN: Psychosocial integrity; CNS: None; CL: Application

74. A nurse works with the family of a client diagnosed with schizoid personality disorder, helping them to assist him in making decisions. Which outcome indicates the nurse's interventions have been successful?
1. The family prevents the client from experiencing disappointments.
2. The family encourages the client to talk about specific issues and concerns.
3. The family removes alcohol and unnecessary prescription drugs from the house.
4. The family doesn't let the client obtain secondary gains from illness.

75. A nurse discusses job possibilities with a client diagnosed with schizoid personality disorder. Which suggestion by the nurse should be helpful?
1. "You could work in a family restaurant part-time on the weekends and holidays."
2. "Maybe your friend could get you that customer service job where you work only in the evenings."
3. "Your idea of applying for the position of filing and organizing records is worth pursuing."
4. "Being an introvert limits the employment opportunities you can pursue."

76. A client with borderline personality disorder is learning how to verbalize, rather than act on, the desire to hurt himself. What is the most appropriate nursing intervention?
1. Explain how pain triggers intense anger and causes the client to act out.
2. Determine how problems with the client's family cause him to act aggressively.
3. Teach the client that being volatile is a normal reaction to unfair events.
4. Have the client work on identifying speech and behavior that accompany anger.

77. A client with borderline personality disorder states that he doesn't know how to deal with his impulsive behavior. Which intervention should the nurse implement?
1. Teach the client that impulsive behavior is part of his illness.
2. Explore how depression influences impulsive situations.
3. Select an example of an impulsive situation and explore it.
4. Decrease interactions in which impulsive behavior occurs.

When trying to answer question 75, think about the type of activities this client prefers.

Three more hurdles...I mean questions...to go!

In question 77, focus on the client's impulsive behavior.

74. 2. A client with schizoid personality disorder typically is vague and has difficulty with self-expression; encouraging the client to talk about specific issues and concerns shows that the nurse's interventions were successful. It's neither realistic nor helpful for the family to protect the client from disappointments. Clients with schizoid personality disorder aren't at high risk for substance abuse and don't seek secondary gains from illness.
CN: Psychosocial integrity; CNS: None; CL: Application

75. 3. Clients with schizoid personality disorder prefer solitary activities, such as filing, to working with others. Working as a cashier or customer service representative would involve interacting with many people. Not all jobs require extensive interpersonal contact.
CN: Psychosocial integrity; CNS: None; CL: Analysis

76. 4. Aggressive speech and inappropriate behaviors indicate that the client is angry or upset; these feelings may trigger acting out. Pain rarely triggers intense anger or makes a client act out. Blaming one's family of origin for inappropriate handling of anger isn't helpful. Being volatile isn't a normal reaction to unfair life events. The client needs to express anger in safe and appropriate ways.
CN: Psychosocial integrity; CNS: None; CL: Analysis

77. 3. By selecting an impulsive situation to explore with the client, the nurse can help him begin to understand the causes and consequences of his behavior and learn how to modify it. Although impulsive behavior is part of borderline personality disorder, the nurse's intervention needs to address ways to handle it. Anxiety, not depression, is strongly related to impulsive behavior. Decreasing social interactions is unrealistic; it's more useful to address the impulsive behavior.
CN: Psychosocial integrity; CNS: None; CL: Analysis

78. A nurse is monitoring a client who appears to be hallucinating. The nurse notes paranoid content in the client's speech and that he appears agitated. The client is gesturing at a figure on the television. Which nursing interventions are appropriate? Select all that apply.
1. In a firm voice, instruct the client to stop the behavior.
2. Reinforce that the client is not in any danger.
3. Acknowledge the presence of the hallucinations.
4. Instruct other team members to ignore the client's behavior.
5. Immediately implement physical restraint procedures.
6. Use a calm voice and simple commands.

79. When assessing a client diagnosed with impulse control disorder, the nurse observes violent, aggressive, and assaultive behavior. Which assessment data is the nurse also likely to find? Select all that apply.
1. The client functions well in other areas of his life.
2. The degree of aggressiveness is out of proportion to the stressor.
3. The violent behavior is most often justified by the stressor.
4. The client has a history of parental alcoholism and chaotic, abusive family life.
5. The client has no remorse about the inability to control his behavior.

78. 2, 3, and 6. Using a calm voice, the nurse should reassure the client that he's safe. She shouldn't challenge the client; rather, she should acknowledge his hallucinatory experience. It's not appropriate to request that the client stop the behavior. Implementing restraints isn't warranted at this time. Although the client is agitated, no evidence exists that he is at risk for harming himself or others.

CN: Psychosocial integrity; CNS: None; CL: Application

79. 1, 2, and 4. A client with an impulse control disorder who displays violent, aggressive, and assaultive behavior generally functions well in other areas of his life. The degree of aggressiveness is typically out of proportion with the stressor. Such a client commonly has a history of parental alcoholism and a chaotic family life, and often verbalizes sincere remorse and guilt for the aggressive behavior.

CN: Psychosocial integrity; CNS: None; CL: Application

An incredible job! You've finished another big chapter! That's music to my ears!

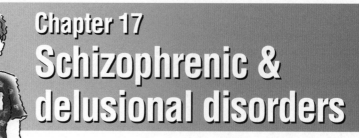

Chapter 17
Schizophrenic & delusional disorders

So I'm talking to Queen Elizabeth the other day, and she said you'd do spectacularly well on this chapter. (I'm kidding. What, do I look delusional?) Personally, I think you'll do even better than that. Go for it!

Therapeutic intervention is the key.

1. A schizophrenic client tells his primary nurse that he's scheduled to meet the King of Samoa at a special time, making it impossible for the client to leave his room for dinner. Which response by the nurse is <u>most appropriate</u>?
1. "It's mealtime. Let's go so you can eat."
2. "The King of Samoa told me to take you to dinner."
3. "Your physician expects you to follow the unit's schedule."
4. "People who don't eat on this unit aren't being cooperative."

2. During breakfast, a client announces that he is still the President of the United States. What is the <u>best</u> response from the nurse?
1. "How are you, Mr. President?"
2. "The real president was on TV last night."
3. "How is your breakfast?"
4. "Is this the Oval Office then?"

3. A 40-year-old client with a diagnosis of chronic, undifferentiated schizophrenia lives in a rooming house that has a weekly nursing clinic. He scratches while he tells the nurse he feels creatures eating away at his skin. Which intervention should be done <u>first</u>?
1. Talk about his hallucinations and fears.
2. Refer him for anticholinergic adverse reactions.
3. Assess for possible physical problems such as rash.
4. Call his physician to get his medication increased to control his psychosis.

1. **1.** A delusional client is so wrapped up in his false beliefs that he tends to disregard activities of daily living, such as nutrition and hydration. He needs clear, concise, firm directions from a caring nurse to meet his needs. The second option belittles and tricks the client, possibly evoking mistrust on the part of the client. The third option evades the issue of meeting his basic needs. The last option is demeaning and doesn't address the delusion.
CN: Health promotion and maintenance; CNS: None; CL: Application

2. **3.** Asking about breakfast redirects the client and focuses him on a structured activity or reality-based task. The other responses focus attention on or support the client's delusion.
CN: Psychosocial integrity; CNS: None; CL: Application

3. **3.** Clients with schizophrenia generally have poor visceral recognition because they live so fully in their fantasy world. They need to have an in-depth assessment of physical complaints that may spill over into their delusional symptoms. Talking with the client won't provide an assessment of his itching, and itching isn't an adverse reaction of antipsychotic drugs. Calling the physician to get the client's medication increased doesn't address his physical complaints.
CN: Safe, effective care environment; CNS: Management of care; CL: Application

CN: Client needs category   CNS: Client needs subcategory   CL: Cognitive level

4. A 22-year-old schizophrenic client was admitted to the psychiatric unit during the night. The next morning, he began to misidentify the nurse and call her by his sister's name. Which intervention is best?
1. Assess the client for potential violence.
2. Take the client to his room, where he'll feel safer.
3. Assume the misidentification makes the client feel more comfortable.
4. Correct the misidentification and orient the client to the unit and staff.

Orienting a new client to the staff and the surroundings can help him feel in control.

5. The nurse is aware that a schizophrenic client who is experiencing prolonged isolation is at risk for developing:
1. delusions.
2. hallucinations.
3. lack of volition.
4. waxy flexibility.

6. A client diagnosed with schizophrenia several years ago tells a nurse that he feels "very sad." The nurse observes that he's smiling when he says it. The nurse interprets the behavior as which of the following?
1. Inappropriate affect
2. Extrapyramidal
3. Insight
4. Inappropriate mood

7. A disorganized schizophrenic's symptoms include the distressing triad of extreme social withdrawal, odd mannerisms, and other regressive behaviors. What is the most appropriate intervention by the nurse?
1. Require the client to attend one group activity each day.
2. Suggest that the client keeps up with his same gender peer group.
3. Interact with the client often and briefly, in a friendly manner.
4. Allow the client to come out when he is ready.

The word disorganized refers to a type of schizophrenia, and to me!

4. 4. Misidentification can contribute to anxiety, fear, aggression, and hostility. Orienting a new client to the hospital unit, staff, and other clients, along with establishing a nurse–client relationship, can decrease these feelings and help the client feel in control. Assessing for potential violence is an important nursing function for any psychiatric client, but a perceived supportive environment reduces the risk for violence. Withdrawing to his room, unless interpersonal relationships have become nontherapeutic for him, encourages the client to remain in his fantasy world.
CN: Psychosocial integrity; CNS: None; CL: Application

5. 2. Prolonged isolation can produce sensory deprivation, manifested by hallucinations. A delusion is a false, fixed belief that has no basis in reality. Lack of volition is a symptom associated with type I negative symptoms of schizophrenia. Waxy flexibility is a motor disturbance that's a predominant feature of catatonic schizophrenia.
CN: Psychosocial integrity; CNS: None; CL: Application

6. 1. Affect refers to behaviors such as facial expression that can be observed when a person is expressing and experiencing feelings. If the client's affect doesn't reflect the emotional content of the statement, the affect is considered inappropriate. Extrapyramidal symptoms are adverse effects of some categories of medication. Insight is a component of the mental status examination and is the ability to perceive oneself realistically and understand if a problem exists. Mood is an extensive and sustained feeling tone.
CN: Psychosocial integrity; CNS: None; CL: Application

7. 3. Interacting with the client often and in a friendly manner suggests planned, short, frequent, and undemanding interactions. Clients with disorganized schizophrenia require one-on-one nonthreatening activities and should not remain in social isolation.
CN: Psychosocial integrity; CNS: None; CL: Application

8. A client on the psychiatric unit is copying and imitating the movements of his primary nurse. During recovery, he says, "I thought the nurse was my mirror. I felt connected only when I saw my nurse." The nurse identifies this behavior as which of the following?
 1. Modeling
 2. Echopraxia
 3. Ego-syntonicity
 4. Ritualism

9. The teenage son of a father with schizophrenia is worried that he might have schizophrenia as well. Which behavior would be an indication that he should be evaluated for signs of the disorder?
 1. Moodiness
 2. Preoccupation with his body
 3. Spending more time away from home
 4. Changes in sleep patterns

10. The nurse is teaching the family of a client with a psychiatric disorder about <u>traditional</u> antipsychotic drugs and their effect on symptoms. Which of the following symptoms would be most responsive to these types of drugs?
 1. Apathy
 2. Delusions
 3. Social withdrawal
 4. Attention impairment

> Pay attention to the key word in questions 10 and 11.

11. A client was hospitalized after his son filed a petition for involuntary hospitalization for safety reasons. The son seeks out the nurse because his father is angry and refuses to talk with him. He's frustrated and feeling very guilty about his decision. What is the <u>most appropriate</u> response by the nurse?
 1. "Your father is here because he needs help."
 2. "He'll feel differently about you as he gets better."
 3. "It sounds like you're feeling guilty about leaving your father here."
 4. "This is a stressful time for you, but you'll feel better as he gets well."

8. **2.** Echopraxia is the copying of another's behaviors and is the result of the loss of ego boundaries. Modeling is the conscious copying of someone's behaviors. Ego-syntonicity refers to behaviors that correspond with the individual's sense of self. Ritualistic behaviors are repetitive and compulsive.

CN: Psychosocial integrity; CNS: None; CL: Application

9. **4.** In conjunction with other signs, changes in sleep patterns are distinctive initial signs of schizophrenia. Other signs include changes in personal care habits and social isolation. Moodiness, preoccupation with the body, and spending more time away from home are normal adolescent behaviors.

CN: Health promotion and maintenance; CNS: None; CL: Application

10. **2.** Positive symptoms, such as delusions, hallucinations, thought disorder, and disorganized speech, respond to traditional antipsychotic drugs. The other options are part of the category of negative symptoms, including affective flattening, restricted thought and speech, apathy, anhedonia, asociality, and attention impairment, and are more responsive to the new atypical antipsychotics, such as clozapine (Clozaril), risperidone (Risperdal), and olanzapine (Zyprexa).

CN: Physiological integrity CNS: Pharmacological and parenteral therapies; CL: Application

11. **3.** This response focuses on the son and helps him discuss and deal with his feelings. Unresolved feelings of guilt, shame, isolation, and loss of hope impact on the family's ability to manage the crisis and be supportive to the client. The other options offer premature reassurance and cut off the opportunity for the son to discuss his feelings.

CN: Psychosocial integrity; CNS: None; CL: Application

12. A client has followed her antipsychotic medication regimen for a number of years. Her physician has prescribed antibiotic therapy for a newly acquired urinary tract infection. What is the most important nursing intervention?
1. Arrange for possible hospitalization.
2. Have a visiting nurse give the medication.
3. Give instructions on the medication, possible adverse effects, and a return demonstration for teaching effectiveness.
4. Develop a psychoeducational program to address the client's emotional and physical problems arising from physiological problems.

13. A client begins to display some bothersome and dismaying new symptoms from his antipsychotic medicine. He is concerned because he has noted improvement of his psychotic symptoms but is now experiencing uncontrollable restlessness of his limbs and head. The client calls the clinic to ask what is happening and how he can stop it. What is the best response by the nurse?
1. Tell the client to ignore these symptoms because they will go away.
2. Explain that he should try to experiment with different dosages to see how he feels.
3. Inform him that if he develops blurred vision or a fever that he must go to the nearest emergency room.
4. Reassure him that he is experiencing signs of tardive dyskinesia and should see his psychiatric provider to begin a medication that helps resolve these symptoms.

Signs and symptoms are big on NCLEX examinations.

14. A client approaches a nurse and tells her that he hears voices telling him that he's evil and deserves to die. Which response by the nurse is most appropriate?
1. "The voices aren't real, so ignore them."
2. "I don't see anyone in the room."
3. "I don't hear any voices, but I understand that you do."
4. "Tell the voices you won't listen to them."

15. A 49-year-old client is admitted to the emergency department frightened and reporting that he's hearing voices telling him to do bad things. Which intervention should be the nurse's priority?
1. Tell the client he's safe and that the voices aren't real.
2. Tell the client he's safe now and promise the staff will protect him.
3. Assess the nature of the commands by asking the client what the voices are saying.
4. Administer a neuroleptic medication.

Remember to prioritize!

12. 3. The client has been successful and reliable in carrying out her current medication regimen. The nurse should assume the competency includes self-administration of antibiotics if the instructions are understood. No evidence exists that the client is having a relapse as a result of the infection, so she wouldn't need a psychoeducational program or hospitalization. Having a community nurse give the medication encourages dependency as opposed to self-care.
CN: Safe, effective care environment; CNS: Management of care; CL: Application

13. 4. Symptoms of tardive dyskinesia include tongue protrusion, lip smacking, chewing, blinking, grimacing, choreiform movements of limbs and trunk, and foot tapping. Primary prevention of tardive dyskinesia is achieved by using the lowest effective dose of a neuroleptic for the shortest time. However, with diseases of chronic psychosis such as schizophrenia, this strategy must be balanced with the fact that increased dosages of neuroleptics are more beneficial in preventing recurrence of psychosis. If tardive dyskinesia is diagnosed, the causative drug should be discontinued. Blurred vision is a common adverse reaction of antipsychotic drugs and usually disappears after a few weeks of therapy. Restlessness is associated with akathisia. Sudden fever is a symptom of a malignant neurological disorder. The prescribing authority will make appropriate changes to meet the client's need.
CN: Physiological integrity; CNS: Reduction of risk potential; CL: Application

14. 3. The nurse should let the client know that although she can't hear the voices, she understands that they are real to him. She should keep communication open and encourage him to talk. Telling the client that the voices aren't real may make him hold tighter to his belief and doesn't promote trust. Telling him to talk back to the voices validates their reality.
CN: Psychosocial integrity; CNS: None; CL: Application

15. 3. Safety is the priority. The nurse should directly ask the client about the nature of the auditory commands to adequately assess the safety of the client and staff. The nurse should never make promises to the client that she may not be able to fulfill. The physician may order a neuroleptic, but the nurse's priority is to address safety.
CN: Safe, effective care environment; CNS: Management of care; CL: Application

16. A client admitted to an inpatient unit approaches a nursing student saying he descended from a long line of people of a "superrace." What is the most appropriate response by the nursing student?
1. Smile and walk into the nurses' station.
2. Challenge the client's false belief.
3. Listen for hidden messages in themes of delusion, indicating unmet needs.
4. Introduce herself, shake hands, and sit down with the client in the dayroom.

Teach nursing students the importance of genuine interest and concern for client's needs.

16. 4. The first goal is to establish a relationship with the client, which includes creating psychological space for the creation of trust. The student should sit and make herself available, reflecting concern and interest. Walking into the nurses' station would indicate disinterest and lack of concern about the client's feelings. After establishing a relationship and lessening the client's anxiety, the student can orient the client to reality, listen to his concerns and fears, and try to understand the feelings reflected in the delusions. Delusions are firmly maintained false beliefs, and attempts to dismiss them don't work.
CN: Safe, effective care environment; CNS: Management of care; CL: Application

17. Which nursing diagnosis is most appropriate for a client with acute schizophrenic reaction?
1. Social isolation related to impaired ability to trust
2. Impaired physical mobility related to fear of hostile impulses
3. Disturbed sleep patterns related to impaired thinking ability
4. Risk for other-directed violence related to perceptual distortions

An accurate nursing diagnosis helps all nurses better understand the client.

17. 1. Clients with schizophrenia are mistrustful, which results in withdrawal and social isolation. Mobility isn't a common problem for persons with schizophrenia. Sleep disturbance may be present but isn't the most common symptom. Contrary to popular belief, persons with schizophrenia usually aren't violent.
CN: Safe, effective care environment; CNS: Management of care; CL: Analysis

18. A nurse is assisting with morning care when a client suddenly throws off the covers and starts shouting, "My body is changing and disintegrating because I'm not of this world." The nurse describes this behavior as which of the following?
1. Depersonalization
2. Ideas of reference
3. Looseness of association
4. Paranoid ideation

18. 1. Depersonalization is a state in which the client feels unreal or believes parts of the body are being distorted. Ideas of reference are beliefs unrelated to situations and hold special meaning for the individual. The term loose associations refer to sentences that have vague connections to each other. Paranoid ideations are beliefs that others intend to harm the client in some way.
CN: Psychosocial integrity; CNS: None; CL: Analysis

19. A 16-year-old client with a diagnosis of undifferentiated schizophrenia has become very clingy and begins sucking her thumb while interacting with the nurse. The nurse interprets this behavior as which of the following?
1. Repression
2. Regression
3. Rationalization
4. Projection

20. What is the most appropriate assessment technique for the nurse to implement when interviewing a client with paranoia?
1. Using indirect questions
2. Using direct questions
3. Using lead-in remarks
4. Using open-ended sentences

21. A nurse on a psychiatric unit observes a client in the corner of the room moving his lips as if he were talking to himself. What is the <u>most appropriate</u> intervention?
1. Ask him why he's talking to himself.
2. Leave him alone until he stops talking.
3. Tell him it isn't good for him to talk to himself.
4. Invite him to join in a card game with the nurse.

22. A client makes vague statements with no logical connections. He asks whether the nurse understands. What is the best response by the nurse?
1. "Why don't we wait until later to talk about it?"
2. "You're not making sense, so I won't talk about this topic."
3. "Yes, I understand the overall sense of the logical connections from the idea."
4. "I want to understand what you're saying, but I'm having difficulty following you."

23. A client asks a nurse if she hears the voice of the nonexistent man speaking to him. What is the most appropriate response by the nurse?
1. "No one is in your room except you."
2. "Yes, I hear him, but I won't listen to him."
3. "What has he told you? Is it helpful advice?"
4. "No, I don't hear him, but I know you do. What is he saying?"

Any way you measure it, you're doing great.

I'm trying to understand but sometimes it's difficult.

Do you hear what I hear?

19. 2. Regression, a return to earlier behavior in order to reduce anxiety, is the basic defense mechanism in schizophrenia. Repression is the blocking of unacceptable thoughts or impulses from the consciousness. Rationalization is a defense mechanism used to justify one's behavior. Projection is a defense mechanism in which one blames others and attempts to justify actions.
CN: Psychosocial integrity; CNS: None; CL: Application

20. 2. Direct questioning is the most appropriate technique to use when interviewing a client with paranoid schizophrenia. Specific questions (such as, "Are you hearing voices right now?") provide the nurse with useful information. The other forms of communication may be misunderstood by the client, and his responses may be vague.
CN: Psychosocial integrity; CNS: None; CL: Application

21. 4. Being with the nurse provides stimulation that competes with the hallucinations. The client doesn't think he's talking to himself; he's responding only to the voices he hears. Being alone keeps the client in his fantasy world. Telling the client that he shouldn't talk to himself fails to understand how real his fantasy world and hallucinations are.
CN: Psychosocial integrity; CNS: None; CL: Application

22. 4. The nurse needs to communicate that she wants to understand without blaming the client for the lack of understanding. Asking the client to wait because he's too confused cuts off an attempt to communicate and asks the client to do what he can't at present. Telling the client that he isn't making sense is judgmental and could impair the therapeutic relationship. Pretending to understand is a violation of trust and can damage the therapeutic relationship.
CN: Psychosocial integrity; CNS: None; CL: Application

23. 4. This response points out reality and shows concern and support. Attempting to argue the client out of the belief might entrench him more firmly in his belief, making him feel more out of control because of the negative and fearful nature of hallucinations. The other two options violate the trust of the therapeutic relationship.
CN: Safe, effective care environment; CNS: Management of care; CL: Application

24. The nurse is providing information to a client who is taking chlorpromazine. What is the most important information for the nurse to provide?
1. Reduce the dosage if you feel better.
2. Occasional social drinking isn't harmful.
3. Stop taking the drug immediately if adverse reactions develop.
4. Schedule routine medication checks.

25. A 34-year-old male client is referred to a mental health clinic by the court. The client harassed a couple next door to him with charges that the wife was in love with him. He wrote love notes and called her on the telephone throughout the night. The client is employed and has had no problems in his job. Which disorder is suspected?
1. Major depression
2. Paranoid schizophrenia
3. Delusional disorder
4. Bipolar affective disorder

26. A homebound client taking clozapine (Clozaril) tells the nurse he has been feeling tired for 5 days. His temperature is 99.6° F; pulse, 110 beats/minute; and respirations, 20 breaths/minute. What is the best information for the nurse to tell the client?
1. Take the medication with milk.
2. Stop the medication at once and see the physician immediately.
3. Understand that the symptoms will disappear as soon as you get more rest.
4. Stop the medication gradually and see the physician next week.

27. A client who is delusional approaches the nurse and states, "You are my aunt and you live with my family." What is the most appropriate response by the nurse?
1. "I'm not your aunt."
2. "I don't live here."
3. "I'm honored."
4. "This is my name. What is your aunt's name?"

Do the client's symptoms suggest an emergency situation?

24. 4. Ongoing assessment by a primary health care provider is important to assess for adverse reactions and continued therapeutic effectiveness. The dosage should be changed only after checking with the primary care provider. Alcoholic beverages are contraindicated while taking an antipsychotic drug. Adverse reactions should be reported immediately to determine if the drug should be discontinued.

CN: Physiological integrity; CNS: Pharmacological and parenteral therapies; CL: Application

25. 3. The client has a delusional disorder with erotomanic delusions as his primary symptom and believes he's loved intensely by a married person showing no interest in him. No symptoms of major depression exist. The client doesn't believe someone is trying to harm him, the hallmark characteristic of paranoia. Bipolar affective disorder is characterized by cycles of extreme emotional highs (mania) and lows (depression).

CN: Psychosocial integrity; CNS: None; CL: Application

26. 2. The client should stop the medication and see his physician immediately because fever can be a sign of agranulocytosis, which is a medical emergency. Taking antipsychotic medication with milk, nicotine, and caffeine will decrease the effectiveness. Rest will have no effect on this client's symptoms. Drowsiness and fatigue usually disappear with continued therapy.

CN: Physiological integrity; CNS: Pharmacological and parenteral therapies; CL: Application

27. 4. By the nurse stating her name and asking the name of the client's aunt, the nurse acknowledges the client is speaking of family, while basing it in a realistic interaction. The other responses all focus on and respond directly to the client's fixed delusional system.

CN: Psychosocial integrity; CNS: None; CL: Application

28. A client tells the nurse that he can only drink bottled water since the water from his sink has been poisoned. The nurse understands that the client is exhibiting which of the following?
1. Paranoia
2. Auditory hallucinations
3. Delusions of grandeur
4. Perseveration

29. A client with a diagnosis of schizophrenia is receiving an antipsychotic medication. His physician has just prescribed benztropine (Cogentin). The nurse determines that this medication was <u>most likely</u> prescribed which adverse reaction?
1. Tardive dyskineas
2. Hypertensive crisis
3. Acute dystonia
4. Orthostatic hypotension

The words most likely can help you focus on the answer.

30. What is the most appropriate nursing intervention for a client experiencing hallucinations?
1. Confine him in his room until he feels better.
2. Provide a competing stimulus that distracts from the hallucinations.
3. Discourage attempts to understand what precipitates his hallucinations.
4. Support perceptual distortions until he gives them up of his own accord.

31. A client with schizophrenia reports that her hallucinations have decreased in frequency. What is the most appropriate nursing intervention to address the client's problem with social isolation?
1. Have the client join in a group game.
2. Name the client as the leader of the client support group.
3. Have the client play solitaire.
4. Ask the client to participate in a group sing-along.

Music can be very therapeutic.

28. 1. This client is exhibiting extreme suspiciousness and distrust of others. Auditory hallucinations occur when a client hears voices that are often threatening or violent. Delusions of grandeur are an exaggerated sense of self-importance. A client with perseveration involuntarily repeats words.
CN: Psychosocial integrity; CNS: None; CL: Application

29. 3. Benztropine is used as adjunctive therapy in parkinsonism and for all conditions and medications that produce extrapyramidal symptoms except tardive dyskinesia. Its anticholinergic effect reduces the extrapyramidal effects associated with antipsychotic drugs. Hypertensive crisis and orthostatic hypotension aren't associated with extrapyramidal symptoms.
CN: Psychosocial integrity; CNS: Pharmacological and parenteral therapies; CL: Analysis

30. 2. Providing competing stimuli acknowledges the presence of the hallucination and teaches ways to decrease the frequency of hallucinations. The other options support and maintain hallucinations or deny their existence.
CN: Psychosocial integrity; CNS: None; CL: Application

31. 4. Having the client participate in a noncompetitive group activity that doesn't require individual participation won't present a threat to the client. Games can become competitive and lead to anxiety or hostility. The client probably lacks sufficient social skills to lead a group at this time. Playing solitaire doesn't encourage socialization.
CN: Psychosocial integrity; CNS: None; CL: Application

32. A single 24-year-old client is admitted with acute schizophrenic reaction. The nurse anticipates that which of the following is the most appropriate therapy for the client?
1. Counseling to produce insight into behavior
2. Biofeedback to reduce agitation associated with schizophrenia
3. Drug therapy to reduce symptoms associated with acute schizophrenia
4. Electroconvulsive therapy to treat the mood component of schizophrenia

33. A client tells a nurse voices are telling him to do "terrible things." What is the best response by the nurse?
1. Find out what the voices are telling him.
2. Let him go to his room to decrease his anxiety.
3. Begin talking to the client about an unrelated topic.
4. Tell the client the voices aren't real.

34. A client is preoccupied with his belief that the CIA has been planning to take him away to save the agency from his influence. These delusions are a defense against which underlying feeling?
1. Aggression
2. Guilt
3. Inferiority
4. Persecution

35. A client has started taking haloperidol (Haldol). What is the most important instruction for the nurse to give the client?
1. "You should report feelings of restlessness or agitation at once."
2. "Use a sunscreen outdoors on a year-round basis."
3. "Be aware you'll feel increased energy taking this drug."
4. "This drug will indirectly control essential hypertension."

32. 3. Drug therapy is usually successful in normalizing behavior and reducing or eliminating hallucinations, delusions, thought disorder, affect flattening, apathy, and asociality. Counseling isn't appropriate at this time. Electroconvulsive therapy might be considered for schizoaffective disorder, which has a mood component, and is a treatment of choice for clinical depression. Biofeedback reduces anxiety and modifies behavioral responses but isn't the major component in the treatment of schizophrenia.
CN: Psychosocial integrity; CNS: None; CL: Application

33. 1. For safety purposes, the nurse must find out whether the voices are directing the client to harm himself or others. Further assessment can help identify appropriate therapeutic interventions. Isolating a person during this intense sensory confusion often reinforces the psychosis. Changing the topic indicates that the nurse isn't concerned about the client's fears. Dismissing the voices shuts down communication between the client and the nurse.
CN: Psychosocial integrity; CNS: None; CL: Application

34. 3. The delusional system contains grandiose ideation that allows the client to feel important rather than inferior. Feelings of aggression will appear as violent or hostile thoughts. Guilt results in beliefs that the person deserves to be punished. Persecution is the fear that others are trying to harm you.
CN: Psychosocial integrity; CNS: None; CL: Application

35. 1. Agitation and restlessness are adverse effects of haloperidol and can be treated with anticholinergic drugs. Haloperidol isn't likely to cause photosensitivity or control essential hypertension. Although the client may experience increased concentration and activity, these effects are due to a decrease in symptoms, not the drug itself.
CN: Physiological integrity; CNS: Pharmacological and parenteral therapies; CL: Application

I have important information to tell you.

36. A 45-year-old client experiencing delusions has been admitted to the crisis center. When assessing the content of the delusions, the nurse should look for which aspect of the delusions?
1. Logic
2. Religious beliefs
3. Themes
4. True experiences

37. The nurse is caring for a 58-year-old male client diagnosed with paranoid schizophrenia. The client says, "The earth and the roof of the house rule the political structure with particles of rain." The nurse interprets this statement as which of the following?
1. Tangentiality
2. Perseveration
3. Loose association
4. Thought blocking

38. Which symptom indicates that schizophrenia is a thought disorder?
1. Faulty logic
2. Distorted but organized thinking
3. Organized but disruptive thoughts
4. Appropriate perception but difficulty responding appropriately to people and events

39. A client with schizophrenia tells the nurse that the President consults with him before making major decisions. What is the best response by the nurse?
1. "How long have you known the President?"
2. "You're fortunate to know the President."
3. "How will you speak with the President from the hospital?"
4. "You must feel important. Now let's make your bed."

36. 3. Understanding the themes inherent in the client's psychotic symptoms may help the nurse learn what stresses trigger the symptoms. A delusion is a false, fixed belief that misrepresents perceptions or experiences and isn't open to rational argument. Assessing for logic, religious beliefs, or true experiences draws the nurse into the delusional thinking and therefore isn't therapeutic.
CN: Psychosocial integrity; CNS: None; CL: Analysis

37. 3. Loose association refers to changing ideas from one unrelated theme to another, as exhibited by the client. Tangentiality is the wandering from topic to topic. Perseveration is involuntary repetition of the answer to a question in response to a new question. Thought blocking is having difficulty articulating a response or stopping midsentence.
CN: Psychosocial integrity; CNS: None; CL: Application

38. 1. Thought disorders are characterized by problems in the form and organization of thinking. They appear as loose associations, word salad, tangentiality, illogicality, circumstantiality, pressure of speech, and poverty of speech that impairs communication. Thinking is disorganized, and perceptions are often misinterpreted. The other options are inaccurate characteristics of schizophrenia.
CN: Psychosocial integrity; CNS: None; CL: Analysis

39. 4. Acknowledging that the client feels important addresses the underlying reason for the delusion. The other options reinforce the reality of the delusion.
CN: Psychosocial integrity; CNS: None; CL: Analysis

40. A client is admitted after being found on a highway, hitting at cars and yelling at motorists. When approached by the nurse, the client shouts, "You're the one who stole my husband from me!" The nurse interprets the behavior as:
1. hallucinatory experience.
2. delusional experience.
3. disorientation to the environment.
4. phobic experience.

41. The nurse is teaching the family of a client with schizophrenia about symptoms of remission. Which of the following responses would be the most accurate?
1. The disease is in the prodromal phase.
2. The client no longer has prominent psychotic symptoms.
3. The client is free from all signs of illness and is no longer on medication.
4. The client is free from all signs of illness whether or not he's on medication.

42. A client with schizophrenia is huddled on the floor and appears to be interacting with someone underneath the bed. The nurse notes that the client appears afraid. Which assessment by the nurse is most likely correct?
1. The client is having hallucinations.
2. The client is having suicidal ideations.
3. The client is having nightmares.
4. The client is having delusions.

43. A nurse on an inpatient unit is having a discussion with a client diagnosed with schizophrenia about his schedule for the day. The client comments that he was highly active at home and then explains the volunteer job he held. The nurse interprets the client's response as reflecting which of the following?
1. Circumstantiality
2. Loose associations
3. Referential
4. Tangentiality

I'd be remiss if I didn't advise you to read this question carefully.

40. 2. A delusion is a false, fixed belief manufactured without appropriate or sufficient evidence to support it. The client's statements don't represent hallucinations because they aren't perceptual disorders. No information in the question addresses orientation. The client's statements don't represent a phobia because they don't represent an irrational fear.
CN: Psychosocial integrity; CNS: None; CL: Application

41. 2. Schizophrenia is a chronic disorder with periods of remission and exacerbation. The prodromal phase is the precursor to an exacerbation. Clients aren't usually cured but are treated over time with case management, medication, symptom management skills, social skill training, network support, vocational training, and health-promoting practices.
CN: Psychosocial integrity; CNS: None; CL: Application

42. 1. The client appears to be having auditory hallucinations and is hearing voices that he perceives to be coming from under the bed. There is no evidence that the client is having suicidal ideations, nightmares, or delusions.
CN: Psychosocial integrity; CNS: None; CL: Analysis

43. 4. Tangentiality describes thought patterns loosely connected but not directly related to the topic. In circumstantiality, the person digresses with unnecessary details. Loose associations are rapid shifts in the expression of ideas from one subject to another in an unrelated manner. Referential thinking is when an individual incorrectly interprets neutral incidents and external events as having a particular or special meaning for him.
CN: Psychosocial integrity; CNS: None; CL: Application

44. While talking to a client with schizophrenia, a nurse notes the client frequently uses unrecognizable words with no common meaning. The nurse identifies this as which of the following?
1. Echolalia
2. Clang association
3. Neologisms
4. Word salad

45. While caring for a hospitalized client diagnosed with schizophrenia, a nurse observes the client watching television. The client tells the nurse the television is speaking directly to him. Which term describes this belief?
1. Autistic thinking
2. Concrete thinking
3. Paranoid thinking
4. Referential thinking

46. A nurse is talking with the family of a client diagnosed with schizophrenia. The mother asks, "What causes this disorder?" What is the <u>best</u> response by the nurse?
1. Prenatal or postpartum central nervous system damage
2. Bacterial infections in the mother during pregnancy or delivery
3. A biological predisposition exacerbated by environmental stressors
4. Lack of bonding and attachment during infancy, which leads to depression in later life

47. What is the most appropriate action for a nurse to implement when caring for a client who is having a delusion?
1. Ask the client to describe his delusion.
2. Explain to the client that the delusion isn't real.
3. Act as if the delusion is real to reduce the client's anxiety.
4. Engage the client in an organized activity.

Are you talking to me?

Pay attention to the key words.

44. 3. Neologisms are newly coined words with personal meanings to the client with schizophrenia. Echolalia is parrotlike echoing of spoken words or sounds. Clang association is the linking of words by sound rather than meaning. A word salad is stringing words in sequence that have no connection to one another.
CN: Psychosocial integrity; CNS: None; CL: Application

45. 4. Referential, or primary process thinking, is a belief that incidents and events in the environment have special meaning for the client. Autistic thinking is a disturbance in thought due to the intrusion of a private fantasy world, internally stimulated, resulting in abnormal responses to people. Concrete thinking is the literal interpretation of words and symbols. Paranoid thinking is the belief that others are trying to harm you.
CN: Psychosocial integrity; CNS: None; CL: Application

46. 3. The holistic theory, currently the most widely accepted theory of its type, states that an interaction between biological predisposition and environmental stressors is the cause of schizophrenia. The biological explanation states that schizophrenia is caused by a brain disease, a bacterial infection in utero, or early brain damage. The psychoanalytic perspective involves the belief that the mother–infant bond is the source of the schizophrenia.
CN: Physiological integrity; CNS: Physiological adaptation; CL: Application

47. 4. Engaging the client in an organized activity reinforces reality. Asking the client to describe the delusion and acting as if the delusion is real reinforce the delusion's reality. Explaining that the delusion isn't real won't help and may make the client hold tighter to the delusion.
CN: Psychosocial integrity; CNS: Physiological adaptation; CL: Application

48. During the initial interview, a schizophrenic client states to the nurse, "I don't enjoy things anymore. I used to love to read mystery books but even that isn't enjoyable now." The nurse determines the client is experiencing which of the following?
1. Avolition
2. Anhedonia
3. Alogia
4. Flat affect

49. In preparation for discharge, a client diagnosed with schizophrenia was taught symptom self-management as part of a relapse prevention program. Which statement indicates to the nurse that the client understands symptom monitoring?
1. "When I hear voices, I become afraid I'll relapse."
2. "My parents aren't involved enough to be aware if I begin to relapse."
3. "My family is more protected from stress if I keep them out of my illness process."
4. "When I'm feeling stressed, I go to a quiet room by myself and do imagery."

50. A client diagnosed with schizophrenia has been taking haloperidol (Haldol) for 1 week when a nurse observes that the client's eyeball is fixated on the ceiling. Which specific condition is the client exhibiting?
1. Akathisia
2. Neuroleptic malignant syndrome
3. Oculogyric crisis
4. Tardive dyskinesia

51. A client who is taking antipsychotic medications becomes agitated, fearful, and panicky that people are staring at him. He paces with his neck twisted to one side, and his eyes forcefully drawn upward toward the ceiling. The nurse recognizes the need for intervention. What is the most appropriate medication for the nurse to administer?
1. I.M. benztropine (Cogentin)
2. Haloperidol (Haldol)
3. Paliperidone (Invega)
4. Diazepam (Valium)

48. 2. Anhedonia is the loss of pleasure in things that are usually pleasurable. Avolition is the lack of motivation. Alogia, also called poverty of speech, is a decrease in the amount of richness of speech. A flat affect is the absence of emotional expression.
CN: Physiological integrity; CNS: None; CL: Application

49. 4. This statement indicates the client has learned a technique for coping with stress with the use of imagery technique. The other options don't show an understanding of symptom self-monitoring and may result in symptom intensification and possible relapse.
CN: Psychosocial integrity; CNS: None; CL: Application

50. 3. An oculogyric crisis involves a fixed positioning of the eyes, typically in an upward gaze. Neuroleptic malignant syndrome causes increased body temperature, muscle rigidity, and altered consciousness. Akathisia is a restlessness that can cause pacing and tapping of the fingers or feet. Stereotyped involuntary movements (tongue protrusion, lip smacking, chewing, blinking, and grimacing) characterize tardive dyskinesia.
CN: Physiological integrity; CNS: Pharmacological and parenteral therapies; CL: Application

51. 1. Benztropine and trihexyphenidyl are anticholinergic drugs used to counteract the dystonic reactions and adverse reactions of antipsychotic drugs. Haloperidol is an antipsychotic medication. It also is used to control tics and vocal utterances that are part of Tourette's syndrome. Paliperidone is used to treat mania and at lower doses as maintenance for bipolar disorder. It is also used for schizophrenia and schizoaffective disorder. Diazepam is a benzodiazepine.
CN: Physiological integrity; CNS: Pharmacological and parenteral therapies; CL: Application

52. A 50-year-old schizophrenic client becomes agitated and confronts the nurse with clenched fists. What is the <u>most appropriate</u> intervention by the nurse?
1. Take the client by the hand and lead him to the activity room for cards.
2. Step up to the client and tell him his behavior is inappropriate.
3. Call for security to take him to a seclusion room.
4. Speak to him in a quiet voice and offer him medication to help him calm down.

53. A 20-year-old client has been diagnosed with schizophrenia. He presently lives by himself; doesn't bathe or dress himself; and is erratic with eating, drinking, and taking prescribed medications. Which nursing diagnosis for this client has <u>priority</u>?
1. Ineffective role performance related to isolation
2. Activity intolerance related to perceptual distortions
3. Ineffective coping
4. Imbalanced nutrition: Less than body requirements related to symptoms of schizophrenia

54. As a nurse approaches the nursing station, a client with the diagnosis of delusional disorder raises his voice and says, "You're following me. What do you want?" What is the best response by the nurse?
1. "Are you frightened?"
2. "You know I'm not following you."
3. "You'll have to go into seclusion if you continue to threaten me."
4. "I'm sorry if I frightened you. I was returning to the nursing station after going out for lunch."

55. Which action by a client with stable schizophrenia is <u>most important</u> for preventing relapse?
1. Attending group therapy sessions
2. Participating in family support meetings
3. Attending social skills training sessions
4. Consistently taking prescribed medications

For question 52, you're looking for the most appropriate action.

They're all important, but which one takes priority?

The words most important in question 55 indicate the need to prioritize. As a matter of fact, there's lots of prioritizing on this page.

52. 4. Always use the least restrictive means to calm a client. Never touch an agitated client; touch can be misinterpreted as a threat and can further escalate the situation. Stepping up to an agitated client can be seen as an aggressive act. Seclusion is a last resort.

CN: Physiological integrity; CNS: Reduction of risk potential; CL: Application

53. 4. The deterioration of the client undergoing a schizophrenic crisis is manifested in multiple self-care deficits. Adequate nutrition in these instances is the primary concern of the nurse. The other problems can be addressed after the client has been stabilized.

CN: Safe, effective care environment; CNS: Management of care; CL: Application

54. 4. Being clear in communication, remaining calm, and showing concern increases the chance the client will cooperate, lessening potential for violence. The first option tries to identify the client's feelings but doesn't convey warmth and concern. The second option isn't empathic and shows no indication of trying to reach the client at a level beyond content of communication. The third option may increase the client's anxiety, fear, and mistrust when the nurse engages in a power struggle and triggers competitiveness within the client.

CN: Psychosocial integrity; CNS: None; CL: Application

55. 4. Although all of the choices are important for preventing relapse, compliance with the medication regimen is central to the treatment of schizophrenia, a brain disease.

CN: Safe, effective care environment; CNS: Management of care; CL: Application

56. A client approaches the nurse and points at the sky, showing her where the men would be coming from to get him. What is the <u>best</u> response by the nurse?
1. "Why do you think the men are coming here?"
2. "You're safe here; we won't let them harm you."
3. "It seems like the world is pretty scary for you, but you're safe here."
4. "There are no bad men in the sky because no one lives that close to earth."

57. A client is brought to the crisis response center by his family. During evaluation, he reports being depressed for the last month and complains about voices constantly whispering to him. Which diagnosis is the <u>most likely</u>?
1. Catatonic schizophrenia
2. Disorganized schizophrenia
3. Paranoid schizophrenia
4. Schizoaffective disorder

58. What is the <u>most appropriate</u> nursing intervention for a nurse to implement when caring for a client with paranoid schizophrenia?
1. Defend yourself when the client is verbally hostile toward you.
2. Provide a warm approach by touching the client.
3. Explain everything you're doing before you do it.
4. Clarify the content of the client's delusions.

59. The nurse is interviewing a client with a delusional disorder. Which of the following conditions would the nurse expect from this client?
1. Bizarre behavior
2. Agitation
3. Impaired short-term memory
4. Apparently normal functioning

56. 3. This response acknowledges the client's fears, listens to his feelings, and offers a sense of security as the nurse tries to understand the concerns behind the symbolism. She reflects these concerns to the client, along with reassurance of safety. The first option validates the delusion, not the feelings and fears, and doesn't orient the client to reality. The second option gives false reassurance. Because the nurse isn't sure of the symbolism, she can't make this promise. The last option rejects the client's feelings and doesn't address the client's fears.
CN: Safe, effective care environment; CNS: Management of care; CL: Application

57. 4. A client with a major depressive episode who begins to hear voices and at times thinks someone is after him is most likely schizoaffective. The client who repeats phrases and shows waxy flexibility or stupor with prominent grimaces is most likely catatonic. The client with disorganized speech and behavior and a flat or inappropriate affect most likely has disorganized schizophrenia. The client who expresses thoughts of people spying on him, attributes ulterior motives to others, and has a flat affect is most likely paranoid schizophrenic.
CN: Psychosocial integrity; CNS: None; CL: Analysis

58. 3. Explaining everything you do will prevent misinterpretation of your actions. A nondefensive stance provides an atmosphere in which the client's angry feelings can be explored. Touching the paranoid client should be avoided because it can be interpreted as threatening. The content of delusions should not be the focus of your care because the content is illogical.
CN: Psychosocial integrity: CNS: None; CL: Analysis

59. 4. The psychosocial functioning of the person with a delusional disorder may be relatively unimpaired. Another common characteristic of the client with a delusional disorder is the apparent normality of his behavior and appearance when his delusional ideas aren't being discussed or acted on. The client with delusional disorder doesn't have such symptoms as concrete thinking, bizarre or agitated behavior, and impaired memory, typical of a client with schizophrenia who functions at a lower level.
CN: Psychosocial integrity; CNS: None; CL: Application

60. A client is admitted to a psychiatric unit for a delusional disorder. He explains to a nurse that he made a contract with God to be the best minister on earth. Now that he has achieved the goal, most of his friends have stopped seeing him out of envy. On mental status examination, there is little impairment in psychosocial functioning. Which condition is expected?
1. Nonbizarre delusions
2. Fragmentary delusions
3. Regressive behavior
4. Regressive delusions

61. Which statement made by a client taking fluphenazine tells the nurse that the client understands his discharge instructions?
1. "I need to stay out of the sun."
2. "I need to drink plenty of fluids."
3. "I can't eat cheese."
4. "I need to plan rest periods throughout the day."

62. The nurse is teaching the family of a client who has been prescribed thiothixene (Navane). Which of the following adverse reactions concerning this medication would be the <u>most</u> accurate for the nurse to discuss?
1. Akinesia
2. Hypotension
3. Sedation
4. Weight gain

63. Inability to carry out daily responsibilities typically occurs during the prodromal phase of schizophrenia. Which symptom may also occur during this phase?
1. Increased energy and motivation
2. Increased social interaction
3. Impaired role functioning and neglect of personal hygiene
4. Heightened work performance

You've finished 60 questions. The rest of this test should be a snap.

SNAP

I didn't intend to cause any adverse reactions.

60. 1. The essential feature of delusional disorder is the presence of one or more nonbizarre delusions that persist for at least 1 month. The most common delusions by subtypes are erotomanic, grandiose, jealousy, persecutory, and somatic. Bizarre delusions are patently absurd beliefs with absolutely no foundation in reality. Fragmentary delusions are unconnected delusions not organized around a coherent theme. Regressive behaviors revert back to a less mature state and aren't associated with a mental disorder.
CN: Psychosocial integrity; CNS: None; CL: Application

61. 1. Fluphenazine is an antipsychotic drug that can cause photosensitivity and sunburn. Clients taking this drug don't need to increase fluid intake, avoid cheeses, or plan rest periods.
CN: Physiological integrity; CNS: Pharmacological and parenteral therapies; CL: Analysis

62. 1. Thiothixene is a high-potency agent with a high affinity for the dopamine-2 receptors, resulting in the increased likelihood of akinesia, a form of extrapyramidal symptoms. Although thiothixene targets other neurotransmitters responsible for hypotension, sedation, and weight gain, their affinity to these receptors is weak and more likely to occur with low-potency psychotropics.
CN: Physiological integrity; CNS: Pharmacological and parenteral therapies; CL: Application

63. 3. Prodromal (early) signs and symptoms of schizophrenia can occur 1 month to 1 year before the first psychotic break and represent a clear deterioration in functioning. They may include impaired role functioning and neglect of personal hygiene as well as social withdrawal and depression. Increases in energy and social interaction and heightened work performance don't occur during the prodromal phase.
CN: Psychosocial integrity; CNS: None; CL: Application

64. The daughter of a client with schizophrenia states, "I'm afraid I may develop this disease, too." The nurse explains that schizophrenia is associated with which of the following?
1. Sexual abuse
2. A combination of genetic and other factors
3. Both parents having schizophrenia
4. Emotional trauma during childhood

Families often search for the link to their loved one's disease.

65. A nurse teaches a class of caregivers about the positive and negative behaviors of schizophrenia. The nurse explains positive behaviors as:
1. limited spontaneous speech.
2. inability to initiate and persist in goal-directed activities.
3. misinterpretation of experiences and altered sensory input.
4. extremely brief replies to questions.

66. A nurse is facilitating a group of schizophrenic clients when one client says, "I like to drive my car, bar, tar, far." This pattern of speech is known as which disorder?
1. Clang association
2. Echolalia
3. Echopraxia
4. Neologisms

Which pattern of speech is the client using?

67. A schizophrenic client who is receiving antipsychotic medication reports that he feels nervous. He paces, fidgets, and can't seem to stay still. The primary cause of these behaviors is most likely which disorder?
1. Akathisia
2. Tardive dyskinesia
3. Akinesia
4. Anxiety

64. **2.** Experts believe schizophrenia results from a combination of genetic, environmental, and other factors—such as viruses, birth injuries, and nutritional factors. Schizophrenia incidence is higher among relatives of persons with the disease. It can occur even if both parents don't have schizophrenia. Emotional trauma during childhood hasn't been linked to schizophrenia.

CN: Psychosocial integrity; CNS: None; CL: Application

65. **3.** Positive behaviors of schizophrenia include attention-getting behaviors, which can result from misinterpretation of experiences and altered sensory input (such as hallucinations, delusions, and bizarre behavior). Negative behaviors are those that render the client inert and unmotivated, such as lack of spontaneous speech, poverty of thought, apathy, and poor social functioning.

CN: Psychosocial integrity; CNS: None; CL: Application

66. **1.** Linking together words based on their sounds rather than their meanings is called clang association. Echolalia is the involuntary parrotlike repetition of words spoken by others. Echopraxia refers to meaningless imitation of others' motions. Neologisms are new words that a person invents.

CN: Psychosocial integrity; CNS: None; CL: Application

67. **1.** Akathisia is an extrapyramidal adverse effect of some antipsychotic medications, manifested by restlessness and an inability to stay still. Tardive dyskinesia refers to involuntary abnormal movements of the mouth, tongue, face, and jaw. Anxiety is an unpleasant state of inner turmoil, often accompanied by nervous behavior, somatic complaints, and rumination. Akinesia is absence of movement.

CN: Physiological integrity; CNS: Pharmacological and parenteral therapies; CL: Analysis

68. Which nursing diagnosis is <u>most appropriate</u> for a client diagnosed with schizophrenia, disorganized type?
1. Feeding self-care deficit
2. Disturbed sleep pattern
3. Impaired verbal communication
4. Social isolation

69. A client with paranoid schizophrenia tells the nurse that two people talking in the hall are planning to kidnap and kill him. The client's thought pattern reflects which of the following?
1. Auditory hallucinations
2. Delusions of grandeur
3. Ideas of reference
4. Echolalia

70. A client with schizophrenia is taking clozapine (Clozaril). The nurse determines the client is experiencing adverse effects of the medication when the client exhibits which symptoms? Select all that apply.
1. Sore throat
2. Pill-rolling movements
3. Polyuria
4. Fever
5. Polydipsia
6. Orthostatic hypotension

71. Clients with serious mental illness are not limited to a single symptom or diagnosis. Adult or elderly schizophrenics sometimes present with petulance and temper tantrums. How can the nurse best understand this childish behavior in the context of a complex psychotic person?
1. The client is malingering.
2. The client is intellectually challenged.
3. The client is employing regression to reduce his anxiety.
4. The client is spoiled and angry.

68. 3. Schizophrenia, disorganized type, is characterized by disorganized speech, disorganized behavior, and inappropriate or flat affect. Feeding self-care deficit, disturbed sleep pattern, and social isolation aren't classic manifestations of this type of schizophrenia.
CN: Psychosocial integrity; CNS: None; CL: Analysis

69. 3. A client with ideas of reference mistakenly believes that other people's thoughts, speech, and behaviors refer to the client. Auditory hallucinations are sounds that aren't based in reality. Delusions of grandeur are false beliefs that arise without appropriate external stimuli. Echolalia refers to involuntary repetition of words spoken by others.
CN: Psychosocial integrity; CNS: None; CL: Application

70. 1 and 4. Sore throat, fever, and sudden onset of other flulike symptoms are signs of agranulocytosis. The condition is caused by a lack of sufficient granulocytes (a type of white blood cell), which causes the client to be susceptible to infection. The client's white blood cell count should be monitored at least weekly throughout the course of treatment. Pill-rolling movements can occur in those experiencing extrapyramidal adverse effects associated with antipsychotic medication that has been prescribed for a much longer time frame than clozapine. Polydipsia (excessive thirst) and polyuria (increased urine output) are common adverse effects of lithium. Orthostatic hypotension is an adverse effect of tricyclic antidepressants.
CN: Physiological integrity; CNS: Pharmacological and parenteral therapies; CL: Application

71. 2. Clients who have impaired or ineffective communication skills may communicate instead through their behavior. A sense of powerlessness may be related to perceived or real threats that they are unable to express. The particular behavior exhibited may be related to the level of Maslow's Hierarchy of Needs that they perceive as being threatened. Having this need met, even temporarily or briefly, reduces the anxiety for these persons.
CN: Psychosocial integrity; CNS: None; CL: Application

You finished! Job well done!

Chapter 18
Substance abuse disorders

1. Family members of an alcoholic client ask the nurse to help them intervene. Which action is essential for a successful intervention?
1. All family members must tell the client they're powerless.
2. All family members must describe how the addiction affects them.
3. All family members must come up with their share of financial support.
4. All family members must become caregivers during the detoxification period.

2. A client who abuses alcohol tells a nurse, "I'm sure I can become a social drinker." What is the <u>most appropriate</u> response by the nurse?
1. "When do you think you can become a social drinker?"
2. "What makes you think you'll learn to drink normally?"
3. "Does your alcohol use cause major problems in your life?"
4. "How many alcoholic beverages can a social drinker consume?"

3. A client asks a nurse not to tell his parents about his alcohol problem. What is the most appropriate response by the nurse?
1. "How can you not tell them? Is that being honest?"
2. "Don't you think you'll need to tell them someday?"
3. "Do alcohol problems run in either side of your family?"
4. "What do you think will happen if you tell your parents?"

The words most appropriate help clarify the correct answer.

1. 2. After the family is taught about addiction, they must write down examples of how the addiction has affected each of them and use this information during the intervention. It isn't necessary to tell the client the family is powerless. The family is empowered through this intervention experience. In many cases, a third-party payer will help with treatment costs. Doing an intervention doesn't make family members responsible for financial support or providing care and support during the detoxification period.
CN: Psychosocial integrity; CNS: None; CL: Analysis

2. 3. This question may help the client recall the problematic results of using alcohol and the reasons the client began treatment. Asking when he believes he can become a social drinker will only encourage the addicted person to deny the problem and develop an unrealistic, self-defeating goal. Asking how many alcoholic beverages a social drinker can consume and why the client thinks he can drink normally will encourage the addicted person to defend himself and deny the problem.
CN: Psychosocial integrity; CNS: None; CL: Application

3. 4. Clients who struggle with addiction problems often believe people will be judgmental, rejecting, and uncaring if they are told that the client is recovering from alcohol abuse. The first option challenges the client and will put him on the defensive. The second option will make the client defensive and construct rationalizations as to why his parents don't need to know. The third option is a good assessment question, but it isn't an appropriate question to ask a client who's afraid to tell others about his addiction.
CN: Psychosocial integrity; CNS: None; CL: Analysis

4. The nurse is caring for a client who is experiencing alcohol withdrawal. The nurse would be most concerned if the client exhibited which of the following?
1. Hallucinations
2. Nervousness
3. Diaphoresis
4. Nausea

5. When assessing a client with prolonged, chronic alcohol intake, the nurse would expect to find which of the following?
1. Enlarged liver
2. Nasal irritation
3. Muscle wasting
4. Limb paresthesia

6. A client is receiving chlordiazepoxide (Librium) as needed for signs and symptoms of alcohol withdrawal. The nurse assesses the client and determines the need for medication when the client displays:
1. mild tremors, hypertension, tachycardia.
2. bradycardia, hyperthermia, sedation.
3. hypotension, decreased reflexes, drowsiness.
4. hypothermia, mild tremors, slurred speech.

7. A client who abuses alcohol tells a nurse, "Alcohol helps me sleep." What is the most appropriate response by the nurse?
1. "Alcohol doesn't help promote sleep."
2. "Continued alcohol use causes insomnia."
3. "One glass of alcohol at dinnertime can induce sleep."
4. "Sometimes, alcohol can make one drowsy enough to fall asleep."

A disease can have many "stages," each with its own symptoms.

What I would give for a good night's sleep.

4. 1. Hallucinations are a sign of late alcohol withdrawal. The nurse should stay with the client, have someone notify the physician, and institute seizure precautions. Nervousness, diaphoresis, and nausea are signs of early withdrawal.
CN: Physiological integrity; CNS: Reduction of risk potential; CL: Analysis

5. 1. A major effect of alcohol on the body is liver impairment, and an enlarged liver is a common physical finding. Nasal irritation is commonly seen with clients who snort cocaine. Muscle wasting and limb paresthesia don't tend to occur with clients who abuse alcohol.
CN: Physiological integrity; CNS: Physiological adaptation; CL: Application

6. 1. Chlordiazepoxide is given during alcohol withdrawal. Symptoms that indicate a need for this drug include tremors, hypertension, tachycardia, and elevated body temperature. Bradycardia, sedation, hypotension, decreased reflexes, hypothermia, and slurred speech aren't symptoms of alcohol withdrawal.
CN: Physiological integrity; CNS: Pharmacological and parenteral therapies; CL: Application

7. 1. Alcohol use may initially promote sleep, but with continued use, it causes insomnia. Evidence shows that alcohol doesn't facilitate sleep. One glass of alcohol at dinnertime won't induce sleep. The last option doesn't give information about how alcohol affects sleep. It makes the client think alcohol use to induce sleep is an appropriate strategy to try.
CN: Physiological integrity; CNS: Physiological adaptation; CL: Analysis

8. A client who is withdrawing from alcohol is being given lorazepam (Ativan). The client's family asks the nurse about the medication. What is the best response by the nurse?
1. "Short-term use of lorazepam can lead to dependence."
2. "The lorazepam will reduce the symptoms of withdrawal."
3. "The lorazepam will make him forget about symptoms of withdrawal."
4. "The lorazepam will also help with his heart disease."

9. A client who abuses alcohol tells the nurse that everyone in his family has an alcohol problem and nothing can be done about it. What is the most appropriate response by the nurse?
1. "You're right; it's much harder to become a recovering person."
2. "This is just an excuse for you so you don't have to work on becoming sober."
3. "Sometimes, nothing can be done, but you may be the exception in this family."
4. "Alcohol problems can occur in families, but you can decide to take the steps to become and stay sober."

10. The nurse is caring for a client with a history of chronic alcoholism and is aware that the client may be predisposed to which of the following?
1. Arteriosclerosis
2. Heart failure
3. Heart valve damage
4. Pericarditis

11. A young, depressed adult woman with a history of alcohol abuse is admitted to the hospital after a motor vehicle accident. The nurse performs the admission assessment of the client and anticipates that the history will include which of the following?
1. Defiant responses
2. Infertility
3. Memory loss
4. Sexual abuse

It's important to teach the family *and* the client.

I feel like I'm failing fast.

8. 2. Lorazepam is a short-acting benzodiazepine usually given for 1 week to help the client in alcohol withdrawal. Long-term (not short-term) use of lorazepam can lead to dependence. The medication isn't given to help forget the experience; it lessens the symptoms of withdrawal. It isn't used to treat coexisting cardiovascular problems.
CN: Physiological integrity; CNS: Pharmacological and parenteral therapies; CL: Application

9. 4. This statement challenges the client to become proactive and take the steps necessary to maintain a sober lifestyle. The first option agrees with the client's denial and isn't a useful response. The second option confronts the client and may make him more adamant in defense of this position. The third option agrees with the client's denial and isn't a useful response.
CN: Psychosocial integrity; CNS: None; CL: Application

10. 2. Heart failure is a severe cardiac consequence associated with long-term alcohol use. Arteriosclerosis, heart valve damage, and pericarditis aren't medical consequences of alcoholism.
CN: Physiological integrity; CNS: Reduction of risk potential; CL: Application

11. 4. Many women diagnosed with substance abuse problems also have a history of physical or sexual abuse. Alcohol abuse isn't a common finding in a young woman showing defiant behavior or experiencing infertility. Memory loss isn't a common finding in a young woman experiencing alcohol abuse.
CN: Psychosocial integrity; CNS: None; CL: Analysis

12. A client with a history of alcohol abuse has been diagnosed with nutritional deficits. What is the best intervention for the nurse to implement?
1. Encourage the client to eat a diet high in calories.
2. Help the client recognize and follow a balanced diet.
3. Have the client drink liquid protein supplements daily.
4. Have the client monitor the calories consumed each day.

I am the best at taking this test.

12. 2. Clients who abuse alcohol are usually malnourished and need help to follow a balanced diet. Increasing calories may cause the client to just eat empty calories. The client must be involved in the decision to supplement the daily dietary intake. The nurse can't force the client to drink liquid protein supplements. Having the client monitor calorie intake could be done only after the client recognizes the need to maintain a balanced diet. Calorie counts usually aren't needed in most recovering clients who begin to eat from the basic food groups.

CN: Physiological integrity; CNS: Basic care and comfort; CL: Application

13. A client with a history of alcohol abuse tells the nurse that he refuses to take his vitamins. What is the most appropriate response by the nurse?
1. "It's important to take vitamins to stop your craving."
2. "Prolonged use of alcohol can cause vitamin depletion."
3. "For every vitamin you take, you'll help your liver heal."
4. "By taking vitamins, you don't need to worry about your diet."

13. 2. Chronic alcoholism interferes with the metabolism of many vitamins. Vitamin supplements can prevent deficiencies from occurring. Taking vitamins won't stop a person from craving alcohol or help a damaged liver heal. A balanced diet is essential in addition to taking multivitamins.

CN: Health promotion and maintenance; CNS: None; CL: Application

14. The nurse determines further teaching about nutrition is necessary when an alcoholic client makes which statement?
1. "I should avoid foods high in fat."
2. "I should eat only one balanced meal per day."
3. "I should take vitamin and mineral supplements."
4. "I should eat large portions of food containing fiber."

Three square meals a day, please.

14. 2. If the client eats only one adequate meal each day, there will be a deficit of essential nutrients. It's appropriate for the client to take vitamin and mineral supplements to prevent deficiency in these nutrients. Avoiding foods high in fat content and consuming large portions of foods containing fiber indicate the client has good knowledge about nutrition.

CN: Health promotion and maintenance; CNS: None; CL: Analysis

15. A client tells the nurse, "I have been drinking ever since they told me I had learning disabilities." How does the nurse interpret this response?
1. The client is self-medicating.
2. The client has an excuse to drink.
3. The client isn't a productive person.
4. The client will be unable to stop drinking.

15. 1. A client with learning disabilities may experience frustration, depression, or overall feelings of low self-esteem and may self-medicate with alcohol. Many people with learning disabilities don't resort to alcohol but develop other coping skills to handle the disability. People with learning disabilities can be very productive. A person with a learning disability can successfully recover from alcohol addiction.

CN: Psychosocial integrity; CNS: None; CL: Application

16. A nurse is caring for a client undergoing treatment for acute alcohol dependence. The client tells the nurse, "I don't have a problem. My wife made me come here." Which defense mechanism does the nurse interpret the client's statement as representing?
1. Projection and suppression
2. Denial and rationalization
3. Rationalization and repression
4. Suppression and denial

17. During a family therapy session, an alcoholic client tells a family member, "You made it easy for me to use alcohol. You always made excuses for my behavior." What should the nurse encourage the family to do?
1. Give up enabling behaviors
2. Manage the client's self-care
3. Deal with negative behaviors
4. Evaluate the home environment

I'll take "Defense mechanisms" for $200, Alex.

18. What is the <u>most important</u> short-term goal for a client with a knowledge deficit about the effects of alcohol on the body?
1. Test blood chemistries daily.
2. Verbalize the results of substance use.
3. Talk to a pharmacist about the substance.
4. Attend a weekly aerobic exercise program.

19. An alcoholic client tells the nurse, "I feel so depressed about what I've done to my family that I feel like giving up." It is <u>most important</u> for the nurse to assess the client for which of the following?
1. Family support
2. A plan for self-harm
3. A sponsor for the client
4. Other ambivalent feelings

You need to know how to prioritize!

16. 2. The client is using denial and rationalization. Denial is the unconscious disclaimer of unacceptable thoughts, feelings, needs, or certain external factors. Rationalization is the unconscious effort to justify intolerable feelings, behaviors, and motives. The client isn't using projection, suppression, or repression.
CN: Psychosocial integrity; CNS: None; CL: Application

17. 1. Enabling the behaviors of family members allows the client to continue the addiction by rationalizing, denying, or otherwise excusing the problem. Managing the client's self-care isn't an issue that needs to be addressed based on the client's statement. Dealing with negative behaviors and evaluating the home environment don't address the client's statement about the family's enabling behavior.
CN: Psychosocial integrity; CNS: None; CL: Application

18. 2. It's important for the client to talk about the health consequences of the continued use of alcohol. Testing blood chemistries daily gives the client minimal knowledge about the effects of alcohol on the body and isn't the most useful information in a teaching plan. A pharmacist isn't the appropriate health care professional to educate the client about the effects of alcohol use on the body. Although exercise is an important goal of self-care, it doesn't address the client's knowledge deficit about the effects of alcohol on the body.
CN: Safe, effective care environment; CNS: Management of care; CL: Application

19. 2. When a client talks about giving up, the nurse must explore the potential for suicidal behavior. Although questioning the client about family support, the availability of a sponsor, or ambivalent feelings is important, the priority action is to assess for suicide.
CN: Psychosocial integrity; CNS: None; CL: Application

20. A client withdrawing from alcohol tells the nurse that he is worried about periodic hallucinations. What is the most appropriate intervention by the nurse?
1. Point out that the sensation doesn't exist.
2. Allow the client to talk about the experience.
3. Encourage the client to wash the body areas well.
4. Determine if the client has a cognitive impairment.

21. A client who has been drinking alcohol for 30 years asks a nurse if permanent damage has occurred to his immune system. What is the best response by the nurse?
1. "There is often less resistance to infections."
2. "Sometimes, the body's metabolism will increase."
3. "Put your energies into maintaining sobriety for now."
4. "Drinking puts you at high risk for disease later in life."

Alcohol can make me more susceptible to infections.

22. A client experiencing alcohol withdrawal tells the nurse she is upset about going through detoxification. What is the <u>most important</u> goal for this client?
1. The client will commit to a drug-free lifestyle.
2. The client will work with the nurse to remain safe.
3. The client will drink plenty of fluids on a daily basis.
4. The client will make a personal inventory of strengths.

In this case, the "S" stands for "safety."

23. A client recovering from alcohol abuse needs to develop effective coping skills to handle daily stressors. What is the most appropriate nursing intervention for this client?
1. Determine the client's level of verbal skills.
2. Help the client avoid areas that cause conflict.
3. Discuss examples of successful coping behavior.
4. Teach the client to accept uncomfortable situations.

20. **2.** The client needs to talk about the periodic hallucinations to prevent them from becoming triggers to acting out behaviors and possible self-injury. The client's experience of sensory-perceptual alterations must be acknowledged; therefore, denying that the client's hallucinations exist isn't a helpful strategy. Determining if the client has a cognitive impairment and encouraging the client to wash the body areas well don't address the problem of periodic hallucinations.
CN: Psychosocial integrity; CNS: None; CL: Application

21. **1.** Chronic alcohol use depresses the immune system and causes increased susceptibility to infections. A nutritionally well-balanced diet that includes foods high in protein and B vitamins will help develop a strong immune system. The potential damage to the immune system doesn't increase the body's metabolism. The third option negates the client's concern and isn't an appropriate or caring response. Drinking alcohol may put the client at risk for immune system problems at any time in life.
CN: Psychosocial integrity; CNS: None; CL: Analysis

22. **2.** The priority goal is for client safety. Although drinking enough fluids, identifying personal strengths, and committing to a drug-free lifestyle are important goals, the nurse's first priority must be to promote client safety.
CN: Safe, effective care environment; CNS: Management of care; CL: Application

23. **3.** The client needs help to identify successful coping behavior and develop ways to incorporate that behavior into daily functioning. There are many skills for coping with stress, and determining the client's level of verbal skills may not be important. Encouraging the client to avoid conflict prevents him from learning skills to handle daily stressors.
CN: Psychosocial integrity; CNS: None; CL: Analysis

24. The nurse is caring for a client struggling with alcohol dependence. It is most important for the nurse to do which of the following?
1. Speak briefly and directly.
2. Avoid blaming or preaching to the client.
3. Confront feelings and examples of perfectionism.
4. Determine if nonverbal communication will be more effective.

25. A nurse is working with a client on recognizing the relationship between alcohol abuse and interpersonal problem. Which of the following is the priority intervention?
1. Help the client identify personal strengths.
2. Help the client decrease compulsive behaviors.
3. Examine the client's use of defense mechanisms.
4. Have the client work with peers who can serve as role models.

Remember to prioritize!

26. The nurse has just completed an assessment of a client recovering from alcohol addiction who has limited coping skills. During the assessment, the nurse also identified that the client is experiencing relationship problems. This assessment is supported by which finding?
1. The client is prone to panic attacks.
2. The client doesn't pay attention to details.
3. The client has poor problem-solving skills.
4. The client ignores the need to relax and rest.

27. A nurse suggests to a client struggling with alcohol addiction that keeping a journal may be helpful. The goal of this nursing intervention is to help the client do what?
1. Identify stressors and responses to them.
2. Understand the diagnosis.
3. Help others by reading the journal to them.
4. Develop an emergency plan for use in a crisis.

24. 2. Blaming or preaching to the client causes negativity and prevents the client from hearing what the nurse has to say. Speaking briefly to the client may not allow time for adequate communication. Perfectionism doesn't tend to be an issue. Determining if nonverbal communication will be more effective is better suited for a client with cognitive impairment.
CN: Psychosocial integrity; CNS: None; CL: Analysis

25. 3. Defense mechanisms can impede the development of healthy relationships and cause the client pain. After identifying barriers to relationship problems, it would be appropriate to identify or clarify personal strengths. Compulsive behavior doesn't tend to be a problem for alcoholic clients who struggle with interpersonal problems. Working with peers who are role models would be useful after the client recognizes and gains some insight into the problems. It isn't the priority intervention.
CN: Safe, effective care environment; CNS: Management of care; CL: Analysis

26. 3. To have satisfying relationships, a person must be able to communicate and problem solve. Relationship problems don't predispose people to panic attacks more than other psychosocial stressors. Paying attention to details isn't a major concern when addressing the client's relationship difficulties. Although ignoring the need for rest and relaxation is unhealthy, it shouldn't pose a major relationship problem.
CN: Psychosocial integrity; CNS: None; CL: Analysis

27. 1. Keeping a journal enables the client to identify problems and patterns of coping. From this information, the difficulties the client faces can be addressed. A journal isn't necessarily kept to promote better understanding of the client's illness, but it helps the client understand himself better. Journals aren't read to other people unless the client wants to share a particular part. Journals aren't typically used for identifying an emergency plan for use in a crisis.
CN: Psychosocial integrity; CNS: None; CL: Application

28. The nurse is preparing a teaching plan for a client who abused alcohol. What is the <u>most important</u> information for the nurse to include?
1. Personal needs
2. Illness exacerbation
3. Cognitive distortions
4. Communication skills

It is *most important* that you read this question carefully.

28. 4. Addicted clients typically have difficulty communicating their needs in an appropriate way. Learning appropriate communication skills is a major goal of treatment. Next, behavior that focuses on the self and meeting personal needs will be addressed. The identification of cognitive distortions would be difficult if the client has poor communication skills. Teaching about illness exacerbation isn't a skill, but it is essential for relaying information about relapse.

CN: Psychosocial integrity; CNS: None; CL: Analysis

29. What is the most important assessment for a nurse to implement before starting a teaching session for a client who abuses alcohol?
1. Sleep patterns
2. Decision making
3. Note-taking skills
4. Readiness to learn

29. 4. It's important to know if the client's current situation helps or hinders the potential to learn. Decision making and sleep patterns aren't factors that must be assessed before teaching about addiction. Note-taking skills aren't a factor in determining whether the client will be receptive to teaching.

CN: Psychosocial integrity; CNS: None; CL: Application

30. The nurse is developing interventions to prevent a client who abused alcohol from relapsing. What is the most important intervention for the client?
1. Avoid taking over-the-counter medications.
2. Limit monthly contact with the family of origin.
3. Refrain from becoming involved in group activities.
4. Avoid people, places, and activities from the former lifestyle.

Congratulations! You've finished 30 questions!

30. 4. Changing the client's old habits is essential for sustaining a sober lifestyle. Certain over-the-counter medications that don't contain alcohol will probably need to be used by the client at certain times. It's unrealistic to have the client abstain from all such medications. Contact with the client's family of origin may not be a trigger to relapse, so limiting contact wouldn't be useful. Refraining from group activities isn't a good strategy to prevent relapse. Going to Alcoholics Anonymous and other support groups will help prevent relapse.

CN: Psychosocial integrity; CNS: None; CL: Analysis

31. A client recovering from alcohol abuse tells the nurse, "I get nothing out of Alcoholics Anonymous (AA) meetings." What is the best response by the nurse?
1. "What were you told about going to AA meetings?"
2. "What do you want to get out of the AA meetings?"
3. "When do you think you'll stop going to the meetings?"
4. "Do you think you can control what happens in a meeting?"

31. 2. This response puts some of the responsibility for staying sober on the client and encourages the client to take a more active role. Asking what the client was told about AA meetings opens up a discussion that allows the client to continue to discuss disappointments rather than taking a proactive stand to support the value of AA meetings. The third option condones the client's desire to stop going to the meetings. The fourth option changes the issue from being responsible for staying sober to focusing on what the client can't control.

CN: Psychosocial integrity; CNS: None; CL: Analysis

32. A client asks the nurse, "Why does it matter if I talk to my peers in group therapy?" What is the <u>most appropriate</u> response by the nurse?
1. "Group therapy lets you see what you're doing wrong in your life."
2. "Group therapy acts as a defense against your disorganized behavior."
3. "Group therapy provides a way to ask for support as well as to support others."
4. "In group therapy, you can vent your frustrations and others will listen."

All answers may seem right, but choose the most appropriate one.

33. The nurse is facilitating a family meeting for a client who abuses alcohol. During the meeting, the nurse observes the communication and determines an unhealthy pattern of:
1. use of descriptive jargon.
2. disapproval of behaviors.
3. avoidance of conflicting issues.
4. unlimited expression of nonverbal communication.

34. A client addicted to alcohol is scheduled to begin individual therapy with the nurse. What is the <u>most important</u> nursing intervention for the client?
1. Learn to express feelings.
2. Establish new roles in the family.
3. Determine strategies for socializing.
4. Decrease preoccupation with physical health.

35. A client recovering from alcohol addiction asks the nurse how to talk to his children about the impact of addiction on them. What is the best response by the nurse?
1. "Try to limit references to the addiction and focus on the present."
2. "Talk about all the hardships you've had in working to remain sober."
3. "Tell them you're sorry and emphasize that you're doing so much better now."
4. "Talk to them by acknowledging the difficulties and pain your drinking caused."

32. 3. The best response addresses how group therapy provides opportunities to communicate, learn, and give and get support. Group members will give a client feedback, not just point out what a client is doing wrong. Group therapy isn't a defense against disorganized behavior. People can express all kinds of feelings and discuss a variety of topics in group therapy. Interactions are goal oriented and not just vehicles to vent one's frustrations.
CN: Psychosocial integrity; CNS: None; CL: Application

33. 3. The interaction pattern of a family with a member who abuses alcohol often revolves around denying the problem, avoiding conflict, or rationalizing the addiction. Health care providers are more likely to use jargon. The family might have problems setting limits and expressing disapproval of the client's behavior. Nonverbal communication often gives the nurse insight into family dynamics.
CN: Psychosocial integrity; CNS: None; CL: Analysis

34. 1. The client must address issues, learn ways to cope effectively with life stressors, and express his needs appropriately. After the client establishes sobriety, the possibility of taking on new roles can become a reality. Determining strategies for socializing isn't the priority intervention for an addicted client. Usually, these clients need to change former socializing habits. Clients addicted to alcohol don't tend to be preoccupied with physical health problems.
CN: Safe, effective care environment; CNS: Management of care; CL: Analysis

35. 4. Part of the healing process for the family is to acknowledge the pain, embarrassment, and overall difficulties the client's drinking problem caused family members. The first option facilitates the client's ability to deny the problem. The second option prevents the client from acknowledging the difficulties the children endured. The third option leads the client to believe only a simple apology is needed. The addiction must be addressed and the children's pain acknowledged.
CN: Psychosocial integrity; CNS: None; CL: Application

36. The nurse is preparing a client with the diagnosis of alcohol dependency for discharge from the hospital. What is the <u>most important</u> goal for the client?
1. Find a way to drink socially.
2. Allow self to grieve recent losses.
3. Work to bring others into treatment.
4. Develop relapse-prevention strategies.

37. A client addicted to alcohol tells a nurse, "Making friends used to be hard for me." The nurse determines that client teaching about relationships has been successful when the client makes which statement?
1. "I've set limits on my behaviors toward others."
2. "I need to be judgmental of others."
3. "I won't become intimately involved with others."
4. "I can't bear to see myself hurt again in a relationship."

38. A client who abused alcohol for more than 20 years is diagnosed with cirrhosis of the liver. The nurse determines that teaching about the disease has been successful when the client makes which statement?
1. "If I decide to stop drinking, I won't kill myself."
2. "If I watch my blood pressure, I should be okay."
3. "If I take vitamins, I can undo some liver damage."
4. "If I use nutritional supplements, I won't have problems."

39. A client tells a nurse, "I'm not going to have problems from smoking marijuana." What is the most appropriate response by the nurse?
1. "Evidence shows it can cause major health problems."
2. "Marijuana can cause reproductive problems later in life."
3. "Smoking marijuana isn't as dangerous as smoking cigarettes."
4. "Some people have minor or no reactions to smoking marijuana."

Your client teaching stems in part from an understanding of the severity of disease.

36. 4. The primary goal for a client in outpatient treatment is to focus on strategies that prevent relapse. Finding ways to drink socially and working to bring others into treatment aren't goals of outpatient therapy. Allowing self to grieve the losses the addiction caused is a part of the early work of inpatient therapy and may be continued in outpatient therapy.
CN: Safe, effective care environment; CNS: Management of care; CL: Analysis

37. 1. When the client can set personal limits and maintain boundaries, the ability to have successful interpersonal relationships can occur. Being judgmental is contraindicated if a client wants to have successful relationships. Setting arbitrary limits on relationships indicates the client needs to learn more interpersonal relationship skills. The universal truth about relationships is that they bring both joy and pain. The last statement indicates a need to learn more about relationships.
CN: Psychosocial integrity; CNS: None; CL: Application

38. 1. This statement reflects the client's perception of the severity of the condition and the life-threatening complications that can result from continued use of alcohol. Aggressive treatment is required, not merely watching one's blood pressure. At this point in the illness, there is little likelihood that liver damage from cirrhosis can be altered. The fourth option denies the severity of the problem and negates the life-threatening complications common with a diagnosis of cirrhosis.
CN: Psychosocial integrity; CNS: None; CL: Analysis

39. 2. Marijuana causes cardiac, respiratory, immune, and reproductive health problems. Most people who smoke marijuana don't have major health problems. All people who smoke marijuana have symptoms of intoxication. The residues from marijuana are more toxic than those from cigarettes.
CN: Psychosocial integrity; CNS: None; CL: Application

40. The nurse is performing an assessment of a client with a history of polysubstance abuse. What is the <u>most important</u> information for the nurse to obtain?
1. Oral administration of any drug
2. Time of last use of each drug
3. How the drug was obtained
4. The place the drug was used

41. A client says, "I started using cocaine as a recreational drug, but now I can't seem to control the use." The nurse interprets the client's statement as most consistent with which drug behavior?
1. Toxic dose
2. Dual diagnosis
3. Cross-tolerance
4. Compulsive use

42. A client tells the nurse that he used amphetamines to be productive at work. The nurse is aware that abrupt discontinuation of the drug will produce which symptom?
1. Severe anxiety
2. Increased yawning
3. Altered perceptions
4. Amotivational syndrome

43. A 20-year-old client is admitted with bone marrow depression. He tells the nurse he's been abusing drugs since age 13. The nurse reviews the client's history for use of which drug?
1. Amphetamines
2. Cocaine
3. Inhalants
4. Marijuana

44. A client has stopped using phencyclidine (PCP). It is most important for the nurse to monitor the client's behavior for which reason?
1. Fatigue can cause feelings of being overwhelmed.
2. Agitation and mood swings can occur during withdrawal.
3. Bizarre behavior can be a precursor to a psychotic episode.
4. Memory loss and forgetfulness can cause unsafe conditions.

Remember to prioritize!

You should know which drugs cause which adverse effects!

40. 2. The time of last use gives information about expected withdrawal symptoms of the drugs and what immediate treatment is necessary. How the drugs were obtained and the places the drugs were used aren't essential information for treatment, nor is administration.
CN: Psychosocial integrity; CNS: None; CL: Application

41. 4. Compulsive drug use involves taking a substance for a period of time significantly longer than intended. A toxic dose is the amount of a drug that causes a poisonous effect. Dual diagnosis is the coexistence of a drug problem and a mental health problem. Cross-tolerance occurs when the effects of a drug are decreased and the client takes larger amounts to achieve the desired drug effect.
CN: Psychosocial integrity; CNS: None; CL: Application

42. 1. When amphetamines are abruptly discontinued, the client may experience severe anxiety or agitation. Increased yawning is a symptom of opioid withdrawal. Altered perceptions occur when a client is withdrawing from hallucinogens. Amotivational syndrome is seen with clients using marijuana.
CN: Psychosocial integrity; CNS: None; CL: Application

43. 3. Inhalants cause severe bone marrow depression. Marijuana, cocaine, and amphetamines don't cause bone marrow depression.
CN: Physiological integrity; CNS: Pharmacological and parenteral therapies; CL: Application

44. 3. Bizarre behavior and speech are associated with PCP withdrawal and can indicate psychosis. Fatigue isn't necessarily a problem when a client stops using PCP. Agitation, mood swings, memory loss, and forgetfulness don't tend to occur when a client has stopped using PCP.
CN: Psychosocial integrity; CNS: None; CL: Analysis

45. A nurse is caring for a client who is experiencing amphetamine withdrawal. The nurse should assess the client for which of the following?
1. Disturbed sleep
2. Increased yawning
3. Psychomotor agitation
4. Inability to concentrate

46. A client has been admitted to the emergency department and states he just used cocaine. The nurse monitors the client for which condition?
1. Tachycardia
2. Hyperthermia
3. Hypotension
4. Bradypnea

47. What is the most important teaching information for the nurse to provide a client who abuses prescription drugs?
1. Herbal substitutes are safer to use.
2. Medication should be used only for the reason prescribed.
3. The client should consult a physician before using a drug.
4. Consider if family members influence the client to use drugs.

48. The family of an adolescent who smokes marijuana asks a nurse if the use of marijuana leads to abuse of other drugs. What is the <u>most appropriate</u> response by the nurse?
1. "Use of marijuana is a stage your child will go through."
2. "Many people use marijuana and don't use other street drugs."
3. "Use of marijuana can lead to abuse of more potent substances."
4. "It's difficult to answer that question as I don't know your child."

45. 1. It's common for a person withdrawing from amphetamines to experience disturbed sleep and unpleasant dreams. Increased yawning is seen with clients withdrawing from opioids. Psychomotor agitation is seen in cocaine withdrawal, and the inability to concentrate is seen in caffeine withdrawal.
CN: Psychosocial integrity; CNS: None; CL: Application

46. 1. Tachycardia is common because cocaine increases the heart's demand for oxygen. Cocaine doesn't cause hyperthermia (elevated temperature), hypotension (decreased blood pressure), or bradypnea (decreased respiratory rate).
CN: Psychosocial integrity; CNS: None; CL: Application

47. 2. People often take prescribed drugs for reasons other than those intended, primarily to self-medicate or experience a sense of euphoria. The safety and efficacy of most herbal remedies haven't been established. Sometimes, over-the-counter medications are necessary for minor problems. There may be a family history of substance abuse, but it isn't a priority when planning nursing care.
CN: Psychosocial integrity; CNS: None; CL: Application

48. 3. Marijuana is considered a "gateway drug" because it tends to lead to the abuse of more potent drugs. People who use marijuana tend to use or at least experiment with more potent substances. Marijuana isn't a part of a developmental stage that adolescents go through. It isn't important that the nurse knows the child.
CN: Psychosocial integrity; CNS: None; CL: Application

49. A pregnant client is thinking about stopping cocaine use. The nurse determines that teaching about drug use and pregnancy has been effective when the client makes which statement?
1. "Right after birth, I'll give the baby up for adoption."
2. "I'll help the baby get through the withdrawal period."
3. "I don't want the baby to have withdrawal symptoms."
4. "It's scary to think the baby may have Down syndrome."

50. A client with a history of cocaine abuse exhibits behavior changes following return from an inpatient treatment facility. The nurse anticipates that the physician will order which test?
1. Antibody screen
2. Glucose screen
3. Hepatic screen
4. Urine screen

51. A nurse is assessing a client with a history of substance abuse who has pinpoint pupils, a heart rate of 56 beats/minute, a respiratory rate of 6 breaths/minute, and temperature of 96.4° F. The nurse determines that which is the most likely cause of the client's symptoms?
1. Opioids
2. Amphetamines
3. Cannabis
4. Alcohol

52. A nurse is caring for a client recovering from cocaine abuse. The <u>priority</u> intervention for this client would be?
1. Skin care
2. Suicide precautions
3. Frequent orientation
4. Nutrition consultation

53. The nurse is assessing a client who repeatedly abuses cocaine. It is important for the nurse to observe the client for which of the following?
1. Panic attacks
2. Bipolar cycling
3. Attention deficits
4. Expressive aphasia

My highest priority is getting to question 80.

49. 3. Neonates born to mothers addicted to cocaine have withdrawal symptoms at birth. If the client says she'll give the baby up for adoption after birth or help the baby get through the withdrawal period, the teaching was ineffective because the mother doesn't see the impact of her drug use on the child. Use of cocaine during pregnancy doesn't contribute to the baby having Down syndrome.
CN: Psychosocial integrity; CNS: None; CL: Analysis

50. 4. A urine toxicology screen would show the presence of cocaine in the body. Glucose, hepatic, or antibody screening wouldn't show the presence of cocaine in the body.
CN: Psychosocial integrity; CNS: None; CL: Application

51. 1. Opioids, such as morphine and heroin, can cause pinpoint pupils and a reduced heart rate, respiratory rate, and body temperature with intoxication. Amphetamine intoxication can lead to tachycardia, euphoria, and irritability. Cannabis (marijuana) intoxication can cause slowed reflexes, lethargy, and tachycardia. Alcohol intoxication leads to slurred speech, unsteady gait, and uncoordination.
CN: Psychosocial integrity; CNS: None; CL: Application

52. 2. Clients recovering from cocaine use are prone to "postcoke depression" and have a likelihood of becoming suicidal if they can't take the drug. Frequent orientation and skin care are routine nursing interventions but aren't the most immediate considerations for this client. Nutrition consultation isn't the most pressing intervention for this client.
CN: Safe, effective care environment; CNS: Management of care; CL: Analysis

53. 2. Clients who frequently use cocaine will experience the rapid cycling effect of excitement and then severe depression. They don't tend to experience panic attacks, expressive aphasia, or attention deficits.
CN: Psychosocial integrity; CNS: None; CL: Analysis

54. A client who uses cocaine finally admits he also abused other drugs to <u>equalize the effect</u> of cocaine. The nurse is aware that the client's drug history may include which substance?
1. Alcohol
2. Amphetamines
3. Caffeine
4. Phencyclidine

55. A group of teenagers tell the school nurse they used cocaine because they were bored. What is the <u>most important</u> goal for the nurse?
1. Prepare a drug lecture.
2. Restrict school privileges.
3. Establish an activity schedule.
4. Report the incident to their parents.

56. The nurse determines that teaching about cocaine has been effective when the client makes which statement?
1. "I wasn't using cocaine to feel better about myself."
2. "I started using cocaine more and more until I couldn't stop."
3. "I'm not addicted to cocaine because I don't use it every day."
4. "I'm not going to be a chronic user; I only use it on holidays."

57. A client who formerly used lysergic acid diethylamide (LSD) is seeking counseling. The nurse anticipates that the assessment of the client will include which finding?
1. Lack of trust
2. Panic attacks
3. Recurrent depression
4. Loss of ego boundaries

What would have the opposite effect?

Don't panic now. Just attack this question with your eyes wide open.

54. 1. A cocaine addict will commonly use alcohol to decrease or equalize the stimulating effects of cocaine. Caffeine, phencyclidine, and amphetamines aren't used to equalize the stimulating effects of cocaine.
CN: Psychosocial integrity; CNS: None; CL: Application

55. 3. Having an activity schedule enables the adolescents to develop coping skills to make better choices about what to do with their free time. Preparing a drug lecture or restricting school privileges won't be seen as useful by the adolescents and may inadvertently contribute to their inappropriate behavior. As the nurse works with the adolescents, it would be more effective to have the children talk to their parents about their drug use.
CN: Psychosocial integrity; CNS: None; CL: Application

56. 2. This statement reflects the trajectory or common pattern of cocaine use and indicates successful teaching. The first option reflects the client's denial. People gravitate to the drug and continue its use because it gives them a sense of well-being, competency, and power. Cocaine abusers tend to be binge users and can be drug free for days or weeks between use, but they still have a drug problem. The fourth option indicates the client is in denial about the drug's potential to become a habit. Effective teaching didn't occur.
CN: Psychosocial integrity; CNS: None; CL: Analysis

57. 2. Clients who used LSD typically have a history of panic attacks or psychotic behavior. This is often referred to as a "bad trip." Loss of ego boundaries, recurrent depression, and lack of trust don't tend to be problems for this type of client.
CN: Psychosocial integrity; CNS: None; CL: Analysis

58. The nurse is developing a plan of care for a client who has been using phencyclidine (PCP). What is the priority assessment for this client?
1. Cardiac arrest
2. Seizure disorder
3. Violent behavior
4. Delirium reaction

59. A client who smoked marijuana daily for 10 years tells a nurse, "I don't have any goals, and I just don't know what to do." What is the <u>most appropriate</u> nursing intervention for this client?
1. Focus the interaction.
2. Use nonverbal methods.
3. Use reflection techniques.
4. Ask open-ended questions.

You're almost at question 60. That should motivate you to keep moving!

60. A nurse is performing a physical assessment on a client who uses heroin. It is most important for the nurse to assess the client for which of the following?
1. Hepatitis
2. Peptic ulcers
3. Hypertension
4. Chronic pharyngitis

I feel so abused.

61. The family of a client in rehabilitation following heroin withdrawal asks a nurse why the client is receiving naltrexone (ReVia). What is the best response by the nurse?
1. To help reverse withdrawal symptoms
2. To keep the client sedated during withdrawal
3. To take the place of detoxification with methadone
4. To decrease the client's memory of the withdrawal experience

58. 3. When a client is using phencyclidine, an acute psychotic reaction can occur. The client is capable of sudden, explosive, violent behavior. Phencyclidine doesn't tend to cause cardiac arrest or a seizure disorder. Delirium is associated with inhalant intoxication.
CN: Physiological integrity; CNS: Reduction of risk potential; CL: Application

59. 1. A client with amotivational syndrome from chronic use of marijuana tends to talk in tangents and needs the nurse to focus the conversation. Nonverbal communication or reflection techniques wouldn't be useful as this client must focus and learn to identify and accomplish goals. Using only open-ended questions won't allow the client to focus and establish specific goals.
CN: Psychosocial integrity; CNS: None; CL: Application

60. 1. Hepatitis is the most common medical complication of heroin abuse. Peptic ulcers are more likely to be a complication of caffeine use, hypertension is a complication of amphetamine use, and chronic pharyngitis is a complication of marijuana use.
CN: Physiological integrity; CNS: Physiological adaptation; CL: Application

61. 1. Naltrexone is an opioid antagonist and helps the client stay drug free. Keeping the client sedated during withdrawal isn't the reason for giving this drug. The drug doesn't decrease the client's memory of the withdrawal experience and isn't used in place of detoxification with methadone.
CN: Psychosocial integrity; CNS: None; CL: Application

62. What is the <u>priority</u> nursing intervention for a client recovering from cocaine addiction?
1. Help the client find ways to be happy and competent.
2. Foster the creative use of self in community activities.
3. Teach the client to handle stresses in the work setting.
4. Help the client acknowledge the current level of dependency.

Maybe we should be called priority engineers instead of nurses.

62. **1.** The major component of a treatment program for a client with cocaine addiction is to have the client feel happy and competent. Cocaine addiction is difficult to treat because the drug actions reinforce its use. There are often perceived positive effects. Clients often credit the drug with giving them creative energy instead of looking within themselves. Fostering the creative use of self may inadvertently reinforce the client's drug use. Teaching the client to handle stresses is appropriate but isn't the most immediate nursing action. Examining the client's level of dependency isn't the immediate choice, as the client needs to work on remaining drug free.
CN: Safe, effective care environment; CNS: Management of care; CL: Application

63. A client tells a nurse, "I've been clean from drugs for the past 5 years, but my life really hasn't changed." The nurse determines that further discussion should include which concept?
1. Further education
2. Conflict resolution
3. Career development
4. Personal development

63. **4.** True recovery involves changing the client's distorted thinking and working on personal and emotional development. Before the client pursues further education, career development, or conflict resolution skills, it's imperative the client devotes energy to emotional and personal development.
CN: Psychosocial integrity; CNS: None; CL: Analysis

A journey of a thousand miles starts with one step.

64. A client discusses with the nurse how drug addiction has made life unmanageable. The nurse determines that information to assist the client with coping would include:
1. how peers have committed to sobriety.
2. how to accomplish family of origin work.
3. the addiction process and tools for recovery.
4. how environmental stimuli serve as drug triggers.

64. **3.** When the client admits life has become unmanageable, the best strategy is to teach about the addiction, how to obtain support, and how to develop new coping skills. Information about how peers committed to sobriety would be shared with the client as the treatment process begins. Identification of how environmental stimuli serve as drug triggers would be a later part of the treatment process and family of origin work. Initially, the client must commit to sobriety and learn skills for recovery.
CN: Psychosocial integrity; CNS: None; CL: Analysis

65. A nurse is assessing a client with a history of cocaine abuse. The nurse is aware that the assessment may include which finding?
1. Glossitis
2. Pharyngitis
3. Bilateral ear infections
4. Perforated nasal septum

65. **4.** When cocaine is snorted frequently, the client often develops a perforated nasal septum. Bilateral ear infections, pharyngitis, and glossitis aren't common physical findings for a client with a history of cocaine abuse.
CN: Psychosocial integrity; CNS: None; CL: Application

66. A client recovering from cocaine abuse is participating in group therapy. The nurse determines that the client has benefited from the therapy when the client makes which statement?
  1. "I think the laws about drug possession are too strict in this country."
  2. "I'll be more careful about talking about my drug use to my children."
  3. "I finally realize the short high from cocaine isn't worth the depression."
  4. "I can't understand how I could get all these problems that we talked about in group."

I'm flying high— but not for long!

67. A family tells the nurse that they are concerned about a family member who stopped using amphetamines 3 months ago and is now acting paranoid. What is the best response by the nurse?
  1. "A person gets symptoms of paranoia with polysubstance abuse."
  2. "When a person uses amphetamines, paranoid tendencies may continue for months."
  3. "Sometimes, family dynamics and a high suspicion of continued drug use make a person paranoid."
  4. "Amphetamine abusers may have severe anxiety and paranoid thinking."

68. The nurse is trying to determine if a client who abuses heroin has any drug-related problems. What is the most appropriate question for the nurse to ask?
  1. "When did your spouse become aware of your use of heroin?"
  2. "Do you have a probation officer that you report to periodically?"
  3. "Have you experienced any legal violations while being intoxicated?"
  4. "Do you have a history of frequent visits with the employee assistance program manager?"

And the verdict is—the most appropriate answer.

69. A nurse is caring for a client addicted to heroin who is experiencing withdrawal symptoms. The nurse is aware that the withdrawal symptoms may be affected by which factor?
  1. Ego strength
  2. Liver function
  3. Seizure history
  4. Kidney function

66. 3. This is a realistic appraisal of a client's experience with cocaine and how harmful the experience is. The first option indicates the client was distracting self from personal issues and isn't working on goals in the group setting. Talking about drugs to children must be reinforced with nonverbal behavior, and not talking about drugs may give children the wrong message about drug use. The fourth option indicates the client is in denial about the consequences of cocaine use.
CN: Psychosocial integrity; CNS: None; CL: Analysis

67. 2. After a client uses amphetamines, there may be long-term effects that exist for months after use. Two common effects are paranoia and ideas of reference. Even with polysubstance abuse, the paranoia comes from the chronic use of amphetamines. The third option blames the family when the paranoia comes from the drug use. Severe anxiety isn't typically manifested in paranoid thinking.
CN: Psychosocial integrity; CNS: None; CL: Analysis

68. 3. This question focuses on obtaining direct information about drug-related legal problems. When a spouse becomes aware of a partner's substance abuse, the first action isn't necessarily to institute legal action. Even if the client reports to a probation officer, the offense isn't necessarily a drug-related problem. Asking if the client has a history of frequent visits with the employee assistance program manager isn't useful. It assumes any visit to the employee assistance program manager is related to drug issues.
CN: Psychosocial integrity; CNS: None; CL: Analysis

69. 2. Liver function status is an important variable that can be used to indicate the severity of a client's drug withdrawal. Ego strength, seizure history, and kidney function aren't variables that can be used to predict the severity of withdrawal symptoms.
CN: Physiological integrity; CNS: Reduction of risk potential; CL: Analysis

70. A client who uses cocaine denies that drug use is a problem. What is the best intervention by the nurse?
1. State ways to cope with stress.
2. Repeat the drug facts as needed.
3. Identify the client's ambivalence.
4. Use open-ended, factual questions.

Think therapeutic.

71. A nurse is working with parents of an adolescent client who abuses inhalants. What is the most important information for the nurse to provide?
1. Consequences must be enforceable.
2. Everything can become a consequence.
3. When setting consequences, be verbally forceful.
4. Consequences are seldom needed with adolescents.

72. A nurse is caring for a very pessimistic client undergoing treatment for cocaine abuse. The nurse anticipates the client may make which statement?
1. "I'll never get better. This is useless."
2. "I don't think I want to see my family anymore. They're not supportive."
3. "I'm fatigued all the time. My energy is low."
4. "I want to get better now. Can't we rush the treatment?"

73. A nurse is working with a client addicted to cocaine who is in denial. What is the most appropriate intervention for the nurse to implement?
1. Ask whether the client sees the drug use as a problem.
2. Focus on the pain the client is having during withdrawal.
3. Reinforce the connection between drug use and harmful results.
4. Help the client recognize reality by pointing out withdrawal symptoms.

Only a handful of questions to go!

70. 4. The use of open-ended, factual questions will help the client acknowledge that a drug problem is present. Stating ways to cope with stress and identifying the client's ambivalence won't be effective for breaking through a client's denial. Repeating drug facts won't be effective, as the client will perceive it as preaching or nagging.
CN: Psychosocial integrity; CNS: None; CL: Application

71. 1. Consequences must be specific and enforceable. Sometimes, parents are prone to make consequences that are too difficult to enforce or that actually become a punishment for the parents. Everything can't be made into a consequence. Being verbally forceful isn't appropriate because the consequence can occur in a civil tone of voice. A consequence can be used with every person regardless of developmental stage.
CN: Psychosocial integrity; CNS: None; CL: Analysis

72. 1. Clients withdrawing from drugs such as cocaine frequently experience depression. It's common for drug-addicted clients to experience fatigue without becoming pessimistic. Being impulsive or having feelings of estrangement aren't necessarily related to a client becoming pessimistic about treatment.
CN: Psychosocial integrity; CNS: None; CL: Analysis

73. 3. To deal with the client's denial, the nurse must confront the drug use and point out the results of the behavior. Asking if the client sees the drug use as a problem will only reinforce the client's denial and provide a forum to intellectualize the problem or provide excuses for it. Pain isn't associated with withdrawal from cocaine. Pointing out withdrawal symptoms may not be the most effective strategy, as the client often downplays the significance of the problem.
CN: Psychosocial integrity; CNS: None; CL: Analysis

74. The nurse is caring for a client who uses cocaine and has been admitted to an intensive outpatient rehabilitation program. It is most important for the nurse to assess the client for which finding?
1. GI distress
2. Blurred vision
3. Perceptual distortions
4. Increased appetite

75. A client who abuses alcohol is admitted to an outpatient drug and alcohol treatment facility. The nurse determines that which of the following is the most objective way to determine if the client is still using alcohol?
1. Having the client walk a straight line
2. Smelling the client's breath
3. Giving the client a breath alcohol test
4. Asking the client if he has been drinking

76. The nurse anticipates that a client undergoing nicotine withdrawal may make which statement?
1. "I sometimes feel like I'm seeing things."
2. "I feel lousy, and I'm grumpy with everybody."
3. "I can't believe I feel fine after just having stopped smoking."
4. "I'm always yawning now."

77. A polyaddicted client is hospitalized for withdrawal complications. What is the <u>most important</u> goal for this client?
1. The client will remain safe during the detoxification period.
2. The client will develop an accurate perception of his drug problem.
3. The client will abstain from mood-altering drugs.
4. The client will learn coping strategies to help him stop relying on drugs.

Which finding should you expect in question 74?

This isn't one of my better moments.

74. 4. Increased appetite is typical during cocaine or nicotine withdrawal. GI distress (especially nausea and vomiting) occurs during alcohol or opioid withdrawal. Blurred vision isn't typical in cocaine withdrawal. Perceptual distortions are common during withdrawal from phencyclidine (PCP, or "angel dust"), amphetamines, and hallucinogens.
CN: Physiological integrity; CNS: Physiological adaptation; CL: Application

75. 3. A breath alcohol test is the most objective way to determine if the client is still using alcohol. Having him walk a straight line and smelling his breath aren't objective tests. Asking him if he has been drinking may not elicit an honest answer (many clients who abuse alcohol deny alcohol use).
CN: Psychosocial integrity; CNS: None; CL: Application

76. 2. During nicotine withdrawal, the client is typically irritable and nervous. Seeing things (hallucinations) isn't linked to nicotine withdrawal. A client going through nicotine withdrawal is unlikely to "feel fine." Yawning is associated with withdrawal from opioids, not nicotine.
CN: Physiological integrity; CNS: Physiological adaptation; CL: Application

77. 1. Client safety takes highest priority during detoxification. During this time, it's unrealistic to expect clients to perceive their drug problems accurately; typically, they experience cognitive impairment or deny their addiction. In the hospital, the client usually doesn't have access to drugs and should be drug free; the goal of abstaining from mood-altering drugs takes highest priority after discharge. Learning coping strategies is an appropriate goal immediately after withdrawal and when medical care is completed.
CN: Safe, effective care environment; CNS: Management of care; CL: Application

78. A client with an alcohol addiction requests a prescription for disulfiram (Antabuse). To determine the client's ability to take the drug appropriately, the nurse should assess which of the following?
  1. Whether the client will take a prescription drug
  2. Whether the client's family accepts the use of this treatment strategy
  3. Whether the client is willing to follow the necessary dietary restrictions
  4. Whether the client is motivated to stay sober

79. A nurse has developed a relationship with a client who has an addiction problem. The nurse determines that the therapeutic interaction is in the working stage when the client does what? Select all that apply.
  1. The client addresses how the addiction has contributed to family distress.
  2. The client reluctantly shares the family history of addiction.
  3. The client verbalizes difficulty identifying personal strengths.
  4. The client discusses financial problems related to the addiction.
  5. The client expresses uncertainty about meeting with the nurse.
  6. The client acknowledges the addiction's effects on the children.

80. A client has received chlordiazepoxide (Librium) to control the symptoms of alcohol withdrawal. The chlordiazepoxide has been ordered as needed. The nurse assesses the client and determines an additional dose of medication is needed when the client displays which symptoms? Select all that apply.
  1. Tachycardia
  2. Mood swings
  3. Elevated blood pressure and temperature
  4. Piloerection
  5. Tremors
  6. Increasing anxiety

78. 4. A client with a strong craving for alcohol (and a lack of impulse control) isn't a good candidate for disulfiram therapy. Disulfiram is a prescription drug. Accepting the treatment strategy is a decision that the client and health care provider make; although family input may be welcome, family members don't make the final decision. Significant dietary restrictions aren't necessary during disulfiram therapy (except for alcohol and foods prepared or cooked in it).
CN: Psychosocial integrity; CNS: None; CL: Analysis

79. 1, 3, and 6. These statements are indicative of the nurse–client working phase, in which the client explores, evaluates, and determines solutions to identified problems. The remaining statements address what happens during the introductory phase of the nurse–client interaction.
CN: Psychosocial integrity; CNS: None; CL: Analysis

80. 1, 3, 5, and 6. Benzodiazepines are usually administered based on elevations in heart rate, blood pressure, and temperature as well as on the presence of tremors and increasing anxiety. Mood swings are expected during the withdrawal period and are not an indication for further medication administration. Piloerection is not a symptom of alcohol withdrawal.
CN: Physiological integrity; CNS: Pharmacological and parenteral therapies; CL: Analysis

You've finished chapter 18. You deserve a standing ovation!

For more information on dissociative disorders, check this independent Web site: www.mentalhealth.com.

Chapter 19
Dissociative disorders

1. The nurse is assessing a client experiencing dissociative identify disorder (DID). The nurse anticipates the client to make which statement?
1. "My father wasn't around much."
2. "I feel good about myself."
3. "I can recall many traumatic events from childhood."
4. "My father loved me one day and hit me the next day."

2. A nursing care plan for a client experiencing dissociative identity disorder (DID) should address which of the following?
1. Ritualistic behavior
2. Out-of-body experiences
3. History of severe childhood abuse
4. Ability to give a thorough personal history

3. What is the most appropriate diagnostic statement for a client experiencing dissociative identity disorder (DID)?
1. Disturbed personal identity related to delusional ideations
2. Risk for self-directed violence related to suicidal ideations or gestures
3. Deficient diversional activity related to lack of environmental stimulation
4. Disturbed sensory perception: visual hallucinations related to altered sensory reception of visual stimulation

1. 4. Repeated exposure to a childhood environment that alternates between highly stressful and then loving and supportive can be a factor in the development of DID. Many children grow up in a household without a father but don't develop DID. Clients with DID commonly have low self-esteem. Because of dissociation from the trauma, a client with DID usually can't recall childhood traumatic events.
CN: Psychosocial integrity; CNS: None; CL: Application

2. 3. DID is theorized to develop as a protective response to such traumatic experiences as severe child abuse. Ritualistic behavior is seen with obsessive-compulsive disorders. Out-of-body experiences are more commonly associated with depersonalization disorder. Because of the dissociative response to personal experiences, people with DID are usually unable to give a thorough personal history.
CN: Psychosocial integrity; CNS: None; CL: Application

3. 2. A common reason clients with DID are admitted to a psychiatric facility is because one of the alter personalities is trying to kill another personality. Hallucinations, delusions, and personal identity disturbances are commonly associated with schizophrenic disorders. Because of the assortment of alter personalities controlling the client with DID, diversional activity deficit is rarely a problem.
CN: Safe, effective care environment; CNS: Management of care; CL: Application

Nursing diagnoses standardize client care.

4. Which nursing intervention is most important for a client experiencing dissociative identity disorder (DID)?
1. Give antipsychotic medications as prescribed.
2. Maintain consistency when interacting with the client.
3. Confront the client about the use of alter personalities.
4. Prevent the client from interacting with others when one of the alter personalities is in control.

5. A nurse notes a change in voice and mannerisms of a client experiencing dissociative identity disorders (DID) after he learns that his wife has filed for divorce. What is the <u>most appropriate</u> nursing intervention?
1. Avoid discussing the client's feelings.
2. Force the client to discuss his feelings.
3. Offer encouragement to the client.
4. Encourage the client to verbalize his feelings.

6. A nurse determines therapeutic interactions have been successful when a client with dissociative identity disorder (DID) displays which behavior?
1. Confronting the abuser
2. Attending the unit's milieu meetings
3. Preventing alter personalities from emerging
4. Reporting no longer having feelings of anger

7. The nurse identifies which behavior as most indicative of a client experiencing dissociative identity disorder (DID)?
1. Complaining of physical health problems with no organic basis
2. Being unable to account for certain times on a day-to-day basis
3. Participating in discussions about abusive incidents that occurred in the past
4. Being able to form a therapeutic relationship with the nurse after meeting twice

8. A nurse is caring for a client experiencing a dissociative disorder. What is the priority intervention by the nurse?
1. Plan activities in which the client will attain success.
2. Offer praise whether or not the client has been successful.
3. Have the client engage in repetitive activities to reduce stress.
4. Encourage the client to keep a journal to recognize unsuccessful coping strategies.

Understanding the client's problem allows you to provide more effective care.

Sometimes I just can't remember anything.

4. 2. Establishing trust and support is important when interacting with a client with DID. Many of these clients have had few healthy relationships. Medication hasn't proven effective in the treatment of DID. Confronting the client about the alter personalities would be ineffective because the client has little, if any, knowledge of the presence of these other personalities. Isolating the client wouldn't be therapeutically beneficial.
CN: Safe, effective care environment; CNS: Management of care; CL: Analysis

5. 4. Encouraging a client with DID to verbalize his feelings will help him cope with his anxieties. Forcing the client to discuss his feelings can increase his level of anxiety. Avoiding discussion of feelings doesn't reduce anxiety and avoids the issue. Offering encouragement that the client will be able to cope with the divorce gives false reassurance and can erode the client's trust in the nurse.
CN: Psychosocial integrity; CNS: None; CL: Analysis

6. 2. Attending milieu meetings decreases feelings of isolation and shows the client has begun to trust the nurse. Often, the abuser was a part of the client's childhood, and confrontation in adulthood may not be possible or therapeutic. The client is often unaware of an alter personality and thus can't prevent these alter personalities from emerging. Clients with DID have dissociated from painful experiences, so the host personality often doesn't have negative feelings about such experiences.
CN: Psychosocial integrity; CNS: None; CL: Analysis

7. 2. When alter personalities are in control, periods of amnesia are common for clients with DID. Complaining of physical health problems with no organic basis describes clients with somatoform disorder. The client doesn't have memories of the abusive episodes, so he's unable to participate in discussions. These clients typically are slow in forming trusting relationships because many past relationships have been hurtful.
CN: Psychosocial integrity; CNS: None; CL: Application

8. 1. The care plan should include activities that will help the client be successful and feel a sense of accomplishment. Offering false praise can harm the nurse–client relationship and erode any sense of trust that develops. Keeping a journal of successes helps promote the self-esteem of the individual.
CN: Psychosocial integrity; CNS: None; CL: Application

9. A hospitalized client with dissociative identity disorder (DID) reports hearing voices. What is the <u>most appropriate</u> nursing intervention?
1. Instruct the client to lie down.
2. Give an as-needed dose of haloperidol (Haldol).
3. Encourage the client to continue with his daily activities.
4. Notify the physician that the client is having a psychotic episode.

Which way is *most appropriate?*

9. 3. Because many clients with DID hear voices, it's appropriate to have the client continue with daily activities. Having the client lie down and rest would have no therapeutic value. The voices the client hears are probably alter personalities communicating. This doesn't indicate a psychotic episode, so the physician wouldn't be notified to prescribe such antipsychotic medication as haloperidol. Although you can instruct the client to rest, it does not take priority over resumption of activities.
CN: Safe, effective care environment; CNS: Management of care; CL: Application

10. Which goal should the nurse implement for a client experiencing dissociative disorder?
1. Learning how to control periods of mania
2. Learning how to integrate all the alternate personalities
3. Developing coping strategies to deal with the traumatic childhood
4. Determining what is causing them to feel they have periods of "lost time"

10. 4. The initial symptom many clients with DID experience, prompting them to seek health care, is the sensation of lost time. These are times the alter personalities are in control. Before therapeutic interventions, clients with DID may not even be aware of childhood trauma because of dissociation from the event. Initially, the client with DID isn't aware of the presence of alternate personalities. Depression, not mania, may be another early symptom of clients with DID.
CN: Psychosocial integrity; CNS: None; CL: Application

Think therapeutic here.

11. A client who is experiencing symptoms of dissociative identity disorder reports hearing voices and asks the nurse, "Am I crazy?" What is the <u>most appropriate</u> response by the nurse?
1. "What do the voices tell you?"
2. "Why would you think you're crazy?"
3. "Clients with DID often report hearing voices."
4. "Hearing voices is often a symptom of schizophrenia."

11. 3. The most therapeutic answer is to give correct information. Asking what the voices tell the client would be changing the topic without answering the question. Asking "why" questions can put the client on the defensive. Schizophrenia isn't the only cause of hearing voices, and this response suggests the client may be schizophrenic.
CN: Psychosocial integrity; CNS: None; CL: Analysis

12. The nurse is preparing to admit a client diagnosed with dissociative identity disorder (DID) to the inpatient psychiatric unit. What is the most appropriate intervention by the nurse?
1. Arrange to have staff check on the client every 15 to 30 minutes.
2. Prevent all family from visiting until the third day of hospitalization.
3. Make sure the staff understands the client will be on seizure precautions.
4. Place the client in a quiet room away from the noise of the nurse's station.

12. 1. A common reason for clients with DID to be hospitalized is for suicidal ideations or gestures. For the client's safety, frequent checks should be done. Family interactions might be therapeutic for the client, and the family may be able to provide a more thorough history because of the client's dissociation from traumatic events. Seizure activity isn't an expected symptom of DID. Because of the possibility of suicide, the client's room should be close to the nurse's station.
CN: Psychosocial integrity; CNS: None; CL: Application

It helps to know what symptoms to watch for.

13. A client is being treated at a community mental health clinic. The nurse has been instructed to observe for any behaviors indicating dissociative identity disorder (DID). The nurse should observe the client for which of the following?
1. Delusions of grandeur
2. Reports of often being very tired
3. Changes in dress, mannerisms, and voice
4. Refusal to make a follow-up appointment

13. 3. When alter personalities are in control, the person will have complete personality changes. Delusions of grandeur are more frequently associated with disorders such as manic states and schizophrenia. Complaints of fatigue aren't a main symptom of DID. The refusal to make a follow-up appointment could indicate many problems, including noncompliance.
CN: Psychosocial integrity; CNS: None; CL: Application

CN: Client needs category   CNS: Client needs subcategory   CL: Cognitive level

14. The nurse has implemented a teaching plan for a client with dissociative identity disorder (DID). The nurse determines that teaching was successful when the client makes which statement?
1. "I will never marry."
2. "I won't get better, even with treatment."
3. "I need to take my pills for anxiety."
4. "I need to attend my therapy sessions faithfully."

15. When interacting with a client experiencing dissociative identity disorder, a nurse observes that one of the alter personalities is in control. What is the <u>most appropriate</u> intervention?
1. Give recognition to the alter personality.
2. Notify the physician.
3. Immediately stop interacting with the client.
4. Ignore the alter personality and ask to speak to the host personality.

Stay focused on therapeutic interventions.

16. A client diagnosed with dissociative identity disorder (DID) understands the need to continue therapy when the client makes which statement?
1. "Therapy will help eliminate my family problems."
2. "I must continue going to outpatient treatment for the next 2 months."
3. "I understand that I need to integrate all my alter personalities into one."
4. "Once therapy is complete, I won't have the traits of my alter personalities."

17. A family member of a client diagnosed with dissociative identity disorder (DID) asks a nurse if hypnotic therapy might help the client. What is the <u>most appropriate</u> response by the nurse?
1. "What would make you think that?"
2. "No, hypnosis is rarely used in the treatment of psychiatric conditions."
3. "Yes, but this treatment is used only after other types of therapy have failed."
4. "Yes, often the client doesn't have conscious awareness of alter personalities."

It's important to understand how the other person feels.

18. Which nursing intervention is most appropriate when caring for a client with dissociative identity disorder?
1. Remind the alter personalities they're part of the host personality.
2. Interact with the client only when the host personality is in control.
3. Establish an empathetic relationship with each emerging personality.
4. Provide positive reinforcement to the client when calm alter personalities are present instead of angry ones.

14. 4. Most clients diagnosed with DID can be successfully treated with long-term therapy. For many of the conditions, pharmacological therapy has little effect. Many clients with DID marry.
CN: Psychosocial integrity; CNS: None; CL: Application

15. 1. By giving recognition to the alter personalities, the nurse conveys to the client that she believes the alter personalities exist. The physician doesn't need to be notified because this is an expected occurrence. Asking to speak to the host personality or immediately stopping interaction with the client won't stop the client from being controlled by alter personalities.
CN: Psychosocial integrity; CNS: None; CL: Application

16. 3. The main goal of therapy for clients with DID is to integrate, not eliminate, the alter personalities. Therapy is often long-term. Through therapy, the client can learn how to cope with family problems.
CN: Psychosocial integrity; CNS: None; CL: Application

17. 4. Because of dissociation from painful events, hypnosis is often very effective in the treatment of clients with DID. It may be under hypnosis that alter personalities start to emerge. Hypnosis is used in a variety of psychiatric conditions. The first option could place the family member on the defensive. Hypnosis is often a first-line treatment for the client with DID.
CN: Psychosocial integrity; CNS: None; CL: Application

18. 3. Establishing an empathetic relationship with each emerging personality provides a therapeutic environment to care for the client. Interacting with the client only when the host personality is in control would be useless because the client has limited, if any, control or awareness when alter personalities are in control.
CN: Psychosocial integrity; CNS: None; CL: Application

19. While interacting with a client experiencing dissociative identity disorder (DID), a nurse observes one of the alter personalities take over. The client goes from being very calm to angry and shouting. What is the best response by the nurse?
1. "Is one of you upset?"
2. "Why have you become angry?"
3. "Tell me what you're feeling right now."
4. "Let me speak to someone who isn't angry."

20. A client with dissociative identity disorder has been in therapy for 2 years. The client just learned that her father who sexually abused her throughout childhood has passed away. The nurse determines that which is the most appropriate intervention?
1. Have the client seek inpatient therapy.
2. Encourage the client's verbalization of feelings of anger and guilt.
3. Encourage the client's alter personalities to emerge during this stressful time.
4. Stress to the client that the death of the abuser should be very helpful in her healing process.

21. The nurse is developing a teaching plan for a client experiencing dissociative identity disorder (DID). Which activity is <u>most</u> appropriate?
1. Group therapy with only clients who have DID
2. Inpatient therapy groups led by a psychologist
3. Support group with adult survivors of child abuse
4. Group therapy with clients who have a variety of diagnoses

22. A nurse observes that the alter personality of a client with a dissociative identity disorder is in control. The client is sitting in the dayroom, interacting with others. His voice becomes louder and more intense, and he's tearful and confused. What is the priority intervention by the nurse?
1. Allow the client to continue interacting with clients in the dayroom.
2. Ask to speak to one of the adult alter personalities of the host personality.
3. Remove the client from the dayroom and allow the client to play with toys.
4. Remove the client from the dayroom and reorient him that he's in a safe place.

Keep it up, you're doing great!

19. 3. This response encourages integration and discourages dissociation. When interacting with clients with DID, the nurse always wants to remind the client that the alter personalities are a component of one person. Responses reinforcing interaction with only one alter personality instead of trying to interact with the individual as a single person aren't appropriate. Asking "why" questions can put the client on the defensive and impede further communication.
CN: Psychosocial integrity; CNS: None; CL: Application

20. 2. The death of the abuser may cause the client to experience feelings of anger and guilt. Unless the client becomes suicidal or rapidly deteriorates, inpatient treatment won't be necessary. Encouraging the client's alter personalities to emerge could result in further dissociation. The death of the abuser can be a very stressful event and can leave the client with unresolved feelings.
CN: Health promotion and maintenance; CNS: None; CL: Analysis

21. 1. Homogenous group therapy has proven to be the most beneficial for clients with DID. In other groups, the members may find interacting on such an intimate level with a client with DID overwhelming and frightening. Not all victims of child abuse develop DID. Unless the client with DID is suicidal, hospitalization isn't required.
CN: Psychosocial integrity; CNS: None; CL: Application

22. 4. Removing the client at this time may protect him from future embarrassment. Asking to speak to an alter personality encourages dissociation. Allowing the client to play with toys also reinforces and encourages dissociation. Reorienting the client discourages dissociation and encourages integration.
CN: Safe, effective care environment; CNS: Safety and infection control; CL: Analysis

23. A nurse on the psychiatric unit is caring for a 51-year-old male client who has suicidal ideations. Which nursing intervention takes <u>priority</u>?
1. Discouraging sleep except at bedtime
2. Making a verbal contract with the client to notify the staff of suicidal thoughts
3. Limiting time spent alone by encouraging the client to participate in group activities
4. Creating a safe physical and interpersonal environment

24. A 14-year-old client is admitted to an inpatient adolescent unit. The treatment team believes the client has dissociative identity disorder (DID). Based on this assessment data, which nursing intervention should the nurse anticipate using?
1. Request a social work consultation.
2. Institute elopement precautions.
3. Confront the parents about the staff's suspicion of child abuse.
4. Prevent the client from interacting with other clients on the unit.

25. The nurse determines that therapy has been effective for a client with dissociative identity disorder (DID) when:
1. the client is forgetful.
2. the client sleeps through the night.
3. the client has had several unsuccessful relationships.
4. the client hears voices.

26. A client diagnosed with dissociative identity disorder (DID) is admitted to an inpatient psychiatric unit. The unit nurse-manager asks all staff members to attend a meeting. Which reason for the meeting is the <u>most likely</u>?
1. To review the restraint protocol with the staff
2. To inform the staff that no one should refuse to work with the client
3. To warn the staff that this client may be difficult and challenging to work with
4. To allow staff members to discuss concerns about working with a client with DID

27. A 26-year-old man is reported missing after being the victim of a violent crime. Two months later, a family member finds him working in a city 100 miles from his home. The man does not recognize the family member or recall being the victim of a crime. The client is <u>most likely</u> exhibiting which condition?
1. Depersonalization disorder
2. Dissociative amnesia
3. Dissociative fugue
4. Dissociative identity disorder

Take note: the question is asking which intervention has the priority.

Know when to request a consultation from other medical professionals.

23. **4.** Creating a safe environment, including removing obvious hazards, recognizing nonobvious hazards, maintaining close observation, serving as a client advocate in interpersonal situations, and communicating concern to the client in verbal and nonverbal ways, is the nurse's highest priority. Other interventions, such as discouraging sleep except at bedtime, making a verbal contract, and encouraging participation in group activities, should be included in the client's plan, but these don't have top priority.
CN: Psychosocial integrity; CNS: None; CL: Application

24. **1.** In many cases, clients with DID have been subjected to child abuse. The social worker is the appropriate person to investigate the child's home setting. The client isn't at any more risk for elopement than the other adolescent clients. Until there has been an investigation into the client's home setting, confrontation wouldn't be appropriate or therapeutic. Clients with DID are always encouraged to interact with other clients on the unit.
CN: Safe, effective care environment; CNS: Management of care; CL: Application

25. **2.** Because clients with DID often have sleep disorders, sleeping through the night is a sign of effective therapy. Forgetfulness, difficulty forming relationships, and hallucinations are signs of unsuccessful treatment.
CN: Psychosocial integrity; CNS: None; CL: Analysis

26. **4.** Allowing all staff members to meet together may prevent the staff from splitting into groups of those who believe the validity of this diagnosis and those who don't. Unless this client shows behaviors harmful to himself or others, restraints aren't needed. Telling the staff no one should refuse to work with the client or this client will probably be very difficult, and challenging sets a very negative tone as staff plan and provide care for the client.
CN: Safe, effective care environment; CNS: Management of care; CL: Application

27. **3.** Dissociative fugue is sudden flight after a traumatic event. During the episode, the person may assume a new identity and not recognize people from his past. Depersonalization disorder is the sudden loss of the sense of one's own reality. Dissociative amnesia doesn't involve flight from work or home. Dissociative identity disorder is the coexistence of two or more personalities in one person.
CN: Psychosocial integrity; CNS: None; CL: Application

28. A client has just had an episode of dissociative fugue. What is the <u>most appropriate</u> nursing intervention?
1. Let the client verbalize the fear and anxiety he feels.
2. Encourage the client to share his experiences during the episode.
3. Have the client sign a contract stating he won't leave the premises again.
4. Tell the client he won't resolve his problems by running away from them.

29. The nurse has provided teaching for family members of a client with a dissociative disorder. The nurse determines that teaching was effective when the family makes which statement about dissociative disorders?
1. "They occur as a result of incest."
2. "They occur as a result of substance abuse."
3. "They occur in more than 40% of all people."
4. "They occur as a result of the brain trying to protect the person from severe stress."

30. What is the <u>most appropriate</u> nursing intervention for a client who experienced a recent episode of dissociative fugue?
1. Place the client on elopement precautions.
2. Help the client identify resources to deal with stressful situations.
3. Allow the client to share his experiences about the dissociative fugue episode.
4. Confront the client about his running away from problems instead of dealing with them.

31. A 32-year-old client tells the nurse his home was lost in a flood last month. When questioned about his feelings about the loss, he doesn't remember being in a flood or owning a home. What is the client most likely exhibiting?
1. Depersonalization disorder
2. Dissociative amnesia
3. Dissociative fugue
4. Dissociative identity disorder

32. The nurse is assessing a client with dissociative amnesia. Which circumstance would most likely contribute to this condition?
1. Binge drinking
2. A hostage situation
3. A closed-head injury
4. A fight with a family member

I'm feeling slightly overwhelmed—but it helps to tell someone.

Helping the client help himself is an important aspect of teaching.

I feel like I'm a mess from all this stress!

28. 1. An episode of dissociative fugue can be a very frightening experience. The client rarely remembers the events during the episode. Signing a contract would have little effect because a dissociative fugue episode isn't something the client consciously wanted to do. Because the client isn't conscious of "running away," this response isn't helpful.
CN: Psychosocial integrity; CNS: None; CL: Analysis

29. 4. Dissociative disorders are thought to be a form of coping with an extreme stressor or event that occurred in the client's life. Incest is only one of many reasons dissociative disorders occur. Typically, substance abuse isn't a cause (but may be an effect) of a dissociative disorder. Dissociative disorders are actually very rare.
CN: Psychosocial integrity; CNS: None; CL: Analysis

30. 2. Dissociative fugue is precipitated by stressful situations. Helping the client identify resources could prevent recurrences. Once the dissociative fugue episode is over, the client returns to normal functioning; he wouldn't be an elopement risk. The client usually has amnesia about the events during the dissociative fugue episode, which limits his ability to share the experience. The client doesn't realize that he's running away from his problems.
CN: Psychosocial integrity; CNS: None; CL: Analysis

31. 2. Dissociative amnesia commonly occurs after a person has been in a traumatic event. Depersonalization disorder is characterized by recurrent sensations of loss of one's own reality. Dissociative fugue is the sudden departure from one's home or work. Dissociative identity disorder is the coexistence of two or more personalities within the same individual.
CN: Psychosocial integrity; CNS: None; CL: Analysis

32. 2. Dissociative amnesia typically occurs after the person has experienced a very stressful, traumatic situation. Binge drinking doesn't cause dissociative amnesia. A closed-head injury could result in physiological but not dissociative amnesia. Having a fight with a family member typically wouldn't be stressful enough to cause dissociative amnesia.
CN: Psychosocial integrity; CNS: None; CL: Application

33. A client was the driver in an automobile accident in which a 3-year-old boy was killed. The client is diagnosed with dissociative amnesia. He verbalizes understanding of his treatment plan when he makes which statement?
1. "I won't drive a car again for at least a year."
2. "I'll take my Ativan (lorazepam) anytime I feel upset about this situation."
3. "I'll visit the child's grave as soon as I'm released from the hospital."
4. "I'll attend my hypnotic therapy sessions prescribed by my psychiatrist."

34. A client with dissociative amnesia shows understanding of the condition when which statement is made?
1. "I'll probably never be able to regain my memories of the fire."
2. "I have problems with my memory due to my abuse of tranquilizers."
3. "If I concentrate hard enough, I'll be able to bring up memories of the car accident."
4. "To protect my mental well-being, my brain has temporarily hidden my memories of the rape from me."

35. A client is admitted for a diagnostic workup for possible dissociative amnesia. What is the <u>most appropriate</u> nursing intervention for this client?
1. Restrain the client if he attempts to wander off the unit.
2. Question the client every hour about orientation to time, place, and person.
3. Provide teaching on computed tomography scans and other imaging tests.
4. Encourage the client not to dwell on the traumatic event that lead to his memory loss.

36. Amobarbital (Amytal) has been prescribed for a client with dissociative amnesia. The nurse determines that teaching about the medication has been successful when the client makes which statement?
1. "This medication helps me sleep."
2. "This medication helps me control my anxiety."
3. "I must take this drug once a day after discharge if the drug is to be therapeutically beneficial."
4. "I'm given this medication during therapy sessions to increase my ability to remember forgotten events."

37. A client experiencing dissociative amnesia says, "You must think I'm really stupid because I have no recollection of the accident." What is the <u>best</u> response by the nurse?
1. "Why would I think you're stupid?"
2. "Have I acted like I think you're stupid?"
3. "What kind of grades did you get in school?"
4. "As a protective measure, the brain sometimes doesn't let us remember traumatic events."

Hmm! Which intervention is most appropriate?

Sometimes a simple explanation is the best one.

33. 4. Hypnosis can be beneficial to this client because it allows repressed feelings and memories to surface. The client may be ready to drive again, and circumstances may dictate that he drives again before a year has passed. The client needs to learn other coping mechanisms besides taking a highly addictive drug such as lorazepam (Ativan). Visiting the child's grave on release from the hospital may be too traumatic and encourage continuation of the amnesia.
CN: Psychosocial integrity; CNS: None; CL: Application

34. 4. One of the cardinal features of dissociative amnesia is that the person has loss of memory of a traumatic event. With therapy and time, the person will probably be able to recall the traumatic event. This type of amnesia isn't related to substance abuse. With this disorder, the loss of memory is a protective function performed by the brain and isn't within the person's conscious control.
CN: Psychosocial integrity; CNS: None; CL: Analysis

35. 3. Clients with a type of memory problem commonly have a diagnostic workup to rule out any physical cause. Clients with dissociative amnesia typically don't have a problem with wandering. Frequent attempts to assess the client's orientation level could easily make the client more distressed and agitated. In many cases, the client doesn't have memories of the traumatic events before amnesia.
CN: Health promotion and maintenance; CNS: None; CL: Application

36. 4. This drug is given to the client with dissociative amnesia to help her remember forgotten events. It isn't prescribed as a sleep aid or anti-anxiety agent. Because the drug is given during therapy to recall forgotten events, there would be no therapeutic benefit to taking this drug at home.
CN: Physiological integrity; CNS: Pharmacological and parenteral therapies; CL: Analysis

37. 4. This provides a simple explanation for the client. The use of "why" can put someone on the defensive. The second option takes the focus off the client. The third option changes the topic.
CN: Psychosocial integrity; CNS: None; CL: Application

38. What is the most important intervention to implement when caring for a client with a dissociative disorder?
  1. Encourage the client to participate in unit activities and meetings.
  2. Question the client about the events triggering the dissociative disorder.
  3. Allow the client to remain in his room anytime he's experiencing feelings of dissociation.
  4. Encourage the client to form friendships with other clients in his therapy groups to decrease his feelings of isolation.

38. 1. Attending unit activities and meetings helps decrease the client's sense of isolation. Often, the client can't recall the events that triggered the dissociative disorder, so questioning him would not be helpful. The client would need to be isolated from others only if he's unable to interact appropriately. A client with a dissociative disorder has typically had few healthy relationships. Forming friendships with others in therapy could be setting the client up to continue in unhealthy relationships.

CN: Safe, effective care environment; CNS: Management of care; CL: Application

39. The nurse is performing an assessment on a client diagnosed with depersonalization disorder. The nurse anticipates the client will display which of the following?
  1. Disorientation to time, place, and person
  2. Sensation of detachment from body or mind
  3. Unexpected and sudden travel to another location
  4. A feeling that one's environment will never change

How can you tell when your client understands your instructions?

39. 2. In depersonalization disorder, the person feels detached from his body and mental processes. The person is usually oriented to time, place, and person. Unexpected and sudden travel to another location is one of the characteristics of dissociative fugue. Clients with depersonalization disorder often feel the outside world has changed.

CN: Psychosocial integrity; CNS: None; CL: Application

40. A client with depersonalization disorder verbalizes understanding of the ways to decrease his symptoms when he makes which statement?
  1. "I'll avoid any stressful situation."
  2. "Meditation will help control my symptoms."
  3. "I'll need to practice relaxation exercises regularly."
  4. "I may need to remain on antipsychotic medication for the rest of my life."

40. 3. Relaxation can lead to a decrease in maladaptive responses. Although stress can be a predisposing factor in depersonalization disorder, it's impossible to avoid all stressful situations. Meditation is the voluntary induction of the sensation of depersonalization. This isn't a psychotic disorder, so antipsychotic medication wouldn't be therapeutic or beneficial.

CN: Psychosocial integrity; CNS: None; CL: Analysis

41. A client with depersonalization disorder spends much of his day in a dreamlike state during which he ignores personal care needs. Which nursing diagnosis is <u>most appropriate</u> for this client?
  1. Disturbed personal identity related to organic brain damage
  2. Impaired memory related to frequently being in a dreamlike state
  3. Dressing self-care deficit related to perceptual impairment
  4. Deficient knowledge related to performance or personal care needs due to lack of information

Making the right nursing diagnosis is critical for effective nursing care.

41. 3. Because of time spent in a dreamlike state, many clients with depersonalization disorder ignore self-care needs. There's no known organic brain damage with this disorder. Memory impairment is more of a problem with other dissociative disorders, such as dissociative identity disorder and dissociative amnesia. The dreamlike state can lead to problems meeting personal care needs, not a knowledge deficit.

CN: Safe, effective care environment; CNS: Safety and infection control; CL: Application

42. A client tells the nurse that he frequently feels that he's floating above his body. During these times, he says he's aware of who he is and where he's located. The nurse determines that this client is experiencing:
1. depersonalization disorder.
2. dissociative amnesia.
3. dissociative identity disorder.
4. dissociative fugue.

43. The nurse is teaching the family of a client with depersonalization disorder. The family wants to know which setting has the <u>most</u> success in treating this disorder. What is the best response by the nurse?
1. Inpatient psychiatric hospital
2. Community mental health clinic
3. Family practice physician's office
4. Support group for clients with depersonalization disorder

44. A client with depersonalization disorder tells the nurse, "I feel like such a freak when I have an out-of-body experience." What is the <u>most appropriate</u> response by the nurse?
1. "How often do you have these feelings?"
2. "I don't understand what you mean by a freak."
3. "Tell me more about these out-of-body experiences."
4. "How does your husband feel about you having these experiences?"

45. The nurse is assessing a client diagnosed with dissociative disorder. Which of the following characteristics would the nurse most likely observe?
1. A group of disorders with the common symptom of hallucinations
2. A group of disorders with a rapid disruption of the client's memory
3. A group of disorders with impairment of memory or identity due to the development of organic changes in the brain
4. A group of disorders with impairment of memory or identity due to an unconscious attempt to protect the person from emotional pain or traumatic experiences

46. A client diagnosed with depersonalization disorder tells the nurse, "I feel like my arm isn't attached to my body." What is the most appropriate response by the nurse?
1. "Do you know where you are?"
2. "What makes you feel that way?"
3. "Don't worry because I can see your arm is attached to your body."
4. "This disorder causes people to feel that body parts may be unattached to the rest of the body."

Which kinds of questions tend to encourage discussion?

Don't stop now. You're almost there!

42. 1. One of the cardinal symptoms of depersonalization disorder is feeling detached from one's body or mental processes. During the feelings of detachment, the person doesn't become disoriented. Dissociative amnesia is defined as one or more episodes of being unable to recall important information. Dissociative identity disorder is the existence of two or more personalities that take control of the person's behavior. In a dissociative fugue, the person has no memory of his life before the flight.
CN: Psychosocial integrity; CNS: None; CL: Analysis

43. 2. Most clients with depersonalization disorder can be treated successfully on an outpatient basis. These clients only need to be hospitalized if they become suicidal or have severe depression or anxiety. Because no organic basis for the disorder usually exists, these clients aren't treated in a family practice physician's office. Because the disorder is rare, few support groups are composed only of clients with this disorder.
CN: Psychosocial integrity; CNS: None; CL: Application

44. 3. This open-ended response allows the client to focus and expand on this topic. Asking how often the experiences occur is a closed-ended question that doesn't encourage discussion of the experience. The second option could cause the client to focus too narrowly on only one aspect of the topic. Asking how the client's husband feels makes it appear that the nurse wants to change the topic.
CN: Psychosocial integrity; CNS: None; CL: Analysis

45. 4. A group of disorders in which there's impairment of memory or identity due to an unconscious attempt to protect the client from emotional pain or traumatic experiences describes dissociative disorders. Hallucinations are associated with schizophrenic disorders. The onset of dissociative disorders may be gradual, sudden, or chronic. There's no known organic cause for dissociative disorders.
CN: Psychosocial integrity; CNS: None; CL: Application

46. 4. Reinforcing that what the client feels is an expected result of the disease process would be most appropriate. Asking if the client knows where he is changes the topic. Asking why he feels that way could put the client on the defensive. Stating that his arm is attached to his body belittles the client's feelings.
CN: Psychosocial integrity; CNS: None; CL: Application

47. A client experiencing a dissociative disorder suddenly wanders away from the facility. When the nurse finds him, he can't recall what happened. The nurse interprets this behavior as which of the following?
1. Repression
2. Depersonalization
3. Derealization
4. Dissociative fugue

48. A nurse conducts an admission assessment on a client diagnosed with dissociative identity disorder. Which sign or symptom supports this diagnosis?
1. A sense of being in a dream
2. Inability to remember a particular event
3. Having two or more personalities
4. Ritualistic behavior

49. The nurse has just completed an assessment of a client. Which assessment findings place the client at the <u>highest</u> risk of suicide?
1. Suicide plan, handy means of carrying out plan, and history of previous attempt
2. Preoccupation with morbid thoughts and limited support system
3. Suicidal ideation, active suicide planning, and family history of suicide
4. Threats of suicide, recent job loss, and intact support system

50. A nurse finds a client experiencing suicidal ideation. The client attempted to hang themselves. What is the most important intervention for the nurse to implement?
1. Place the client in seclusion with checks every 15 minutes.
2. Assign a nursing staff member to remain with the client at all times.
3. Make the client stay with the group at all times.
4. Refuse to let the client in his room.

My mind keeps wandering to another place.

47. 4. Dissociative fugue is characterized by suddenly wandering away from one's usual place, accompanied by amnesia for all or part of the past. Repression is a defense mechanism in which thoughts and feelings are kept from consciousness. Depersonalization is a feeling of detachment or separation from one's self. Derealization is a feeling that the external world is unreal.
CN: Psychosocial integrity; CNS: None; CL: Application

48. 3. Dissociative identity disorder is characterized by having two or more distinct personalities, often in conflict with one another. A sense of being in a dream is common in depersonalization disorders. Selective amnesia refers to an inability to recall certain events that occurred during a specified period and is more common in traumatic stress disorders. Ritualistic behavior is seen in obsessive-compulsive disorders.
CN: Psychosocial integrity; CNS: None; CL: Application

49. 1. A lethal plan with a handy means of carrying it out poses the highest risk and requires immediate intervention. Although all of the remaining risk factors can lead to suicide, they aren't considered as high a risk as a formulated, lethal plan and the means at hand. However, a client exhibiting any of these risk factors should be taken seriously and considered at risk for suicide.
CN: Psychosocial integrity; CNS: None; CL: Application

50. 2. Implementing a one-on-one, staff-to-client ratio is the nurse's highest priority. Doing so allows the client to maintain his self-esteem and keeps him safe. Seclusion would damage the client's self-esteem. Forcing the client to stay with the group and refusing to let him in his room don't guarantee his safety.
CN: Psychosocial integrity; CNS: None; CL: Application

51. A client with a dissociative identity disorder experiences amnesia. Which nursing diagnosis is most appropriate?
1. Powerlessness
2. Ineffective coping
3. Disturbed sensory perception, visual
4. Risk for self-directed violence

52. After taking a potentially lethal drug overdose, a client tells the nurse that his alter "did it." Which nursing diagnosis takes highest priority?
1. Posttrauma syndrome
2. Anxiety
3. Risk for self-directed violence
4. Disturbed personal identity

53. A severely depressed client who has made multiple suicide attempts matter-of-factly tells the nurse that her family life was normal and uneventful. Which behaviors would lead the nurse to suspect a diagnosis of a dissociative identity disorder (DID) in this client? Select all that apply.
1. Inability to recall important personal information too severe to be explained by ordinary forgetfulness
2. Absence of any physiological effects of a substance, such as alcohol or drugs
3. Ability to selectively and consciously choose to avoid certain painful topics
4. A sense of grandiosity, that she's special and has a particular mission for mankind
5. Posttraumatic symptoms, such as flashbacks, nightmares, and an exaggerated startle response

54. A client with dissociative identity disorder experiences frequent periods of memory loss. What is the most appropriate nursing intervention for this client?
1. Orienting the client to time, place, person, and situation
2. Explaining to the client the circumstances surrounding the memory loss
3. Assessing for cues that the client is ready to discuss the memory loss
4. Telling the client not to worry because the memory loss has no physiological base

I know my highest priority at the moment.

Congratulations! You should feel on top of the world!

51. **2.** Amnesia may result from an inability to cope with anxiety. Powerlessness, disturbed sensory perception, and risk for self-directed violence aren't appropriate in this situation.
CN: Psychosocial integrity; CNS: None; CL: Analysis

52. **3.** Taking a potentially lethal drug overdose indicates that the client poses a danger to himself. Because the alter may act again, the risk for self-directed violence persists. The other nursing diagnoses either aren't relevant or take lower priority.
CN: Psychosocial integrity; CNS: None; CL: Analysis

53. **1, 2, and 5.** A dissociative disorder is a persistent state of being disconnected from the totality of one's personhood, particularly painful emotions. With dissociative disorder, the inability to recall personal information is far more extensive than ordinary forgetfulness; the symptoms occur apart from any chemical inducement, and the individual doesn't have the ability to consciously make a decision to separate from painful emotions or topics. A sense of grandiosity isn't characteristic of this disorder. Posttraumatic symptoms, such as flashbacks, nightmares, and an exaggerated startle response, are also signs and symptoms of DID.
CN: Psychosocial integrity; CNS: None; CL: Analysis

54. **3.** Memory loss serves as a protective mechanism for many clients with dissociative identity disorder; the nurse should wait until the client is ready to discuss the problem, as shown by certain cues. Orienting the client may force the client out of the protective mechanism of the memory loss (which the client may not be ready for and can result in further harm). Explaining the circumstances surrounding the memory loss and telling the client not to worry aren't therapeutic interventions.
CN: Psychosocial integrity; CNS: None; CL: Application

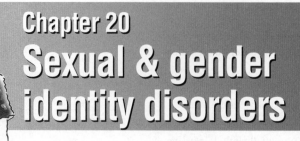

Chapter 20
Sexual & gender identity disorders

1. A client has undergone surgery for the repair of an abdominal aortic aneurysm. The client's wife asks the nurse if her husband will be impotent. What is the <u>most appropriate</u> response by the nurse?
1. "Don't worry, he'll be all right."
2. "He has other problems to worry about."
3. "We'll cross that bridge when we come to it."
4. "There is a chance of impotence after repair of an abdominal aortic aneurysm."

2. The nurse is preparing discharge instructions for a female client who has suffered a spinal cord injury at the C4 level. What is the most important information for the nurse to include?
1. After a spinal cord injury, women usually remain fertile; therefore, you may consider contraception if you don't want to become pregnant.
2. After a spinal cord injury, women usually are unable to conceive a child.
3. Sexual intercourse shouldn't be different for you.
4. After a spinal cord injury, menstruation usually stops.

3. A nurse is caring for a 39-year-old male client who recently underwent surgery and is having difficulty accepting changes in his body image. Which nursing intervention is most appropriate?
1. Actively listening to the client as he expresses positive and negative feelings about his body image
2. Restricting the client's opportunity to view the incision and dressing because it's upsetting
3. Assisting the client to focus on future plans for recovery
4. Assisting the client to repress anger while discussing the body image alteration

Therapeutic communication involves demonstrating sensitivity to your client's and his family's concerns.

Note that question 3 is asking you which action is appropriate.

1. 4. Impotence and retrograde ejaculation are sexual dysfunctions commonly experienced by male clients after abdominal aortic aneurysm. Telling a family member that the client will be all right is offering false assurance. Stating that he has other problems isn't therapeutic and doesn't address the wife's concern. Telling the client's wife to "cross that bridge when we come to it" ignores her concerns and isn't therapeutic.
CN: Psychosocial integrity; CNS: None; CL: Application

2. 1. After a spinal cord injury, women remain fertile and can conceive and deliver a child. If a woman doesn't want to become pregnant, she must use contraception. Menstruation isn't affected by a spinal cord injury, but sexual functioning may be different.
CN: Physiological integrity; CNS: Physiological adaptation; CL: Application

3. 1. The nurse must observe for any indication that the client is ready to address his body image change. The client should be allowed to look at the incision and dressing if he wants to do so. It's too soon to focus on the future with this client. The nurse should allow the client to express his feelings and not repress them because repression prolongs recovery.
CN: Psychosocial integrity; CNS: None; CL: Application

4. A female client with chronic obstructive pulmonary disease (COPD) tells a nurse, "I no longer have enough energy to make love to my husband." What is the <u>most appropriate</u> nursing intervention?
1. Refer the couple to a sex therapist.
2. Advise the woman to seek a gynecological consult.
3. Suggest methods and measures that facilitate sexual activity.
4. Tell the client, "If you talk this over with your husband, he'll understand."

5. A client with an ileostomy tells the nurse he is unable to have an erection. The nurse is aware that:
1. the client will never regain functioning.
2. the client needs an abdominal X-ray.
3. the client has no problem with self-control.
4. impotence is uncommon following an ileostomy.

6. A recently divorced 40-year-old client who has undergone radiation therapy for testicular cancer tells the nurse he is unable to achieve an erection. Which nursing diagnosis is <u>most appropriate</u>?
1. Ineffective coping related to radiation therapy
2. Sexual dysfunction related to the effects of radiation therapy
3. Disturbed body image related to the effects of radiation therapy
4. Imbalanced nutrition: Less than body requirements related to radiation therapy

7. A nurse is preparing the teaching plan for a newly married female client with a cervical spinal cord injury. The client does not want to become pregnant at this time. What is the most important intervention by the nurse?
1. Provide the client with brochures on sexual practice.
2. Provide the client's husband with material on vasectomy.
3. Instruct the client on the rhythm method of contraception.
4. Instruct the client's husband on inserting a diaphragm with contraceptive jelly.

Several answers are possible. But which one is the most appropriate?

There's that phrase most appropriate again.

4. 3. Sexual dysfunction in COPD clients is the direct result of dyspnea and reduced energy levels. Measures to reduce physical exertion, enhance oxygenation, and accommodate decreased energy levels may aid sexual activity. If the problem persists, a consult with a sex therapist might be necessary. A gynecological consult isn't necessary. Discussing this with her husband may not resolve the problem.
CN: Physiological integrity; CNS: Reduction of risk potential; CL: Application

5. 4. Sexual dysfunction is uncommon after an ileostomy. Psychological causes of impotence should be explored. An abdominal X-ray isn't indicated for sexual dysfunction. An ileostomy can change a person's self-control, making sexual functioning difficult.
CN: Physiological integrity; CNS: Physiological adaptation; CL: Analysis

6. 2. Radiation or chemotherapy may cause sexual dysfunction. Libido may only be temporarily affected, and the client should be provided with emotional support. The client may experience alopecia or skin changes as well as weight loss, but he isn't verbalizing concern in this area. The client hasn't verbalized fear or concern related to the cancer. Nutrition hasn't been mentioned.
CN: Psychosocial integrity; CNS: None; CL: Analysis

7. 4. Because the client experienced a cervical spinal cord injury, she won't be able to insert any form of contraception protection by herself; therefore, it's vital to provide her husband with instruction on insertion of a diaphragm. Providing the couple with literature on sexual practice doesn't address the client's concerns. During this time of crisis, the couple doesn't wish to have children, but they may reconsider, so providing information on vasectomy isn't appropriate. The rhythm method isn't the most effective way to prevent pregnancy.
CN: Psychosocial integrity; CNS: None; CL: Application

8. A female client tells the nurse she is having her menstrual period every 2 weeks and it lasts for 1 week. The nurse interprets this as which pattern?
1. Amenorrhea
2. Dyspareunia
3. Menorrhagia
4. Metrorrhagia

9. The nurse anticipates that which of the following is a major stressor for a couple being treated for infertility?
1. Examinations
2. Giving specimens
3. Scheduling intercourse
4. Finding out which partner is infertile

10. A 38-year-old female client has been diagnosed with uterine cancer and must undergo a hysterectomy. What is the most important nursing intervention?
1. Ask her if she is having pain.
2. Refer her to a psychotherapist.
3. Don't discuss the subject with her.
4. Encourage her to verbalize her feelings.

11. A 50-year-old male client who had a myocardial infarction 8 weeks ago tells a nurse, "My wife wants to make love, but I don't think I can. I'm worried that it might kill me." What is the most appropriate response by the nurse?
1. "Tell me about your feelings."
2. "Let's increase your rehabilitation schedule."
3. "Let me call the primary health care provider for you."
4. "Tell your wife when you're able you'll make love."

What's the difference between menorrhagia and metrorrhagia?

Let's put together a plan of care that will meet all of your needs.

8. 3. Menorrhagia is an excessive menstrual period. Amenorrhea is lack of menstruation. Dyspareunia is painful intercourse. Metrorrhagia is uterine bleeding from another cause other than menstruation.

CN: Physiological integrity; CNS: Reduction of risk potential; CL: Application

9. 3. The major cause of stress in infertile couples is planning sexual intercourse to correlate to fertility cycles. The inconvenience and discomfort of producing specimens and receiving examinations isn't a major stressor. Most couples undergoing fertility treatment understand that one partner is usually infertile.

CN: Health promotion and maintenance; CNS: None; CL: Application

10. 4. Encourage the client to verbalize her feelings because loss of one's reproductive organs may bring on feelings of loss of sexuality. Pain is a concern after surgery, but it has no bearing on body image. Referring her to a psychotherapist may be premature; the client should be given time to work through her feelings. Avoidance of the subject isn't a therapeutic nursing intervention.

CN: Psychosocial integrity; CNS: None; CL: Application

11. 1. The nurse should address the client's concerns. Asking the client to verbalize his feelings will permit the nurse to gain insight into the problem. The rehabilitation schedule shouldn't be increased until the nurse assesses the situation and is sure no harm will come to the client. Calling the primary health care provider before a complete assessment is made is inappropriate. Telling the wife that eventually the client will make love may place strain on the marriage.

CN: Psychosocial integrity; CNS: None; CL: Application

12. A 55-year-old female client who is in cardiac rehabilitation tells a nurse that she's unable to make love to her husband because she often feels fatigued and has a sense of doom. What is the most appropriate information for the nurse to provide?
1. Instruct her not to have intercourse until she is ready.
2. Instruct her to take a nitroglycerin tablet prior to intercourse.
3. Encourage her to learn additional methods to use for sexual intercourse.
4. Encourage her to verbalize her feelings while you perform a physical examination on her.

13. A 33-year-old female client tells the nurse that she has never had an orgasm. Her partner is upset that he is unable to meet her needs. What is the best intervention by the nurse?
1. Ask the client if she desires intercourse.
2. Assess the couple's perception of the problem.
3. Tell the client that most women don't reach orgasm.
4. Refer the client to a therapist because she has sexual aversion disorder.

14. A 20-year-old female client is in the emergency department after being sexually assaulted by a stranger. Which nursing intervention has the highest priority?
1. Assisting the client in identifying which of her behaviors placed her at risk for the attack
2. Making an appointment for the client in 6 weeks at a local sexual assault crisis center
3. Encouraging discussion of the client's early childhood experiences
4. Assisting the client in identifying family or friends who could provide immediate support for her

15. A 50-year-old client has been taking antihypertensive medication that the physician prescribed. During a routine office visit for blood pressure monitoring, the client tells the nurse that he is unable to have sexual intercourse with his wife anymore. The nurse determines that this is most likely the result of his:
1. advancing age.
2. blood pressure.
3. stressful lifestyle.
4. blood pressure medication.

I know all about feeling fatigued.

The NCLEX may include sexual identity questions for clients of different ages.

12. 4. Because the client has a complaint of fatigue, she should be examined and her feelings should be explored. Instructing her not to have intercourse doesn't address her concerns. She shouldn't take nitroglycerin before intercourse until her fatigue is evaluated. Before recommending alternative methods for intercourse, the client should be assessed physically and psychologically.
CN: Psychosocial integrity; CNS: None; CL: Application

13. 2. Assessing the couple's perception of the problem will define the problem and assist the couple and the nurse in understanding it. When assessing the client, the nurse should be professional and matter-of-fact and shouldn't make the client feel inadequate or defensive by asking if she desires intercourse. Most individuals can be taught to reach orgasm if there is no underlying medical condition. A nurse can't make a medical diagnosis such as sexual aversion disorder.
CN: Psychosocial integrity; CNS: None; CL: Application

14. 4. The client needs a lot of support to help her through this ordeal. Assisting the client in identifying behaviors that place her at risk for the attack places the blame on the client. Waiting 6 weeks to make an appointment is incorrect—the local crisis center must be called immediately. Some psychiatric disorders are related to early childhood experiences, but rape isn't.
CN: Psychosocial integrity; CNS: None; CL: Application

15. 4. Antihypertensive medication may cause impotence in men. Blood pressure itself doesn't cause impotence but its treatment does. Stress may cause erectile dysfunction, but there's no evidence that the client is under stress. Men are usually able to have an erection throughout their lives.
CN: Physiological integrity; CNS: Pharmacological and parenteral therapies; CL: Application

16. Adult victims of childhood sexual abuse need to be monitored for signs and symptoms of which disorder?
 1. Depression and substance abuse disorders
 2. Bipolar and somatization disorders
 3. Narcissistic disorders and bulimia nervosa
 4. Obsessive-compulsive and posttraumatic stress disorders

Don't despair over answering this question—focus on this disorder's symptoms.

17. Which nursing intervention is important for a client who engages in sexual acts with animals (zoophilia)?
 1. Place the client in the seclusion room.
 2. Assess triggers that stimulate the behaviors.
 3. Have the primary health care provider order antidepressant medication.
 4. Counsel the client not to discuss his sexual behaviors with anyone.

18. A 25-year-old client convicted of raping a female college student has completed his parole and has been attending a sex offenders group for 5 years. The client tells the nurse that he no longer wishes to participate in the group. What is the most important intervention by the nurse?
 1. Insist that the client remain in therapy.
 2. Perform a self-evaluation and assess the discomfort level.
 3. Call the parole board and tell them of the client's decision.
 4. Call the client's family and tell them of his decision and progress.

19. A 32-year-old client who engages in voyeurism has come to the hospital for treatment so his family and friends don't find out. The nurse planning care for this client should include which intervention?
 1. Encourage the client to inform his family and friends so that he isn't living a lie.
 2. Suggest individual therapy to discuss socially unacceptable behavior.
 3. Develop the care plan without input from the client.
 4. Evaluate the client's defense mechanism.

You've really set sail on this chapter.

16. 1. Childhood sexual abuse is closely linked to the development of depression and substance abuse disorders. It's also linked to the development of somatization and posttraumatic stress disorders and bulimia nervosa. Victims of childhood sexual abuse aren't predisposed to developing bipolar, narcissistic, or obsessive-compulsive disorders.
CN: Psychosocial integrity; CNS: None; CL: Analysis

17. 2. Assessing the triggers that stimulate inappropriate sexual behavior helps to prevent recurrence. The seclusion room should be used only to ensure the safety of the client and staff. Antidepressants aren't indicated for sexual disorders; hormonal therapy is the usual drug treatment. Clinical support and group therapy are used to teach sexually acceptable behavior.
CN: Psychosocial integrity; CNS: None; CL: Analysis

18. 2. If the client has successfully completed therapy, then the nurse must evaluate her own value system. Insisting that the client remain in therapy may not prove to be successful, as he must be motivated to undergo therapy. Calling the parole board may be an inappropriate decision, especially if the client has met all of his requirements. A nurse can't release confidential information to the client's family without his permission and consent.
CN: Psychosocial integrity; CNS: None; CL: Analysis

19. 2. Discussing inappropriate sexual behavior with the client increases compliance with treatment and decreases the risk of relapse. Informing family and friends isn't an initial intervention; disclosure to family and friends is usually delayed until the client acknowledges his behavior. All care planning should involve the client. An initial evaluation should focus on the antecedents to the inappropriate behavior.
CN: Psychosocial integrity; CNS: None; CL: Application

20. A client is admitted to the psychiatric unit for paraphiliac coercive disorder: rape. What is the most important question for the nurse to ask the client?
1. "Tell me what you're feeling."
2. "Do you have any lifestyle problems?"
3. "What brings you to the hospital for treatment?"
4. "Do you believe you're here for a sexual disorder?"

21. A 38-year-old female client was returning home from the store late in the evening and was sexually assaulted. She is brought to the emergency department and is crying. What is the most important intervention by the nurse?
1. Filing a police report
2. Calling the client's family
3. Encouraging the client to enroll in a self-defense class
4. Remaining with the client and assisting her through the crisis

22. A client is admitted to the psychiatric unit as part of his probation period for exhibitionism and fetishism. The client seems to be adjusting well, but several clients report that their undergarments are missing. Which action would be most appropriate?
1. Notify the primary health care provider.
2. Search the client's room.
3. Call a community meeting and let the clients settle the matter.
4. Privately assess whether the client is engaging in sexual activities on the unit.

23. A client is admitted to the hospital for scatophilia and tells the nurse that he doesn't want to talk to her about his sexual behaviors. Which response from the nurse is the most appropriate?
1. "I need to ask you the questions on the database."
2. "It's your right not to answer my questions."
3. "I know this must be difficult for you."
4. "OK, I'll just write 'no comment.'"

Prioritizing correctly is extremely important for question 21.

Clients with sexual disorders may be ashamed and unwilling to discuss the problem.

20. 4. If a client had a cognitive disorder, then he would be using denial as a defense mechanism and would deny having a sexual disorder. Asking what a client is feeling is important, but it doesn't provide information on the use of defense mechanisms. Asking about lifestyle problems will provide the nurse with information related to problems with relationships. Asking why the client is at the hospital will tell the nurse if the client has insight into his illness.
CN: Psychosocial integrity; CNS: None; CL: Application

21. 4. Sexual assault is treated as a medical emergency, and the client requires constant attention and assistance during the crisis. Filing a police report wouldn't take precedence over a medical emergency. Comforting the client by contacting family should be carried out after the client's injuries are treated. Encouraging the client to enroll in a self-defense class isn't appropriate during crisis.
CN: Psychosocial integrity; CNS: None; CL: Application

22. 4. Meeting with the client privately establishes trust. This client needs to be assessed for what triggers might be present to prompt this behavior. Notification of the primary health care provider shouldn't be done without assessment of the client. Searching the client's room without discussion is a violation of a trusting milieu. It isn't therapeutic to encourage the unit to confront one member of the community.
CN: Psychosocial integrity; CNS: None; CL: Application

23. 3. Stating "I know this must be difficult for you" acknowledges the client's feelings and opens communications. Insisting that the form needs to be completed doesn't open up communications or acknowledge the client's feelings. Clients have rights, but data collection is necessary so that help with the problem can be offered. Writing "no comment" alone would be inappropriate.
CN: Psychosocial integrity; CNS: None; CL: Application

24. Which therapy may be used with a client who admits to frottage?
1. Electroconvulsive therapy
2. Relaxation therapy
3. Administration of psychotropic agents
4. Positive reinforcement and group therapy

24. 4. Frottage involves rubbing against someone in a public place. Positive reinforcement and group therapy are used to assist a client with frottage to develop new sexual response patterns. Electroconvulsive therapy and relaxation therapy aren't indicated for this condition. Psychotropic medications are used for dangerous and compulsive practices and aren't indicated for this condition.
CN: Psychosocial integrity; CNS: None; CL: Analysis

Keep going; you're doing great!

25. When treating a client admitted to the psychiatric unit for transvestic fetishism, the nurse should develop a care plan based on which nursing diagnosis?
1. Ineffective health maintenance
2. Ineffective sexuality patterns
3. Complicated grieving
4. Bathing self-care deficit

25. 2. Ineffective sexuality patterns would be appropriate because transvestic fetishism refers to intense sexual arousal with cross-dressing. Ineffective health maintenance is an appropriate diagnosis for someone experiencing a health problem. Complicated grieving refers to the inability to recover from a loss. The client hasn't exhibited any problems with health, self-care, or loss. Bathing self-care deficit is a diagnosis for the inability to meet self-care needs.
CN: Psychosocial integrity; CNS: None; CL: Application

26. The nurse is caring for a client with a paraphiliac disorder. What is the most important goal for the client?
1. To attend all meetings on the unit
2. To use triggers to initiate sexual behaviors
3. To inform his employer of the reason for hospitalization
4. To verbalize appropriate methods to meet sexual needs upon discharge

26. 4. Upon discharge, the client should verbalize an alternative appropriate method to meet his sexual needs and effective strategies to prevent relapse. It isn't imperative that the client attend all meetings on the unit, but it's important that he attend the prescribed group sessions. A client with a paraphiliac disorder should recognize triggers that initiate inappropriate sexual behaviors and learn ways to direct his impulses. The client may wish to discuss the disorder with his spouse but not necessarily his employer.
CN: Psychosocial integrity; CNS: None; CL: Analysis

Effective care may involve managing interactions between clients.

27. A client admitted to the hospital with a diagnosis of pedophilia tells his roommate about his problems. His roommate runs down the hall yelling at the nurse, "I don't want to be in here with a child molester." Which response from the nurse is <u>most appropriate</u>?
1. "Stop acting out."
2. "Calm down and go back to your room."
3. "Your roommate isn't a child molester."
4. "I can see you're upset. Sit down and we'll talk."

27. 4. Acknowledging that the client is upset and sitting down and talking with him will allow the client to verbalize his feelings. If a client were agitated or anxious over his roommate, it wouldn't be therapeutic or safe to keep those clients together without intervention. Telling the client to stop acting out or to calm down isn't a therapeutic response. Stating that the pedophile isn't a child molester doesn't acknowledge the client's feelings.
CN: Psychosocial integrity; CNS: None; CL: Application

28. When assigning rooms, a nurse should <u>not</u> place a client who has a diagnosis of sexual sadism with which other client?
1. A client with a diagnosis of sexual masochism
2. A client with a diagnosis of voyeurism
3. A client who's an exhibitionist
4. A client who's a homosexual

28. 1. A client who's admitted with a diagnosis of sexual masochism is aroused through suffering and, therefore, shouldn't be placed with a client who's diagnosed with sexual sadism, who's aroused by inflicting pain. A voyeur is aroused by secretly observing someone who's naked or engaged in sexual activity. An exhibitionist is aroused through the exposure of one's genitals to an unsuspecting person. A homosexual enjoys relationships with someone of the same sex.
CN: Safe, effective care environment; CNS: Management of care; CL: Application

29. A nurse is obtaining a health history from a client who states he has been diagnosed with voyeurism. Which of the following actions would the nurse expect to assess in this client?
1. Observing others while they disrobe
2. Wearing clothing of the opposite sex
3. Rubbing against a nonconsenting person
4. Using rubber sheeting for sexual arousal

29. 1. Voyeurism is sexual arousal from secretly observing someone who is disrobing. Transvestic fetishism describes someone who enjoys crossdressing. Rubbing against someone who is nonconsenting is frottage. Using objects for sexual arousal is fetishism.
CN: Psychosocial integrity; CNS: None; CL: Application

Hello, information? Do you know the answer to question 30?

30. The nurse is teaching the family of a client with scatophilia. Which response by the nurse is <u>most</u> accurate in teaching about the characteristics of this disorder?
1. The client uses the telephone for sexual arousal.
2. The client uses nonliving objects such as women's underwear for sexual gratification.
3. The client is aroused through contact with children.
4. The client is aroused by rubbing against a nonconsenting person.

30. 1. Telephone scatophilia is a paraphilia in which a person derives sexual arousal by engaging in lewd conversations on the telephone. Fetishism involves the use of nonliving objects whose presence is required or preferred for sexual excitement. Pedophiles engage in fondling or sexual activities with children under 13 years of age. Frottage is rubbing against a nonconsenting person for sexual arousal.
CN: Psychosocial integrity; CNS: None; CL: Application

31. A female being treated for infertility confides to the nurse that she hasn't told her partner she has been treated for a sexually transmitted disease in the past. What is the best response by the nurse?
1. "Do you think withholding this information is the basis for a trusting relationship?"
2. "Don't you think your partner deserves to know?"
3. "What concerns do you have about sharing this information?"
4. "I can understand why you would want to keep this information from him."

31. 3. This response encourages the client to verbalize her concerns in a safe environment and begin to choose a course of action for how to deal with this issue now. Telling the client that she's withholding information that may cause distrust in her relationship or that her partner deserves to know conveys negative judgments. The fourth response doesn't encourage discussion or problem solving.
CN: Psychosocial integrity; CNS: None; CL: Application

32. A client has learned that his gay roommate has tested positive for human immunodeficiency virus (HIV). The client asks the nurse about moving to another room on the psychiatric unit because the client doesn't feel "safe" now. What is the <u>most appropriate</u> action by the nurse?
1. Move the client to another room.
2. Ask the client to describe any fears.
3. Move the client's roommate to a private room.
4. Explain that such a move wouldn't be therapeutic for the client or his roommate.

33. A nurse lecturing on paraphilias informs her audience that recidivism is high for clients with paraphilias. Which definition best describes recidivism?
1. Insight into treatment
2. Aggressive sexual assault
3. Behaviors associated with sexual deviation
4. Continued inappropriate behavior after treatment

34. Which nursing diagnosis is most appropriate for a client with sexual masochism?
1. Risk for self-mutilation
2. Ineffective role performance
3. Ineffective coping
4. Risk for other-directed violence

35. Which statement made by a client with paraphilia indicates a potential for relapse?
1. "I am going to outpatient therapy."
2. "I am going to try to attend all therapy sessions."
3. "I don't need this, and I can't imagine why the judge sent me here."
4. "The physician wants me to take leuprolide acetate (Lupron). I think that will help."

36. A female client taking antidepressant medication complains to the nurse that she has a decreased desire for sex, which is causing significant marital stress. What is the <u>most appropriate</u> response by the nurse?
1. "Don't stop taking the medication."
2. "What are your thoughts on how you should handle this?"
3. "Doesn't your husband understand the importance of your medication?"
4. "Have you discussed this with your physician?"

I predict you will be able to select which action is most appropriate.

The NCLEX often tests your ability to educate accurately.

More than one answer may seen correct, but choose the most appropriate.

32. 2. To intervene effectively, the nurse must first understand the client's fears. After exploring the client's fears, the nurse may move the client or his roommate or explain why such a move wouldn't be therapeutic.

CN: Psychosocial integrity; CNS: None; CL: Application

33. 4. Recidivism is defined as continuing in an unacceptable behavior after completing treatment to correct that behavior. High level of insight isn't connected with any specific disorder. Aggressive sexual assault is a type of paraphilia. Sexually deviant behaviors are known as paraphilias.

CN: Psychosocial integrity; CNS: None; CL: Analysis

34. 1. A person with sexual masochism is sexually aroused by being the receiver of pain and, therefore, may injure himself. A person diagnosed with transvestic fetishism may have ineffective role performance. There is no evidence that this client isn't coping. A sexual sadist would be a danger to others.

CN: Psychosocial integrity; CNS: None; CL: Analysis

35. 3. A lack of insight to the problem may indicate a potential for relapse. Attending all therapy sessions and outpatient therapy demonstrates compliance with the treatment plan. Leuprolide acetate is an antiandrogenic that lowers testosterone levels and decreases the libido.

CN: Psychosocial integrity; CNS: None; CL: Analysis

36. 2. Encouraging the client to verbalize her thoughts will help the client to problem solve and identify feelings related to different choices. The first response is too directive and doesn't encourage exploration on the part of the client. The third response conveys negative judgment. The fourth response might be appropriate, but it also may give the impression that the nurse doesn't want to discuss this issue with the client.

CN: Psychosocial integrity; CNS: None; CL: Application

CN: Client needs category   CNS: Client needs subcategory   CL: Cognitive level

37. A mother brings her 14-year-old son to the psychiatric crisis room. The client's mother states, "He's always dressing in female clothing. There must be something wrong with him." Which response from the nurse would be most appropriate?
1. "Your son will be evaluated shortly."
2. "I'll tell your son that this isn't appropriate."
3. "I know you're upset. Would you like to talk?"
4. "I wouldn't want my son to dress in girl's clothing."

38. A 17-year-old female who enjoys playing ball with boys and is most comfortable in jeans tells her mother she doesn't want to go to the prom if she has to wear a frilly dress. Her mother asks, "What should I do with my daughter?" What is the best response by the nurse?
1. Tell the client's mother, "She'll grow out of it."
2. Offer to speak to the client about her dressing habits.
3. Ask the client's mother to talk about her fears for her daughter.
4. Tell the client's mother to make her go to the prom but not wear a dress.

39. A 39-year-old male client tells the nurse he wants to undergo a sex reassignment operation because he feels trapped in his male body. The nurse anticipates that a priority intervention of the client's treatment plan would be which of the following?
1. Telling his family and friends
2. Attending psychotherapy
3. Visiting transsexual bars
4. Seeing a surgeon

40. Estrogen therapy has been prescribed for a male client who wishes to undergo sexual reassignment surgery. The nurse determines that the client understands the therapy when he states its purpose is to accomplish which of the following?
1. "To develop breasts"
2. "To cause menstruation"
3. "To assist with cross-dressing"
4. "To develop body hair and lack of menstruation"

I want to make sure you understand.

37. 3. Acknowledging the mother's feelings and offering her an opportunity to verbalize her concerns provides a forum for open communication. Telling the client's mother that he'll be evaluated shortly doesn't address her concerns. Telling the client that this behavior isn't appropriate doesn't assess his feelings nor does it analyze the behavior. The nurse shouldn't offer an opinion by stating she wouldn't want her son dressing in female clothing.
CN: Psychosocial integrity; CNS: None; CL: Application

38. 3. Asking the client's mother to verbalize her fears will permit the nurse to accurately assess the mother's distress. The client's mother may be upset over the behavior or the fact that her daughter doesn't wish to go to the prom. Telling the client's mother that her daughter will grow out of it may be offering the mother false reassurance. The nurse shouldn't speak to the client about her behavior as this implies a value judgment on the part of the nurse. Forcing her to go to the prom isn't therapeutic and doesn't address the mother's fears.
CN: Psychosocial integrity; CNS: None; CL: Application

39. 2. Before having a sex reassignment operation, the client should have several years of psychotherapy. The family, as well as friends, should be told of the client's plans. Visiting transsexual bars has no bearing on having a sex reassignment operation. Seeing a surgeon isn't usually done on a regular basis until after the completion of psychotherapy.
CN: Psychosocial integrity; CNS: None; CL: Analysis

40. 1. A male who receives long-term estrogen therapy will develop female secondary sexual characteristics such as breasts. A male on estrogen won't menstruate because he doesn't have a uterus. Estrogen has no bearing on cross-dressing. Androgens would be taken by a female to develop body hair and stop menstruation.
CN: Psychosocial integrity; CNS: None; CL: Analysis

41. A nurse is caring for several clients with gender identity disorders. Which client category is at highest risk for anxiety related to transsexualism?
1. Elderly
2. Adolescent
3. Young adult
4. Prepubescent child

42. What is the gender identity disorder that results in the person believing he or she is the opposite sex?
1. Exhibitionism
2. Homosexuality
3. Transsexualism
4. Transvestitism

43. A transsexual client wishes to have a sexual reassignment operation and tells the nurse he's ready to begin hormonal therapy. Which fact about the client must be true <u>before</u> estrogen therapy is administered?
1. He has cross-dressed and lived as the opposite sex for several years.
2. He has decided against undergoing the operation.
3. He has decided he needs more psychotherapy.
4. He has been functioning sexually as a female.

44. An adolescent who is suffering from gender identity disorder is unable to progress through which developmental task?
1. Initiative versus guilt
2. Intimacy versus isolation
3. Industry versus inferiority
4. Identity versus role confusion

A client's age can affect his anxiety related to gender identity disorders.

I remember reading about Erik Erikson. But now I'm confused.

41. 2. Adolescents who are transsexuals are usually very distraught over the changes occurring within their body. Elderly persons, young adults, and young children aren't experiencing rapidly developing secondary sexual characteristics in their bodies; therefore, they aren't at high risk for anxiety.
CN: Psychosocial integrity; CNS: None; CL: Analysis

42. 3. A client who is diagnosed with transsexual disorder believes they're really of the opposite sex. An exhibitionist is someone who's sexually aroused by displaying one's genitals in a public place. A homosexual enjoys sexual relations with a person of the same sexual orientation. A transvestite enjoys cross-dressing.
CN: Psychosocial integrity; CNS: None; CL: Application

43. 1. Before a sexual reassignment operation, the client should live as the opposite sex after undergoing several years of psychotherapy. A client wishing to take hormonal therapy is in the final step before receiving the operation and therefore hasn't decided against the surgery. Psychotherapy is an ongoing modality for someone requesting a sexual reassignment operation. A male doesn't have female reproductive organs, so he couldn't have been functioning sexually as a female.
CN: Psychosocial integrity; CNS: None; CL: Analysis

44. 4. According to developmentalist Erik Erikson, adolescence is a time when role identity is found as a result of independence and sexual maturity; role confusion would result from the inability to integrate all experiences. Initiative versus guilt is when a child begins to conceptualize and interpersonalize relationships. Intimacy versus isolation is a stage in which the adult meets other adults and establishes relationships. Industry versus inferiority is when a child incorporates and acquires social skills.
CN: Health promotion and maintenance; CNS: None; CL: Analysis

45. A 35-year-old client who has been married for 10 years arrives at the psychiatric clinic stating, "I can't live this lie any more. I wish I were a woman. I don't want my wife. I need a man." What is the priority intervention by the nurse?
  1. Call the primary health care provider.
  2. Encourage the client to speak to his wife.
  3. Have the client admitted.
  4. Sit down with the client and talk about his feelings.

What should you do first?

46. A 14-year-old female client admits to having transsexual feelings and states, "I would rather die than live in this body." What is the most appropriate <u>initial</u> intervention by the nurse?
  1. Explain to her that she is too young to have these feelings.
  2. Call her parents and let them know about her feelings.
  3. Encourage her to verbalize her feelings.
  4. Ask her if she plans to kill herself.

47. A female client enjoys wearing men's clothing. Her sister tells the nurse that the client wishes for a sexual reassignment operation. The client tells the nurse she just wants to be left alone. Which initial nursing intervention is most appropriate?
  1. Tell the client she is repressing her true feelings.
  2. Encourage the client to verbalize her feelings.
  3. Tell the client's sister to mind her own business.
  4. Encourage the client to avoid her sister.

48. A mother is concerned about her son and says he's 10 years old and has been playing with dolls since he was 2. Which initial strategy should be included in his care plan?
  1. Providing counseling for his mother
  2. Instructing the mother to throw away the dolls
  3. Instructing the mother on play that's age-appropriate
  4. Exploring with the child his feelings related to the dolls

Keep going! Fewer than 10 questions to go!

45. 4. Sitting down with the client and exploring his feelings will allow the nurse to assess him. The primary health care provider shouldn't be notified until an assessment is made. The client shouldn't speak to his wife until he has processed his feelings. An assessment of the client should be made before admitting the client to the unit.

CN: Psychosocial integrity; CNS: None; CL: Application

46. 4. Whenever a client verbalizes feelings of preferring death to life, the nurse should always make sure that the client doesn't have a plan. Transsexual tendencies usually arise during the adolescent years, so it is appropriate for the client to have these feelings. Calling her parents wouldn't be a priority until after a psychological safety assessment is completed. Encouraging her to verbalize her feelings isn't an initial action for the nurse.

CN: Psychosocial integrity; CNS: None; CL: Application

47. 2. The client needs to verbalize her feelings regarding wearing male attire as well as her desire to be left alone. Telling the client she is repressing her true feelings is judgmental. It's inappropriate for a nurse to tell a family member to mind her own business or to tell the client to avoid her sister.

CN: Psychosocial integrity; CNS: None; CL: Application

48. 4. It's important to assess the child's feelings as well as to explore his preference for dolls rather than sports. The mother may need to be instructed on methods to cope with his behaviors but only after the child is permitted to verbalize. Until proper assessment is made, it's inappropriate to remove the dolls. There's no evidence of age-inappropriate play.

CN: Psychosocial integrity; CNS: None; CL: Application

49. A new graduate nurse expresses concern to the nurse-manager about working with clients who want to discuss sexual problems. What is the best response by the nurse-manager?
  1. "It's part of the job. You'll get used to it."
  2. "You can refer those types of questions to other health care professionals."
  3. "If you've graduated from nursing school and passed the NCLEX, you qualify as a sex counselor."
  4. "Tell me more about your concern."

49. 4. The nurse-manager would need to explore more what the nurse's specific concerns were before she could counsel her appropriately. Telling the nurse she'll get used to it doesn't allow the nurse to express her feelings or validate her concerns. Option 2 may be a possibility, but the nurse-manager needs to understand the problem first. Passing the NCLEX doesn't qualify the nurse as a sex counselor. Sex therapists have additional training and education.

CN: Safe effective care environment; CNS: Management of care; CL: Analysis

50. A 57-year-old male client who has a history of hypertension expresses concern about his sexual functioning to the nurse. What is the <u>most important</u> assessment data for the nurse to review?
  1. Medication history
  2. Sexual practices
  3. Medical conditions
  4. Family history

We have a history together.

50. 1. Many antihypertensive medications can affect sexual functioning; the nurse must assess if the client is taking other medications that may also alter sexual functioning. Sexual practices are part of the nursing assessment, as are other medical conditions and family history. However, obtaining a thorough medication history and reviewing effects on the client may help alleviate misconceptions and easily identify the source of the problem.

CN: Physiological integrity; CNS: Pharmacological and parenteral therapies; CL: Application

51. A male client brings a list of his prescribed medications to the clinic. During the initial assessment, he tells the nurse that he has been experiencing delayed ejaculation. Which of the following drug classes would <u>most likely</u> be associated with this condition?
  1. Anticoagulants
  2. Antibiotics
  3. Antihypertensives
  4. Steroids

51. 3. Antihypertensive agents can cause or contribute to sexual dysfunction. Anticoagulants, antibiotics, and steroids have no known effect on sexual function.

CN: Physiological integrity; CNS: Pharmacological and parenteral therapies; CL: Application

52. After a myocardial infarction (MI), a client tells the nurse he's afraid he'll have another heart attack if he attempts sexual intercourse. Which nursing diagnosis is <u>most</u> appropriate?
  1. Deficient knowledge related to sexual dysfunction
  2. Disturbed body image related to lifestyle changes
  3. Sexual dysfunction related to disturbances in self-esteem
  4. Disturbed body image related to effects of treatment

I just want to know what's safe.

52. 1. After an MI, many clients fear that engaging in sex will trigger another one. The nurse should teach the client about when he can safely resume sexual activity and which positions to use during intercourse to conserve energy. The client's fears result from lack of knowledge, not disturbances in self-esteem or body image.

CN: Psychosocial integrity; CNS: None; CL: Application

53. A 42-year-old female client complains of painful intercourse. Which nursing <u>diagnosis</u> is most appropriate in planning the client's care?
1. Ineffective coping
2. Disturbed body image
3. Ineffective sexuality patterns
4. Sexual dysfunction

54. A 46-year-old female client is diagnosed with a problem in sexual functioning. When planning her care, which nursing intervention takes <u>highest</u> priority?
1. Assessing the client's sexual functioning
2. Assessing the client's role in her sexual relationship
3. Determining the nurse's own beliefs and feelings about this issue
4. Interviewing the client's sexual partner

55. A 35-year-old male client states he has little or no sexual desire. He also states that this is causing great distress in his marriage. What further information would be the <u>most useful</u> in assessing the situation? Select all that apply.
1. The client's age when he had his first girlfriend
2. When the problem first appeared and potential contributing factors
3. Medications and dosages
4. Report of recent bladder or prostate problems
5. Age of the client's wife

56. Pedophilia is diagnosed by the presence of specifically defined behaviors and characteristics. Which statements regarding pedophilia are correct? Select all that apply.
1. A strong sexual attraction to prepubescent children exists.
2. Male children are more commonly the focus of attention than female children.
3. The pedophile is usually very attentive to a child's needs in order to gain the child's attention.
4. The disorder generally begins in early adulthood.
5. The pedophile must be age 16 or older or at least 5 years older than the child.

53. 4. Sexual dysfunction is the most useful nursing diagnosis for this client because she has identified painful intercourse as a physical problem, which can alter the giving and receiving of pleasure and satisfaction. Ineffective coping would apply if the client stated she avoids intercourse or expresses alternative coping mechanisms. Disturbed body image isn't appropriate because the client hasn't stated she feels uncomfortable in some way about herself. Ineffective sexuality patterns would apply if the client stated that she doesn't engage in intercourse or have the ability to relate to others sexually.
CN: Psychosocial integrity; CNS: None; CL: Application

54. 3. The nurse must first identify her own beliefs and feelings about the issue and remain nonjudgmental. The other actions may be relevant but take lower priority.
CN: Safe, effective care environment; CNS: Management of care; CL: Application

55. 2 and 3. Option 2 is correct and provides opportunity to gather useful information in better understanding the client's current condition. Option 3 is correct because certain medications can have a profound effect on sexual desire. The client's age when he started dating has no bearing on the current problem. Reporting previous problems is useful but wouldn't provide a sufficient explanation for the lack of sexual desire. The age of the client's wife is irrelevant and doesn't provide assessment data.
CN: Psychosocial integrity; CNS: None; CL: Analysis

56. 1, 3, and 5. Pedophilia is a disorder characterized by a strong sexual attraction to prepubescent children that generally begins to manifest itself in adolescence, not early adulthood. By definition, the pedophile must be age 16 or older or at least 5 years older than the child. The pedophile generally is attentive to the needs of children in order to gain their trust, loyalty, and attention. Female, not male, children are more commonly the focus of attention.
CN: Psychosocial integrity; CNS: None; CL: Application

Time to celebrate! You finished chapter 20!

New information about eating disorders is released almost continuously. For the latest about disorders of critical importance for young people, check the Web site of the National Eating Disorders Association at **www.nationaleatingdisorders.org**.

Chapter 21
Eating disorders

1. A parent with a daughter who was diagnosed with bulimia nervosa asks a nurse, "How can my child have an eating disorder when she isn't underweight?" What is the <u>most appropriate</u> response by the nurse?
1. "A person with bulimia nervosa can maintain a normal weight."
2. "It's hard to face this type of problem in a person you love."
3. "At first, there is no weight loss; it comes later in the disease."
4. "This is a serious problem even though there is no weight loss."

Choose the most appropriate answer!

2. A 15-year-old female is brought to the clinic by her parents because of a significant amount of weight loss in the past 4 months. The nurse suspects the client may have anorexia nervosa. The nurse would assess the client for which of the following?
1. Hypertension
2. Amenorrhea
3. Hyperthermia
4. Diarrhea

3. Which statement made by the client about the binge-purge cycle that occurs with bulimia nervosa indicates understanding of the disorder?
1. "There are emotional triggers connected to bingeing."
2. "Over time, people usually grow out of bingeing behaviors."
3. "Bingeing isn't the problem; purging is the issue to address."
4. "When a person gets too hungry, there's a tendency to binge."

Help your client understand her behavior.

4. Which of the following would the nurse expect to find in the psychological history of a client who has an eating disorder? Select all that apply.
1. Flexibility
2. Ritualism
3. Feelings of helpfulness
4. Depression
5. Separation and individuation conflicts
6. Distorted body image

1. 1. A client with bulimia nervosa may be of normal weight, overweight, or underweight. Weight loss isn't a clinical criterion for bulimia nervosa. The second option doesn't address the need for information about the relationship between weight change and bulimia nervosa. The third option is incorrect because there may be little or no weight loss. The fourth option doesn't address the issue of weight change in a client with bulimia nervosa.
CN: Psychosocial integrity; CNS: None; CL: Application

2. 2. Anorexia nervosa is characterized by profound weight loss caused by severe restriction of food intake by the client. If severe enough, it causes amenorrhea in females, along with decreased—not increased—body temperature. It usually doesn't produce diarrhea, but it may produce constipation because decreased oral intake leads to decreased GI motility.
CN: Physiological integrity; CNS: Reduction of risk potential; CL: Application

3. 1. It's important for the client to understand the emotional triggers to bingeing, such as disappointment, depression, and anxiety. People don't outgrow eating behaviors. This leads a person to believe binge eating is a normal part of growth and development when it definitely isn't. The third option negates the seriousness of bingeing and leads the client to believe only vomiting is a problem, not overeating. Physiological hunger doesn't predispose a client to binge behaviors.
CN: Physiological integrity; CNS: Reduction of risk potential; CL: Application

4. 2, 4, 5, and 6. Flexibility and feelings of helpfulness are not in the psychological profile of a client with an eating disorder. Rigidity and feelings of helplessness are seen.
CN: Psychosocial integrity; CNS: None; CL: Application

CN: Client needs category   CNS: Client needs subcategory   CL: Cognitive level

5. A client with a diagnosis of bulimia nervosa is working on relationship issues. Which nursing intervention is the most important?
1. Have the client work on developing social skills.
2. Focus on how relationships cause bulimic behavior.
3. Help the client identify feelings about relationships.
4. Discuss how to prevent getting overinvolved in relationships.

6. A young female client with bulimia nervosa tells the nurse she wants to lessen her feelings of powerlessness. What is the <u>most important</u> short-term goal?
1. Learn problem-solving skills.
2. Decrease symptoms of anxiety.
3. Perform self-care activities daily.
4. Verbalize how to set limits with others.

Question 6 is asking you to prioritize.

7. Which of the following responses from a client should the nurse address first?
1. "My life is over if I gain weight."
2. "I feel dizzy and light-headed when I get up."
3. "My teeth hurt."
4. "I don't have the same hard grip with my hands as I used to."

8. The nurse is developing interventions to prevent a client with an eating disorder from developing refeeding syndrome. Which interventions are appropriate? Select all that apply.
1. Monitor the client three times a week in an outpatient clinic.
2. Monitor serum electrolytes.
3. Refeed the client over a period of 3 days.
4. Administer fluid replacement as prescribed.
5. Monitor the client's vital signs frequently.

9. The nurse is aware that which of the following is a <u>life-threatening</u> complication of bulimia nervosa?
1. Serum calcium 10.1 mg/dl
2. Heart rate 56 beats/minute
3. Serum potassium 2.9 mEq/L
4. Respiratory rate 16 breaths/minute

Read carefully! You need to select all.

5. 3. The client needs to address personal feelings, especially uncomfortable ones because they may trigger bingeing behavior. Social skills are important to a client's well-being, but they aren't typically a major problem for the client with bulimia nervosa. Relationships don't cause bulimic behaviors. It's the inability to handle stress or conflict that arises from interactions that causes the client to be distressed. The client isn't necessarily overinvolved in relationships; the issue may be the lack of satisfying relationships in the person's life.
CN: Psychosocial integrity; CNS: None; CL: Application

6. 1. If the client can learn effective problem-solving skills, she'll gain a sense of control and power over her life. Anxiety is commonly caused by feelings of powerlessness. Performing daily self-care activities won't reduce one's sense of powerlessness. Verbalizing how to set limits and protect self from the intrusive behavior of others is a necessary life skill, but problem-solving skills take priority.
CN: Psychosocial integrity; CNS: None; CL: Analysis

7. 2. The priority intervention by the nurse would be to address the cardiovascular status of the client by assessing the clients vital signs (B/p, pulse, and respiratory rate) to note any alterations. The first answer choice is an example of catastrophizing. Dental erosion and caries are commonly found in a client with an eating disorder; muscle weakness is also commonly found in a client with an eating disorder.
CN: Safe, effective care environment; CNS: Management of care; CL: Application

8. 2, 4, and 5. It is important to monitor the electrolytes, fluid replacement, and vitals. The client needs to be hospitalized during the refeeding phase of recovery from an eating disorder. The refeeding must be carried out over 7 days.
CN: Physiological integrity; CNS: Reduction of risk potential; CL: Analysis

9. 3. Electrolyte imbalance such as hypokalemia (normal serum potassium is 3.5 to 4.5 mEq/L) can be a life-threatening complication of bulimia nervosa due to purging behaviors. A serum calcium level of 10.1 mg/dl is within normal range. A heart rate of 56 beats/minute indicates bradycardia but isn't life threatening. A respiratory rate of 16 breaths/minute is within the normal range (16 to 20 breaths/minute) and not life threatening.
CN: Physiological integrity; CNS: Reduction of risk potential; CL: Application

10. A nurse is talking to a client with bulimia nervosa about the complications of laxative abuse. Which statement by the client indicates that the client understands the risks?
1. "I don't really have much taste for food, so there's no loss in getting it out of my system more quickly."
2. "Laxatives help me get rid of extra calories before they're added to my body. I know I just shouldn't eat the extra calories to begin with."
3. "Laxatives are over-the-counter medications that have no harmful effect."
4. "Using laxatives prevents my body from absorbing essential nutrients, such as protein, fat, and calcium."

11. The nurse is aware that which assessment finding distinguishes bulimia nervosa from binge-eating disorder?
1. Binge-eating disorder is not associated with the regular use of inappropriate compensatory behaviors (such as purging, fasting, and excessive exercise).
2. Binge eating occurs at least two times a week in bulimia nervosa but not in binge-eating disorder.
3. Bulimia nervosa clients eat food within a 2-hour time frame in amounts that surpass any amount most people would eat in a similar period of time.
4. A sense of lack of control over eating during the episode is found in a client with a binge-eating disorder.

12. A female client is talking to a nurse about her binge-purge cycle. What is the most appropriate question for the nurse to ask the client?
1. "Do you know how to stop the binge-purge cycle?"
2. "Does the binge-purge cycle help you lose weight?"
3. "Can the binge-purge cycle take away your anxiety?"
4. "How often do you go through the binge-purge cycle?"

13. A nurse is assessing a client with bulimia nervosa for possible substance abuse. What is the <u>most important</u> question for the nurse to ask the client?
1. "Have you ever used diet pills?"
2. "Where would you go to buy drugs?"
3. "At what age did you start drinking?"
4. "Do your peers ever offer you drugs?"

You're doing great! It looks like all your studying is paying off.

Consider all the answers. Then choose the most important one.

10. 4. A serious complication of laxative abuse is malabsorption of nutrients, such as proteins, fats, and calcium. Laxative abuse doesn't tend to affect the client's sense of taste. Clients with bulimia nervosa need to change their negative thinking with respect to calories and the use of laxatives.
CN: Physiological integrity; CNS: Reduction of risk potential; CL: Application

11. 1. In binge-eating disorder, there is no compensatory behavior associated with the binge eating; hence, the client is at risk of developing obesity. The other listed characteristics are found in both disorders.
CN: Psychosocial integrity; CNS: None; CL: Analysis

12. 4. This is an important question because there's often a range of frequencies, such as from a once-a-week pattern to multiple times per day. The frequency of binge-purge cycles may also alert the nurse to the degree of risk from fluid and electrolyte imbalances. Asking the client if she knows how to stop the binge-purge cycle isn't appropriate as it will generate feelings of self-blame and shame. It's common for clients to experience daily fluctuations in weight (some report variations of up to 10 lb). Although the binge-purge behavior may decrease anxiety initially, it tends to generate overall negative feelings about self.
CN: Psychosocial integrity; CNS: None; CL: Application

13. 1. Some clients with bulimia nervosa have a history of using or actively use amphetamines to control weight. The use of alcohol and street drugs is also common. The second and fourth questions could be answered by the client without revealing drug use. The age the client started drinking may not show current substance use.
CN: Psychosocial integrity; CNS: None; CL: Application

CN: Client needs category   CNS: Client needs subcategory   CL: Cognitive level

14. A female client with bulimia nervosa is discussing her abnormal eating behaviors with the nurse. Which statement by the client indicates an understanding of the disorder?
1. "When my loneliness gets to me, I start to binge."
2. "I know that when my life gets better, I'll eat right."
3. "I know I waste food and waste my money on food."
4. "After my parents' divorce, I'll talk about bingeing and purging."

15. Which of the following would a nurse most likely observe in an anorexic client? Select all that apply.
1. Preoccupation with food
2. Amenorrhea
3. Body weight within normal range
4. Lanugo
5. Bradycardia
6. Hypertension
7. Hyperthermia

16. A mother of a female client with bulimia nervosa asks a nurse if bulimia nervosa will stop her daughter from menstruating. What is the best response by the nurse?
1. "All women with anorexia nervosa or bulimia nervosa will have amenorrhea."
2. "When your daughter is bingeing and purging, she won't have normal periods."
3. "The eating disorder must be ongoing for your daughter's menstrual cycle to change."
4. "Women with bulimia nervosa may have a normal or abnormal menstrual cycle, depending on the severity of the problem."

17. Which nursing diagnosis should have the highest priority in the plan of care for a client with an eating disorder?
1. Interrupted family processes
2. Imbalanced nutrition: Less than body requirements
3. Disturbed body image
4. Ineffective coping

18. A female client with bulimia nervosa tells a nurse her major problem is eating too much food in a short period of time and then vomiting. Which short-term goal is the <u>most important</u>?
1. Help the client understand every person has a satiety level.
2. Encourage the client to verbalize fears and concerns about food.
3. Determine the amount of food the client will eat without purging.
4. Obtain a therapy appointment to look at the emotional causes of bulimia nervosa.

Remember to look closely for all that apply.

Help the client see the importance of reaching a short-term goal.

14. 1. Binge eating is a way to handle the uncomfortable feelings of frustration, loneliness, anger, and fear. The second option indicates the client is experiencing denial of the eating disorder. The third option addresses the client's guilt feelings; it doesn't reflect knowledge of her eating disorder. The fourth option shows the client isn't ready to discuss her eating disorder.

CN: Psychosocial integrity; CNS: None; CL: Analysis

15. 1, 2, 4, and 5. Body weight is below 85% of expected normal weight in anorexic clients. Hypotension and hypothermia are symptoms that the nurse could also expect to find in an anorexic client.

CN: Psychosocial integrity; CNS: None; CL: Application

16. 4. Women with bulimia nervosa may have a normal or abnormal menstrual cycle, depending on the severity of the eating disorder. Not all women with eating disorders have amenorrhea. The eating disorder can disrupt the menstrual cycle at any point in the illness.

CN: Health promotion and maintenance; CNS: None; CL: Analysis

17. 2. The most immediate priority is to meet the nutritional needs of the client to prevent complications. The other nursing diagnoses are all important long-term goals that can be addressed once the client's immediate physiological needs have been met.

CN: Safe, effective care environment; CNS: Management of care; CL: Analysis

18. 3. The client must meet her nutritional needs to prevent further complications, so she must identify the amount of food she can eat without purging as her first short-term goal. Binge eaters can't recognize their satiety level or their feelings of fullness. Obtaining knowledge or verbalizing her fears and feelings about food are not priority goals for this client. After meeting immediate physiological needs, therapy is an important part of dealing with this disorder.

CN: Physiological integrity; CNS: Reduction of risk potential; CL: Application

19. Which statement indicates to the nurse that a female client with bulimia nervosa is making progress in interrupting the binge-purge cycle?
1. "I called my friend the last two times I got upset."
2. "I know I'll have this problem with eating forever."
3. "I started asking my mother or sister to watch me eat each meal."
4. "I can have my boyfriend bring me home from parties if I want to purge."

20. A client with bulimia nervosa asks a nurse, "How can I ask for help from my family?" What is the most appropriate response by the nurse?
1. "When you ask for help, make sure you really need it."
2. "Have you ever asked for help before?"
3. "Ask family members to spend time with you at mealtime."
4. "Think about how you can handle this situation without help."

21. A female client with bulimia nervosa tells a nurse that she doesn't eat during the day, but after 5:00 p.m., she begins to binge and vomit. What is the most appropriate nursing intervention?
1. Help the client stop eating the foods on which she binges.
2. Discuss the effects of fasting on the client's pattern of eating.
3. Encourage the client to become involved in food preparation.
4. Teach the client to eat earlier in the day and decrease intake at night.

22. A female client with bulimia nervosa tells a nurse she was doing well until last week, when she had a fight with her father. Which nursing intervention is most appropriate?
1. Examine the relationship between feelings and eating.
2. Discuss the importance of therapy for the entire family.
3. Encourage the client to avoid certain family members.
4. Identify daily stressors and learn stress management skills.

23. Which statement from a bulimic client shows that she understands the concept of relapse?
1. "If I can't maintain control over things, I'll have problems."
2. "If I have problems, then that says I haven't learned much."
3. "If this illness becomes chronic, I won't be able to handle it."
4. "If I have problems, I can start over again and not feel hopeless."

Is most appropriate the same as "prioritize?"

If at first you don't succeed, try again—to choose the correct answer.

19. 1. A sign of progress is when the client begins to verbalize feelings and interact with people instead of going to food for comfort. The second option indicates the client needs more information on how to handle the disorder. Having another person watch the client eat isn't a helpful strategy as the client will depend on others to help control food intake. The last option indicates the client is in denial about the severity of the problem.
CN: Psychosocial integrity; CNS: None; CL: Analysis

20. 2. Determine whether the client has ever been successful in asking for help. Previous experiences affect the client's ability to ask for help now. The client needs to ask for help anytime without analyzing the level of need. Having other people around at mealtime isn't the only way to ask for help. Developing a support system is imperative for this client.
CN: Psychosocial integrity; CNS: None; CL: Analysis

21. 2. If a person fasts for most of the day, it's common to become extremely hungry, overeat by bingeing, and then feel the need to purge. Restricting food intake can actually trigger the binge-purge cycle. In treatment, the client is taught to identify foods that trigger eating, discuss the feelings associated with these foods, and work to eat them in normal amounts. Involvement in food preparation won't promote changes in the client's behaviors. The last option doesn't address how fasting can trigger the binge-purge cycle.
CN: Psychosocial integrity; CNS: None; CL: Application

22. 1. The client needs to understand her feelings and develop healthy coping skills to handle unpleasant situations. Family therapy may be indicated but shouldn't be an immediate intervention. Avoidance isn't a useful coping strategy; eventually, the underlying issues need to be explored. All clients can benefit from stress management skills, but for this client, care must focus on the relationship between feelings and eating behaviors.
CN: Psychosocial integrity; CNS: None; CL: Application

23. 4. This statement indicates that the client knows a relapse is just a slip, and positive gains made from treatment haven't been lost. Negative self-statements can lead to relapse. Control issues relate to powerlessness, which contributes to relapse.
CN: Psychosocial integrity; CNS: None; CL: Application

24. What is the treatment team's <u>priority</u> in planning the care of a client with an eating disorder?
1. Preventing the client from performing any muscle-building exercises
2. Keeping the client on bed rest until she attains a specified weight
3. Meeting daily to discuss manipulation and countertransference
4. Monitoring the client's weight and vital signs daily

25. A nurse is caring for a client with bulimia nervosa. It is most important for the nurse to assess the client for which of the following? Select all that apply.
1. Severe electrolyte imbalances
2. Damaged teeth due to the eroding effects of gastric acids on tooth enamel
3. Pneumonia from aspirated stomach contents
4. Cessation of menses
5. Esophageal tears and gastric rupture
6. Intestinal inflammation

26. A client with anorexia nervosa attended psychoeducational sessions on principles of adequate nutrition. Which statement by the client indicates the teaching was effective?
1. "I eat while I'm doing things to distract myself."
2. "I eat all my food at night right before I go to bed."
3. "I eat small amounts of food slowly at every meal."
4. "I eat only when I'm with my family and trying to be social."

27. A client with anorexia nervosa tells a nurse, "I'll never have the slender body I want." What is the <u>most appropriate</u> intervention by the nurse?
1. Call a family meeting to get help from the parents.
2. Help the client work on developing a realistic body image.
3. Make an appointment to see the dietitian on a weekly basis.
4. Develop an exercise program the client can do twice a week.

Remember to prioritize!

All options may be good, but choose the most appropriate one.

24. 3. Clients with eating disorders commonly use manipulative ploys and countertransference to resist weight gain (if they restrict food intake) or to maintain purging practices (if they're bulimic). Such clients commonly play staff members against one another. Muscle building is acceptable because it burns relatively few calories. Keeping the client on bed rest until a specified weight is reached may result in power struggles and prevent focusing on pertinent issues. Monitoring the client's weight and vital signs is important but not on a daily basis unless the client's condition warrants such scrutiny.
CN: Psychosocial integrity; CN: None; CL: Application

25. 1, 2, 4, and 5. Constant bingeing and purging behaviors can result in severe electrolyte imbalances, erosion of tooth enamel from constant exposure to gastric acids, menstrual irregularities, esophageal tears, and, in severe cases, gastric rupture. Aspiration pneumonia is unlikely because the vomiting is controlled. Intestinal inflammation isn't typically associated with bulimia nervosa.
CN: Physiological integrity; CNS: Physiological adaptation; CL: Application

26. 3. Slowly eating small amounts of food facilitates adequate digestion and prevents distention. Healthy eating is best accomplished when a person isn't doing other things while eating. Eating right before bedtime isn't a healthy eating habit. If a client eats only when the family is present or when trying to be social, eating is tied to social or emotional cues rather than nutritional needs.
CN: Health promotion and maintenance; CNS: None; CL: Application

27. 2. With anorexia nervosa, the client pursues thinness and has a distorted view of self. A family meeting may not help the client develop a more realistic view of the body. Although meeting with a dietitian might be helpful, it isn't a priority. Clients with anorexia nervosa typically exercise excessively.
CN: Psychosocial integrity; CNS: None; CL: Application

28. A client with anorexia nervosa tells a nurse, "My parents never hug me or say I've done anything right." What is the <u>most appropriate</u> nursing intervention?
1. Teach the family principles of assertive behavior.
2. Discuss the difficulties the family has in social situations.
3. Help the family convey a positive attitude toward the client.
4. Explore the family's ability to express affection appropriately.

29. A client with anorexia nervosa is having problems with peer relationships. The nurse determines that which of the following is the best communication strategy?
1. Use concrete language and maintain a focus on reality.
2. Direct the client to talk about what is causing the anxiety.
3. Teach the client to communicate feelings and express self appropriately.
4. Confront the client about being depressed and self-absorbed.

30. A nurse plans to include the parents of a client with anorexia nervosa in therapy sessions along with the client. What fact should the nurse remember about parents of clients with anorexia?
1. They tend to overprotect their children.
2. They usually have a history of substance abuse.
3. They maintain emotional distance from their children.
4. They alternate between loving and rejecting their children.

31. The nurse has instructed a client with an eating disorder about Prozac (fluoxetine). The nurse determines that teaching has been effective when the client makes which statement?
1. "I can eat anything and anytime I want. This medication will control my eating."
2. "I can drive my car as soon as I get home"
3. "I should call my provider if I have cravings for large amounts of food."
4. "It may take 1 to 3 weeks for this medication to be effective for me."

Keep going! You've got all my support!

28. 4. There's often a lack of affection and warmth in families who have a member with an eating disorder. Although assertiveness is an important skill, the family member needs to realize assertiveness isn't always rewarded. Difficulties in social situations are important to address, but the intervention must focus on how to express positive feelings and affection. A positive attitude helps a person become better able to handle the pressures of life, but it may not change the family's display of affection.
CN: Psychosocial integrity; CNS: None; CL: Application

29. 3. Clients with anorexia nervosa often communicate on a superficial level and avoid expressing feelings. Identifying feelings and learning to express them are initial steps in decreasing isolation. Clients with anorexia nervosa are usually able to discuss abstract and concrete issues. Discussions shouldn't be limited to the client's feelings of anxiety as the client may not be aware of the cause of the anxiety, which may result in misdirected self-reflection. Confrontation usually isn't an effective communication strategy as it may cause the client to withdraw and become more depressed.
CN: Psychosocial integrity; CNS: None; CL: Application

30. 1. Clients with anorexia nervosa typically come from a family with parents who are controlling and overprotective. These clients use eating to gain control of an aspect of their lives. Having a history of substance abuse, maintaining an emotional distance, and alternating between love and rejection aren't typical characteristics of parents of children with anorexia nervosa.
CN: Psychological integrity; CNS: None; CL: Application

31. 4. Prozac does not control eating. Operating hazardous equipment and/or driving should be done after individual effects are determined. Providers are to be notified if sexual dysfunction occurs or is intolerable.
CN: Safe, effective care environment; CNS: Management of care; CL: Application

32. A nurse is working with a female client with anorexia nervosa who has acrocyanosis in her extremities. Which short-term goal is most important for the client?
1. Do daily range-of-motion exercises.
2. Eat some fatty foods daily.
3. Check neurological reflexes.
4. Promote adequate circulation.

33. A female client with anorexia nervosa is discharged from the hospital after gaining 12 lb. Which statement by the client best indicates that the nurse's discharge teachings have been effective?
1. "I plan to eat two small meals a day."
2. "I feel that this is scary, but I'm not going to write about it in my journal."
3. "I have to diet because I've gained 12 lb."
4. "I'll need to attend therapy for support to stay healthy."

34. Prozac (fluoxetine) is a selective serotonin reuptake inhibitor (SSRI) commonly prescribed for clients with eating disorders. Which of the following manifestations of serotonin syndrome would the nurse expect to see as soon as 2 hours after the start of treatment? Select all that apply.
1. Sleepiness
2. Hallucinations
3. Fever
4. Anxiety
5. Hypertension
6. Tremors
7. Diaphoresis

35. Monoamine oxidase inhibitors (MAOIs) have been prescribed for a client with bulimia nervosa. What is the most important information for the nurse to give the client?
1. "Drink several glasses of water with each dose."
2. "Do not eat foods that contain tyramine, such as cheese, cottage cheese, pickled herring, and salami."
3. "Watch for bleeding and bruising."
4. "Call your provider if you have tremors or feel anxious or agitated."

Fatty foods are almost never the right answer!

Clients with anorexia nervosa have an intense fear of gaining weight.

32. 4. Circulation changes will cause extremities to be cold, numb, and have dry and flaky skin. Exercise may help prevent contractures and muscle atrophy, but it may have only a limited secondary effect on promoting circulation. Intake of fatty foods won't have an impact on the client's skin problems. Checking neurological reflexes won't necessarily assist with handling skin problems.
CN: Physiological integrity; CNS: Reduction of risk potential; CL: Application

33. 4. The client is planning to attend therapy after discharge, which shows an understanding of the need for continued counseling. Eating only two small meals a day is an unrealistic plan for meeting nutritional needs. Feeling insecure when leaving a controlled environment is a common response to discharge. Gaining 12 lb indicates that the client's nutritional needs are being met at the present caloric intake.
CN: Psychosocial integrity; CNS: None; CL: Analysis

34. 2, 3, 4, 6, and 7. Other symptoms of serotonin syndrome include mental confusion, difficulty concentrating, agitation, hyperreflexia, and incoordination.
CN: Safe, effective care environment; CNS: Management of care; CL: Application

35. 2. The ingestion of tyramine results in a hypertensive crisis. Answer choices 1, 3, and 4 do not create or affect a hypertensive crisis.
CN: Safe, effective care environment; CNS: Management of care; CL: Analysis

36. A nurse is analyzing the need for health teaching in a female client with anorexia nervosa who lives in a chaotic family situation. What is the <u>most</u> important question for the nurse to ask the client?
1. "For how many months have your periods been irregular?"
2. "How often do you think about food in a 24-hour period?"
3. "What were the circumstances before your eating disorder?"
4. "How much and what kinds of exercise do you engage in every day?"

37. An adolescent female client with anorexia nervosa tells a nurse about her outstanding academic achievements and her thoughts about suicide. Which factor must the nurse consider when making a care plan for this client?
1. Self-esteem
2. Physical illnesses
3. Paranoid delusions
4. Relationship avoidance

38. A nurse is developing a care plan for a family with a member who has anorexia nervosa. What is the most important information for the nurse to include?
1. Coping mechanisms used in the past
2. Concerns about changes in lifestyle and daily activities
3. Rejection of feedback from family and significant others
4. Appropriate eating habits and social behaviors centering on eating

39. Which goal is best to help a client with anorexia nervosa recognize self-distortions?
1. Identify the client's misperceptions of self.
2. Acknowledge immature and childlike behaviors.
3. Determine the consequences of a faulty support system.
4. Recognize the age-appropriate tasks to be accomplished.

40. Parents of a client with anorexia nervosa ask the nurse for information about the risk factors for this disorder. The nurse determines understanding of the information when the parents make which statement?
1. "Risk factors include the inability to be still and emotional lability."
2. "Risk factors include a high level of anxiety and disorganized behavior."
3. "Risk factors include low self-esteem and problems with family relationships."
4. "Risk factors include a lack of life experience and no opportunities to learn skills."

Care plans encourage staff to work toward the same goals.

I don't doubt that you'll choose the correct answer.

36. 3. This question lets the nurse get information about the family and background situations that influenced the client's needs and distorted eating. The other options deal with menstrual history, exercise patterns, and food obsessions. Although they're relevant, they don't provide information related to the family situation.
CN: Psychosocial integrity; CNS: None; CL: Analysis

37. 1. The client lacks self-esteem, which contributes to her level of depression and feelings of personal ineffectiveness, which in turn may lead to suicidal thoughts. Physical illnesses are common with clients with anorexia nervosa, but they don't relate to this situation. Paranoid delusions refer to false ideas that others want to harm you. No evidence exists that this client is socially isolated.
CN: Psychosocial integrity; CNS: None; CL: Analysis

38. 1. Examination of positive and negative coping mechanisms used by the family allows the nurse to build a care plan specific to the family's strengths and weaknesses. The way the family copes with concerns is more important than the concerns themselves. Feedback from the family and significant others is vital when building a care plan. Eating habits and behaviors are symptoms of the way people cope with problems.
CN: Psychosocial integrity; CNS: None; CL: Application

39. 1. Questioning the client's misperceptions and distortions will create doubt about how the client views himself. Acknowledging immature behaviors or determining the consequences of a faulty support system won't promote client recognition of self-distortions. Recognizing the age-appropriate tasks to be accomplished by the client won't help the client recognize distortions.
CN: Psychosocial integrity; CNS: None; CL: Analysis

40. 3. There are several risk factors for eating disorders, including low self-esteem, history of depression, substance abuse, and dysfunctional family relationships. Restlessness and emotional lability are symptoms of manic depressive illness. Anxiety and disorganized behavior could be signs of a psychotic disorder. A lack of life experiences and an absence of opportunities to learn life skills may be a result of anorexia nervosa.
CN: Psychosocial integrity; CNS: None; CL: Analysis

CN: Client needs category   CNS: Client needs subcategory   CL: Cognitive level

41. A client with anorexia nervosa has started taking fluoxetine hydrochloride (Prozac). The nurse should closely monitor the client for which of the following?
1. Drowsiness
2. Dry mouth
3. Light-headedness
4. Nausea

42. A client who has been hospitalized during the past week for an eating disorder is quite concerned about being discharged today. Which response(s) by the nurse is (are) most appropriate? Select all that apply.
1. "I have set up a structured and inflexible eating schedule for you that you need to adhere to when you get home."
2. "You need to have someone closely monitor you when you eat and right after you eat."
3. "I have set up follow-up treatment for you at the nearby outpatient clinic."
4. "I encourage you to participate in the eating disorder support group."
5. "Let's create a maintenance plan for you."

43. A female client with anorexia nervosa tells a nurse that she has developed hair on most of her body. Which of the following disorders would the nurse most likely expect to be associated with the client's anorexia nervosa?
1. Anemia
2. Osteoporosis
3. Dehydration
4. Electrolyte imbalance

44. A female client with anorexia nervosa is talking to a nurse about her group therapy. Which statement shows the group experience has <u>helped</u> the client?
1. "I feel I'm different and I don't need a lot of friends."
2. "I'll tell my parents it's not just me who has problems."
3. "I can see how to do things better and become the best."
4. "I think I have some unrealistic expectations of myself."

Knowing adverse reactions to key drugs is important.

You're heading down the home stretch! Keep going!

My plan to study all night is starting to seem unrealistic.

41. 4. Nausea is an adverse reaction to the drug that compounds the eating disorder problem, and the client must be closely monitored. Although the adverse reactions of drowsiness, dry mouth, or light-headedness may occur, they aren't likely to interfere with treatment.
CN: Physiological integrity; CNS: Pharmacological and parenteral therapies; CL: Application

42. 3, 4, and 5. Selections 1 and 2 are done when the client is still hospitalized.
CN: Psychosocial integrity; CNS: None; CL: Application

43. 3. When a client with anorexia nervosa has fine hair all over her body (lanugo), the nurse would perform a more extensive assessment of the skin. Lanugo indicates dehydration due to starvation. Anemia is associated with hematological complications. Osteoporosis is associated with the musculoskeletal system. Electrolyte imbalance is associated with body metabolism.
CN: Health promotion and maintenance; CNS: None; CL: Application

44. 4. A goal of group therapy is to provide methods to assess whether personal expectations are unrealistic. Other goals are to learn to handle problems, not to blame parents or others, decrease perfectionist tendencies, and decrease isolation and learn to have healthy peer relationships.
CN: Psychosocial integrity; CNS: None; CL: Application

45. A nurse is caring for a client who has anorexia nervosa. They are working on the goal of developing social relationships. The nurse determines the client is meeting the goal when the client does which of the following?
1. The client talks about the value of peer relationships.
2. The client decides to talk to her parents about her friends.
3. The client expresses the need to establish trust relationships.
4. The client attends an activity without prompting from others.

46. What is the initial action a nurse should take when a young female client with anorexia nervosa says, "I'll try to eat something"?
1. Provide a small portion of a healthy food.
2. Weigh the client before and after eating.
3. Ask the client what she thinks she can eat.
4. Suggest the client drink something before eating.

47. A client with anorexia nervosa tells a nurse, "I feel so awful and inadequate." What is the best response by the nurse?
1. "You're being too hard on yourself."
2. "Someday, you'll feel better about things."
3. "Tell me something you like about yourself."
4. "Maybe relaxing by yourself will help you feel better."

48. What is the <u>priority</u> nursing assessment of a client with an eating disorder?
1. Cultural and gender needs
2. Substance abuse history
3. Academic achievement and performance
4. Level of danger to self or others

49. An adolescent female client with anorexia nervosa starts outpatient treatment. Which client statement indicates an understanding of the eating disorder?
1. "I'm not worried because no one ever dies from anorexia."
2. "I still feel fat even though I'm told that I'm not."
3. "My old school friends aren't important to me anymore."
4. "I don't feel right unless I do an intense workout every day."

The client must agree to the goal or it won't work.

The term priority indicates that you should select the answer which would be of first concern during assessment.

45. 4. When a client with anorexia nervosa attends an activity without prompting from others, it's a positive sign the client is working toward developing social relationships. Talking about the value of relationships is also beneficial but is only the first step in establishing them. Talking to parents about friends is a start but doesn't necessarily indicate that the client can establish relationships. Expressing the need to establish trust relationships is a first step, but an indication of success would be actually initiating such a relationship.
CN: Psychosocial integrity; CNS: None; CL: Application

46. 1. Small amounts of food won't overwhelm the client when given at frequent intervals. They also won't overtax the GI and cardiac systems. Weighing the client before and after meals is a useless, stress-provoking action. Asking the client questions may provoke anxiety. It's better to give the client food when she asks. Drinking something before eating isn't necessary; the fluid may prevent the client from being able to eat a sufficient amount of the food.
CN: Physiological integrity; CNS: Reduction of risk potential; CL: Application

47. 3. This statement redirects the client to talk about positive aspects of self. The other options minimize her feelings or don't address the client's concerns or encourage the client to change her self-image.
CN: Psychosocial integrity; CNS: None; CL: Application

48. 4. The priority in assessment should be to determine if the client is a danger to herself or to others. Cultural and gender needs, substance abuse history, and academic performance are an important part of assessment but not the priority.
CN: Safe, effective care environment; CNS: Management of care; CL: Analysis

49. 2. A client with anorexia nervosa shows a basic understanding of the disorder if she can talk about feeling fat even though she's actually underweight, or if she expresses an intense fear of gaining weight. Anorexia nervosa has a mortality of approximately 10% to 15%. People with eating disorders tend to isolate themselves from friends and family members because of their intense focus on food, weight, and exercise. A client with anorexia nervosa may exercise compulsively to prevent weight gain; this behavior indicates continuing presence of the eating disorder.
CN: Psychosocial integrity; CNS: None; CL: Analysis

CN: Client needs category   CNS: Client needs subcategory   CL: Cognitive level

50. What is the <u>most</u> important question for the nurse to ask when assessing the self-esteem of a client with anorexia nervosa?
1. "How would you describe yourself to others?"
2. "What activities do you enjoy doing with your friends?"
3. "Do you play any sports at school or in your community?"
4. "How do you decide how to spend your free time?"

51. Which psychosocial finding should a nurse expect when assessing a client with anorexia nervosa?
1. Avoidant behavior
2. Antisocial behavior
3. Introverted behavior
4. Hypervigilant behavior

52. A nurse notes severe hypocalcemia in a client with anorexia nervosa. Which history finding supports a diagnosis of osteoporosis?
1. Eating a vegetarian diet
2. Drinking well water
3. Going scuba diving
4. Smoking cigarettes

53. A female client with anorexia nervosa is receiving care from her family after successfully completing the refeeding stage of treatment. Which nursing intervention takes <u>priority</u> at this time?
1. Providing a strong support system and opportunities to do reality testing
2. Teaching the family stress-reduction skills to help promote family harmony
3. Promoting anticipatory grieving over the loss each family member is experiencing
4. Assisting the family to work on the issues of autonomy and separation

Do others see me as I see myself?

50. 1. Clients with anorexia nervosa tend to have low self-esteem even if they're high achievers in school, activities, and sports; asking for a self-description can uncover the client's distorted body image and low self-esteem. Questions about activities with friends, involvement in sports, or how the client decides to spend her free time don't necessarily elicit information about self-esteem.
CN: Psychosocial integrity; CNS: None; CL: Analysis

51. 3. Clients with anorexia nervosa typically demonstrate introverted behavior. Clients with bulimia, not anorexia nervosa, tend to show avoidant and dependent behaviors. Clients with eating disorders don't necessarily demonstrate antisocial behavior. Hypervigilant behavior is common in clients with posttraumatic stress disorder, not eating disorders.
CN: Psychosocial integrity; CNS: None; CL: Analysis

52. 4. Hypocalcemia and cigarette smoking increase the risk for osteoporosis. Eating a vegetarian diet, drinking well water, and going scuba diving don't predispose the client to osteoporosis.
CN: Physiological integrity; CNS: Reduction of risk potential; CL: Analysis

53. 4. When a client with anorexia nervosa successfully completes the refeeding stage of treatment, the family must work on separation and individuation of the client and on decreasing family rigidity and overprotectiveness. Although the client needs a strong support system, developing a sense of self is more important at this time; also, reality testing isn't a typical problem in clients with eating disorders. All families can benefit from learning stress-reduction skills; however, at this time, these skills take lower priority than developing client independence. Anticipatory grieving isn't particularly relevant for family members of a client with an eating disorder.
CN: Psychosocial integrity; CNS: None; CL: Application

54. A client with bulimia nervosa has a history of severe GI problems caused by excessive purging. The nurse is aware that the client is at risk for which of the following?
1. Renal calculi
2. Esophageal tears
3. Focal seizures
4. Muscle atrophy

55. A nurse is caring for an anorexic client with a nursing diagnosis of imbalanced nutrition: less than body requirements related to dysfunctional eating patterns. Which interventions would be appropriate for this client? Select all that apply.
1. Provide small, frequent meals.
2. Monitor weight gain.
3. Allow the client to skip meals until the antidepressant levels are therapeutic.
4. Encourage the client to keep a journal.
5. Encourage the client to eat three substantial meals per day.

Good for you! It looks like you really measure up!

54. 2. A bulimic client with severe GI problems from excessive purging is at increased risk for esophageal tears and irritation or esophagitis. Although clients with eating disorders may develop renal calculi, this client is at greater risk for developing esophageal tears. Focal seizures and muscle atrophy aren't related to severe GI problems.
CN: Physiological integrity; CNS: Reduction of risk potential; CL: Analysis

55. 1, 2, and 4. Due to self-starvation, clients with anorexia can rarely tolerate large meals three times per day. Small, frequent meals may be tolerated better by the anorexic client, and they provide a way to gradually increase daily caloric intake. The nurse should monitor the client's weight carefully because a client with anorexia may try to hide weight loss. The client may be emotionally restrained and afraid to express her feelings; therefore, keeping a journal can serve as an outlet for these feelings, which can assist recovery. An anorexic client is already underweight and shouldn't be permitted to skip meals.
CN: Health promotion and maintenance; CNS: None; CL: Analysis

Part IV

Maternal-neonatal care

Chapter 22
Antepartum care

Looking for information about antepartum care before tackling this chapter? Visit **www.obgyn.net**, an independent Web site dedicated to obstetric and gynecologic health problems.

1. During an examination, a client who's 32 weeks pregnant becomes dizzy, light-headed, and pale. While the client is lying supine, which nursing intervention should take <u>priority</u>?
1. Listen to fetal heart tones.
2. Take the client's blood pressure.
3. Ask the client to breathe deeply.
4. Turn the client on her left side.

2. A nurse is assessing a client at 33 weeks' gestation. Leopold's maneuvers indicate that the fetus is in a breech position. What is the best location for the nurse to auscultate fetal heart tones?
1. Midway between the symphysis pubis and the umbilicus
2. Right lower quadrant of the abdomen
3. Right upper quadrant of the abdomen
4. Above the level of the umbilicus

3. In twin-to-twin transfusion syndrome, the arterial circulation of one twin is in communication with the venous circulation of the other twin. One fetus is considered the "donor" twin, and one becomes the "recipient" twin. Assessment of the recipient twin would most likely show which condition?
1. Anemia
2. Oligohydramnios
3. Polycythemia
4. Small fetus

Which intervention is of primary importance?

Careful. Question 3 asks about the recipient twin, not the donor.

1. 4. As the enlarging uterus increases pressure on the inferior vena cava, it compromises venous return, which can cause dizziness, light-headedness, and pallor when the client is supine. The nurse can relieve these symptoms by turning the client on her left side, which relieves pressure on the vena cava and restores venous return. Although they're valuable assessments, fetal heart tone and maternal blood pressure measurements don't correct the problem. Because deep breathing has no effect on venous return, it can't relieve the client's symptoms.
CN: Safe, effective care environment; CNS: Management of care; CL: Analysis

2. 4. When the fetus is in the breech position, fetal heart tones are best heard at or above the level of the umbilicus.
CN: Health promotion and maintenance; CNS: None; CL: Application

3. 3. The recipient twin in twin-to-twin transfusion syndrome is transfused by the other twin. The recipient twin then becomes polycythemic and often has heart failure due to circulatory overload. The donor twin becomes anemic. The recipient twin has polyhydramnios, not oligohydramnios. The recipient twin is usually large, whereas the donor twin is often small.
CN: Physiological integrity; CNS: Physiological adaptation; CL: Analysis

4. A pregnant client who reports painless vaginal bleeding at 28 weeks' gestation is diagnosed with placenta previa. The placental edge reaches the internal os. The nurse would suspect the client has which type of placenta previa?
1. Low-lying placenta previa
2. Marginal placenta previa
3. Partial placenta previa
4. Total placenta previa

5. Expectant management of the client with a placenta implanted in the lower uterine segment includes which procedure or treatment?
1. Stat culture and sensitivity
2. Antenatal steroids after 34 weeks' gestation
3. Ultrasound examination every 2 to 3 weeks
4. Scheduled delivery of the fetus before fetal maturity in a hemodynamically stable mother

The NCLEX is not exactly what I expected.

6. A client with painless vaginal bleeding at 28 weeks' gestation has just been diagnosed as having placenta previa. Which statement by the client indicates that she understands the nurse's teaching?
1. "I am still able to have sexual intercourse with my husband."
2. "I can continue to go to exercise class three times a week."
3. "I will still be able to fly to Florida for the holidays."
4. "I need to limit my activity and rest."

I feel like I'm attached at the hip to these books.

7. The nurse is teaching a client with placenta previa who has developed placenta accreta. Which statement concerning this condition would be the most correct?
1. The placenta invades the myometrium.
2. The placenta covers the cervical os.
3. The placenta penetrates the myometrium.
4. The placenta attaches to the myometrium.

4. 2. A marginal placenta previa is characterized by implantation of the placenta in the margin of the cervical os, not covering the os. A low-lying placenta is implanted in the lower uterine segment but doesn't reach the cervical os. A partial placenta previa is the partial occlusion of the cervical os by the placenta. The internal cervical os is completely covered by the placenta in a total placenta previa.
CN: Physiological integrity; CNS: Physiological adaptation; CL: Analysis

5. 3. Placenta previa occurs when the placenta is implanted in the lower uterine segment. Fetal surveillance through ultrasound examination every 2 to 3 weeks is indicated to evaluate fetal growth, amniotic fluid, and placental location in clients with placenta previa being expectantly managed. A stat culture and sensitivity would be done for severe bleeding or maternal or fetal distress and isn't part of expectant management. Antenatal steroids may be given to clients between 24 and 34 weeks' gestation to enhance fetal lung maturity. In a hemodynamically stable mother, delivery of the fetus should be delayed until fetal lung maturity is attained.
CN: Physiological integrity; CNS: Reduction of risk potential; CL: Analysis

6. 4. The client with placenta previa needs to restrict her activities and may be placed on bed rest. She should avoid sexual intercourse, strenuous activity, and long-distance travel.
CN: Physiological integrity; CNS: Reduction of risk potential; CL: Analysis

7. 4. Placenta accreta is the abnormal attachment of the placenta to the myometrium of the uterus. When the placenta invades the myometrium, it's called placenta increta. When the placenta covers the cervical os, it's called placenta previa. Placenta percreta occurs when the villi of the placenta penetrate the myometrium to the serosa level.
CN: Physiological integrity; CNS: Physiological adaptation; CL: Application

8. The nurse is caring for a client suspected of having a hydatidiform mole. Which signs and symptoms would confirm this diagnosis?
1. Heavy, bright red bleeding every 21 days
2. Fetal cardiac motion after 6 weeks' gestation
3. Benign tumors found in the smooth muscle of the uterus
4. "Snowstorm" pattern on ultrasound with no fetus or gestational sac

Sometimes, it's hard to keep your symptoms straight, isn't it?

9. A 21-year-old client who has just been diagnosed with having a hydatidiform mole asks the nurse about risk factors. What is the best response by the nurse?
1. Age in 20s or 30s
2. High socioeconomic status
3. Primigravida
4. Prior molar gestation

10. A 21-year-old female client arrives at the emergency department with complaints of cramping, abdominal pain, and mild vaginal bleeding. Pelvic examination shows a left adnexal mass that is tender when palpated. Culdocentesis shows blood in the cul-de-sac. The nurse suspects this client may have which condition?
1. Abruptio placentae
2. Ectopic pregnancy
3. Hydatidiform mole
4. Pelvic inflammatory disease (PID)

Now you're getting up to speed. Way to go!

11. The nurse assesses a client at 34 weeks' gestation who arrives at the emergency department with severe abdominal pain, uterine tenderness, and an increased uterine tone. The client denies vaginal bleeding. The external fetal monitor shows fetal distress with severe, variable decelerations. The client most likely has which condition?
1. Abruptio placentae
2. Ectopic pregnancy
3. Molar pregnancy
4. Placenta previa

8. 4. Ultrasound is the technique of choice in diagnosing a hydatidiform mole. The chorionic villi of a molar pregnancy resemble a "snowstorm" pattern on ultrasound. Bleeding with a hydatidiform mole is often dark brown and may occur erratically for weeks or months. There's no cardiac activity because there's no fetus. Benign tumors found in the smooth muscle of the uterus are leiomyomas or fibroids.
CN: Physiological integrity; CNS: Reduction of risk potential; CL: Analysis

9. 4. A previous molar gestation increases a woman's risk for developing a subsequent molar gestation by four to five times. Adolescents and women age 40 years and older are at increased risk for molar pregnancies. Multigravidas, especially women with a prior pregnancy loss, and women with lower socioeconomic status are at an increased risk for this problem.
CN: Health promotion and maintenance; CNS: None; CL: Analysis

10. 2. Most ectopic pregnancies don't appear as obvious life-threatening medical emergencies. Ectopic pregnancies must be considered in any sexually active woman of childbearing age who complains of menstrual irregularity, cramping abdominal pain, and mild vaginal bleeding. The client with an ectopic pregnancy who is experiencing blood loss will have blood in the cul-de-sac. PID, abruptio placentae, and hydatidiform moles won't show blood in the cul-de-sac.
CN: Physiological integrity; CNS: Reduction of risk potential; CL: Analysis

11. 1. A client with severe abruptio placentae will often have severe abdominal pain. The uterus will have increased tone with little to no return to resting tone between contractions. The fetus will start to show signs of distress, with decelerations in the heart rate or even fetal death with a large placental separation. An ectopic pregnancy, which usually occurs in the fallopian tubes, would rupture well before 34 weeks. A molar pregnancy generally would be detected before 34 weeks' gestation, and no fetal heart sounds would be present. Placenta previa usually involves painless vaginal bleeding without uterine contractions.
CN: Physiological integrity; CNS: Reduction of risk potential; CL: Analysis

12. During a routine visit to the clinic, a client tells the nurse that she thinks she may be pregnant. The physician orders a pregnancy test. The nurse is aware that pregnancy would <u>most</u> accurately be confirmed by which of the following?
1. Increase in human chorionic gonadotropin (HCG)
2. Decrease in HCG
3. Increase in luteinizing hormone (LH)
4. Decrease in LH

13. A nurse is assessing a pregnant client. Which symptom should the nurse expect to observe?
1. Increased tidal volume
2. Increased expiratory volume
3. Decreased inspiratory capacity
4. Decreased oxygen consumption

14. A client is scheduled for amniocentesis. What is the most important intervention for the nurse to implement?
1. Tell the client to drink 1 L of water.
2. Have the client void.
3. Instruct the client to fast for 12 hours.
4. Place the client on her left side.

15. A nurse is taking an initial history on a pregnant client, who asks about the chances of having dizygotic twins. Which statement by the nurse is correct?
1. "They occur most frequently in Asian women."
2. "There's a decreased risk with increased parity."
3. "There's an increased risk with increased maternal age."
4. "There's no increased risk with the use of fertility drugs."

So many hormones to learn; so little time!

Which statement is true about dizygotic twins?

12. 1. HCG increases in a woman's blood and urine to fairly large concentrations until the 15th week of pregnancy. The other hormone values aren't indicative of pregnancy.

CN: Health promotion and maintenance; CNS: None; CL: Application

13. 1. A pregnant client breathes deeper, which increases the tidal volume of gas moved in and out of the respiratory tract with each breath. The expiratory volume and residual volume decrease as the pregnancy progresses. The inspiratory capacity increases during pregnancy. The increased oxygen consumption in the pregnant client is 15% to 20% greater than in the nonpregnant state.

CN: Health promotion and maintenance; CNS: None; CL: Application

14. 2. Before amniocentesis, the client should void to empty the bladder, reducing the risk of bladder perforation. The client doesn't need to drink fluids before amniocentesis nor does she need to fast. The client should be placed in a supine position for the procedure.

CN: Health promotion and maintenance; CNS: None; CL: Application

15. 3. Dizygotic twinning is influenced by race (most frequent in Black women and least frequent in Asian women), age (increased risk with increased maternal age), parity (increased risk with increased parity), and fertility drugs (increased risk with the use of fertility drugs, especially ovulation-inducing drugs). The incidence of monozygotic twins isn't affected by race, age, parity, heredity, or fertility medications.

CN: Health promotion and maintenance; CNS: None; CL: Application

16. A client in her fifth month of pregnancy is having a routine clinic visit. The nurse should assess the client for which common <u>second</u> trimester condition?
1. Mastitis
2. Metabolic alkalosis
3. Physiological anemia
4. Respiratory acidosis

A pregnant client's needs may vary in each trimester.

16. 3. Hemoglobin and hematocrit values decrease during pregnancy as the increase in plasma volume exceeds the increase in red blood cell production. Mastitis is an infection in the breast characterized by a swollen tender breast and flulike symptoms. This condition is most frequently seen in breastfeeding clients. Alterations in acid–base balance during pregnancy result in a state of respiratory alkalosis, compensated by mild metabolic acidosis.

CN: Health promotion and maintenance; CNS: None; CL: Application

17. A 21-year-old client at 6 weeks' gestation is diagnosed with hyperemesis gravidarum. The nurse is aware that the client is at risk for which condition?
1. Bowel perforation
2. Electrolyte imbalance
3. Miscarriage
4. Gestational hypertension

17. 2. Excessive vomiting in clients with hyperemesis gravidarum often causes weight loss and fluid, electrolyte, and acid–base imbalances. Clients with severe hyperemesis may have a low-birth-weight infant, but the disorder generally isn't life threatening to the fetus. Gestational hypertension and bowel perforation aren't related to hyperemesis. The effects of hyperemesis on the fetus depend on the severity of the disorder.

CN: Physiological integrity; CNS: Reduction of risk potential; CL: Analysis

18. A 29-year-old client has gestational diabetes. The nurse is teaching her about managing her glucose levels. Which therapy would be most appropriate for this client?
1. Diet
2. Long-acting insulin
3. Oral hypoglycemic drugs
4. Glucagon

Clients with gestational diabetes need nutritional counseling.

18. 1. Clients with gestational diabetes are usually managed by diet alone to control their glucose intolerance. Long-acting insulin usually isn't needed for blood glucose control in the client with gestational diabetes. Oral hypoglycemic drugs are contraindicated in pregnancy. Glucagon raises blood glucose and is used to treat hypoglycemic reactions.

CN: Health promotion and maintenance; CNS: None; CL: Application

19. A client who is pregnant and has developed preeclampsia asks the nurse why magnesium sulphate has been prescribed for her. What is the best response by the nurse?
1. "It prevents hemorrhage."
2. "It prevents hypertension."
3. "It prevents hypomagnesemia."
4. "It prevents seizures."

19. 4. The anticonvulsant mechanism of magnesium is believed to depress seizure foci in the brain and peripheral neuromuscular blockade. Magnesium doesn't help prevent hemorrhage in preeclamptic clients. Antihypertensive drugs other than magnesium are preferred for sustained hypertension. Hypomagnesemia isn't a complication of preeclampsia.

CN: Physiological integrity; CNS: Pharmacological and parenteral therapies; CL: Analysis

20. While assessing a client in her 24th week of pregnancy, the nurse learns that the client has been experiencing signs and symptoms of pregnancy-induced hypertension, or preeclampsia. Which sign or symptom helps differentiate preeclampsia from eclampsia?
1. Seizures
2. Headaches
3. Blurred vision
4. Weight gain

21. A pregnant client has a negative contraction stress test (CST). How does the nurse interpret this result?
1. Persistent late decelerations in fetal heartbeat occurred, with at least three contractions in a 10-minute window.
2. Accelerations of fetal heartbeat occurred, with at least 15 beats/minute, lasting 15 to 30 seconds in a 20-minute period.
3. Accelerations of fetal heartbeat were absent or didn't increase by 15 beats/minute for 15 to 30 seconds in a 20-minute period.
4. There was good fetal heart rate (FHR) variability and no decelerations from contraction in a 10-minute period in which there were three contractions.

22. A pregnant client with sickle cell anemia is at an increased risk for having a sickle cell crisis during pregnancy. The nurse anticipates that aggressive management of a sickle cell crisis would include which treatment?
1. Antihypertensive agents
2. Diuretic agents
3. I.V. fluids
4. Acetaminophen (Tylenol) for pain

23. A nurse is performing a cardiac assessment on a pregnant client and determines normal findings to include which of the following?
1. Cardiac tamponade
2. Heart failure
3. Endocarditis
4. Systolic murmur

I didn't mean to cause a crisis.

I think I hear the answer to question 23.

20. 1. The primary difference between pre-eclampsia and eclampsia is the occurrence of seizures, which occur when the client becomes eclamptic. Headaches, blurred vision, weight gain, increased blood pressure, and edema of the hands and feet are all indicative of preeclampsia.

CN: Physiological integrity; CNS: Physiological adaptation; CL: Application

21. 4. A CST measures the fetal response to uterine contractions. A client must have three contractions in a 10-minute period. A negative CST shows good FHR variability with no decelerations from uterine contractions. Persistent late decelerations with contractions indicate a positive CST. Reactive nonstress tests (NSTs) have accelerations in the fetal heartbeat of at least 15 beats/minute lasting 15 to 30 seconds in a 20-minute period. No accelerations in the heartbeat of at least 15 beats/minute for 15 to 30 seconds in a 20 minute period indicate a nonreactive NST.

CN: Physiological integrity; CNS: Reduction of risk potential; CL: Analysis

22. 3. A sickle cell crisis during pregnancy is usually managed by exchange transfusion, oxygen, and I.V. fluids. Antihypertensive drugs usually aren't necessary. Diuretics wouldn't be used unless fluid overload resulted. The client usually needs a stronger analgesic than acetaminophen to control the pain of a crisis.

CN: Physiological integrity; CNS: Reduction of risk potential; CL: Analysis

23. 4. Systolic murmurs are heard in up to 90% of pregnant clients, and the murmur disappears soon after the delivery. Cardiac tamponade, which causes effusion of fluid into the pericardial sac, isn't normal during pregnancy. Despite the increases in intravascular volume and workload of the heart associated with pregnancy, heart failure isn't normal in pregnancy. Endocarditis is most often associated with I.V. drug use and isn't a normal finding in pregnancy.

CN: Health promotion and maintenance; CNS: None; CL: Application

24. A 42-year-old pregnant client presents for her first prenatal visit at 16 weeks' gestation. She has severe morning sickness and no fetal heart tones. Her blood pressure is 150/100 mm Hg. Fundal height is 24 cm. The nurse interprets this assessment as most likely indicative of which condition?
1. Abruptio placenta
2. Placenta previa
3. Normal pregnancy
4. Hydatidiform mole

The words most likely can help you focus on the correct answer.

25. A client with gestational hypertension is receiving magnesium sulfate to prevent seizure activity. The nurse reviews the magnesium level and identifies a therapeutic level as:
1. 4 to 7 mEq/L.
2. 8 to 10 mEq/L.
3. 10 to 12 mEq/L.
4. greater than 15 mEq/L.

26. A client is receiving I.V. magnesium sulfate for severe preeclampsia. It is most important for the nurse to assess the client for which of the following?
1. Anemia
2. Decreased urine output
3. Hyperreflexia
4. Increased respiratory rate

With the right drug, I can get rid of that extra magnesium.

27. The nurse is planning care for a client receiving magnesium sulfate intravenously. The nurse recognizes the need to have which medication available for emergency use?
1. Calcium gluconate (Kalcinate)
2. Hydralazine
3. Naloxone
4. Rh₀(D) immune globulin (RhoGAM)

24. 4. The incidence of hydatidiform mole, also known as gestational trophoblastic disease, is higher in women who are older than 35 years of age, have low protein intake, or are of Asian heritage. Molar pregnancy should be suspected in clients who have bleeding during the first half of pregnancy, hyperemesis, pregnancy-induced hypertension, absent fetal heart tones, and enlarged uterus for the time of pregnancy. The signs and symptoms do not pertain to the other conditions.

CN: Health promotion and maintenance; CNS: None; CL: Application

25. 1. The therapeutic level of magnesium for clients with gestational hypertension is 4 to 7 mEq/L. A serum level of 8 to 10 mEq/L may cause the absence of reflexes in the client. Serum levels of 10 to 12 mEq/L may cause respiratory depression, and a serum level of magnesium greater than 15 mEq/L may result in respiratory paralysis.

CN: Physiological integrity; CNS: Pharmacological and parenteral therapies; CL: Application

26. 2. Decreased urine output may occur in clients receiving I.V. magnesium and should be monitored closely to keep urine output at greater than 30 ml/hour because magnesium is excreted through the kidneys and can easily accumulate to toxic levels. Anemia isn't associated with magnesium therapy. Magnesium infusions may cause depression of deep tendon reflexes or hyporeflexia. The client should be monitored for respiratory depression and paralysis when serum magnesium levels reach approximately 15 mEq/L.

CN: Physiological integrity; CNS: Pharmacological and parenteral therapies; CL: Analysis

27. 1. Calcium gluconate is the antidote for magnesium toxicity. Ten milliliters of 10% calcium gluconate is given I.V. push over 3 to 5 minutes. Hydralazine is given for sustained elevated blood pressures in preeclamptic clients. Naloxone is used to correct narcotic toxicity. Rh₀(D) immune globulin is given to women with Rh-negative blood to prevent antibody formation from Rh-positive conceptions.

CN: Physiological integrity; CNS: Pharmacological and parenteral therapies; CL: Analysis

28. A pregnant client is screened for tuberculosis during her first prenatal visit. An intradermal injection of purified protein derivative (PPD) of the tuberculin bacilli is administered by the nurse. The client is considered to have a positive test when which event occurs?
1. An indurated wheal under 10 mm in diameter appears in 6 to 12 hours.
2. An indurated wheal over 10 mm in diameter appears in 48 to 72 hours.
3. A flat circumcised area under 10 mm in diameter appears in 6 to 12 hours.
4. A flat circumcised area over 10 mm in diameter appears in 48 to 72 hours.

29. A 23-year-old client who is at 27 weeks' gestation arrives at her physician's office with complaints of fever, nausea, vomiting, malaise, unilateral flank pain, and costovertebral angle tenderness. Which diagnosis is most likely?
1. Asymptomatic bacteriuria
2. Bacterial vaginosis
3. Pyelonephritis
4. Urinary tract infection (UTI)

30. Clients with which condition would be appropriate for a trial of labor after a prior cesarean delivery?
1. Complete placenta previa
2. Invasive cervical cancer
3. Premature rupture of membranes
4. Prior classical cesarean delivery

31. A nurse is teaching a client who received a dose of Rh$_0$(D) immune globulin (RhoGAM) at 28 weeks' gestation to prevent Rh isoimmunization. Which statement is most accurate about the development of this condition?
1. Rh-positive maternal blood crosses into fetal blood, stimulating fetal antibodies.
2. Rh-positive fetal blood crosses into maternal blood, stimulating maternal antibodies.
3. Rh-negative fetal blood crosses into maternal blood, stimulating maternal antibodies.
4. Rh-negative maternal blood crosses into fetal blood, stimulating fetal antibodies.

A mysterious wheal will appear within the next few days.

This isn't my kind of trial.

28. 2. A positive PPD result would be an indurated wheal over 10 mm in diameter that appears in 48 to 72 hours. The area must be a raised wheal, not a flat circumcised area, to be considered positive.
CN: Physiological integrity; CNS: Reduction of risk potential; CL: Application

29. 3. The symptoms indicate acute pyelonephritis, a serious condition in a pregnant client. Asymptomatic bacteriuria doesn't cause symptoms. Bacterial vaginosis causes milky white vaginal discharge but no systemic symptoms. UTI symptoms include dysuria, urgency, frequency, and suprapubic tenderness.
CN: Physiological integrity; CNS: Reduction of risk potential; CL: Analysis

30. 3. Clients with premature rupture of membranes are permitted a trial of labor after a previous cesarean delivery. Clients with placenta previa or a prior classical cesarean delivery shouldn't be given a trial of labor due to the risk of uterine rupture or severe bleeding. A client with invasive cervical cancer should be scheduled for a cesarean delivery.
CN: Physiological integrity; CNS: Physiological adaptation; CL: Analysis

31. 2. Rh isoimmunization occurs when Rh-positive fetal blood cells cross into the maternal circulation and stimulate maternal antibody production. In subsequent pregnancies with Rh-positive fetuses, maternal antibodies may cross back into the fetal circulation and destroy the fetal blood cells.
CN: Physiological integrity; CNS: Reduction of risk potential; CL: Application

32. Which dose of $Rh_o(D)$ immune globulin (RhoGAM) is appropriate for a pregnant client at 28 weeks' gestation?
1. 50 mcg in a sensitized client
2. 50 mcg in an unsensitized client
3. 300 mcg in a sensitized client
4. 300 mcg in an unsensitized client

33. A client hospitalized for preterm labor tells the nurse she's having occasional contractions. Which nursing intervention would be the <u>most</u> <u>appropriate</u>?
1. Teach the client the possible complications of preterm birth.
2. Tell the client to walk to see if she can get rid of the contractions.
3. Encourage her to empty her bladder and drink plenty of fluids and give I.V. fluids.
4. Notify anesthesia for immediate epidural placement to relieve the pain associated with contractions.

34. A client's prenatal history shows her to be a 23-year-old gravida 4, para 2. The nurse has correctly interpreted this information when she makes which statement?
1. "The client has been pregnant four times and has had two miscarriages."
2. "The client has been pregnant four times and has had two children born after 20 weeks' gestation."
3. "The client has been pregnant four times and has had two cesarean deliveries."
4. "The client has been pregnant four times and has had two spontaneous abortions."

35. A nurse is planning the care of a pregnant client. Which condition would require more frequent visits?
1. Blood type O positive
2. First pregnancy at age 33 years
3. History of allergy to honey bee pollen
4. History of insulin-dependent diabetes mellitus

It may be premature. But I think you're doing great!

Nobody told me that I'd have to know Latin!

32. 4. An Rh-negative unsensitized woman should be given 300 mcg of RhoGAM at 28 weeks' gestation after an indirect Coombs test is done to verify that sensitization hasn't occurred. For a first trimester abortion or ectopic pregnancy, 50 mcg of RhoGAM is given. The administration of RhoGAM to a sensitized client isn't effective.
CN: Physiological integrity; CNS: Pharmacological and parenteral therapies; CL: Analysis

33. 3. An empty bladder and adequate hydration may help decrease or stop labor contractions. Teaching the potential complications is likely to increase the client's anxiety rather than help her relax. Walking may encourage contractions to become stronger. It would be inappropriate to call anesthesia and have an epidural placed because further assessment of contractions is necessary.
CN: Physiological integrity; CNS: Reduction of risk potential; CL: Application

34. 2. Gravida refers to the number of times a client has been pregnant; para refers to the number of viable children born after 20 weeks' gestation. Therefore, the client who is gravida 4, para 2 has been pregnant four times and had two live-born children.
CN: Health promotion and maintenance; CNS: None; CL: Analysis

35. 4. A woman with a history of diabetes has an increased risk for perinatal complications, including hypertension, preeclampsia, and neonatal hypoglycemia and, therefore, needs to be more closely monitored. The age of 33 years without other risk factors doesn't increase risk, nor does type O positive blood or environmental allergens.
CN: Safe, effective care environment; CNS: Management of care; CL: Application

36. To detect life-threatening complications as early as possible in a client receiving a tocolytic agent, the nurse should be alert for which finding?
1. Serum blood glucose level of 140 mg/dl
2. Maternal heart rate of 54 beats/minute
3. Bilateral crackles on lung auscultation
4. Weakened carotid pulse

37. What would be the most appropriate medication to administer for a client who has been in early labor (contractions every 10 to 12 minutes) for 12 hours without progression to help stimulate uterine contractions?
1. Estrogen
2. Fetal cortisol
3. Oxytocin
4. Progesterone

38. A pregnant client asks the nurse about the pregnancy stage in which maternal and fetal blood are exchanged. Which response by the nurse would be most accurate?
1. Conception
2. 9 weeks' gestation, when the fetal heart is well developed
3. 32 to 34 weeks' gestation (third trimester)
4. Maternal and fetal blood are never exchanged.

39. A pregnant client asks the nurse why she should lie on her left side when resting or sleeping in the later stages of pregnancy. What is the best response by the nurse?
1. To facilitate digestion
2. To facilitate bladder emptying
3. To prevent compression of the vena cava
4. To avoid the development of fetal anomalies

Some complications require prompt action.

The resting or sleeping position is important in the later stages of pregnancy.

36. 3. Tocolytics are used to stop labor contractions. The most common adverse effect associated with the use of these drugs is pulmonary edema. Therefore, bilateral crackles on lung auscultation, a sign of pulmonary edema, require prompt action. A serum glucose level of 140 mg/dl is elevated and should be reported; however, it isn't life threatening. Tocolytics may cause tachycardia and increased cardiac output with bounding arterial pulsations.
CN: Physiological integrity; CNS: Pharmacological and parenteral therapies; CL: Analysis

37. 3. Oxytocin is the hormone responsible for stimulating uterine contractions. Pitocin, the synthetic form, may be given to clients to induce or augment uterine contractions. Although estrogen has a role in uterine contractions, it isn't given in a synthetic form to help uterine contractility. Fetal cortisol is believed to slow the production of progesterone by the placenta. Progesterone has a relaxing effect on the uterus.
CN: Physiological integrity; CNS: Pharmacological and parenteral therapies; CL: Application

38. 4. Only nutrients and waste products are transferred across the placenta. Blood exchange never occurs. Complications and some medical procedures can cause an exchange to occur accidentally.
CN: Physiological integrity; CNS: Physiological adaptation; CL: Application

39. 3. The weight of the pregnant uterus is sufficiently heavy to compress the vena cava, which could impair blood flow to the uterus, possibly decreasing oxygen to the fetus. The side-lying position hasn't been shown to prevent fetal anomalies, nor does it facilitate bladder emptying or digestion.
CN: Physiological integrity; CNS: Reduction of risk potential; CL: Analysis

40. A pregnant client is concerned about lack of fetal movement. What is the best response by the nurse?
1. Start taking two prenatal vitamins.
2. Take a warm bath to facilitate fetal movement.
3. Eat foods that contain a high sugar content to enhance fetal movement.
4. Lie down once a day and count the number of fetal movements for 15 to 30 minutes.

Client teaching is an important role for the nurse.

40. 4. Having the client lie down once during the day will allow her to concentrate on detecting fetal movement, which can be reassuring. Additionally, when the mother is up and actively walking around, it tends to be soothing to the fetus, resulting in sleep promotion. Lying down will make it easier for the client to detect movement. Instructing her to take additional prenatal vitamins isn't recommended as vitamins can be toxic when taken in excess. Taking a warm bath is also likely to be soothing to the fetus. There's also a risk for hyperthermia if the water is too warm or the client is immersed too long. Eating additional sugary foods isn't recommended as some pregnant clients are more susceptible to cavities.

CN: Health promotion and maintenance; CNS: None; CL: Application

41. What is the <u>most appropriate</u> intervention for the nurse to recommend for a pregnant client who complains of swelling in her feet and ankles?
1. Limit fluid intake.
2. Buy walking shoes.
3. Sit and elevate the feet.
4. Start taking a diuretic as needed daily.

This recommendation works for me!

41. 3. Sitting down and putting up her feet will promote venous return and therefore decrease edema. Limiting fluid intake isn't recommended unless there are additional medical complications such as heart failure. Buying walking shoes won't necessarily decrease edema. Diuretics aren't recommended during pregnancy because it's important to maintain an adequate circulatory volume.

CN: Physiological integrity; CNS: Basic care and comfort; CL: Application

42. Which intervention should a nurse recommend to a client having severe heartburn during her pregnancy?
1. Eat several small meals daily.
2. Eat crackers on waking every morning.
3. Drink a preparation of salt and vinegar.
4. Drink orange juice frequently during the day.

42. 1. Eating small, frequent meals will place less pressure on the esophageal sphincter, reducing the likelihood of the regurgitation of stomach contents into the lower esophagus. None of the other suggestions have been shown to decrease heartburn.

CN: Physiological integrity; CNS: Basic care and comfort; CL: Application

43. Which maternal complication is associated with obesity in pregnancy?
1. Mastitis
2. Placenta previa
3. Preeclampsia
4. Rh isoimmunization

43. 3. The incidence of preeclampsia in obese clients is about seven times higher than that in nonobese pregnant clients. Mastitis, placenta previa, and Rh isoimmunization aren't associated with increased incidence in obese pregnant clients.

CN: Physiological integrity; CNS: Reduction of risk potential; CL: Analysis

44. A nonstress test (NST) is ordered for a client with preeclampsia. The nurse is aware that the test will be performed to assess which of the following?
1. Anemia
2. Fetal well-being
3. Intrauterine growth retardation (IUGR)
4. Oligohydramnios

It's important to know the recommended fasting blood sugar level during pregnancy.

45. A client is at 33 weeks' gestation and has had diabetes since she was 21. When checking her fasting blood sugar level, which value would indicate to the nurse that the client's disease was controlled?
1. 45 mg/dl
2. 85 mg/dl
3. 120 mg/dl
4. 136 mg/dl

46. A client with diabetes, who is in the late third trimester, has a nonstress test twice weekly. The 20-minute test showed three fetal heart rate accelerations that exceeded the baseline by 15 beats/minute and that lasted longer than 15 seconds. The nurse knows these results are consistent with which interpretation of a nonstress test?
1. Reactive test
2. Nonreactive test
3. Positive test
4. Negative test

You're almost at question 50 and you're doing great.

47. A client is diagnosed with preterm labor at 28 weeks' gestation. Later, she comes to the emergency department saying, "I think I'm in labor." The nurse should expect her physical examination to show which condition?
1. Painful contractions with no cervical dilation
2. Regular uterine contractions with cervical dilation
3. Irregular uterine contraction with no cervical dilation
4. Irregular uterine contractions with cervical effacement

44. 2. An NST is based on the theory that a healthy fetus will have transient fetal heart rate accelerations with fetal movement. A fetus with compromised uteroplacental circulation usually won't have these accelerations, which indicates a nonreactive NST. An NST can't detect anemia in a fetus. Serial ultrasounds will detect IUGR and oligohydramnios in a fetus.
CN: Health promotion and maintenance; CNS: None; CL: Analysis

45. 2. Recommended fasting blood sugar levels in pregnant clients with diabetes are 60 to 90 mg/dl. A fasting blood sugar level of 45 mg/dl is low and may result in symptoms of hypoglycemia. A blood sugar level below 120 mg/dl is recommended for 1-hour postprandial values. A blood sugar level above 136 mg/dl in a pregnant client indicates hyperglycemia.
CN: Health promotion and maintenance; CNS: None; CL: Analysis

46. 1. The nonstress test is the preferred antepartum heart rate screening test for pregnant clients with diabetes. A reactive nonstress test is two or more fetal heart rate accelerations that exceed the baseline by at least 15 beats/minute and that last longer than 15 seconds within a 20-minute period. A nonreactive nonstress test lacks accelerations in the fetal heart rate with fetal movement. The terms positive and negative aren't used to describe the interpretation of nonstress tests.
CN: Physiological integrity; CNS: Reduction of risk potential; CL: Analysis

47. 2. Regular uterine contractions (every 10 minutes or more) along with cervical dilation change before 36 weeks is considered preterm labor. No cervical change with uterine contractions isn't considered preterm labor.
CN: Health promotion and maintenance; CNS: None; CL: Application

CN: Client needs category   CNS: Client needs subcategory   CL: Cognitive level

48. A client at 18 weeks' gestation reports fluttering sensations in her abdomen. Which statement made by the client indicates that the nurse's teaching was successful?
1. "This is my baby moving."
2. "I will seek prompt medical attention if this happens again."
3. "This is an early sign of labor."
4. "I will avoid spicy foods."

49. A pregnant client is visiting the clinic and complains about the tiny, blanched, slightly raised end arterioles on her face, neck, arms, and chest. The nurse should explain that these are normal during pregnancy and referred to as which finding?
1. Epulis
2. Linea nigra
3. Striae gravidarum
4. Telangiectasias

Oh my! I think your baby just moved.

50. Which nursing intervention for a pregnant adolescent client has the highest priority during the first trimester?
1. Schedule the client for a screening glucose tolerance test.
2. Refer the client to a dietitian for nutritional counseling.
3. Tell the client that she will most likely need a cesarean delivery due to the head size of the fetus.
4. Assess the client for signs and symptoms of placenta previa.

51. A nurse is discussing nutrition with a prima gravida client. The client states that she knows that calcium is important during pregnancy; however, she and her family don't consume many milk or dairy products. What advice should the nurse give?
1. "The prenatal vitamins that are recommended will satisfy all dietary requirements."
2. "You could supplement your diet with 1,800 mg of over-the-counter calcium tablets."
3. "You should consume other nondairy foods that are high in calcium."
4. "After the first trimester, calcium intake isn't significant because all fetal organ structures are formed."

48. 1. Fluttering in the abdomen, also called quickening, begins between 16 and 22 weeks' gestation and is caused by fetal movement. It doesn't require medical attention, nor is it a sign of early labor. Eating spicy foods has no effect on quickening.

CN: Health promotion and maintenance; CNS: None; CL: Analysis

49. 4. The dilated arterioles that occur during pregnancy are due to the elevated level of circulating estrogen and are called telangiectasias. An epulis is a red raised nodule on the gums that may develop at the end of the first trimester and continue to grow as the pregnancy progresses. The linea nigra is a pigmented line extending from the symphysis pubis to the top of the fundus during pregnancy. Striae gravidarum, or stretch marks, are slightly depressed streaks that commonly occur over the abdomen, breast, and thighs during the second half of pregnancy.

CN: Health promotion and maintenance; CNS: None; CL: Application

50. 2. Adolescent clients are at risk for delivering low-birth-weight neonates, not macrosomic neonates. Nutritional counseling should be included as part of prenatal care for adolescent clients. The final head size of the fetus is unknown at this time. Adolescents aren't at increased risk for developing gestational diabetes or placenta previa.

CN: Health promotion and maintenance; CNS: None; CL: Analysis

51. 3. Food is considered the ideal source of nutrients. However, milk and dairy aren't the only sources of calcium. While prenatal vitamins are generally recommended, they don't satisfy all requirements. The calcium requirement for pregnancy is 1,300 mg/day, and over-the-counter supplements aren't always safe and should be specifically recommended by the health care practitioner. While it's true that all fetal organs are formed by the end of the first trimester, development continues throughout pregnancy.

CN: Health promotion and maintenance; CNS: None; CL: Application

52. Which drug should a nurse choose to use as an antagonist for magnesium sulfate?
1. Oxytocin (Pitocin)
2. Terbutaline
3. Calcium gluconate
4. Naloxone

Who are you calling an antagonist?

52. 3. Calcium gluconate should be kept at the bedside while a client is receiving a magnesium infusion. If magnesium toxicity occurs, calcium gluconate is administered as an antidote. Oxytocin is the synthetic form of the naturally occurring pituitary hormone used to initiate or augment uterine contractions. Terbutaline is a β_2-adrenergic agonist that may be used to relax the smooth muscle of the uterus, especially for preterm labor and uterine hyperstimulation. Naloxone is an opiate antagonist administered to reverse the respiratory depression that may follow administration of opiates.

CN: Physiological integrity; CNS: Pharmacological and parenteral therapies; CL: Analysis

53. A nurse receives an order to start an infusion of blood for a client who's hemorrhaging due to a placenta previa. It is most important for the nurse to obtain which of the following?
1. Y tubing, normal saline solution, and a 20G catheter
2. Y tubing, lactated Ringer's solution, and an 18G catheter
3. Y tubing, normal saline solution, and an 18G catheter
4. Y tubing, lactated Ringer's solution, and a 20G catheter

53. 3. Blood transfusions require Y tubing, normal saline solution to mix with the blood product, and an 18G catheter to avoid lysing (breaking) the red blood cells. A 20G catheter lumen isn't large enough for a blood transfusion. Lactated Ringer's solution isn't the I.V. solution of choice with a blood transfusion.

CN: Physiological integrity; CNS: Pharmacological and parenteral therapies; CL: Application

54. A nurse is assessing a client who is experiencing a normal pregnancy. The nurse would anticipate the assessment to include which finding?
1. A 10 beat/minute drop in heart rate
2. A 2 breath/minute increase in respiratory rate
3. A 15 mm Hg increase in systolic blood pressure
4. A 2,000/µl drop in leukocyte count

54. 2. During pregnancy there is a slight increase (2 breaths/minute) in respiratory rate. Heart rate may increase up to 15 beats/minute by the end of pregnancy. Systolic and diastolic pressures may decrease by 5 to 10 mm Hg. The leukocyte count rises in pregnancy and may range from 10,000 to 12,000/µl.

CN: Physiological integrity; CNS: Reduction of risk potential; CL: Application

55. The nurse is teaching a student nurse about the GTPAL system, which documents a client's previous pregnancies. Which statement most accurately describes this system?
1. Total neonates, Preterm neonates, Anencephalic neonates, and Live births
2. Total neonates, Problem pregnancies, Abortions, and Live births
3. Term neonates, Preterm neonates, Anencephalic neonates, and Live births
4. Term neonates, Preterm neonates, Abortions, and Living children

56. The nurse is reviewing the glucose tolerance test results of a client who is at 26 weeks' gestation. The nurse determines further intervention is necessary when the results identify:
1. a glucose level of 120 mg/dl during a 1-hour glucose tolerance test.
2. a 1-hour glucose level of 160 mg/dl during a 3-hour glucose tolerance test.
3. a 2-hour glucose level of 180 mg/dl during a 3-hour glucose tolerance test.
4. a 3-hour glucose level of 130 mg/dl during a 3-hour glucose tolerance test.

57. A 32-year-old woman is at 15 weeks' gestation when admitted to the labor unit. According to the GTPAL system, she is a G5 P1212. Which description does this indicate?
1. Total of 5 pregnancies, 1 full-term pregnancy, 2 problem pregnancies, 1 spontaneous abortion, and 2 live births
2. Total of 5 children, 1 full-term pregnancy, 2 preterm pregnancies, 1 abortion, and 2 live births
3. Total of 5 pregnancies, 1 full-term pregnancy, 2 preterm pregnancies, 1 abortion, and 2 living children
4. Total of 5 pregnancies, 1 full-term pregnancy, 2 problem pregnancies, 1 abortion, and 2 living children

58. The nurse is assessing a 32-year-old woman who is 15 weeks' pregnant and has a history of hypertension. The nurse is aware that the client is most at risk for which condition?
1. Abruptio placentae
2. Preterm labor
3. Spontaneous abortion
4. Anemia

Hmm. Let me think. "G" is for gravida; T is for…

It's important to know the medical history of a pregnant client.

55. **4.** In GTPAL, G stands for gravida; T denotes the number of term neonates born after 37 weeks' gestation; P, the number of preterm neonates born before 37 weeks' gestation; A, the number of pregnancies ending with spontaneous or therapeutic abortion; and L, the number of children currently living.

CN: Health promotion and maintenance; CNS: None; CL: Application

56. **3.** Gestational diabetes is diagnosed when a 2-hour glucose level is 155 mg/dl or greater during a 3-hour glucose tolerance test. Diagnostic criteria for the 100-g, 3-hour glucose tolerance test for gestational diabetes mellitus include plasma or serum glucose levels of or greater than: fasting, 75 mg/dl; 1 hour, 180 mg/dl; 2 hours, 155 mg/dl; and 3 hours, 140 mg/dl.

CN: Physiological integrity; CNS: Reduction of risk potential; CL: Application

57. **3.** T indicates the number of term neonates born at 37 weeks' gestation or after; P, the number of preterm neonates born before 37 weeks' gestation; A, the number of pregnancies ending with spontaneous or therapeutic abortion; and L, the number of children currently living. In this case, the client has been pregnant five times (including the current pregnancy); has had one pregnancy of at least 37 weeks' gestation, two preterm pregnancies, and one abortion; and has two living children.

CN: Health promotion and maintenance; CNS: None; CL: Application

58. **1.** A history of hypertension predisposes the client for developing abruptio placentae. She isn't at risk for developing preterm labor, spontaneous abortion, or anemia.

CN: Physiological integrity; CNS: Reduction of risk potential; CL: Analysis

59. A 32-year-old female client has her first prenatal visit at 15 weeks' gestation. Which finding during this visit is abnormal?
 1. Fundal height of 18 cm
 2. Blood pressure of 124/72 mm Hg
 3. Urine negative for protein
 4. Weight of 144 lb (65.3 kg)

60. A 25-year-old primiparous client arrives for her first prenatal visit at 10 weeks' gestation. She seems nervous and has many questions. What is the most important intervention by the nurse?
 1. Assess the client's concerns while taking a comprehensive history.
 2. Ask the client to undress to prepare for the physical examination.
 3. Reassure the client that all her questions will be answered during the visit.
 4. Tell the client there's nothing to worry about; the physician will take care of her.

61. Accompanied by her father, a primiparous 15-year-old client arrives for her first prenatal visit at 30 weeks' gestation. Her father refuses to leave the room and tells the nurse that the girl is shy and he will answer the questions for her. What should the nurse be most concerned?
 1. The possibility of preterm labor with an adolescent pregnancy
 2. Lack of prenatal care until this visit
 3. Possible child abuse or domestic violence
 4. Difficulties of an overprotective parent in dealing with his daughter

Question 59 is asking for an abnormal finding.

What should the nurse be most concerned about? Let me think.

59. 1. Fundal height (in centimeters) should equal the number of weeks of gestation between 18 and 34 weeks; however, it shouldn't be used alone to determine weeks of gestation. This client should have a fundal height of 15 to 16 cm. The blood pressure, urine, and weight findings are within normal limits for the information given.
CN: Physiological integrity; CNS: Reduction of risk potential; CL: Analysis

60. 3. Providing initial reassurance helps set the client's mind at ease. Assessing the client's concerns while taking a history would be appropriate only if the client wrote down her questions in advance. Asking her to disrobe immediately may make the client even more nervous. She should be treated as a partner in her care rather than be told that the physician will take care of everything.
CN: Safe, effective care environment; CNS: Management of care; CL: Application

61. 3. Generally, a father would be somewhat uncomfortable staying in a room while his pregnant daughter is examined. If he insists on staying during the history and physical examination, the nurse should gently but firmly ask him to wait in another room. If the nurse suspects possible child abuse or domestic violence, the father may not want the girl to be alone with the nurse, fearing that she might reveal the abuse or violence. (Typically, a victim of domestic violence says nothing if the perpetrator is in the room with her.) The possibility of preterm labor and lack of prenatal care should be considered—but they aren't the primary concerns in this situation. An overprotective parent can be supported and taught how to let go of a child as time goes by; a social work referral may be warranted.
CN: Psychosocial integrity; CNS: None; CL: Analysis

62. What is the <u>best</u> way for a nurse to determine if a pregnant client is the victim of domestic abuse or violence?
1. Interview the client with her partner in the room.
2. Interview the client with the physician present.
3. Interview the client alone in a nonjudgmental way.
4. Interview the client in a nonjudgmental way, with the partner present.

63. A client with gestational hypertension is experiencing abdominal pain and vaginal bleeding. Which assessment should the nurse perform first?
1. Assess fetal heart tones
2. Assess strength of contractions
3. Assess urinary output
4. Assess serum electrolytes

64. During the second and third trimesters, common pregnancy discomforts may increase in number and severity. During the assessment of a pregnant client, the nurse normally expects to see which findings?
1. Ankle edema, hemorrhoids, nausea and vomiting, and shortness of breath
2. Ankle edema, shortness of breath, leg cramps, and increased vaginal discharge
3. Leg cramps, Braxton Hicks contractions, and nausea and vomiting
4. Leg cramps, ankle edema, and shortness of breath

65. A client with mild preeclampsia is being prepared for discharge from the hospital. The nurse determines an understanding of discharge instructions when the client makes which statement?
1. "I will lie on my left side."
2. "I should increase my sodium intake."
3. "I will take acetaminophen for a headache."
4. "I will monitor my weight each week."

It's up to you to do your best.

Way to go! You're almost there!

62. 3. To help the client feel protected and develop enough trust in the nurse to share her "secret," the nurse should interview her alone in a nonjudgmental way. If the partner is present, the client is likely to clam up for fear of retaliation the next time they're alone together.

CN: Psychosocial integrity; CNS: None; CL: Application

63. 1. Since the findings suggest that the client is experiencing abruptio placentae, fetal heart tones should immediately be assessed to determine fetal well-being. The other interventions should also be implemented, but after the fetus is assessed.

CN: Physiological integrity; CNS: Reduction of risk potential; CL: Analysis

64. 4. Leg cramps, ankle edema, and shortness of breath are normal during the second and third trimesters. The nurse should teach the client how to relieve minor discomforts and what to report if the discomfort becomes unbearable. Nausea and vomiting should subside by the end of the first trimester; if they don't, the nurse should suspect an undiagnosed problem, such as hyperemesis gravidarum or emotional factors that may be exacerbating the nausea and vomiting. Increased vaginal discharge generally occurs during the first trimester and decreases at the end of this period. A yellow, curd-like, or malodorous discharge suggests an abnormal vaginal infection, which should be reported to the physician.

CN: Health promotion and maintenance; CNS: None; CL: Application

65. 1. The client should lie on her left side to improve uterine and renal blood flow and enhance venous return. Sodium intake should be limited in the client with preeclampsia. A headache should be reported to the health care provider since it can signal a worsening of the eclampsia. Weight should be monitored daily to assess for fluid retention.

CN: Physiological integrity; CNS: Reduction of risk potential; CL: Analysis

66. When teaching an antepartum client about the passage of the fetus through the birth canal during labor, the nurse describes the cardinal mechanisms of labor. Place these events in the proper sequence in which they occur.

1. Flexion

2. External rotation

3. Descent

4. Expulsion

5. Internal rotation

6. Extension

66.

3. Descent

1. Flexion

5. Internal rotation

6. Extension

2. External rotation

4. Expulsion

As the fetus moves through the birth canal, it goes through position changes to ensure that the smallest diameter of fetal head presents to the smallest diameter of the birth canal. Termed the cardinal mechanisms of labor, these position changes occur in the following sequence: descent, flexion, internal rotation, extension, external rotation, and expulsion.

CN: Health promotion and maintenance; CNS: None; CL: Application

67. A nurse is palpating the uterus of a client who is at 20 weeks' gestation to measure fundal height. Identify the area of the abdomen where the nurse should expect to feel the uterine fundus.

67. At 20 weeks' gestation, fundal height should be at about the umbilicus. Fundal height should be measured from the symphysis pubis to the top of the uterus. Serial measurements assess fetal growth over the course of the pregnancy. Between weeks 18 and 34, the centimeters measured correlate roughly with the week of gestation.

CN: Health promotion and maintenance; CNS: None; CL: Application

Chapter 23
Intrapartum care

1. A client with a term, uncomplicated pregnancy comes into the labor-and-delivery unit in early labor saying that she thinks her water has broken. Which action by a nurse would be <u>most appropriate</u>?
1. Prepare the woman for delivery.
2. Ask what time this happened and note the color, amount, and odor of the fluid.
3. Immediately contact the physician.
4. Collect a sample of the fluid for microbial analysis.

2. A client who's at 36 weeks' gestation comes into the labor-and-delivery unit with mild contractions. The client states that she has placenta previa. The nurse is aware that this client is at risk for which of the following?
1. Sudden rupture of membranes
2. Vaginal bleeding
3. Emesis
4. Fever

3. A client's labor doesn't progress. After ruling out cephalopelvic disproportion, the physician orders I.V. administration of 1,000 ml normal saline solution with oxytocin (Pitocin) 10 units to run at 2 milliunits/minute. Two milliunits/minute is equivalent to how many ml/minute?
1. 0.002
2. 0.02
3. 0.2
4. 2

Pay attention to the words *most appropriate*. They're the key to the answer.

I need a book on math 101.

1. 2. Noting the color, amount, and odor of the fluid, as well as the time of the rupture, will help guide the nurse in her next action. There's no need to call the client's physician immediately or prepare the client for delivery if the fluid is clear and delivery isn't imminent. Rupture of membranes isn't unusual in the early stages of labor. Fluid collection for microbial analysis isn't routine if there's no concern for infection (maternal fever).
CN: Physiological integrity; CNS: Reduction of risk potential; CL: Application

2. 2. Contractions may disrupt the microvascular network in the placenta of a client with placenta previa and result in bleeding. If the separation of the placenta occurs at the margin of the placenta, the blood will escape vaginally. Sudden rupture of the membranes isn't related to placenta previa. Fever would indicate an infectious process, and emesis isn't related to placenta previa.
CN: Physiological integrity; CNS: Reduction of risk potential; CL: Application

3. 3. The answer is found by setting up a ratio and following through with the calculations, shown below. Each unit of oxytocin contains 1,000 milliunits. Therefore, 1,000 ml of I.V. fluid contains 10,000 milliunits (10 units) of Pitocin. All other options are incorrect.

$$\frac{10,000}{1,000} = \frac{2}{X}$$
$$10,000X = 2,000$$
$$X = \frac{2,000}{10,000}$$
$$X = 0.2 \text{ ml}$$

CN: Physiological integrity; CNS: Pharmacological and parenteral therapies; CL: Analysis

4. A client in labor has been receiving oxytocin (Pitocin) to aid her progress. The nurse caring for her notes that contractions are lasting 100 seconds. Which action should the nurse take <u>first</u>?
1. Stop the oxytocin infusion.
2. Notify the physician.
3. Monitor fetal heart tones as usual.
4. Turn the client on her left side.

Don't underestimate the importance of the word first.

5. A client at term arrives in the labor unit experiencing contractions every 4 minutes. After a brief assessment, she's admitted, and an electronic fetal monitor is applied. Which observation should the nurse be most concerned about?
1. Total weight gain of 30 lb (13.6 kg)
2. Maternal age of 32 years
3. Blood pressure of 146/90 mm Hg
4. Treatment for syphilis at 15 weeks' gestation

6. To detect fetal distress during labor, a nurse should be alert for which finding?
1. Fetal scalp pH of 7.14
2. Fetal heart rate of 144 beats/minute
3. Acceleration of fetal heart rate with contractions
4. Presence of long-term variability

7. During the labor of a client with a breech presentation, the amniotic membranes rupture. Meconium is present in the amniotic fluid. The client asks the nurse what this means. What is the most appropriate response by the nurse?
1. "This often happens during a prolonged delivery."
2. "This indicates a blood incompatibility between the fetus and mother."
3. "This is a sign of fetal distress."
4. "This is normal in a breech delivery."

4. 1. Oxytocin stimulates contractions and should be stopped. A contraction that continues for more than 90 seconds signals tetany and could lead to decreased placental perfusion and, possibly, uterine rupture. The nurse should monitor the fetal heart tones, stop the oxytocin, and notify the physician. The client should be turned on her left side to increase blood flow to the fetus, which can be decreased with tetany. This decreased blood flow can potentially compromise the fetus.
CN: Physiological integrity; CNS: Reduction of risk potential; CL: Application

5. 3. A blood pressure of 146/90 mm Hg may indicate gestational hypertension. Over time, gestational hypertension reduces blood flow to the placenta and can cause intrauterine growth restriction and other problems that make the fetus less able to tolerate the stress of labor. A weight gain of 30 lb is within expected parameters for a healthy pregnancy. A woman over age 30 doesn't have a greater risk of complications if her general condition is healthy before pregnancy. Syphilis that has been treated doesn't pose an additional risk.
CN: Physiological integrity; CNS: Reduction of risk potential; CL: Application

6. 1. A scalp pH below 7.25 indicates acidosis and fetal hypoxia. A fetal heart rate of 144 beats/minute, acceleration of the fetal heart rate with contractions, and long-term variability are normal responses of a healthy fetus to labor.
CN: Physiological integrity; CNS: Reduction of risk potential; CL: Application

7. 4. Meconium in a breech presentation may be caused by compression of the fetus's intestinal tract during descent. Meconium in the amniotic fluid is a sign of fetal distress in a cephalic presentation and isn't a normal finding, even during a prolonged delivery. Yellow-stained amniotic fluid is a sign of a possible blood incompatibility between fetus and mother and is due to bilirubin from the breakdown of red blood cells.
CN: Physiological integrity; CNS: Reduction of risk potential; CL: Analysis

8. A client at 42 weeks' gestation is 3 cm dilated, 30% effaced, with membranes intact and the fetus at −2 (minus 2) station. Fetal heart rate (FHR) is 140 beats/minute. After 2 hours, the nurse notes on the external fetal monitor that, for the past 10 minutes, the FHR ranged from 160 to 190 beats/minute. The client states that her baby has been extremely active. Uterine contractions are strong, occurring every 3 to 4 minutes and lasting 40 to 60 seconds. Which finding would indicate fetal hypoxia?
1. Abnormally long uterine contractions
2. Abnormally strong uterine intensity
3. Excessively frequent contractions, with rapid fetal movement
4. Excessive fetal activity and fetal tachycardia

9. A client at 33 weeks' gestation and leaking amniotic fluid is placed on an external fetal monitor. The monitor indicates uterine irritability, and contractions are occurring every 4 to 6 minutes. The physician orders terbutaline. What is the most important information for the nurse to tell the client?
1. "This medicine will make you breathe better."
2. "You may feel a fluttering or tight sensation in your chest."
3. "This will dry your mouth and make you feel thirsty."
4. "You'll need to replace the potassium lost by this drug."

10. A 17-year-old primigravida with severe hypertension of pregnancy has been receiving magnesium sulfate I.V. for 3 hours. The latest assessment reveals deep tendon reflexes (DTR) of +1, blood pressure of 150/100 mm Hg, a pulse of 92 beats/minute, a respiratory rate of 10 breaths/minute, and urine output of 20 ml/hour. Which action would be most appropriate?
1. Continue monitoring per standards of care.
2. Stop the magnesium sulfate infusion.
3. Increase the infusion rate by 5 gtt/minute.
4. Decrease the infusion rate by 5 gtt/minute.

Remember that every piece of information provided may not be necessary to answer the question.

Sometimes you have to think fast on your feet.

8. 4. Fetal tachycardia and excessive fetal activity are the first signs of fetal hypoxia. The duration of uterine contractions is within normal limits. Uterine intensity can be mild to strong and still be within normal limits. The frequency of contractions is within the normal limits for the active phase of labor.
CN: Physiological integrity; CNS: Reduction of risk potential; CL: Analysis

9. 2. A fluttering or tight sensation in the chest is a common adverse reaction to terbutaline. Terbutaline relieves bronchospasm, but the client is receiving it to reduce uterine motility. Mouth dryness and thirst occur with the inhaled form of terbutaline but are unlikely with the subcutaneous form. Hypokalemia is a potential adverse reaction following large doses of terbutaline but not at doses of 0.25 mg.
CN: Health promotion and maintenance; CNS: None; CL: Application

10. 2. Magnesium sulfate should be withheld if the client's respiratory rate or urine output falls or if reflexes are diminished or absent, all of which are true for this client. The client also shows other signs of impending toxicity, such as flushing and feeling warm. Inaction won't resolve the client's suppressed DTRs and low respiratory rate and urine output. The client is already showing central nervous system depression because of excessive magnesium sulfate, so increasing the infusion rate is inappropriate. Impending toxicity indicates that the infusion should be stopped rather than just slowed down.
CN: Physiological integrity; CNS: Pharmacological and parenteral therapies; CL: Application

11. During a vaginal examination of a client in labor, the nurse palpates the fetus's larger, diamond-shaped fontanelle toward the anterior portion of the client's pelvis. The nurse interprets this assessment as indicating that:
1. the client can expect a brief and intense labor with potential for lacerations.
2. the client is at risk for uterine rupture and needs constant monitoring.
3. the client may need interventions to ease back pain and change the fetal position.
4. the fetus will be delivered using forceps or a vacuum extractor.

12. The cervix of a 26-year-old primigravida in labor is 5 cm dilated and 75% effaced, and the fetus is at 0 station. The physician prescribes an epidural regional block. Into which position should the nurse place the client when the epidural is administered?
1. Lithotomy
2. Supine
3. Prone
4. Lateral

13. A nurse administers oxytocin (Pitocin) to a client to induce labor. The nurse determines that immediate intervention is necessary when the client presents with which finding?
1. Contractions longer than 70 seconds, occurring every 2 minutes or less
2. Dry mucous membranes and decreased skin turgor
3. Fetal heart rate of 160 beats/minute
4. Maternal heart rate of 56 beats/minute

14. Which fetal position is <u>most favorable</u> for birth?
1. Vertex presentation
2. Transverse lie
3. Frank breech presentation
4. Posterior position of the fetal head

Be careful of the words will be in option 4. They indicate an absolute, a near rarity in health care.

Question 14 is asking for the optimal birthing position.

11. 3. The fetal position is occiput posterior (OP), a position that commonly produces intense back pain during labor. Most of the time, the fetus rotates during labor to occiput anterior position. Positioning the client on her side can facilitate this rotation. An occiput posterior position would most likely result in prolonged labor. Occiput posterior alone doesn't create a risk of uterine rupture. The fetus would be delivered with forceps or vacuum extractor only if its presenting part doesn't rotate and descend spontaneously.
CN: Health promotion and maintenance; CNS: None; CL: Analysis

12. 4. The client should be placed on her left side or sitting upright, with her shoulders parallel and legs slightly flexed. Her back shouldn't be flexed because this position increases the possibility that the dura may be punctured and the anesthetic will accidentally be given as spinal, not epidural, anesthesia. None of the other positions allows proper access to the epidural space.
CN: Physiological integrity; CNS: Reduction of risk potential; CL: Application

13. 1. Oxytocin, given to induce labor, may cause uterine tetany, which increases the risk of uterine rupture. Therefore, the infusion should be stopped and the physician notified if contractions last greater than 70 seconds and occur every 2 minutes or less. Oxytocin has an antidiuretic effect and can cause fluid overload, not dehydration indicated by dry mucous membranes and decreased skin turgor. A normal fetal heart rate is 120 to 160 beats/minute. Oxytocin may cause maternal tachycardia, not bradycardia.
CN: Physiological integrity; CNS: Pharmacologic parenteral therapies; CL: Application

14. 1. Vertex presentation (flexion of the fetal head) is the optimal presentation for passage through the birth canal. Transverse lie is an unacceptable fetal position for vaginal birth and requires a cesarean birth delivery. Frank breech presentation, in which the buttocks present first, is a high-risk situation, and cesarean birth is recommended. Posterior positioning of the fetal head can make it difficult for the fetal head to pass under the maternal symphysis pubis bone.
CN: Physiological integrity; CNS: Reduction of risk potential; CL: Analysis

15. A nurse has admitted a client to the labor-and-delivery unit and is teaching her about the stages of labor. The client demonstrates an understanding of these stages when she states that birth occurs during which stage?
1. First stage of labor
2. Second stage of labor
3. Third stage of labor
4. Fourth stage of labor

Take the stage please!

16. A nurse is reviewing laboratory data on a client admitted to the labor-and-delivery unit. What is the most important laboratory value for the nurse to obtain?
1. Blood type
2. Calcium
3. Iron
4. Oxygen saturation

17. The nurse is assessing the fetal heart rate of a laboring woman who is full term. What does the nurse anticipate the fetal heart rate to be?
1. 80 to 100 beats/minute
2. 100 to 120 beats/minute
3. 120 to 160 beats/minute
4. 160 to 180 beats/minute

18. A nurse has connected a laboring client to an external electronic fetal monitor. What data can the nurse expect to obtain from the monitor?
1. Gender of the fetus
2. Fetal position
3. Labor progress
4. Oxygenation

What can the fetal heart rate strip tell you?

19. The nurse is preparing a client in labor for the administration of an epidural. What is the most important intervention by the nurse?
1. Give a fluid bolus of 500 ml.
2. Check for maternal pupil dilation.
3. Assess maternal reflexes.
4. Assess maternal gait.

15. 2. The second stage of labor begins with complete dilation (10 cm) and ends with the expulsion of the fetus. The first stage of labor is the stage of dilation, which is divided into three distinct phases: latent, active, and transition. The third stage of labor begins with the birth of the infant and ends with the expulsion of the placenta. The fourth stage of labor is the first 4 hours after placental expulsion, in which the client's body begins the recovery process.
CN: Health promotion and maintenance; CNS: None; CL: Application

16. 1. Blood type is a critical value to have because the risk of blood loss is always a potential complication during the labor-and-delivery process. Approximately 40% of a woman's cardiac output is delivered to the uterus; therefore, blood loss can occur quite rapidly in the event of uncontrolled bleeding. Calcium and iron aren't critical values, and oxygen saturation isn't a laboratory value.
CN: Physiological integrity; CNS: Reduction of risk potential; CL: Analysis

17. 3. A rate of 120 to 160 beats/minute in the fetal heart is appropriate for filling the heart with blood and pumping it out to the system. Faster or slower rates don't accomplish perfusion adequately and could indicate fetal compromise.
CN: Health promotion and maintenance; CNS: None; CL: Knowledge

18. 4. Oxygenation of the fetus may be indirectly assessed through fetal monitoring by closely examining the fetal heart rate strip. Accelerations in the fetal heart rate strip indicate good oxygenation, while decelerations in the fetal heart rate sometimes indicate poor fetal oxygenation. The fetal heart rate strip can't determine the gender of the fetus or assess fetal position. Labor progress can be directly assessed only through cervical examination.
CN: Physiological integrity; CNS: Reduction of risk potential; CL: Application

19. 1. One of the major adverse effects of epidural administration is hypotension. Therefore, a 500-ml fluid bolus is usually administered to help prevent hypotension in the client who wishes to receive an epidural for pain relief. Assessments of maternal reflexes, pupil response, and gait aren't necessary.
CN: Physiological integrity; CNS: Reduction of risk potential; CL: Analysis

20. A client required an episiotomy for the delivery of her baby. The nurse is aware that the client may be at risk for which of the following?
1. Blood loss
2. Uterine disfigurement
3. Prolonged dyspareunia
4. Hormonal fluctuation postpartum

21. A client in early labor tells the nurse that she has a thick, yellow discharge from both of her breasts. What is the most appropriate intervention by the nurse?
1. Tell her that her milk is starting to come in because she's in labor.
2. Complete a thorough breast examination and document the results in the chart.
3. Perform a culture on the discharge and inform the client that she might have mastitis.
4. Inform the client that the discharge is colostrum, normally present after the fourth month of pregnancy.

22. While performing an admission nursing assessment of a client in early labor, the nurse observes a brown, raised lesion resembling a mole 2.5 in. (5 cm) below the left breast. What is the most appropriate response by the nurse?
1. "That looks like a mole and is clinically insignificant."
2. "That looks like seborrhea keratosis and is a precancerous lesion."
3. "That's a supernumerary nipple, a common finding."
4. "That's a skin tag and is clinically insignificant."

23. A client in early labor is concerned about the pinkish "stretch marks" on her abdomen. Which statement by the client indicates that the nurse's teaching has been effective?
1. "My stretch marks will completely fade away within 6 weeks."
2. "My stretch marks will fade but not disappear after delivery."
3. "An emollient cream will help fade my stretch marks."
4. "A regular exercise program will help my stretch marks go away."

It's important to know the adverse effects of a procedure and how to offset them.

Teaching is an important part of a nurse's role.

Stretch marks are yet another reminder of the joy of giving birth!

20. 3. Prolonged dyspareunia (painful intercourse) may result when complications such as infection interfere with wound healing. Minimal blood loss occurs when an episiotomy is performed. The uterus isn't affected by episiotomy because it's the perineum that is cut to accommodate the fetus. Hormonal fluctuations that occur during the postpartum period aren't the result of an episiotomy.
CN: Physiological integrity; CNS: Reduction of risk potential; CL: Analysis

21. 4. After the fourth month, colostrum may be expressed. The breasts normally produce colostrum for the first few days after delivery. Milk production begins 1 to 3 days postpartum. A clinical breast examination isn't usually indicated in the intrapartum setting. Although a culture may be indicated, it requires advanced assessment as well as a medical order.
CN: Health promotion and maintenance; CNS: None; CL: Application

22. 3. Supernumerary nipples are common in men and women and are usually located 2.5 to 3 in. (5 to 6 cm) below the breast near the midline. A supernumerary nipple resembles a mole, although closer inspection will reveal a small nipple and areola and is clinically insignificant. A mole (nevus) may be macular or papular, tan to brown in color, and usually has smooth borders. Keratosis lesions are raised, thickened areas of pigmentation that look scaly and warty. They don't become cancerous. Skin tags (acrochordons) are overgrowths of normal skin that form a stalk and are polyp-like.
CN: Health promotion and maintenance; CNS: None; CL: Analysis

23. 2. Striae are wavy, depressed streaks that may occur over the abdomen, breasts, or thighs as pregnancy progresses. They fade with time to a silvery color but won't disappear. Creams may soften the skin but won't remove the striae. Regular exercise won't affect the stretch marks.
CN: Health promotion and maintenance; CNS: None; CL: Application

24. Which position increases cardiac output and stroke volume of a client in labor?
1. Supine
2. Sitting
3. Side-lying
4. Semi-Fowler's

25. A nurse is caring for a full-term pregnant client in active labor. The electronic fetal monitor reveals a fetal heart rate of less than 70 beats/minute. The nurse interprets this as which of the following?
1. Severe fetal bradycardia
2. Normal fetal heart rate
3. Fetal tachycardia
4. Moderate fetal bradycardia

26. A nurse is performing Leopold's maneuvers on a client in the early stages of labor. The nurse is most concerned when which of the following occurs?
1. Palpation of the upper fundus reveals a firm, round shape.
2. Palpation of the upper fundus reveals a soft, less-defined shape.
3. Palpation of the side of the fundus reveals a smooth, firm shape.
4. Palpation of the lower fundus reveals a firm, round shape.

27. A client who's at 35 weeks' gestation arrives at a labor-and-delivery unit leaking clear fluid from her vagina. What is the <u>most appropriate</u> intervention?
1. Perform a cervical examination.
2. Obtain a catheterized urine specimen.
3. Encourage the client to ambulate.
4. Obtain a sterile speculum sample of the fluid.

28. A client at 35 weeks' gestation tells the nurse she's having occasional abdominal contractions that started occurring irregularly. The contractions have remained irregular. What is the best information for the nurse to tell the client?
1. "These contractions will disappear when you walk."
2. "These contractions will increase in frequency and intensity."
3. "These contractions will become regular."
4. "These contractions will move to the lower back."

Things are sure getting slow around here.

Ah, the sweet sound of most appropriate.

Walking is a great way to relieve stress and other things!

24. 3. In the side-lying position, cardiac output increases, stroke volume increases, and the pulse rate decreases. In the supine position, the blood pressure can drop severely, due to the pressure of the fetus and enlarged uterus on the vena cava, resulting in supine hypotensive or vena caval syndrome. Neither the sitting nor semi-Fowler's position increases cardiac output or stroke volume.
CN: Health promotion and maintenance; CNS: None; CL: Application

25. 1. A fetal heart rate (FHR) below 70 beats/minute is considered severe fetal bradycardia and is associated with rapidly occurring fetal acidosis. FHR from 70 to 100 beats/minute is considered moderate fetal bradycardia. Normal FHR for a full-term fetus is 120 to 160 beats/minute. Fetal tachycardia is an FHR above 160 beats/minute.
CN: Health promotion and maintenance; CNS: None; CL: Application

26. 1. Palpation of the upper fundus reveals a firm, round head in a breech presentation and a soft, less-defined shape in a cephalic delivery. The firm, smooth back of the fetus is palpated on the side of the fundus and may be palpated with cephalic and breech presentations. In a cephalic presentation, palpation of the lower fundus reveals a firm, round head.
CN: Health promotion and maintenance; CNS: None; CL: Application

27. 4. A sterile speculum examination is performed to identify ruptured membranes. Confirmation is done with Nitrazine paper and a positive ferning test. With premature rupture of membranes in a client under 37 weeks' gestation, cervical examinations are contraindicated to reduce the incidence of infection. Clean catch urine specimens, not catheterized specimens, would be appropriate to rule out infection. The client should ambulate only after a thorough nursing assessment and examination to determine the safety of walking for the client and fetus.
CN: Physiological integrity; CNS: Reduction of risk potential; CL: Application

28. 1. Braxton Hicks contractions begin and remain irregular. They're felt in the abdomen and remain confined to the abdomen and groin. They commonly disappear with ambulation. True contractions begin irregularly but become regular and predictable increasing in frequency and intensity, causing cervical effacement and dilation. True contractions are felt initially in the lower back and radiate to the abdomen in a wavelike motion.
CN: Physiological integrity; CNS: Physiological adaptation; CL: Analysis

29. While in the first stages of labor, a client with active genital herpes is admitted to the labor-and-delivery area. Which type of birth should the nurse anticipate for this client?
1. Midforceps
2. Low forceps
3. Induction
4. Cesarean

30. A nurse is monitoring a client in labor and notes on the external fetal monitor that the fetal heart rate (FHR) drops with the start of each contraction. What is the priority action by the nurse?
1. Turn the client to the left side.
2. Continue to observe FHR.
3. Administer oxygen by face mask.
4. Place the client in Trendelenburg position.

31. The nurse is teaching the stages of labor to a 26-year-old pregnant client. The client would demonstrate that teaching has been effective when she states that crowning occurs during which stage of labor?
1. First
2. Second
3. Third
4. Fourth

32. A nurse suspects that the laboring client may have been physically abused by her male partner. What is the <u>most appropriate</u> intervention by the nurse?
1. Confront the male partner.
2. Question the woman in front of her partner.
3. Contact hospital security.
4. Collaborate with the interprofessional team, including the physician, to make a referral to social services.

Would you like to know when my crowning took place?

Did you notice the words *most appropriate* in question 32? Another hint!

29. 4. For a client with active genital herpes, cesarean delivery helps avoid infection transmission to the neonate, which could occur during a vaginal birth. Midforceps and low forceps are types of vaginal births that could transmit the herpes infection to the neonate. Induction is used only during vaginal birth; therefore, it's inappropriate for this client.
CN: Physiological integrity; CNS: Reduction of risk potential; CL: Application

30. 2. Decelerations in FHR, called early decelerations, occur with the onset of uterine contractions. They're caused by head compression during the contraction and aren't a sign of fetal distress. Therefore, no action is necessary, and the nurse should continue to monitor the FHR.
CN: Physiological integrity; CNS: Reduction of risk potential; CL: Application

31. 2. The second stage of labor begins at full cervical dilation (10 cm) and ends when the infant is born. Crowning is present during this stage as the fetal head, pushed against the perineum, causes the vaginal introitus to open, allowing the fetal scalp to be visible. The first stage begins with true labor contractions and ends with complete cervical dilation. The third stage is from the time the infant is born until the delivery of the placenta. The fourth stage is the first 1 to 4 hours following delivery of the placenta.
CN: Health promotion and maintenance; CNS: None; CL: Application

32. 4. Collaborating with others in the health care team and the physician to make a referral to social services will create a plan and provide support for the client. Additionally, by law, the nurse or nursing supervisor must report the suspected abuse to the police and follow up with a written report. Although confrontation can be used therapeutically, this action will most likely provoke anger in the suspected abuser. Questioning the woman in front of her partner doesn't allow her the privacy required to address this issue and may place her in greater danger. If the woman isn't in imminent danger, there's no need to call hospital security.
CN: Physiological integrity; CNS: Reduction of risk potential; CL: Analysis

CN: Client needs category   CNS: Client needs subcategory   CL: Cognitive level

33. During a vaginal examination of a client in labor, it is determined that the biparietal diameter of the fetal head has reached the level of the ischial spines. What is the <u>most accurate</u> documentation of this fetal station?
1. −1
2. 0
3. +1
4. +2

34. A client who developed diabetes mellitus during the pregnancy has just been admitted in the labor-and-delivery unit by the nurse. It is most important for the nurse to do what?
1. Ask the client about her most recent blood glucose levels.
2. Prepare oral hypoglycemic medications for administration during labor.
3. Notify the neonatal intensive care unit that a client with diabetes has been admitted.
4. Prepare the client for cesarean delivery.

35. A client is admitted to the labor-and-delivery unit with a known anencephalic fetus. What is the most appropriate intervention by the nurse?
1. Assess fetal heart tones.
2. Reassure the client that she'll get pregnant again soon.
3. Avoid talking about the baby.
4. Provide privacy.

36. A 30-year-old multiparous client admitted to the labor-and-delivery unit has not received prenatal care for this pregnancy. What is the most important data for the nurse to obtain?
1. Date of last menstrual period (LMP)
2. Family history of sexually transmitted diseases (STDs)
3. Name of insurance provider
4. Number of siblings

The words *most accurate* help clarify the correct answer.

The estimated date of delivery can be determined with the proper information.

33. 2. When the largest diameter of the presenting part (typically the biparietal diameter of the fetal head) is level with the ischial spines, the fetus is at station 0. A station of −1 indicates that the fetal head is 1 cm above the ischial spines. At +1, it's 1 cm below the ischial spines. At +2, it's 2 cm below the ischial spines.
CN: Health promotion and maintenance; CNS: None; CL: Application

34. 1. As part of the history, asking about the client's most recent blood glucose levels will indicate how well her diabetes has been controlled. Oral hypoglycemic drugs are never used during pregnancy because they cross the placental barrier, stimulate fetal insulin production, and are potentially teratogenic. Plans to admit the infant to the neonatal intensive care unit are premature. Cesarean delivery is no longer the preferred delivery for clients with diabetes. Vaginal birth is preferred and presents a lower risk to the mother and fetus.
CN: Physiological integrity; CNS: Reduction of risk potential; CL: Application

35. 4. Providing privacy is an appropriate therapeutic intervention for the client and family to grieve their loss. Fetal heart tones are rarely assessed in a client with an anencephalic fetus; most fetuses won't survive due to lack of cerebral function. Reassuring the client that she will get pregnant again dismisses how she is feeling about her current loss and also provides false reassurance. The nurse should take the lead from the client and family as some people want to talk about their loss and others don't.
CN: Psychosocial integrity; CNS: None; CL: Application

36. 1. The date of the LMP is essential to estimate the date of delivery. The nursing history would also include subjective information, such as personal (but not necessarily family) history of STDs, gravidity, and parity. Although beneficial to the hospital for financial reimbursement, the insurance provider has no bearing on the nursing history. Likewise, the number of siblings isn't pertinent to the assessment.
CN: Health promotion and maintenance; CNS: None; CL: Analysis

37. The nurse is caring for a laboring client who developed hypertension of pregnancy. The nurse is concerned when the client displays which finding?
1. Decreasing blood pressure
2. Increasing oliguria
3. Decreasing edema
4. Trace levels of protein in the urine

38. While performing a cervical examination, a nurse's fingertips feel pulsating tissue. What would be the most appropriate nursing intervention?
1. Leave the client and call the physician.
2. Put the client in a semi-Fowler's position.
3. Ask the client to push with the next contraction.
4. Leave the fingers in place and press the nurse call light.

39. A client is admitted to the labor-and-delivery unit in labor, with blood flowing down her legs. Which nursing intervention would be <u>most appropriate</u>?
1. Place an indwelling catheter.
2. Monitor fetal heart tones.
3. Perform a cervical examination.
4. Prepare the client for cesarean delivery.

Question 39 is asking you to prioritize!

37. 2. Renal plasma flow and glomerular filtration are decreased in gestational hypertension, so increasing oliguria indicates a worsening condition. Blood pressure increases (not decreases) as a result of increased peripheral resistance. Increasing (not decreasing) edema would suggest a worsening condition. Trace levels to +1 proteinuria are acceptable levels. Higher levels would indicate a worsening condition.
CN: Health promotion and maintenance; CNS: None; CL: Application

38. 4. When the umbilical cord precedes the fetal presenting part, it's known as a prolapsed cord. Leaving the fingers in place and calling for assistance is the safest intervention for the fetus, as you'll need to keep the fetus off the cord to reduce cord compression. The nursing staff will contact the physician, and the client will probably need a cesarean delivery because of the risk of fetal demise with the fetus pressing against the cord during delivery. Placing the client in the semi-Fowler's position would increase the pressure of the fetus on the umbilical cord. Asking the client to push with the next contraction would be contraindicated, as it would also force the presenting part against the cord, causing severe bradycardia and possible fetal demise.
CN: Physiological integrity; CNS: Reduction of risk potential; CL: Application

39. 2. Monitoring fetal heart tones would be the first step because it's necessary to establish fetal well-being due to a possible placenta previa or abruptio placentae. Although an indwelling catheter may be placed, it isn't an early intervention. Performing a cervical examination would be contraindicated because any agitation of the cervix with a previa can result in hemorrhage and death for the mother or fetus. Preparing the client for a cesarean delivery may not be indicated. A sonogram will need to be performed to determine the cause of bleeding. If the diagnosis is a partial placenta previa, the client may still be able to deliver vaginally.
CN: Physiological integrity; CNS: Reduction of risk potential; CL: Application

40. A client in labor is receiving magnesium sulfate to treat hypertension of pregnancy. How should this drug be administered?
   1. As a loading dose of 4 g in normal saline solution, followed by a continuous infusion of 1 to 2 g/hour
   2. As a loading dose of 2 g in normal saline solution, followed by a continuous infusion of 2 g/hour
   3. As a loading dose of 4 g in dextrose 5% in water (D5W), followed by a continuous infusion of 1 to 2 g/hour
   4. As a loading dose of 4 g in D5W, followed by a continuous infusion of 4 g/hour

41. A multiparous client who has been in labor for 2 hours states that she feels the urge to move her bowels. How should the nurse respond?
   1. Let the client get up to use the toilet.
   2. Allow the client to use a bedpan.
   3. Perform a pelvic examination.
   4. Check the fetal heart rate (FHR).

You're really "delivering" the right answers. Keep going!

42. The physician has ordered an I.V. of 5% dextrose in lactated Ringer's solution at 125 ml/hour. The I.V. tubing delivers 10 drops per ml. How many drops per minute should fall into the drip chamber?
   1. 10 to 11
   2. 12 to 13
   3. 20 to 21
   4. 22 to 24

43. An amniotomy is performed on a client in labor. Following this procedure, what is the priority nursing intervention?
   1. Encourage the client to use breathing exercises as contractions increase.
   2. Assess fetal heart tones.
   3. Assist the client to ambulate to promote labor.
   4. Position the client on her left side.

Your math skills are being tested on this one! You can do it!

40. 3. A loading dose of magnesium sulfate should be given as a 4-g bolus, followed by a continuous infusion of 1 to 2 g/hour in D5W for maintenance. Magnesium sulfate shouldn't be administered in normal saline solution.

CN: Physiological integrity; CNS: Pharmacological and parenteral therapies; CL: Application

41. 3. A complaint of rectal pressure usually indicates a low presenting fetal part, signaling imminent delivery. The nurse should perform a pelvic examination to assess the dilation of the cervix and station of the presenting fetal part. Don't let the client use the toilet or a bedpan before she's examined because she could deliver on the toilet or in the bedpan. Checking the FHR is important but comes after the nurse evaluates the client's complaint.

CN: Health promotion and maintenance; CNS: None; CL: Application

42. 3. Multiply the number of milliliters to be infused (125) by the drop factor (10); $125 \times 10 = 1{,}250$. Then divide the answer by the number of minutes to run the infusion (60); $1{,}250/60 = 20.83$, or 20 to 21 gtt/minute.

CN: Physiological integrity; CNS: Pharmacological and parenteral therapies; CL: Application

43. 2. The nurse's priority is to assess fetal heart tones. When the amniotic membrane is ruptured, the umbilical cord may enter the birth canal with the gush of fluid and the presenting part may cause cord compression. After amniotomy, contractions may intensify; however, helping the client with her breathing should be done after fetal well-being is assessed. Ambulation may also promote labor but should only be done after fetal well-being is established. While the left lateral position enhances blood flow, it isn't a priority until fetal heart tones are assessed.

CN: Physiological integrity; CNS: Reduction of risk potential; CL: Application

44. The effectiveness of drug therapy for a client at 34 weeks' gestation with hypertension of pregnancy can be determined by which finding?
  1. Absence of seizures
  2. Weight gain of 4 lb (1.8 kg)/week
  3. Blood pressure of 154/90 mm Hg
  4. Urinary output of 25 ml/hour

45. A laboring client in the latent stage of labor begins complaining of pain in the epigastric area, blurred vision, and a headache. The nurse knows that which medication should be prepared for administration?
  1. Terbutaline
  2. Oxytocin (Pitocin)
  3. Magnesium sulfate
  4. Calcium gluconate

46. A nurse is assisting in monitoring a client in labor. Which monitoring data are indicative of fetal well-being?
  1. Fetal heart rate of 145 to 155 beats/minute with 15-second accelerations to 160
  2. Fetal heart rate of 130 to 140 beats/minute with late decelerations to 110
  3. Fetal heart rate of 110 to 120 beats/minute with variable deceleration to 90
  4. Fetal heart rate of 165 to 175 beats/minute with late decelerations to 140

47. A nurse is examining a client in active labor who has had spontaneous rupture of the amniotic membrane and notes a protruding umbilical cord. What is the priority nursing action the nurse should take?
  1. Push the umbilical cord into the uterus.
  2. Place the client in Trendelenburg position.
  3. Instruct the client to begin to push.
  4. Wrap the cord in a dry sterile dressing.

It's important to know how to measure a drug's effectiveness.

Remembering when different decelerations occur is important!

44. 1. Therapeutic effects of drugs used to treat hypertension of pregnancy in a client at 34 weeks' gestation, such as magnesium sulfate, include an absence of seizures, a weight gain of 2 lb (0.9 kg)/week, a normal blood pressure, and a urinary output greater than 30 ml/hour.
CN: Physiological integrity; CNS: Pharmacological and parenteral therapies; CL: Analysis

45. 3. Magnesium sulfate is the drug of choice to treat hypertension of pregnancy because it reduces edema by causing a shift from the extracellular spaces into the intestines. It also depresses the central nervous system, which decreases the incidence of seizures. Terbutaline is a smoothmuscle relaxant used to relax the uterus. Oxytocin is the synthetic form of the pituitary hormone used to stimulate uterine contractions. Calcium gluconate is the antagonist for magnesium toxicity.
CN: Physiological integrity; CNS: Pharmacological and parenteral therapies; CL: Analysis

46. 1. Accelerations of up to 15 beats/minute above baseline for a duration of 15 seconds are signs of fetal well-being. Decelerations initiated 30 to 40 seconds after the onset of the contraction are termed late decelerations and are due to uteroplacental insufficiency from decreased blood flow during uterine contractions. Variable decelerations are an indication of cord compression. Variable decelerations can occur with or without contractions.
CN: Physiological integrity; CNS: Physiological adaptation; CL: Analysis

47. 2. A Trendelenburg or knee-chest position takes the weight of the fetus off the umbilical cord, allowing blood to flow. The cord should never be pushed back into the uterus, as this could damage the cord, obstruct the flow of blood through the cord to the fetus, or introduce infection into the uterus. The client shouldn't be instructed to push as she is only in active labor and emergency surgery may be necessary. The cord should be wrapped in a sterile saline–soaked gauze.
CN: Physiological integrity; CNS: Reduction of risk potential; CL: Application

48. The first day of a client's last menstrual period (LMP) was October 10. Using Nägele's rule, what is the estimated date of delivery?
1. July 10
2. July 17
3. August 10
4. August 17

49. At 1 minute of life, a neonate is crying vigorously, has a heart rate of 98, is active with normal reflexes, and has a pink body and blue extremities. Which Apgar score would be correct for this neonate?
1. 6
2. 7
3. 8
4. 9

50. A client in labor suddenly sits upright, clutches her chest, and gasps for breath. Which laboratory finding indicates that the client's condition is worsening?
1. Increased fibrinogen level
2. Increased platelet count
3. Prolonged prothrombin time
4. Reduced partial thromboplastin time

51. Immediately after delivery, a nurse assesses the neonate's respiratory effort as slow. The neonate is actively moving but grimaces in response to stimulation. His fingers and toes are bluish, and his heart rate is 130 beats/minute. Which step should the nurse take next?
1. Tell the physician that the neonate appears abnormal.
2. Assign an Apgar score of 8.
3. Assign an Apgar score of 10.
4. Provide oxygen and stimulate the baby to cry.

Can you figure out this little one's estimated time of arrival?

48. 2. After determining the first day of the LMP, the nurse would subtract 3 months and add 7 days. If the client's LMP was October 10, subtracting 3 months is July 10, and adding 7 days brings the date to July 17.
CN: Health promotion and maintenance; CNS: None; CL: Analysis

49. 3. Heart rate, respiratory effort, muscle tone, reflex irritability, and color are used to assess the Apgar score. Each of the signs is assigned a score of 0, 1, or 2. The highest possible score is 10. This neonate lost 1 point for a heart rate less than 100 beats/minute and 1 point for its acrocyanosis, a common finding in which the trunk is pink but the extremities are bluish.
CN: Health promotion and maintenance; CNS: None; CL: Analysis

50. 3. The client most likely has an amniotic fluid embolism. Disseminated intravascular coagulation is a life-threatening complication of this condition and is marked by a decreased platelet count and fibrinogen level and a prolonged prothrombin time and partial thromboplastin time.
CN: Physiological integrity; CNS: Reduction of risk potential; CL: Analysis

51. 4. The nurse should stimulate the baby to cry, provide oxygen, and call the physician to evaluate reflex irritability. It would be inappropriate to tell the physician that the neonate appears abnormal. The neonate's Apgar score is 7. Of a maximum possible score of 10, the nurse deducts 1 point for acrocyanosis, 1 point for slow respiratory effort, and 1 point for the grimace (indicating reflex irritability).
CN: Safe, effective care environment; CNS: Management of care; CL: Application

52. A pregnant client has a total hemoglobin level of 9 g/dl. Which risk is <u>greatest</u> during the intrapartum period?
1. Small-for-gestational-age neonate
2. Fetal distress
3. Excessive postpartum bleeding
4. Shortness of breath

What do you think is the greatest risk?

52. 2. Fetal distress is more common in women with anemia than in the general nonanemic population. A small-for-gestational-age neonate and excessive postpartum bleeding are diagnosed after the intrapartum period. Shortness of breath occurs more commonly antepartally; the risk for developing shortness of breath doesn't increase during the intrapartum period.

CN: Physiological integrity; CNS: Reduction of risk potential; CL: Application

53. Which is the <u>most common</u> and popular method for assessing fetal status throughout labor?
1. Fetal heart rate (FHR) auscultation using a stethoscope
2. FHR auscultation and recording using electronic fetal monitoring
3. Asking the client how she feels and whether the fetus is moving
4. Doing pelvic examinations to check the location of the fetal presenting part

53. 2. The most common and popular method for fetal assessment throughout labor is electronic monitoring, which records the FHR and maternal contractions and shows how the fetus reacts to the stress of contractions. Although FHR auscultation can be done with a stethoscope, it's less common because it requires advanced skills. Asking the client how she feels and whether the fetus is moving are important but don't provide specifics about fetal well-being. A pelvic examination reveals cervical dilation and fetal station but doesn't reveal fetal well-being.

CN: Health promotion and maintenance; CNS: None; CL: Analysis

54. Which finding in a client who is at 36 weeks' gestation indicates that premature rupture of the membranes has occurred?
1. Fernlike pattern when vaginal fluid dries on a glass slide.
2. Nitrogen paper indicates acidic pH of fluid.
3. Cervical dilation of 8 cm
4. Contractions occurring every 3 minutes

There are three main fetal presentations: cephalic, breech, and shoulder.

54. 1. A fernlike pattern that forms when vaginal fluid is dried on a glass slide is a sign of ruptured membranes. Amniotic fluid is alkaline when tested with nitrogen paper. Cervical dilation and length of contractions don't indicate the condition of the membranes.

CN: Physiological integrity; CNS: Reduction of risk potential; CL: Application

55. The nurse is teaching an intrapartum client about fetal presentation. Which statement about fetal presentation would be the most accurate?
1. Fetal body part that enters the maternal pelvis first
2. Relationship of the presenting part to the maternal pelvis
3. Relationship of the long axis of the fetus to the long axis of the mother
4. A classification according to the fetal part

55. 1. Presentation is the fetal body part that enters the pelvis first; it's classified by the presenting part; the three main presentations are cephalic, breech, and shoulder. The relationship of the presenting fetal part to the maternal pelvis refers to fetal position. The relationship of the long axis of the fetus to the long axis of the mother refers to fetal lie; the three possible lies are longitudinal, transverse, and oblique.

CN: Physiological integrity; CNS: Physiological adaptation; CL: Application

56. A client with gestational diabetes has just delivered a 10-lb, 2-oz neonate at 39 weeks' gestation. Which priority nursing intervention should be included in the care plan?
1. Teach the mother about the nutritional needs of the neonate.
2. Obtain a serum neonatal glucose level.
3. Obtain a serum neonatal bilirubin level.
4. Prepare to administer insulin to the neonate.

56. 2. The priority nursing intervention is to monitor the neonate's serum glucose level due to the increased risk of hypoglycemia. During pregnancy, the fetus secretes high levels of insulin to counteract the high maternal glucose levels. This elevated insulin secretion in the neonate can lead to severe hypoglycemia after birth. While it is important to discuss the neonate's nutritional needs with the mother, it isn't an immediate priority. The newborn of a mother with diabetes may develop hyperbilirubinemia but not as quickly as hypoglycemia may develop. Since the neonate is at risk for hypoglycemia, insulin wouldn't be appropriate.
CN: Safe, effective care environment; CNS: Management of care; CL: Application

57. The nurse is caring for a client in labor. Which components of labor contractions would be the most accurate for the nurse to assess with this client?
1. Pelvic type, duration, and frequency
2. Contraction type and frequency and pelvic type
3. Contraction duration, frequency, and intensity
4. Contraction type, duration, and intensity

57. 3. The three components of a contraction that the nurse must evaluate are the duration, frequency, and intensity of each contraction. Pelvic type has no bearing on contractions.
CN: Health promotion and maintenance; CNS: None; CL: Application

The Lamaze method of prepared childbirth uses breathing techniques to ease delivery.

58. A client in labor is using the Lamaze method of prepared childbirth. Her cervix is dilated 5 cm, with contractions occurring 2 to 3 minutes apart. The nurse should instruct the client to breathe at which level?
1. Level 1
2. Level 2
3. Level 3
4. Level 4

58. 2. Level 2 breathing techniques are useful when cervical dilation is between 4 and 6 cm. Level 1 breathing techniques are useful for early contractions; level 3 and level 4 breathing techniques are used in the transition stage of labor.
CN: Health promotion and maintenance; CNS: None; CL: Application

59. A client has received dinoprostone (Prostin E2) for cervical ripening. It is most important for the nurse to assess the client for which of the following?
1. Vomiting
2. Euphoria
3. Uterine inversion
4. Constipation

59. 1. Headache, nausea and vomiting, chills, fever, and hypertension are adverse effects of dinoprostone. Euphoria and uterine inversion are rare adverse effects of this drug. Diarrhea, not constipation, is a possible adverse effect.
CN: Physiological integrity; CNS: Pharmacological and parenteral therapies; CL: Analysis

60. A nurse is caring for a client with short, mild contractions and cervical dilation of 4 cm. Using an external fetal monitor, the nurse observes variable decelerations. Which action should the nurse take first?
1. Prepare for imminent delivery.
2. Place the client on her left side.
3. Administer oxygen by face mask.
4. Prepare the client for a stillbirth.

61. At 39 weeks' gestation, a primiparous client arrives at the labor-and-delivery unit complaining of lower back pain that started 6 hours ago. A pelvic examination reveals that her cervix is dilated 3 cm and 75% effaced. Which action would be appropriate for the nurse to take?
1. Instruct the client to push.
2. Determine the Apgar score.
3. Monitor the fetal heart rate.
4. Assess the lochia.

62. A nurse is assisting in monitoring a client who's receiving oxytocin (Pitocin) to induce labor. The nurse should be alert to which maternal adverse reactions? Select all that apply.
1. Hypertension
2. Jaundice
3. Dehydration
4. Fluid overload
5. Uterine tetany
6. Bradycardia

Don't give up now. Only three questions left!

63. A client is admitted to the labor-and-delivery unit at 36 weeks' gestation. She has a history of cesarean delivery and complains of severe abdominal pain that started less than 1 hour earlier. When the nurse palpates tetanic contractions, the client again complains of severe pain. After the client vomits, she states that the pain is better and then passes out. Which nursing intervention takes the highest priority?
1. Assess the client's level of pain.
2. Place the client in a left lateral position.
3. Administer I.V. antibiotics.
4. Prepare the client for immediate surgery.

Keep up the good work!

60. 2. Variable decelerations in fetal heart rate are caused by compression of the umbilical cord. Typically, variable decelerations are corrected by placing the client in a left lateral position to alleviate cord pressure. Since variable decelerations are usually transient and correctable, the nurse wouldn't prepare for an imminent or stillbirth. If other measures have been ineffective in correcting the variable deceleration, oxygen may be administered.

CN: Physiological integrity; CNS: Reduction of risk potential; CL: Analysis

61. 3. This client is in the latent phase of the first stage of labor. The nurse should monitor the fetal heart in this stage and all stages of labor. Pushing is appropriate during the second stage of labor when the cervix is fully dilated. The nurse determines the Apgar score on the neonate immediately after delivery. During the fourth stage, the nurse assesses the amount, color, and consistency of lochia.

CN: Health promotion and maintenance; CNS: None; CL: Application

62. 1, 4, and 5. Adverse effects of oxytocin in the mother include hypertension, fluid overload, and uterine tetany. Oxytocin's antidiuretic effect increases renal reabsorption of water, leading to fluid overload, not dehydration. Jaundice and bradycardia are adverse effects that may occur in the neonate. Tachycardia, not bradycardia, is a maternal adverse effect.

CN: Physiological integrity; CNS: Pharmacology and parenteral therapies; CL: Application

63. 4. Uterine rupture is a medical emergency that may occur before or during labor. Signs and symptoms typically include abdominal pain that may ease after uterine rupture, vomiting, vaginal bleeding, hypovolemic shock, and fetal distress. The client should be prepared for immediate surgery to save her life and that of the fetus. While assessing and relieving pain are important interventions, they aren't priorities in this life-threatening situation. Placing the client in a left lateral position won't affect her condition. Antibiotics may be administered but aren't the highest priority in this situation.

CN: Safe, effective care environment; CNS: Management of care; CL: Application

64. Which illustration represents a right occiput posterior (ROP) fetal position?

1.

2.

3.

4.

65. The nurse is evaluating an external fetal monitoring strip of a client in labor. What condition is the nurse concerned about?
1. Cephalopelvic disproportion
2. Oligohydramnios
3. Uteroplacental insufficiency
4. Hydramnios

64. 1. Fetal positioning is determined by how the fetus presents in relation to the mother's pelvis, which is divided into four quadrants: right anterior, left anterior, right posterior, and left posterior. In a ROP position, the fetus' occiput points to the maternal right posterior quadrant. Option 2 shows a right occiput anterior (ROA) position, option 3 shows a left occiput posterior (LOP), and option 4 shows a left occiput anterior (LOA).

CN: Health promotion and maintenance; CNS: None; CL: Application

65. 3. This fetal monitoring strip illustrates a late deceleration. The decrease in fetal heart rate begins after the peak of the contraction and doesn't return to baseline until the contraction is over. Late decelerations are associated with uteroplacental insufficiency, shock, or fetal metabolic acidosis. Cephalopelvic disproportion may cause early, not late, decelerations early in labor. Oligohydramnios (less than the normal amount of amniotic fluid) may be associated with variable decelerations. Hydramnios (excessive amniotic fluid) may be associated with uterine rupture.

CN: Physiological integrity; CNS: Reduction of risk potential; CL: Analysis

1. When completing the morning postpartum assessment, a nurse notices a client's perineal pad is completely saturated with lochia rubra. What is the <u>priority</u> action of the nurse?
  1. Vigorously massage the fundus.
  2. Immediately call the physician.
  3. Have the charge nurse review the assessment.
  4. Ask the client when she last changed her perineal pad.

Question 1 is asking you what to do first! What a way to start!

2. A postpartum mother asks the nurse what would cause a decreased supply of breast milk. What is the best response by the nurse?
  1. Supplemental feedings with formula
  2. Maternal diet high in vitamin C
  3. An alcoholic drink
  4. Frequent feedings

Which of these options would promote comfort best?

3. A breastfeeding mother is experiencing engorged breasts and asks the nurse if there is anything she can do to get relief. What is the best intervention for the nurse to implement?
  1. Applying ice
  2. Applying a breast binder
  3. Teaching the client how to express her breasts in a warm shower
  4. Administering bromocriptine (Parlodel)

1. 4. If the morning assessment is done relatively early, it's possible that the client hasn't yet been to the bathroom, in which case her perineal pad may have been in place all night. Secondly, her lochia may have pooled during the night, resulting in a heavy flow in the morning. Vigorous massage of the fundus isn't recommended for heavy bleeding or hemorrhage. The nurse wouldn't want to call the physician unnecessarily. If the nurse were uncertain, it would be appropriate to have another qualified individual check the client but only after a complete assessment of the client's status.
CN: Safe, effective care environment; CNS: Management of care; CL: Analysis

2. 1. Routine formula supplementation may interfere with establishing an adequate milk volume because suckling by the baby at the breast stimulates prolactin production, the hormone responsible for milk production. Vitamin C levels haven't been shown to influence milk volume. One drink containing alcohol generally tends to relax the mother, facilitating letdown. Excessive consumption of alcohol may block letdown of milk to the infant, although supply isn't necessarily affected. Frequent feedings are likely to increase milk production.
CN: Health promotion and maintenance; CNS: None; CL: Application

3. 3. Teaching the client how to express her breasts in a warm shower aids with letdown and will give temporary relief. Ice can promote comfort by decreasing blood flow (vasoconstriction), numbing, and discouraging further letdown of milk; however, this is followed by a rebound reaction of more letting down once the ice is removed. Breast binders aren't effective in relieving the discomforts of engorgement. Bromocriptine is no longer indicated for lactation suppression.
CN: Physiological integrity; CNS: Basic care and comfort; CL: Application

4. A new graduate nurse is being oriented to the care of clients on a postpartum unit. The preceptor explains that routine assessment includes which of the following?
1. Antibody screen
2. Babinski's reflex
3. Homans' sign
4. Patellar reflex

5. A nurse determines that teaching about Kegel exercises has been effective when the client makes which statement?
1. "They assist with lochia removal."
2. "They promote the return of normal bowel function."
3. "They promote blood flow, allowing for healing and strengthening the musculature."
4. "They assist the woman in burning calories for rapid postpartum weight loss."

6. To detect pulmonary embolus in a client in the immediate postpartum period, a nurse should be alert to which symptoms?
1. Sudden dyspnea and chest pain
2. Chills and fever
3. Bradycardia and hypertension
4. Confusion and bradypnea

7. The nurse is preparing a plan of care for a client who has had a cesarean delivery. What is the most important intervention for the nurse to include?
1. Frequent douching after she's discharged
2. Coughing and deep-breathing exercises
3. Sit-ups at 2 weeks postoperatively
4. Side-rolling exercises

If you know what Kegel exercises are, you should get question 5 correct easily.

4. 3. Homans' sign, or pain on dorsiflexion of the foot, may indicate deep vein thrombosis (DVT). Postpartum women are at increased risk of DVT because of changes in clotting mechanisms to control bleeding at delivery. An antibody screen wouldn't be classified as an assessment technique. Both Babinski's reflex and the patellar reflex need not be routinely assessed in the postpartum woman.
CN: Health promotion and maintenance; CNS: None; CL: Analysis

5. 3. Exercising the pubococcygeal muscle increases blood flow to the area. The increased blood flow brings oxygen and other nutrients to the perineal area to aid in healing. Additionally, these exercises help to strengthen the musculature, thereby decreasing the risk of future complications, such as incontinence and uterine prolapse. Performing Kegel exercises may assist with lochia removal, but that isn't their main purpose. Bowel function isn't influenced by Kegel exercises. Kegel exercises don't expend sufficient energy to burn many calories.
CN: Health promotion and maintenance; CNS: None; CL: Analysis

6. 1. Signs of pulmonary embolus include sudden dyspnea and chest pain. Chills and fever signal an infection. The client with a pulmonary embolus would have tachycardia, hypotension, confusion, and tachypnea.
CN: Physiological integrity; CNS: Reduction of risk potential; CL: Analysis

7. 2. As for any postoperative client, coughing and deep-breathing exercises should be taught to keep the alveoli open and prevent infection. Frequent douching isn't recommended for women and is contraindicated in women who have just given birth. Sit-ups at 2 weeks postpartum could potentially damage the healing of the incision. Side-rolling exercises aren't an accepted medical practice.
CN: Physiological integrity; CNS: Reduction of risk potential; CL: Application

8. A student nurse asks why a client would express disappointment after having a cesarean delivery instead of a vaginal delivery. What is the best response by the nurse?
1. "Cesarean deliveries cost more."
2. "Depression is more common after a cesarean delivery."
3. "The client is usually more fatigued after cesarean delivery."
4. "The client may feel a loss for not having experienced a 'normal' birth."

Remember to be sensitive to your postpartum client's needs.

9. The nurse reviews the assessment findings of a postpartum client who has experienced a vaginal birth. The nurse determines that which finding is normal?
1. Redness or swelling in the calves
2. A palpable uterine fundus beyond 10 days postpartum
3. Vaginal dryness after the lochial flow has ended
4. Dark red lochia for approximately 6 weeks after the birth

10. On completing a fundal assessment, the nurse notes the fundus is situated on the client's left abdomen. Which action is appropriate?
1. Ask the client to empty her bladder.
2. Straight catheterize the client immediately.
3. Call the client's primary health care provider for direction.
4. Straight catheterize the client for half of her urine volume.

Make sure a client with HIV is aware of the risks of breastfeeding.

11. A client who is positive for human immunodeficiency virus (HIV) tells a nurse she would like to breastfeed. Which is the best response by the nurse?
1. "Breastfeeding will help reduce the risk of hemorrhage."
2. "Breast milk is better than formula for the baby."
3. "Breastfeeding will help with bonding."
4. "Breast milk can transmit HIV to the baby."

8. 4. Clients occasionally feel a loss after a cesarean delivery especially if it was unplanned. They may feel they're inadequate because they couldn't deliver their infant vaginally. The cost of cesarean delivery doesn't generally apply because the woman isn't directly responsible for payment. No conclusive studies support the theory that depression is more common after cesarean delivery when compared to vaginal delivery. Although clients are usually more fatigued after a cesarean delivery, fatigue hasn't been shown to cause feelings of disappointment over the method of delivery.
CN: Psychosocial integrity; CNS: None; CL: Analysis

9. 3. Vaginal dryness is a normal finding during the postpartum period due to hormonal changes. Redness or swelling in the calves may indicate thrombophlebitis. The fundus shouldn't be palpable beyond 10 days. Dark red lochia (indicating fresh bleeding) should only last 2 to 3 days postpartum.
CN: Health promotion and maintenance; CNS: None; CL: Application

10. 1. A full bladder may displace the uterine fundus to the left or right side of the abdomen. A straight catheterization is unnecessarily invasive if the woman can urinate on her own. Nursing interventions should be completed before notifying the primary health care provider in a nonemergency situation.
CN: Physiological integrity; CNS: Reduction of risk potential; CL: Application

11. 4. Since HIV can be transmitted to the baby through breast milk, the client shouldn't breastfeed. Breastfeeding does stimulate uterine contractions, but in this case, breastfeeding should be discouraged. It wouldn't be appropriate to tell a client who shouldn't breastfeed that breast milk is best for the baby. In this case, formula is best. The client should be shown other ways to bond with her baby, such as holding, playing, and talking to the baby.
CN: Physiologic integrity; CNS: Reduction of risk potential; CL: Analysis

12. A client had a spontaneous vaginal delivery after 18 hours of labor. Her excessive vaginal bleeding has now become a postpartum hemorrhage. <u>Immediate</u> nursing care of this client should include which intervention?
1. Avoiding massaging the uterus
2. Monitoring vital signs every hour
3. Placing the client in Trendelenburg's position
4. Elevating the head of the bed to increase blood flow

This question requires your immediate attention.

13. A nurse is assessing a client with type 1 diabetes mellitus whose delivery was complicated by polyhydramnios and macrosomia. The nurse is aware that this client is at risk for which of the following?
1. Postpartum mastitis
2. Increased insulin needs
3. Postpartum hemorrhage
4. Gestational hypertension

14. The nurse is caring for a diabetic, postpartum client who has developed an infection. The nurse is aware that infections in diabetic clients tend to be more severe and can quickly lead to complications. The nurse should assess this client for which condition?
1. Anemia
2. Ketoacidosis
3. Respiratory acidosis
4. Respiratory alkalosis

Uh oh. It's time to feed the baby again.

15. Which client action should alert a nurse to a potential problem in a client with mastitis?
1. Breastfeeding every 6 hours
2. Breastfeeding on the affected breast first
3. Increasing daily fluid intake
4. Emptying the affected breast completely with each feeding

12. 3. The client should be placed in Trendelenburg's position to prevent or control hypovolemic shock. The uterus should be palpated to determine if it's contracting and should be massaged if it's boggy or not contracting. Vital signs should be monitored continuously, or at least every 10 to 15 minutes until the client's condition stabilizes. The head of the bed should not be elevated because this will further lower the blood pressure.
CN: Safe, effective care environment; CNS: Management of care; CL: Analysis

13. 3. The client is at risk for a postpartum hemorrhage from the overdistention of the uterus because of the extra amniotic fluid and the large baby. The uterus may not be able to contract as well as it would normally. The diabetic mother usually has decreased insulin needs for the first few days postpartum. Neither polyhydramnios nor macrosomia would increase the client's risk of mastitis or gestational hypertension.
CN: Physiological integrity; CNS: Reduction of risk potential; CL: Application

14. 2. Diabetic clients who become pregnant tend to become sicker and develop illnesses quicker than pregnant women without diabetes. Severe infections in diabetes can lead to diabetic ketoacidosis. Anemia, respiratory acidosis, and respiratory alkalosis aren't generally associated with infections in diabetic clients.
CN: Physiological integrity; CNS: Reduction of risk potential; CL: Analysis

15. 1. Mastitis is an infection of the breast characterized by flulike symptoms, along with redness and tenderness in the breast. Since mastitis may be due to milk stasis, the breastfeeding client should breastfeed every 2 to 3 hours. Other measures that the client with mastitis should follow include breastfeeding on the affected side first, drinking plenty of fluids, and completely emptying the affected breast with each feeding, expressing milk by hand or using a pump, if necessary.
CN: Physiological integrity; CNS: Physiological adaptation; CL: Analysis

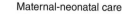

16. A nurse caring for clients on a postpartal unit is aware that a condition requiring immediate intervention would be?
1. Blood loss in excess of 200 ml, occurring 24 hours to 6 weeks after delivery
2. Blood loss in excess of 400 ml, occurring 24 hours to 6 weeks after delivery
3. Blood loss in excess of 500 ml, occurring 24 hours to 6 weeks after delivery
4. Blood loss in excess of 100 ml, occurring 24 hours to 6 weeks after delivery

17. The nurse is prioritizing care of a client in the immediate postpartum period (first 2 hours). What is the most important assessment for the nurse to perform?
1. Blood glucose level
2. Electrocardiogram (ECG)
3. Height of fundus
4. Stool test for occult blood

Question 17 requires your *immediate* attention.

18. A nurse is performing an assessment of a postpartum client 2 hours after delivery and notes heavy bleeding with large clots. What is the most appropriate initial action by the nurse?
1. Massaging the fundus firmly
2. Performing bimanual uterine compressions
3. Administering ergonovine (Ergotrate)
4. Notifying the physician

First things first! The word *initial* is a clue in this one.

19. A nurse is about to give a client with type 2 diabetes mellitus her insulin before breakfast on her first day postpartum. Which statement by the client indicates an understanding of insulin requirements immediately postpartum?
1. "I will need less insulin now than during my pregnancy."
2. "I will need more insulin now than during my pregnancy."
3. "I will need less insulin now than before I was pregnant."
4. "I will need more insulin now than before I was pregnant."

16. 3. Postpartum hemorrhage involves blood loss in excess of 500 ml. Most delayed postpartum hemorrhages occur between the fourth and ninth days postpartum. The most frequent causes of a delayed postpartum hemorrhage include retained placental fragments, intrauterine infection, and fibroids.
CN: Physiological integrity; CNS: Reduction of risk potential; CL: Application

17. 3. A focused physical assessment should be performed every 15 minutes for the first 1 to 2 hours postpartum, including assessment of the fundus, lochia, perineum, blood pressure, pulse, and bladder function. A blood glucose level needs to be obtained only if the woman has risk factors for an unstable blood glucose level or if she has symptoms of an altered blood glucose level. An ECG would be necessary only if the woman is at risk for cardiac difficulty. A stool test for occult blood generally wouldn't be valid during the immediate postpartum period; it's difficult to sort out lochial bleeding from rectal bleeding.
CN: Health promotion and maintenance; CNS: None; CL: Application

18. 1. Initial management of excessive postpartum bleeding is firm massage of the fundus along with a rapid infusion of oxytocin or lactated Ringer's solution. Bimanual compression is performed by a physician. Ergotrate should be used only if the bleeding doesn't respond to massage and oxytocin. The physician should be notified if the client doesn't respond to fundal massage, but other measures can be taken in the meantime.
CN: Safe, effective care environment; CNS: Management of care; CL: Analysis

19. 3. Postpartum insulin requirements are usually significantly lower than prepregnancy requirements. Occasionally, clients may require little to no insulin during the first 24 to 48 hours postpartum.
CN: Physiological integrity; CNS: Reduction of risk potential; CL: Analysis

20. Which assessment finding in a postpartum client requires further nursing assessment?
1. Fundus at the umbilicus 1 hour postpartum
2. Fundus 3 cm below the umbilicus on postpartum day 3
3. Fundus not palpable in the abdomen at 2 weeks postpartum
4. Fundus slightly to right; 2 cm above umbilicus on postpartum day 2

21. Which condition should the nurse look for in a client's history that may explain an increase in the severity of afterpains?
1. Bottle feeding
2. Diabetes
3. Multiple gestation
4. Primiparity

22. When giving a postpartum client self-care instructions, a nurse instructs her to report heavy or excessive bleeding. Which statement by the client indicates she understands the nurse's instructions?
1. "I will call the doctor if I saturate a pad in 1 hour or less."
2. "I will call the doctor if I partially saturate a pad in 1 hour."
3. "I will call the doctor if I saturate a pad in 4 to 6 hours."
4. "I will call the doctor if I saturate a pad in 8 hours."

23. The nurse is assessing a postpartum client who has lochia serosa. When the client asks the nurse how long to expect this type of bleeding, how should the nurse respond?
1. Days 3 to 4 postpartum
2. Days 3 to 10 postpartum
3. Days 10 to 14 postpartum
4. Days 14 to 42 postpartum

You're doing great! Keep up the good work!

Remember: There are 3 types of lochia. Which type is this question referring to?

20. 4. A uterus that isn't midline or is above the umbilicus on postpartum day 2 might be caused by a full, distended bladder or a uterine infection, requiring further assessment by the nurse. Within the first 12 hours postpartum, the fundus usually is at or below the umbilicus. The fundus should descend approximately 1 cm/day thereafter. The fundus shouldn't be palpated in the abdomen after day 10.

CN: Health promotion and maintenance; CNS: None; CL: Analysis

21. 3. Multiple gestation, breastfeeding, multiparity, and conditions that cause overdistention of the uterus will increase the intensity of afterpains. Bottle feeding and diabetes aren't directly associated with increasing severity of afterpains, unless the client has delivered a macrosomic infant.

CN: Health promotion and maintenance; CNS: None; CL: Analysis

22. 1. Bleeding is considered heavy when a woman saturates a sanitary pad in 1 hour. Excessive bleeding occurs when a postpartum client saturates a pad in 15 minutes. Moderate bleeding occurs when the bleeding saturates less than 6 in. (15 cm) of a pad in 1 hour.

CN: Health promotion and maintenance; CNS: None; CL: Application

23. 2. On the third and fourth postpartum days, the lochia becomes a pale pink or brown and contains old blood, serum, leukocytes, and tissue debris. This type of lochia usually lasts until postpartum day 10. Lochia rubra usually lasts for the first 3 to 4 days postpartum and consists of blood, decidua, and trophoblastic debris. Lochia alba, which contains leukocytes, decidua, epithelial cells, mucus, and bacteria, may continue for 2 to 6 weeks postpartum.

CN: Health promotion and maintenance; CNS: None; CL: Application

24. A client and her neonate have a blood incompatibility, and the neonate has had a positive direct Coombs' test. Which nursing intervention is appropriate?
1. Because the woman has been sensitized, give Rh₀(D) immune globulin (RhoGAM).
2. Because the woman hasn't been sensitized, give RhoGAM.
3. Because the woman has been sensitized, don't give RhoGAM.
4. Because the woman hasn't been sensitized, don't give RhoGAM.

25. The nurse is teaching a client with newly diagnosed mastitis about her condition. The client asks the nurse about what caused her to develop the condition. What is the <u>best</u> response by the nurse?
1. *Escherichia coli* (*E. coli*)
2. Group B beta-hemolytic streptococci (GBS)
3. *Staphylococcus aureus* (*S. aureus*)
4. *Staphylococcus pyogenes* (*S. pyogenes*)

26. A nurse should expect to observe which behavior in a client on the fourth postpartum day?
1. The client asks many questions about the baby's care.
2. The client wants to relate her birth experience.
3. The client asks the nurse to select her meals for her.
4. The client asks the nurse to help her bathe herself.

27. Which verbalization should be cause for concern to a nurse treating a postpartum client within a few days of delivery?
1. The client is nervous about taking the baby home.
2. The client feels empty since she delivered the baby.
3. The client would like to watch the nurse give the baby her first bath.
4. The client would like the nurse to take her baby to the nursery so she can sleep.

Blood incompatibility between a client and her neonate is serious business.

It's important to listen to the feelings and concerns of a postpartum client.

24. 3. A positive Coombs' test means that the Rh-negative woman is now producing antibodies to the Rh-positive blood of the neonate. RhoGAM shouldn't be given to a sensitized client because it won't be able to prevent antibody formation.

CN: Physiological integrity; CNS: Reduction of risk potential; CL: Analysis

25. 3. The most common cause of mastitis is *S. aureus*, transmitted from the neonate's mouth. Mastitis isn't harmful to the neonate. *E. coli*, GBS, and *S. pyogenes* aren't associated with mastitis. GBS infection is associated with neonatal sepsis and death.

CN: Health promotion and maintenance; CNS: None; CL: Analysis

26. 1. The taking-hold phase usually lasts from days 3 to 10 postpartum. During this stage, the mother strives for independence and autonomy; she also becomes curious and interested in the care of the baby and is most ready to learn. During the taking-in phase, which usually lasts 2 to 3 days, the mother is passive and dependent and expresses her own needs rather than the neonate's needs. During this taking-in phase, the client may ask the nurse to help her with self-care, wants to talk about the birth experience, and lets others make decisions for her.

CN: Psychosocial integrity; CNS: None; CL: Application

27. 2. A mother experiencing postpartum blues may say she feels empty now that the infant is no longer in her uterus. She may also verbalize that she feels unprotected now. Many first-time mothers are nervous about caring for their neonates by themselves after discharge. New mothers may want a demonstration before doing a task themselves. A client may want to get some uninterrupted sleep, so she may ask that the baby be taken to the nursery.

CN: Psychosocial integrity; CNS: None; CL: Analysis

CN: Client needs category   CNS: Client needs subcategory   CL: Cognitive level

28. During the assessment of a postpartum client, the nurse notes continuous seepage of blood from the vagina and a firm uterus 1 cm below the umbilicus. The nurse suspects that the client may have experienced which of the following?
1. Retained placental fragments
2. Urinary tract infection (UTI)
3. Cervical laceration
4. Uterine atony

29. The nurse determines further teaching is necessary when a client on anticoagulant therapy for deep vein thrombosis makes which statement?
1. "I will continue to take my iron replacement therapy."
2. "I will take aspirin for headaches."
3. "I will avoid restrictive clothing."
4. "I will report shortness of breath immediately."

30. A pregnant client is very upset when she hears that her TORCH panel has returned positive. She is distraught and says, "This means the baby has HIV!" The nurse replies that the H in TORCH represents which of the following disorders?
1. Hemophilia
2. Hepatitis B virus
3. Herpes simplex virus
4. Human immunodeficiency virus

31. The nurse is concerned that a client who experienced a perinatal loss 3 days ago may being exhibiting signs of dysfunctional grieving. It is important to assess the client for which sign?
1. Lack of appetite
2. Denial of the death
3. Blaming herself
4. Frequent crying spells

32. A nurse is assessing the fundus of a client who is 12 hours postpartum and finds that the fundus is boggy. Which action should the nurse take first?
1. Prepare the client for surgery.
2. Administer blood replacement products.
3. Massage the fundus.
4. Administer methylergonovine (Methergine), as ordered.

Why is everyone avoiding me?

A good massage is just what the doctor, or in this case the nurse, ordered.

28. 3. Continuous seepage of blood may be due to cervical or vaginal lacerations if the uterus is firm and contracting. Retained placental fragments and uterine atony may cause subinvolution of the uterus, making it soft, boggy, and larger than expected. UTI won't cause vaginal bleeding, although hematuria may be present.
CN: Physiological integrity; CNS: Reduction of risk potential; CL: Application

29. 2. Discharge teaching should include informing the client to avoid salicylates, which may potentiate the effects of anticoagulant therapy. Iron won't affect anticoagulation therapy. Restrictive clothing should be avoided to prevent the recurrence of thrombophlebitis. Shortness of breath should be reported immediately because it may be a symptom of pulmonary embolism.
CN: Physiological integrity; CNS: Reduction of risk potential; CL: Analysis

30. 3. TORCH represents the following maternal infections: **T**oxoplasmosis; **O**thers, such as gonorrhea, syphilis, varicella, hepatitis, and human immunodeficiency virus; **R**ubella; **C**ytomegalovirus; and **H**erpes simplex virus. Hemophilia is a clotting disorder in which factors VII and X are deficient.
CN: Physiological integrity; CNS: Reduction of risk potential; CL: Application

31. 2. Denial of the perinatal loss is dysfunctional grieving in the client. Lack of appetite, blaming oneself, and frequent crying spells are part of a normal grieving process.
CN: Psychosocial integrity; CNS: None; CL: Application

32. 3. The nurse should first massage the boggy uterus to stimulate it to contract. The client may need surgery but only if other measures fail to cause the uterus to contract and control bleeding. Blood replacement products may be given if the client has a significant blood loss. Methylergonovine (Methergine) may be ordered if massage fails to firm the uterus.
CN: Physiological integrity; CNS: Reduction of risk potential; CL: Analysis

33. An Rh-positive client has just delivered a 6 lb, 10 oz neonate vaginally after 17 hours of labor. What factor may place this client at risk?
1. Length of labor
2. Maternal Rh status
3. Method of delivery
4. Size of the baby

34. A nurse is caring for a breastfeeding client who delivered by cesarean section. What is the most important information for the nurse to teach the client?
1. Delay breastfeeding until 24 hours after delivery.
2. Breastfeed frequently during the day and every 4 to 6 hours at night.
3. Use the cradle hold position to avoid incisional discomfort.
4. Use the football hold position to avoid incisional discomfort.

35. Which client behavior indicates an understanding of the nurse's teaching plan for breastfeeding?
1. The client washes her nipples with soap and water.
2. The client lets her nipples air dry.
3. The client lets the baby attach to the nipple only.
4. The client pulls the baby off the nipple when feeding is done.

36. A client with mastitis tells the nurse she is concerned about breastfeeding her neonate. What is the best response by the nurse?
1. Stop breastfeeding until completing the antibiotic.
2. Supplement feeding with formula until the infection resolves.
3. Do not use analgesics because they aren't compatible with breastfeeding.
4. Continue to breastfeed; mastitis won't infect the infant.

33. 1. A prolonged length of labor places the mother at increased risk for developing an infection. The average size of the baby, vaginal delivery, and Rh status of the client do not place the mother at increased risk.
CN: Physiological integrity; CNS: Physiological adaptation; CL: Analysis

34. 4. When breastfeeding after a cesarean delivery, the client should be encouraged to use the football hold to avoid incisional discomfort. Breastfeeding should be initiated as soon after birth as possible. The mother should be encouraged to breastfeed her infant every 2 to 3 hours throughout the night as well as during the day to increase the milk supply.
CN: Health promotion and maintenance; CNS: None; CL: Analysis

35. 2. The nipples should be allowed to air dry after breastfeeding to keep them dry and prevent irritation. Only water should be used to wash the nipples since soap removes natural oils and dries out the nipples. When breastfeeding, the baby should grasp both the nipple and areola. When the baby is done with a breast, the baby's grasp on the nipple should be released before removing the baby from the breast.
CN: Health promotion and maintenance; CNS: None; CL: Application

36. 4. The client with mastitis should be encouraged to continue breastfeeding while taking antibiotics for the infection. No supplemental feedings are necessary because breastfeeding doesn't need to be altered and actually encourages resolution of the infection. Analgesics are safe and should be administered as needed.
CN: Health promotion and maintenance; CNS: None; CL: Analysis

37. The nurse is assessing a 6-week postpartum client in the obstetrician's office. In the exam room, the nurse asks the client how she's feeling. The client bursts into tears and reports she can barely get out of bed to dress, is crying most of the time, and feels like a failure. The nurse suspects the client is experiencing which condition?
1. Postpartum blues
2. Postpartum depression
3. Postpartum neurosis
4. Postpartum psychosis

I wish I didn't feel so inadequate.

38. A client who is breastfeeding reports pain, redness, and swelling in her right breast. What is the most important information for the nurse to give the client?
1. Wear a tight-fitting brassiere while breastfeeding.
2. Breastfeeding should be stopped permanently.
3. Continue antibiotic until pain, redness, and swelling subside.
4. Apply moist heat compresses to the right breast.

39. A 6-week postpartum client is being assessed by the nurse at the obstetrician's office. The nurse notes that the uterus is enlarged and soft and that the client is experiencing vaginal bleeding. The nurse suspects the client has which condition?
1. Cervical laceration
2. Clotting deficiency
3. Perineal laceration
4. Uterine subinvolution

All I did was stand up, and I'm so light-headed!

40. A client needs to void 3 hours after a vaginal delivery. Which risk factor necessitates assisting her out of bed?
1. Chest pain
2. Breast engorgement
3. Orthostatic hypotension
4. Separation of episiotomy incision

37. 2. Postpartum depression occurs in approximately 10% to 15% of all postpartum women. This depression is characterized by disabling feelings of inadequacy and an inability to cope that can last up to 3 years. The client is often tearful and despondent. The client with postpartum blues experiences crying and sadness, generally between 3 and 5 days postpartum, but this condition resolves itself quickly. Postpartum neurosis includes neurotic behavior during the initial 6 weeks after birth. Postpartum psychosis includes hallucinations, delusions, and phobias.
CN: Psychosocial integrity; CNS: None; CL: Application

38. 4. Moist heat compresses reduce inflammation and swelling of the affected area and relieve pain. The client shouldn't wear a tight or constrictive brassiere while breastfeeding to allow the milk to flow freely and empty the breast. There's no need to stop breastfeeding permanently. Antibiotics should be taken for the prescribed cause of therapy and shouldn't be stopped when symptoms subside.
CN: Health promotion and maintenance; CNS: None; CL: Application

39. 4. Late postpartum bleeding is typically the result of subinvolution of the uterus. Retained products of conception or infection often cause subinvolution. Cervical or perineal lacerations can cause an immediate postpartum hemorrhage. A client with a clotting deficiency may also have an immediate postpartum hemorrhage, if the deficiency isn't corrected at the time of delivery.
CN: Physiological integrity; CNS: Physiological adaptation; CL: Application

40. 3. The rapid decrease in intra-abdominal pressure occurring after birth causes splanchnic engorgement. The client is at risk for orthostatic hypotension when standing due to the blood pooling in this area. Breast engorgement is caused by vascular congestion in the breast before true lactation. The client shouldn't experience separation of the episiotomy incision or chest pain when standing.
CN: Health promotion and maintenance; CNS: None; CL: Analysis

41. Prior to administration of the rubella vaccine, what is the most important information for the nurse to teach the client?
1. The vaccine is safe in clients with egg allergies.
2. Breastfeeding isn't compatible with the vaccine.
3. Transient arthralgia and rash are uncommon adverse effects.
4. The client should avoid getting pregnant for 3 months after the vaccination because the vaccine has teratogenic effects.

42. The nurse is caring for a postpartum client who develops preeclampsia. Which medication should the nurse expect to administer?
1. Diazepam (Valium)
2. Hydralazine
3. Magnesium sulfate
4. Nifedipine (Procardia)

43. Which complication is associated with magnesium sulfate therapy?
1. Hypotension
2. Postpartum depression
3. Postpartum hemorrhage
4. Uterine infection

44. A nurse is reviewing the plan of care for a client with an episiotomy on the third postpartum day. It is most important for the plan to include which instruction?
1. Apply ice to the perineum.
2. Encourage the use of sitz baths.
3. Avoid tightening the pelvic muscles.
4. Massage the perineal area.

Don't lose your focus.

41. 4. The client must understand that she must not become pregnant for 2 to 3 months after the vaccination because of its potential teratogenic effects. The rubella vaccine is made from duck eggs so an allergic reaction may occur in clients with egg allergies. The virus isn't transmitted into the breast milk, so clients may continue to breast-feed after vaccination. Transient arthralgia and rash are common adverse effects of the vaccine.

CN: Health promotion and maintenance; CNS: None; CL: Application

42. 3. Magnesium sulfate is commonly used in the treatment of preeclampsia to prevent seizures. It also produces a smooth-muscle depression effect, which can lower blood pressure. Diazepam may also be given for seizure activity. Nifedipine and hydralazine are used for severely hypertensive preeclamptic women.

CN: Physiological integrity; CNS: Pharmacological and parenteral therapies; CL: Application

43. 3. Because magnesium sulfate relaxes smooth muscle, the uterus should be assessed for uterine atony, which would increase the risk of postpartum hemorrhage. Postpartum depression and uterine infection aren't associated with magnesium sulfate therapy. Magnesium sulfate is considered more of an anticonvulsant than an antihypertensive.

CN: Physiological integrity; CNS: Pharmacological and parenteral therapies; CL: Comprehension

You're making great strides. Keep going!

44. 2. A sitz bath reduces inflammation and relaxes the perineum, promoting healing and reducing discomfort. Ice should only be used for the first 24 hours following delivery. Kegel exercises, which involve tightening and relaxing the pelvic muscles, improve circulation and reduce edema. Massaging the perineum may disrupt the suture line and cause more pain.

CN: Physiological integrity; CNS: Physiological adaptation; CL: Analysis

CN: Client needs category   CNS: Client needs subcategory   CL: Cognitive level

45. A mother with diabetes tells the nurse she wants to breastfeed but is concerned about the effects of breastfeeding on her health. What is the best response by the nurse?
1. Mothers with diabetes who breastfeed have a hard time controlling their insulin needs.
2. Mothers with diabetes shouldn't breastfeed because of potential complications.
3. Mothers with diabetes shouldn't breastfeed; insulin requirements are doubled.
4. Mothers with diabetes may breastfeed; insulin requirements may decrease from breastfeeding.

46. Which activity by a client indicates that a nurse's teaching about perineal care has been effective?
1. The client uses a spray bottle to cleanse the perineum after urination and bowel movements.
2. The client wipes the perineum from back to front after urinating or a bowel movement.
3. The client douches after urination or a bowel movement.
4. The client changes perineal pads three times a day.

47. A nurse is assessing a multiparous client on her first postpartum day. Which assessment finding indicates that the client is at risk for hemorrhage?
1. Hemoglobin level of 12 g/dl
2. Uterine atony
3. Thrombophlebitis
4. Moderate amount of lochia rubra

48. On the first postpartum night, a client requests that her baby be sent back to the nursery so she can get some sleep. The client is most likely in which phase?
1. Depression phase
2. Letting-go phase
3. Taking-hold phase
4. Taking-in phase

To breastfeed or not to breastfeed, that is the question.

Remember, when you're dealing with a postpartum client, you've got two clients to think about.

45. 4. Breastfeeding has an antidiabetogenic effect. Insulin needs are decreased because carbohydrates are used in milk production. Breastfeeding mothers are at a higher risk of hypoglycemia in the first postpartum days after birth because the glucose levels are lower. Mothers with diabetes should be encouraged to breastfeed.
CN: Physiological integrity; CNS: Pharmacological and parenteral therapies; CL: Application

46. 1. The client should cleanse the perineal area after urinating or a bowel movement using a spray or peri-bottle. The client should wipe from front to back after urination or a bowel movement to avoid contaminating the perineal area. Perineal pads should be changed when they are soiled to keep the perineum clean.
CN: Health promotion and maintenance; CNS: None; CL: Application

47. 2. Multiparous women often experience a loss of uterine tone due to frequent distentions of the uterus from past pregnancies. As a result, this client is also at higher risk for hemorrhage. Thrombophlebitis doesn't increase the risk of hemorrhage during the postpartum period. The hemoglobin level and lochia flow are within acceptable limits.
CN: Health promotion and maintenance; CNS: None; CL: Analysis

48. 4. The taking-in phase occurs in the first 24 hours after birth. The mother is concerned with her own needs and requires support from staff and relatives. The depression phase isn't an appropriate answer. The letting-go phase begins several weeks later, when the mother incorporates the new infant into the family unit. The taking-hold phase occurs when the mother is ready to take responsibility for her care as well as her infant's care.
CN: Health promotion and maintenance; CNS: None; CL: Analysis

49. Four clients each gave birth 12 hours ago. The nurse determines that which client would most likely suffer complications after birth?
1. Gravida 2 Para 2002, cesarean birth, incisional site intact, hemoglobin level 9.8 g/dl
2. Gravida 2 Para 1011, cesarean birth, incisional site intact, pulse 84 beats/minute
3. Gravida 1 Para 1001, vaginal delivery, midline episiotomy, temperature 99.8° F (37.7° C)
4. Gravida 1 Para 1001, vaginal delivery, ruptured membranes 10 hours before delivery

50. Which statement by a client shows an understanding of how to prevent breast engorgement while breastfeeding?
1. "I will apply moist heat to my breasts three times a day."
2. "I will breastfeed every 1 to 3 hours."
3. "I will use a breast pump to obtain milk for feedings."
4. "I will wear a tight bra continually."

51. A client has delivered twins. What is the most important intervention for a nurse to implement?
1. Assess fundal tone and lochia flow.
2. Apply a cold pack to the perineal area.
3. Administer analgesics, as ordered.
4. Encourage voiding by offering the bedpan.

52. The nurse considers which of the following to be a <u>normal</u> physiological response in the early postpartum period?
1. Urinary urgency and dysuria
2. Rapid diuresis
3. Decrease in blood pressure
4. Increased motility of the GI system

Which client is at the greatest risk for complications?

Question 52 is looking for a *normal* response.

49. 1. Women who are anemic in pregnancy (defined as a hemoglobin <10 g/dl) may experience more complications, such as poor wound healing and inability to tolerate activity. The vital signs in answers 2 and 3 are within normal limits. Dehydration can cause a slightly elevated temperature. Women whose membranes are ruptured more than 24 hours before birth are more prone to developing chorioamnionitis.

CN: Health promotion and maintenance; CNS: None; CL: Analysis

50. 2. Frequent breastfeeding empties the breast, decreasing the risk of engorgement. Moist heat can stimulate the let-down reflex, leading to engorgement. A breast pump isn't necessary if a baby is able to breastfeed regularly. A tight brassiere may prevent the breasts from emptying completely when breastfeeding, increasing the risk of engorgement.

CN: Health promotion and maintenance; CNS: None; CL: Application

51. 1. Women who deliver twins are at a higher risk for postpartum hemorrhage due to overdistention of the uterus, which causes uterine atony. Assessing fundal tone and lochia flow helps to determine risks for hemorrhage. Applying cold packs to the perineum, administering analgesics as ordered, and offering the bedpan are all significant nursing interventions but not as important as preventing postpartum hemorrhage.

CN: Health promotion and maintenance; CNS: None; CL: Analysis

52. 2. In the early postpartum period, there's an increase in the glomerular filtration rate and a drop in progesterone levels, which result in rapid diuresis. There should be no urinary urgency, although a woman may feel anxious about voiding. There's minimal change in blood pressure following childbirth and a residual decrease in GI motility.

CN: Physiological integrity; CNS: Physiological adaptation; CL: Application

53. During the third postpartum day, which observation about a client should the nurse be <u>most likely</u> to make?
1. The client appears interested in learning more about neonatal care.
2. The client talks a lot about her birth experience.
3. The client sleeps whenever the neonate isn't present.
4. The client requests help in choosing a name for the neonate.

54. The nurse is aware that which of the following is the most likely cause of uterine atony that may lead to postpartum hemorrhage?
1. Hypertension
2. Cervical and vaginal tears
3. Urine retention
4. Endometritis

What's the nurse's most likely observation?

55. Which assessment finding of a client 22 hours after a cesarean delivery requires immediate action by the nurse?
1. Heart rate of 132 beats/minute and blood pressure of 84/60 mm Hg
2. Oral temperature of 100.2° F
3. A gush of blood from the vagina when the client stands up
4. Complaints of abdominal pain and cramping

56. Which percentage of postpartum clients experiences "postpartum blues"?
1. 20% to 25%
2. 50% to 80%
3. 30% to 45%
4. 100%

Have you ever heard the postpartum blues?

53. 1. By the third postpartum day, the client should be in the taking-hold phase, in which the new mother strives for independence and is eager for her neonate. The other options describe the phase in which the mother relives her birth experience.
CN: Health promotion and maintenance; CNS: None; CL: Analysis

54. 3. Urine retention causes a distended bladder to displace the uterus above the umbilicus and to the side, which prevents the uterus from contracting. The uterus needs to remain contracted if bleeding is to stay within normal limits. Cervical and vaginal tears can cause postpartum hemorrhage but are less common occurrences in the postpartum period. Maternal hypertension and endometritis don't cause postpartum hemorrhage.
CN: Health promotion and maintenance; CNS: None; CL: Application

55. 1. Tachycardia (heart rate of 132 beats/minute) and hypotension (blood pressure of 84/60 mm Hg) may be signs of hemorrhage. An oral temperature of 100.2° F may be due to dehydration, when it occurs on the first postpartum day. A gush of blood from the vagina when a client stands is a normal finding on the first postpartum day. Complaints of abdominal pain and cramping are expected following cesarean delivery.
CN: Physiological integrity; CNS: Reduction of risk potential; CL: Application

56. 2. The "postpartum blues"—a transient mood alteration that arises during the first 3 weeks postpartum and is typically self-limiting—affect 50% to 80% of postpartum clients. A more severe mood alteration, seen in approximately 20% of clients, involves changes that occur within a few days after delivery and may last for a few days to more than 1 year.
CN: Psychosocial integrity; CNS: None; CL: Application

57. When performing a <u>comprehensive</u> fundal check during a postpartum assessment, a nurse evaluates which fundal state?
1. Fundal consistency, location, and height
2. Fundal consistency and height
3. Fundal location and potential fundal distention
4. Fundal location and height

Don't sweat it! You're almost there!

57. **1.** A comprehensive fundal check includes evaluation of fundal consistency, height, and location. Normal results are a firm fundus that's at the correct height for the postpartum day and located in the center of the pelvis. Options 2, 3, and 4 don't reflect a comprehensive fundal check because they're missing valuable components.

CN: Physiological integrity; CNS: Physiological adaptation; CL: Analysis

58. A nurse is performing an assessment on a postpartum client. The assessment reveals that the fundus is firm. The nurse interprets this as indicating:
1. a firm tumor at the top of the uterus.
2. contraction of the uterus.
3. continuing labor contractions.
4. bladder distention.

58. **2.** A firm postpartum fundus means that the uterus has contracted and is constricting blood vessels, thereby decreasing lochial flow. A uterine tumor doesn't necessarily cause a firm fundus. The client wouldn't experience labor contractions during the postpartum period. Bladder distention restricts the uterus from contracting downward, resulting in a soft, boggy uterus and increased vaginal bleeding.

CN: Physiological integrity; CNS: Physiological adaptation; CL: Analysis

59. A primipara who is $Rh_o(D)$ negative has just given birth to an Rh-positive baby. Which <u>priority</u> nursing intervention should be included in the plan of care?
1. Administer $Rh_o(D)$ immune globulin to the neonate within 3 days.
2. Administer $Rh_o(D)$ immune globulin to the client within 3 days.
3. Administer $Rh_o(D)$ immune globulin to the client at her first postpartum visit in 6 weeks.
4. Administer $Rh_o(D)$ immune globulin to the neonate at the first well-baby visit.

Discharge teaching is important. Which instruction should you include for your clients with DVT?

59. **2.** Administering $Rh_o(D)$ immune globulin to the client within 72 hours of delivery prevents antibodies from forming that can destroy fetal blood cells in the next pregnancy. $Rh_o(D)$ immune globulin isn't given to the baby. The client shouldn't wait 6 weeks to receive $Rh_o(D)$ immune globulin as antibodies will already have formed.

CN: Safe, effective care environment; CNS: Management of care; CL: Application

60. A postpartum client is receiving anticoagulant therapy for deep vein thrombophlebitis. What is the most important information for the nurse to include in discharge teaching?
1. Avoid iron replacement therapy.
2. Wear a girdle and knee-high stockings whenever possible.
3. Avoid over-the-counter salicylates.
4. Be aware that shortness of breath is a common adverse effect of anticoagulants.

60. **3.** Discharge teaching should include an instruction to avoid salicylates, which may magnify the effects of anticoagulant therapy. Iron doesn't affect anticoagulant therapy. The client should avoid restrictive clothing to prevent recurrence of thrombophlebitis. She should report shortness of breath immediately because it may indicate pulmonary embolus.

CN: Health promotion and maintenance; CNS: Reduction of risk potential; CL: Application

61. The nurse is assessing a breastfeeding client on the fourth postpartum day. The nurse documents which findings as normal?
1. Soft, nontender breasts
2. Engorged breasts with inflamed, radiating areas that are sore to the touch
3. Slightly tender, cracked nipples; slightly firm, nontender breasts; transitional milk
4. Tender, intact nipples; firm, tender breasts; transitional milk

62. Which client statement should alert the nurse to a potential problem in a breastfeeding primiparous client?
1. "I will consume an additional 500 calories/day."
2. "I will increase my intake of protein."
3. "I will limit my fluid intake."
4. "I will eat foods high in vitamins and minerals."

63. A nurse is teaching a breastfeeding primiparous client how to prevent sore nipples. The nurse determines further teaching is necessary when the client makes which statement?
1. "I should breastfeed for only 3 to 4 minutes at a time until my milk flow is established."
2. "I should position the baby properly during feedings."
3. "I should pull the baby gently away from my nipple after the feeding."
4. "I should prevent the baby from feeding after my breast has been emptied."

64. A client is 2 days postpartum and is talking with her nurse about the bleeding she's having, asking, "Will it always be so heavy?" Which statement by the nurse would be the <u>most accurate</u>?
1. "This is lochia alba and will last 4 weeks."
2. "This is lochia serosa and will last 2 days."
3. "This is lochia rubra and will last 3 to 4 days."
4. "This is your menstrual cycle, and it will last 6 weeks."

I need to determine which findings are normal for this client.

Only 7 more questions to go!

61. 4. Tender, intact nipples; firm, tender breasts; and transitional milk are normal in a breastfeeding client on the fourth postpartum day. Engorged, inflamed breasts signal mastitis. Tender, cracked nipples aren't a normal finding; they require intervention and client teaching to help the nipples heal and help the client avoid the problem in the future.
CN: Physiological integrity; CNS: Physiological adaptation; CL: Application

62. 3. A breastfeeding client who states that fluid intake should be limited should alert the nurse that more education is needed. Increased fluids are needed for milk production. The breastfeeding client should consume an additional 500 calories/ day, increase protein intake, and eat foods high in vitamins and minerals.
CN: Health promotion and maintenance; CNS: None; CL: Application

63. 1. In some cases, it takes 7 minutes for the letdown reflex to cause milk to fill the breast. The other answers indicate that the client understands the nurse's instructions.
CN: Physiological integrity; CNS: Reduction of risk potential; CL: Application

64. 3. Lochia rubra, which is made up of blood, mucus, and tissue debris, lasts 3 to 4 days. Lochia serosa, which consists of blood, mucus, and leukocytes, lasts from day 3 to day 10 postpartum. Lochia alba, which consists largely of mucus, lasts from day 10 to day 14 postpartum. Lochia alba may last up to 6 weeks postpartum. Postpartum bleeding is not the menstrual cycle.
CN: Physiological integrity; CNS: Physiological adaptation; CL: Application

65. On examining a client who gave birth 3 hours ago, the nurse finds that the client has completely saturated a perineal pad within 15 minutes. Which actions should the nurse take? Select all that apply.
1. Begin an I.V. infusion of lactated Ringer's solution.
2. Assess the client's vital signs.
3. Palpate the client's fundus.
4. Place the client in high Fowler's position.
5. Administer a pain medication.

66. Which characteristic of lochia should a nurse expect in a client who is 2 weeks postpartum?
1. It's creamy white to brown and may have a stale odor.
2. It's creamy white to brown, contains decidual cells, and may have a stale odor.
3. It's brown to red, contains tissue fragments, and may have an odor.
4. It's brown to red and contains decidual cells and leukocytes.

67. In a client 1 week postpartum with retained placental fragments, which finding should alert a nurse of a common complication?
1. Puerperal infection
2. Postpartum depression
3. Postpartum hemorrhage
4. Uterine subinvolution

68. The nurse is assisting in developing a care plan for a client who had an episiotomy. Which interventions would be included for the nursing diagnosis of acute pain related to perineal sutures? Select all that apply.
1. Apply an ice pack intermittently to the perineal area for 3 days.
2. Avoid the use of topical pain gels.
3. Administer sitz baths three to four times per day.
4. Encourage the client to do Kegel exercises.
5. Limit the number of times the perineal pad is changed.

Stay with it! Just a few more to go!

65. 2 and 3. Assessing vital signs provides information about the client's circulatory status and identifies significant changes to report to the physician. By palpating the client's fundus, the nurse also gains valuable assessment data. A boggy uterus may lead to excessive bleeding. Starting an I.V. infusion requires a physician's order. Placing the client in high Fowler's position may lower blood pressure and be harmful to the client. Administration of a pain medication doesn't address the current problem.

CN: Physiological integrity; CNS: Reduction of risk potential; CL: Application

66. 2. Lochia alba occurs from 1 to 3 weeks postpartum. Lochia alba is creamy white to brown, contains decidual cells, and may have a stale odor. It also contains leukocytes. Lochia alba shouldn't contain tissue fragments or have a foul odor.

CN: Physiological integrity; CNS: Physiological adaptation; CL: Application

67. 3. Retained placental fragments, which prevent the uterus from contracting properly, increase postpartum blood loss. This loss may be dramatic and lead to postpartum hemorrhage of 500 ml of blood or more. Although retained placental fragments may also lead to uterine subinvolution or infection, these are less common complications. Postpartum depression is a psychiatric disorder not related to retained placental fragments.

CN: Health promotion and maintenance; CNS: None; CL: Application

68. 3 and 4. Sitz baths help decrease inflammation and tension in the perineal area. Kegel exercises improve circulation to the area and help reduce edema. Ice packs should be applied to the perineum for the first 24 hours only; after that time, heat should be used. Topical pain gels should be applied to the suture area to reduce discomfort, as ordered. The perineal pad should be changed frequently to prevent irritation caused by the discharge.

CN: Physiological integrity; CNS: Basic care and comfort; CL: Application

69. A nurse is palpating the uterine fundus of a client who delivered a baby 8 hours ago. At what level in the abdomen would the nurse expect to feel the fundus?

69. The uterus should be felt at the level of the umbilicus from 1 hour after birth and for about the next 24 hours.

CN: Physiological integrity;
CNS: Reduction of risk potential;
CL: Application

70. A mother with a past history of varicose veins has just delivered her first baby. A nurse suspects that the mother has developed pulmonary embolus. Which of the data below would lead to this nursing judgment? Select all that apply.
1. Sudden dyspnea
2. Chills, fever
3. Diaphoresis
4. Bradycardia
5. Confusion

70. 1, 3, and 5. Sudden dyspnea along with diaphoresis and confusion are classic symptoms that develop when a thrombus (stationary blood clot) from a varicose vein becomes an embolus (moving clot) that lodges in the pulmonary circulation. Chills and fever would indicate infection. A client with an embolus usually develops tachycardia.

CN: Physiological integrity; CNS: Physiological adaptation;
CL: Analysis

71. A nurse observes several interactions between a mother and her neonate son. Which maternal behaviors should the nurse identify as evidence of mother–infant attachment? Select all that apply.
1. Talks and coos to her son.
2. Cuddles her son close to her.
3. Doesn't make eye contact with her son.
4. Requests that the nurse take the baby to the nursery for feedings.
5. Encourages the father to hold the baby.
6. Takes a nap when the baby is sleeping.

71. 1 and 2. Talking, cooing, and cuddling with her son are positive signs of mother–infant attachment. Avoiding eye contact is a nonbonding behavior. Eye contact, touching, and speaking help establish attachment with a neonate. Feeding a neonate is an important role of a new mother and facilitates attachment. Encouraging the father to hold the neonate will facilitate attachment. Resting while the neonate is sleeping will conserve needed energy and allow the mother to be alert.

CN: Psychosocial integrity; CNS: None; CL: Analysis

You did it! A star is born (no pun intended)!

Neonates depend on you for *everything*. Let's show 'em you've got what it takes for neonatal care!

1. A client has given birth to a preterm neonate. The client tells the nurse that she still wants to breastfeed her neonate. The nurse should explain to the mother that:
1. breast milk contains antibodies that help protect her neonate.
2. commercial formula will provide better nutrition for the neonate.
3. breastfeeding can be started when the neonate is ready for discharge.
4. the neonate will be less likely to develop an infection on commercial formula.

2. The parents of a neonate admitted to the neonatal intensive care unit ask why the physician has ordered surfactant therapy. Which statement would be most accurate for parent education?
1. Surfactant will help regulate the baby's breathing pattern.
2. Surfactant helps clear mucus and fluid from the respiratory system to make breathing easier.
3. Surfactant helps mature the upper airways to make breathing easier.
4. Surfactant helps in keeping the lungs expanded after the baby starts breathing on its own.

3. While assessing a 2-hour-old neonate, a nurse observes the neonate to have acrocyanosis. Which nursing action should be performed <u>initially</u>?
1. Activate the code blue or emergency system.
2. Do nothing because acrocyanosis is normal in the neonate.
3. Immediately take the neonate's temperature according to facility policy.
4. Notify the physician of the need for a cardiac consult.

You need to keep the parents informed of the whats and whys of their baby's care.

What do you need to do first?

1. 1. Studies have proven that breast milk provides preterm neonates with better protection from infection, such as necrotizing enterocolitis, because of the antibodies contained in breast milk. Commercial formula doesn't provide any better nutrition than breast milk. Breast milk feedings can be started as soon as the neonate is stable. The neonate is more likely to develop infections when fed formula rather than breast milk.

CN: Health promotion and maintenance; CNS: None; CL: Application

2. 4. Surfactant works by reducing surface tension in the lung. It allows the lung to remain slightly expanded, decreasing the amount of work required for inspiration. Surfactant hasn't been shown to influence upper airway maturation, regulate the neonate's breathing pattern, or clear the respiratory tract.

CN: Physiological integrity; CNS: Pharmacological and parental therapies; CL: Application

3. 2. Acrocyanosis, or bluish discoloration of the hands and feet in the neonate (also called peripheral cyanosis), is a normal finding and shouldn't last more than 24 hours after birth. The other choices are inappropriate.

CN: Physiological integrity; CNS: Physiological adaptation; CL: Application

CN: Client needs category CNS: Client needs subcategory CL: Cognitive level

4. When teaching parents of a neonate the proper position for the neonate's sleep, a nurse stresses the importance of placing the neonate on his back to reduce the risk of which of the following?
1. Aspiration
2. Sudden infant death syndrome (SIDS)
3. Suffocation
4. Gastroesophageal reflux (GER)

5. A nurse is caring for a client with gestational diabetes. Which complication is the neonate most at risk of developing?
1. Anemia
2. Hypoglycemia
3. Nitrogen loss
4. Thrombosis

Knowing the risk factors can help guide your assessment.

6. The nurse is aware that preterm neonates who receive prolonged mechanical ventilation at birth are at risk for which condition?
1. Chronic lung disease
2. Esophageal atresia
3. Hydrocephalus
4. Renal failure

7. The nurse is performing a neonatal assessment. What is the <u>best</u> indication of adequate hydration?
1. Soft, smooth skin
2. A sunken fontanel
3. Bradycardia
4. No urine output in the first 24 hours of life

Here's to you! You're the best!!

4. 2. Supine positioning is recommended to reduce the risk of SIDS in infancy. The risk of aspiration is slightly increased with the supine position. Suffocation would be less likely with an infant supine than prone, and the position for GER requires the head of the bed to be elevated.
CN: Health promotion and maintenance; CNS: None; CL: Application

5. 2. Neonates of mothers with diabetes are at risk for hypoglycemia due to increased insulin levels. During gestation, an increased amount of glucose is transferred to the fetus through the placenta. The neonate's liver cannot initially adjust to the changing glucose levels after birth. This may result in an overabundance of insulin in the neonate, resulting in hypoglycemia. Neonates of mothers with diabetes aren't at increased risk for anemia, nitrogen loss, or thrombosis.
CN: Physiological integrity; CNS: Physiological adaptation; CL: Analysis

6. 1. Chronic lung disease following prematurity commonly results from the high pressures that must sometimes be used to maintain adequate oxygenation. Esophageal atresia, a structural defect in which the esophagus and trachea communicate with each other, doesn't relate to mechanical ventilation. Hydrocephalus and renal failure don't typically occur in these clients.
CN: Physiological integrity; CNS: Physiological adaptation; CL: Analysis

7. 1. Soft, smooth skin is a sign of adequate hydration. A sunken fontanel and no urine output in the first 24 hours of life are signs of poor hydration. In the case of no urine output, kidney dysfunction would also be a concern. Tachycardia, not bradycardia, may occur with dehydration.
CN: Physiological integrity; CNS: Physiological adaptation; CL: Analysis

8. The nurse is performing a neurological assessment on a neonate and considers which sign as a normal finding?
1. Doll eyes
2. "Sunset" eyes
3. Positive Babinski's sign
4. Pupils that don't react to light

Question 8 asks what's normal versus what's abnormal. Be careful!

9. A nurse is caring for four clients on an antepartum unit. Which client would be carrying a viable conceptus at the earliest stage?
1. A client at 9 weeks' gestation
2. A client at 14 weeks' gestation
3. A client at 24 weeks' gestation
4. A client at 30 weeks' gestation

10. A client's mother asks the nurse why her newborn grandson is getting an injection of vitamin K. Which statement best explains why this drug is given to neonates?
1. Vitamin K assists with coagulation.
2. Vitamin K assists the gut to mature.
3. Vitamin K initiates the immunization process.
4. Vitamin K protects the brain from excess fluid production.

I'm very important to the well-being of a neonate. Do you know why?

11. A neonate is born to a woman infected with hepatitis B. Which treatment should be administered to this neonate?
1. Hepatitis B vaccine at birth and 1 month
2. Hepatitis B immune globulin at birth; no hepatitis B vaccine
3. Hepatitis B immune globulin within 48 hours of birth and hepatitis B vaccine at 1 month
4. Hepatitis B immune globulin within 12 hours of birth and hepatitis B vaccine at birth, 1 month, and 6 months

8. 3. A positive Babinski's sign is present in infants until approximately age 1. A positive Babinski's reflex is normal in neonates but abnormal in adults. Doll eyes are a neurological response, but this sign is also noted in adults. The appearance of "sunset" eyes, in which the sclera is visible above the iris, results from cranial nerve palsies and may indicate increased intracranial pressure. A neonate's pupils normally react to light as in an adult.
CN: Health promotion and maintenance; CNS: None; CL: Analysis

9. 3. At approximately 23 to 24 weeks' gestation, the lungs are developed enough to sometimes maintain extrauterine life. The lungs are the most immature system during the gestational period. Medical care for premature labor begins much earlier (aggressively at 21 weeks' gestation).
CN: Health promotion and maintenance; CNS: None; CL: Analysis

10. 1. Vitamin K, deficient in the neonate, is needed to activate clotting factors II, VII, IX, and X. In the event of trauma, the neonate would be at risk for excessive bleeding. Vitamin K doesn't assist the gut to mature, but the gut produces vitamin K after maturity is achieved. Vitamin K doesn't influence fluid production in the brain or the immunization process.
CN: Physiological integrity; CNS: Pharmacological and parenteral therapies; CL: Application

11. 4. Hepatitis B immune globulin should be given as soon as possible after birth but within 12 hours. Neonates should also receive hepatitis B vaccine at regularly scheduled intervals. This sequence of care has been determined as superior to the others provided.
CN: Health promotion and maintenance; CNS: None; CL: Analysis

CN: Client needs category   CNS: Client needs subcategory   CL: Cognitive level

12. When a neonate is delivered with meconium staining in the amniotic fluid, which sequence of events will most effectively <u>decrease</u> the risk of meconium aspiration?
1. Deliver the thorax; then suction the nose.
2. Clamp the umbilical cord; then suction the neonate's mouth.
3. Deliver the head; then suction the mouth and then the nose.
4. Deliver the thorax; then suction the nose and then the mouth.

13. Erythromycin ointment is administered to a neonate's eyes shortly after birth. The neonate's mother asks the nurse why this is done. The best response by the nurse would be that the medication prevents which condition?
1. Cataracts
2. Diabetic retinopathy
3. Ophthalmia neonatorum
4. Strabismus

An ounce of prevention is worth a pound of cure!

14. A client with group AB blood whose husband has group O blood has just given birth. Which signs would indicate ABO blood incompatibility in the neonate?
1. Negative Coombs' test
2. Bleeding from the nose or ear
3. Jaundice after the first 24 hours of life
4. Jaundice within the first 24 hours of life

That's 15 questions down. Keep it up!

15. Which circumstance of delivery would predispose a neonate to respiratory distress syndrome (RDS)?
1. Preterm birth
2. Vaginal delivery
3. First born of twins
4. Postdate pregnancy

12. 3. To minimize the risk of aspiration of meconium after delivery, the neonate's mouth and then nose should be suctioned after delivery of the head. This suctioning shouldn't be delayed until after delivery of the thorax because the neonate will take its first breath with meconium in its mouth.
CN: Physiological integrity; CNS: Reduction of risk potential; CL: Analysis

13. 3. Eye prophylaxis is administered to the neonate immediately or soon after birth to prevent ophthalmia neonatorum often due to *Neisseria gonorrhoeae* or *Chlamydia trachomatis*. Cataracts are opacity of the lens of the eye associated with children with congenital rubella, galactosemia, and cortisone therapy. Diabetic retinopathy occurs in clients with diabetes when the retina bleeds into the vitreous, causing scarring, after which neovascularization occurs. Strabismus is neuromuscular incoordination of the eye alignment.
CN: Physiological integrity; CNS: Pharmacological and parenteral therapies; CL: Application

14. 4. The neonate with an ABO blood incompatibility with its mother generally will have jaundice within the first 24 hours of life. The neonate would have a positive Coombs' test result. Bleeding from the nose and ear should be investigated for possible causes but probably isn't related to ABO incompatibility. Jaundice after the first 24 hours of life is physiological jaundice.
CN: Physiological integrity; CNS: Reduction of risk potential; CL: Analysis

15. 1. Preterm birth is the single most important risk factor for developing RDS. The second born of twins and neonates born by cesarean delivery are also at increased risk for RDS. Surfactant deficiency, which commonly results in RDS, isn't a problem for postdate neonates.
CN: Physiological integrity; CNS: Physiological adaptation; CL: Analysis

16. Two days after circumcision, a nurse notes a yellow-white exudate around the head of the neonate's penis. What would be the <u>most</u> appropriate nursing intervention?
  1. Leave the area alone.
  2. Report the findings to the physician.
  3. Take the neonate's temperature.
  4. Remove the exudate with a warm washcloth.

> The color of an exudate helps determine its cause.

17. A client has just given birth at 42 weeks' gestation. When assessing the neonate, which physical finding is expected by the nurse?
  1. A sleepy, lethargic baby
  2. Lanugo covering the body
  3. Desquamation of the epidermis
  4. Vernix caseosa covering the body

18. A client delivers a small-for-gestation neonate. The nurse is aware that this neonate is most at risk for developing which of the following?
  1. Anemia probably due to chronic fetal hypoxia
  2. Hyperthermia due to decreased glycogen stores
  3. Hyperglycemia due to decreased glycogen stores
  4. Polycythemia probably due to chronic fetal hypoxia

19. The nurse is assessing a neonate with a suspected infection. Which finding would the nurse anticipate?
  1. Flushed cheeks
  2. Increased appetite
  3. Decreased temperature
  4. Increased activity level

> The test-taking expertise you're gaining from answering these questions will be well worth the effort you're putting in. Keep at it!

16. 1. The yellow-white exudate is part of the granulation process and a normal finding for a healing penis after circumcision. Therefore, notifying the physician isn't necessary. There's no indication of an infection that would necessitate taking the neonate's temperature. The exudate shouldn't be removed.
CN: Health promotion and maintenance; CNS: None; CL: Analysis

17. 3. Postdate fetuses lose the vernix caseosa, and the epidermis may become desquamated. These neonates are usually very alert. Lanugo is missing in the postdate neonate.
CN: Health promotion and maintenance; CNS: None; CL: Application

18. 4. The small-for-gestation neonate is at risk for developing polycythemia (not anemia) because of a state of anoxia during intrauterine life. The neonates are also at increased risk for developing hypoglycemia and hypothermia due to decreased glycogen stores.
CN: Health promotion and maintenance; CNS: None; CL: Analysis

19. 3. Temperature instability, especially when it results in a low temperature in the neonate, may be a sign of infection. Term infants with sepsis are more likely to be febrile, whereas the preterm infant is more likely to show signs of hypothermia. The neonate's color commonly changes with an infection process but generally becomes ashen or mottled. The neonate with an infection will usually show a decrease in appetite and a decrease in activity level, or lethargy.
CN: Physiological integrity; CNS: Physiological adaptation; CL: Analysis

20. A neonate has just been delivered without incident. Which symptom would indicate successful adaptation to extrauterine life?
1. Nasal flaring
2. Light audible grunting
3. Respiratory rate of 40 to 60 breaths/minute
4. Apgar score of 5

21. After reviewing the client's maternal history of magnesium sulfate during labor, which condition should the nurse anticipate as a potential problem in the neonate?
1. Hypoglycemia
2. Jitteriness
3. Respiratory depression
4. Tachycardia

22. Which nursing intervention would be helpful for a neonate experiencing drug withdrawal?
1. Place the Isolette in a quiet area of the nursery.
2. Withhold all medication to improve the liver's metabolization of drugs.
3. Dress the neonate in loose clothing so he won't feel restricted.
4. Place the Isolette near the nurses' station for frequent contact with health care workers.

23. A client with gestational diabetes delivers a neonate. The nurse is aware that the neonate is at risk for developing which condition?
1. Atelectasis
2. Microcephaly
3. Pneumothorax
4. Macrosomia

It's time to adapt to the "outside of the womb" world.

I need special interventions... whatever that means.

20. 3. A respiratory rate of 40 to 60 breaths/minute is normal for a neonate during the transitional period. Nasal flaring and audible grunting are signs of respiratory distress. An Apgar score of 5 or less indicates a need for resuscitative efforts.
CN: Health maintenance and promotion; CNS: None; CL: Analysis

21. 3. Magnesium sulfate crosses the placenta, and adverse neonatal effects are respiratory depression, hypotonia, and bradycardia. The serum blood sugar isn't affected by magnesium sulfate. The neonate would be floppy, not jittery.
CN: Physiological integrity; CNS: Pharmacological and parenteral therapies; CL: Analysis

22. 1. Neonates experiencing drug withdrawal commonly have sleep disturbance. The neonate should be moved to a quiet area of the nursery to minimize environmental stimuli. Medications, such as phenobarbital and paregoric, should be given as needed. The neonate should be swaddled to prevent him from flailing and stimulating himself.
CN: Psychosocial integrity; CNS: None; CL: Analysis

23. 4. Neonates of mothers with diabetes are at increased risk for macrosomia (excessive fetal growth) as a result of the combination of the increased supply of maternal glucose and an increase in fetal insulin. Along with macrosomia, neonates of diabetic mothers are at risk for respiratory distress syndrome, hypoglycemia, hypocalcemia, hyperbilirubinemia, and congenital anomalies. They aren't at greater risk for atelectasis or pneumothorax. Microcephaly is usually the result of cytomegalovirus or rubella virus infection.
CN: Health promotion and maintenance; CNS: None; CL: Analysis

24. A neonate is diagnosed with hemorrhagic disease. Which medication should have been given to the neonate as a <u>preventive</u> measure?
1. Vitamin K
2. Heparin
3. Iron
4. Warfarin

25. Which nursing intervention places a neonate at an increased risk for losing heat during the transition period?
1. Placing a cap on the neonate's head immediately after delivery
2. Preheating the radiant warmer prior to delivery
3. Placing the thermometer on the shelf of the radiant warmer
4. Wrapping the neonate in the same blankets used for drying

26. A nursery nurse wraps a neonate in a blanket and keeps the nursery temperature warm. Which type of heat loss is she trying to prevent in the neonate?
1. Conduction
2. Convection
3. Evaporation
4. Radiation

27. A nurse is explaining physiological hyperbilirubinemia to the parents of a neonate. Which statement made by one of the parents would demonstrate a correct understanding of the concept?
1. "The neonate usually also has a medical problem."
2. "In term neonates, it usually appears after 24 hours."
3. "It's caused by elevated conjugated bilirubin levels."
4. "It's usually progressive from the neonate's feet to his head."

Which measure is *preventive*, rather than curative or restorative?

Be careful with this prefix. *Hyper* is almost identical to *hypo*, but its meaning, of course, is vastly different.

24. 1. Neonates have coagulation deficiencies because of a lack of organisms that help produce vitamin K in the intestines, which helps the liver synthesize clotting factors II, VII, IX, and X. Heparin and warfarin are given as anticoagulant therapy, not to prevent hemorrhagic disease in the neonate. Iron is stored in the fetal liver; hemoglobin binds to iron and carries oxygen.
CN: Health promotion and maintenance; CNS: None; CL: Application

25. 4. Wrapping the infant in the previously used wet blankets causes continued heat loss by evaporation. Placing a cap on the neonate's head immediately after delivery, preheating the radiant warmer, and placing objects outside of the crib help prevent heat loss.
CN: Health promotion and maintenance; CNS: None; CL: Application

26. 2. Convection heat loss is the flow of heat from the body surface to cooler air. Conduction is the loss of heat from the body surface to cooler surfaces in direct contact. Evaporation is the loss of heat that occurs when a liquid is converted to a vapor. Radiation is the loss of heat from the body surface to cooler solid surfaces not in direct contact but in relative proximity.
CN: Health promotion and maintenance; CNS: None; CL: Application

27. 2. Physiological jaundice in term neonates first appears after 24 hours. Neonates are otherwise healthy and have no medical problems. Hyperbilirubinemia is caused almost exclusively from unconjugated bilirubin. Jaundice usually appears in a cephalocaudal progression from head to feet.
CN: Physiological integrity; CNS: Reduction of risk potential; CL: Analysis

28. A neonate has been diagnosed with caput succedaneum. Which information should the nurse include while teaching the mother about caput succedaneum?
1. It usually resolves in 3 to 6 weeks.
2. It doesn't cross the cranial suture line.
3. It's a collection of blood between the skull and periosteum.
4. It involves swelling of the tissue over the presenting part of the fetal head.

29. A postpartum client expresses concern about the look of her baby's first stool, which she describes as "dark and slimy." Which is the best statement for the nurse to make for client education?
1. "These types of stools occur when the baby is dehydrated in utero."
2. "The physician will be notified about this abnormal occurrence when he examines the infant."
3. "This bowel movement is called meconium and is considered normal."
4. "The type of first stool for your baby is determined by your diet during pregnancy."

30. A 3-day-old neonate needs phototherapy for hyperbilirubinemia. What is a priority of care for a neonate receiving phototherapy?
1. Tube feedings
2. Feeding the neonate under phototherapy lights
3. Mask over the eyes to prevent retinal damage
4. Temperature monitored every 6 hours during phototherapy

31. A nurse is caring for four neonates. Which neonate is most likely to develop hyperbilirubinemia?
1. Neonate of an African-American mother
2. Neonate of an Rh-positive mother
3. Neonate with ABO incompatibility
4. Neonate with Apgar scores of 9 and 10 at 1 and 5 minutes

When you're teaching a new mom, it helps to know what to expect at each stage in a neonate's development!

You're going strong. Keep at it!

28. **4.** Caput succedaneum is the swelling of tissue over the presenting part of the fetal scalp due to sustained pressure. This boggy edematous swelling is present at birth, crosses the suture line, and most commonly occurs in the occipital area. A cephalohematoma is a collection of blood between the skull and periosteum that doesn't cross cranial suture lines and resolves in 3 to 6 weeks. Caput succedaneum resolves within 3 to 4 days.
CN: Physiological integrity; CNS: Physiological adaptation; CL: Application

29. **3.** Meconium collects in the GI tract during gestation and is initially sterile. Meconium is greenish black because of occult blood and is viscous. Dehydration in utero does not occur. Physician notification is not necessary, as this is a normal occurrence for the first bowel movement. The stool of a neonate is not affected by the mother's antenatal diet.
CN: Health promotion and maintenance; CNS: None; CL: Analysis

30. **3.** The neonate's eyes must be covered with eye patches in addition to the genitalia to prevent damage. The neonate can be removed from the lights and held for feeding. The neonate's temperature should be monitored at least every 2 to 4 hours because of the risk of hyperthermia with phototherapy.
CN: Physiological integrity; CNS: Physiological adaptation; CL: Analysis

31. **3.** The mother's blood type, which is different from the neonate's, has an impact on the neonate's bilirubin level because of the antigen-antibody reaction. African-American neonates tend to have lower mean levels of bilirubin. Chinese, Japanese, Korean, and Greek neonates tend to have higher incidences of hyperbilirubinemia. Neonates of Rh-negative, not Rh-positive, mothers tend to have hyperbilirubinemia. Low Apgar scores may indicate a risk of hyperbilirubinemia.
CN: Physiological integrity; CNS: Physiological adaptation; CL: Analysis

32. A neonate has developed a major infection. Which gram-positive bacteria most likely contributed to this problem?
1. *Escherichia coli*
2. Group B streptococci
3. *Klebsiella* species
4. *Pseudomonas aeruginosa*

33. A neonate develops sepsis 18 hours after birth. Which organism most likely contributed to this problem?
1. *Candida albicans*
2. *Chlamydia trachomatis*
3. *Escherichia coli*
4. Group B beta-hemolytic streptococci

I'm responsible and proud of it!

34. A new mother tells the nurse that although she understands breastfeeding is the best, she will change to formula feeding when she returns to work in a few weeks. What information should the nurse include when teaching about formula feeding? Select all that apply.
1. All babies should be started on soy-based formulas because of the risk of future allergic reactions.
2. When mixing the powdered formula, be sure to follow the manufacturer's directions on the container to ensure proper nutrition.
3. All babies on formula should have an iron-fortified formula to ensure healthy brain growth.
4. Only a brand-name formula should be used because it has the best nutritional value.
5. The client should speak to her baby's doctor about the best formula to use when she plans on changing from breastfeeding to formula feeding.

35. The nurse is attempting to interact with a neonate experiencing drug withdrawal. Which behavior indicates to the nurse that the neonate is willing to interact?
1. Gaze aversion
2. Hiccups
3. Quiet, alert state
4. Yawning

32. 2. GBS are gram-positive cocci that the neonate is exposed to if these bacteria are colonized in the vaginal tract. *E. coli*, *Klebsiella*, and *P. aeruginosa* species are gram-negative rods that can produce bacterial infection in neonates. The incidence of early-onset GBS has declined by 80% with the use of intrapartum antibiotic prophylaxis (IAP); however, GBS and *E. coli* continue to account for approximately two-thirds of early-onset infection.

CN: Physiological integrity; CNS: Physiological adaptation; CL: Analysis

33. 4. Transmission of group B beta-hemolytic streptococci to the fetus results in respiratory distress that can rapidly lead to septic shock. *E. coli* is the second most common cause. Candidiasis may be acquired from the birth canal and causes infection later than 24 hours. *Chlyamydia trachomatis* infection causes neonatal conjunctivitis and pneumonia.

CN: Physiological integrity; CNS: Physiological adaptation; CL: Analysis

34. 2, 3, and 5. Many different brands of formula are available, but all must meet strict U.S. Food and Drug administration (FDA) requirements. The American Academy of Pediatrics recommends that all babies be fed iron-fortified formula unless contraindicated. It is vitally important that parents follow the directions on the package when mixing powdered formula to ensure proper nutrition for the baby. The baby's primary care provider and the parents should decide what the best formula for the baby is. There has not been proven a higher association of allergies for babies who begin a cow milk–based formula.

CN: Physiological integrity; CNS: Reduction of risk potential; CL: Application

35. 3. When caring for a neonate experiencing drug withdrawal, the nurse needs to be alert for distress signals from the neonate. Stimuli should be introduced one at a time when the neonate is in a quiet, alert state. Gaze aversion, yawning, sneezing, hiccups, and body arching are distress signals that the neonate can't handle stimuli at that time.

CN: Psychosocial integrity; CNS: None; CL: Analysis

36. When teaching umbilical cord care to a new mother, a nurse would include which information?
1. Apply alcohol to the cord with each diaper change.
2. Cover the cord with petroleum jelly after bathing.
3. Do nothing but keep it dry and open to air.
4. Wash the cord with soap and water each day during a tub bath.

37. A nurse is caring for an infant of a mother with diabetes. The nurse is aware that which physiological finding would be <u>most</u> indicative of a hypoglycemic episode?
1. Hyperalert state
2. Jitteriness
3. Excessive crying
4. Serum glucose level of 60 mg/dl

38. A mother of a term neonate asks what the thick, white, cheesy coating is on his skin. Which statement by the nurse correctly describes the function of this coating for the neonate?
1. It helps keep the neonate warm after birth.
2. It prevents neonatal dehydration after birth.
3. It serves as a protective coating in utero.
4. It decreases the development of birthmarks.

39. Which drug is <u>routinely</u> given to the neonate within 1 hour of birth?
1. Erythromycin ophthalmic ointment
2. Gentamicin
3. Nystatin
4. Vitamin A

40. A client asks the nurse how lung maturity is determined in the neonate. What is the <u>best</u> response by the nurse?
1. Meconium in the amniotic fluid
2. Glucocorticoid treatment just before delivery
3. Lecithin-to-sphingomyelin ratio more than 2:1
4. Absence of phosphatidylglycerol in amniotic fluid

The stump of the umbilical cord will fall off later.

What can I say? I'm just part of the normal routine.

Why do they think I'm immature?

36. 3. Research has found that there is no difference in infection rates between cords treated with antiseptics such as alcohol and dry or natural cord care. In addition, antiseptics may prolong the time to cord separation. Petroleum jelly prevents the cord from drying and encourages infection. Infants aren't given tub baths but are sponged off until the cord falls off.

CN: Health promotion and maintenance; CNS: None; CL: Application

37. 2. Hypoglycemia in a neonate is expressed as jitteriness, lethargy, diaphoresis, and a serum glucose level below 40 mg/dl. A hyperalert state in a neonate is more suggestive of neurological irritability and has no correlation to blood glucose levels. Excessive crying isn't found in hypoglycemia. A serum glucose level of 60 mg/dl is a normal level.

CN: Physiological integrity; CNS: Physiological adaptation; CL: Analysis

38. 3. Vernix caseosa is a white, cheesy material present on the neonate's skin at birth. The purpose of the vernix caseosa is to protect the fetus in utero. It does not prevent dehydration or keep the neonate warm after birth. There is no association between vernix caseosa and birthmarks.

CN: Health promotion and maintenance; CNS: None; CL: Analysis

39. 1. Erythromycin ophthalmic ointment is given for prophylactic treatment of ophthalmic neonatorum. Gentamicin is an antibiotic used in the treatment of an infection of the neonate. Nystatin is used for treatment of neonate thrush. Vitamin K, not vitamin A, is given.

CN: Physiological integrity; CNS: Pharmacological and parenteral therapies; CL: Analysis

40. 3. Lecithin and sphingomyelin are phospholipids that help compose surfactant in the lungs; lecithin peaks at 36 weeks, and sphingomyelin concentrations remain stable. Meconium is released because of fetal stress before delivery, but it's chronic fetal stress that matures lungs. Glucocorticoids must be given at least 48 hours before delivery. The presence of phosphatidylglycerol indicates lung maturity.

CN: Physiological integrity; CNS: Physiological adaptation; CL: Analysis

41. Which assessment finding would place the neonate at the least risk for developing respiratory distress syndrome (RDS)?
1. Second born of twins
2. Neonate born at 34 weeks
3. Neonate of a diabetic mother
4. Chronic maternal hypertension

Congratulations! You're halfway through this chapter.

42. A nurse is performing an assessment on a neonate. Which finding is considered common in the healthy neonate?
1. Single palmar (Simian) crease
2. Conjunctival hemorrhages
3. Cystic hygroma
4. Bulging fontanelle

43. When performing nursing care for a neonate after a birth, which intervention has the highest nursing priority?
1. Obtain a Dextrostix.
2. Give the initial bath.
3. Give the vitamin K injection.
4. Cover the neonate's wet head with a cap.

Which one of these actions is a priority right after birth?

44. When assessing a neonate's skin, the nurse observes small, white papules surrounded by erythematous dermatitis. Which most accurately describes this condition?
1. Cutis marmorata
2. Epstein's pearls
3. Erythema toxicum
4. Mongolian spots

41. 4. Chronic maternal hypertension is an unlikely factor because chronic fetal stress tends to increase lung maturity. The second born of twins may be prone to greater risk of asphyxia leading to RDS. Premature neonates younger than 36 weeks are associated with RDS. Even with a mature lecithin-to-sphingomyelin ratio, neonates of mothers with diabetes may still develop respiratory distress.
CN: Physiological integrity; CNS: Physiological adaptation; CL: Analysis

42. 2. Conjunctival hemorrhages are commonly seen in neonates secondary to the cranial pressure applied during the birth process. Single palmar (Simian) creases are present in 40% of the neonates with trisomy 21. Cystic hygroma is a neck mass that can affect the airway. Bulging fontanelles are a sign of intracranial pressure.
CN: Health promotion and maintenance; CNS: None; CL: Analysis

43. 3. The American Academy of Pediatrics recommends that vitamin K be given in the delivery room within 1 hour of birth. Dextrostix tests, appropriate for neonates with risk factors, are obtained at 30 minutes to 1 hour of age. Initial baths aren't given until the neonate's temperature is stable. The head shouldn't be covered until the hair is dried under a radiant warmer.
CN: Safe, effective care environment; CNS: Management of care; CL: Analysis

44. 3. Erythema toxicum has lesions that come and go on the face, trunk, and limbs. They're small, white or yellow papules or vesicles with erythematous dermatitis and resemble flea bites. Cutis marmorata is bluish mottling of the skin. Epstein's pearls, found in the mouth, are similar to facial milia. Mongolian spots are large macules or patches that are gray or blue green.
CN: Health promotion and maintenance; CNS: None; CL: Application

45. Which nursing consideration is <u>most important</u> when giving a neonate his initial bath?
1. Give a tub bath.
2. Use water and mild soap.
3. Give it right after delivery.
4. Use hexachlorophene soap.

46. The nurse is teaching the parents of a neonate about the Centers for Disease Control and Prevention (CDC) recommendations for hepatitis B vaccine. Which statement by the nurse would be the most accurate concerning these recommendations?
1. "It should be given to all neonates."
2. "It should be given to neonates exposed to hepatitis B only."
3. "It should be given to neonates showing symptoms of hepatitis B."
4. "It should be given to neonates whose mothers have human immunodeficiency virus."

47. A male neonate has just been circumcised. Which nursing intervention is part of the initial care of a circumcised neonate?
1. Apply alcohol to the site.
2. Change the diaper as needed.
3. Keep the neonate in the supine position.
4. Apply petroleum gauze to the site for 24 hours.

48. The nurse is performing an assessment on a neonate. Which assessment finding is <u>most suggestive</u> of hypothermia?
1. Bradycardia
2. Hyperglycemia
3. Metabolic alkalosis
4. Shivering

49. Which nursing intervention helps <u>prevent</u> evaporative heat loss in the neonate immediately after birth?
1. Administering warm oxygen
2. Controlling the drafts in the room
3. Immediately drying the neonate
4. Placing the neonate on a warm, dry towel

What's most important for baby's first bath?

I'm sure to stay warm now.

45. 2. Use only water and mild soap on a neonate to prevent drying out the skin. The initial bath is given when the neonate's temperature is stable. Tub baths are delayed until the umbilical cord falls off. Hexachlorophene soaps should be avoided; they're neurotoxic and may be absorbed through a neonate's skin.
CN: Health promotion and maintenance; CNS: None; CL: Application

46. 1. The CDC recommends that the hepatitis B vaccine be given to all neonates, including those born to hepatitis B surface antigen–negative mothers, before hospital discharge.
CN: Health promotion and maintenance; CNS: None; CL: Application

47. 4. Petroleum gauze is applied to the site for the first 24 hours to prevent the skin edges from sticking to the diaper (unless a Plastibell procedure was used). Alcohol is contraindicated for circumcision care. Diapers are changed more frequently to inspect the site. Neonates are initially kept in the prone position.
CN: Health promotion and maintenance; CNS: None; CL: Application

48. 1. Hypothermic neonates become bradycardic proportional to the degree of core temperature. Hypoglycemia is seen in hypothermic neonates. Metabolic acidosis, not alkalosis, is seen as a result of slowed respirations. Neonates use nonshivering thermogenesis.
CN: Health promotion and maintenance; CNS: None; CL: Analysis

49. 3. Immediately drying the neonate decreases evaporative heat loss from his moist body from birth. Controlling the drafts in the room and administering warmed oxygen help reduce convective loss. Placing the neonate on a warm, dry towel decreases conductive losses.
CN: Health promotion and maintenance; CNS: None; CL: Analysis

50. A nurse is performing an assessment on a neonate. Which assessment finding would indicate a metabolic response to cold stress?
1. Arrhythmias
2. Hypoglycemia
3. Increase in liver function
4. Increase in blood pressure

51. Which would be the <u>highest priority</u> in regulating the temperature of a neonate?
1. Supply extra heat sources to the neonate.
2. Keep the ambient room temperature less than 100° F (37.8° C).
3. Minimize the energy needed for the neonate to produce heat.
4. Block radiant, convective, conductive, and evaporative losses.

52. Which neonate would be <u>most</u> at risk for a problem with thermoregulation?
1. A term neonate born to a diabetic mother.
2. A neonate born at 36 weeks' gestation.
3. A neonate born at 39 weeks' gestation.
4. A term neonate with signs of jaundice at 36 hours of age.

53. Which clinical finding is <u>most suggestive</u> to the nurse of physiological hyperbilirubinemia in a neonate?
1. Clinical jaundice before 36 hours of age
2. Clinical jaundice lasting beyond 14 days
3. Bilirubin levels of 12 mg/dl by 3 days of life
4. Serum bilirubin level increasing by more than 5 mg/dl/day

The word highest is a clue to the answer!

Sometimes, timing is everything!

50. 2. Hypoglycemia occurs as the consumption of glucose increases with the increase in metabolic rate. Arrhythmias and increases in blood pressure occur because of cardiorespiratory manifestations. Liver function declines in cold stress.
CN: Health promotion and maintenance; CNS: None; CL: Analysis

51. 4. Prevention of heat loss is always the first goal in thermoregulation to avoid hypothermia. The second goal is to minimize the energy necessary for neonates to produce heat. Adding extra heat sources is a means of correcting hypothermia. The ambient room temperature should be kept at approximately 100° F.
CN: Safe, effective care environment; CNS: Management of care; CL: Application

52. 2. Preterm neonates are not able to thermoregulate due to the lack of brown fat. The more premature the infant, the more immature the thermoregulation system. Infants born to diabetic mothers and those with jaundice are not more at risk for problems with thermoregulation than a premature infant.
CN: Physiological integrity; CNS: Reduction of risk potential; CL: Analysis

53. 3. Increased bilirubin levels in the liver usually cause bilirubin levels of 12 mg/dl by the third day of life. This is from the impaired conjugation and excretion of bilirubin and difficulty clearing bilirubin from plasma. The other answers suggest pathological jaundice.
CN: Physiological integrity; CNS: Reduction of risk potential; CL: Analysis

54. A nurse is caring for a full-term neonate who's receiving phototherapy for hyperbilirubinemia. The nurse determines immediate intervention is necessary when the neonate exhibits which of the following?
1. Maculopapular rash
2. Absent Moro reflex
3. Greenish stools
4. Bronze-colored skin

55. The nurse is aware that a neonate undergoing phototherapy treatment needs to be monitored for which of the following?
1. Hyperglycemia
2. Increased insensible water loss
3. Severe decrease in platelet count
4. Increased GI transit time

56. Which assessment finding might be seen in a neonate suspected of having early breast-milk jaundice?
1. History of being a poor feeder
2. Decreased bilirubin level around day 3 of life
3. Clinical jaundice evident after 24 hours
4. Interruption of breastfeeding resulting in decreased bilirubin levels between 24 and 72 hours

57. The nurse is aware that which sign is the <u>earliest</u> indication of respiratory distress syndrome (RDS) in a neonate?
1. Bilateral crackles
2. Pale gray color
3. Tachypnea more than 60 breaths/minute
4. Poor capillary filling time (3 to 4 seconds)

58. A nurse is caring for a neonate with respiratory problems. Which condition is most likely to be caused by fluid remaining in the lungs of the neonate after delivery?
1. Choanal atresia
2. Meconium aspiration
3. Pulmonary hemorrhage
4. Transient tachypnea of a newborn

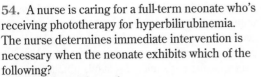

The signs are pointing to a dangerous situation.

It's important to recognize the earliest clue.

54. 2. An absent Moro reflex, lethargy, and seizures are symptoms of bilirubin encephalopathy, which can be life threatening. A maculopapular rash, greenish stools, and bronze-colored skin are minor side effects of phototherapy that should be monitored but don't require immediate intervention.
CN: Physiological integrity; CNS: Physiological adaptation; CL: Analysis

55. 2. Increased insensible water loss is due to absorbed photon energy from the lights. Hyperglycemia isn't a characteristic effect of phototherapy treatment. There may be a mild decrease in platelet count. GI transit time may decrease with use of phototherapy.
CN: Health promotion and maintenance; CNS: None; CL: Analysis

56. 4. The exact cause of early breast-milk jaundice is unknown. If bilirubin levels don't decrease after 3 days, human milk is eliminated as a cause. These babies are typically good eaters with good weight gain. Bilirubin levels increase, rather than decrease, at day 3. Jaundice in the first 24 hours of life is characteristic of hemolytic disease.
CN: Health promotion and maintenance; CNS: None; CL: Analysis

57. 3. Tachypnea and expiratory grunting occur early in RDS to help improve oxygenation. Crackles occur as the respiratory distress progressively worsens. A pale gray skin color obscures earlier cyanosis as respiratory distress symptoms persist and worsen. Poor capillary filling time, a later manifestation, occurs if signs and symptoms aren't treated.
CN: Health promotion and maintenance; CNS: None; CL: Analysis

58. 4. Transient tachypnea of a newborn is caused by a delay in removing excessive amounts of lung fluid. Choanal atresia is caused by a protrusion of bone or membrane into nasal passages, causing blockage or narrowing. Meconium aspiration is meconium aspirated into the lungs during birth. Pulmonary hemorrhage is bleeding into the alveoli.
CN: Physiological integrity; CNS: Physiological adaptation; CL: Analysis

59. A neonate is admitted to the neonatal intensive care unit with persistent pulmonary hypertension. The nurse anticipates the neonate will receive which medication?
1. Dobutamine
2. Isoproterenol (Isuprel)
3. Prostaglandin E2
4. Inhaled nitric oxide

60. Which neonatal respiratory disorder is usually mild and runs a self-limited course?
1. Pneumonia
2. Meconium aspiration syndrome
3. Transient tachypnea of newborn
4. Persistent pulmonary hypertension

You've reached question 60. Outstanding!

61. Which procedure should be <u>avoided</u> in a neonate born with diaphragmatic hernia?
1. Chest X-ray
2. Mask ventilation
3. Placement of orogastric tube
4. Immediate endotracheal intubation

62. A nurse is preparing to administer Survanta (beractant) to a preterm infant. The order is for 4 ml/kg. The neonate weighs 2,000 g. How many total milliliters will be used for one dose? Record your answer as a whole number:

_____ milliliters

63. A nurse is caring for a neonate with fetal alcohol syndrome (FAS). Which craniofacial change is most indicative of FAS?
1. Macrocephaly
2. Microphthalmia
3. Wide palpebral fissures
4. Well-developed philtrum

59. 4. Inhaled nitric oxide is a potent selective pulmonary vasodilator. Dobutamine is a vasopressor, not a vasodilator. Isoproterenol dilates pulmonary arteries but doesn't decrease pulmonary vascular resistance. Prostaglandin E2 is an oxytocic substance used to induce abortion and doesn't affect pulmonary vasodilation.

CN: Physiological integrity; CNS: Pharmacological and parenteral therapies; CL: Analysis

60. 3. Transient tachypnea has an invariably favorable outcome after several hours to several days. The outcome of pneumonia depends on the causative agent involved and may have complications. Meconium aspiration, depending on severity, may have long-term adverse effects. In persistent pulmonary hypertension, the mortality rate is more than 50%.

CN: Physiological integrity; CNS: Physiological adaptation; CL: Analysis

61. 2. Mask ventilation should be avoided to prevent air from being introduced into the GI tract by this technique. An emergency chest X-ray will help in diagnosing this defect. An orogastric tube is needed to decompress the bowel and stomach within the chest. Intubation is needed to ventilate the neonate because of the defect.

CN: Physiological integrity; CNS: Physiological adaptation; CL: Application

62. 8. The answer is 8 ml.

First, convert the weight from grams to kilograms using the conversion:

1,000 g = 1 kg
1,000 g/1 kg = 2,000 g/X kg
X = 2 kg

Then, determine how many milliliters are needed by using the following formula:

4 ml × 2 kg = 8 ml total dose.

CN: Physiological integrity; CNS: Pharmacological and parenteral therapies; CL: Application

63. 2. Distinctive facial dysmorphology of children with FAS most commonly involves the eyes (microphthalmia). Microcephaly is generally seen, as are short palpebral fissures, thin lips, and a poorly developed philtrum.

CN: Physiological integrity; CNS: Physiological adaptation; CL: Analysis

64. A 36-week neonate born weighing 1,800 g has microcephaly and microphthalmia. Based on these findings, which risk factor might be <u>expected</u> in the maternal history?
1. Use of alcohol
2. Use of marijuana
3. Gestational diabetes
4. Positive group B streptococci

65. Which condition requires intervention when displayed by a neonate born to a mother with a history of chronic alcohol abuse?
1. Hypoactivity
2. High birth weight
3. Poor wake and sleep patterns
4. High threshold of stimulation

The mother's history may be the key to the neonate's current condition.

66. A neonate is admitted to rule out a diagnosis of cystic fibrosis. Which GI disorder <u>most likely</u> indicates this diagnosis?
1. Duodenal obstruction
2. Jejunal atresia
3. Malrotation
4. Meconium ileus

67. The nurse is providing discharge instructions to the parents of a neonate regarding safety. What is the most important information for the nurse to include? Select all that apply.
1. "Heavy blankets or stuffed animals can be placed in the crib."
2. "The car seat used should be a front-facing model."
3. "Never leave your infant alone in the tub."
4. "Verify that you babysitter knows CPR."
5. "The car seat used should be a rear-facing model."

Keep reading each question carefully and you'll do well.

68. A neonate has an imperforate anus, tracheo-esophageal fistula, and a single umbilical artery. A nurse suspects that the neonate might have which congenital disorder?
1. Beckwith-Wiedemann syndrome
2. Trisomy 13
3. Turner's syndrome
4. VATER association

64. 1. The most common sign of the effects of alcohol on fetal development is retarded growth in weight, length, and head circumference. Intrauterine growth retardation isn't characteristic of marijuana use. Gestational diabetes usually produces large-for-gestational-age neonates. Positive group B *Streptococcus* isn't a relevant risk factor.
CN: Health promotion and maintenance; CNS: None; CL: Analysis

65. 3. Altered sleep patterns are caused by disturbances in the central nervous system from alcohol exposure in utero. Hyperactivity is a characteristic deficit generally associated with fetal alcohol syndrome (FAS). Low birth weight is a physical defect seen in neonates with FAS. Neonates with FAS generally have a low threshold for stimulation.
CN: Physiological integrity; CNS: Physiological adaptation; CL: Application

66. 4. Meconium ileus is a luminal obstruction of the distal small intestine by abnormal meconium seen in neonates with cystic fibrosis. Duodenal obstruction, jejunal atresia, and malrotation aren't characteristic findings in neonates with cystic fibrosis.
CN: Physiological integrity; CNS: Physiological adaptation; CL: Analysis

67. 3, 4, and 5. Infants should never be left alone in the tub, as they can easily drown. All caretakers should be trained in CPR. Car seats should be rear-facing models, not front-facing models, until the infant is 2 years old or reaches the maximum height and weight for that seat. Heavy blankets or stuffed animals in the crib increase the risk of sudden infant death syndrome (SIDS).
CN: Health promotion and maintenance; CNS: None; CL: Application

68. 4. VATER association clinically presents with three or more defects, including the three mentioned. These defects aren't associated with Beckwith-Wiedemann syndrome. Trisomy 13 and Turner's syndrome (45XO) are chromosomal aberrations that aren't typically seen with the other defects. VATER association includes: Vertebral anomalies, Anal atresia, Tracheal-Esophageal fistula, and Renal anomalies.
CN: Physiological integrity; CNS: Physiological adaptation; CL: Analysis

69. An initial assessment of a female neonate shows pink-streaked vaginal discharge. This finding indicates which condition?
1. Cystitis
2. Birth trauma
3. Neonatal candidiasis
4. Withdrawal of maternal hormones

70. When assessing for congenital anomalies in a neonate, which symptom is seen <u>first</u> with tracheoesophageal atresia?
1. Torticollis
2. Nasal stuffiness
3. Oligohydramnios
4. Excessive oral secretions

71. A new mother states to the nurse, "My baby spits up after every feeding." Which intervention would be appropriate to teach the mother initially for this problem?
1. Feed the baby every hour.
2. Change the infant to a soy formula.
3. Lay the infant on its stomach after every feeding.
4. Burp the infant more frequently during each feeding.

72. The nurse is aware that cold stress in the neonate can lead to which condition?
1. Anemia
2. Hyperglycemia
3. Metabolic alkalosis
4. Increased oxygen consumption

73. Which initial nursing intervention best addresses the needs of a term neonate with adequate respiratory and heart rates but who has central cyanosis?
1. Provide tactile stimulation.
2. Give supplemental free-flow oxygen.
3. Assist ventilation with a bag and mask.
4. Intubate and suction the lower airway.

69. 4. Withdrawal of maternal estrogen can produce pseudomenstruation. Cystitis or a urinary tract infection in a neonate would show generalized signs of sepsis. Birth trauma may cause surface abrasions but not vaginal discharge. Neonates with candidal infections usually have oral lesions (thrush) or monilial diaper rash.
CN: Health promotion and maintenance; CNS: None; CL: Application

70. 4. Accumulated secretions are copious in neonates with this disorder because the neonate can't swallow. Torticollis would be present only if there was a defect of muscle or bone. Nasal stuffiness is very common in neonates and doesn't indicate esophageal abnormalities. Atresia will produce polyhydramnios because the fetus can't swallow the amniotic fluid.
CN: Physiological integrity; CNS: Physiological adaptation; CL: Analysis

71. 4. Frequent burping decreases the amount of air the infant has in its stomach. Laying an infant on its back or side after feeding is preferred. Formula may have to be changed if it is determined that the spitting is related to milk intolerance, but this is not the initial reaction. Infants should be fed every 2 to 4 hours.
CN: Health promotion and maintenance; CNS: None; CL: Analysis

72. 4. The neonate's metabolic rate increases as a result of cold stress, which leads to an increased oxygen requirement. Cold stress doesn't increase erythrocyte destruction. Cold stress leads to anaerobic glycolysis, which results in metabolic acidosis. The increased metabolic rate leads to the use of glycogen stores and produces hypoglycemia.
CN: Physiological integrity; CNS: Reduction of risk potential; CL: Analysis

73. 2. Room air is currently insufficient, seen by the central cyanosis. Tactile stimulation is needed only if the neonate is apneic or gasping. Bag and mask ventilation is indicated only if the heart rate is less than 100 beats/minute. Intubation is indicated only in special circumstances, such as prematurity or a diaphragmatic hernia.
CN: Health promotion and maintenance; CNS: None; CL: Application

74. A woman delivers a 3,250-g neonate at 42 weeks' gestation. Which physical finding is <u>expected</u> during an examination of this neonate?
1. Abundant lanugo
2. Absence of sole creases
3. Breast bud of 1 to 2 mm in diameter
4. Leathery, cracked, and wrinkled skin

75. While performing an initial assessment on a term neonate with an Asian mother, the nurse notes a bluish marking across the neonate's lower back. The nurse interprets this as:
1. a sign of birth trauma.
2. a telangiectatic hemangioma.
3. a typical marking in dark-skinned races.
4. an indication that hyperbilirubinemia may follow.

76. A nurse in the neonatal nursery is serving as preceptor for a student nurse. The student asks the nurse why a neonate's head is cone shaped. Which response is accurate?
1. "It results from caput succedaneum. The difficult labor caused bruising and swelling of the neonate's head."
2. "It results from molding. Overriding of the cranial sutures allows the neonate's head to pass though the birth canal."
3. "It results from cephalohematoma. Some blood has collected between the skull bone and periosteum."
4. "It results from hydrocephalus. Either too much cerebrospinal fluid (CSF) is being formed or too little is being absorbed."

Question 74 asks about an expected finding, not necessarily an abnormal one.

Your role as a preceptor is to help "mold" future nurses.

74. 4. Neonatal skin thickens with maturity and is typically peeling by postterm. Lanugo disappears as pregnancy progresses, with very little remaining on the postterm neonate. Because sole creases increase in number and depth with gestational age, a postterm neonate would have deep sole creases. A postterm neonate would have a well-developed breast bud of 5 to 10 mm in diameter.
CN: Health promotion and maintenance; CNS: None; CL: Analysis

75. 3. This is a Mongolian spot, commonly found over the lumbosacral area in neonates of Black, Asian, Latin American, or Native American origin. They may be found on any part of the body. The coloration is due to the deposition of melanocytes, not erythrocytes, and, without other findings, isn't a bruise resulting from a birth trauma. A telangiectatic hemangioma is a salmon pink coloration found at the nape of the neck, eyelids, and forehead. A Mongolian spot is a deep dermal infiltration of melanocytes, so there would be no breakdown of erythrocytes to cause hyperbilirubinemia. Mongolian spots may sometimes be confused with bruising, so thorough documentation of their presence is a must.
CN: Health promotion and maintenance; CNS: None; CL: Analysis

76. 2. Molding refers to overlapping of the cranial sutures, which causes the neonate's head to appear cone shaped. Caput succedaneum, cephalohematoma, and hydrocephalus don't result in a cone-shaped head. Caput succedaneum is an area of localized swelling and bruising over a presenting part. Cephalohematoma is a collection of blood between the skull bone and periosteum. Hydrocephalus is an increase in the size of the entire head as a result of increased CSF volume.
CN: Health promotion and maintenance; CNS: None; CL: Analysis

77. A neonate who has been receiving formula feedings is discharged from the neonate nursery. Twenty-four hours later, the mother calls the hospital, stating that the neonate is vomiting most of his feedings. The nurse determines further instruction is necessary when the mother makes which statement?
1. "Every time I feed him, he spits up about a teaspoonful of formula onto his bib."
2. "I'm using prepared formula, and he takes ½ oz to 1 oz every 3 to 4 hours."
3. "I feed him every time he cries. Sometimes, he eats 4 oz at a time every couple of hours."
4. "I burp him after each ½ oz of formula."

78. A healthy term neonate born by cesarean delivery was admitted to the transitional nursery 30 minutes ago and placed under a radiant warmer. The neonate has an axillary temperature of 99.5° F (37.5° C), a respiratory rate of 80 breaths/minute, and a heelstick glucose value of 60 mg/dl. Which action should the nurse take?
1. Wrap the neonate warmly and place him in an open crib.
2. Administer an oral glucose feeding of dextrose 10% in water.
3. Increase the temperature setting on the radiant warmer.
4. Obtain an order for I.V. fluid administration.

79. A home health nurse assesses a neonate who is 48 hours old and was discharged from the hospital 24 hours ago. Which assessment finding indicates a potential problem?
1. The neonate cries but no tears appear.
2. Small papules appear all over the neonate's skin.
3. The neonate doesn't turn his head in the direction that his cheek is stroked.
4. The neonate produces a greenish-brown stool.

You're doing great! You've almost finished the chapter!

77. 3. Feeding the neonate every time he cries results in overfeeding. A neonate's crying doesn't always signal hunger; sometimes, it means his diaper is wet, he needs to suck, or he wants to be held. A neonate who's spitting up should be burped after every ounce of formula or less. For the first few days, the neonate's normal stomach capacity is 15 ml, so he should be fed every 3 to 4 hours. All neonates spit up a small amount because of an immature cardiac sphincter.
CN: Physiological integrity; CNS: Basic care and comfort; CL: Application

78. 4. Assessment findings indicate that the neonate is in respiratory distress—most likely from transient tachypnea, which is common after cesarean delivery. The normal respiratory rate is 30 to 60 breaths/minute; a neonate with a rate of 80 breaths/minute shouldn't be fed but should receive I.V. fluids until the respiratory rate returns to normal. To allow close observation for worsening respiratory distress, the neonate should be kept unclothed in the radiant warmer. Temperature is in the normal range; raising the warmer's temperature setting would cause overheating and worsen the neonate's respiratory distress.
CN: Physiological integrity; CNS: Basic care and comfort; CL: Application

79. 3. A normal, healthy neonate turns in the direction that the cheek is stroked. Failure to do so may indicate a neurological problem, which the nurse should report to the physician. A neonate's lacrimal glands are immature, resulting in tearless crying for up to 2 months. Erythema toxicum neonatorum causes a transient maculopapular rash—a normal finding in all neonates. Greenish-brown stools at 48 hours are normal and indicate that the neonate is eliminating formula or breast milk instead of meconium.
CN: Health promotion and maintenance; CNS: None; CL: Application

80. A nurse is administering vitamin K (AquaMEPHYTON; phytonadione) to a preterm neonate following delivery. The medication comes in a concentration of 2 mg/ml, and the ordered dose is 0.5 mg to be given subcutaneously. How many milliliters should the nurse administer? Record your answer using two decimal points.

_____ milliliters

80. 0.25. Use the following formula to calculate drug dosages: Dose on hand/Quantity on hand = Dose desired/X. Plug in the values, and the equation is as follows: 2 mg/ml = 0.5 mg/X. X = 0.25 ml.

CN: Physiological integrity; CNS: Pharmacological and parenteral therapies; CL: Application

81. A nurse is eliciting reflexes in a neonate during a physical examination. Identify the area the nurse would touch to elicit a plantar grasp reflex.

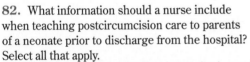

81. To elicit a plantar grasp reflex, the nurse should touch the sole of the foot near the base of the digits, causing flexion or grasping. This reflex disappears around age 9 months.

CN: Health promotion and maintenance; CNS: None; CL: Application

82. What information should a nurse include when teaching postcircumcision care to parents of a neonate prior to discharge from the hospital? Select all that apply.
1. The infant must void before being discharged.
2. Petroleum jelly should be applied to the glans of the penis with each diaper change.
3. The infant can take tub baths while the circumcision heals.
4. Any blood noted on the front of the diaper should be reported.
5. The circumcision will require care for 2 to 4 days after discharge.

82. 1, 2, and 5. It's necessary for the infant to void prior to discharge to ensure that the urethra isn't obstructed. A lubricating ointment is appropriate and is applied with each diaper change (unless a Plastibell procedure was used). Typically, the penis heals within 2 to 4 days, and circumcision care is required for that period only. To prevent infection, avoid giving the infant tub baths until the circumcision is healed; sponge baths are appropriate. A small amount of bleeding is expected following a circumcision; parents should report only a large amount of bleeding.

CN: Health promotion and maintenance; CNS: None; CL: Application

Part V — Care of the child

Chapter 26
Growth & development

1. A mother tells a nurse that her 22-month-old child says "no" to everything. When scolded, the toddler becomes angry and starts crying loudly but then immediately wants to be held. How does the nurse best interpret this behavior?
   1. The toddler isn't effectively coping with the stress.
   2. The toddler's need for affection isn't being met.
   3. This is normal behavior for a 2-year-old child.
   4. This behavior suggests the need for counseling.

Question 1 wants you to read the rest but go with the best.

2. The mother of a 12-month-old infant expresses concern about the effect of frequent thumb sucking on her child's teeth. After the nurse teaches her about this matter, which response by the mother indicates that the teaching has been effective?
   1. "Thumb sucking should be discouraged at 12 months."
   2. "I'll give the baby a pacifier instead."
   3. "Sucking is important to the baby."
   4. "I'll wrap the thumb in a bandage."

3. An adolescent client has just had surgery and has a dressing on the abdomen. Which question should the nurse expect the client to ask initially?
   1. "Did the surgery go OK?"
   2. "Will I have a large scar?"
   3. "What complications can I expect?"
   4. "When can I return to school?"

4. For an 8-month-old infant, the nurse should plan to provide which toy to promote the child's cognitive development?
   1. Blocks to stack
   2. Jack-in-the-box
   3. Small rubber ball
   4. Play gym strung across the crib

1. **3.** Toddlers are confronted with the conflict of achieving autonomy yet relinquishing the much-enjoyed dependence on—and affection of—others. As a result, their negativism is a necessary part of their growth and development. Nothing about this behavior indicates that the child is under stress, isn't receiving sufficient affection, or requires counseling.
CN: Health promotion and maintenance; CNS: None; CL: Analysis

2. **3.** Sucking is the infant's chief pleasure. However, thumb sucking can cause malocclusion if it persists after age 4. Many fetuses begin sucking their fingers in utero and, as infants, refuse a pacifier as a substitute. A young child is likely to chew on a bandage, which could lead to airway obstruction.
CN: Health promotion and maintenance; CNS: None; CL: Analysis

3. **2.** Adolescents are deeply concerned about their body image and how they appear to others. An adolescent probably wouldn't ask how the surgery went or what complications to expect, although an adult would. Although an adolescent may be curious as to when he can return to school, it probably wouldn't be his primary concern.
CN: Health promotion and maintenance; CNS: None; CL: Application

4. **2.** According to Piaget's theory of cognitive development, an 8-month-old child will look for an object after it disappears from sight to develop the cognitive skill of object permanence. Stacking blocks and small balls are inappropriate because infants frequently put their fingers or objects into their mouth. Anything strung across an infant's crib is a safety hazard, especially to a child who may use it to pull to a standing position.
CN: Health promotion and maintenance; CNS: None; CL: Application

5. A 14-month-old is admitted to the pediatric unit with a diagnosis of croup. Which characteristics would the nurse expect the toddler to demonstrate if he's developing normally? Select all that apply.
1. Strong hand grasp
2. Tendency to hold one object while looking for another
3. Recognition of familiar voices (smiles in recognition)
4. Presence of Moro reflex
5. Weight that's triple his birth weight
6. Closed anterior fontanel

6. The school nurse overhears a conversation between two 7-year-old boys. Which comment by a 7-year-old boy to his friend best typifies his developmental stage?
1. "Girls are so yucky."
2. "My mommy and I are always together."
3. "I can't decide if I like Amy or Heather better."
4. "I can turn into Batman when I come out of my closet."

7. A nurse should expect a 3-year-old child to be able to perform which action?
1. Ride a tricycle
2. Tie shoelaces
3. Roller skate
4. Jump rope

8. A 6-month-old infant is admitted to the pediatric unit for a 2-week course of antibiotics. His parents can visit only on weekends. Which action indicates that the nurse understands the infant's emotional needs?
1. The nurse places the infant in a four-bed unit.
2. The nurse places the infant in a room away from other children.
3. The nurse assigns the infant to a different nurse each day.
4. The nurse assigns the infant to the same nurse as often as possible.

> You had better treat me with "kid" gloves.

> Which action indicates that the nurse understands?

5. 1, 2, 3, and 5. A strong hand grasp is demonstrated within the first month of life. Holding one object while looking for another is accomplished by the 20th week. Within the first year of life, the toddler masters smiling at familiar faces and voices, the toddler's birth weight triples, and the Moro reflex disappears. The anterior fontanel closes at approximately age 18 months.

CN: Health promotion and maintenance; CNS: None; CL: Application

6. 1. During the school-age years, the most important social interactions typically are those with peers. Peer-to-peer interactions lead to the formation of intimate friendships between same-sex children. Friendships with opposite-sex children are uncommon. At this age, children socialize more frequently with friends than with parents. Interest in peers of the opposite sex generally doesn't begin until ages 10 to 12. Magical thinking and fantasy play are more characteristic during the preschool years.

CN: Health promotion and maintenance; CNS: None; CL: Application

7. 1. At age 3, gross motor development and refinement in hand–eye coordination enable a child to ride a tricycle. The fine motor skills required to tie shoelaces and the gross motor skills required for roller skating and jumping rope develop around age 5.

CN: Health promotion and maintenance; CNS: None; CL: Application

8. 4. Building a sense of trust is crucial with an infant at this stage of growth and development. Consistent caregivers will promote a sense of trust. Placing him in a four-bed unit isn't the best choice because a 6-month-old child doesn't play with other children. Placing him in a room away from other children would isolate him from others, which is neither necessary nor helpful.

CN: Health promotion and maintenance; CNS: None; CL: Application

9. A term neonate weighs 7.5 lb (3 kg) at birth. The parents ask the nurse how much the child should weigh when he is 1 year old. What is the best response by the nurse?
1. 16 lb (7.3 kg)
2. 22 lb (10 kg)
3. 28 lb (12.7 kg)
4. 32 lb (14.5 kg)

10. Which behavior by a preschool child indicates to the nurse that the child is in the appropriate stage of growth and development?
1. He cries in protest when his mother leaves.
2. He asks for a bandage after having blood drawn.
3. He's upset about having a scar after surgery.
4. He wants to know why his friends don't visit.

11. A nurse observes parents playing with their 10-month-old daughter. Which behavior indicates that the infant is developing object permanence?
1. She looks for the toy that her parents hid under the blanket.
2. She returns the play blocks to the same spot on the table.
3. She recognizes that a ball of clay is the same object even when it's flattened out.
4. She bangs two cubes in her hands and throws them to the floor.

12. A nurse is teaching the parents of a 6-month-old infant about age-specific growth and development. Which statement is true regarding infant development? Select all that apply.
1. A 6-month-old infant has trouble holding objects.
2. A 6-month-old infant can usually roll from prone to supine and supine to prone positions.
3. A teething ring is appropriate for a 6-month-old infant.
4. Head lag is commonly noted in infants at age 6 months.
5. Lack of visual coordination usually resolves by age 6 months.

9. 2. A term neonate who weighs 7.5 lb at birth should triple his birth weight by age 1 year; therefore, he should weigh approximately 22 to 23 lb. A weight of 16 lb is roughly a doubling of birth weight, which should occur by 6 months. A weight of 28 or 32 lb indicates a gain that exceeds three times the birth weight.
CN: Health promotion and maintenance; CNS: None; CL: Analysis

10. 2. A preschooler typically asks for a bandage after having blood drawn because he has poorly defined body boundaries and believes he will lose all of his blood from the hole the needle has made. A toddler cries in protest when the parent leaves. An adolescent might be upset about a surgical scar because he's concerned about body image. A school-age child might ask why his friends don't visit because peers become important by that age.
CN: Heath promotion and maintenance; CNS: None; CL: Analysis

11. 1. Object permanence is exhibited by the infant looking for objects that have been hidden from sight. Returning the blocks to the same spot on the table is imitative behavior. Recognizing that a ball of clay is the same object even when flattened out is an example of the theory of conservation, which occurs in early-school-age children. Banging two cubes in her hands and throwing them to the floor is normal behavior for a 10-month old but doesn't indicate object permanence.
CN: Health promotion and maintenance; CNS: None; CL: Application

12. 2, 3, and 5. Gross motor skills of the 6-month-old infant include rolling from front to back and back to front. Teething usually begins around age 6 months, and therefore, a teething ring is appropriate. Visual coordination is usually resolved by age 6 months. At age 6 months, fine motor skills include purposeful grasps. The 6-month-old infant should have good head control and should no longer display head lag when pulled up to a sitting position.
CN: Health promotion and maintenance; CNS: None; CL: Application

13. A nurse is conducting a physical examination on an infant. Identify the anatomical landmark she should use to measure chest circumference.

14. The nurse is examining the breasts of an adolescent girl. She classifies her sexual maturity as Tanner stage 3. Which graphic depicts this stage?

1.

2.

3.

4.

Super job! You finished this chapter in record time! Way to go!

13. Chest circumference is most accurately measured by placing the measuring tape around the infant's chest with the tape covering the nipples. If measured above or below the nipples, a false measurement is obtained.

CN: Health promotion and maintenance; CNS: None;
CL: Application

14. 2. In Tanner stage 3, the entire breast enlarges and the nipple doesn't protrude. Option 1 shows Tanner stage 5: an adult breast has developed, the nipple protrudes, and the areola no longer appears separate from the breast. Option 3 shows Tanner stage 4: the breast enlarges and the nipple and papilla protrude and appear as a secondary mound. Option 4 shows Tanner stage 2: breast buds appear and the areola is slightly widened and appears as a small mound.

CN: Physiological integrity; CNS: Reduction of risk potential;
CL: Application

You've reached our test on cardiovascular disorders in children. Before taking this comprehensive test, why not bolster yourself with a heart-healthy snack of celery and low-fat cream cheese? Yum!

Chapter 27
Cardiovascular disorders

1. The nurse auscultates the first heart sound, interpreting this sound as occurring:
  1. late in diastole.
  2. early in diastole.
  3. with closure of the mitral and tricuspid valves.
  4. with closure of the aortic and pulmonic valves.

2. A nurse is performing a cardiac assessment on a child. Which characteristic would indicate a diagnosis of a grade 1 heart murmur?
  1. The murmur is equal to the heart sounds.
  2. The murmur is softer than the heart sounds.
  3. The murmur can be heard with the naked ear.
  4. The murmur is associated with a precordial thrill.

You might have a lot of questions ahead of you, but I know you can do it!

3. A graduate nurse has started working in a pediatric intensive care unit and is measuring the client's cardiac output. The nurse recognizes which of the following as determinants of cardiac output. Select all that apply.
  1. Contractility
  2. Preload
  3. Afterload
  4. Urine output
  5. Heart rate

1. 3. The S$_1$ occurs during systole with closure of the mitral and tricuspid valves. The fourth heart sound is heard late in diastole and may be a normal finding in children. The third heart sound is heard early in diastole. The second heart sound occurs during diastole with closure of the aortic and pulmonic valves.

CN: Health promotion and maintenance; CNS: None; CL: Analysis

2. 2. A grade 1 heart murmur is commonly difficult to hear and softer than the heart sounds. A grade 2 murmur is usually equal to the heart sounds. A grade 6 murmur can be heard with the naked ear or with the stethoscope off the chest. A grade 4 murmur is associated with a precordial thrill. A thrill is a palpable manifestation associated with a loud murmur.

CN: Health promotion and maintenance; CNS: None; CL: Analysis

3. 1, 2, 3, and 5. Cardiac output is calculated by taking heart rate times the stroke volume. Stroke volume is the amount of blood ejected by the heart in any one contraction. It's influenced by preload, afterload, and contractility. Preload is the amount of blood returning to the heart. Contractility is the ability of the cardiac muscle to act as an efficient pump. Afterload is the resistance the ventricles pump against when ejecting blood. Urine output is used to assess cardiac output, not determine it.

CN: Physiological integrity; CNS: Physiological adaptation; CL: Application

4. A child is diagnosed with cardiogenic shock. Which of the following manifestations would the nurse expect to find in this child? Select all that apply.
1. Decreased urine output
2. Bradycardia
3. Tachypnea
4. Bounding peripheral pulses
5. Capillary refill of less than 2 seconds

5. Which assessment would the nurse consider as a <u>late</u> sign of shock in a 6-month-old infant?
1. Heart rate of 172 beats/minute
2. Blood pressure of 64/36 mm Hg in right arm
3. Capillary refill of 4 seconds
4. Pale, cool, mottled skin

6. A 2-year-old child is showing signs of shock. A 10 ml/kg bolus of normal saline solution is ordered. The child weighs 40 lb. How many milliliters should be administered?
1. 18.2 ml
2. 182 ml
3. 40 ml
4. 400 ml

7. The following are found during the assessment of a 1-month-old child. Which of the following would lead the nurse to suspect a cardiac defect?
1. Weight gain
2. Hyperactivity
3. Poor nutritional intake
4. Pink mucous membranes

8. A nurse is reviewing the waveforms of an electrocardiogram of an infant with a nursing student. The student asks the nurse which waveform indicates ventricular depolarization and contraction. What would be the best response by the nurse?
1. P wave
2. PR interval
3. QRS complex
4. T wave

Yikes! Is this what they mean by cardiogenic shock?

Yes, this is a math question. Stay cool, and you'll do great!

4. 1 and 3. Cardiogenic shock occurs when cardiac output is decreased and tissue oxygen needs aren't adequately met. Signs of cardiogenic shock include apprehension, irritability, pallor, decreased urine output, tachycardia, tachypnea, weak pulses, cool extremities, and poor capillary refill.
CN: Physiological integrity; CNS: Physiological adaptation; CL: Analysis

5. 2. Hypotension is considered a late sign of shock in children. This represents a decompensated state and impending cardiopulmonary arrest. Tachycardia; delayed capillary refill; and pale, cool, mottled skin are earlier indicators of shock that may show compensation.
CN: Physiological integrity; CNS: Physiological adaptation; CL: Analysis

6. 2. The correct formula for this calculation is 10 ml/kg × 18.18. Convert pounds to kilograms (40 divided by 2.2 = 18.18 kg) and then multiply that by 10. Answer 2 is correct. The other options are incorrect.
CN: Physiological integrity; CNS: Pharmacological and parenteral therapies; CL: Analysis

7. 3. Infants and children with heart defects tend to have poor nutritional intake and weight loss, indicating poor cardiac output, heart failure, or hypoxemia. The child appears lethargic or tired because of the heart failure or hypoxia. Pink, moist mucous membranes are normal.
CN: Health promotion and maintenance; CNS: None; CL: Analysis

8. 3. The QRS complex reflects ventricular depolarization and contraction. The P wave represents atrial depolarization and contraction. The PR interval represents the time it takes an impulse to trace from the atrioventricular node to the bundle of His. The T wave represents repolarization of the ventricles.
CN: Physiological integrity; CNS: Reduction of risk potential; CL: Application

9. Which of the following is a noninvasive method of evaluating cardiac status in a child?
1. Transthoracic echocardiogram
2. Cardiac enzyme levels
3. Cardiac catheterization
4. Transesophageal pacing

I think I detect the correct statement.

10. An echocardiogram has been ordered for a child. What is the <u>most</u> accurate information for the nurse to tell the parents?
1. The child must be sedated in order to get an accurate result.
2. It uses sound waves to measure and evaluate cardiac structures and function.
3. The transthoracic method of echocardiogram is an invasive procedure.
4. It is the most definitive method of evaluating cardiac function.

11. A cardiac catheterization has been scheduled for an 8-year-old child. Prior to the procedure, what would be the <u>most appropriate</u> nursing intervention for the child and his parents?
1. Supplying a map of the hospital
2. Limiting visitors to parents only
3. Offering a guided tour of the hospital and catheterization laboratory
4. Explaining that the child can't eat or drink for 1 to 2 days postoperatively

What can you do to ease the family's fears?

12. The nurse is teaching the parents of a child who is scheduled for a cardiac catheterization. Which statement by the nurse is the most accurate regarding cardiac catheterization?
1. It is a noninvasive procedure.
2. General anesthesia is required.
3. It uses high-frequency sound waves to produce an image of the heart in motion.
4. It provides visualization of the heart and great vessels with radiopaque dye.

9. 1. A transthoracic echocardiogram is a noninvasive procedure to visualize the anatomy of the heart. Blood testing determines cardiac enzyme levels. Cardiac catheterization involves passing a catheter into the chambers of the heart for direct visualization of the heart and great vessels. Transesophageal pacing requires a probe to be placed in the esophagus for high-frequency ultrasound.
CN: Physiological integrity; CNS: Reduction of risk potential; CL: Analysis

10. 2. Echocardiograms use sound waves to measure and evaluate cardiac structures and function. The transthoracic method is not an invasive procedure; however, the transesophageal method is considered invasive. The child does not have to be sedated, but lying quietly is preferred. While an echocardiogram gives the physician a good idea of cardiac function, a cardiac catheterization is the definitive method for a complete and accurate picture.
CN: Physiological integrity; CNS: Reduction of risk potential; CL: Application

11. 3. A guided tour will help minimize fears and allay anxieties for the child and parents. It gives the opportunity for questions and teaching. A map of the hospital is helpful, but a tour provides the family with more information. Visitors should include all significant others and siblings as part of the preoperative teaching. The child will be able to start clear liquids and advance as tolerated after the procedure is completed and the child is fully awake.
CN: Physiological integrity; CNS: Physiological adaptation; CL: Analysis

12. 4. Cardiac catheterization provides visualization of the heart and great vessels. It's an invasive procedure in which a thin catheter is passed into the chambers of the heart through a peripheral vein or artery. General anesthesia may be used for more complex catheterizations or procedures that place the child at greater risk. High-frequency sound waves describe ultrasound and echocardiography. Conscious sedation is usually given before cardiac catheterization.
CN: Physiological integrity; CNS: Reduction of risk potential; CL: Application

13. Which nursing intervention would be <u>most appropriate</u> for a nurse to implement when caring for a 2-year-old child immediately after cardiac catheterization?
1. Allow the child to sit on the parent's lap.
2. Allow the parent to lie in bed with the child to keep him flat.
3. Assess vital signs every 2 to 4 hours.
4. Replace a bloody groin dressing with a new dressing.

14. The nurse is preparing to discharge a child after cardiac catheterization. What is the most important information for the nurse to provide?
1. The child should drink fluids and eat a regular diet.
2. The child may participate in sports once home.
3. The child can routinely bathe after returning home.
4. The child may return to school the next day.

15. A 2-year-old child is being monitored after cardiac surgery. The nurse is aware that the assessment findings representing a decrease in cardiac output would be which of the following? Select all that apply.
1. Hypotension
2. Decreased urine output
3. Weak peripheral pulses
4. Capillary refill less than 2 seconds
5. Warm fingers and toes

16. The nurse is monitoring a 3-year-old child who is experiencing distress after having cardiac surgery. Which of the following signs indicate cardiac tamponade? Select all that apply.
1. Hypertension
2. Muffled heart sounds
3. Widened pulse pressure
4. Decreased chest tube drainage
5. Dyspnea

You've already answered 15 questions! See how time flies when you're taking a test?

Which signs indicate cardiac tamponade?

13. 2. During recovery, the child should remain flat in bed, keeping the punctured leg straight for the prescribed time. The child should avoid raising the head, sitting, straining the abdomen, or coughing. Vital signs are taken every 15 minutes until the child is awake and stable, then every half hour, and then hourly as ordered. If bleeding occurs at the insertion site, the nurse should mark the margins with a pen and monitor for changes.
CN: Physiological integrity; CNS: Physiological adaptation; CL: Analysis

14. 1. A regular diet and increased fluids are encouraged after catheterization. Increased fluids may flush the injected dyes out of the system. Normal activities may be resumed, but strenuous physical activities or sports should be avoided for about 3 days. Prolonged bathing can be resumed in 3 days. A sponge bath is encouraged until then. The child may return to school 3 days after discharge.
CN: Physiological integrity; CNS: Physiological adaptation; CL: Analysis

15. 1, 2, and 3. Signs of decreased cardiac output include weak peripheral pulses, hypotension, low urine output, delayed capillary refill, and cool extremities.
CN: Physiological integrity; CNS: Physiological adaptation; CL: Analysis

16. 2, 4, and 5. Symptoms of cardiac tamponade include muffled heart sounds, hypotension, a narrowing pulse pressure, tachycardia, dyspnea, apprehension/fear, elevated right atrial and left atrial filling pressures, and sudden cessation of chest tube drainage. Cardiac tamponade occurs when a large volume of fluid or clots interferes with ventricular filling and pumping and collects in the pericardial sac, decreasing cardiac output.
CN: Physiological integrity; CNS: Physiological adaptation; CL: Analysis

17. A nurse is monitoring fluid and electrolyte balance in a child after cardiac surgery requiring cardiopulmonary bypass. Which of the following are expected findings? Select all that apply.
   1. Urine output of 5 ml/kg/hour
   2. Glucose level of 153 mg/dL
   3. Glucose level of 59 mg/dL
   4. Potassium level of 5.5 mEq/L
   5. Potassium level of 3.2 mEq/L

17. 2 and 5. In response to surgery and cardio-pulmonary bypass, the body secretes aldosterone and antidiuretic hormone. This in turn increases sodium levels and decreases urine output, which is defined as less than 1 to 2 ml/kg/hour. Hyperglycemia results from the body's decreased release of insulin and stimulation of glycogenolysis. It may also result from the administration of corticosteroids that occurs during the surgery. Hypokalemia is a result of intracellular fluid shifts that occur during bypass.
CN: Physiological integrity; CNS: Physiological adaptation; CL: Analysis

18. A nurse is teaching wound care to parents after cardiac surgery. Which statement made by the nurse is <u>most appropriate</u>?
   1. It is okay to apply lotions and powders to the incision area when you go home.
   2. Your child may take a tub bath tomorrow.
   3. Your child may complain of tingling, itching, or numbness at the incision site.
   4. If the adhesive strips over the incision fall off, call the physician.

I'm itching to get question 18 correct.

18. 3. As the area heals, tingling, itching, and numbness are normal sensations and will eventually go away. Lotions and powders should be avoided during the first 2 weeks after surgery. A complete bath should be delayed for the first week, although sponge baths are allowed. Adhesive strips may loosen or fall off on their own. This is a common and normal occurrence.
CN: Physiological integrity; CNS: Physiological adaptation; CL: Analysis

19. Parents ask a nurse about their 8-year-old son's activity level after cardiac surgery. Which would be the best response by the nurse?
   1. There are no exercise limitations.
   2. Your child may go back to school in 3 days.
   3. You should encourage a balance of rest and exercise.
   4. Climbing and contact sports are restricted for 1 week.

19. 3. Activity should be increased gradually each day, allowing for a sensible balance of rest and exercise. School and large crowds should be avoided for at least 2 weeks to prevent exposure to people with active infections. Sports and contact activities should be restricted for about 6 weeks, giving the sternum enough time to heal.
CN: Physiological integrity; CNS: Physiological adaptation; CL: Analysis

20. The nurse is providing discharge instructions for the parents of an infant who has recently undergone cardiac surgery. The nurse determines that teaching was effective when the parents state: Select all that apply.
   1. "I should not stop giving my baby any of its medicines until the doctor tells me to."
   2. "I need to find low-sodium formula to feed to my baby."
   3. "I am going to take my baby to church on Sunday so that everyone can see her."
   4. "I should not schedule an appointment for my baby to get its immunizations right away."

It's important that a child's family understands all discharge instructions.

20. 1 and 4. Drugs, such as digoxin and furosemide, shouldn't be stopped abruptly. There are no diet restrictions, and the child may resume her regular diet. Parents are encouraged to keep their child away from crowds for the first few weeks after surgery in order to prevent exposure to infections such as colds or respiratory syncytial virus bronchiolitis. Immunizations are delayed at least 6 weeks after surgery.
CN: Physiological integrity; CNS: Reduction of risk potential; CL: Analysis

21. The nurse is caring for a 4-year-old client with a chest tube that has been placed on water seal. The nurse assesses the chest tube and determines that it is functioning correctly when which of the following occurs?
1. The water level rises with inhalation.
2. Bubbling is seen in the suction chamber.
3. Bubbling is seen in the water seal chamber.
4. Water seal is obtained by clamping the tube.

21. 1. The water seal chamber is functioning appropriately when the water level rises in the chamber with inhalation and falls with expiration. This shows that negative pressure required in the lung is being maintained. Bubbling in the suction chamber should be seen only when suction is being used. Bubbling in the water seal chamber generally indicates the presence of an air leak. The chest tube should never be clamped; a tension pneumothorax may occur. Water seal is activated when the suction is disconnected.

CN: Physiological integrity; CNS: Reduction of risk potential; CL: Application

22. A child's chest tube becomes dislodged. Place a number by the interventions in the order that they should be performed by the nurse.
_____ Monitor vital signs.
_____ Place petroleum gauze dressing over the insertion site.
_____ Prepare for re-insertion of the chest tube.
_____ Call the physician.
_____ Document the incident.

22.
___3___ Monitor vital signs.
___1___ Place petroleum gauze dressing over the insertion site.
___4___ Prepare for reinsertion of the chest tube.
___2___ Call the physician.
___5___ Document the incident.

Petroleum gauze should be placed over the site immediately to prevent a pneumothorax. The physician should be notified after this step. Vital signs will be continuously monitored until physician arrives and/or during reinsertion. The patient should be prepped for reinsertion of the tube. The incident will then need to be documented within the patient's medical record.

CN: Physiological integrity; CNS: Reduction of risk potential; CL: Application

23. What are the expected assessment findings of an infant with heart failure? Select all that apply.
1. Heart rate of 100 beats/minute
2. Respiratory rate of 62 breaths/minute
3. Gallop murmur
4. +3 pulses in all extremities
5. Liver palpated at level of umbilicus

Question 23 is a milestone. Way to go!

23. 2, 3, and 5. Tachycardia, not bradycardia or low normal heart rates, occurs as a compensatory mechanism to the decrease in cardiac output. It also reflects the body's attempt to increase the force and rate of myocardial contraction and increase oxygen consumption of the heart. The respiratory rate increases, not decreases, in an attempt to increase oxygenation. Pulses are usually weak and thready. When the heart stretches beyond efficiency, an extra heart sound or S_3 gallop murmur may be audible. This is related to excessive preload and ventricular dilation. The liver becomes edematous (hepatomegaly) due to fluid retention.

CN: Physiological integrity; CNS: Physiological adaptation; CL: Analysis

24. An emergency room nurse is assessing a pediatric client in heart failure. Which symptom is consistent with a diagnosis of left-sided heart failure?
1. Weight gain
2. Peripheral edema
3. Neck vein distention
4. Tachypnea and dyspnea

25. Which nursing intervention is most appropriate when caring for an infant with heart failure?
1. Limit fluid intake.
2. Avoid using infant seats.
3. Cluster nursing activities.
4. Place the infant prone or supine.

Do you know what happens when my left side isn't working properly?

26. Which diet plan is recommended for an infant with heart failure?
1. Restriction of fluids
2. Weigh infant once a week.
3. Use of low-sodium formula
4. Increase the caloric content per ounce.

What's the diet plan?

27. A boy with patent ductus arteriosus was delivered 6 hours earlier and is being held by his mother. As the nurse enters the room to assess the neonate's vital signs, the mother says, "The physician says that my baby has a heart murmur. Does that mean he has a bad heart?" Which response by the nurse would be the most appropriate?
1. "He'll need more tests to determine his heart condition."
2. "He'll require oxygen therapy at home for a while."
3. "He'll be fine. Don't worry about him."
4. "The murmur is caused by the natural opening, which can take a day or two to close. It's a normal part of your baby's transition."

24. 4. Respiratory symptoms, such as tachypnea and dyspnea, are seen as a result of pulmonary congestion. Peripheral edema, jugular vein distention, and weight gain are seen with systemic venous congestion or right-sided heart failure. Fluid accumulates in the interstitial spaces because of blood pooling in the venous circulation.

CN: Physiological integrity; CNS: Physiological adaptation; CL: Application

25. 3. Energy expenditures need to be limited to reduce metabolic and oxygen needs. Nursing care should be clustered, followed by long periods of undisturbed rest. Fluid may be restricted in older children, but infants' nutritional requirements depend on fluid needs. Infants should be placed in the semi-Fowler's or upright position. Infant seats help maintain an upright position. This facilitates lung expansion, provides less restrictive movement of the diaphragm, relieves pressure from abdominal organs, and decreases pulmonary congestion.

CN: Physiological integrity; CNS: Physiological adaptation; CL: Analysis

26. 4. Formulas with increased caloric content are given to meet the greater caloric requirements from the overworked heart and labored breathing. Fluid restriction and low-sodium formulas aren't recommended. An infant's nutritional needs depend on fluid. Daily weights at the same time of the day on the same scale before feedings are recommended to follow trends in nutritional stability and diuresis. Low-sodium formulas may cause hyponatremia and can lead to decreased bone development.

CN: Physiological integrity; CNS: Basic care and comfort; CL: Application

27. 4. Although the nurse may want to tell the client not to worry, the most appropriate response would be to explain the neonate's present condition to relieve the mother and to acknowledge an awareness of the condition. A neonate's vascular system changes with birth; certain factors help to reverse the flow of blood through the ductus and ultimately favor its closure. This closure typically begins within the first 24 hours after birth and ends within a few days after birth. Diagnostic tests, especially invasive ones such as a cardiac catheterization, are reserved for when the infant becomes symptomatic. Oxygen is contraindicated in infants with this condition as it lowers the pulmonary vascular resistance and will lead to too much blood flow through the lungs.

CN: Health promotion and maintenance; CNS: None; CL: Analysis

28. A teenage client with heart failure is prescribed digoxin (Lanoxin) and asks the nurse, "What's the drug supposed to do?" The best response(s) by the nurse would be which of the following? Select all that apply.
1. "Improve the way your heart works."
2. "Keep you from getting an infection in your heart."
3. "Help you to not retain fluid."
4. "Lower your blood pressure."
5. "Slow your heart rate down."

29. Which assessment finding would lead the nurse to suspect a child has a digoxin level greater than 2 mcg/ml?
1. Weight gain
2. Tachycardia
3. Nausea and vomiting
4. Seizures

30. An 11-month-old infant with heart failure weighs 10 kg. Digoxin is prescribed as 10 mcg/kg/day in divided doses every 12 hours. How much is given per dose?
1. 10 mcg
2. 50 mcg
3. 100 mcg
4. 500 mcg

31. A child with heart failure is taking captopril (Capoten). What are the desired effects of this medication? Select all that apply.
1. Increased blood pressure
2. Decreased blood pressure
3. Decreased preload
4. Improved urine output

32. The parents of a newborn child have just been told that he has a heart defect known as patent ductus arteriosus. Which statement made by the parents indicates that teaching has been effective?
1. "Heart failure is uncommon in this defect."
2. "The ductus normally closes completely by age 6 weeks."
3. "An open ductus arteriosus causes decreased blood flow to the lungs."
4. "It represents a cyanotic defect with decreased pulmonary blood flow."

Knowing the classification of a drug can help you remember its actions.

I don't think this ace will inhibit me.

28. 1, 3, and 5. Digoxin is a cardiac glycoside. Its effects include increasing the force of contraction, decreasing the heart rate, slowing conduction through the atrioventricular node, and indirectly promoting dieresis by increasing perfusion to the kidneys. Digoxin will not keep one from getting an infection, and it does not have a significant effect on blood pressure.
CN: Physiological integrity; CNS: Pharmacological and parenteral therapies; CL: Application

29. 3. Digoxin toxicity in infants and children may present with nausea, vomiting, anorexia, or a slow, irregular apical heart rate. Weight gain, tachycardia, or seizures wouldn't be seen in digoxin toxicity.
CN: Physiological integrity; CNS: Pharmacological and parenteral therapies; CL: Analysis

30. 2. 10 kg × 10 mcg/kg/day = 100 mcg/day divided by 2 doses = 50 mcg/dose.
CN: Physiological integrity; CNS: Pharmacological and parenteral therapies; CL: Analysis

31. 2, 3, and 4. Angiotensin-converting enzyme (ACE) inhibitors block the conversion of angiotensin I to angiotensin II in the kidney. This causes vasodilation and decreased secretion of aldosterone. This leads to lowered blood pressure and decreased preload. Renal perfusion is also enhanced, which leads to improved diuresis (or urine output) and, therefore, also decreased preload.
CN: Physiological integrity; CNS: Pharmacological and parenteral therapies; CL: Application

32. 2. At birth, oxygenated blood normally causes the ductus to constrict, and the vessel closes completely by age 6 weeks. This defect is considered an acyanotic defect with increased pulmonary blood flow. The open ductus arteriosus can cause an excessive blood flow to the lungs because of the high pressure in the aorta. Heart failure is common in premature infants with a patent ductus arteriosus.
CN: Physiological integrity; CNS: Physiological adaptation; CL: Analysis

33. Which intervention or drug is recommended initially for preterm neonates to close a patent ductus arteriosus?
1. Indomethacin
2. Prostaglandin E₁
3. Surgical ligation
4. Cardiac catheterization

34. A nurse is caring for a client with patent ductus arteriosus. Which of the following assessment findings are consistent with this diagnosis? Select all that apply.
1. Weak peripheral pulses
2. Machinelike murmur
3. Widened pulse pressure
4. Tachypnea
5. Cyanosis

Question 34 asks which finding you expect, not necessarily one that may or may not occur.

35. During observation of a child who has undergone cardiac catheterization, the nurse notes significant bleeding from the percutaneous femoral catheterization site. Place the following interventions in their order of priority.
_____ Apply direct, continuous pressure.
_____ Reapply a pressure dressing.
_____ Seek the assistance of another nurse.
_____ Check the pulses in the affected leg.

How did I get into a chapter on cardiovascular disorders?

36. Which finding is expected by the nurse when assessing a child with an acyanotic heart defect?
1. Overweight
2. Bradycardia
3. Hepatomegaly
4. Decreased respiratory rate

33. 1. Preterm neonates with good renal function may receive oral indomethacin, a prostaglandin inhibitor, to encourage ductal closure. If this isn't effective, surgery is suggested. Prostaglandin E₁ will ensure patency of a patent ductus arteriosus for infants dependent on an open ductus arteriosus. Surgical ligation and a cardiac catheterization procedure may also be performed in infants and children.
CN: Physiological integrity; CNS: Physiological adaptation; CL: Analysis

34. 2, 3, and 4. The continuous, turbulent flow of blood from the aorta through the patent ductus arteriosus to the pulmonary artery produces a machinelike murmur. There's a widened pulse pressure and bounding peripheral pulses from the runoff of blood from the aorta to the pulmonary artery. Tachypnea is a common finding in all infants and children with heart defects. Cyanosis is not a common finding in children with defects that have increased pulmonary blood flow, such as ductus arteriosus. Cyanosis is common in defects that result in decreased pulmonary blood flow.
CN: Physiological integrity; CNS: Physiological adaptation; CL: Analysis

35. ___1___ Apply direct, continuous pressure.
___4___ Reapply a pressure dressing.
___2___ Seek the assistance of another nurse.
___3___ Check the pulses in the affected leg.

Bleeding from a major vessel must be stopped immediately to prevent massive hemorrhage. Vital signs would be taken after bleeding control measures are instituted. Calling for help is important, but pressure on the site must be applied and maintained while help is found. Pulses would be checked after bleeding is controlled or while pressure is being applied. A new dressing can be applied after bleeding is controlled.
CN: Physiological integrity; CNS: Reduction of risk potential; CL: Application

36. 3. Hepatomegaly may result from blood backing up into the liver due to the difficulty of entering the right side of the heart. The increase in blood flow to the lungs may cause tachycardia (not bradycardia) and increased respiratory rates to compensate. Poor growth and development, not excess weight gain, may be seen because of the increased energy required for breathing.
CN: Physiological integrity; CNS: Physiological adaptation; CL: Analysis

37. During observation of a child who has undergone cardiac catheterization, the nurse notes significant bleeding from the percutaneous femoral catheterization site. Which action should be taken <u>first</u>?
1. Apply direct, continuous pressure.
2. Assess the pulse and blood pressure.
3. Seek the assistance of another nurse.
4. Check the pulses in the affected leg.

38. Which signs may be seen in a child with a ventricular septal defect? Select all that apply.
1. Tachypnea
2. Plots at 95th percentile for height on growth chart
3. Plots at the 10th percentile for weight on growth chart
4. Bradycardia
5. Increased length of time to finish a bottle or breastfeeding

39. When caring for a child diagnosed with a ventricular septal defect, which description would the nurse incorporate when teaching the parents about this condition?
1. It is a narrowing of the aortic arch.
2. It is a failure of a septum to develop completely between the atria.
3. It is a narrowing of the valves at the entrance of the pulmonary artery.
4. It is a failure of a septum to develop completely between the ventricles.

40. The nurse is caring for a newborn who has been diagnosed with a ventricular septal defect. The newborn is not exhibiting any signs of heart failure. The parents ask the nurse why the doctors do not want to perform surgery immediately on the newborn. Which is the most appropriate response?
1. "The baby is just too little to have surgery right now."
2. "Waiting will allow you time to bond with your new baby."
3. "The doctor wants to wait and see if the hole in your baby's heart will close on its own."
4. "Your baby is not sick enough to require surgery at this point in time."

You can see these signs without a magnifying glass!

37. 1. Bleeding from a major vessel must be stopped immediately to prevent massive hemorrhage. Vital signs would be taken after bleeding control measures are instituted. Calling for help is important, but pressure on the site must be applied and maintained while help is found. Pulses would be checked after bleeding is controlled.
CN: Physiological integrity; CNS: Reduction of risk potential; CL: Application

38. 1, 3, and 5. Children with ventricular septal defect usually present with symptoms of heart failure (tachypnea and tachycardia, for example), poor growth and development, and failure to thrive. They also have difficulties in feeding due to their decreased cardiac output and tachypnea.
CN: Physiological integrity; CNS: Physiological adaptation; CL: Analysis

39. 4. Failure of a septum to develop between the ventricles results in a left-to-right shunt, which is noted as a ventricular septal defect. The narrowing of the aortic arch describes coarctation of the aorta. Narrowing of the valves at the pulmonary artery describes pulmonic stenosis. When the septum fails to develop between the atria, it's considered an atrial septal defect.
CN: Physiological integrity; CNS: Physiological adaptation; CL: Application

40. 3. This is the most appropriate response as 20% to 60% of ventricular septal defects will close spontaneously. While older, bigger infants do have better surgical outcomes, you would not say the baby is too little for surgery. Surgery is not delayed in order to add more bonding time; it is dependent on the infant's symptoms and size. Again, whereas statement 4 is technically correct, statement 3 is the more appropriate response.
CN: Physiological integrity; CNS: Physiological adaptation; CL: Analysis

CN: Client needs category   CNS: Client needs subcategory   CL: Cognitive level

41. A child with a ventricular septal defect repair is receiving dopamine (Intropin) postoperatively. The parents ask the nurse why the child is getting the medication. What is the best response by the nurse?
1. "To decrease heart rate"
2. "To decrease urine output"
3. "To increase cardiac output"
4. "To decrease cardiac contractility"

42. An infant returns to his room after a cardiac catheterization. What would be the most important information for the nurse to teach the parents about mobility? Select all that apply.
1. The infant may sit in an infant swing.
2. The infant may be held as long as the affected extremity is immobilized.
3. The infant may be maintained on bed rest with the affected extremity immobilized.
4. The infant may be held upright in arms in order to eat.

43. A client with Down syndrome (trisomy 21) comes to the pediatric clinic for a well visit. Which cardiac anomaly would this child be at risk for?
1. Atrial septal defect
2. Pulmonic stenosis
3. Ventricular septal defect
4. Atrioventricular canal defect

44. The nurse is assessing a child after a cardiac catheterization. Which of the following findings requires an immediate phone call to a physician?
1. Weak, thready pulse in dorsalis pedis pulse
2. Oral temperature of 99° F
3. Urine output of 2 ml/kg
4. Slightly bloody drainage around catheterization site dressing

You know more about drugs than you realize!

Question 42 already? Wow! You're making great strides!

We both think you're doing great!

41. 3. Dopamine stimulates β_1- and β_2-adrenergic receptors. It's a selective cardiac stimulant that will increase cardiac output, heart rate, and cardiac contractility. Urine output increases in response to dilation of the blood vessels to the mesentery and kidneys.

CN: Physiological integrity; CNS: Pharmacological and parenteral therapies; CL: Application

42. 2 and 3. The goal is to keep the leg immobilized in order to prevent hemorrhage. The child should be maintained on bed rest with the affected extremity immobilized after cardiac catheterization to prevent hemorrhage. Allowing the infant to sit in a swing, even with the affected extremity immobilized, places him at risk for hemorrhage. Infants may be held, especially if that keeps the infant calm and the leg remains immobilized. The infant should not be held upright as that will increase risk of hemorrhage.

CN: Physiological integrity; CNS: Reduction of risk potential; CL: Application

43. 4. Atrioventricular canal defects (or endocardial cushion defects) are seen most in children with Down syndrome. Atrial septal defects account for about 10% of all cardiac anomalies. Pulmonic stenosis is responsible for about 8% of all cardiac anomalies. Ventricular septal defects are the most common cardiac anomaly.

CN: Health promotion and maintenance; CNS: None; CL: Application

44. 1. The pulse below the catheterization site should be strong and equal to the unaffected extremity. A weakened pulse may indicate vessel obstruction or perfusion problems. Slightly elevated temperature and low normal urine output (normal urine output is 1 to 2 ml/kg/hour) are relatively normal findings after catheterization and may be the result of decreased oral fluids. A small amount of bloody drainage is normal; however, the site must be assessed frequently for increased bleeding, and the margins of the drainage should be marked on the dressing.

CN: Physiological integrity; CNS: Reduction of risk potential; CL: Application

45. Which cardiac anomaly produces a left-to-right shunt?
1. Atrial septal defect
2. Pulmonic stenosis
3. Tetralogy of Fallot
4. Total anomalous pulmonary venous return

My shunt is left to right. How about yours?

46. The nurse is aware that the assessment findings associated with a child who has a defect resulting in a left-to-right shunt include which of the following? Select all that apply.
1. Weight gain
2. Edema in extremities
3. Tachypnea
4. Retractions
5. Hepatomegaly
6. Decreased activity tolerance

47. A nurse is caring for a 3-year old child who is one day postoperative after having undergone a ventricular septal defect repair. The child weighs 15 kg. The most appropriate outcome for this child is:
1. capillary refill will be greater than 3 seconds.
2. pain score will be greater than 5.
3. urine output will be 25 ml/hour.
4. heart rate will be less than 70 beats/minute.

48. A 6-month-old infant with uncorrected tetralogy of Fallot suddenly becomes increasingly cyanotic and diaphoretic with weak peripheral pulses and an increased respiratory rate. Prioritize the following interventions.
_____ Administer oxygen.
_____ Administer morphine sulfate.
_____ Place the infant in a knee-chest position.
_____ Calm or comfort the infant.

45. 1. Atrial septal defects shunt from left to right because pressures are greater on the left side of the heart. Pulmonic stenosis, tetralogy of Fallot, and total anomalous pulmonary venous return will show a right-to-left shunting of blood.
CN: Health promotion and maintenance; CNS: None; CL: Analysis

46. 3, 4, and 6. Left-to-right shunting leads to increased pulmonary blood flow or blood flow to the lungs. The child will generally present with symptoms mimicking respiratory difficulties. Weight gain, extremity edema, and hepatomegaly are more commonly found in children with systemic venous congestion, not pulmonary congestion. Children with left-to-right shunts tend to be small for age because the work of breathing increases metabolic demand and children's caloric intake is used for the work of breathing and the work of the heart; thus, few calories are left for the child to grow.
CN: Health promotion and maintenance; CNS: None; CL: Analysis

47. 3. The patient needs to have a urine output of 1 to 2 ml/kg/hour. The capillary refill should be less than 3 seconds. The nurse should help the patient have a lower pain score than 5 as this is moderate pain and can have an impact on the child's recovery. The heart rate should be greater than 70 beats/minute; the normal range for this child is 70 to 110 beats/minute.
CN: Physiological integrity; CNS: Physiological adaptation; CL: Analysis

48. __**3**__ Administer oxygen.
__**4**__ Administer morphine sulfate.
__**1**__ Place the infant in a knee-chest position.
__**2**__ Calm or comfort the infant.

The knee-chest position reduces the workload of the heart by increasing the blood return to the heart and keeping the blood flow more centralized. Calming and comforting the infant will help to relax the infant, thereby helping to decrease the pressure in the lungs, which will therefore promote more blood flow through the lungs and improve oxygen saturation levels. Oxygen should be administered quickly but only after placing the infant in the knee-chest position and attempting to calm the infant. Morphine should be administered after repositioning and oxygen administration are completed. It will help to calm the infant and helps to relieve the infundibular spasm associated with hypercyanotic spells.
CN: Safe effective care environment; CNS: Management of care; CL: Application

49. A 15-year-old client is diagnosed with coarctation of the aorta. Which of the following would be expected assessment findings? Select all that apply.
1. Blood pressure of 120/76 mm Hg in the right arm
2. Blood pressure of 172/98 mm Hg in the left arm
3. Blood pressure of 84/46 mm Hg in the right leg
4. Complaints of headache
5. +3 pulses in both arms
6. +3 pulses in both legs

50. Which of the following are important to assess in a child who has undergone surgical repair of a coarctation of the aorta? Select all that apply.
1. Urine output
2. Neuromuscular function of the lower extremities
3. Lung sounds
4. Bowel sounds

51. The nurse is preparing to assess a child with a possible cardiac anomaly. It is most important for the nurse to assess which of the following?
1. Skin turgor
2. Temperature
3. Pupil size and reaction to light
4. Blood pressure in all four extremities

52. Which intervention is recommended postoperatively for a client with a surgical repair of coarctation of the aorta?
1. Administration of dopamine (Intropin)
2. Maintaining hypothermia
3. Administering sodium nitroprusside (Nipride)
4. Administering a bolus of I.V. fluids

I've heard of "go with the flow," but this is ridiculous!

Hint: Cardiac anomalies can be extreme.

49. 2, 3, 4, and 6. As blood is pumped from the left ventricle to the aorta some blood flows to the head and upper extremities, while the rest meets obstruction and jets through the constricted area. Pressures and pulses are greater in the upper extremities. Decreased or absent pulses are found in the lower extremities. Children who are diagnosed during their adolescent years present with hypertension, headaches, dizziness, fainting, and epistaxis.

CN: Physiological integrity; CNS: Physiological adaptation; CL: Analysis

50. 1, 2, 3, and 4. All are extremely important to assess. Due to the surgical approach in which the surgeon performs a thoracotomy and cross-clamps the aorta while repairing the area of defect, there is lack of blood flow to the lower extremities for a short period of time. Urine output must be closely monitored as well as reflexes, movement, and sensation of the lower extremities. Lung and bowel sounds are important for all postoperative assessments.

CN: Physiological integrity; CNS: Physiological adaptation; CL: Analysis

51. 4. Measuring blood pressure in all four extremities is necessary to document hypertension and the blood pressure gradient between the upper and lower extremities. Temperature, skin turgor, and pupillary assessment are also important but are not as specific for cardiac assessment as the blood pressure.

CN: Physiological integrity; CNS: Physiological adaptation; CL: Application

52. 3. Blood pressure is tightly managed and kept low so that there is no excessive pressure on the fresh suture lines, which could lead to rupture and postoperative hemorrhage. Sodium nitroprusside is a potent vasodilator and is used to keep the blood pressure on the lower side of normal, or even slightly decreased. Vasoconstrictors, such as dopamine and epinephrine, would be contraindicated because they would elevate blood pressure. Normothermia is maintained, and diuretics may be given to decrease fluid volume.

CN: Physiological integrity; CNS: Physiological adaptation; CL: Analysis

53. Which assessment is expected by the nurse when assessing a child with tetralogy of Fallot?
1. Machinelike murmur
2. Eisenmenger's complex
3. Increasing cyanosis with crying or activity
4. Higher pressures in the upper extremities than with the lower extremities

When it comes to assessment, practice makes perfect!

54. A child with tetralogy of Fallot has clubbing of the fingers and toes. The nurse is aware that the clubbing is most likely to be caused by:
1. polycythemia.
2. chronic hypoxia.
3. pansystolic murmur.
4. abnormal growth and development.

55. A child with tetralogy of Fallot may assume which position of comfort during exercise?
1. Prone
2. Semi-Fowler's
3. Side-lying
4. Squatting

I'll bet you already know the answer!

56. A nurse is describing tetralogy of Fallot to a child's parents. Which statement by the parents demonstrates that the teaching has been effective?
1. "The condition is commonly referred to as 'blue tets'."
2. "A child with this condition experiences hypercyanotic, or 'tet,' spells."
3. "A child with this condition experiences frequent respiratory infections."
4. "A child with this condition experiences decreased or absent pulses in the lower extremities."

53. 3. A child with tetralogy of Fallot will be mildly cyanotic at rest and have increasing cyanosis with crying, activity, or straining, as with a bowel movement. A machinelike murmur is a characteristic of patent ductus arteriosus. Eisenmenger's complex is a complication of pulmonary pressure exceeding systemic pressure. Higher pressures in the upper extremities are characteristic of coarctation of the aorta.
CN: Physiological integrity; CNS: Physiological adaptation; CL: Application

54. 2. Chronic hypoxia longer than 6 months causes clubbing of the fingers and toes when untreated. Hypoxia varies with the degree of pulmonic stenosis. Polycythemia is an increased number of red blood cells as a result of the chronic hypoxemia. A pansystolic murmur is heard at the middle to lower left sternal border but has no impact on clubbing. Growth and development may appear normal.
CN: Physiological integrity; CNS: Physiological adaptation; CL: Analysis

55. 4. A child may squat or assume a knee-chest position to reduce venous blood flow from the lower extremities and to increase systemic vascular resistance, which diverts more blood flow into the pulmonary artery. Prone, semi-Fowler's, and side-lying positions won't produce this effect.
CN: Physiological integrity; CNS: Physiological adaptation; CL: Analysis

56. 2. Hypercyanotic, or "tet," spells may occur as a result of increasing obstruction of right ventricular outflow, resulting in decreased pulmonary blood flow and increased right-to-left shunting. Infants with mild obstruction to blood flow have little or no right-to-left shunting and appear pink, or "pink tets." Frequent respiratory infections are seen in defects with increased pulmonary blood flow, such as a patent ductus arteriosus. Decreased or absent pulses in the lower extremities are a sign of coarctation of the aorta.
CN: Physiological integrity; CNS: Physiological adaptation; CL: Analysis

57. A child diagnosed with tetralogy of Fallot has been ordered to undergo testing. Which test would best indicate the direction and amount of shunting in this child?
1. Chest radiography
2. Echocardiography
3. Electrocardiography (ECG)
4. Cardiac catheterization

Hello? Is anybody there? I must have a bad connection.

58. A nurse is teaching parents about tricuspid atresia. Which statement indicates that the parents understand this disorder?
1. "There's a narrowing at the aortic outflow tract."
2. "The pulmonary veins don't return to the left atrium."
3. "There's a narrowing at the entrance of the pulmonary artery."
4. "There's no communication between the right atrium and right ventricle."

59. Which of the following are likely characteristics of a child diagnosed with tricuspid atresia? Select all that apply.
1. Cyanosis
2. Machinelike murmur
3. Decreased respiratory rate
4. Capillary refill more than 2 seconds
5. Clubbed fingers

Tricuspid atresia always makes me blue.

60. The nurse is caring for a child with tricuspid atresia who develops polycythemia. Which statement(s) is (are) most accurate concerning this manifestation? Select all that apply.
1. The red blood cell count is normal.
2. There is an increased ability for the oxygen to carry blood.
3. There is an increased risk of developing a thrombus.
4. The viscosity of the blood is unchanged.

57. 4. Cardiac catheterization provides specific information about the direction and amount of shunting, coronary anatomy, and each portion of the heart defect. Chest radiographs will show right ventricular hypertrophy pushing the heart apex upward, resulting in a boot-shaped silhouette. Echocardiogram scans define such defects as large ventricular septal defects, pulmonic stenosis, and malposition of the aorta. While an echocardiogram can show direction of blood flow, a cardiac catheterization can give more accurate information regarding the flow of blood and the amount of shunting. ECG shows right ventricular hypertrophy with tall R waves and does not show direction of blood flow.
CN: Physiological integrity; CNS: Reduction of risk potential; CL: Application

58. 4. Tricuspid atresia is failure of the tricuspid valve to develop, leaving no communication between the right atrium and right ventricle. Narrowing at the aortic outflow tract is aortic stenosis. Total anomalous pulmonary venous return is a defect in which the pulmonary veins don't return to the left atrium but abnormally return to the right side of the heart. The narrowing at the entrance of the pulmonary artery represents pulmonic stenosis.
CN: Physiological integrity; CNS: Physiological adaptation; CL: Analysis

59. 1, 4, and 5. Cyanosis is the most consistent clinical sign of tricuspid atresia. Tachypnea and dyspnea are commonly present because of the decreased pulmonary blood flow and right-to-left shunting. Tricuspid atresia doesn't have a characteristic murmur. A machinelike murmur is characteristic of a patent ductus arteriosus. Decreased oxygenation would increase capillary refill time. Clubbed fingers in children result from chronic hypoxia and may be seen in children with this defect.
CN: Physiological integrity; CNS: Physiological adaptation; CL: Analysis

60. 2 and 3. Polycythemia is an increased number of red blood cells, thereby increasing the ability of the blood to carry oxygen to the cells. It is the body's attempt at compensating for the chronic hypoxia associated with this heart defect. Due to this clinical manifestation, the viscosity of the blood increases, which leaves the child at risk for developing a thrombus, particularly when dehydrated. There is also not as much room for clotting factors, which can leave the child at risk for blood clotting disorders.
CN: Physiological integrity; CNS: Physiological adaptation; CL: Application

61. An infant has been diagnosed with tricuspid atresia. Which surgical intervention should a nurse expect the physician to recommend?
1. Blalock-Taussig operation
2. Fontan procedure
3. Jatene procedure
4. Patch closure

61. 1. The Blalock-Taussig operation is used to palliate infants with tricuspid atresia and is often the initial surgical procedure. It is performed to increase pulmonary blood flow. A bidirectional Glenn procedure is performed next when the child is approximately 4 to 8 months old. The Fontan procedure is the last surgical procedure performed. The child is usually 2 to 3 years old at the time of this procedure. Both the Glenn and the Fontan close septal defects and redirect systemic venous return to the lungs, thereby eliminating the ventricular pumping of blood between the atrium and the pulmonary artery. The Jatene procedure is used to correct a mixed defect such as transposition of the great arteries. Patch closures are used for defects such as a ventricular or atrial septal defect.
CN: Physiological integrity; CNS: Physiological adaptation; CL: Application

Read this question carefully to make sure you know what's being asked.

62. The nurse is preparing to administer digoxin (Lanoxin) to an infant. What is the most important intervention by the nurse?
1. Mix the digoxin with the infant's food.
2. Double the subsequent dose if a dose is missed.
3. Give the digoxin with antacids when possible.
4. Withhold the dose if the apical pulse rate is less than 90 beats/minute.

62. 4. Digoxin is used to decrease heart rate; however, the apical pulse must be carefully monitored to detect a severe reduction. Administering digoxin to an infant with a heart rate of less than 90 beats/minute could further reduce the rate and compromise cardiac output. Mixing digoxin with food may interfere with accurate dosing. Double-dosing should never be done. Antacids may decrease drug absorption.
CN: Physiological integrity; CNS: Pharmacological and parenteral therapies; CL: Application

63. A nurse is assessing a child who has undergone complete repair of total anomalous pulmonary venous connection. The nurse is most concerned when the child experiences which of the following?
1. Decreased work of breathing
2. Decreasing respiratory rate
3. Decreasing oxygenation saturation levels
4. Increasing urine output

63. 3. A child who has pulmonary venous obstruction will exhibit signs of increasing respiratory distress, such as increased respiratory rate, dyspnea, and shortness of breath. Oxygen saturation levels will decrease. Urine output will decrease as the heart fails.
CN: Physiological integrity; CNS: Physiological adaptation; CL: Application

You're halfway there. Fantastic!

64. The nurse is assessing a child with a total anomalous pulmonary venous return defect. The nurse would expect the assessment to include which finding?
1. Hypertension
2. Frequent respiratory infections
3. Normal growth and development
4. Above-average weight gain on the growth chart

64. 2. Children with total anomalous pulmonary venous return defects are prone to repeated respiratory infections due to increased pulmonary blood flow. Hypertension usually occurs with coarctation of the aorta, an acyanotic defect with obstructive flow. Poor feeding and failure to thrive are also signs of this defect. Infants look thin and malnourished.
CN: Physiological integrity; CNS: Physiological adaptation; CL: Application

65. The nurse is aware that a client who had a repair of total anomalous pulmonary venous return is at risk for which of the following?
1. Hypotension
2. Pulmonary hypertension
3. Ventricular arrhythmias
4. Pulmonary vein dilatation

66. The parents of an infant recently diagnosed with tricuspid atresia have been told that their child will need a series of three-staged surgeries during the first few years of life. Which statements indicate that the parents have an understanding of the procedures? Select all that apply.
1. "My child will have this dusky color for the rest of his life."
2. "These procedures will make my child have a normal heart."
3. "Once fixed, my baby will not have to take any more medicine."
4. "My baby will be just like all of the other children once the surgeries are all done."
5. "My child will have to be closely monitored for signs of a stroke."

67. Which assessment finding would the nurse commonly assess in a child with truncus arteriosus?
1. Weak, thready pulses
2. Narrowed pulse pressure
3. Pink and moist mucous membranes
4. Harsh, systolic regurgitant murmur

Listen closely and you'll hear the answer to question 67.

68. The nurse is preparing to administer digoxin and diuretics to an infant diagnosed with truncus arteriosus. What is best method of administration?
1. Use of a measuring spoon
2. Use of a graduated dropper
3. Use of an oral syringe
4. Mixing the drug in a bottle with juice or milk

If it doesn't taste good, I don't want it.

65. 2. Pulmonary hypertension, atrial arrhythmias, and pulmonary vein obstruction are complications that may result postoperatively. The left atrium is small and sensitive to fluid volume loading. An increase in the pressure in the right atrium is required to ensure left atrial filling.
CN: Physiological integrity; CNS: Physiological adaptation; CL: Analysis

66. 1 and 5. The child will be dusky, particularly around mucous membranes and nail beds, for the rest of his life as a result of chronic hypoxemia. The resultant polycythemia and increased blood viscosity increase the child's chances of developing a thrombus, leading to a cerebrovascular accident or stroke. The three surgeries do not make the child have a "normal" heart, as they do not fix the original defect. The child will more than likely be on medications for the rest of his life, and the child will more than likely be smaller in stature than other children.
CN: Physiological integrity; CNS: Physiological adaptation; CL: Analysis

67. 4. As a result of the ventricular septal defect, a harsh systolic regurgitant murmur is heard along the left sternal border and is usually accompanied by a thrill. Increasing pulmonary blood flow causes bounding pulses and a widened pulse pressure. Systemic and pulmonary blood mixing leads to mild or moderate cyanosis, so mucous membranes may appear dull or gray.
CN: Physiological integrity; CNS: Physiological adaptation; CL: Analysis

68. 3. Use of a syringe, particularly for doses that are less than 1 ml in volume, provide the most accurate way of drawing up and administering the medication. The volume of the drop administered with a dropper can vary, depending on the viscosity of the medication. While some medications may come with a dropper, that dropper is designed for that medication alone, and the oral syringe is still more accurate. A measuring spoon, such as a teaspoon that bakers use, is not as accurate as a syringe. Mixing drugs with juice, milk, or food may cause a problem if the child doesn't completely finish the meal because then how much the child received isn't definite. In addition, this action may lead to food aversions, which prevent the child from drinking or eating for fear of tasting the drug.
CN: Physiological integrity; CNS: Pharmacological and parenteral therapies; CL: Application

69. Which change would the nurse expect after administering oxygen to an infant with uncorrected tetralogy of Fallot?
1. Disappearance of the murmur
2. No evidence of cyanosis
3. Improvement of finger clubbing
4. Less agitation

70. Which statement about transposition of the great arteries is correct?
1. Electrocardiography will always show arrhythmias.
2. Diagnosis can be made in utero.
3. A chest X-ray can show an accurate view of the defect.
4. Heart failure is not a related complication.

71. A nurse is assessing a child with transposition of the great arteries. Which associated defect should the nurse expect to see in this client?
1. Mitral atresia
2. Pulmonic stenosis
3. Patent foramen ovale
4. Hypoplasia of the left ventricle

72. Administration of which medication would be the <u>most important</u> in treating unrepaired transposition of the great arteries?
1. Digoxin (Lanoxin)
2. Furosemide (Lasix)
3. Enalapril (Vasotec)
4. Prostaglandin E$_1$ (Alprostadil)

73. What surgical procedure is recommended for repair of transposition of the great arteries?
1. Jatene procedure
2. Fontan procedure
3. Balloon atrial septostomy
4. Blalock-Taussig operation

You're almost up to question 75! Way to go!

It's most important that you read each question carefully.

69. 4. Supplemental oxygen will help the infant breathe more easily and feel less anxious or agitated. Disappearance of the murmur, no evidence of cyanosis, and improvement of finger clubbing would not occur as a result of supplemental oxygen administration.
CN: Physiological integrity; CNS: Physiological adaptation; CL: Application

70. 2. Echocardiography done by a fetal cardiologist can diagnose transposition of the great arteries in utero. The other defects associated with this defect include a patent foramen ovale and a ventricular septal defect that contribute to developing heart failure. Electrocardiography may or may not reveal arrhythmias. Chest X-ray can show cardiomegaly and pulmonary vascular markings only. Echocardiography or cardiac catheterization may be required preoperatively to show the coronary artery anatomy before surgical repair.
CN: Physiological integrity; CNS: Physiological adaptation; CL: Analysis

71. 3. A patent foramen ovale, patent ductus arteriosus, and ventricular septal defect are associated defects related to transposition of the great arteries. A patent foramen ovale is the most common and is necessary to provide adequate mixing of blood between the two circulations. Pulmonic stenosis is associated with tetralogy of Fallot. Hypoplasia of the left ventricle and mitral atresia are two defects associated with hypoplastic left heart syndrome.
CN: Physiological integrity; CNS: Physiological adaptation; CL: Analysis

72. 4. Prostaglandin E$_1$ is necessary to maintain patency of the patent ductus arteriosus and improve systemic arterial flow in children with inadequate intracardiac mixing. Digoxin, diuretics (such as furosemide), and angiotensin-converting enzyme (ACE) inhibitors (such as enalapril) will treat heart failure when present.
CN: Physiological integrity; CNS: Pharmacological and parenteral therapies; CL: Application

73. 1. The Jatene procedure involves transposing the great arteries and mobilizing and reimplanting the coronary arteries. The Fontan procedure is recommended for repair of tricuspid atresia. Balloon atrial septostomy is a palliative procedure used during cardiac catheterization for children without a coexisting lesion. Blalock-Taussig operation is used to palliate tricuspid atresia and pulmonic atresia.
CN: Physiological integrity; CNS: Physiological adaptation; CL: Application

CN: Client needs category   CNS: Client needs subcategory   CL: Cognitive level

74. Which statement by the nurse best describes a characteristic of valvular pulmonic stenosis?
1. "The valve is normal."
2. "The right ventricle is hypoplastic."
3. "Left ventricular hypertrophy develops."
4. "Divisions between the cusps are fused."

75. During the assessment of a child with pulmonic stenosis, the nurse would anticipate observing which of the following?
1. Hyperactivity
2. Normal respiratory rate
3. Systolic ejection murmur
4. Capillary refill more than 2 seconds

76. Which finding is seen during cardiac catheterization of a child with pulmonic stenosis?
1. Right-to-left shunting
2. Left-to-right shunting
3. Decreased pressure in the right side of the heart
4. Increased oxygenation in the left side of the heart

I know what I am looking for!

Keep going! You're doing great!

77. A nurse is caring for a 16-year-old client with aortic stenosis. The nurse anticipates that during periods of activity the child may experience which of the following? Select all that apply.
1. Chest pain
2. Dizziness
3. Inability to run as long as his peers
4. Dusky lips and fingernail beds

78. A nurse is teaching the parents of a child newly diagnosed with aortic stenosis. Which statements should the nurse include in her teaching about this disorder? Select all that apply.
1. "The aortic valve is typically tricuspid, but it is commonly bicuspid in aortic stenosis."
2. "It causes an increase in cardiac output."
3. "Your child needs to be encouraged to immediately report any chest pain or nausea and vomiting."
4. "Your child will have blue lips and nail beds as he gets older."

74. 4. Blood flow through the valve is restricted by fusion of the divisions between the cusps. The valve may be normal or malformed. Right ventricular hypertrophy develops due to resistance to blood flow.
CN: Physiological integrity; CNS: Physiological adaptation; CL: Analysis

75. 3. A systolic ejection murmur, which may be accompanied by a thrill, can be heard at the upper left sternal border. The decrease in pulmonary blood flow causes fatigue and dyspnea. Systemic cyanosis may result from right ventricular failure that increases the capillary refill time.
CN: Physiological integrity; CNS: Physiological adaptation; CL: Analysis

76. 1. Right-to-left shunting develops through a patent foramen ovale, an atrial septal defect, or a ventricular septal defect due to right ventricular failure and an increase in pressure in the right side of the heart. Decreased oxygenation in the left side of the heart is noted because of the right-to-left shunt and decreased pulmonary blood flow.
CN: Physiological integrity; CNS: Physiological adaptation; CL: Analysis

77. 1, 2, and 3. Children with aortic stenosis may develop chest pain similar to angina when they are active. They also may complain of dizziness, exercise intolerance or decreased endurance, fatigue, syncope, dyspnea, and palpitations. They do not experience symptoms of cyanosis such as dusky lips or mucous membranes.
CN: Physiological integrity; CNS: Physiological adaptation; CL: Application

78. 1 and 3. Aortic stenosis is often caused by a malformation in the cusps of the valve itself. While the valve is supposed to be tricuspid, it is often bicuspid. Children with this defect should not participate in strenuous activity as it can predispose them to myocardial infarction or sudden death. Chest pain or nausea and vomiting are signs of myocardial ischemia and need to be reported immediately. There is decreased cardiac output as the left ventricle becomes hypertrophied due to trying to pump against the stenotic valve. Children with this defect are not cyanotic and have pink mucous membranes.
CN: Physiological integrity; CNS: Physiological adaptation; CL: Analysis

79. The <u>most appropriate</u> information for the nurse to give the parents of a child with aortic stenosis would be?
1. Restrict exercise.
2. Avoid dental procedures
3. Avoid digoxin.
4. Restrict fluid intake.

Is it OK if I run around?

80. The nurse is planning care for a 9-year-old male child with heart failure. Which nursing diagnosis should receive <u>priority</u>?
1. Risk for decreased cardiac tissue perfusion related to sympathetic response to heart failure
2. Imbalanced nutrition: Less than body requirement related to rapid tiring while feeding
3. Anxiety (parent) related to unknown nature of child's illness
4. Decreased cardiac output related to cardiac defect

81. Which nursing diagnosis is the <u>most appropriate</u> to include in a family-centered plan of care when caring for an infant newly diagnosed with hypoplastic left heart syndrome?
1. Death anxiety
2. Delayed growth and development
3. Deficient diversional activity
4. Risk for activity intolerance

82. A child is receiving prednisone after undergoing a heart transplant. The parents of the child ask the nurse what the purpose of the medication is. The best response by the nurse would be?
1. "It stimulates the appetite."
2. "It suppresses the body's immune response."
3. "It improves wound healing."
4. "It prevents fluid retention."

79. 1. Exercise should be restricted because of low cardiac output and left ventricular failure. Strenuous activity has been reported to result in sudden death from the development of myocardial ischemia. Dental procedures are not contraindicated and are in fact advised. The child may need prophylactic antibiotics to prevent bacterial endocarditis. Digoxin may be needed if the child develops heart failure. Fluid restriction is not necessary unless the child develops severe heart failure.
CN: Physiological integrity; CNS: Physiological adaptation; CL: Application

80. 4. The primary nursing diagnosis for a child with heart failure is decreased cardiac output related to cardiac defect. The most common cause of heart failure in children is congenital heart defects. Some defects result from the blood being pumped from the left side of the heart to the right side of the heart. The heart can't manage the extra volume, resulting in the pulmonary system becoming overloaded. Risk for decreased cardiac tissue perfusion, imbalanced nutrition, and anxiety don't take priority over decreased cardiac output.
CN: Physiological integrity; CNS: Physiological adaptation; CL: Application

81. 1. Without intervention, death usually occurs within the first few days of life as a result of progressive hypoxia, acidosis, and shock as the ductus closes and systemic perfusion diminishes. If the parents choose cardiac transplantation, the child may die waiting for a donor heart. For those who choose surgery, the child may not survive the three stages of the surgery. The other three choices will apply as the infant becomes older and are not the most appropriate at this time.
CN: Physiological integrity; CNS: Physiological adaptation; CL: Analysis

82. 2. The goal of prednisone for this client is to suppress the immune system, thereby preventing organ rejection. Prednisone is often used in combination with other immunosuppressant medications in order to prevent rejection. While corticosteroids do stimulate appetite, that is not the desired effect for this child. Prednisone and other corticosteroids cause decreased ability of wounds to heal; fluid retention is one of the side effects.
CN: Physiological integrity; CNS: Pharmacological and parenteral therapies; CL: Application

83. A child who received a heart transplant has been taking prednisone. The nurse is most concerned when the child experiences which of the following?
1. Weight loss
2. Hyperpyrexia
3. Anorexia
4. Poor wound healing

84. A child is given 0.5 mg/kg/day of prednisone divided into two doses. The child weighs 10 kg. How much is given in each dose?
1. 2.5 mg
2. 5 mg
3. 10 mg
4. 1.5 mg

85. The nurse is caring for 3-year-old client who has a high red blood cell count and polycythemia. The most important intervention for the nurse to include in the plan of care would be?
1. Encouragement of fluid intake
2. Administration of analgesics
3. Sodium-restricted diet
4. Use of a soft toothbrush

86. Which statement by the nurse about bacterial or infective endocarditis is <u>most</u> accurate?
1. "Bacteria invade only the tissues of the heart."
2. "It is an infection of the valves and inner lining of the heart."
3. "It is an inappropriate fusion of the endocardial cushions during fetal life."
4. "It is caused by alterations in cardiac preload, afterload, or contractility."

87. A child with suspected bacterial endocarditis arrives at the emergency department. The nurse would anticipate the assessment findings to include which of the following? Select all that apply.
1. Weight gain
2. Murmur
3. Low-grade fever
4. Malaise
5. Headache

83. 4. Common adverse reactions to prednisone include poor wound healing, weight gain, delayed temperature response, increased appetite, delayed sexual maturation, growth impairment, and a cushingoid appearance. The school-age child who has received prednisone is usually overweight and has a moon-shaped face.

CN: Physiological integrity; CNS: Pharmacological and parenteral therapies; CL: Application

84. 1. The child should receive 2.5 mg/dose. Use the following equations:

$$0.5 \text{ mg/kg} \times 10 \text{ kg} = 5 \text{ mg};$$
$$5 \text{ mg}/2 \text{ doses} = 2.5 \text{ mg/dose}$$

CN: Physiological integrity; CNS: Pharmacological and parenteral therapies; CL: Analysis

85. 1. Dehydration needs to be prevented. The blood of a child with polycythemia is thicker and more viscous, which leaves it prone to thrombus development. Dehydration makes the blood even thicker, leading to increased risk of clot formation. Analgesics are good to include in the plan of care of a child, especially if the child is experiencing pain, but they will not prevent thrombus formation. A soft toothbrush is used when the child is at risk for bleeding and will not be useful in preventing thrombus formation. A sodium-restricted diet will have no effect on clotting and is not recommended in infants and children.

CN: Physiological integrity; CNS: Reduction of risk potential; CL: Application

86. 2. Bacterial or infective endocarditis is an infection of the valves and inner lining of the heart. It's usually caused by the bacteria *Streptococcus viridans* and commonly affects children with acquired or congenital anomalies of the heart or great vessels. Bacteria may grow into adjacent tissues and may break off and embolize elsewhere, such as the spleen, kidney, lung, skin, and central nervous system. Endocardial cushion defects represent inappropriate fusion of the endocardial cushions in fetal life. Alterations in preload, afterload, contractility, or heart rate refer to heart failure.

CN: Physiological integrity; CNS: Physiological adaptation; CL: Application

87. 2, 3, 4, and 5. Symptoms may include a low-grade intermittent fever, decrease in hemoglobin level, tachycardia, anorexia, weight loss, malaise, headache, joint and muscle pain, and decreased activity level. Bacteremia leads to these signs of an infection. The murmur is due to damage to the cardiac valves or myocardium.

CN: Physiological integrity; CNS: Physiological adaptation; CL: Application

Hey, I'm just along for the ride.

Are you blaming me for this, or what?

88. Which factor may lead to bacterial endocarditis in a child with underlying heart disease?
1. History of a cold for 3 days
2. Dental work pretreated with antibiotics
3. Peripheral I.V. catheter in place for 1 day
4. Indwelling urinary catheter for 2 days leading to a urinary tract infection

89. Erythromycin (E-Mycin) is given to a 6-year-old child before dental work to prevent endocarditis. The child weighs 44 lb. The order is for 20 mg/kg by mouth 2 hours before the procedure. The bottle comes concentrated as 400 mg/5 ml. How many milliliters should the child receive?
1. 2.5 ml
2. 5 ml
3. 5.5 ml
4. 10 ml

90. What is the <u>most</u> common adverse reaction a nurse might observe after administering enteric-coated erythromycin (Ery-tab)?
1. Weight gain
2. Constipation
3. Increased appetite
4. Nausea and vomiting

91. A child is hospitalized with bacterial endocarditis. Which nursing diagnosis is <u>most appropriate</u>?
1. Constipation
2. Excess fluid volume
3. Deficient diversional activity
4. Imbalanced nutrition: More than body requirements

Wow! You finished question 90! The rest should be a snap!

Nursing diagnoses: Share the knowledge!

88. 4. Bacterial organisms can enter the bloodstream from any site of infection such as a urinary tract infection. Gram-negative bacilli are common causative agents. Colds are usually viral, not bacterial. Dental work is a common portal of entry if not pretreated with antibiotics. A peripheral I.V. catheter is an entry site but only if signs and symptoms of infection are present. Long-term indwelling catheters pose a higher risk for infection.
CN: Physiological integrity; CNS: Physiological adaptation; CL: Analysis

89. 2. The child should receive 5 ml. Use the following equations:
Convert pounds to kilograms:
44 lb/2.2 kg = 20 kg
Then, determine how many milligrams to give:
20 mg/kg × 20 kg = 400 mg
Next, determine how many milliliters to give:
400 mg/400 mg × 5 ml = 5 ml
(desired/have × amount on hand = amount to administer)
CN: Physiological integrity; CNS: Pharmacological and parenteral therapies; CL: Analysis

90. 4. Erythromycin is an antibiotic. Common adverse effects include nausea, vomiting, diarrhea, abdominal pain, and anorexia. It should be given with a full glass of water and after meals or with food to lessen gastrointestinal symptoms.
CN: Physiological integrity; CNS: Pharmacological and parenteral therapies; CL: Application

91. 3. Treatment for bacterial endocarditis requires long-term hospitalization or home care for I.V. antibiotics. Children may be bored and depressed, needing age-appropriate activities. Excess fluid volume, constipation, and imbalanced nutrition: more than body requirements may be possible nursing diagnoses related to the adverse reactions of antibiotics, such as gastrointestinal upset.
cn: Physiological integrity; cns: Physiological adaptation; cl: Analysis

92. The nurse would expect a child with Kawasaki disease to exhibit which of the following? Select all that apply.
1. Low-grade fever
2. Strawberry tongue
3. Desquamation of hands and feet
4. Bilateral conjunctival infection with yellow exudates
5. Irritability

92. 2, 3, and 5. Characteristics of Kawasaki disease (mucocutaneous lymph node syndrome) include a high fever of 5 or more days unresponsive to antibiotics and antipyretics; dry, red eyes without exudates; inflammation of the pharynx and oral mucosa; strawberry tongue (caused by sloughing of the coating of the tongue); perineal rash; desquamation of the hands and feet; arthritis; cervical lymphadenopathy; and extreme irritability. The cardiac symptoms, such as myocarditis and coronary artery aneurysms, are often subclinical and are diagnosed with further investigation, such as echocardiogram.

CN: Physiological integrity; CNS: Physiological adaptation; CL: Application

Which statement is most appropriate?

93. A nurse is teaching the parents of a child with Kawasaki disease. Which statement should the nurse include in her teaching about this disorder?
1. "It mostly occurs in the summer and fall."
2. "Diagnosis can be made with laboratory testing."
3. "It's an acute systemic vasculitis of unknown cause."
4. "It manifests in two different stages: acute and subacute."

93. 3. Kawasaki disease can best be described as an acute systemic vasculitis of unknown cause. Most cases are geographic and seasonal, with most occurring in the late winter and early spring. Diagnosis is based on clinical findings of five of the six diagnostic criteria and associated laboratory results. There's no specific laboratory test for diagnosis. There are three stages: acute, subacute, and convalescent.

CN: Physiological integrity; CNS: Physiological adaptation; CL: Application

94. The nurse determines that a child with Kawasaki disease has entered the <u>subacute</u> phase when the assessment includes which of the following?
1. Polymorphous rash
2. Normal blood values
3. Cervical lymphadenopathy
4. Desquamation of the hands and feet

What happens during the subacute phase of this disease?

94. 4. The subacute phase shows characteristic desquamation of the hands and feet. Blood values return to normal at the end of the convalescent phase. Cervical lymphadenopathy and a polymorphous rash can be seen in the acute phase due to the onset of inflammation and fever.

CN: Physiological integrity; CNS: Physiological adaptation; CL: Analysis

95. A nurse is caring for a child with Kawasaki disease. Which symptom should concern the nurse the most?
1. Mild diarrhea
2. Pain in the joints
3. Abdominal pain with vomiting
4. Increased erythrocyte sedimentation rate (ESR)

95. 3. The most serious complication of this disease is cardiac involvement. Abdominal pain, vomiting, and restlessness are the main symptoms of an acute myocardial infarction in children. Mild diarrhea can be treated with oral fluids. Pain in the joints is an expected sign of arthritis that usually occurs in the subacute phase. An increased ESR is a reflection of the inflammatory process and may be seen for 2 to 4 weeks after the onset of symptoms.

CN: Physiological integrity; CNS: Physiological adaptation; CL: Analysis

96. A child is undergoing testing to rule out a diagnosis of Kawasaki disease. Which test results may lead to this diagnosis? Select all that apply.
1. Hematuria
2. Leukocytosis
3. Thrombocytopenia
4. Decreased erythrocyte sedimentation rate
5. Elevated C-reactive protein levels

97. Therapy for Kawasaki disease includes a single dose of I.V. gamma globulin, prescribed at 2 g/kg. The child weighs 14.5 kg. How many grams should this child receive?

98. A child is receiving 8 g of I.V. gamma globulin for treatment of Kawasaki disease. The child weighs 20 kg. The order is for 8 g of gamma globulin over 12 hours. The concentration is 8 g in 300 ml of normal saline. How many milliliters per hour will this child receive?
1. 12 ml/hour
2. 25 ml/hour
3. 50 ml/hour
4. 40 ml/hour

99. A child is prescribed aspirin as part of the therapy for Kawasaki disease. The order is for 80 mg/kg/day orally in four divided doses until the child is afebrile. The child weighs 15 kg. How much is given in one dose?
1. 60 mg
2. 300 mg
3. 320 mg
4. 1,200 mg

100. A nurse is giving discharge instructions to the parents of a child with Kawasaki disease. Which statement by the parents shows an understanding of the treatment plan?
1. "A regular diet can be resumed at home."
2. "Black, tarry stools are considered normal."
3. "My child should use a soft-bristled toothbrush."
4. "My child can return to playing soccer next week."

Here's another dosing question. You can do it!

The numbers just keep coming!

Listen for feedback to find out if your instructions were understood.

96. **2 and 5.** Inflammation of the small vessels, along with pancarditis, leads to an elevated leukocyte count, increased platelet count, increased erythrocyte sedimentation rate, and elevated C-reactive protein levels. Urinalysis shows proteinuria or sterile pyuria.
CN: Physiological integrity; CNS: Physiological adaptation; CL: Analysis

97. 29. 14.5 kg × 2 g = 29 g
CN: Physiological integrity; CNS: Pharmacological and parenteral therapies; CL: Analysis

98. **2.** The child should receive 25 ml/hour. Use the following equation: 300 ml/12 hours = 25 ml/hour.
CN: Physiological integrity; CNS: Pharmacological and parenteral therapies; CL: Analysis

99. **2.** The child should receive 300 mg in one dose. Use the following equation:
First, determine how many milligrams should be given in 1 day:
80 mg/kg × 15 kg = 1,200 mg
Then, determine how many milligrams should be given in one dose:
1,200 mg/4 doses = 300 mg/dose
CN: Physiological integrity; CNS: Pharmacological and parenteral therapies; CL: Analysis

100. **3.** Because of the anticoagulant effects of aspirin therapy, a soft-bristled toothbrush will prevent bleeding of the gums. A low-cholesterol diet should be followed until coronary artery involvement resolves. Black, tarry stools are abnormal and are signs of bleeding that should be reported to the physician immediately. Contact sports should be avoided because of the cardiac involvement and excessive bruising that may occur as a result of aspirin therapy.
CN: Physiological integrity; CNS: Physiological adaptation; CL: Analysis

101. A nurse is preparing the family of a client with Kawasaki disease for discharge. What is the most appropriate information for the nurse to include?
1. Stop the aspirin when you return home.
2. Immunizations can be given in 2 weeks.
3. The child may return to school in 1 week.
4. Frequent echocardiography will be needed.

102. A nurse is teaching the parents of a child with <u>acute</u> rheumatic fever about the disorder. Which statement would be the most accurate concerning this condition?
1. It is a progressive inflammation of the small vessels of the body.
2. It is a mucocutaneous lymph node syndrome.
3. It is a serious infection of the endocardial surface of the heart.
4. It is a sequela of group A beta-hemolytic streptococcal infections.

103. Which assessment findings are expected in a child with acute rheumatic fever? Select all that apply.
1. Aschoff bodies
2. Arthritis affecting one joint
3. High fever for 5 or more days
4. Nonpruritic rash
5. Murmur
6. Irregular movements of the extremities

104. Which of the following are required to establish a diagnosis of acute rheumatic fever?
1. Laboratory tests
2. Fever and four Jones criteria
3. Positive blood cultures for *Staphylococcus* organisms
4. Use of Jones criteria and presence of a streptococcal infection

Read carefully. Question 102 asks about acute rheumatic fever, not chronic.

101. 4. Because of the risk of coronary artery involvement and possible aneurysm development, repeat echocardiography and electrocardiography will be required the first few weeks and at 6 months. Aspirin therapy may be continued for 2 weeks after the onset of symptoms. If signs of coronary artery involvement are present, aspirin therapy may be continued indefinitely. Live-virus vaccines should be avoided for 6 to 11 months after gamma globulin therapy because of an increased risk of a cross-sensitivity reaction to the antibodies found in the dose given. Returning to school should be avoided until cleared by the physician.
CN: Physiological integrity; CNS: Physiological adaptation; CL: Analysis

102. 4. Acute rheumatic fever is a multisystem disorder caused by group A beta-hemolytic streptococcal infections. It may involve the heart, joints, central nervous system, and skin. Kawasaki disease is also known as a mucocutaneous lymph node syndrome characterized by a progressive inflammation of the small vessels. Endocarditis describes a serious infection of the endocardial surface of the heart.
CN: Health promotion and maintenance; CNS: None; CL: Application

103. 1, 4, 5, and 6. Clinical manifestations associated with rheumatic fever include Aschoff bodies (inflammatory, hemorrhagic bullous lesions), murmur, pericardial rub, polyarthritis that moves to different joints every 1 to 2 days, erythema marginatum (macular rash), subcutaneous nodules, and chorea (irregular movements of the extremities, facial grimaces, and speech disturbances). A low-grade fever is a minor manifestation. A high fever of 5 or more days may represent Kawasaki disease.
CN: Physiological integrity; CNS: Physiological adaptation; CL: Application

104. 4. Two major or one major and two minor manifestations from Jones criteria and the presence of a streptococcal infection justify the diagnosis of rheumatic fever. There's no single laboratory test for diagnosis. Fever and four diagnostic criteria are required to diagnose Kawasaki disease. Blood cultures would be positive for *Streptococcus*, not *Staphylococcus*, organisms.
CN: Physiological integrity; CNS: Physiological adaptation; CL: Analysis

105. Which diagnostic criterion is considered a major Jones criterion for acute rheumatic fever?
1. Carditis
2. Prolonged PR interval
3. Low-grade fever
4. Previous heart disease

106. A nurse is caring for a child with acute rheumatic fever. Which symptom would indicate Sydenham's chorea?
1. Cardiomegaly
2. Regurgitant murmur
3. Pericardial friction rubs
4. Involuntary muscle movements

107. Criteria for rheumatic fever are being discussed with parents. A nurse determines that the parents understand chorea when they make which statement?
1. "My child may not be able to walk."
2. "Long movies may help for relaxation."
3. "My child might have difficulty in school."
4. "Many activities and visitors are recommended."

108. A 3-year-old child has a positive culture for a *Streptococcus* organism. The <u>most important</u> discharge instruction for the nurse to give the parents would be?
1. Administer aspirin as needed for the fever.
2. Administer antibiotics until the fever goes away.
3. Administer antibiotics for the prescribed amount of time.
4. Encourage the child to drink while he is awake.

109. A nurse is preparing a child for discharge after being diagnosed with rheumatic fever without carditis. What instructions should the nurse give the parents?
1. "Give aspirin for signs of chorea."
2. "Give penicillin for 1 month total."
3. "Only give penicillin for dental work."
4. "It isn't necessary to give penicillin before dental procedures."

I was just trying to "keep up with the Jones."

Question 108 is asking for the most important discharge instruction.

Don't sweat it! You're almost there.

105. 1. Carditis is a major diagnostic criterion of acute rheumatic fever. It's the only manifestation that can lead to death or long-term sequelae. Prolonged PR interval, low-grade fever, and previous heart disease are considered minor Jones diagnostic criteria.
CN: Physiological integrity; CNS: Physiological adaptation; CL: Application

106. 4. Sydenham's chorea is an involvement of the central nervous system by the rheumatic process. This is seen as muscular incoordination; purposeless, involuntary movements; and emotional lability. A regurgitant murmur, cardiomegaly, and a pericardial friction rub are clinical signs of rheumatic carditis.
CN: Physiological integrity; CNS: Physiological adaptation; CL: Application

107. 3. Chorea may last 1 to 6 months. Central nervous system involvement contributes to a shortened attention span, so children might have difficulty learning in school. A quiet environment is required for treatment. Muscle incoordination may cause the child to be more clumsy than usual when walking.
CN: Physiological integrity; CNS: Physiological adaptation; CL: Analysis

108. 3. Infection caused by *Streptococcus* organisms is treated with antibiotics, mainly penicillin. The antibiotics need to be administered for the entire course of therapy and should not be stopped when symptoms go away. Antipyretics, such as acetaminophen, may be given for fever. Aspirin is not recommended due to the risk of Reye's syndrome. Fluid intake is encouraged to prevent dehydration from decreased oral intake due to the sore throat or to replace fluids lost because of possible diarrhea from the antibiotics.
CN: Physiological integrity; CNS: Physiological adaptation; CL: Analysis

109. 4. Children who might benefit from prophylactic penicillin include those with unrepaired congenital heart defects, heart defects repaired with synthetic material, or prior infective endocarditis, and some children with heart transplants. Prophylactic antibiotic therapy isn't otherwise recommended.
CN: Physiological integrity; CNS: Pharmacological and parenteral therapies; CL: Application

CN: Client needs category   CNS: Client needs subcategory   CL: Cognitive level

110. Which nursing diagnosis is <u>most appropriate</u> for a child with rheumatic fever?
1. Imbalanced nutrition: More than body requirements
2. Risk for injury
3. Delayed growth and development
4. Impaired gas exchange

111. A nurse is teaching the parents of a child who was diagnosed with sinus bradycardia. Which statement about the condition is the most correct?
1. "It is a heart rate less than normal for age."
2. "It is a heart rate greater than normal for age."
3. "It is a variation of the normal cardiac rhythm."
4. "It is an increase in sinus node impulse formation."

112. In which condition or group is sinus bradycardia a <u>normal</u> finding?
1. Hypoxia
2. Hypothermia
3. Growth-delayed adolescent
4. Physically conditioned adolescent

Sometimes, abnormal is *normal*, and vice versa!

113. Treatment for a child with symptomatic bradycardia includes atropine 0.02 mg/kg/dose. If the child weighs 20 kg, how much is given per dose?
1. 0.02 mg
2. 0.04 mg
3. 0.2 mg
4. 0.4 mg

114. Atropine is being administered to a child with sinus bradycardia. Which statement is the most accurate about the administration of this medication?
1. It increases heart rate.
2. It raises blood pressure.
3. It dilates bronchial tubes.
4. It decreases heart rate.

110. 2. Because of symptoms of chorea, safety measures should be taken to prevent falls or injury. There may be imbalanced nutrition: less than body requirements due to a sore throat and dysphagia. Growth and development usually aren't delayed. Impaired gas exchange usually isn't an issue unless the condition worsens with carditis and heart failure is present.
CN: Physiological integrity; CNS: Physiological adaptation; CL: Analysis

111. 1. Sinus bradycardia can best be described as a heart rate less than normal for age. Sinus tachycardia refers to a heart rate greater than normal for age or an increase in sinus node impulse formation. A sinus arrhythmia is a variation of the normal cardiac rhythm.
CN: Physiological integrity; CNS: Physiological adaptation; CL: Application

112. 4. A physically conditioned adolescent might have a lower than normal heart rate; this is of no significance. Hypoxia and hypothermia are pathological states in which a slow heart rate may produce a compromised hemodynamic state. Growth-delayed adolescents won't have bradycardia as a normal finding.
CN: Physiological integrity; CNS: Physiological adaptation; CL: Analysis

113. 4. The child should receive 0.4 mg. Use the following equation:
$$0.02 \text{ mg/kg} \times 20 \text{ kg} = 0.4 \text{ mg}$$
CN: Physiological integrity; CNS: Pharmacological and parenteral therapies; CL: Analysis

114. 1. Atropine blocks vagal impulses to the myocardium and stimulates the cardioinhibitory center in the medulla, thereby increasing heart rate and cardiac output. Atropine is not given to directly increase blood pressure or dilate the bronchial tubes.
CN: Physiological integrity; CNS: Pharmacological and parenteral therapies; CL: Application

115. A nurse has administered atropine to an 11-month-old infant for the treatment of sinus bradycardia. The nurse would be most concerned if the infant displayed which <u>adverse reaction</u>?
1. Lethargy
2. Diarrhea
3. No tears when crying
4. Increased urine output

What's an adverse reaction?

116. A child has a defect resulting in a right-to-left shunt. The nurse would anticipate assessment of the child to include which of the following findings? Select all that apply.
1. Cyanosis of lips and nail beds
2. Auscultation of crackles in lung fields
3. Clubbed fingers
4. Tachypnea
5. Bradycardia

117. The nurse is developing a plan of care for a child with heart failure. It is most important for the nurse to include which of the following? Select all that apply.
1. Cluster all care.
2. Weigh the child weekly.
3. Maintain the child in a supine position.
4. Offer small, frequent feedings.
5. Maintain a cool environment.

115. 3. Atropine dries up secretions and also lessens the response of ciliary and iris sphincter muscles in the eye, causing mydriasis. It usually causes paradoxical excitement in children. Constipation and urinary retention can be seen due to a decrease in smooth-muscle contractions of the gastrointestinal and genitourinary tracts.
CN: Physiological integrity; CNS: Pharmacological and parenteral therapies; CL: Application

116. 1, 3, and 4. Children who have a defect that results in blood shunting from the right side of the heart to the left are cyanotic and often have pulse oximeter readings in the 70% to 90% range. This is due to blood being shunted from the right side of the heart to the left side of the heart and not going through the lungs. With long-term cyanosis, there are clubbed fingers. Children are often tachypneic in an attempt to improve oxygenation. They are often tachycardic in order to increase cardiac output. Crackles are usually heard in children with defects that have increased pulmonary blood flow.
CN: Physiological integrity; CNS: Physiological adaptation; CL: Analysis

117. 1 and 4. Nursing assessments and interventions should be clustered in order to allow the child opportunities to rest and conserve energy. Small, frequent feedings (such as every 3 hours) allow for rest periods yet allow the child an ample opportunity to take in enough calories without having to take in a large volume of formula or food. The child should be weighed daily with the same clothes and the same scale. The child should be placed in an upright position, usually at a 30- to 45-degree angle in order to optimize chest expansion and decrease work of breathing. Children with heart failure need a normothermic environment because anything too hot or too cold will lead to unnecessary expenditure of calories.
CN: Physiological integrity; CNS: Physiological adaptation; CL: Application

118. Which condition may lead to sinus arrest or sinus pause in a child?
1. Hypokalemia
2. Hyperthermia
3. Valsalva's maneuver
4. Decreased intracranial pressure

119. The nurse is aware that amiodarone (Cordarone) is used to treat which of the following?
1. Atrial dysrhythmias
2. Ventricular dysrhythmias
3. Both atrial and ventricular dysrhythmias
4. Heart failure

120. List three common reversible causes of tachycardia in children with their associated interventions.
1. _____
2. _____
3. _____

121. Which finding would the nurse anticipate in a 1-year-old child with supraventricular tachycardia?
1. Heart rate of 100 beats/minute
2. Heart rate of 180 beats/minute
3. Heart rate of less than 80 beats/minute
4. Heart rate of more than 240 beats/minute

118. 3. Sinus arrest may occur in children when vagal tone is increased such as during Valsalva's maneuver in vomiting, gagging, or straining during a bowel movement. This represents a failure of the sinoatrial node to generate an impulse. A straight line or pause occurs, indicating the absence of electrical activity. After the pause, another impulse will be generated and a cardiac complex will appear. Hyperkalemia, hypothermia, and increased intracranial pressure are pathological conditions that may also produce sinus arrest.
CN: Physiological integrity; CNS: Physiological adaptation; CL: Analysis

119. 3. Amiodarone is used to treat both atrial and ventricular dysrhythmias. It is not used in the treatment of heart failure.
CN: Physiological integrity; CNS: Pharmacological and parenteral therapies; CL: Application

120. Possible answers include:
1. Pain — analgesics
2. Fever — antipyretics such as acetaminophen or ibuprofen
3. Dehydration — fluid replacement, either with oral or I.V. fluids
4. Anxiety or fear — comfort with holding, parental presence, answering of questions, comfort object such as a stuffed animal or blanket, or diversional activities such as games or singing

121. 4. Supraventricular tachycardia may be related to increased automaticity of an atrial cell other than the sinoatrial node, or as a reentry mechanism. The rhythm is regular and can occur at rates of 240 beats/minute or more. A heart rate of 100 beats/minute is a normal finding for a 1-year-old child. A heart rate around 180 beats/minute may represent sinus tachycardia. A heart rate of less than 80 beats/minute can be characterized as sinus bradycardia.
CN: Physiological integrity; CNS: Physiological adaptation; CL: Analysis

122. A 2-year-old child is experiencing supraventricular tachycardia. The nurse determines that the <u>first</u> intervention to implement is:
1. administration of digoxin.
2. administration of adenosine.
3. synchronized cardioversion.
4. immersion of the child's hands in cold water.

In question 122, the word *first* is your clue to the right answer.

123. A 2-month-old infant arrives in the emergency department with a heart rate of 180 beats/minute and a temperature of 103.18° F (39.58° C) rectally. What is the <u>most appropriate</u> nursing intervention?
1. Give acetaminophen (Tylenol).
2. Encourage fluid intake.
3. Apply carotid massage.
4. Place the infant's hands in cold water.

124. A critically ill 4-year-old is in the pediatric intensive care unit. Telemetry monitoring reveals junctional tachycardia. Identify where this arrhythmia originates.

122. **4.** Vagal maneuvers such as immersion of the hands in cold water are commonly tried first as a mechanism to decrease the heart rate. Other vagal maneuvers include breath-holding, carotid massage, gagging, and placing the head lower than the rest of the body. Synchronized cardioversion may be required if vagal maneuvers and drugs are ineffective. If a child has low cardiac output, cardioversion may be used instead of drugs. Verapamil isn't recommended. Digoxin is one of the most common drugs given to help decrease heart rate by increasing myocardial contractility and automaticity and reducing excitability.
CN: Physiological integrity; CNS: Reduction of risk potential; CL: Application

123. **1.** Acetaminophen should be given first to decrease the temperature. A heart rate of 180 beats/minute is normal in an infant with a fever. A tepid sponge bath may be given to help decrease the temperature and calm the infant. Carotid massage is an attempt to decrease the heart rate as a vagal maneuver. This won't work in this infant because the source of the increased heart rate is fever. Fluid intake is encouraged after the acetaminophen is given to help replace insensible fluid losses.
CN: Physiological integrity; CNS: Physiological adaptation; CL: Application

124. In junctional tachycardia, the atrioventricular node rapidly fires.
CN: Physiological integrity; CNS: Physiological adaptation; CL: Analysis

125. An infant who weighs 8 kg is to receive ampicillin 25 mg/kg I.V. every 6 hours. How many milligrams should the nurse administer per dose? Record your answer using a whole number.

_____ milligrams

126. The nurse is caring for an infant with a heart defect that involves increased pulmonary blood flow. Which illustration shows a congenital heart disorder with increased pulmonary blood flow?

1.

2.

3.

4.

125. 200. The nurse should calculate the correct dose using the following equation: 25 mg/kg × 8 kg = 200 mg.

CN: Physiological integrity; CNS: Pharmacological and parenteral therapies; CL: Application

126. **2.** In patent ductus arteriosus, an accessory fetal structure that connects the pulmonary artery to the aorta fails to close at birth. This allows blood to shunt from the aorta to the pulmonary artery. Option 1 depicts aortic stenosis (narrowed aortic valve), and option 3 shows pulmonic stenosis (narrowed pulmonic valve); both are obstruction to blood flow disorders. Option 4 shows tricuspid atresia (failure of the tricuspid valve to develop), a decreased pulmonary blood flow disorder.

CN: Physiological integrity; CNS: Physiological adaptation; CL: Analysis

This chapter covers sickle cell disease, varicella, Rocky Mountain spotted fever, leukemia, and many other blood and immune system disorders in kids. It's a whopper of a chapter on a critically important area. If you're ready, let's begin!

Chapter 28
Hematologic & immune disorders

1. A child comes to the emergency department feeling feverish and lethargic. Which assessment finding suggests Reye's syndrome to the nurse?
 1. Fever, profoundly impaired consciousness, and hepatomegaly
 2. Fever, splenomegaly, and hyperactive reflexes
 3. Afebrile, intractable vomiting, and rhinorrhea
 4. Malaise, cough, and sore throat

Early diagnosis is crucial to treating Reye's syndrome.

2. Which aspect is <u>most important</u> for successful management of the child with Reye's syndrome?
 1. Early diagnosis
 2. Initiation of antibiotics
 3. Isolation of the child
 4. Staging of the illness

3. A child with Reye's syndrome is in stage I of the illness. Which measure can be taken to prevent further progression of the illness?
 1. Invasive monitoring
 2. Endotracheal intubation
 3. Hypertonic glucose solution
 4. Pancuronium bromide (Pavulon)

1. 1. Reye's syndrome is defined as toxic encephalopathy, characterized by fever, profoundly impaired consciousness, and disordered hepatic function. Intractable vomiting occurs during the first stage of Reye's syndrome, but rhinorrhea usually precedes the onset of the illness. Reye's syndrome doesn't affect the spleen but causes fatty degeneration of the liver. Hyperactive reflexes occur with central nervous system involvement. Malaise, cough, and sore throat are viral symptoms that commonly precede the illness.
CN: Physiological integrity; CNS: Physiological adaptation; CL: Analysis

2. 1. Early diagnosis and therapy are essential because of the rapid clinical course of the disease and its high mortality. Reye's syndrome is associated with a viral illness, and antibiotic therapy isn't crucial to preventing the initial progression of the illness. Isolation isn't necessary because the disease isn't communicable. Staging, although important to therapy, occurs after a differential diagnosis is made.
CN: Physiological integrity; CNS: Reduction of risk potential; CL: Application

3. 3. For children in stage I of Reye's syndrome, treatment is primarily supportive and directed toward restoring blood glucose levels and correcting acid–base imbalances. I.V. administration of dextrose solutions with added insulin helps to replace glycogen stores. Noninvasive monitoring is adequate to assess status at this stage. Endotracheal intubation may be necessary later. Pancuronium bromide is used as an adjunct to endotracheal intubation and wouldn't be used in this stage of Reye's syndrome.
CN: Physiological integrity; CNS: Reduction of risk potential; CL: Application

CN: Client needs category   CNS: Client needs subcategory   CL: Cognitive level

4. The nurse is reviewing lab results of a newly admitted client. Which group of laboratory results, along with the clinical manifestations, <u>establishes</u> a diagnosis of Reye's syndrome?
1. Elevated liver enzymes and prolonged prothrombin and partial thromboplastin times
2. Increased serum glucose and insulin levels
3. Increased bilirubin and alkaline phosphatase levels
4. Decreased serum glucose and ammonia levels

5. The nurse is caring for a client who is in the latter stages of Reye's syndrome. What is the most important intervention by the nurse to prevent or reduce cerebral edema?
1. Noninvasive pressure monitoring
2. Paralysis and sedation
3. Liberal fluid replacement
4. Nonassisted ventilation

6. The nurse is assessing a child acutely ill with Reye's syndrome. Which assessment change would the nurse be most concerned about?
1. Irritability and quick pupil response
2. Increased blood pressure and decreased heart rate
3. Decreased blood pressure and increased heart rate
4. Sluggish pupil response and decreased blood pressure

7. A client with Reye's syndrome is exhibiting increased intracranial pressure (ICP). Which nursing intervention would be the <u>most</u> appropriate for this client?
1. Position the child with the head elevated and the neck in a neutral position.
2. Maintain the child in the prone position.
3. Cluster together interventions that may be perceived as noxious.
4. Position the child in the supine position, with the child's head turned to the side.

The word *establishes* is a big hint.

Read this question carefully.

4. 1. Reye's syndrome causes fatty degeneration of the liver, altering results of liver function studies. Decreased serum glucose levels, with reduced insulin levels, occur secondary to dehydration caused by intractable vomiting. Serum bilirubin and alkaline phosphatase usually aren't affected.
CN: Physiological integrity; CNS: Physiological adaptation; CL: Analysis

5. 2. Skeletal muscles are paralyzed with the administration of pancuronium (Pavulon). This prevents activity, especially coughing, that might increase intracranial pressure (ICP). Invasive monitoring is essential to detect increased ICP. Liberal fluid replacement may increase cerebral edema and should be strictly monitored. Tracheal intubation is performed as soon as possible to prevent hypoventilation and increased carbon dioxide levels.
CN: Physiological integrity; CNS: Reduction of risk potential; CL: Analysis

6. 2. A marked increase in intracranial pressure (ICP) will trigger the pressure response; increased ICP produces an elevation in blood pressure with a reflex slowing of the heart rate. Irritability is commonly an early sign, but pupillary response becomes more sluggish in response to increased ICP.
CN: Physiological integrity; CNS: Physiological adaptation; CL: Application

7. 1. Positioning the child with the head elevated and neck in the neutral position helps decrease ICP. The prone and supine positions cause increased ICP. Interventions that may be perceived as noxious should be spaced over time because, if clustered together, they may have a cumulative effect in increasing ICP. Turning the head to the side may impede venous return from the head and increase ICP.
CN: Physiological integrity; CNS: Physiological adaptation; CL: Application

8. The goal of nursing care for a client with Reye's syndrome is to minimize intracranial pressure (ICP). Which nursing intervention helps to meet this goal?
   1. Keeping the head of the bed flat
   2. Frequent position changes
   3. Positioning to avoid neck flexion
   4. Suctioning and chest physiotherapy

Stay calm when encountering NCLEX questions you're unsure about. That's what I do.

9. The nurse is caring for an unconscious child with Reye's syndrome. What is the most appropriate nursing intervention?
   1. Keeping the arms and legs flexed
   2. Placing the child on a sheepskin
   3. Avoiding the use of lotions on the skin
   4. Placing the client in a supine position

10. A parent asks the nurse if medications can cause Reye's syndrome. The most appropriate response by the nurse is that Reye's syndrome has been connected to:
   1. acetaminophen (Tylenol).
   2. aspirin.
   3. ibuprofen (Motrin).
   4. guaifenesin (Robitussin).

OK. OK. So I'm to blame.

11. A nurse should tell parents to stop the administration of acetylsalicylic acid (aspirin) and notify a physician if their child is exposed to which of the following?
   1. Stress
   2. Scabies
   3. Influenza
   4. Environmental allergies

8. **3.** Jugular vein compression can increase ICP by interfering with venous return. The head of the bed should be elevated to help promote venous return. Nursing procedures such as frequent positioning tend to cause overstimulation; therefore, care should be taken to avoid such procedures to prevent increased ICP. Suctioning and percussion are poorly tolerated and are contraindicated, unless concurrent respiratory problems are present.
CN: Physiological integrity; CNS: Physiological adaptation; CL: Application

9. **2.** Placing the child on a sheepskin helps to prevent pressure on prominent areas of the body. Keeping extremities in a flexed position can lead to contractures. Rubbing the extremities with lotion stimulates circulation and helps prevent drying of the skin. Placing the child supine would be contraindicated because of the risk of aspiration and increasing intracranial pressure. The supine position puts undue pressure on the sacral and occipital areas.
CN: Physiological integrity; CNS: Physiological adaptation; CL: Application

10. **2.** Aspirin administration is associated with the development of Reye's syndrome. Acetaminophen, ibuprofen, and guaifenesin haven't been associated with the development of Reye's syndrome. In fact, there has been a decreased incidence of Reye's syndrome with the increased use of acetaminophen and ibuprofen for management of fevers in children.
CN: Physiological integrity; CNS: Pharmacological and parenteral therapies; CL: Application

11. **3.** A strong association exists between influenza and aspirin administration and the development of Reye's syndrome. There's no contraindication with the other conditions.
CN: Physiological integrity; CNS: Pharmacological and parenteral therapies; CL: Application

12. The nurse is caring for a client with Reye's syndrome who's receiving pancuronium (Pavulon). What is the most important intervention for the nurse to include in the plan of care?
1. Applying artificial tears as needed
2. Providing regular tactile stimulation
3. Performing active range-of-motion (ROM) exercises
4. Placing the client in a supine position

You're doing so well I'm going to cry.

13. Which goal should be achieved by performing a craniotomy on a client with Reye's syndrome?
1. Decreasing carbon dioxide levels
2. Determining the extent of brain injury
3. Reducing pressure from an edematous brain
4. Allowing continuous monitoring of intracranial pressure (ICP)

Be sensitive not only to your client's needs but also to the family's needs as well.

14. The nurse is aware that parents of a child with Reye's syndrome need a great deal of emotional support. What is the most important intervention for the nurse to include in the plan of care?
1. Not accepting aggressive behavior from the parents
2. Encouraging the parents not to overreact and to hope for the best
3. Letting the parents interpret the child's behaviors and responses
4. Explaining therapies and clarifying or reinforcing the information given

15. The nurse is caring for a client in stage V of Reye's syndrome. The nurse documents which assessment data?
1. Vomiting, lethargy, and drowsiness
2. Seizures, flaccidity, and respiratory arrest
3. Hyperventilation and coma
4. Disorientation, aggressiveness, and combativeness

12. 1. Pancuronium suppresses the corneal reflex, making the eyes prone to irritation. Artificial tears prevent drying. Tactile stimulation isn't appropriate because it may elicit a pressure response. Active ROM exercises may cause an increase in pressure. The head of the bed should be elevated slightly, with the paralyzed client in a side-lying or semiprone position to prevent aspiration and minimize intracranial pressure.
CN: Physiological integrity; CNS: Pharmacological and parenteral therapies; CL: Application

13. 3. In severe cases of cerebral edema, creating bilateral bone flaps (craniotomy) is most effective in decreasing ICP. Carbon dioxide levels can be decreased through mechanical ventilation. Most clients with Reye's syndrome recover without any resulting brain injury. Continuous monitoring of ICP is implemented through central venous pressure lines.
CN: Physiological integrity; CNS: Reduction of risk potential; CL: Analysis

14. 4. Explaining treatments and therapies will help to alleviate undue stress in the parents. An awareness of the potential for aggressive behaviors provides nurses with the understanding that helps them support the parents in their grief. Being too quick to reassure may block a parent's expression of fears. Parents may need help interpreting their child's behavior to avoid assigning erroneous meanings to the many signs their child exhibits.
CN: Psychosocial integrity; CNS: None; CL: Application

15. 2. Staging criteria were developed to help evaluate the client's progress and to evaluate the efficacy of therapies. The clinical manifestations of stage V include seizures, loss of deep tendon reflexes, flaccidity, and respiratory arrest. Vomiting, lethargy, and drowsiness occur in stage I. Hyperventilation and coma occur in stage III. Disorientation and aggressive behavior occur in stage II.
CN: Physiological integrity; CNS: Physiological adaptation; CL: Analysis

16. A nurse is administering an immunization to a 2-month-old child. Which immunity will the child form?
1. Acquired immunity
2. Active immunity
3. Natural immunity
4. Passive immunity

17. The parent of a neonate asks the nurse what is the recommended age for beginning hepatitis B immunization. Which response is the <u>most</u> accurate?
1. Birth
2. 4 months
3. 6 months
4. 1 year

18. It would be most appropriate for which infant to begin receiving the measles vaccine?
1. A 6-month old
2. A 12-month old
3. An 18-month old
4. A 24-month old

19. Which immunizations should a healthy 2-month-old infant receive?
1. Measles, mumps, rubella (MMR), and inactivated polio (IPV)
2. MMR and varicella
3. Diphtheria, tetanus, and pertussis (DTP), and influenza nasal mist
4. DTP and IPV

20. The child who's diagnosed with thalassemia major (Cooley's anemia) typically suffers complications from the disease and from the treatment. The nurse is aware that this child is at risk for which of the following?
1. Hypertrophy of the thyroid
2. Hypertrophy of the thymus
3. Polycythemia vera and thrombosis
4. Chronic hypoxia and iron overload

What's with all the shots?

Test-taking tip: Read every question and all the options carefully before selecting your answer.

16. 2. Active immunity occurs when the individual forms immune bodies against certain diseases, either by having the disease or by the introduction of a vaccine into the individual. Acquired immunity results from exposure to the bacteria, virus, or toxins. Natural immunity is resistance to infection or toxicity. Passive immunity is a temporary immunity caused by transfusion of immune plasma proteins.
CN: Health promotion and maintenance; CNS: None; CL: Application

17. 1. According to the American Academy of Pediatrics, birth to age 2 months is the recommended time for beginning hepatitis B immunizations.
CN: Health promotion and maintenance; CNS: None; CL: Application

18. 2. According to the American Academy of Pediatrics, the first dose of the measles vaccine should be administered at age 12 to 15 months.
CN: Health promotion and maintenance; CNS: None; CL: Application

19. 4. At age 2 months, DTP and IPV are the recommended immunizations. DTP and IPV are given again at 4 months, and DTP is given again alone at 6 months. MMR is given at age 12 months. Influenza nasal mist is a weakened live vaccine that should be given to healthy individuals over 2 years of age.
CN: Health promotion and maintenance; CNS: None; CL: Application

20. 4. In thalassemia major, increased destruction of red blood cells (RBCs) causes anemia. RBCs also have a shortened life span. The body responds by increasing the production of RBCs, but it can't adequately produce enough mature cells to meet the body's demands. This process results in chronic hypoxia. Children with the disorder are given multiple transfusions of packed RBCs. The combination of excessive RBC destruction and multiple transfusions causes too much iron to be deposited in organs and tissues and results in damage to the involved organs. The thymus and thyroid aren't involved. Polycythemia vera refers to excessive RBC production, which can result in thrombosis.
CN: Physiological integrity; CNS: Reduction of risk potential; CL: Analysis

CN: Client needs category   CNS: Client needs subcategory   CL: Cognitive level

21. Which is the treatment of choice for severe aplastic anemia?
  1. Liver transplantation
  2. Exchange transfusion
  3. Bone marrow transplantation
  4. Administration of intravenous immunoglobulins

21. 3. Aplastic anemia refers to either a congenital or an acquired condition in which severe pancytopenia, or decrease in cellular components of the blood, occurs. Children with the condition have profound anemia, are susceptible to infections, and risk bleeding. When a good match of donor bone marrow is available, transplantation is the treatment of choice. Liver transplantation, exchange transfusion, and the administration of intravenous immunoglobulins aren't treatments for aplastic anemia.

CN: Physiological integrity; CNS: Physiological adaptation; CL: Application

22. A nurse is caring for a child with sickle cell anemia. The nurse anticipates that which type of transfusion is most likely to be given to the child?
  1. Plasma
  2. Platelets
  3. Whole blood
  4. Packed red blood cells (RBCs)

22. 4. Packed RBCs are given to children when their hemoglobin is dangerously low. Severe anemia decreases oxygen perfusion and leads to increased sickling of cells. Packed cells are RBCs with plasma removed. If enough whole blood were given to reach the desired hemoglobin level, fluid overload could occur. Thus, the plasma is removed, and packed RBCs are infused. The RBCs are needed to transport oxygen. Platelets are given to children with low platelets, not anemia.

CN: Physiological integrity; CNS: Pharmacological and parenteral therapies; CL: Analysis

23. What information is <u>most important</u> for the nurse to be aware of when administering immunizations?
  1. Properly store the vaccine, and follow the recommended procedure for injection.
  2. Monitor clients for approximately 1 hour after administration for adverse reactions.
  3. Take the vaccine out of refrigeration 1 hour before administration.
  4. Inject multiple vaccines at the same injection site.

Stop and think: Which direction would be of primary importance?

23. 1. Vaccines must be properly stored to ensure their potency. The nurse must be familiar with the manufacturer's directions for storage and reconstitution of the vaccine. Faulty refrigeration is a major cause of primary vaccine failure. It isn't necessary to monitor the clients, but the nurse should teach parents to call the physician and report any adverse effects. Taking the vaccine out of refrigeration too early can affect its potency. If more than one vaccine is to be administered, different injection sites should be used. The nurse should note which vaccine is given and at what site in case of a local reaction.

CN: Health promotion and maintenance; CNS: None; CL: Application

24. A child is admitted to the hospital with a diagnosis of severe combined immunodeficiency disease (SCID). During the admission interview and assessment, the nurse should observe the child for which symptom?
1. Bruising
2. Failure to thrive
3. Prolonged bleeding
4. Susceptibility to infection

25. A child is admitted to the hospital for an asthma exacerbation. The nursing history reveals this client was exposed to chickenpox 1 week ago. The nurse is correct in her assessment of room assignment when she determines that:
1. isolation isn't required.
2. immediate isolation is required.
3. isolation would be required 10 days after exposure.
4. isolation would be required 12 days after exposure.

26. On assessment of a child's skin, the nurse notes a papular, pruritic rash with some vesicles. The rash is profuse on the trunk and sparse on the distal limbs. Based on this assessment, which illness does the client have?
1. Measles
2. Mumps
3. Roseola
4. Chickenpox

27. A parent calls the school nurse to ask when her child who developed chickenpox can return to school. What is the most appropriate response by the nurse?
1. When the child is afebrile
2. When all vesicles have dried
3. When vesicles begin to crust over
4. When lesions and vesicles are gone

Here's to you! Twenty-five questions, and you're doing great.

Chickenpox is highly contagious. Teach parents how to assess when it's safe to send kids back to school.

24. 4. SCID is characterized by absence of both humoral and cell-mediated immunity. The most common manifestation is susceptibility to infection early in life, most often by age 3 months. SCID is characterized by chronic infection, failure to completely recover from an infection, and frequent reinfection. The history reveals no logical source for infection. Failure to thrive is a consequence of persistent illnesses. Prolonged bleeding and bruising indicate abnormalities in the clotting system.
CN: Physiological integrity; CNS: Physiological adaptation; CL: Analysis

25. 2. The incubation period for chickenpox is 2 to 3 weeks, commonly 13 to 17 days. A client is commonly isolated 1 week after exposure to avoid the risk of an earlier breakout. A person is infectious from 1 day before eruption of lesions to 6 days after the vesicles have formed crusts.
CN: Safe, effective care environment; CNS: Safety and infection control; CL: Application

26. 4. Chickenpox rash is highly pruritic. The rash begins as a macule, rapidly progresses to a papule, and then becomes a vesicle. All three stages are present in varying degrees at one time. Measles begins as an erythematous maculopapular eruption on the face; the eruption gradually spreads downward. Mumps isn't associated with a skin rash. Roseola rash is nonpruritic and is described as discrete rose-pink macules, appearing first on the trunk and then spreading to the neck, face, and extremities.
CN: Health promotion and maintenance; CNS: None; CL: Analysis

27. 2. Chickenpox is contagious. It's transmitted through direct contact, droplet spread, and contact with contaminated objects. Vesicles break open; therefore, a person is potentially contagious until all vesicles have dried. It isn't necessary to wait until dried lesions have disappeared. Some vesicles may be crusted over, and new ones may have formed. Macules, papules, vesicles, and crusting are present in varying degrees at one time. A child may be free from fever but continue to have vesicles. Isolation is usually necessary only for about 1 week after the onset of the disease.
CN: Health promotion and maintenance; CNS: None; CL: Analysis

28. A parent calls the nurse "hotline" to ask about the clinical manifestations associated with roseola. What is the best response by the nurse?
1. "Apparent sickness, fever, and rash"
2. "Fever for 3 to 4 days, followed by rash"
3. "Rash, without history of fever or illness"
4. "Rash for 3 to 4 days, followed by high fevers"

29. The nurse is assessing a child with suspected roseola. The nurse determines the child has a roseola rash when she observes which finding?
1. Maculopapular red spots
2. Macular and pruritic, with papules and vesicles
3. Rose-pink macules that fade on pressure
4. Red maculopapular eruption, beginning on the face

Read each question carefully and don't do anything rash.

30. A parent asks the nurse if it is alright to let his child scratch the chickenpox on his abdomen. The nurse explains that if the child scratches the chickenpox, he may be at risk for developing which condition?
1. Myocarditis
2. Neuritis
3. Obstructive laryngitis
4. Secondary bacterial infection

31. A child with suspected pertussis is admitted to the hospital. During assessment of the child, the nurse observes a cough with which characteristics?
1. Dry, hacking, and more frequent on awakening
2. Loose and nonproductive
3. Occurring more frequently during the day
4. Harsh and associated with a high-pitched crowing sound

Think before you respond: Can I contract rubella?

32. A preschool teacher has just found out she is pregnant. She asks the school nurse if there is any communicable disease that requires isolating an infected child from pregnant women. What is the most appropriate response by the nurse?
1. Pertussis
2. Roseola
3. Rubella
4. Scarlet fever

33. The nurse would expect the physician to order which medication as the treatment of choice for scarlet fever?
1. Acyclovir (Zovirax)
2. Amphotericin B
3. Ibuprofen (Motrin)
4. Penicillin

28. **2.** Roseola is manifested by persistent high fever for 3 to 4 days in a child who appears well. Fever precedes the rash. When the rash appears, a precipitous drop in fever occurs and the temperature returns to normal.
CN: Health promotion and maintenance; CNS: None; CL: Analysis

29. **3.** Roseola rashes are discrete, rose-pink macules or maculopapules that fade on pressure and usually last 1 to 2 days. Maculopapular red spots may indicate fifth disease. Chickenpox rash is macular, with papules and vesicles. Roseola isn't pruritic. Measles begin as a maculopapular eruption on the face.
CN: Health promotion and maintenance; CNS: None; CL: Application

30. **4.** Secondary bacterial infections can occur as a complication of chickenpox. Irritation of skin lesions can lead to cellulitis or even an abscess. Myocarditis isn't considered a complication of chickenpox but has been noted as a complication of mumps. Neuritis has been associated with diphtheria. Obstructive laryngitis occurs as a complication of measles.
CN: Physiological integrity; CNS: Reduction of risk potential; CL: Application

31. **4.** The cough associated with pertussis is a harsh series of short, rapid coughs, followed by a sudden inspiration and a high-pitched crowing sound. Cheeks become flushed or cyanotic, eyes bulge, and the tongue protrudes. Paroxysm may continue until a thick mucus plug is dislodged. This cough occurs most commonly at night.
CN: Physiological integrity; CNS: Physiological adaptation; CL: Analysis

32. **3.** Rubella (German measles) has a teratogenic effect on the fetus. An infected child must be isolated from pregnant women. Pertussis, roseola, and scarlet fever don't have any teratogenic effects on a fetus.
CN: Safe, effective care environment; CNS: Safety and infection control; CL: Application

33. **4.** The causative agent of scarlet fever is group A beta-hemolytic streptococci, which is susceptible to penicillin. Erythromycin is used for penicillin-sensitive children. Anti-inflammatory drugs, such as ibuprofen, aren't indicated for these clients. Acyclovir is used in the treatment of herpes infections. Amphotericin B is used to treat fungal infections.
CN: Physiological integrity; CNS: Pharmacological and parenteral therapies; CL: Application

34. A child enrolled in a private preparatory school has been diagnosed with scarlet fever. Several parents have called the school and voiced concern over the risk of their children becoming infected. The parents are requesting that the infected child be isolated for one month. It is most appropriate for the nurse to tell the parents that respiratory isolation of an infected child is necessary:
1. until the associated rash disappears.
2. until completion of antibiotic therapy.
3. until the client is fever-free for 24 hours.
4. until 24 hours after initiation of treatment.

35. Which instruction should the nurse include when teaching parents about the care of a child with chickenpox?
1. Administer penicillin or erythromycin as ordered.
2. Administer local or systemic antipruritics as ordered.
3. Offer periods of interaction with other children to provide distraction.
4. Avoid administering varicella-zoster immune globulin to children receiving long-term salicylate therapy.

36. A child is admitted with scarlet fever. Which causative agent does the nurse identify as a contributor to this infection?
1. Roseola
2. Staphylococcal parotitis
3. Streptococcal pharyngitis
4. Chickenpox

37. A mother infected with human immunodeficiency virus (HIV) inquires about the possibility of breastfeeding her newborn. What is the most appropriate response by the nurse?
1. "Breastfeeding isn't an option."
2. "Breastfeeding would be best for your baby."
3. "Breastfeeding is only an option if the mother is taking zidovudine (Retrovir)."
4. "Breastfeeding is an option if milk is expressed and fed by a bottle."

38. Which subjective assessment finding helps diagnose human immunodeficiency virus (HIV) infection in children?
1. Excessive weight gain
2. Arrhythmia
3. Intermittent diarrhea
4. Tolerance of feedings

So this is what they mean by "highly pruritic."

In which body fluids has HIV been isolated?

34. 4. A child requires respiratory isolation until 24 hours after initiation of treatment. Rash may persist for 3 weeks. It isn't necessary to wait until the end of treatment. Fever usually breaks 24 hours after therapy has begun. It isn't necessary to maintain isolation for an additional 24 hours.
CN: Safe, effective care environment; CNS: Safety and infection control; CL: Application

35. 2. Chickenpox is highly pruritic. Preventing the child from scratching is necessary to prevent scarring and secondary infection caused by irritation of lesions. Penicillin and erythromycin aren't usually used in the treatment of chickenpox. Interaction with other children would be contraindicated because of the risk of communication, unless the other children previously have had chickenpox or been immunized. Varicella-zoster immune globulin should be administered to exposed children who are on long-term aspirin therapy because of the possible risk of Reye's syndrome.
CN: Physiological integrity; CNS: Pharmacological and parenteral therapies; CL: Application

36. 3. The causative agent of scarlet fever is group A beta-hemolytic streptococci; therefore, scarlet fever may follow a strep throat infection. Roseola, parotitis, and chickenpox aren't strep infections and don't contribute to scarlet fever.
CN: Physiological integrity; CNS: Reduction of risk potential; CL: Analysis

37. 1. Mothers infected with HIV are unable to breastfeed because HIV has been isolated in breast milk and could be transmitted to the infant. Taking zidovudine doesn't prevent transmission. The risk of breastfeeding isn't associated with direct contact with the breast but with the possibility of HIV contained in the breast milk.
CN: Health promotion and maintenance; CNS: None; CL: Application

38. 3. A differential diagnosis may be based on the presence of an underlying cellular immunodeficiency-related disease; symptoms include intermittent episodes of diarrhea, repeated respiratory infections, and the inability to tolerate feedings. Poor weight gain and failure to thrive are objective assessment findings that result from intolerance of feedings and frequent infections. Arrhythmia isn't associated with HIV.
CN: Physiological integrity; CNS: Physiological adaptation; CL: Analysis

39. Which approach should be included in the diagnostic workup for a 12-month-old infant who's suspected of having acquired immunodeficiency syndrome (AIDS)?
1. Sputum culture
2. Esophageal biopsy
3. Parental counseling prior to testing
4. Human immunodeficiency syndrome (HIV) enzyme-linked immunosorbent assay (ELISA)

Which approach should the nurse include in the diagnostic workup?

40. Parents of a child with Kawasaki disease should be taught the importance of keeping follow-up appointments to monitor and prevent which complication?
1. Encephalitis
2. Glomerulonephritis
3. Myocardial infarction (MI)
4. Idiopathic thrombocytopenia

41. The nurse has just admitted a client with sickle cell crisis. What is the priority intervention by the nurse?
1. Giving blood transfusions
2. Giving antibiotics
3. Increasing fluid intake and giving analgesics
4. Preparing the client for a splenectomy

42. The nurse is assessing a client in the emergency department suspected of being in vaso-occlusive crisis. Which assessment findings would indicate that the client is having a vaso-occlusive crisis?
1. Hypotension and thready pulse
2. Pallor and poor capillary refill
3. Anemia, jaundice, and reticulocytosis
4. Acute leg pain and hand-foot syndrome

Question 42 is testing your knowledge of the four types of episodic crisis.

Caution

39. 3. AIDS and HIV are devastating diagnoses. Before testing, parents should be counseled regarding the disease, reasons for the tests, confidentiality, and benefits of early treatment. Sputum culture might help diagnose an upper respiratory infection associated with AIDS but isn't a diagnostic test for AIDS. Esophageal biopsy isn't indicated. ELISA isn't used diagnostically for children younger than 18 months because of the maternal antibodies in the child's blood.
CN: Psychosocial integrity; CNS: None; CL: Application

40. 3. In Kawasaki disease, inflammation of small and medium blood vessels can result in weakening of the vessels and aneurysm formation, especially in the heart. Blood flow through damaged vessels can cause thrombus formation and MI. Encephalitis, glomerulonephritis, and idiopathic thrombocytopenia aren't associated with Kawasaki disease.
CN: Health promotion and maintenance; CNS: None; CL: Application

41. 3. The primary therapy for sickle cell crisis is to increase fluid intake according to age and to give analgesics. Blood transfusions are only given conservatively to avoid iron overload. Antibiotics are given to clients with fever. Routine splenectomy isn't recommended. Splenectomy in clients with sickle cell anemia is controversial.
CN: Physiological integrity; CNS: Physiological adaptation; CL: Application

42. 4. Vaso-occlusive crises are the result of sickled cells obstructing the blood vessels. The major symptoms are fever, acute pain from visceral hypoxia, hand-foot syndrome, and arthralgia. A precipitous drop in blood volume is indicative of a splenic sequestration crisis and is exhibited by hypotension and a thready pulse. Aplastic crisis exhibits pallor and poor capillary refill and may result in symptoms of shock. Hyperhemolytic crisis is characterized by anemia, jaundice, and reticulocytosis and may also produce symptoms of shock.
CN: Physiological integrity; CNS: Physiological adaptation; CL: Analysis

43. A parent is inquiring about their child who tested positive for <u>sickle cell trait</u>. What is the most appropriate response by the nurse?
1. "Your child has sickle cell anemia."
2. "Your child is a carrier of the disorder but doesn't have sickle cell anemia."
3. "Your child is a carrier of the disease and will pass the disease to any offspring."
4. "Your child doesn't have the disease at present but may show evidence of the disease as he gets older."

44. The nurse is preparing a treatment plan for a child with sickle cell anemia in vaso-occlusive crisis. What is the most important nursing intervention for the nurse to include?
1. Managing pain
2. Providing a cool environment
3. Immobilizing the affected part
4. Restricting fluids

45. The nurse is being observed by a group of student nurses while assessing a child in vaso-occlusive crisis. A student asks the nurse why she did not palpate the child's abdomen. What is the most appropriate response by the nurse?
1. Risk of splenic rupture
2. Risk of inducing vomiting
3. Increase in abdominal pain
4. Risk of blood cell destruction

46. The nurse is reviewing the interventions listed in the plan of care for a child in vaso-occlusive crisis. What is the most important intervention for the nurse to implement?
1. Administering analgesics
2. Monitoring fluid restrictions
3. Encouraging activity as tolerated
4. Administering oxygen as prescribed

Know the difference between a positive test for sickle cell trait and a positive test for sickle cell anemia.

Which nursing intervention will help me keep going?

43. 2. A child with sickle cell trait is only a carrier and may never show any symptoms, except under special hypoxic conditions. A child with sickle cell trait doesn't have the disease and will never test positive for sickle cell anemia. Sickle cell anemia would be transmitted to offspring only as the result of a union between two individuals who are positive for the trait.
CN: Health promotion and maintenance; CNS: None; CL: Application

44. 1. Pain management is an important aspect in the care of a client with sickle cell anemia in vaso-occlusive crisis. The goal is to prevent sickling. This can be accomplished by promoting tissue oxygenation, hydration, and rest, which minimize energy expenditure and oxygen utilization. A cool environment can cause vasoconstriction and thus more sickling and pain. Immobilization can promote stasis and increase sickling.
CN: Physiological integrity; CNS: Basic care and comfort; CL: Analysis

45. 1. Palpating a child's abdomen in vaso-occlusive crisis should be avoided because sequestered red blood cells may precipitate splenic rupture. Abdominal pain alone wouldn't be a reason to avoid palpation. Vomiting or blood cell destruction wouldn't occur from palpation of the abdomen.
CN: Physiological integrity; CNS: Reduction of risk potential; CL: Application

46. 4. Administering oxygen is the most effective way to maximize tissue perfusion. Short-term oxygen therapy helps to prevent hypoxia, which leads to metabolic acidosis, causing sickling. Long-term oxygen therapy will depress erythropoiesis. Analgesics are used to control pain. Hydration is essential to promote hemodilution and maintain electrolyte balance. Bed rest should be promoted to reduce oxygen utilization.
CN: Physiological integrity; CNS: Reduction of risk potential; CL: Application

47. The nurse is providing postoperative care to a client with sickle cell anemia. What is the most important intervention for the nurse to include in the plan of care?
1. Increasing fluids
2. Preparing the child psychologically
3. Discouraging coughing
4. Limiting the use of analgesics

48. The parents of a child with sickle cell anemia ask the nurse what would be a <u>priority</u> factor in the prevention of infection for their child. What is the most appropriate response by the nurse?
1. Providing adequate nutrition
2. Avoiding emotional stress
3. Visiting the physician when sick
4. Avoiding strenuous physical exertion

49. Which schedule is recommended for the immunization of normal infants and children in the first year of life?
1. Birth, 2 months, 4 months, 6 months, 12 months
2. 1 month, 3 months, 5 months, 9 months, 18 months
3. 2 months, 6 months, 9 months, 12 months, 14 months
4. 2 months, 4 months, 6 months, 12 to 15 months

50. Which assessment finding would indicate vaso-occlusive crisis in a child with sickle cell anemia?
1. Painful urination
2. Pain with ambulation
3. Complaints of throat pain
4. Fever with associated rash

Don't let question 48 trip you up! It's asking you to prioritize.

You've reached question 50! You're doing great!

47. 1. The main surgical risk of anesthesia is hypoxia; however, emotional stress, demands of wound healing, and the potential for infection can each increase the sickling phenomenon. Increased fluids are encouraged because keeping the child well hydrated is important for hemodilution to prevent sickling. Preparing the child psychologically to decrease fear will minimize undue emotional stress. Deep coughing is encouraged to promote pulmonary hygiene and prevent respiratory tract infection. Analgesics are used to control wound pain and to prevent abdominal splinting and decreased ventilation.
CN: Physiological integrity; CNS: Reduction of risk potential; CL: Application

48. 1. The nurse must stress adequate nutrition. Avoiding strenuous physical exertion and emotional stress are important aspects to prevent sickling, but adequate nutrition remains a priority. Frequent medical supervision is imperative to prevention because infection is commonly a predisposing factor toward development of a crisis.
CN: Health promotion and maintenance; CNS: None; CL: Application

49. 1. The nurse needs to be aware of the schedule for immunizations as well as the latest recommendations for their use. According to the American Academy of Pediatrics, the recommended age for beginning primary immunizations of normal infants is at birth.
CN: Health promotion and maintenance; CNS: None; CL: Application

50. 2. Bone pain is one of the major symptoms of vaso-occlusive crisis in clients with sickle cell anemia. Hand-foot syndrome, characterized by edematous painful extremities, is usually exhibited in the refusal of the child to bear weight and ambulate. Painful urination doesn't occur, but sickle cell anemia can cause kidney abnormalities. Throat pain isn't a symptom of vaso-occlusive crisis. Fever commonly accompanies vaso-occlusive crisis but isn't associated with rash.
CN: Physiological integrity; CNS: Physiological adaptation; CL: Analysis

51. The nurse is assessing a child with sickle cell anemia. Which bone-related complication would the nurse be alert for during assessment?
  1. Arthritis
  2. Osteoporosis
  3. Osteogenic sarcoma
  4. Spontaneous fractures

52. What is a nurse's role with the parents of a child who has been diagnosed with sickle cell anemia?
  1. Encouraging selective birth methods or abortion
  2. Referring only sickle cell–positive parents for counseling
  3. Rendering support to parents of newly diagnosed children
  4. Reinforcing the idea that transmission is unlikely in subsequent pregnancies

53. A 14-year-old girl is admitted for sickle cell crisis. Which nursing intervention would be the most important?
  1. Gathering information about the child's ability to cope with this condition
  2. Monitoring the child's temperature every 2 hours
  3. Providing adequate oxygenation, hydrations, and pain management
  4. Making sure the family is involved in every step of the child's care

54. A nurse is administering a blood transfusion to a client with sickle cell anemia. Which assessment findings would indicate that the client is having a transfusion reaction?
  1. Diaphoresis and hot flashes
  2. Urticaria, flushing, and wheezing
  3. Fever, urticaria, and red raised rash
  4. Fever, disorientation, and abdominal pain

I was minding my own business when things got really complicated.

One wrong part of an option makes the entire option wrong.

51. 2. Sickle cell anemia causes hyperplasia and congestion of the bone marrow, resulting in osteoporosis. Arthritis doesn't occur secondary to sickle cell anemia; however, a crisis can cause localized swelling over joints, resulting in arthralgia. Bones do become weakened, but spontaneous fractures don't occur as a result. Osteogenic sarcoma is bone cancer; sickle cell anemia isn't a contributing factor to bone cancer.

CN: Physiological integrity; CNS: Physiological adaptation; CL: Application

52. 3. The nurse can be instrumental in providing genetic counseling. She can give parents correct information about the disease and render support to parents of newly diagnosed children. Alternative birth methods are discussed, but parents make their own decisions. All heterozygous, or trait-positive, parents should be referred for genetic counseling. The risk of transmission in subsequent pregnancies remains the same.

CN: Health promotion and maintenance; CNS: None; CL: Application

53. 3. The most critical need of a client in sickle cell crisis is to provide adequate oxygenation, hydrations, and pain management until the crisis passes. Obtaining a temperature every 2 hours would not be the priority intervention. While assessing the client's ability to cope and involving the family in the child's care are important, they aren't the priority interventions during a sickle cell crisis.

CN: Safe, effective care environment; CNS: Management of care; CL: Analysis

54. 2. Allergic reactions may occur when the recipient reacts to allergens in the donor's blood; this reaction causes urticaria, flushing, and wheezing. A febrile reaction can occur, causing fever and urticaria, but it isn't accompanied by rash. Diaphoresis, hot flashes, disorientation, and abdominal pain aren't symptoms of a transfusion reaction.

CN: Physiological integrity; CNS: Reduction of risk potential; CL: Analysis

55. A mother brings her 5-year-old child to the clinic and asks the nurse how often a child should receive the influenza virus vaccine. Which response would be the most accurate?
1. Annually
2. Twice a year
3. Never; contraindicated in children
4. Only with the outbreak of illness

56. A 3-year-old sister of a neonate is diagnosed with pertussis. The mother has a history of having been immunized as a child. Which information should be included in teaching the mother about possible infection of her neonate?
1. The baby will inevitably contract pertussis.
2. Immune globulin is effective in protecting the infant.
3. The risk to the infant depends on the mother's immune status.
4. Erythromycin should be administered prophylactically to the infant.

57. A child has recently been admitted to the pediatric unit with laboratory values indicating an increase in hemoglobin A_2. Based on this finding, the nurse should expect to follow a care plan based on which condition?
1. Beta-thalassemia trait
2. Iron deficiency
3. Lead poisoning
4. Sickle cell anemia

58. A 4-year-old child has a petechial rash but is otherwise well. The platelet count is 20,000/ml, and the hemoglobin level and white blood cell (WBC) count are normal. Which diagnosis is most likely?
1. Acute lymphoblastic leukemia (ALL)
2. Disseminated intravascular coagulation (DIC)
3. Idiopathic thrombocytopenic purpura (ITP)
4. Systemic lupus erythematosus (SLE)

59. Which instruction should be included in a nurse's discharge teaching for the parents of a newborn diagnosed with sickle cell anemia?
1. Stressing the importance of iron supplementation
2. Stressing the importance of monthly vitamin B_{12} injections
3. Reviewing signs of abdominal pain in infants and demonstrating how to take a temperature
4. Explaining that immunizations are contraindicated

Prevention is commonly the best medicine!

55. 1. The influenza virus vaccine is usually administered annually. The vaccine isn't contraindicated in children but is targeted at clients with chronic cardiac, pulmonary, hematologic, and neurological problems. The vaccine is given to prevent the onset of illness before an outbreak occurs.

CN: Health promotion and maintenance; CNS: None; CL: Application

56. 4. In exposed, high-risk persons such as neonates, erythromycin may be effective in preventing or lessening severity of the disease if administered during the preparoxysmal stage. Immune globulin isn't indicated because it's used as an immunization against hepatitis A. Neonates exposed to pertussis are at considerable risk for infections, regardless of the mother's immune status; however, infection isn't inevitable.

CN: Health promotion and maintenance; CNS: None; CL: Application

57. 1. The concentration of hemoglobin A_2 is increased with beta-thalassemia trait. In severe iron deficiency, hemoglobin A_2 may be decreased. The hemoglobin A_2 level is normal in lead poisoning and sickle cell anemia.

CN: Physiological integrity; CNS: Reduction of risk potential; CL: Application

58. 3. The onset of ITP typically occurs between ages 1 and 6 years. Clients look well, except for a petechial rash. ALL is associated with a low platelet count but an abnormal hemoglobin level and WBC count. DIC is secondary to a severe underlying disease. SLE is rare in a 4-year-old child.

CN: Physiological integrity; CNS: Physiological adaptation; CL: Analysis

59. 3. Acute splenic sequestration is a serious complication of sickle cell anemia. Early detection of splenomegaly by parents is an important aspect of client management. Parents should be able to take the temperature and identify abdominal pain. A temperature of 101.3° F to 102.2° F (38.5° C to 39° C) calls for emergency evaluation, even if the child appears well. Folic acid requirement is increased; therefore, supplementation may be indicated. Vitamin B_{12} supplementation and iron supplementation aren't necessary. Parents should be encouraged to keep immunizations up to date.

CN: Health promotion and maintenance; CNS: None; CL: Application

60. Which finding yields a poor prognosis for a child with leukemia?
1. Presence of a mediastinal mass
2. Late central nervous system (CNS) leukemia
3. Normal white blood cell (WBC) count at diagnosis
4. Disease presents between ages 2 and 10 years

61. A 1-year-old boy in the pediatrician's office for an examination is noted to be pale. He's in the 75th percentile for weight and the 25th percentile for length. His physical examination is normal, but his hematocrit is 24%. Which question would be <u>most</u> <u>helpful</u> in establishing a diagnosis of anemia?
1. Is the child on any medications?
2. What's the child's usual daily diet?
3. Did the child receive phototherapy for jaundice?
4. What's the pattern and appearance of bowel movements?

62. A nurse is teaching the parents of a child newly diagnosed with Hodgkin's disease. Which statement should the nurse include in her teaching?
1. Staging laparotomy is mandatory for every client.
2. Excessive weight gain can be a symptom.
3. Hodgkin's disease is rare before age 5 years.
4. Incidence of Hodgkin's disease peaks between ages 11 and 15 years.

63. The nurse is caring for a child with perinatally acquired human immunodeficiency virus. The nurse is aware that children usually demonstrate symptoms of acquired immunodeficiency syndrome (AIDS) at what age?
1. Within the first month of life
2. At 1 to 3 months of age
3. At 18 to 24 months of age
4. At 3 to 5 years of age

64. Which factors can place adolescent girls at risk for iron deficiency anemia? Select all that apply.
1. Menses
2. Vegetarian diet
3. Weight-loss diets
4. Skipping meals
5. Poverty

Question 60 asks about a prognosis, not a diagnosis.

These questions are tough! Hang in there!

60. **1.** The presence of a mediastinal mass indicates a poor prognosis for children with leukemia. The prognosis is poorer if age at onset is younger than 2 years or older than 10 years. A WBC count of 100,000/ml or higher and early CNS leukemia also indicate a poor prognosis for a child with leukemia.
CN: Physiological integrity; CNS: Physiological adaptation; CL: Analysis

61. **2.** Iron deficiency anemia is the most common nutritional deficiency in children between ages 9 months and 15 months. Anemia in a 1-year-old child is mostly nutritional in origin, and its cause will be suggested by a detailed nutritional history. None of the other selections would be helpful in diagnosing anemia.
CN: Health promotion and maintenance; CNS: None; CL: Analysis

62. **3.** Hodgkin's disease is rare before age 5 years. Staging laparotomy is not recommended for clients who have obvious intra-abdominal disease by noninvasive studies. Systemic symptoms of Hodgkin's disease include fever, night sweats, malaise, weight loss, and pruritus. The peak incidence of Hodgkin's disease occurs in late adolescence and young adulthood (ages 15 to 34 years).
CN: Physiological integrity; CNS: Physiological adaptation; CL: Analysis

63. **3.** The majority of children with perinatally transmitted AIDS appear normal in early infancy. Symptoms usually develop at 18 to 24 months of age.
CN: Physiological integrity; CNS: Physiological adaptation; CL: Application

64. **1, 2, 3, 4,** and **5.** All of the options place adolescent girls, who are still growing, at risk for iron deficiency anemia. That's because these girls lose blood monthly with menstrual periods, and they typically consume inadequate amounts of nutrients because of their eating patterns, which include hurried meals, vegetarian diets, weight-loss diets, and skipping meals. Poverty also increases the risk of iron deficiency anemia because of the inability to purchase meats and other iron-rich foods.
CN: Health promotion and maintenance; CNS: None; CL: Analysis

65. Which treatment would be most appropriate for a child diagnosed with iron deficiency anemia?
1. Blood transfusion
2. Oral ferrous sulfate
3. An iron-fortified cereal
4. Intramuscular iron dextran

I can help with iron deficiency anemia.

65. 2. A prompt rise in hemoglobin level and hematocrit follows the administration of oral ferrous sulfate. Blood transfusion is rarely indicated unless a child becomes symptomatic or is further compromised by a superimposed infection. Dietary modifications are appropriate long-term measures, but they won't make enough iron available to replenish iron stores. Intramuscular dextran is reserved for situations in which compliance can't be achieved because it's expensive, painful, and no more effective than oral iron.
CN: Physiological integrity; CNS: Physiological adaptation; CL: Application

66. A child is admitted to the hospital with flulike symptoms. Diagnostic testing reveals the IgM antibody parvovirus B19 is present. The nurse interprets this finding as being indicative of which condition?
1. Roseola
2. Fifth disease
3. Varicella
4. Mumps

66. 2. Fifth disease is known to be caused by human parvovirus B19. Roseola is thought to be caused by the human herpes virus 6. Varicella is caused by the varicella-zoster virus. Mumps is caused by the paramyxovirus.
CN: Physiological integrity; CNS: Reduction of risk potential; CL: Application

67. A 6-year-old child has been diagnosed with Rocky Mountain spotted fever. In teaching the parents about the cause of the illness, a nurse would be correct in telling them that a bite by which animal or insect caused the illness?
1. Cat
2. Mosquito
3. Spider
4. Tick

Bug bites really *tick* me off!

67. 4. Rocky Mountain spotted fever is caused by *Rickettsia rickettsii*, which is transmitted by the bite of a tick. Mosquito, spider, and cat bites haven't been known to transmit *R. rickettsii*.
CN: Safe, effective care environment; CNS: Safety and infection control; CL: Application

68. An iron dextran (INFeD) injection has been ordered for an 8-month-old child with iron deficiency anemia whose parents haven't been compliant with oral supplements. How should the nurse administer the injection?
1. Intradermally
2. Subcutaneously
3. Intramuscularly
4. Intramuscularly using the Z-track method

68. 4. If iron dextran is ordered, it must be injected deeply into a large muscle mass, using the Z-track method to minimize skin staining and irritation. Neither a subcutaneous nor an intradermal injection would inject the dextran into the muscle. The Z-track method is preferred over a normal intramuscular injection.
CN: Physiological integrity; CNS: Pharmacological and parenteral therapies; CL: Application

69. The nurse has provided dietary instruction to a client for the prevention of nutritional anemia. The nurse determines that further instruction is not necessary when the client selects which food?
1. Citrus fruits
2. Fish
3. Green vegetables
4. Milk products

69. 3. Green vegetables are good sources of iron. Citrus foods aren't sources of iron but help with the absorption of iron. Fish isn't a good source of dietary iron. Milk is deficient in iron and should be limited in cases of nutritional anemia.
CN: Physiological integrity; CNS: Basic care and comfort; CL: Application

70. Liquid oral iron supplements have been prescribed for a child. The parents tell the nurse they are apprehensive to administer the medication. What is the most important information for the nurse to provide?
1. Give the supplements with food.
2. Stop the medication if vomiting occurs.
3. Decrease the dose if constipation occurs.
4. Give the medicine via a dropper or through a straw.

71. Which symptom is the primary clinical manifestation of hemophilia?
1. Petechiae
2. Prolonged bleeding
3. Decreased clotting time
4. Decreased white blood cell (WBC) count

72. The nurse would be alert for signs and symptoms of internal bleeding <u>most commonly</u> at which site for a client with hemophilia?
1. Brain tissue
2. GI tract
3. Joint cavities
4. Spinal cord

73. The nurse is teaching parents of a hemophilic child about the immediate treatment for bleeding. The nurse determines that teaching has been effective when the parents make which statement?
1. "Apply heat to the area."
2. "Withhold factor replacement."
3. "Apply pressure for at least 5 minutes."
4. "Immobilize and elevate the affected area."

74. A 2-year-old child with hemophilia who sustains a joint injury is <u>best</u> treated promptly at which location?
1. Home
2. Clinic
3. Hospital unit
4. Emergency department

You're already at number 70? Super! You're really something!

Careful! All of these answers may be accurate, but this question is asking for the most common site.

70. 4. Liquid iron preparations may temporarily stain the teeth; therefore, the drug should be given by dropper or through a straw. Supplements should be given between meals, when the presence of free hydrochloric acid is greatest. If vomiting occurs, supplementation shouldn't be stopped; instead, it should be administered with food. Constipation can be decreased by increasing intake of fruits and vegetables.

CN: Physiological integrity; CNS: Pharmacological and parenteral therapies; CL: Application

71. 2. The effect of hemophilia is prolonged bleeding, anywhere from or within the body. With severe deficiencies, hemorrhage can occur as a result of minor trauma. Petechiae are uncommon in persons with hemophilia because repair of small hemorrhages depends on platelet function, not on blood clotting mechanisms. Clotting time is increased in a client with hemophilia. A decrease in WBCs is not indicative of hemophilia.

CN: Physiological integrity; CNS: Physiological adaptation; CL: Analysis

72. 3. The joint cavities, especially the knees, ankles, and elbows, are the most common site of internal bleeding. This bleeding typically results in bone changes and crippling, disabling deformities. Intracranial hemorrhage occurs less commonly than expected because the brain tissue has a high concentration of thromboplastin. Hemorrhage along the GI tract and spinal cord can occur but are less common.

CN: Physiological integrity; CNS: Physiological adaptation; CL: Application

73. 4. Elevating the area above the level of the heart will decrease blood flow. Cold, not heat, should be applied to promote vasoconstriction. Factor replacement should not be delayed. Pressure should be applied to the area for at least 10 to 15 minutes to allow clot formation.

CN: Physiological integrity; CNS: Physiological adaptation; CL: Application

74. 1. Prompt treatment to prevent joint injury and other complications is best delivered in the home. After the child reaches age 2 or 3 years, parents can learn venipuncture techniques so treatment can be done at home and further injury avoided. The life of the child and family is also less disrupted. The child may be transfused on a regular basis to prevent bleeding and will be given additional doses of the missing factor when an injury occurs. By mid- to late-school age, children can learn to administer their own treatment.

CN: Physiological integrity; CNS: Reduction of risk potential; CL: Application

CN: Client needs category   CNS: Client needs subcategory   CL: Cognitive level

75. Which nursing measure is an important aid in <u>prevention</u> of the crippling effects of joint degeneration caused by hemophilia?
1. Avoiding the use of analgesics
2. Using aspirin for pain relief
3. Administering replacement factor
4. Using active range-of-motion (ROM) exercises

Read carefully. This question is looking for a preventive measure.

76. When comparing bleeding disorders, an increased tendency to bleed in which area differentiates von Willebrand's disease from hemophilia?
1. Brain tissue
2. GI tract
3. Mucous membranes
4. Spinal cord

77. Which nursing measure should be implemented for a client with von Willebrand's disease who's having <u>epistaxis</u>?
1. Lying the child supine
2. Avoiding packing of the nostrils
3. Avoiding pressure to the nose
4. Applying pressure to the nose

Epistaxis is a term from early in your program. Remember?

78. A nurse is teaching the parents of a child with acute lymphoblastic leukemia. The parents ask for information about what helps determine long-term survival. The nurse discusses which of the following as the three most important prognostic factors?
1. Histologic type of disease, initial platelet count, and type of treatment
2. Type of treatment, stage at diagnosis, and child's age at diagnosis
3. Histologic type of disease, initial white blood cell (WBC) count, and client's age at diagnosis
4. Progression of illness, WBC count at time of diagnosis, and client's age at diagnosis

75. 3. Prevention of bleeding is the goal and is achieved by factor replacement therapy. Active ROM exercises are contraindicated after a bleeding episode because the joint capsule can be stretched, causing bleeding. Acetaminophen should be used for pain relief because aspirin has anticoagulant effects. Analgesics should be administered before physical therapy to control pain and provide the maximum benefit.
CN: Physiological integrity; CNS: Physiological adaptation; CL: Application

76. 3. The most characteristic clinical feature of von Willebrand's disease is an increased tendency to bleed from mucous membranes, which may be seen as frequent nosebleeds or menorrhagia. In hemophilia, the joint cavities are the most common site of internal bleeding. Bleeding into the GI tract, spinal cord, and brain tissue can occur, but these are not the most common sites for bleeding.
CN: Physiological integrity; CNS: Physiological adaptation; CL: Application

77. 4. Applying pressure to the nose may stop bleeding because most bleeds occur in the anterior part of the nasal septum. Encourage mouth breathing at this time. The child should be instructed to sit up and lean forward to avoid aspiration of blood. Packing with tissue or cotton may be used to help stop bleeding, although care must be taken in removing packing to avoid dislodging the clot. Pressure should be maintained for at least 10 minutes to allow clotting to occur.
CN: Physiological integrity; CNS: Physiological adaptation; CL: Application

78. 3. Histologic type of leukemia is the factor whose prognostic value is considered to be of greatest significance in determining long-range outcome. Children with a normal or low WBC count appear to have a much better prognosis than those with a high WBC count. Children diagnosed between ages 2 and 10 years have consistently demonstrated a better prognosis than those diagnosed before age 2 or after age 10 years.
CN: Physiological integrity; CNS: Physiological adaptation; CL: Analysis

79. Which complications are the three main consequences of leukemia?
1. Bone deformities, spherocytosis, and infection
2. Anemia, infection, and bleeding tendencies
3. Lymphocytopoiesis, growth delays, and hirsutism
4. Polycythemia, decreased clotting time, and infection

You, my friend, are doing extraordinarily well. Keep up the good work!

80. A child is seen in the pediatrician's office for complaints of bone and joint pain. Which other assessment finding may suggest leukemia?
1. Abdominal pain
2. Increased activity level
3. Increased appetite
4. Petechiae

81. The nurse is assessing a client with leukemia. What assessment findings would indicate that the cancer has invaded the brain?
1. Headache and vomiting
2. Restlessness and tachycardia
3. Hypervigilant and anxious behavior
4. Increased heart rate and decreased blood pressure

82. A student nurse asks the nurse on the hematology unit which type of leukemia has the best prognosis. Which response by the nurse would be the most accurate?
1. Acute lymphoblastic leukemia
2. Acute myelogenous leukemia
3. Basophilic leukemia
4. Eosinophilic leukemia

79. 2. The three main consequences of leukemia are anemia, caused by decreased erythrocyte production; infection secondary to neutropenia; and bleeding tendencies, from decreased platelet production. Bone deformities don't occur with leukemia, although bones may become painful because of the proliferation of cells in the bone marrow. Spherocytosis refers to erythrocytes taking on a spheroid shape and isn't a feature in leukemia. Lymphocytopoiesis is production of lymphocytes with leukemia. Mature cells aren't produced in adequate numbers. Hirsutism and growth delay can be a result of large doses of steroids but aren't common in leukemia. Anemia, not polycythemia, occurs. Clotting times would be prolonged.
CN: Physiological integrity; CNS: Physiological adaptation; CL: Application

80. 4. The most common signs and symptoms of leukemia are a result of infiltration of the bone marrow. These include fever, pallor, fatigue, anorexia, and petechiae, along with bone and joint pain. Abdominal pain may be caused by areas of inflammation from normal flora within the GI tract or any number of other causes. Increased appetite can occur, but it usually isn't a presenting symptom.
CN: Physiological integrity; CNS: Physiological adaptation; CL: Application

81. 1. The usual effect of leukemic infiltration of the brain is increased intracranial pressure. The proliferation of cells interferes with the flow of cerebrospinal fluid in the subarachnoid space and at the base of the brain. The increased fluid pressure causes dilation of the ventricles, which creates symptoms of severe headache, vomiting, irritability, lethargy, increased blood pressure, decreased heart rate, and, eventually, coma. Children with a variety of illnesses are typically hypervigilant and anxious when hospitalized.
CN: Physiological integrity; CNS: Physiological adaptation; CL: Analysis

82. 1. Acute lymphoblastic leukemia, which accounts for more than 80% of all childhood cases, carries the best prognosis. Acute myelogenous leukemia, with several subtypes, accounts for most of the other leukemias affecting children. Basophilic and eosinophilic leukemia are named for the specific cells involved. These are much rarer and carry a poorer prognosis.
CN: Physiological integrity; CNS: Physiological adaptation; CL: Application

83. The nurse is preparing a client diagnosed with leukemia for a spinal tap. The nurse determines that the client understands the reason for the procedure when the client states that the procedure is done:
1. to rule out meningitis.
2. to decrease intracranial pressure (ICP).
3. to aid in classification of the leukemia.
4. to assess for central nervous system (CNS) infiltration.

84. The nurse reviews the treatment plan for a child recently diagnosed with leukemia who is being evaluated for treatment with chemotherapy. Before the initiation of chemotherapy, the nurse anticipates that which of the following tests will be performed?
1. Lumbar puncture
2. Liver function studies
3. Complete blood count (CBC)
4. Peripheral blood smear

85. Which statement by the nurse most accurately explains the need for a child with pauciarticular juvenile rheumatoid arthritis (JRA) to have an annual eye exam?
1. "Detached retinas are commonly associated with the disease."
2. "Painless iritis (inflammation of the iris) is commonly seen with the disease."
3. "Glaucoma is commonly seen with the disease."
4. "Strabismus is commonly seen with the disease."

86. Which medication would the nurse expect the physician to order <u>most</u> commonly for a client with leukemia as prophylaxis against *Pneumocystis carinii* pneumonia?
1. Co-trimoxazole (Bactrim)
2. Oral nystatin suspension
3. Prednisone
4. Vincristine

Think back to basic physiology. Which organs metabolize drugs?

Here's a prescription for the drug of choice. Do you know which one it is?

83. **4.** A spinal tap is performed to assess for CNS infiltration. A spinal tap can be done to rule out meningitis, but this isn't the indication for the test on a leukemic client. It wouldn't be done to decrease ICP, nor does it aid in the classification of the leukemia. Spinal taps can result in brain stem herniation in cases of increased ICP.
CN: Physiological integrity; CNS: Physiological adaptation; CL: Application

84. **2.** Liver and kidney function studies are done before initiation of chemotherapy to evaluate the child's ability to metabolize the chemotherapeutic agents. A lumbar puncture is performed to assess for central nervous system infiltration. A CBC is performed to assess for anemia and white blood cell count. A peripheral blood smear is done to assess the maturity and morphology of red blood cells.
CN: Physiological integrity; CNS: Pharmacological and parenteral therapies; CL: Analysis

85. **2.** Painless iritis may be found in 75% of children with pauciarticular JRA. If it's not detected and is left untreated, permanent scarring in the anterior chamber of the eye may occur, with loss of vision. Children should have annual slit lamp examinations by an ophthalmologist. Detached retinas, glaucoma, and strabismus aren't commonly associated with the disease.
CN: Health promotion and maintenance; CNS: None; CL: Application

86. **1.** The most common cause of death from leukemia is overwhelming infection. *P. carinii* infection is lethal to a child with leukemia. As prophylaxis against *P. carinii* pneumonia, continuous low dosages of co-trimoxazole are typically prescribed. Oral nystatin suspension would be indicated for the treatment of thrush. Prednisone isn't an antibiotic and increases susceptibility to infection. Vincristine is an antineoplastic agent.
CN: Physiological integrity; CNS: Pharmacological and parenteral therapies; CL: Application

Care of the child

87. A 4-year-old child is diagnosed as having acute lymphocytic leukemia. His white blood cell (WBC) count, especially the neutrophil count, is low. What is the most important intervention the nurse should teach the parents?
1. Protect the child from falls because of his increased risk of bleeding.
2. Protect the child from infections because his resistance to infection is decreased.
3. Provide rest periods because the oxygen-carrying capacity of the child's blood is diminished.
4. Treat constipation, which frequently accompanies a decrease in WBC.

88. A child with leukemia has been exposed to chickenpox. The mother calls the doctor's office and asks the nurse if the child needs to have anything done. What is the most appropriate response by the nurse?
1. No treatment is indicated.
2. Acyclovir (Zovirax) should be started on exposure.
3. Varicella-zoster immune globulin (VZIG) should be given with evidence of the disease.
4. VZIG should be given within 72 hours of exposure.

89. The client tells the nurse that she frequently experiences nausea and vomiting after receiving radiation and chemotherapy. The nurse adapts the plan of care to include antiemetics. What is the most appropriate time for the administration of the medication?
1. 30 minutes before initiation of therapy
2. With the administration of therapy
3. Immediately after nausea begins
4. When therapy is completed

90. A child is admitted to the pediatric unit with an unknown mass in her lower left abdomen. Which action should be the nurse's <u>priority</u>?
1. Obtain the history of the illness.
2. Place a "Do not palpate abdomen" sign over the child's bed.
3. Obtain a complete set of vital signs.
4. Schedule a hemoglobin and hematocrit test for early morning.

Sometimes, timing is everything!

87. 2. One of the complications of both acute lymphocytic leukemia and its treatment is a decreased WBC count, especially a decreased absolute neutrophil count. Because neutrophils are the body's first line of defense against infection, the child must be protected from infection. Bleeding is a risk factor if platelets or other coagulation factors are decreased. A decreased hemoglobin level, hematocrit, or both would reduce the oxygen-carrying capacity of the child's blood. Constipation isn't related to the WBC count.
CN: Safe, effective care environment; CNS: Safety and infection control; CL: Application

88. 4. Varicella is a lethal organism to a child with leukemia. VZIG, given within 72 hours, may favorably alter the course of the disease. Giving the vaccine at the onset of symptoms wouldn't likely decrease the severity of the illness. Acyclovir may be given if the child develops the disease but not if the child has just been exposed.
CN: Health promotion and maintenance; CNS: None; CL: Analysis

89. 1. Antiemetics are most beneficial if given before the onset of nausea and vomiting. To calculate the optimum time for administration, the first dose is given 30 minutes to 1 hour before nausea is expected, and then every 2, 4, or 6 hours for approximately 24 hours after chemotherapy. If the antiemetic was given with the medication or after the medication, it could lose its maximum effectiveness when needed.
CN: Physiological integrity; CNS: Pharmacological and parenteral therapies; CL: Application

90. 2. The nurse must take measures to prevent palpation of the mass, if possible. If the mass is a malignant tumor, a do-not-palpate warning will help prevent trauma and rupture of the suspected tumor capsule. Rupture of the tumor capsule may cause seeding of cancer cells throughout the abdomen. Obtaining the history and vital signs and scheduling laboratory work are important but not the priority.
CN: Physiological integrity; CNS: Physiological adaptation; CL: Analysis

91. Which nursing measure is helpful when mouth ulcers develop as an adverse effect of chemotherapy?
1. Using lemon glycerin swabs
2. Administering milk of magnesia
3. Providing a bland, moist, soft diet
4. Frequently washing the mouth with full-strength hydrogen peroxide

91. 3. Oral ulcers are red, eroded, and painful. Providing a bland, moist, soft diet will make chewing and swallowing less painful. The use of lemon glycerin swabs and milk of magnesia should be avoided. Glycerin, a trihydric alcohol, absorbs water and dries the membranes. Milk of magnesia also has a drying effect because unabsorbed magnesium salts exert an osmotic pressure on tissue fluids. Many children also find the taste unpleasant. Frequent mouthwashes without alcohol are indicated. Peroxide shouldn't be used because it's irritating to tissues.
CN: Physiological integrity; CNS: Basic care and comfort; CL: Application

Don't stop now! You're doing a great job!

92. The parents of a child undergoing irradiation are taught about postirradiation somnolence. Which statement, if made by the parents, indicates that the teaching has been effective?
1. "This neurological syndrome will occur immediately."
2. "This neurological syndrome usually occurs within 1 to 2 weeks."
3. "This neurological syndrome usually occurs within 5 to 8 weeks."
4. "This neurological syndrome usually occurs within 3 to 6 months."

92. 3. Postirradiation somnolence may develop 5 to 8 weeks after CNS irradiation and may last 3 to 15 days. It's characterized by somnolence with or without fever, anorexia, nausea, and vomiting. Although the syndrome isn't thought to be clinically significant, parents should be prepared to expect such symptoms and encouraged to allow the child needed rest.
CN: Physiological integrity; CNS: Physiological adaptation; CL: Application

93. The nurse is providing discharge instructions for a client who is receiving chemotherapeutic medications. The nurse is aware that which intervention is most important to prevent hemorrhagic cystitis?
1. Giving antacids
2. Giving antibiotics
3. Restricting fluid intake
4. Increasing fluid intake

93. 4. Sterile hemorrhagic cystitis is an adverse effect of chemical irritation of the bladder from cyclophosphamide. It can be prevented by liberal fluid intake (at least 1½ times the recommended daily fluid requirement). Antibiotics don't aid in the prevention of sterile hemorrhagic cystitis. Restricting fluids would only increase the risk of developing cystitis. Antacids wouldn't be indicated for treatment.
CN: Physiological integrity; CNS: Reduction of risk potential; CL: Application

94. The parents of a child diagnosed with leukemia have stated that they'll give aspirin to their child for pain relief. What is the <u>most</u> appropriate response by the nurse?
1. "It's contraindicated because it decreases platelet production."
2. "It's contraindicated because it promotes bleeding tendencies."
3. "It's not a strong enough analgesic."
4. "It decreases the effects of methotrexate (Trexall)."

What other conditions is aspirin used for?

94. 2. Aspirin would be contraindicated because it promotes bleeding. Aspirin use has also been associated with Reye's syndrome in children. For home use, acetaminophen (Tylenol) is recommended for mild to moderate pain. Aspirin enhances the effects of methotrexate and has no effect on platelet production. Nonopioid analgesia has been effective for mild to moderate pain in clients with leukemia.
CN: Physiological integrity; CNS: Pharmacological and parenteral therapies; CL: Application

95. A child has been diagnosed with cancer and is scheduled for chemotherapy. The parents ask the nurse how they should explain the side effect of hair loss to the child. What is the best response by the nurse?

1. Introduce the idea of a wig after hair loss occurs.
2. Explain that hair typically begins to regrow in 6 to 9 months.
3. Stress that hair loss during a second treatment with the same medication will be more severe.
4. Explain that, as hair thins, keeping it clean, short, and fluffy may camouflage partial baldness.

96. A nurse is discussing childhood cancer with the parents of a child in an oncology unit. Which statement by the nurse would be the <u>most</u> accurate?

1. "The most common site for children's cancer is the bone marrow."
2. "All childhood cancers have a high mortality rate."
3. "Children with leukemia have a higher survival rate if they're older than 11 years when diagnosed."
4. "The prognosis for children with cancer isn't affected by treatment strategies."

97. Which condition assessed by the nurse would be an early warning sign of childhood cancer?

1. Difficult in swallowing
2. Nagging cough or hoarseness
3. Slight change in bowel and bladder habits
4. Swellings, lumps, or masses anywhere on the body

Know the early warning signs of childhood cancer.

95. 4. The nurse must prepare parents and children for possible hair loss. Cutting the hair short lessens the impact of seeing large quantities of hair on bed linens and clothing. Sometimes, keeping the hair short and fuller can make a wig unnecessary. Hair usually regrows in 6 months, depending on the treatment protocol. A child should be encouraged to pick out a wig similar to his own hair style and color before the hair falls out to foster adjustment to hair loss. Hair loss during a second treatment with the same medication is usually less severe.

CN: Psychosocial integrity; CNS: None; CL: Application

96. 1. Childhood cancers occur most commonly in rapidly growing tissue, especially in the bone marrow. Mortality depends on the time of diagnosis, the type of cancer, and the age at which the child was diagnosed. Children who are diagnosed between the ages of 2 and 9 consistently demonstrate a better prognosis. Treatment strategies are tailored to produce the most favorable prognosis.

CN: Physiological integrity; CNS: Physiological adaptation; CL: Application

97. 4. By being aware of early signs of childhood cancer, nurses can refer children for further evaluation. Swellings, lumps, or masses anywhere on the body are early warning signals of childhood cancer. Difficulty swallowing, cough, and hoarseness are early signs of cancer in adults. Usually, there's also a marked change in bowel or bladder habits, not associated with dietary intake.

CN: Health promotion and maintenance; CNS: None; CL: Application

98. Which nursing intervention helps to decrease the adverse effects of radiation therapy on the GI tract?
1. Avoiding the use of antispasmodics
2. Encouraging fluids and a soft diet
3. Giving antiemetics when nausea or vomiting occurs
4. Avoiding mouthwashes to prevent irritation of mouth ulcers

98. 2. Radiation therapy can cause adverse effects such as nausea and vomiting, anorexia, mucosal ulceration, and diarrhea. Antispasmodics are used to help reduce diarrhea. Encouraging fluids and a soft diet will help with anorexia. Antiemetics should be given before the onset of nausea. Frequent mouthwashes are indicated to prevent mycosis.
CN: Physiological integrity; CNS: Physiological adaptation; CL: Application

99. Short-term steroid therapy is used in clients with leukemia to promote which of the following?
1. Increased appetite
2. Altered body image
3. Increased platelet production
4. Decreased susceptibility to infection

99. 1. Short-term steroid therapy produces no acute toxicities and results in two beneficial reactions: increased appetite and a sense of well-being. Physical changes, such as "moon face," a result of steroid use, can cause alterations in body image and can be extremely distressing to children. Prednisone (steroid therapy) has no effect on platelet production but may increase susceptibility to infection.
CN: Physiological integrity; CNS: Pharmacological and parenteral therapies; CL: Application

One hundred questions! You must be proud!

100. Teaching children with leukemia and their families should include potential adverse effects of treatments. Which of the following is an adverse effect of prednisone?
1. Decreased appetite
2. Increased blood glucose
3. Decreased risk of infection
4. Decreased hair growth

100. 2. Prednisone may cause an increase in blood glucose requiring doses of insulin, especially when other factors are involved. Increased appetite, increased risk of infection, and increased hair growth are also adverse effects of prednisone.
CN: Physiological integrity; CNS: Pharmacological and parenteral therapies; CL: Application

101. Which nursing intervention is a <u>priority</u> for a hemophilic child who has fallen and badly bruised his leg?
1. Appropriate dose of aspirin and rest
2. Immobilization of the leg and a dose of ibuprofen
3. Heating pad and administration of factor VIII concentrate
4. Pressure on the site and administration of the required clotting factor

The pressure is really on to prioritize.

101. 4. With any bleeding injury in a client with hemophilia, the first line of treatment is always to replace the clotting factor. Pressure is applied along with cool compresses, and the extremity is immobilized. Aspirin isn't used because of its anticoagulant properties and the risk of Reye's syndrome in children. Immobilizing the leg and giving ibuprofen would be done after applying pressure and administering the necessary clotting factor. Heat isn't used because it increases bleeding.
CN: Safe, effective care environment; CNS: Management of care; CL: Application

102. When teaching an adolescent with iron deficiency anemia about diet choices, which menu selection would indicate that more instruction is necessary?
1. Caesar salad and pretzels
2. Cheeseburger with milkshake
3. Red beans and rice with sausage
4. Egg sandwich and snack peanuts

103. A nurse is speaking to the mother of a child with leukemia who wants to know why her child is so susceptible to infection if he has too many white blood cells (WBCs). Which response by the nurse would be most accurate?
1. This is an adverse effect of the medication he has to take.
2. He hasn't been able to eat a proper diet since he's been sick.
3. Leukemia is a problem of tumors in the internal organs that prevent his ability to fight infection.
4. Leukemia causes production of too many immature WBCs, which can't fight infection very well.

104. A nurse is developing a teaching plan for parents of a toddler who was just diagnosed with sickle cell anemia. Which statement is important to emphasize in the teaching plan?
1. If they have any more children, those children will also have sickle cell anemia.
2. Knowing how to prevent vaso-occlusive crisis is an important part of the parent's role.
3. The child will have a greater tendency to bleed and should avoid contact sports.
4. Vaso-occlusive crisis will occur eventually, requiring medical care.

Good diet choices are important for clients of all ages.

Prevention is the key to not ending up like me.

102. **1.** Caesar salad and pretzels aren't foods high in iron and protein. Meats (especially organ meats), eggs, and nuts have high protein and iron.
CN: Physiological integrity; CNS: Basic care and comfort; CL: Analysis

103. **4.** Leukemia is an unrestricted proliferation of immature WBCs, which don't function properly and are a poor defense against infection. Diet contributes to overall health but doesn't cause the overproduction of WBCs. There are no solid tumors in the internal organs in leukemia. Medications such as chemotherapy can diminish the immune system's effectiveness; however, they don't cause the overproduction of immature WBCs and the poor resistance to infection that the mother asked about.
CN: Physiological integrity; CNS: Physiological adaptation; CL: Application

104. **2.** Prevention is the key to teaching a family of a child with sickle cell anemia. The nurse should emphasize the daily use of prescribed oral antibiotics and avoidance of dehydration, high altitudes, and cold. These interventions can dramatically reduce the incidence of crisis. The disease is autosomal recessive, so each pregnancy has a one in four chance of the child having the disease, a one in four chance of not having the disease, and a two in four chance of carrying the trait. Abnormal bleeding and the need to avoid contact sports are associated with hemophilia.
CN: Health promotion and maintenance; CNS: None; CL: Application

105. A grandmother calls the pediatric children's clinic to find out whether her 3-year-old grandson can get shingles from her. Which response by the nurse would be most appropriate?
1. No, shingles don't occur in small children.
2. Yes, the grandson can get shingles from her. Shingles are caused by the herpes zoster virus.
3. The grandson could develop shingles if the lesions are on exposed skin areas and are weeping.
4. No, but the grandson would be exposed to the varicella-zoster virus, which could lead to the development of chickenpox.

Which response would be appropriate?

106. A child with idiopathic thrombocytopenic purpura is admitted to the hospital with a platelet count of 20,000/μl. The nurse is aware that the child should be closely monitored for which condition?
1. Hyperactivity
2. Proteinuria
3. Hand-foot syndrome
4. Change in level of consciousness (LOC)

107. The nurse is caring for a 1-month-old infant with signs of increased intracranial pressure (ICP). The nurse is aware that a priority intervention will be necessary if the infant displays which of the following?
1. Bulging fontanels, a high-pitched cry, vomiting
2. Frequent crying, sunken fontanel, pulse rate above 120 beats/minute
3. Blood-tinged vomitus, legs flexed to the abdomen, frequent crying
4. Falling asleep during feeding, pulse rate above 120 beats/minute when fussing, irregular arm and leg movements

I can't tell you what's wrong, so look for the signs.

105. 4. Shingles occur when a dormant varicella-zoster virus in a nerve becomes inflamed. The vesicles of shingles contain the virus and would expose others to it. The grandson couldn't develop shingles from such exposure. A herpes virus doesn't cause shingles. Shingles can occur in children but only if they have previously had chickenpox. The impetus for the inflammation is internal, not external.
CN: Safe, effective care environment; CNS: Safety and infection control; CL: Analysis

106. 4. When the platelet count drops to 20,000/μl, the child is at risk for spontaneous bleeding, including intracranially. A change in LOC is an important sign of increased intracranial pressure. This child is likely to become somnolent and difficult to arouse—not hyperactive. Proteinuria is more common in glomerulonephritis. With blood in the urine, protein also increases—but this isn't the primary concern. Hand-foot syndrome occurs in a child with sickle cell disease.
CN: Physiological integrity; CNS: Reduction of risk potential; CL: Application

107. 1. Because fontanels haven't closed by the age of 1 month, they bulge with increasing ICP. A high-pitched cry and vomiting also signal increased ICP. Quality of the cry is an important sign in an infant. Vomiting should be distinguished from a small amount of formula regurgitation, which is normal. Frequent crying may result from various stressors, and quality of the cry should be assessed. Blood-tinged vomitus, flexed legs, and crying indicate an abdominal disorder and pain. Infants normally have irregular arm and leg movements. A pulse rate of 120 beats/minute is normal for a 1-month-old infant at rest; in fact, the pulse may increase to 200 beats/minute during stress.
CN: Physiological integrity; CNS: Reduction of risk potential; CL: Analysis

108. The nurse has just completed discharge teaching for the family of a school-age child with idiopathic thrombocytopenia. The nurse determines that teaching was effective when the family identifies that which activity should be restricted?
1. Swimming
2. Bicycle riding
3. Computer games
4. Exposure to large crowds

Let' see. Which activity should be restricted?

108. 2. When routine blood counts reveal the platelet level is 100,000/µl or less, the child shouldn't engage in contact sports, bicycle or scooter riding, climbing, or other activities that could lead to injury (especially to the head). Swimming releases energy, builds muscle, and allows the child to compete without risking injury, as long as she follows normal safety precautions. Computer games don't cause physical injury. This child need not avoid large crowds because idiopathic thrombocytopenia doesn't suppress the immune system.
CN: Safe, effective care environment; CNS: Safety and infection control; CL: Application

109. A 17-year-old boy with classic hemophilia (hemophilia A) is admitted to the hospital for surgery. His preoperative preparation should include which treatment?
1. Bed rest
2. Transfusion of clotting factor VIII
3. I.V. analgesics given around the clock
4. Hydration at 50% above the normal fluid requirement

109. 2. In classic hemophilia or hemophilia A, clotting factor VIII is deficient. This factor must be transfused before surgery and at intervals afterward to prevent bleeding during and after surgery. Analgesics would be indicated if the child experienced bleeding, especially into the joints. Hydration above the normal requirement isn't needed. Because the child wasn't admitted for bleeding, bed rest isn't necessary.
CN: Physiological integrity; CNS: Reduction of risk potential; CL: Application

110. A child with hemophilia is hospitalized with bleeding into the knee. Which action should the nurse take <u>first</u>?
1. Prepare to administer a whole blood transfusion.
2. Prepare to administer a plasma transfusion.
3. Perform active range-of-motion (ROM) exercise on the affected part.
4. Elevate the affected part.

Hint! It's the first action the nurse should take.

110. 4. Bleeding into the joints is the most common type of bleeding episode in the more severe hemophilia forms. Elevating the affected part and applying pressure and cold are indicated. The nurse should anticipate transfusing the missing clotting factor—not whole blood or plasma, which won't stop the bleeding promptly and may pose a risk of fluid overload. Active ROM exercises are contraindicated because they may cause more bleeding, injury, and pain.
CN: Physiological integrity; CNS: Reduction of risk potential; CL: Application

111. Which intervention is indicated for a child in sickle cell vaso-occlusive crisis?
1. Immobilizing the affected part
2. Applying warm packs to the affected part
3. Applying cool packs to the affected part
4. Performing active range-of-motion (ROM) exercises to the affected part

111. 2. Applying warm packs promotes vasodilation and perfusion and provides pain relief and comfort. Immobilization leads to stasis, which promotes sickling. Cool packs are contraindicated because they cause vasoconstriction and may precipitate red blood cell sickling. A child in vaso-occlusive crisis experiences acute pain and limits movement of the affected part. After the acute crisis passes, the child should be encouraged to ambulate. Active ROM exercises increase pain in the affected part.
CN: Physiological integrity; CNS: Basic care and comfort; CL: Application

112. A 4-year-old child has recently been diagnosed with acute lymphocytic leukemia (ALL). What information about ALL should the nurse provide when educating the client's parents? Select all that apply.
1. Leukemia is a rare form of childhood cancer.
2. ALL affects all blood-forming organs and systems throughout the body.
3. The child shouldn't brush his teeth because of the increased risk of bleeding.
4. Adverse effects of treatment include sleepiness, alopecia, and stomatitis.
5. There's a 95% chance of remission with treatment.
6. The child shouldn't be disciplined during this difficult time.

112. 2, 4, and 5. In ALL, abnormal white blood cells proliferate, but they don't mature past the blast stage. These blast cells crowd out the healthy white blood cells, red blood cells, and platelets in the bone marrow, leading to bone marrow depression. The blast cells also infiltrate the liver, spleen, kidneys, and lymph tissue. Common adverse effects of chemotherapy and radiation include nausea, vomiting, diarrhea, sleepiness, alopecia, anemia, stomatitis, mucositis, pain, reddened skin, and increased susceptibility to infection. There's a 95% chance of obtaining remission with treatment. Leukemia is the most common form of childhood cancer. The child still needs appropriate discipline and limits. A lack of consistent parenting may lead to negative behaviors and fear.

CN: Physiological integrity; CNS: Reduction of risk potential; CL: Application

113. A child with sickle cell anemia is being treated for a crisis. The physician orders morphine sulfate (Duramorph) 2 mg I.V. The concentration of the vial is 10 mg/1 ml of solution. How many milliliters of solution should the nurse administer? Record your answer using one decimal point.

_____ milliliters

113. 0.2. The nurse should calculate the volume to be given using this equation: $2 \text{ mg}/X \text{ ml} = 10 \text{ mg}/1 \text{ ml}; 10X = 2; X = 0.2 \text{ ml}$.

CN: Physiological integrity; CNS: Pharmacological and parenteral therapies; CL: Application

114. A child with sickle cell anemia is being discharged after treatment for a crisis. Which instructions for avoiding future crises should the nurse provide to the client and his family? Select all that apply.
1. Avoid foods high in folic acid.
2. Drink plenty of fluids.
3. Use cold packs to relieve joint pain.
4. Report a sore throat to an adult.
5. Restrict activity to quiet board games.
6. Wash hands before meals and after playing.

Congratulations! You finished! Great job!

114. 2, 4, and 6. Fluids should be encouraged to prevent stasis in the bloodstream, which can lead to sickling. Sore throats, and any other cold symptoms, should be reported because they may indicate the presence of an infection, which can precipitate a crisis (red blood cells sickle and obstruct blood flow to tissues). Children with sickle cell anemia should learn appropriate measures to prevent infection, such as proper hand-washing techniques and good nutrition practices. Folic acid intake should be encouraged to help support new cell growth because new cells replace fragile, sickled cells. Warm packs should be applied to provide comfort and relieve pain; cold packs cause vasoconstriction. The child should maintain an active, normal life. When the child experiences a pain crisis, he limits his own activity according to his pain level.

CN: Physiological integrity; CNS: Reduction of risk potential; CL: Application

Chapter 29
Respiratory disorders

1. Following the death of an infant from sudden infant death syndrome (SIDS), which response by a nurse to the grieving parents is most appropriate?
1. "You didn't cause your infant's death."
2. "An autopsy will confirm the cause of your infant's death."
3. "Don't worry, you'll have more children."
4. "Be sure to place your next infant on his back to sleep."

2. Which child has an increased risk of sudden infant death syndrome (SIDS)?
1. A neonate born at 32 weeks' gestation weighing 4 lb (1.8 kg)
2. A 2-year old with a broken arm
3. An infant hospitalized with a temperature of 103.4° F (39.7° C)
4. A first-born child

3. A 6-week-old infant is brought to the emergency department not breathing; a preliminary finding of sudden infant death syndrome (SIDS) is made to the parents. Which intervention should the nurse take <u>initially</u>?
1. Call their spiritual advisor.
2. Explain the etiology of SIDS.
3. Allow them to see their infant.
4. Collect the infant's belongings and give them to the parents.

Cool! You made it to chapter 29. Keep up the good work!

Careful. This question is asking you to prioritize.

1. 1. The nurse can best support grieving parents by correcting the common falsehood that they could have prevented the infant's death. While an autopsy may need to be performed, it isn't a supportive response to grieving parents. Telling the parents that they will have more children minimizes the death of this infant and belittles the parent's feelings of grief. Instructing the parents to position future infants on their back suggests that the parents could have prevented this child's death.

CN: Psychosocial integrity; CNS: None; CL: Analysis

2. 1. Premature infants, especially those with low birth weight, have an increased risk for SIDS. Infants with apnea, central nervous system disorders, or respiratory disorders have a higher risk of SIDS. Peak age for SIDS is 2 to 4 months. Hospitalization for fever is insignificant. There's an increased risk of SIDS in subsequent siblings of two or more SIDS victims.

CN: Physiological integrity; CNS: Reduction of risk potential; CL: Analysis

3. 3. The parents need time with their infant to assist with the grieving process. Calling their pastor and collecting the infant's belongings are also important steps in the plan of care but aren't priorities. The parents will be too upset to understand an explanation of SIDS at this time.

CN: Psychosocial integrity; CNS: None; CL: Application

4. The family of an infant that died from sudden infant death syndrome (SIDS) asks the nurse what risk factors could have predisposed their child to SIDS. Which response would be the <u>most</u> accurate?
1. Breastfeeding the infant
2. Gestational age of 42 weeks
3. Immunizations
4. Low birth weight

5. An infant is brought to the emergency department (ED) and pronounced dead with the preliminary finding of sudden infant death syndrome (SIDS). Which question to the parents is appropriate?
1. Did you hear the infant cry out?
2. Was the infant's head buried in a blanket?
3. Were any of the siblings jealous of the new baby?
4. How did the infant look when you found him?

6. Which diagnostic test should be included in the care plan for children with an increased risk of sudden infant death syndrome (SIDS)?
1. Pulmonary function tests at regular intervals
2. Home apnea monitor
3. Pulse oximetry while sleeping
4. Chest X-ray at age 1 month

7. The nurse is aware that which reaction is usually exhibited by the family of an infant who has died from sudden infant death syndrome (SIDS)?
1. Feelings of blame or guilt
2. Acceptance of the diagnosis
3. Requests for the infant's belongings
4. Questions regarding the etiology of the diagnosis

8. The parents of an infant who just died from sudden infant death syndrome (SIDS) are angry at God and refuse to see any member of the clergy. Which nursing diagnosis is most appropriate?
1. Ineffective coping
2. Spiritual distress
3. Complicated grieving
4. Chronic sorrow

It's important to be sensitive to a family's feelings when they've lost a child to SIDS.

Is NCLEX distress an approved nursing diagnosis?

4. 4. Prematurity, low birth weight, maternal smoking, and multiple births are important risk factors associated with SIDS. Breastfeeding and a gestational age of 42 weeks aren't significant. Immunizations have been disproved to be associated with the disorder.
CN: Physiological integrity; CNS: Reduction of risk potential; CL: Application

5. 4. Only factual questions should be asked during the initial history in the ED. The other questions imply blame, guilt, or neglect.
CN: Physiological integrity; CNS: Physiological adaptation; CL: Application

6. 2. A home apnea monitor is recommended for infants with an increased risk for SIDS. Diagnostic tests, such as pulmonary function tests, pulse oximetry, and chest X-rays, can't diagnose the risk of surviving or dying from SIDS.
CN: Physiological integrity; CNS: Reduction of risk potential; CL: Application

7. 1. During the first few moments, the parents often are in shock and have overwhelming feelings of blame or guilt. Acceptance of the diagnosis and questions regarding the etiology may not occur until the parents have had time to see the child. The infant's belongings are usually packaged for the family to take home, but some parents may see this as a painful reminder.
CN: Psychosocial integrity; CNS: None; CL: Application

8. 2. The defining characteristics of spiritual distress include anger and refusing to interact with spiritual leaders. While anger is part of the grieving process, there's no indication that the parents aren't coping effectively or are experiencing complicated grieving. Since chronic sorrow, as the name implies, occurs over a period of time and may be cyclical, this isn't an appropriate nursing diagnosis since the death has just occurred.
CN: Psychosocial integrity; CNS: None; CL: Analysis

9. Which plan is most appropriate for a nurse scheduling a home visit to parents who lost an infant to sudden infant death syndrome (SIDS)?
1. One visit in 2 weeks
2. No visit is necessary
3. As soon after death as possible
4. One visit with parents only, no siblings

Make sure you understand the grieving process necessary for SIDS parents.

10. An infant is brought into the emergency room after an apneic episode. It is later determined to be an apparent life-threatening event (ALTE). What statement is incorrect regarding ALTE?
1. There is a causal relationship between ALTE and sudden infant death syndrome (SIDS).
2. Limpness and color change are often features of ALTE.
3. Stimulation or resuscitation is often required to bring about recovery.
4. Most ALTE episodes occur between 8 a.m. and 8 p.m.

11. The nurse is aware that which position is recommended for placing an infant to sleep?
1. Prone position
2. Supine position
3. Side-lying position
4. With head of bed elevated 30 degrees

12. Which activity should the nurse recommend for <u>long-term</u> support of parents with an infant who has died of sudden infant death syndrome (SIDS)?
1. Attending support groups
2. Attending church regularly
3. Attending counseling sessions
4. Discussing feelings with family and friends

9. 3. When parents return home, a visit is necessary as soon after the death as possible. The nurse should assess what the parents have been told, what they think happened, and how they've explained this to the other siblings. Not all of these issues will be resolved in one visit. The number of visits and plan for intervention must be flexible. The needs of the siblings must always be considered.
CN: Psychosocial integrity; CNS: None; CL: Application

10. 1. Studies over the past two decades have not confirmed a causal relationship between preexisting apnea and SIDS. The features of ALTE can be very frightening to the parents. Eighty percent of SIDS deaths occur between midnight and 6 a.m. Gastroesophageal reflux or a central nervous system disorder (presenting as seizure) have been diagnosed in 45% to 50% of infants presenting with ALTE. Recurrent, severe ALTE events requiring cardiopulmonary resuscitation that occur only in the presence of a single caretaker and no reasonable explanation is given after a thorough diagnostic workup should alert the nurse to the possibility of medical child abuse through intentional suffocation (Munchausen's syndrome by proxy).
CN: Physiological integrity; CNS: Reduction of risk potential; CL: Application

11. 2. The American Academy of Pediatrics endorses placing infants face-up in their cribs as a way to reduce sudden infant death syndrome (SIDS). Placing infants on their stomach is thought to make an attack of apnea harder to fight off, but how exactly the sleeping position predisposes a child to SIDS is still unclear. The side-lying position promotes gastric emptying. Raising the head of the bed 30 degrees is recommended for infants with gastroesophageal reflux.
CN: Health promotion and maintenance; CNS: None; CL: Application

12. 1. The best support will come from parents who have had the same experience. Attending church and discussing feelings with family and friends can offer support, but they may not understand the experience. Counseling sessions are usually a short-term support.
CN: Psychosocial integrity; CNS: None; CL: Application

CN: Client needs category   CNS: Client needs subcategory   CL: Cognitive level

13. Which nursing intervention is best to help a 2-year-old child adapt to hospitalization?
1. Allow the child to have favorite toys.
2. Allow the child to play with equipment used on him.
3. Explain procedures in simple terms.
4. Ask one or both parents to stay with the child.

14. A 2-year-old child comes to the emergency department with inspiratory stridor and a barking cough. A preliminary diagnosis of croup has been made. What is the <u>most important</u> intervention for the nurse to provide?
1. Administer I.V. antibiotics.
2. Provide oxygen by facemask.
3. Establish and maintain the airway.
4. Ask the mother to go to the waiting room.

15. The parents of a child ask the nurse what the best intervention is if their child is experiencing an episode of "midnight croup," or acute spasmodic laryngitis. What is the best response by the nurse?
1. Give warm liquids.
2. Raise the heat on the thermostat.
3. Provide humidified air with cool mist.
4. Take the child into the bathroom with a warm running shower.

16. Which sign is <u>most characteristic</u> of a child with croup?
1. Barking cough
2. Fever
3. High heart rate
4. Respiratory distress

Congratulations! You've finished the first 15 questions! Good job!

This question is asking for the symptom most commonly associated with croup.

13. 4. The most important factor in helping a child cope with new and strange surroundings is to have the security of the parents being present. This is the hallmark of family-centered care. Placing the child's favorite toys in the room provides distraction and allows the child to have something of his own with him but may not alleviate fears. Allowing the child to play with the equipment may pose a safety hazard and isn't appropriate. Explaining procedures in simple terms is important, but a 2-year old has limited understanding.
CN: Psychosocial integrity; CNS: None; CL: Application

14. 3. The initial priority is to establish and maintain the airway. Edema and accumulation of secretions may contribute to airway obstruction. Antibiotics aren't indicated for viral illnesses. Oxygen should be administered by tent as soon as possible to decrease the child's distress. Allowing the child to stay with the mother reduces anxiety and distress.
CN: Physiological integrity; CNS: Physiological adaptation; CL: Application

15. 3. High humidity with cool mist provides the most relief. Raising the heat on the thermostat will result in dry, warm air, which may cause secretions to adhere to the airway wall. A warm, running shower provides a mist that may be helpful to moisten and decrease the viscosity of airway secretions and may also decrease laryngeal spasm, but cool liquids would be best for the child. If unable to take liquid, the child needs to be in the emergency department.
CN: Physiological integrity; CNS: Physiological adaptation; CL: Application

16. 1. A resonant cough described as "barking" is the most characteristic sign of croup. The child may present with a low-grade or high fever depending on whether the etiological agent is viral or bacterial. While the child with croup may have a rapid heart rate, it isn't a characteristic sign of croup. The child may have varying degrees of respiratory distress related to swelling or obstruction.
CN: Physiological integrity; CNS: Physiological adaptation; CL: Analysis

17. Which sign should alert a nurse that an 18-month-old child with croup is experiencing increased respiratory distress?
1. A barking cough
2. Intercostal retractions
3. Clubbing of the fingers
4. Increased anterior-posterior chest diameter

18. What is the <u>most important</u> goal for a child with ineffective airway clearance?
1. Reducing the child's anxiety
2. Maintaining a patent airway
3. Providing adequate oral fluids
4. Administering medications as ordered

19. A 19-month-old child with croup is crying as a nurse tries to auscultate breath sounds. Which intervention by the nurse would be most appropriate?
1. Ignore the crying and listen to breaths sounds as best as possible.
2. Tell the parents that they are upsetting the child and to wait outside the room.
3. Tell the child, in a loud and firm voice, that he must sit still and cooperate.
4. Hand the stethoscope to the child to examine before auscultating his lungs.

20. The student nurse asks if any precaution is necessary when caring for children with respiratory infections such as croup. What is the best information for the nurse to provide?
1. Enforce hand washing.
2. Place the child in isolation.
3. Teach children to use tissues.
4. Keep siblings in the same room.

21. The nurse is reviewing orders for the assigned clients. A nebulizer treatment has been ordered for a child with croup. What is the <u>best</u> time for the nurse to administer the treatment?
1. During naptime
2. During playtime
3. After the child eats
4. After the parents leave

I know what's important, but what's the most important?

It's important to gain the child's trust.

17. 2. Intercostal retractions occur as the child's breathing becomes more labored and the use of other muscles is necessary to draw air into the lungs. A barking cough occurs in a child with croup and itself isn't a sign that the condition is worsening. Clubbing of the fingers and a change in chest diameter occur with chronic respiratory conditions.
CN: Physiological integrity; CNS: Physiological adaptation; CL: Analysis

18. 2. The most important goal is to maintain a patent airway. Reducing anxiety and administering medications will follow after the airway is secure. The child shouldn't be allowed to eat or drink anything to prevent the risk of aspiration.
CN: Physiological integrity; CNS: Physiological adaptation; CL: Application

19. 4. Developmentally, children at this age are curious. Therefore, encouraging the child to play with the stethoscope will distract him and help gain trust so that the nurse will be able to auscultate the lungs. Ignoring the child's crying may only get him more upset and won't help the nurse gain his trust. The nurse should use the parents to help quiet and comfort the child. Asking the parents to leave may only upset the child more. The nurse should speak to the child in a soft, comforting tone of voice.
CN: Health promotion and maintenance; CNS: None; CL: Analysis

20. 1. Hand washing helps prevent the spread of infections. Ill children should be placed in separate bedrooms if possible but don't need to be isolated. Teaching children to use tissues properly is important, but the key is disposal and hand washing after use.
CN: Health promotion and maintenance; CNS: None; CL: Application

21. 1. The nurse should administer nebulizer treatments at prescribed intervals. During naptime allows for as little disruption as possible. Administering treatment during playtime will disrupt the child's daily pattern. A child should be given a treatment before eating so the airway will be open and the work of eating will be decreased. Parents are usually helpful when administering treatments. The child can sit on the parents' lap to help decrease anxiety or fear.
CN: Physiological integrity; CNS: Pharmacological and parenteral therapies; CL: Application

22. During the recovery stages of croup, a nurse should explain which intervention to parents?
1. Limiting oral fluid intake
2. Recognizing signs of respiratory distress
3. Providing three nutritious meals per day
4. Allowing the child to go to the playground

Adequate parent teaching is essential for managing a child with croup.

23. Which instruction should a nurse give the parents of a 2-year-old child who wakes in the night with a barking cough?
1. Provide humidified air for the child to breath.
2. Call for an ambulance immediately.
3. Place the child in a warm, dry room.
4. Begin rescue breathing at once.

24. The nurse is assessing a child recently brought to the emergency department. Which observations would cause the nurse to suspect epiglottitis?
1. Decreased secretions
2. Drooling
3. Low-grade fever
4. Spontaneous cough

You're already at question 25. Way to go!

25. Which strategy is the best plan of care for a child with acute epiglottitis?
1. Encourage oral fluids for hydration.
2. Maintain the client in semi-Fowler's position.
3. Administer I.V. antibiotic therapy.
4. Maintain respiratory isolation for 48 hours.

22. 2. Although most children recover without complications, the parents should be able to recognize signs and symptoms of respiratory distress and know how to access emergency services. Oral fluids should be encouraged because fluids help to thin secretions. Although nutrition is important, frequent small nutritious snacks are usually more appealing than an entire meal. Children should have optimal rest and engage in quiet play. A comfortable environment free from noxious stimuli lessens respiratory distress.
CN: Physiological integrity; CNS: Physiological adaptation; CL: Application

23. 1. Humidified air reduces laryngeal irritation and spasm and helps liquefy secretions. The child doesn't need emergency care at this time; however, if the child develops respiratory distress, the parents should be instructed to call emergency medical services and not to drive the child to the hospital themselves. The child shouldn't be placed in a warm, dry room as cool, humidified air is used to reduce laryngospasm. The child doesn't require rescue breathing at the time. Rescue breathing is necessary if the child stops breathing.
CN: Physiological integrity; CNS: Reduction of risk potential; CL: Application

24. 2. Drooling of saliva is common due to the pain of swallowing, excessive secretions, and sore throat. The child usually has a high fever and the absence of a spontaneous cough. The classic picture is the child in a tripod position with mouth open and tongue protruding.
CN: Physiological integrity; CNS: Physiological adaptation; CL: Application

25. 3. The etiological agent for epiglottitis is usually bacterial; therefore, the treatment consists of I.V. antibiotic therapy. The client shouldn't be allowed anything by mouth during the initial phases of the infection to prevent aspiration. The client should be placed in Fowler's position or any position that provides the most comfort and security. Respiratory isolation isn't required.
CN: Physiological integrity; CNS: Physiological adaptation; CL: Application

26. A 2-year-old child is found on the floor next to his toy chest. After first determining unresponsiveness and calling for help, which step should be taken <u>next</u>?
1. Start mouth-to-mouth resuscitation.
2. Begin chest compressions.
3. Check for a pulse.
4. Open the airway.

27. A 10-month-old infant is found in respiratory arrest, and cardiopulmonary resuscitation is started. Which site is best to check for a pulse?
1. Brachial
2. Carotid
3. Femoral
4. Radial

28. When giving rescue breathing to an infant under age 1 year, what is the <u>ratio</u> of breaths per second?
1. 1 breath every 2 to 3 seconds
2. 1 breath every 3 to 5 seconds
3. 1 breath every 4 to 6 seconds
4. 1 breath every 5 to 7 seconds

29. When performing chest compressions on a 2-year-old child, which depth is correct?
1. ½″ to 1″ (1 to 2.5 cm)
2. 1″ to 1½″ (2.5 to 3.5 cm)
3. 1½″ to 2″ (3.5 to 5 cm)
4. 2″ to 2½″ (5 to 6.5 cm)

30. A single nurse rescuer knows that chest compressions must be coordinated with ventilations. Which ratio should the nurse rescuer use for a 3-year-old child?
1. 15 compressions to 1 ventilation
2. 15 compressions to 2 ventilations
3. 30 compressions to 1 ventilation
4. 30 compressions to 2 ventilations

It's important to prioritize in an emergency situation.

The procedure for rescue breathing for infants is different from that for adults.

26. 2. In 2010, the guidelines for cardiopulmonary resuscitation changed. It is now recommended that 30 chest compressions should be done first, followed by 2 breaths. The airway should be opened by using the chin thrust.
CN: Physiological integrity; CNS: Physiological adaptation; CL: Application

27. 1. Palpation of the brachial artery is recommended. The short, chubby neck of infants makes rapid location of the carotid artery difficult. After age 1, the carotid would be used. The femoral pulse, often palpated in a hospital setting, may be difficult to assess because of the infant's position, fat folds, and clothing. The radial pulse isn't a good indicator of central artery perfusion.
CN: Physiological integrity; CNS: Physiological adaptation; CL: Application

28. 2. Rescue breathing should be performed once every 3 to 5 seconds until spontaneous breathing resumes. This provides approximately 20 breaths/minute. One breath every 2 to 3 seconds may cause gastric distention. One breath every 5 to 6 seconds is recommended for adults.
CN: Physiological integrity; CNS: Physiological adaptation; CL: Application

29. 2. The chest compressions should equal approximately one-third to one-half the total depth of the chest. This corresponds to about 1 to 1½″ in a child age 1 to 8, ½″ to 1″ for an infant younger than age 1, and 1½″ to 2″ for an adult.
CN: Physiological integrity; CNS: Physiological adaptation; CL: Application

30. 4. A single health care provider rescuer should use a ratio of 30 chest compressions to 2 ventilations for children ages 1 year to the onset of adolescence. If another rescuer is available, then a ratio of 2 breaths for every 15 chest compressions is used. Ratios of 15:1 and 30:1 won't provide optimal compression and ventilation.
CN: Physiological integrity; CNS: Physiological adaptation; CL: Application

31. A 10-month-old child is found choking and soon becomes unconscious. Which intervention should a nurse attempt <u>first</u> after opening the airway?
1. Look inside the child's mouth for a foreign object.
2. Give five back blows and five chest thrusts.
3. Attempt a blind finger sweep.
4. Attempt rescue breathing.

32. Using which part of the hands is appropriate when performing chest compressions on a child between ages 1 and 8?
1. Heels of both hands
2. Heel of one hand
3. Index and middle fingers
4. Thumbs of both hands

33. A 3-year-old child is brought to the emergency department not breathing, cyanotic, and lethargic. The mother states that she thinks he swallowed a penny. Which intervention should the nurse take <u>first</u>?
1. Give 100% oxygen.
2. Administer five back blows.
3. Attempt a blind finger sweep.
4. Administer abdominal thrusts.

34. Which statement by the parent of a 4-year-old boy who just had a tonsillectomy indicates that a nurse's discharge instruction has been successful?
1. "I will keep him flat on his back in bed."
2. "I will sit him in bed at a 45-degree angle."
3. "I will place him on his stomach with his head to the side."
4. "I will place him on his back with his head on a pillow."

I am going to feel like a real heel if I get this answer wrong.

Again, you're being asked to prioritize.

31. 1. After the airway is open, the nurse should check for a foreign object and remove it with a finger sweep if it can be seen. After this step, 30 quick compressions should be given before rescue breathing is attempted. As soon as the infant is found choking, the nurse should give five back blows and five chest thrusts in an attempt to dislodge the object. Blind finger sweeps should never be performed because this may push the object further back into the airway.
<small>CN: Physiological integrity; CNS: Physiological adaptation; CL: Application</small>

32. 2. The heel of one hand is recommended for performing chest compressions on children between ages 1 and 8. Two hands are used for adult cardiopulmonary resuscitation. Chest thrusts administered with the middle and third fingers, and in some cases, the thumbs of each hand are used on infants younger than age 1.
<small>CN: Physiological integrity; CNS: Physiological adaptation; CL: Application</small>

33. 4. A child between ages 1 and 8 should receive abdominal thrusts to help dislodge the object. Administering 100% oxygen won't help if the airway is occluded. Infants younger than age 1 should receive back blows before chest thrusts. Blind finger sweeps should never be performed because this could push the object further back into the airway.
<small>CN: Physiological integrity; CNS: Physiological adaptation; CL: Application</small>

34. 3. Laying the child on his stomach with the head turned to the side allows blood and other secretions to drain from the mouth and pharynx, reducing the risk of aspiration. Placing the child flat on his back, on his back with a pillow, or at a 45-degree angle doesn't promote drainage and increases the likelihood of aspiration.
<small>CN: Physiological integrity; CNS: Reduction of risk potential; CL: Application</small>

35. A 7-month-old child is diagnosed with otitis media; the physician orders amoxicillin 80 mg/kg/day to be administered twice per day. The child weighs 9 kg. How much amoxicillin should the child receive per dose?
1. 120 mg
2. 180 mg
3. 200 mg
4. 360 mg

36. Children with chronic otitis media commonly require surgery for a myringotomy and ear tube placement. Which management strategy explains the purpose of the ear tubes?
1. To administer antibiotics
2. To flush the middle ear
3. To increase pressure
4. To drain fluid

37. A nurse is discharging a 10-month-old client with a prescription for eardrops. The nurse instructs the parents on the correct administration of the eardrops. It is most important to teach the parents to do which of the following?
1. Pull the earlobe upward.
2. Pull the earlobe up and back.
3. Pull the earlobe down and back.
4. Pull the earlobe down and forward.

38. A child is diagnosed with right chronic otitis media. After the child returns from surgery for myringotomy and placement of ear tubes, which intervention is appropriate?
1. Apply gauze dressings.
2. Position the child on the left side.
3. Position the child on the right side.
4. Apply warm compresses to both ears.

39. To reduce the risk of an infant developing otitis media, a nurse should instruct the parents to:
1. treat all cold symptoms with antibiotics.
2. place the infant in an upright position when feeding from a bottle.
3. avoid washing the ears to keep them dry.
4. swab the outer ear with a cotton-tipped swab.

Make sure you understand this formula. You'll use it again later in this chapter.

You're doing great! Keep it up!

35. 4. The child should receive 360 mg/dose. Here are the calculations: 80 mg × 9 kg = 720 mg/day; 720 mg/2 doses = 360 mg/dose.
CN: Physiological integrity; CNS: Pharmacological and parenteral therapies; CL: Application

36. 4. Ear tubes allow normal fluid to drain (not flush) from the middle ear. They also allow ventilation. The purpose isn't to administer medication. The tubes also allow pressure to equalize in the middle ear.
CN: Physiological integrity; CNS: Physiological adaptation; CL: Application

37. 3. For infants, the parent should be told to gently pull the earlobe down and back to visualize the external auditory canal. For children over age 3 and for adults, the earlobe is gently pulled slightly up and back.
CN: Physiological integrity; CNS: Pharmacological and parenteral therapies; CL: Application

38. 3. The child should be positioned on the right side to facilitate drainage. Gauze dressings aren't necessary after surgery. Some physicians may prefer a loose cotton wick. The left side isn't an area of concern for drainage. Warm compresses may help to facilitate drainage only when used on the affected ear.
CN: Physiological integrity; CNS: Physiological adaptation; CL: Application

39. 2. The risk of otitis media can be reduced by bottle feeding an infant in the upright position. Formula that pools in the nasopharynx is a good medium for bacterial growth, which can move through the shortened, horizontal eustachian tube of the infant. Administering antibiotics with cold symptoms won't reduce the risk of otitis media since colds are due to viral causes. Washing the ears, getting them wet, or swabbing the outer ear doesn't contribute to otitis media.
CN: Health promotion and maintenance; CNS: None; CL: Application

40. The nurse is using an otoscope to assess a child suspected of acute otitis media. Which assessment finding would be indicative of this condition?
  1. Pearl gray tympanic membrane
  2. Bright red, bulging tympanic membrane
  3. Dull gray membrane with fluid behind the eardrum
  4. Bright red or yellow, bulging or retracted, tympanic membrane

40. 4. With acute otitis media, the tympanic membrane may present as bright red or yellow, bulging or retracted. A pearl gray tympanic membrane is a normal finding. Dull gray membrane fluid is consistent with subacute or chronic otitis media.
CN: Physiological integrity; CNS: Physiological adaptation; CL: Application

41. A nurse is teaching the parents of a 1-year-old infant with otitis media. Which statement regarding predisposing factors for otitis media would be the <u>most</u> accurate for the nurse to make?
  1. The cartilage lining is overdeveloped.
  2. When infants sit up, it favors the pooling of fluid.
  3. Humoral defense mechanisms decrease the risk of infection.
  4. Eustachian tubes are short, wide, and straight and lie in a horizontal plane.

Question 41 is asking about a proximate cause of otitis media.

41. 4. In an infant or child, the eustachian tubes are short, wide, and straight and lie in a horizontal plane, allowing them to be more easily blocked by conditions such as large adenoids and infections. Until the eustachian tubes change in size and angle, children are more susceptible to otitis media. Cartilage lining is underdeveloped, making the tubes more distensible and more likely to open inappropriately. The usual lying-down position of infants favors the pooling of fluid such as formula in the pharyngeal cavity. Immature humoral defense mechanisms increase the risk of infection.
CN: Physiological integrity; CNS: Physiological adaptation; CL: Analysis

42. The nurse is aware that which complication is most commonly related to acute otitis media?
  1. Eardrum perforation
  2. Hearing loss
  3. Meningitis
  4. Tympanosclerosis

42. 1. Eardrum perforation is the most common complication as the exudate accumulates and pressure increases. Hearing loss in most cases is conductive in nature and mild in severity but is less common than eardrum perforation. Hearing tests aren't usually performed during episodes of otitis media. Tympanosclerosis and meningitis are possible but uncommon when adequate antibiotic therapy is implemented.
CN: Physiological integrity; CNS: Physiological adaptation; CL: Application

It's important that I stay the course.

43. Which statement by the parent of a child with otitis media indicates an understanding of a nurse's discharge instruction on the use of antibiotics?
  1. "I will give my child the full course of antibiotics."
  2. "I will stop the antibiotics when my child no longer has ear pain."
  3. "I will give the antibiotics whenever my child has ear pain."
  4. "I will put antibiotics in the affected ear."

43. 1. Antibiotics should be given for the full prescribed course of therapy regardless of whether the child has symptoms. Antibiotics are taken at prescribed intervals and not for episodes of ear pain. Oral antibiotics are used to treat otitis media.
CN: Physiological integrity; CNS: Pharmacological and parental therapies; CL: Application

44. A 2-year-old child is diagnosed with epiglottitis. Ceftriaxone is administered. In addition, vancomycin 50 mg/kg/day in three divided doses is ordered. The client weighs 12 kg. How much vancomycin is given per dose?
1. 50 mg
2. 100 mg
3. 200 mg
4. 300 mg

45. A 3-year-old child is receiving vancomycin for acute epiglottitis. Which of the following assessments would lead the nurse to suspect an adverse effect to vancomycin?
1. Constipation
2. Erythematous rash on the face and upper body
3. Increased appetite
4. Increased blood pressure

46. A 3-year-old child is given a preliminary diagnosis of acute epiglottitis. Which nursing intervention is appropriate?
1. Obtain a throat culture immediately.
2. Place the child in a side-lying position.
3. Don't attempt to visualize the epiglottis.
4. Use a tongue blade to look inside the throat.

What did I tell you? Here's that formula again

Vaccines. Who needs them?

47. An infant is brought to the clinic for her 6-month vaccines. The nurse tells the mother that administration of which vaccine is an appropriate step for prevention of epiglottitis?
1. Diphtheria vaccine
2. *Haemophilus influenzae* type B (Hib) vaccine
3. Measles vaccine
4. Inactivated poliovirus vaccine (IPV)

44. 3. The child should receive 200 mg per dose. Here are the calculations:

50 mg × 12 kg = 600 mg/day;
600 mg/3 doses = 200 mg/dose.

CN: Physiological integrity; CNS: Pharmacological and parenteral therapies; CL: Application

45. 2. Some clients may develop an erythematous rash on the face or upper body, often referred to as red man or red neck syndrome. This complication necessitates discontinuing the drug. Epigastric pain and diarrhea are adverse effects that may not necessitate discontinuation of the drug. Hypotension is a serious side effect of vancomycin.

CN: Physiological integrity; CNS: Pharmacological and parenteral therapies; CL: Application

46. 3. The nurse shouldn't attempt to visualize the epiglottis. The use of tongue blades or throat culture swabs may cause the epiglottis to spasm and totally occlude the airway. Throat inspection should be attempted only when immediate intubation or tracheostomy can be performed in the event of further or complete obstruction. The child should always remain in the position that provides the most comfort and security and ease of breathing.

CN: Physiological integrity; CNS: Physiological adaptation; CL: Application

47. 2. Epiglottitis is caused by the bacterial agent *H. influenzae*. The American Academy of Pediatrics recommends that, beginning at age 2 months, children receive the Hib conjugate vaccine. A decline in the incidence of epiglottitis has been seen as a result of this vaccination regimen. The IPV, measles, mumps, and rubella vaccine and diphtheria vaccine are preventive for those diseases.

CN: Health promotion and maintenance; CNS: None; CL: Application

48. Which sign in a 3-year-old child with acute epiglottitis indicates to the nurse that the client's respiratory distress is <u>increasing</u>?
1. Progressive barking cough
2. Increasing irritability
3. Increasing heart rate
4. Productive cough

This question is asking about an increase—not just a presence—of symptoms.

48. 3. Increasing heart rate is an early sign of hypoxia. A progressive barking cough is characteristic of spasmodic croup. A child in respiratory distress will be irritable and restless. As distress increases, the child will become lethargic related to the work of breathing and impending respiratory failure. A productive cough shows that secretions are moving and the child can effectively clear them.
CN: Physiological integrity; CNS: Physiological adaptation; CL: Application

49. While examining a child with acute epiglottitis, a nurse should have which item available?
1. Cool mist tent
2. Intubation equipment
3. Tongue blades
4. Viral culture medium

49. 2. Emergency intubation equipment should be at the bedside to secure the airway if examination precipitates further or complete obstruction. Viral culture medium and cool mist tents are recommended for the diagnosis and treatment of croup. Tongue blades are contraindicated and may cause the epiglottis to spasm.
CN: Physiological integrity; CNS: Physiological adaptation; CL: Application

50. A 2-year-old child is brought to the emergency department in respiratory distress. The child is drooling, sitting upright, and leaning forward with chin thrust out, mouth open, and tongue protruding. Which nursing intervention is most appropriate?
1. Check the child's gag reflex with a tongue blade.
2. Allow the child to cry to keep the lungs expanded.
3. Check the airway for a foreign body obstruction.
4. Support the child in an upright position on the parent's lap.

50. 4. The classic signs of epiglottitis are drooling, sitting upright, and leaning forward with chin thrust out, mouth open, and tongue protruding. The child with epiglottitis should be kept in an upright position to ease the work of breathing and to avoid aspiration of secretions and obstruction of the airway by the swollen epiglottis. Placing the child on the lap of a parent may help reduce the child's anxiety. The gag reflex of a child with epiglottitis should never be checked unless emergency personnel and equipment are immediately available to perform a tracheotomy if the airway should become obstructed by the swollen epiglottis. Likewise, crying and inspecting the airway for a foreign body may also cause entrapment of the epiglottis and obstruction of the airway.
CN: Physiological integrity; CNS: Reduction of risk potential; CL: Application

51. What is the best position for a nurse to place a 3-year-old child with right lower lobe pneumonia?
1. On the right side
2. On the left side
3. Supine
4. Prone

Congratulations! You've finished more than 50 questions! Keep up the good work!

51. 2. The child with right lower lobe pneumonia should be placed on his left side. This places the unaffected left lung in a position so that gravity will promote blood flow to the healthy lung tissue, improving gas exchange. Placing the child on the right side, his back, or his stomach doesn't promote circulation to the unaffected lung.
CN: Physiological integrity; CNS: Physiological adaptation; CL: Application

52. The arterial blood gas analysis of a child with asthma shows a pH of 7.30, P_{CO_2} of 56 mm Hg, and HCO_3^- of 25 mEq/L. The nurse determines that the child has which condition?
1. Metabolic acidosis
2. Metabolic alkalosis
3. Respiratory acidosis
4. Respiratory alkalosis

53. Which neonate is at high risk for developing neonatal chronic lung disease (bronchopulmonary dysplasia)?
1. A neonate born at 38 weeks' gestation receiving 1 to 4 L oxygen during feedings
2. A premature neonate born at 36 weeks' gestation receiving supplemental oxygen
3. A premature neonate born at 28 weeks' gestation on a high-pressure ventilator
4. A neonate born at 42 weeks' gestation who requires treatments for respiratory syncytial virus

54. Which nursing diagnosis is the priority for an infant with neonatal chronic lung disease (bronchopulmonary dysplasia)?
1. Imbalanced nutrition: Less than body requirements
2. Effective breastfeeding
3. Impaired gas exchange
4. Risk for imbalanced fluid volume

55. Which nursing intervention is most appropriate when caring for an infant with neonatal chronic lung disease (bronchopulmonary dysplasia)?
1. Provide frequent playful stimuli.
2. Decrease oxygen during feedings.
3. Place the infant on a set schedule.
4. Place the infant in an open crib.

I think I sense an acid–base disturbance coming on.

Which management strategy is recommended in question 55?

52. 3. Respiratory acidosis is an acid–base disturbance characterized by excess CO_2 in the blood, indicated by a P_{CO_2} greater than 45 mm Hg. The pH level is usually below the normal range of 7.36 to 7.45. The HCO_3^- level is normal in the acute stage and elevated in the chronic stage.
CN: Physiological integrity; CNS: Physiological adaptation; CL: Analysis

53. 3. Premature neonates with low birth weight on high-pressure ventilators are at highest risk for developing neonatal chronic lung disease (bronchopulmonary dysplasia). Supplemental oxygen, respiratory treatments, and 1 to 4 L oxygen for feedings are not high-risk factors for neonatal chronic lung disease (bronchopulmonary dysplasia).
CN: Physiological integrity; CNS: Reduction of risk potential; CL: Application

54. 3. The infant will have impaired gas exchange related to retention of carbon dioxide and borderline oxygenation secondary to fibrosis of the lungs. Although the infant may require increased caloric intake and may have excess fluid volume, imbalanced nutrition: less than body requirements, effective breast-feeding, and risk for imbalanced fluid volume aren't priority nursing diagnoses.
CN: Physiological integrity; CNS: Physiological adaptation; CL: Analysis

55. 3. Timing care activities with rest periods to avoid fatigue and to decrease respiratory effort is essential. Early stimulation activities are recommended, but the infant will have limited tolerance for them because of the illness. Oxygen is usually increased during feedings to help decrease respiratory and energy requirements. Thermoregulation is important because both hypothermia and hyperthermia will increase oxygen consumption and may increase oxygen requirements. These infants are usually maintained on warmer beds or inside Isolettes.
CN: Safe, effective care environment; CNS: Management of care; CL: Application

56. The nurse is planning care for a child admitted to the pediatric unit with neonatal chronic lung disease (bronchopulmonary dysplasia). Which symptom is the nurse most likely to assess?
1. Minimal work of breathing
2. Tachypnea and dyspnea
3. Easily consolable
4. Hypotension

Be sure not to confuse the prefixes hyper and hypo!

56. 2. Tachypnea, dyspnea, and wheezing are intermittently or chronically present secondary to airway obstruction and increased airway resistance. These infants usually show increased work of breathing and increased use of accessory muscles. They're frequently described as irritable and difficult to comfort. Pulmonary hypertension is a common finding resulting from fibrosis and chronic hypoxia.

CN: Physiological integrity; CNS: Physiological adaptation; CL: Application

57. Which nursing intervention is <u>most appropriate</u> for helping parents to cope with a child <u>newly diagnosed</u> with neonatal chronic lung disease (bronchopulmonary dysplasia)?
1. Teach cardiopulmonary resuscitation.
2. Refer them to support groups.
3. Help parents identify necessary lifestyle changes.
4. Evaluate and assess parents' stress and anxiety levels.

57. 4. The emotional impact of neonatal chronic lung disease (bronchopulmonary dysplasia) is clearly a crisis situation. The parents are experiencing grief and sorrow over the loss of a "healthy" child. The other strategies are more appropriate for long-term intervention.

CN: Psychosocial integrity; CNS: None; CL: Application

58. The nursing care plan for an infant with neonatal chronic lung disease (bronchopulmonary dysplasia) includes the nursing diagnosis of impaired gas exchange. Which nursing action would be most appropriate for a nurse to include?
1. Provide chest physiotherapy.
2. Provide enteral feedings.
3. Provide appropriate age-related activities.
4. Promote bonding between parent and child.

58. 1. All these activities are appropriate to include in the care of a child with neonatal chronic lung disease (bronchopulmonary dysplasia); however, providing chest physiotherapy addresses the nursing diagnosis of impaired gas exchange.

CN: Physiological integrity; CNS: Basic care and comfort; CL: Analysis

59. Chlorothiazide is ordered for a 1-year-old client with neonatal chronic lung disease (bronchopulmonary dysplasia). The dosage ordered is 30 mg/kg/day. The client weighs 10 kg. How much is given per dose when administered two times per day?
1. 60 mg/dose
2. 75 mg/dose
3. 150 mg/dose
4. 300 mg/dose

Here's that formula again!

59. 3. The child should receive 150 mg/dose. Here are the calculations:

$$30 \text{ mg/kg} \times 10 \text{ kg} = 300 \text{ mg/day};$$
$$300 \text{ mg/2 doses} = 150 \text{ mg/dose.}$$

CN: Physiological integrity; CNS: Pharmacological and parenteral therapies; CL: Application

60. Infants with neonatal chronic lung disease (bronchopulmonary dysplasia) require frequent, prolonged rest periods. Which sign indicates overstimulation?
1. Increased alertness
2. Good eye contact
3. Cyanosis
4. Lethargy

60. 3. Signs of overstimulation in an immature child include cyanosis, avoidance of eye contact, vomiting, diaphoresis, or falling asleep. The child may also become irritable and show signs of respiratory distress.

CN: Physiological integrity; CNS: Basic care and comfort; CL: Analysis

61. Which outcome should be anticipated of parental care of a child with neonatal chronic lung disease (bronchopulmonary dysplasia)?
1. Reports increased levels of stress
2. Makes safe decisions with professional assistance only
3. Participates in routine, but not complex, caretaking activities
4. Verbalizes the causes, risks, therapy options, and nursing care

62. Neonatal chronic lung disease (bronchopulmonary dysplasia) can be classified into four categories. Which characteristic is noted during the early or <u>first</u> stage of the disease?
1. Interstitial fibrosis
2. Signs of emphysema
3. Hyperexpansion on chest X-ray
4. Resemblance to respiratory distress syndrome

63. Neonatal chronic lung disease (bronchopulmonary dysplasia) can cause increased fluid in the lungs due to disruption of the alveolar-capillary membrane, and the client may begin receiving furosemide (Lasix). Which adverse effect is possible?
1. Hypercalcemia
2. Hyperkalemia
3. Hypernatremia
4. Irregular heart rhythm

64. A pediatric client is to receive furosemide (Lasix) 4 mg/kg/day in one daily dose. The client weighs 20 kg. How many milligrams should be administered in each dose?
1. 20
2. 40
3. 80
4. 160

65. A 2-year-old child with neonatal chronic lung disease (bronchopulmonary dysplasia) is placed on furosemide (Lasix) once per day. The parents are being educated on foods that are rich in potassium. Which food should the nurse recommend?
1. Apples
2. Oranges
3. Peaches
4. Raisins

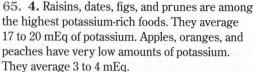

We're raising awareness about our potassium content.

Encourage parents to verbalize their understanding of their infant's disorder.

61. **4.** The parents should understand the causes, risks, and care of their infant by the time of discharge. Having the parents verbalize this information is the only way to assess their understanding. The parents should report decreased levels of stress, be capable of making decisions independently, and participate in routine and complex care.
CN: Physiological integrity; CNS: Basic care and comfort; CL: Analysis

62. **4.** Stage I can be characterized by early interstitial changes and resembles respiratory distress syndrome. Stage IV shows interstitial fibrosis and hyperexpansion on chest X-ray. Stage III shows signs of the beginning of chronic disease with interstitial edema, signs of emphysema, and pulmonary hypertension.
CN: Physiological integrity; CNS: Physiological adaptation; CL: Analysis

63. **4.** An irregular heart rhythm and muscle cramps are adverse effects related to hypokalemia and hypocalcemia and not hypercalcemia or hyperkalemia. Diuretics cause volume depletion by inhibiting reabsorption of sodium and chloride. Hypocalcemia is related to the urinary excretion of calcium. Hypokalemia can occur with excessive fluid loss or as part of contraction alkalosis.
CN: Physiological integrity; CNS: Pharmacological and parenteral therapies; CL: Application

64. **3.** The child should receive 80 mg per dose. Here are the calculations:
$$4 \text{ mg/kg} \times 20 \text{ kg} = 80 \text{ mg}.$$
CN: Physiological integrity; CNS: Pharmacological and parenteral therapies; CL: Application

65. **4.** Raisins, dates, figs, and prunes are among the highest potassium-rich foods. They average 17 to 20 mEq of potassium. Apples, oranges, and peaches have very low amounts of potassium. They average 3 to 4 mEq.
CN: Physiological integrity; CNS: Pharmacological and parenteral therapies; CL: Application

66. Which reason necessitates tracheostomy tube placement in long-term care of infants with neonatal chronic lung disease (bronchopulmonary dysplasia)?
1. Increased risk of tracheomalacia
2. Inability to wean from the ventilator
3. Need to allow for gastrostomy tube feedings
4. Increased signs of respiratory distress

67. A 1-year-old infant with neonatal chronic lung disease (bronchopulmonary dysplasia) has just received a tracheostomy. What is the <u>most appropriate</u> nursing intervention?
1. Keep extra tracheostomy tubes at the bedside.
2. Secure ties at the side of the neck for easy access.
3. Change the tracheostomy tube 2 weeks after surgery.
4. Secure the tracheostomy ties tightly to prevent dislodgment of the tube.

68. An 11-month-old infant with neonatal chronic lung disease (bronchopulmonary dysplasia) and a tracheostomy experiences a decline in oxygen saturation from 97% to 88%. He appears anxious, and his heart rate is 180 beats/minute. Which nursing intervention is most appropriate?
1. Change the tracheostomy tube.
2. Suction the tracheostomy tube.
3. Obtain an arterial blood gas (ABG) level.
4. Increase the oxygen flow rate.

69. Which nursing intervention is appropriate when suctioning a tracheostomy tube?
1. Hypoventilate the child before suctioning.
2. Repeat the suctioning process for two intervals.
3. Insert the catheter 1 to 2 cm below the tracheostomy tube.
4. Inject a small amount of normal saline solution into the tube before suctioning.

Ask yourself what you would need if the worst occurred.

Which intervention is appropriate?

66. 2. Tracheostomy may be required after a child has been ventilator dependent for 6 to 8 weeks and is unable to wean from the ventilator. This will allow for oral feedings and reduce the risks of tracheomalacia and bronchomalacia.
CN: Physiological integrity; CNS: Physiological adaptation; CL: Analysis

67. 1. Extra tracheostomy tubes should be kept at the bedside in case of an emergency, including one size smaller in case the appropriate size doesn't fit due to edema or lack of a tract formation. Ties are usually placed at the back of the neck. The ties should be placed securely but allow the width of a little finger for room to prevent excessive pressure or skin breakdown. The first tracheostomy tube change is usually performed by the physician after 7 days.
CN: Physiological integrity; CNS: Reduction of risk potential; CL: Application

68. 2. Tracheostomy tubes, particularly in small children, require frequent suctioning to remove mucus plugs and excessive secretions. The tracheostomy tube can be changed if suctioning is unsuccessful. Obtaining an ABG level may be beneficial if oxygen saturation remains low and the child appears to be in respiratory distress. Increasing the oxygen flow rate will only help if the airway is patent.
CN: Physiological integrity; CNS: Reduction of risk potential; CL: Analysis

69. 4. Injecting a small amount (1 to 2 drops) of normal saline solution helps to loosen secretions for easier aspiration. Preservative-free normal saline solution should be used. The child should be hyperventilated before and after suctioning to prevent hypoxia. The suctioning process should be repeated until the trachea is clear. If the catheter is inserted too far, it will irritate the carina and may cause blood-tinged secretions. The catheter should be inserted 0.5 cm beyond the tracheostomy tube.
CN: Physiological integrity; CNS: Reduction of risk potential; CL: Application

70. A parent asks the nurse which characteristic distinguishes allergies from colds. What is the best response by the nurse?
1. Skin tests can diagnose a cold.
2. Allergies are accompanied by fever.
3. Colds cause itching of the eyes and nose.
4. Allergies trigger constant and consistent bouts of sneezing.

71. A 2-year old with pneumonia is placed in an oxygen tent with mist. Which nursing action is a priority?
1. Change the child's bed linens and pajamas frequently.
2. Maintain a steady body temperature.
3. Avoid the use of equipment or toys that can produce sparks.
4. Keep the plastic sides of the tent tucked in.

Cold or allergies? That is the (Ah-choo) question!

We really need to watch out for those triggers.

72. A 2-year-old child has been diagnosed with asthma. The parents ask about the most common asthma triggers. What is the best response by the nurse?
1. Weather
2. Peanut butter
3. The cat next door
4. One parent with asthma

73. The nurse is assessing breath sounds of a child admitted with asthma. The nurse would anticipate hearing which sound?
1. Stridor
2. Rhonchi
3. Rales
4. Wheezing

70. 4. Allergies elicit consistent bouts of sneezing, are seldom accompanied by fever, and tend to cause itching of the eyes and nose. Skin testing is performed to determine the client's sensitivity to specific allergens. Colds are accompanied by fever and are characterized by sporadic sneezing.

CN: Health promotion and maintenance; CNS: None; CL: Analysis

71. 3. While all the interventions are appropriate for caring for a child in an oxygen tent with mist, sparks in the presence of oxygen can cause a fire. Therefore, all equipment and toys that may produce a spark should be avoided. Bed linens and pajamas may become damp due to the cool mist and should be changed when needed but only after the risk of fire has been addressed. Keeping the child dry will help promote a steady body temperature, which is important since shivering increases oxygen intake. The sides of the tent should be tucked in since oxygen is heavier than air, making oxygen loss greater at the bottom of the tent.

CN: Safe, effective care environment; CNS: Management of care; CL: Analysis

72. 1. Excessively cold air, wet or humid changes in weather and seasons, and air pollution are some of the most common asthma triggers. Household pets are also a trigger. Evidence suggests that asthma is partly hereditary in nature. Food allergens are rarely responsible for airway reactions in children.

CN: Physiological integrity; CNS: Physiological adaptation; CL: Application

73. 4. Asthma frequently presents with wheezing and coughing. Airway inflammation and edema increase mucous production. Other signs include dyspnea, tachycardia, and tachypnea. Stridor is heard in croup. Rhonchi and rales are not as common in asthma as wheezing.

CN: Physiological integrity; CNS: Physiological adaptation; CL: Application

74. The nurse is aware that a child is at increased risk for an asthma-related death when there has been:
1. use of an inhaler at home.
2. one admission for asthma last year.
3. prior admission to the general pediatric floor.
4. prior admission to an intensive care unit for asthma.

74. 4. Asthma results in varying degrees of respiratory distress. A prior admission to an intensive care unit marks an increased severity and need of immediate therapy. Two or more hospitalizations for asthma, a recent hospitalization or emergency department visit in the past month, or three or more emergency department visits in the past year put a child at high risk for asthma-related death. Current use of systemic steroids would also be a risk factor.

CN: Physiological integrity; CNS: Reduction of risk potential; CL: Analysis

75. During the assessment of a client, the nurse distinguishes that a client has status asthmaticus, instead of asthma, when the client has which characteristic?
1. Several attacks per month
2. Less than six attacks per year
3. Little or no response to bronchodilators
4. Constant and unrelieved by bronchodilators

This question is asking you to distinguish between varying degrees of asthma.

75. 4. Status asthmaticus can best be described as constant and unrelieved by bronchodilators. Moderate asthma is characterized by several attacks per month. Mild asthma is less than six attacks per year. Little or no response to bronchodilators would describe severe asthma.

CN: Physiological integrity; CNS: Physiological adaptation; CL: Application

76. A 2-year-old child with status asthmaticus is admitted to the pediatric unit and begins to receive continuous treatment with albuterol (Proventil), given by nebulizer. The nurse should observe for which of the following?
1. Bradycardia
2. Lethargy
3. Tachycardia
4. Tachypnea

76. 3. Albuterol is a rapid-acting bronchodilator. Common adverse effects include tachycardia, nervousness, tremors, insomnia, irritability, and headache.

CN: Physiological integrity; CNS: Pharmacological and parenteral therapies; CL: Application

77. A 10-year-old child is admitted with asthma. The physician orders a methylprednisolone loading dose of 3 mg/kg. The client weighs 30 kg. How much methylprednisolone is contained in the dose?
1. 60 mg
2. 90 mg
3. 120 mg
4. 180 mg

Do you know why it's called a loading dose?

77. 2. The child should receive 90 mg per dose. Here are the calculations:

$$3 \text{ mg/kg} \times 30 \text{ kg} = 90 \text{ mg}.$$

CN: Physiological integrity; CNS: Pharmacological and parenteral therapies; CL: Application

78. A 10-year-old client with asthma has recently started receiving oral methylprednisolone. He begins to vomit and complains of his stomach hurting. Which nursing intervention is appropriate?
1. Check the methylprednisolone level.
2. Decrease the dose.
3. Take no action; methylprednisolone can cause nausea.
4. Place an I.V. and call the physician.

79. Which finding should a nurse expect on a typical X-ray of a child with asthma?
1. Atelectasis
2. Hemothorax
3. Infiltrates
4. Pneumothoraces

80. The nurse is caring for a client with atelectasis. What is the most important nursing intervention for the nurse to provide?
1. Perform chest physiotherapy.
2. Give increased I.V. fluids.
3. Administer oxygen.
4. Obtain arterial blood gas (ABG) levels.

81. The parents of a 10-year-old child recently diagnosed with asthma ask if the child can continue to play sports. What is the best response by the nurse?
1. Sports don't cause asthma attacks.
2. You should limit activities to quiet play.
3. It's okay to play some sports, but swimming isn't recommended.
4. Physical activity and sports are encouraged, provided the asthma is under control.

78. 4. Nausea and GI upset are adverse effects of methylprednisolone. The treatment of asthma requires treatment of the inflammation that is a hallmark of the disease. If the child cannot tolerate oral corticosteroids, an I.V. dose is warranted.
CN: Physiological integrity; CNS: Pharmacological and parenteral therapies; CL: Analysis

79. 1. Hyperexpansion, atelectasis, and a flattened diaphragm are typical X-ray findings for a child with asthma. Air becomes trapped behind the narrowed airways and the residual capacity rises, leading to hyperinflation. Hypoxemia results from areas of the lung not being well perfused. A hemothorax isn't a finding related to asthma. Infiltrates and pneumothoraces are uncommon.
CN: Physiological integrity; CNS: Physiological adaptation; CL: Analysis

80. 1. Chest physiotherapy and incentive spirometry help to enhance the clearance of mucus and open the alveoli. I.V. and oral fluids are recommended to help liquefy and thin secretions. Administration of oxygen will not give enough pressure to open the alveoli. Obtaining ABG levels isn't necessary.
CN: Physiological integrity; CNS: Physiological adaptation; CL: Application

81. 4. Participation in sports is encouraged but should be evaluated on an individual basis provided the asthma is under control. Exercise-induced asthma is an example of the airway hyperactivity common to asthmatics. Swimming is well tolerated related to the type of breathing and the moisture in the air. Exclusion from sports or activities may hamper peer interaction.
CN: Physiological integrity; CNS: Physiological adaptation; CL: Analysis

You're doing great! Keep up the good work!

82. The nurse is caring for a child with asthma who is being treated with aminophylline after failing to respond to other treatment strategies. The nurse reviews the child's aminophylline level and interprets it as normal when the results show which level?
1. 2 to 4 mcg/ml
2. 5 to 15 mcg/ml
3. 10 to 20 mcg/ml
4. 20 to 30 mcg/ml

83. A nurse is caring for a 2-year-old client with asthma. What is the most appropriate nursing intervention for this client?
1. Give warm liquids.
2. Give cold juice or ice pops.
3. Provide three meals and three snacks.
4. Give I.V. fluid boluses.

Keep this client's age in mind when answering question 83.

84. Which intervention by the parents is appropriate to "allergy proof" the home?
1. Cover floors with carpeting.
2. Designate the basement as the play area.
3. Dust and clean the house thoroughly twice a month.
4. Use foam rubber pillows and synthetic blankets.

"Allergy proofing" a home can be just as important as "kid proofing" it.

85. Which nursing diagnosis is appropriate for a client with acute asthma?
1. Imbalanced nutrition: More than body requirements
2. Excess fluid volume
3. Activity intolerance
4. Constipation

82. 3. The normal therapeutic range of aminophylline is considered to be 10 to 20 mcg/ml. Levels below 10 mcg/ml are considered to be less than therapeutic. Symptoms of toxicity, such as nausea, tachycardia, and irritability, can appear when levels exceed 20 mcg/ml. Levels greater than 30 mcg/ml can cause seizures and arrhythmias.
CN: Physiological integrity; CNS: Pharmacological and parenteral therapies; CL: Application

83. 1. Liquids are best tolerated if they're warm. Cold liquids may cause bronchospasm and should be avoided. Dehydration should be corrected slowly. Small, frequent meals should be provided to avoid abdominal distention that may interfere with diaphragm excursion. Overhydration may increase interstitial pulmonary fluid and exacerbate small airway obstruction.
CN: Physiological integrity; CNS: Physiological adaptation; CL: Application

84. 4. Bedding should be free from allergens with hypoallergenic covers. Unnecessary rugs should be removed, and floors should be bare and mopped a few times a week to reduce dust. Basements or cellars should be avoided to lessen the child's exposure to molds and mildew. Dusting and cleaning should occur daily or at least weekly.
CN: Physiological integrity; CNS: Physiological adaptation; CL: Application

85. 3. Ineffective oxygen supply and demand may lead to activity intolerance. The nurse should promote rest and encourage developmentally appropriate activities. Nutrition may be decreased due to respiratory distress and GI upset. Dehydration is common due to diaphoresis, insensible water loss, and hyperventilation. Medications given to treat asthma may cause nausea, vomiting, and diarrhea, not constipation.
CN: Physiological integrity; CNS: Physiological adaptation; CL: Analysis

86. A nurse is explaining bronchiolitis to the parents of an infant admitted with the condition. Which explanation by the nurse would be the <u>most</u> accurate?
1. Acute inflammation and obstruction of the bronchioles
2. Airway obstruction from aspiration of a solid object
3. Inflammation of the pulmonary parenchyma
4. Acute highly contagious croup-like syndrome

87. A 2-month-old infant is brought to the emergency department, and a preliminary diagnosis of bronchiolitis is given. During assessment of the infant, the nurse would expect to find which of the following?
1. Bradycardia
2. Increased appetite
3. Wheezing on auscultation
4. No signs of an upper respiratory infection

88. In most cases, bronchiolitis is caused by a viral agent, most commonly respiratory syncytial virus (RSV). The nurse should keep in mind which statement regarding RSV infection?
1. It's more prevalent in the summer and fall months.
2. It's most likely to attack the respiratory tract mucosa.
3. It's more commonly seen in children older than age 5.
4. It's not particularly contagious.

89. A student nurse asks the nurse if any precautions are needed when caring for a 2-month-old infant with respiratory syncytial virus (RSV) to <u>prevent</u> the spread of infection. What is the best response by the nurse?
1. Gloves only
2. Gown, gloves, and mask
3. No precautions required; the virus isn't contagious
4. Proper hand washing between clients

90. The nurse teaches parents that which test is used to diagnose respiratory syncytial virus (RSV)?
1. Blood test
2. Nasopharyngeal washings
3. Sputum culture
4. Throat culture

Consider the pathology of bronchiolitis when answering question 87.

You better take precautions if you want to avoid the likes of me.

86. **1.** Bronchiolitis is an infection of the bronchioles, causing the mucosa to become edematous, inflamed, and full of mucus. Lower airway obstruction from a solid object is a form of a foreign body aspiration. Pneumonia is characterized by inflammation of the pulmonary parenchyma. Croup-like syndromes are generally upper airway infections or obstructions.
CN: Physiological integrity; CNS: Physiological adaptation; CL: Application

87. **3.** In bronchiolitis, the bronchioles become narrowed and edematous. This can cause wheezing. These infants typically have a 2- to 3-day history of an upper respiratory infection and feeding difficulties with loss of appetite due to nasal congestion and increased work of breathing. This combination leads to respiratory distress with tachypnea and tachycardia.
CN: Physiological integrity; CNS: Physiological adaptation; CL: Application

88. **2.** RSV attacks the respiratory tract mucosa. The virus is most prevalent in the winter and early spring months. Most children develop the infection between ages 2 and 6 months, and RSV generally occurs during the first 3 years of life. RSV is a highly contagious respiratory virus.
CN: Physiological integrity; CNS: Physiological adaptation; CL: Application

89. **2.** RSV is highly contagious and is spread through direct contact with infectious secretions via hands, droplets, and fomites. Gowns, gloves, and masks should be worn for client care to prevent the spread of infection.
CN: Safe, effective care environment; CNS: Safety and infection control; CL: Application

90. **2.** RSV can only be diagnosed with direct aspiration of nasal secretions or nasopharyngeal washings. Positive identification is accomplished using the enzyme-linked immunosorbent assay. Blood, throat, and sputum cultures can't definitively diagnose RSV.
CN: Physiological integrity; CNS: Physiological adaptation; CL: Application

91. Which child would be at <u>increased risk</u> for a respiratory syncytial virus (RSV) infection?
1. A 2-month-old child managed at home
2. A 2-month-old child with neonatal chronic lung disease (bronchopulmonary dysplasia)
3. A 3-month-old child requiring low-flow oxygen
4. A 2-year-old child

RSV is risky business.

91. 2. Infants with cardiac or pulmonary conditions are at highest risk for RSV. Because of their underlying conditions, they usually require mechanical ventilation. Many infants can be managed at home; few require hospitalization. A 3-month-old infant on low-flow oxygen has some risks of progression but is not at a high risk. A 2-year-old child has built up the immune system and can tolerate the infection without major problems.

CN: Physiological integrity; CNS: Reduction of risk potential; CL: Analysis

92. Parents of a premature infant ask the nurse which medication can help to prevent respiratory syncytial virus (RSV). What is the best response by the nurse?
1. Epinephrine
2. Bronchodilators
3. Corticosteroids
4. Palivizumab

92. 4. Palivizumab is a monoclonal antibody against the RSV F glycoprotein. It can help to prevent serious lower respiratory tract infections caused by RSV. The first dose is given before RSV season, with monthly doses given throughout the season for protection. This agent is indicated for children younger than age 24 months with neonatal chronic lung disease (bronchopulmonary dysplasia) or a history of prematurity (less than 35 weeks) or hemodynamically significant congenital heart disease. Bronchodilators, epinephrine, and corticosteroids are sometimes used for treatment.

CN: Health promotion and maintenance; CNS: None; CL: Analysis

93. Which medication is used to treat bronchiolitis in an immunosuppressed client with severe infection caused by respiratory syncytial virus (RSV)?
1. Albuterol
2. Aminophylline
3. Cromolyn sodium
4. Ribavirin (Virazole)

93. 4. Ribavirin is an antiviral agent that is reserved for use in severely affected immunocompromised clients with RSV. Its efficacy has not been proven for routine use. Aminophylline and albuterol are bronchodilators and haven't been proven effective in viral bronchiolitis. Cromolyn sodium is an inhaled anti-inflammatory agent.

CN: Physiological integrity; CNS: Pharmacological and parenteral therapies; CL: Analysis

Hang in there! You've finished more than 90 questions.

94. The nurse is planning care for an infant with bronchiolitis who requires monitoring for dehydration. What is the <u>most important</u> intervention for the nurse to provide?
1. Measurement of intake and output
2. Blood levels every 4 hours
3. Urinalysis every 8 hours
4. Weighing each diaper

94. 1. Accurate measurement of intake and output is essential to assess for dehydration. Blood levels may be obtained daily or every other day. A urinalysis every 8 hours isn't necessary. Urine specific gravities are recommended but can be obtained with diaper changes. Weighing diapers is a way of measuring output only.

CN: Physiological integrity; CNS: Physiological adaptation; CL: Application

95. Which nursing diagnosis is the priority for an infant with bronchiolitis?
1. Imbalanced nutrition: More than body requirements
2. Deficient diversional activity
3. Impaired gas exchange
4. Social isolation

95. 3. Infants with bronchiolitis will have impaired gas exchange related to bronchiolar obstruction, atelectasis, and hyperinflation. Nutrition may be seen as less than body requirements. If respiratory distress is present, these infants should have nothing by mouth and fluids given I.V. only. Deficient diversional activity and social isolation usually aren't priorities. These infants are too uncomfortable to respond to social stimuli and need quiet, soothing activities that minimize energy.
CN: Physiological integrity; CNS: Physiological adaptation; CL: Analysis

Your hard work is paying off! Keep going!

96. The nurse is teaching parents how to care for a child with bronchiolitis at home. What is the most important information for the nurse to provide?
1. Place the child in a prone position for comfort.
2. Use warm mist to replace insensible fluid loss.
3. Recognize signs of increasing respiratory distress.
4. Engage the child in many activities to prevent developmental delay.

96. 3. It's essential for parents to be able to recognize signs of increasing respiratory distress and know how to count the respiratory rate. The child should be positioned with the head of the bed elevated for comfort and to facilitate removal of secretions. Use of cool mist may help to replace insensible fluid loss. Quiet play activities are required only as the child's energy level permits. These infants show clinical improvement in 3 to 4 days; therefore, developmental delay isn't an issue.
CN: Physiological integrity; CNS: Physiological adaptation; CL: Analysis

97. The nurse is teaching the parents of a child with pneumonia about the condition. Which description is correct?
1. Inflammation of the large airways
2. Severe infection of the bronchioles
3. Inflammation of the pulmonary parenchyma
4. Acute viral infection with maximum effect at the bronchiolar level

97. 3. Pneumonia is an inflammation of the pulmonary parenchyma. Bronchitis is inflammation of the large airways. Bronchiolitis is a severe infection of the bronchioles. Bronchiolitis and respiratory syncytial virus are terms for an acute viral infection with maximum effect at the bronchiolar level.
CN: Physiological integrity; CNS: Physiological adaptation; CL: Application

98. Which organism is the <u>most common</u> causative agent for bacterial pneumonia?
1. *Mycoplasma*
2. Parainfluenza virus
3. *Streptococcus pneumoniae*
4. Respiratory syncytial virus (RSV)

98. 3. *S. pneumoniae* is the most common causative agent of bacterial pneumonia in children. *Mycoplasma* is a causative agent for primary atypical pneumonia. Parainfluenza virus and RSV account for viral pneumonia.
CN: Physiological integrity; CNS: Physiological adaptation; CL: Application

99. The nurse is caring for an 8-year-old child admitted with pneumonia. Based on the child's age, which type of pneumonia would the nurse suspect?
1. Enteric bacilli
2. *Mycoplasma* pneumonia
3. Staphylococcal pneumonia
4. *Chlamydophila* (*Chlamydia*) pneumonia

100. The nurse is monitoring a child with a diagnosis of pertussis. The nurse is most concerned when the child develops which of the following?
1. Barking cough
2. Whooping cough
3. Abrupt high fever
4. Inspiratory stridor

101. A client with a suspected case of tuberculosis (TB) asks the nurse what test will confirm the diagnosis. What is the most appropriate response by the nurse?
1. Chest X-ray
2. Sputum sample
3. Tuberculin test
4. Urine culture

102. The nurse is assessing a child who has been admitted to the emergency department with a diagnosis of tuberculosis. Which symptom would the nurse expect to observe?
1. Chills
2. Hyperactivity
3. Lymphadenitis
4. Weight gain

103. The parents of a 2-year-old child who has been started on rifampin (Rifadin) after testing positive for tuberculosis ask the nurse if there is any important information they need to know about the medication. What is the most important information for the nurse to provide?
1. Hyperactivity
2. Orange body secretions
3. Decreased bilirubin levels
4. Decreased levels of liver enzymes

Whoopee! You reached 100!

Not all adverse effects are serious.

99. **2.** *Mycoplasma* pneumonia is a primary atypical pneumonia seen in children between ages 5 and 12. Enteric bacilli, staphylococcal pneumonia, and *Chlamydophila* (*Chlamydia*) pneumonia are mostly seen in children in the 3-month to 5-year age group.
CN: Physiological integrity; CNS: Physiological adaptation; CL: Application

100. **2.** Pertussis is characterized by consistent short, rapid coughs followed by a sudden inspiration with a high-pitched whooping sound. A barking cough and inspiratory stridor are noted with croup. Pertussis is usually accompanied by a low-grade fever.
CN: Physiological integrity; CNS: Physiological adaptation; CL: Application

101. **2.** A sputum culture is the definitive test. X-rays usually appear normal in children with TB. The tuberculin test isn't necessarily the most reliable test for TB in children. Stool cultures and gastric washings will show positive results on acid-fast smears but aren't specific for *Mycobacterium tuberculosis*. Sputum samples are difficult to obtain from children, so gastric washings commonly replace them.
CN: Physiological integrity; CNS: Physiological adaptation; CL: Analysis

102. **3.** Children are usually asymptomatic and typically don't manifest the usual pulmonary symptoms, but lymphadenitis is more likely in infants and children than in adults. Weight loss, anorexia, night sweats, fatigue, and malaise are general responses to the disease.
CN: Physiological integrity; CNS: Physiological adaptation; CL: Application

103. **2.** Rifampin and its metabolites will turn urine, feces, sputum, tears, and sweat an orange color. This isn't a serious adverse effect. Rifampin may also cause GI upset, headache, drowsiness, dizziness, visual disturbances, and fever. Liver enzyme and bilirubin levels increase because of hepatic metabolism of the drug. Parents should be taught the signs and symptoms of hepatitis and hyperbilirubinemia such as jaundice of the sclera or skin.
CN: Physiological integrity; CNS: Pharmacological and parenteral therapies; CL: Application

104. The school nurse is providing an in-service program about dietary safety to all of the preschool teachers and aides who care for children younger than age 3. What is the most important information for the nurse to provide?
1. Cut hotdogs in half.
2. Limit popcorn and peanuts.
3. Cut grapes into small pieces.
4. Limit hard candy to special occasions.

105. A child is admitted with a possible tracheal foreign body. The nurse anticipates the assessment findings will include which of the following?
1. Cough, dyspnea, and drooling
2. Cough, stridor, and changes in phonation
3. Expiratory wheeze and inspiratory stridor
4. Cough, asymmetrical breath sounds, and wheeze

106. Which activity is recommended to prevent foreign body aspiration during meals?
1. Insist that children are seated.
2. Give children toys to play with.
3. Allow children to watch television.
4. Allow children to eat in a separate room.

107. The nurse is preparing a child for testing for a foreign body aspiration. The nurse explains to the child's parents that the best diagnostic tool for diagnosis of foreign body aspiration is:
1. bronchoscopy.
2. chest X-ray.
3. fluoroscopy.
4. lateral neck X-ray.

The next four questions address foreign body aspiration.

104. 3. Grapes, hotdogs, and sausage should be cut into many small pieces. Hard candy, raisins, popcorn, and peanuts should be avoided for children age 4 and younger.
CN: Physiological integrity; CNS: Reduction of risk potential; CL: Application

105. 3. Expiratory and inspiratory noise indicates that the foreign body is in the trachea. Cough, dyspnea, drooling, and gagging indicate supraglottic obstruction. A cough with stridor and changes in phonation would occur if the foreign body were in the larynx. Asymmetrical breath sounds indicate that the object may be located in the bronchi.
CN: Physiological integrity; CNS: Physiological adaptation; CL: Application

106. 1. Children should remain seated while eating. The risk of aspiration increases if the child is running, jumping, or talking with food in their mouth. Television and toys are a dangerous distraction to toddlers and young children and should be avoided. Children need constant supervision and should be monitored while eating snacks and meals.
CN: Safe, effective care environment; CNS: Safety and infection control; CL: Application

107. 1. Bronchoscopy can give a definitive diagnosis of the presence of foreign bodies and is also the best choice for removal of the object with direct visualization. Chest X-ray and lateral neck X-ray may also be used, but findings vary. Some films may appear normal or show changes such as inflammation related to the presence of the foreign body. Fluoroscopy is valuable in detecting and localizing foreign bodies in the bronchi.
CN: Physiological integrity; CNS: Physiological adaptation; CL: Application

108. Which nursing intervention is <u>most</u> appropriate for a child with cystic fibrosis who is having difficulty clearing secretions?
1. Perform chest physiotherapy four times per day.
2. Administer pancreatic enzymes with meals.
3. Provide oxygen by nasal cannula at all times.
4. Provide a high-calorie, high-protein diet at each meal.

109. Which statement by the parent of a 16-month-old child with cystic fibrosis should alert a nurse to investigate further?
1. "My child is not walking yet."
2. "My child is saying a few words and short phrases."
3. "My child doesn't interact with other 16-month-olds."
4. "My child cries when I leave the room."

110. A nurse is performing an assessment on a newborn with a possible diagnosis of cystic fibrosis. Which of the following is an early sign of the disease?
1. Constipation
2. Decreased appetite
3. Hyperalbuminemia
4. Meconium ileus

Which of these options would be most likely?

108. **1.** Chest physiotherapy should be performed to mobilize secretions so they can be more easily cleared. Pancreatic enzymes should be administered with meals to aid in digestion. Administering oxygen may improve oxygenation but won't help clear secretions. A high-calorie, high-protein diet is important for normal growth and development but won't aid in clearing secretions.

CN: Physiological integrity; CNS: Reduction of risk potential; CL: Application

109. **1.** A toddler should be walking by 15 months. At 10 months, an infant holds on to furniture while walking, walks with support at 11 months, and takes his first steps at 12 months. By 12 months, a child can say a few words, with more words and short phrases being added each month. A child at 16 months engages in solitary play and has little interaction with other children. Separation anxiety is common in toddlers.

CN: Psychosocial integrity; CNS: None; CL: Analysis

110. **4.** Meconium ileus is commonly a presenting sign of cystic fibrosis. Thick, mucilaginous meconium blocks the lumen of the small intestine, causing intestinal obstruction, abdominal distention, and vomiting. Large-volume, loose, frequent, foul-smelling stools are common. These infants may have an increased appetite related to poor absorption from the intestine. The undigested food is excreted, increasing the bulk of feces. Hypoalbuminemia is a common result from the decreased absorption of protein.

CN: Physiological integrity; CNS: Physiological adaptation; CL: Application

111. Which intervention would be most appropriate for a nurse to perform when the parents of a child with cystic fibrosis tell her they are having difficulty coping?
1. Tell the parents they shouldn't expect to have a normal family life.
2. Refer the parents to a cystic fibrosis support group.
3. Show the parents how to perform chest physiotherapy at home.
4. Tell the parents that with good medical care their child can live into adulthood.

112. A toddler with suspected cystic fibrosis is admitted for testing. The nurse explains that the diagnostic criterion for chloride levels is:
1. below 20 mmol/L.
2. below 40 mmol/L.
3. 40 to 60 mmol/L.
4. above 60 mmol/L.

113. The parents of a child with cystic fibrosis ask the nurse which diet is recommended for their child. What is the best response by the nurse?
1. Fat restricted
2. High calorie
3. Low protein
4. Sodium restricted

114. Which statement concerning pancreatic enzymes for a cystic fibrosis client is correct?
1. Capsules may not be opened.
2. Microcapsules can be crushed.
3. Encourage eating throughout the day.
4. Administer enzymes at each meal and with snacks.

In light of the pathology of cystic fibrosis, which is the only diet that makes sense?

111. 2. Support groups can provide the parents with the support they need to cope with their child's condition as well as provide them with accurate information on the disorder. The family shouldn't be discouraged from having as normal a life as possible. Showing the parents how to perform chest physiotherapy is an important intervention but won't help them cope with their child's condition. With good medical care, children with cystic fibrosis can live into adulthood, but telling the parent this doesn't promote the coping skills the parents need.
CN: Physiological integrity; CNS: None; CL: Application

112. 4. A chloride concentration greater than 60 mmol/L is diagnostic of cystic fibrosis. Normal sweat chloride content is less than 40 mmol/L, with the average being 18 mmol/L. Levels between 40 and 60 mmol/L are highly suggestive of cystic fibrosis.
CN: Physiological integrity; CNS: Physiological adaptation; CL: Application

113. 2. A well-balanced, high-calorie, high-protein diet is recommended for a child with cystic fibrosis due to the impaired intestinal absorption. Fat restriction isn't required because digestion and absorption of fat in the intestine are impaired. The child usually increases enzyme intake when high-fat foods are eaten. Low-sodium foods can lead to hyponatremia; therefore, high-sodium foods are recommended, especially during hot weather or when the child has a fever.
CN: Physiological integrity; CNS: Basic care and comfort; CL: Application

114. 4. Enzymes are administered with each feeding, meal, and snack to optimize absorption of the nutrients consumed. Regular capsules may be opened and the contents mixed with a small amount of applesauce or other nonalkaline food. Microcapsules can't be crushed due to the enteric coating. Eating throughout the day should be discouraged. Three meals and two or three snacks per day are recommended.
CN: Physiological integrity; CNS: Physiological adaptation; CL: Application

115. A nurse should include which information on nutrition when teaching the family of a child with cystic fibrosis?
1. Provide a high-calorie, high-protein diet.
2. Place the child on a daily 1,200-ml fluid restriction.
3. Restrict daily intake of sodium to 1.5 g/day.
4. Provide adequate amounts of fat-soluble vitamins.

Teach the family about proper nutrition.

116. A nurse is caring for a client with cystic fibrosis. Ranitidine (Zantac) 4 mg/kg/day every 12 hours is ordered. The child weighs 20 kg. How many milligrams are given per dose?
1. 16
2. 20
3. 40
4. 80

117. Which nursing intervention is appropriate for care of the child with cystic fibrosis?
1. Decrease exercise and limit physical activity.
2. Administer cough suppressants and antihistamines.
3. Administer chest physiotherapy two to four times per day.
4. Administer bronchodilator or nebulizer treatments after chest physiotherapy.

118. Which statement is appropriate for a nurse to make to the parents of a child with cystic fibrosis who are planning to have a second child?
1. "Genetic counseling is recommended."
2. "There's a 50% chance the child will be normal."
3. "There's a 50% chance of the child being affected."
4. "There's a 25% chance the child will only be a carrier."

115. 1. To promote growth and development, the child should eat a high-calorie, high-protein diet. The child with cystic fibrosis should also be encouraged to consume higher than usual amounts of fluids and sodium. The child should be given water-soluble forms of fat-soluble vitamins.
CN: Physiological integrity; CNS: Basic care and comfort; CL: Application

116. 3. The child should receive 40 mg per dose. Here are the calculations:
$$20 \text{ kg} \times 4 \text{ mg/kg} = 80 \text{ mg};$$
$$24 \text{ hr}/12 \text{ hr} = 2 \text{ doses};$$
$$80 \text{ mg}/2 \text{ doses} = 40 \text{ mg}.$$
CN: Physiological integrity; CNS: Pharmacological and parenteral therapies; CL: Application

117. 3. Chest physiotherapy is recommended two to four times per day to help loosen and move secretions to facilitate expectoration. Exercise and physical activity are recommended to stimulate mucous secretion and to establish a good habitual breathing pattern. Cough suppressants and antihistamines are contraindicated. The goal is for the child to be able to cough and expectorate mucous secretions. Bronchodilator or nebulizer treatments are given before chest physiotherapy to help open the bronchi for easier expectoration.
CN: Safe, effective care environment; CNS: Management of care; CL: Application

118. 1. Genetic counseling should be recommended. Cystic fibrosis is an autosomal-recessive disease. Therefore, there's a 25% chance of the child having the disease, a 25% chance of the child being normal, and a 50% chance of the child being a carrier.
CN: Health promotion and maintenance; CNS: None; CL: Application

119. Parents ask the nurse about the cause of their child's cystic fibrosis. Which statement best describes this autosomal-recessive disorder?
1. The genetic disorder is carried on the X chromosome.
2. Both parents must pass the defective gene or set of genes.
3. Only one defective gene or set of genes is passed by one parent.
4. The child has an extra chromosome, resulting in an XXY karyotype.

120. When a nurse enters the room to give an antibiotic elixir to a 3-year-old child, the child says the medication is "yucky" and refuses to take it. Which response by the nurse is best?
1. "Do you want to take the medicine with vanilla ice cream or chocolate ice cream?"
2. "If you don't take the medicine, I will tell your mother."
3. "The doctor says you must take the medicine."
4. "You need to take this medicine to get better."

121. Ceftazidime (Fortaz) has been ordered for a client with cystic fibrosis. The order states to give 40 mg/kg every 8 hours. The child is 2 years old and weighs 38.5 lb. How many milligrams of the ceftazidime are given in one dose?
1. 116
2. 233
3. 260
4. 466

122. A child with cystic fibrosis is placed on an oral antibiotic to be given in four equally divided doses per day for 14 days. Which time schedule is most appropriate?
1. 8 a.m., 12 p.m., 4 p.m., 8 p.m.
2. 8 a.m., 2 p.m., 8 p.m., 2 a.m.
3. 9 a.m., 1 p.m., 5 p.m., 9 p.m.
4. 10 a.m., 2 p.m., 6 p.m., 10 p.m.

They just keep passing me along.

119. 2. In recessive disorders such as cystic fibrosis, both parents must pass the defective gene or set of genes to the child. Sex-linked genetic disorders are carried on the X chromosome. Dominant disorders are characterized by only one defective gene or set of genes passed by one parent. A child with an XXY karyotype would have Klinefelter's syndrome.

CN: Health promotion and maintenance; CNS: None; CL: Application

120. 1. Offering the child a choice of how he wants to take the medication provides the child with some control. Threatening to tell the child's mother won't help and erodes any trust between the child and nurse. Telling the child that the doctor says he must take the medication also isn't helpful. At age 3, trying to reason with the child about why he needs to take the medication won't work because his thinking is still concrete.

CN: Psychosocial integrity; CNS: None; CL: Analysis

121. 2. The child should receive 233 mg per dose. Here are the calculations: 38.5 lb/2.2 kg = 17.5 kg (1 lb equals 2.2 kg); 40 mg/kg × 17.5 kg = 700 mg; 24 hours/8 hours = 3 doses; 700 mg/3 doses = 233 mg.

CN: Physiological integrity; CNS: Pharmacological and parenteral therapies; CL: Application

122. 2. The doses should be given routinely every 6 hours. This helps maintain a therapeutic blood level of the antibiotic. The other answers have doses only every 4 hours during the day and then no doses for 12 hours at night.

CN: Physiological integrity; CNS: Pharmacological and parenteral therapies; CL: Analysis

123. Which complication of cystic fibrosis may eventually lead to death?
1. Rectal prolapse
2. Pulmonary obstruction
3. Gastroesophageal reflux
4. Reproductive system obstruction

124. Which method is best for evaluation of a 6-year-old child with cystic fibrosis who has been placed on an aerosol inhaler?
1. Ask if the parents have any questions.
2. Ask if the child can explain the procedure.
3. Ask the parents if they understand the usage.
4. Ask the client to perform a return demonstration.

125. Which intervention is appropriate for a 2-year-old client with chest trauma who has a left lower chest tube in place?
1. Stripping or milking the tubing
2. Requiring routine dressing changes
3. Clamping the chest tube during transport
4. Inspecting tubing for kinks or obstructions

Which intervention is appropriate?

123. 2. Pulmonary obstruction related to thickened mucous secretions can lead to a progressive pulmonary disturbance and secondary infections that can lead to death. Rectal prolapse is managed with enzyme replacement therapy and manipulation of the rectum back into place. Gastroesophageal reflux can be managed with medications and proper reflux precautions. Obstruction of the reproductive system can lead to infertility due to increased mucus blocking sperm entry in the female or blockage of the vas deferens in the male.

CN: Physiological integrity; CNS: Physiological adaptation; CL: Analysis

124. 4. A return demonstration is the best evaluation. It will show if the client can repeat the steps shown and appropriately use the inhaler. The parents should understand how the inhaler should be used and ask questions, but the child must be able to correctly demonstrate usage first. The child may have difficulty explaining the procedure at age 6.

CN: Physiological integrity; CNS: Pharmacological and parenteral therapies; CL: Application

125. 4. Tubing should be inspected for kinks or obstructions so that drainage can flow freely. Manipulation of the tubing should be avoided. The pressure created from stripping can damage the pleural space or mediastinum. There's no need for routine dressing changes if the dressing isn't soiled and there's no evidence of infection. Inspect and palpate around the dressing routinely. The chest tube should never be clamped because it may lead to a tension pneumothorax. Water seal will protect the client during transit.

CN: Physiological integrity; CNS: Physiological adaptation; CL: Application

126. A toddler in respiratory distress is admitted to the pediatric intensive care unit. When he refuses to keep his oxygen face mask on, his mother tries to help. Which action by a nurse is most appropriate?
 1. Giving the child his favorite toy to play with
 2. Having the mother read the child's favorite book to him
 3. Administering a strong sedative so the child will sleep
 4. Telling the child that the face mask will help him breathe better

127. A 12-year-old boy is discharged from the hospital after an acute asthma attack with a prescription for budesonide (Pulmicort Turbuhaler). Which sign or symptom should the nurse instruct him and his parents to report to the physician immediately?
 1. Diarrhea
 2. Bradycardia
 3. Weight loss
 4. Oral candidiasis

128. A 6-year-old with a history of asthma is being evaluated by an allergist who orders skin testing to be done at the next visit. Which action by a nurse will help ensure accurate skin testing results?
 1. Making sure the child doesn't have a runny nose
 2. Making sure the child hasn't received antihistamines in the past 7 days
 3. Using the child's posterior legs for testing
 4. Limiting testing to environmental allergens

129. Which sign should alert a nurse to a potentially life-threatening complication in a child who received an allergy shot 30 minutes earlier?
 1. Urinary output less than 30 ml/hour
 2. Heart rate of 58 beats/minute
 3. Blood pressure of 82/48 mm Hg
 4. Rash

I know this is one of your favorite books.

Moving along nicely! Keep it up!

126. 2. Having the mother read the child's favorite book will ease his anxiety and provide comfort to the child. Although giving the child a favorite toy is also appropriate, the child needs his mother's comfort because the face mask is frightening. Sedation is contraindicated because it can mask signs of respiratory distress. A toddler is too young to understand that something will make him feel better.
CN: Safe, effective care environment; CNS: Management of care; CL: Application

127. 4. One of the adverse reactions to budesonide is oral candidiasis, and parents should be instructed to monitor the child's mouth for this. Diarrhea, bradycardia, and weight loss are not adverse reactions to this corticosteroid.
CN: Physiological integrity; CNS: Pharmacological and parenteral therapies; CL: Analysis

128. 2. Antihistamines may alter results of skin testing and should be withheld at least 1 week before testing. A runny nose won't alter test results. The forearm and upper back are the best sites for allergy testing. Testing only for environmental allergens precludes diagnosis of allergies to other substances.
CN: Physiological integrity; CNS: Pharmacological and parenteral therapies; CL: Application

129. 3. Anaphylaxis can cause hypotension and tachycardia (not bradycardia). Urinary urgency and incontinence, not anuria, may also be reported. A rash may signal an allergic reaction but not a severe one such as anaphylaxis.
CN: Physiological integrity; CNS: Physiological adaptation; CL: Analysis

130. The nurse is caring for a 17-year-old female client with cystic fibrosis who has been admitted to the hospital to receive I.V. antibiotic and respiratory treatment for exacerbation of a lung infection. The client has many questions about her future and the consequences of the disease. Which statements about the course of cystic fibrosis are true? Select all that apply.
1. Breast development is frequently delayed.
2. The client is at risk for developing diabetes.
3. Pregnancy and childbearing aren't affected.
4. Normal sexual relationships can be expected.
5. Only males carry the gene for the disease.
6. By age 20, the client should be able to decrease the frequency of respiratory treatment.

131. A nurse is preparing to administer the first dose of tobramycin (Nebcin) to an adolescent with cystic fibrosis. The order is for 3 mg/kg I.V. daily in three divided doses. The client weighs 110 lb. How many milligrams should the nurse administer per dose? Record your answer using a whole number.

_____ milligrams

132. A parent is planning to enroll her 9-month-old infant in a day care facility. She asks the nurse what to look for as indicators that the daycare facility is adhering to good infection control measures. How should the nurse reply? Select all that apply.
1. The facility keeps boxes of gloves in the director's office.
2. Diapers are discarded into covered receptacles.
3. Toys are kept on the floor for the children to share.
4. Disposable papers are used on the diaper-changing surfaces.
5. Facilities for hand hygiene are located in every classroom.
6. Soiled clothing and cloth diapers are sent home in labeled paper bags.

130. 1, 2, and 4. Cystic fibrosis delays growth and the onset of puberty. Children with cystic fibrosis tend to be smaller than average size and develop secondary sex characteristics later in life. In addition, clients with cystic fibrosis are at risk for developing diabetes mellitus because the pancreatic duct becomes obstructed as pancreatic tissues are destroyed. Clients with cystic fibrosis can expect to have normal sexual relationships, but fertility becomes difficult because thick secretions obstruct the cervix and block sperm entry. Both men and women carry the gene for cystic fibrosis. Pulmonary disease commonly progresses as the client ages, requiring additional respiratory treatment, not less.

CN: Physiological integrity; CNS: Physiological adaptation; CL: Analysis

131. 50. To perform this dosage calculation, the nurse should first convert the client's weight to kilograms using this formula: 1 kg/2.2 lb = X kg/110 lb; 2.2X = 110; X = 50 kg. Then, she should calculate the client's daily dose using this formula: 50 kg × 3 mg/kg = 150 mg. Finally, the nurse should calculate the divided dose: 150 mg/3 doses = 50 mg/dose.

CN: Physiological integrity; CNS: Pharmacological and parenteral therapies; CL: Application

132. 2, 4, and 5. A parent can assess infection control measures by appraising steps taken by the facility to prevent the spread of potential diseases. Placing diapers in covered receptacles, covering the diaper-changing surfaces with disposable papers, and ensuring that there are hand sanitizers and sinks available for personnel to wash their hands after activities are all indicators that infection control measures are being followed. Gloves should be readily available to personnel and, therefore, should be kept in every room, not in an office. Typically, toys are shared by numerous children; however, this contributes to the spread of germs and infections. All soiled clothing and cloth diapers should be placed in a sealed plastic bag prior to being sent home.

CN: Safe, effective care environment; CNS: Safety and infection control; CL: Application

You finished chapter 29! Now you can breathe easier.

Chapter 30
Neurosensory disorders

Here are two Web sites you can check for more information about neurosensory disorders in children: **www.add.org** (Attention Deficit Disorder Association) and **www.ndss.org** (National Down Syndrome Society).

1. A mother of a 3-year old with a myelomeningocele is thinking about having another baby and asks the nurse if she should make any changes in her diet. What is the best response by the nurse?
1. Increase folic acid to 0.4 mg/day.
2. Increase folic acid to 4 mg/day.
3. Increase ascorbic acid to 0.4 mg/day.
4. Increase ascorbic acid to 4 mg/day.

Most relevant—that's the key phrase for question 2.

2. Which nursing diagnosis is most relevant in the first 12 hours of life for a neonate born with a myelomeningocele?
1. Risk for infection
2. Constipation
3. Impaired physical mobility
4. Delayed growth and development

3. A neonate has been brought to the emergency room by his mother. The nurse assesses the child and suspects that the child may have hydrocephalus. Which observations by the nurse would indicate this condition?
1. Bulging fontanel, low-pitched cry
2. Depressed fontanel, low-pitched cry
3. Bulging fontanel, eyes rotated downward
4. Depressed fontanel, eyes rotated downward

1. 2. The American Academy of Pediatrics recommends that a woman who has had a child with a neural tube defect increase her intake of folic acid to 4 mg/day 1 month before becoming pregnant and continue this regimen through the first trimester. A woman who has no family history of neural tube defects should take 0.4 mg. All women of childbearing age should be encouraged to take a folic acid supplement because the majority of pregnancies in the United States are unplanned. Ascorbic acid hasn't been shown to have any effect on preventing neural tube defects.
CN: Health promotion and maintenance; CNS: None; CL: Application

2. 1. All of these diagnoses are important for a child with a myelomeningocele. However, during the first 12 hours of life, the most life-threatening event would be an infection. The other diagnoses will be addressed as the child develops.
CN: Physiological integrity; CNS: Reduction of risk potential; CL: Application

3. 3. Hydrocephalus is caused from the alteration in circulation of the cerebrospinal fluid (CSF). The amount of CSF increases, causing the fontanel to bulge. This also causes an increase in intracranial pressure. This increase in pressure causes the neonate's eyes to deviate downward (the "setting sun sign"), and the neonate's cry becomes high pitched.
CN: Health promotion and maintenance; CNS: None; CL: Analysis

CN: Client needs category   CNS: Client needs subcategory   CL: Cognitive level

4. The nurse is caring for a child following a shunt insertion on the right side of the head to relieve hydrocephalus. What is the priority intervention for the nurse to include in the plan of care?
1. Place the child flat in bed on the right side.
2. Place the child flat in bed on the left side.
3. Place the child in a semi-Fowler's position.
4. Place the child in an upright position.

5. Which nursing action is <u>appropriate</u> when a child has a seizure?
1. Inserting a nasogastric tube to prevent emesis
2. Restraining the extremities with a pillow or blanket
3. Inserting a tongue blade to prevent injury to the tongue
4. Padding the side rails of the bed to protect the child from injury

6. A mother brings her infant to the emergency department and says he had a seizure. While a nurse is obtaining a history, the mother says she was running out of formula so she stretched the formula by adding three times the normal amount of water. Electrolytes and blood glucose levels are drawn on the infant. The nurse should expect which laboratory value?
1. Blood glucose: 120 mg/dl
2. Chloride: 104 mmol/L
3. Potassium: 4 mmol/L
4. Sodium: 125 mmol/L

7. A child is admitted to the unit with a diagnosis of bacterial meningitis. The nurse is aware that the priority assessment will include which of the following?
1. Hypothermia, irritability, and poor feeding
2. Positive Babinski's reflex, mottling, and pallor
3. Headache, nuchal rigidity, and developmental delays
4. Positive Moro's embrace reflex, hyperthermia, and sunken fontanel

Remember, in emergency situations, your first priority is to ensure the client's safety.

For the NCLEX, you need to be familiar with normal lab values.

4. 2. The child should be flat in bed to avoid rapid decompression of cerebrospinal fluid (CSF) and on the left side or on his back to avoid occlusion of the shunt and blockage of the drainage of CSF. Placing the child in a semi-Fowler's or upright position may promote too rapid decompression of CSF.
CN: Physiological integrity; CNS: Reduction of risk potential; CL: Application

5. 4. A child having a seizure could fall out of bed or injure himself on something, including the side rails of the bed. Attempts to insert anything into the child's mouth may injure the child. Attempting to restrain the child won't stop seizures. In fact, tactile stimulation may increase the seizure activity; therefore, it must be limited as much as possible.
CN: Safe, effective care environment; CNS: Safety and infection control; CL: Application

6. 4. Diluting formula in a different manner than is recommended alters the infant's electrolyte levels. Normal serum sodium for an infant is 135 to 145 mmol/L. When formula is diluted, the infant's sodium is also diluted and will decrease. Hyponatremia is one of the causes of seizures in infants. The other values are all within normal limits.
CN: Physiological integrity; CNS: Reduction of risk potential; CL: Analysis

7. 1. The clinical appearance of a neonate with meningitis is different from that of a child or an adult. Neonates may be either hypothermic or hyperthermic. The irritation to the meninges causes the neonates to be irritable and to have a decreased appetite. They may be pale and mottled with a bulging, full fontanel. Older children and adults with meningitis have headaches, nuchal rigidity, and hyperthermia as clinical manifestations. Normal neonates have positive Moro's embrace and Babinski's reflexes. Developmental delays, if present, would appear when the child was older.
CN: Physiological integrity; CNS: Physiological adaptation; CL: Application

8. Which type of behavior demonstrated by a 6-year-old child would help a school nurse differentiate between attention deficit hyperactivity disorder (ADHD) and a learning disability?
   1. The child reverses letters and words while reading.
   2. The child is easily distracted and reacts impulsively.
   3. The child is always getting into fights during recess.
   4. The child has a difficult time reading a chapter book.

9. Which statement by the parent of a child with cerebral palsy indicates that a nurse's teaching has been successful?
   1. "My child's muscles will get stronger over time."
   2. "My child's condition will get progressively worse."
   3. "My child will have low intelligence."
   4. "My child will need continual therapy to maintain functioning."

10. The nurse is assessing a full-term neonate in the hospital. The nurse is most concerned when the neonate displays which reflex?
   1. A weak sucking reflex
   2. A positive rooting reflex
   3. A positive Babinski's reflex
   4. Startle reflex in response to a loud noise

11. A mother reports that her school-age child has been reprimanded for daydreaming during class. This is a new behavior, and the child's grades are dropping. The nurse should suspect which problem?
   1. The child may have a hearing problem and needs to have his hearing checked.
   2. The child may have a learning disability and needs referral to the special education department.
   3. The child may have attention deficit hyperactivity disorder (ADHD) and needs medication.
   4. The child may be having absence seizures and needs to see his primary health care provider for evaluation.

I'm trying to pay attention. Really I am.

You're through the first 10! Keep going!

8. **2.** Two of the most common characteristics of children with ADHD include inattention and impulsiveness. Children who reverse letters and words while reading have dyslexia. Although aggressiveness may be common in children with ADHD, it isn't a characteristic that will help diagnose this disorder. Six-year-old children aren't usually cognitively ready to read a chapter book.
CN: Health promotion and maintenance; CNS: None; CL: Analysis

9. **4.** The child with cerebral palsy needs continual treatment and therapy to maintain or improve functioning. Without therapy, muscles will get progressively weaker and more spastic. Although some children with cerebral palsy are mentally retarded, many have normal intelligence.
CN: Health promotion and maintenance; CNS: None; CL: Analysis

10. **1.** Normal neonates have a strong, vigorous sucking reflex. The rooting reflex is present at birth and disappears when the infant is between ages 3 and 4 months. A positive Babinski's reflex is present at birth and disappears by the time the infant is age 2 years. The startle reflex is present at birth and disappears when the infant is about age 4 months.
CN: Health promotion and maintenance; CNS: None; CL: Application

11. **4.** Absence seizures are commonly misinterpreted as daydreaming. The child loses awareness, but no alteration in motor activity is exhibited. A mild hearing problem is usually exhibited as leaning forward, talking louder, listening to louder TV and music than usual, and a repetitive "What?" from the child. There isn't enough information to indicate a learning disability. ADHD isn't characterized by episodes of quietness.
CN: Physiological integrity; CNS: Physiological adaptation; CL: Analysis

12. A 2-month-old infant is brought to the well-baby clinic for his first checkup. On initial assessment, the nurse notes the infant's head circumference is at the 95th percentile. What is the <u>most important</u> action by the nurse?
1. Assess vital signs.
2. Measure the head again.
3. Assess neurological signs.
4. Notify the primary health care provider.

13. Which observation indicates to a nurse that the mother of a child with cerebral palsy needs further instruction?
1. The mother gives the child assistive devices for eating.
2. The mother fusses over the mess the child is making.
3. The mother provides adequate time for the child to finish eating.
4. The mother provides finger foods.

14. A 2-year-old child is admitted to the pediatric unit with the diagnosis of bacterial meningitis. Which intervention would be appropriate for a nurse to perform first?
1. Obtain a urine specimen.
2. Draw ordered laboratory tests.
3. Place the toddler in respiratory isolation.
4. Explain the treatment plan to the parents.

15. A 12-year-old child is admitted to the pediatric unit with a diagnosis of possible brain tumor. The nurse would assess the child for which of the following?
1. Bulging fontanel
2. High-pitched cry
3. Behavioral changes
4. Change in vital signs

Now, I should be in the 1,000th percentile.

Take the necessary precautions to protect yourself and others from possible infection.

12. 2. Whenever there's a question about vital signs or assessment data, the first logical step would be to reassess to determine if an error had been made initially. Notifying the primary health care provider and assessing neurological and vital signs are important and would follow the reassessment.
CN: Health promotion and maintenance; CNS: None; CL: Analysis

13. 2. Parents should encourage the child with cerebral palsy to be as independent as possible even if a mess is made while attempting to eat. Assistive devices can help the child with weak or spastic muscles eat independently. The child with cerebral palsy requires more time to bring food to the mouth and to chew and shouldn't be rushed. The parents should provide a calm and stress-free environment for eating. Providing the child with finger foods helps him eat independently.
CN: Physiological integrity; CNS: Basic care and comfort; CL: Analysis

14. 3. Nurses should take necessary precautions to protect themselves and others from possible infection from the bacterial organism causing meningitis. The affected child should immediately be placed in respiratory isolation; then the parents can be informed about the treatment plan. This should be done before laboratory tests are performed.
CN: Safe, effective care environment; CNS: Safety and infection control; CL: Application

15. 3. In a school-age child with a closed cranium, a common symptom of a brain tumor is behavior change due to the increased cranial pressure. A bulging fontanel and high-pitched cry are typical signs in an infant. A change in vital signs is a later sign of increased intracranial pressure.
CN: Physiological integrity; CNS: Physiological adaptation; CL: Application

16. A preschool-age child has just been admitted to the pediatric unit with a diagnosis of bacterial meningitis. What is the most important intervention for the nurse to include in the plan of care?
1. Take vital signs every 4 hours.
2. Monitor temperature every 4 hours.
3. Decrease environmental stimulation.
4. Encourage the parents to hold the child.

17. A child has just returned to the pediatric unit following ventriculoperitoneal shunt placement for hydrocephalus. Which intervention should a nurse perform <u>first</u>?
1. Assess intake and output.
2. Place the child on the side opposite the shunt.
3. Offer fluids because the child has a dry mouth.
4. Administer pain medication by mouth as ordered.

18. An otherwise healthy 18-month-old child has a history of febrile seizures and is in the well-child clinic today. Which statement by the father would indicate to the nurse that additional teaching needs to be done?
1. "I have ibuprofen available in case it's needed."
2. "My child will outgrow these seizures by age 5."
3. "I always keep phenobarbital with me in case of a fever."
4. "The most likely time for a seizure is when the fever is rising."

19. When assessing a 5-month-old infant, which symptom should alert a nurse that the infant needs further follow-up?
1. Absent grasp reflex
2. Rolls from back to side
3. Balances head when sitting
4. Moro's embrace reflex present

The important word in the question is first!

Note that for question 18, you're looking for an incorrect response from the father.

16. 3. A child with the diagnosis of meningitis is much more comfortable with decreased environmental stimuli. Noise and bright lights stimulate the child and can be irritating, causing the child to cry, in turn increasing intracranial pressure. Vital signs would be taken initially every hour and temperature monitored every 2 hours. Children are usually much more comfortable if allowed to lie flat because this position doesn't cause increased meningeal irritation.
CN: Physiological integrity; CNS: Physiological adaptation; CL: Application

17. 2. Following shunt placement surgery, the child should be placed on the side opposite of the surgical site to prevent pressure on the shunt valve. Intake and output will be assessed, but that isn't the priority nursing intervention. The child is usually on nothing-by-mouth status until the nasogastric tube is removed and bowel sounds return. Pain medication should be administered by an I.V. route initially postoperatively.
CN: Physiological integrity; CNS: Basic care and comfort; CL: Application

18. 3. Anticonvulsant drugs, such as phenobarbital, are administered to children with prolonged seizures or neurological abnormalities. Ibuprofen, not phenobarbital, is given for fever. Febrile seizures usually occur after age 6 months and are unusual after age 5 years. Treatment is to decrease the temperature because seizures occur as the temperature rises.
CN: Health promotion and maintenance; CNS: None; CL: Application

19. 4. Moro's embrace reflex should be absent at 4 months. Grasp reflex begins to fade at 2 months and should be absent at 3 months. A 4-month-old infant should be able to roll from back to side and balance his head when sitting.
CN: Health promotion and maintenance; CNS: None; CL: Application

20. The nurse is teaching an adolescent who has just been started on valproic acid (Depakene) for the treatment of seizures about the medication. What is the most important information for the nurse to include?
1. This medication has no adverse effects.
2. A common adverse effect is weight gain.
3. Drowsiness and irritability commonly occur.
4. Early morning dosing is recommended to decrease insomnia.

21. The nurse is teaching parents of a child recently diagnosed with cerebral palsy about the diagnosis. Which statement indicates to the nurse that teaching was effective?
1. "Cerebral palsy is a condition that runs in families."
2. "Cerebral palsy means there will be many disabilities."
3. "Cerebral palsy is a condition that doesn't get worse."
4. "Cerebral palsy occurs because of too much oxygen to the brain."

22. An older child has a craniotomy for removal of a brain tumor. Which statement would be appropriate for a nurse to say to the parents?
1. "Your child really had a close call."
2. "I'm sure your child will be back to normal soon."
3. "I'm so glad to hear your child doesn't have cancer."
4. "What has the physician told you about the tumor?"

23. A 6-month-old infant is being admitted with a diagnosis of bacterial meningitis. A nurse should place the infant in which room?
1. A room with a 12-month-old infant with urinary tract infection
2. A room with an 8-month-old infant with failure to thrive
3. An isolation room near the nurses' station
4. A two-bed room in the middle of the hall

For question 22, keep in mind the difference between the nurse's and physician's roles.

20. 2. Weight gain is a common adverse effect of valproic acid. Drowsiness and irritability are adverse effects more commonly associated with phenobarbital. Felbamate (Felbatol) more commonly causes insomnia.

CN: Physiological integrity; CNS: Pharmacological and parenteral therapies; CL: Application

21. 3. By definition, cerebral palsy is a nonprogressive neuromuscular disorder. It can be mild or quite severe and is believed to be the result of a hypoxia event during the pregnancy or the birth process.

CN: Physiological integrity; CNS: Physiological adaptation; CL: Application

22. 4. When comforting parents, it's best to first ascertain what the physician has told them about the tumor. Since the outcome of the surgery isn't known, it would be inappropriate to indicate that the child had a close call. Usually after a craniotomy, it takes several weeks or longer before the child is back to normal. Final pathology results won't be available for several days, so refrain from making premature statements about whether the tumor is malignant.

CN: Psychosocial integrity; CNS: None; CL: Application

23. 3. A child who has the diagnosis of bacterial meningitis will need to be placed in isolation near the nurses' station until that child has received I.V. antibiotics for 24 hours. The child is considered contagious. Additionally, bacterial meningitis can be quite serious; therefore, the child should be placed near the nurses' station for close monitoring and easier access in case of a crisis.

CN: Safe, effective care environment; CNS: Safety and infection control; CL: Application

24. In caring for a 9-year-old child immediately after a head injury, a nurse notes a blood pressure of 110/60 mm Hg, a heart rate of 78 beats/minute, dilated and nonreactive pupils, minimal response to pain, and slow response to name. Which symptom should cause the nurse the most concern?
  1. Vital signs
  2. Nonreactive pupils
  3. Slow response to name
  4. Minimal response to pain

25. Which assignment made by a charge nurse would be <u>appropriate</u>?
  1. A registered nurse (RN) to an infant newly diagnosed with bacterial meningitis
  2. A student nurse to an adolescent with cystic fibrosis and many medications
  3. A licensed practical nurse (LPN) or a licensed vocational nurse (LVN) to a newly admitted child with acute leukemia who is receiving blood
  4. A nursing assistant to a transfer client with a head injury and frequent seizures

26. An infant has returned to the pediatric unit after repair of a myelomeningocele. A nurse notices that the infant has had no urine output in the past 2 hours. Which nursing intervention would be most appropriate?
  1. Perform Credé's maneuver on the infant's bladder.
  2. Catheterize the infant's bladder.
  3. Ask the mother to breast-feed the infant.
  4. Increase the I.V. fluid rate.

27. A 2-month-old infant who had an L4–L5 myelomeningocele repair comes to the clinic for a well-baby checkup. The mother reports that she catheterizes the infant every 2 to 3 hours. Which aspect of care should a nurse discuss with the mother?
  1. Changing to a special diet
  2. Scheduled immunizations
  3. Normal gross motor function
  4. Possibility of developing a latex allergy

The ability to delegate responsibly is often tested on the NCLEX.

Is this mother doing the correct thing or not?

24. 2. Dilated and nonreactive pupils indicate that anoxia or ischemia of the brain has occurred. If the pupils are also fixed (don't move), then herniation of the brain stem has occurred. The vital signs are normal. Slow response to name can be normal after a head injury. Minimal response to pain is an indication of the child's level of consciousness.
CN: Physiological integrity; CNS: Physiological adaptation; CL: Application

25. 1. An RN would be appropriately assigned to care for an infant with meningitis. The RN would make frequent assessments and provide a high level of care. Student nurses may not be allowed to give medications without supervision, and it may be easier for the RN or LPN to provide care to this client. In many institutions, LPNs (or LVNs) aren't allowed to monitor clients receiving blood or blood products. A transfer client with a head injury would need frequent assessments that only an RN or an LPN would be able to provide.
CN: Safe, effective care environment; CNS: Management of care; CL: Application

26. 2. Swelling around the surgical site may cause transient urinary retention, and catheterization is required to empty the bladder. Credé's maneuver isn't recommended because it can cause renal rupture. Breast-feeding the infant would be inappropriate in this situation. The fluid rate wouldn't be increased because there's no indication that the infant is dehydrated.
CN: Physiological integrity; CNS: Reduction of risk potential; CL: Application

27. 4. Children who are repeatedly exposed to latex products, such as during bladder catheterizations, are at high risk for developing a latex allergy. There's no need for a special diet unless another problem indicates that it would be necessary. This infant would receive the regularly scheduled immunizations. Gross motor function will be abnormal in an infant with an L4–L5 repair.
CN: Health promotion and maintenance; CNS: None; CL: Application

28. The nurse is teaching the parents of a 17-month-old child diagnosed with cerebral palsy how to prevent the scissoring position. What is the most appropriate instruction by the nurse?
1. Keep the child in leg braces 23 hours per day.
2. Let the child lay down as much as possible.
3. Try to keep the child as quiet as possible.
4. Place the child on your hip.

29. The mother of a child with a ventriculoperitoneal shunt says her child has a temperature of 101.2° F (38.4° C), a blood pressure of 108/68 mm Hg, and a pulse of 100 beats/minute. The child is lethargic and vomited the night before. Other children in the family have had similar symptoms. Which nursing intervention is most appropriate?
1. Provide symptomatic treatment.
2. Advise the mother this is a viral infection.
3. Consult the primary health care provider.
4. Have the mother bring the child to the primary health care provider's office.

30. The mother of a 10-year-old child with attention deficit hyperactivity disorder tells the nurse her husband won't allow their child to take more than 5 mg of methylphenidate (Ritalin) every morning. The child isn't doing better in school. What is the best response by the nurse?
1. "Sneak the medication to the child anyway."
2. "Put the child in charge of administering the medication."
3. "Bring the child's father to the clinic to discuss the medication."
4. "Have the school nurse give the child the rest of the medication."

31. A hospitalized child is to receive 75 mg of acetaminophen (Tylenol) for fever control. How much will the nurse administer if the acetaminophen is 40 mg per 0.4 ml?
1. 0.37 ml
2. 0.75 ml
3. 1.12 ml
4. 1.5 ml

Make sure both parents understand the rationale for treatment of a sick child.

28. 4. To interrupt the scissoring position, flex the knees and hips. Placing the child on the hip is an easy way to stop this common spastic positioning. Wearing leg braces 23 hours per day is inappropriate and doesn't allow the child to move freely. Trying to keep the child quiet and flat are inappropriate. This child needs stimulation and movement to reach the goal of development to the fullest potential.
CN: Physiological integrity; CNS: Basic care and comfort; CL: Application

29. 4. One of the complications of a ventriculoperitoneal shunt is a shunt infection. Shunt infections can have similar symptoms as a viral infection, so it's best to have the child examined. These symptoms may be due to the same viral infection that the siblings have, but it's better to have the child examined to rule out a shunt infection because infection can progress quickly to a very serious illness.
CN: Physiological integrity; CNS: Reduction of risk potential; CL: Application

30. 3. Bringing the father to the clinic for a teaching session about the medication should assist him in understanding why it's necessary for the child to receive the full dose. A nurse shouldn't advise dishonesty to a client or family. The father should be included in the treatment as much as possible.
CN: Physiological integrity; CNS: Pharmacological and parenteral therapies; CL: Application

31. 2. The nurse will administer 0.75 ml. Because 10 mg equals 0.1 ml, then 75 mg equals 0.75 ml.
CN: Physiological integrity; CNS: Pharmacological and parenteral therapies; CL: Application

32. The nurse is preparing a toddler for a lumbar puncture. For this procedure, the nurse should place the child in which position?
1. Lying prone, with the neck flexed
2. Sitting up, with the back straight
3. Lying on one side, with the back curved
4. Lying prone, with the feet higher than the head

33. When caring for a school-age child who has had a brain tumor removed, a nurse makes the following assessment: pupils equal and reactive to light; motor strength equal; knows name, date, but not location; and complains of a headache. What is the most appropriate intervention by the nurse?
1. Provide medication for the headache.
2. Immediately notify the primary health care provider.
3. Check what the child's level of consciousness (LOC) has been.
4. Call the child's parents to come and sit at the child's bedside.

34. Following a craniotomy on a child, I.V. fluids are ordered to run at 27 ml/hour. The tubing delivers 60 ml/hour. How many drops per minute should the nurse set the pump for?
1. 14 drops/minute
2. 27 drops/minute
3. 54 drops/minute
4. 60 drops/minute

35. The parents of a 19-month-old child bring their toddler to the clinic for a regular checkup. When palpating the toddler's fontanels, what should the nurse expect to find?
1. Closed anterior fontanel and open posterior fontanel
2. Open anterior fontanel and closed posterior fontanel
3. Closed anterior and posterior fontanels
4. Open anterior and posterior fontanels

I'm happy to accommodate any drip rate that is needed.

32. 3. Lumbar puncture involves placing a needle between the lumbar vertebrae into the subarachnoid space. For this procedure, the nurse should position the client on one side, with the back curved, because curving the back maximizes the space between the lumbar vertebrae, facilitating needle insertion. Prone and seated positions don't achieve separation of the vertebrae.
CN: Physiological integrity; CNS: Reduction of risk potential; CL: Application

33. 3. When there's an abnormality in current assessment data, it's vital to determine what the client's previous status was. Determine whether the status has changed or remained the same. Providing medication for the headache would be done after ascertaining the previous LOC. Contacting the primary health care provider and the child's parents isn't necessary before a final assessment has been made.
CN: Physiological integrity; CNS: Physiological adaptation; CL: Application

34. 2. The pump should be set for 27 drops/minute. Tubing that delivers 60 ml per 60 minutes would deliver 1 ml/minute. To deliver 27 ml/hour, the nurse would set the pump at 27.
CN: Physiological integrity; CNS: Pharmacological and parenteral therapies; CL: Application

35. 3. By age 18 months, the anterior and posterior fontanels should be closed. The diamond-shaped anterior fontanel normally closes between ages 9 and 18 months. The triangular posterior fontanel normally closes between ages 2 and 3 months.
CN: Health promotion and maintenance; CNS: None; CL: Application

36. A 10-year-old child with a concussion is admitted to the pediatric unit. A nurse should place this child in a room with which roommate?
1. A 6-year-old child with osteomyelitis
2. An 8-year-old child with gastroenteritis
3. A 10-year-old child with rheumatic fever
4. A 12-year-old child with a fractured femur

37. A nurse notes that a 4-year-old child with cerebral palsy has a weight at the 30th percentile and a height at the 60th percentile. What is the most important information for the nurse to provide the family?
1. He should eat fewer calories per day.
2. His height and weight are within the normal range.
3. He needs to increase his number of calories per day.
4. He is small for a 4-year-old child and will never be average.

38. After a pathogen compromises the blood-brain and blood-cerebrospinal fluid (CSF) barriers, infection will spread to the meninges for which reason?
1. The spinal fluid has a rich erythrocyte content.
2. Glucose content of the spinal fluid is relatively high.
3. There's a build-up of infectious exudate within the ventricular system.
4. CSF is devoid of the body's major defense systems.

39. A client is experiencing a severe headache as a result of increased intracranial pressure (ICP). The nurse is aware that the headache is caused by which mechanism?
1. Cervical hyperextension
2. Stretching of the meninges
3. Cerebral ischemia related to altered circulation
4. Reflex spasm of the neck extensors to splint the neck against cervical flexion

You've completed almost 40 questions. Looking good!

36. 4. A child with a concussion should be placed with a roommate who's free from infection and close to the child's age. Osteomyelitis, gastroenteritis, and rheumatic fever involve infection.
CN: Safe, effective care environment; CNS: Management of care; CL: Application

37. 2. The height and weight are between the 25th and 75th percentile, so the child is considered normal.
CN: Health promotion and maintenance; CNS: None; CL: Application

38. 4. After an organism compromises the natural barriers, the CSF provides an ideal medium for growth. All of the body's typical major defense systems are essentially absent in normal CSF. The CSF sample in bacterial meningitis typically reveals a decreased glucose level and it has, along with any erythrocytes present, little influence on the spread of infection. Exudate that may be present is the result of the infectious process, not the cause.
CN: Physiological integrity; CNS: Physiological adaptation; CL: Analysis

39. 2. The mechanism producing the headache that accompanies increased ICP may be the stretching of the meninges and pain fibers associated with blood vessels. With nuchal rigidity, cervical flexion is painful due to the stretching of the inflamed meninges, and the pain triggers a reflex spasm of the neck extensors to splint the area against further cervical flexion. It occurs in response to the pain; it doesn't cause it. Cerebral ischemia occurs because of vascular obstruction and decreased perfusion of the brain tissue.
CN: Physiological integrity; CNS: Physiological adaptation; CL: Analysis

40. While assessing the breath sounds of a child admitted with fever, seizures, and vomiting, the nurse notes petechiae on the child's back. What is the most appropriate action by the nurse?
1. Cover the petechiae with dry sterile dressings.
2. Initiate seizure precautions.
3. Suspect that the child has been abused.
4. Assess the child's neurological status.

Signs. Signs. Everywhere signs.

40. 4. Since fever, seizures, vomiting, and petechiae are signs of meningitis, the nurse should promptly assess the child's neurological status and report the findings to the physician. Petechiae are tiny purple or red spots within the dermal or submucosal layers of the skin and do not require dry sterile dressings nor are they signs of abuse. While the nurse should already have initiated seizure precautions, the finding of petechiae wouldn't be a reason to initiate seizure precautions.
CN: Physiological integrity; CNS: Physiological adaptation; CL: Analysis

41. A nurse is assessing a 3-year-old child with suspected nuchal rigidity. Which assessment data indicates nuchal rigidity?
1. Positive Kernig's sign
2. Negative Brudzinski's sign
3. Positive Homans' sign
4. Negative Kernig's sign

41. 1. A positive Kernig's sign indicates nuchal rigidity, caused by an irritative lesion of the subarachnoid space. Brudzinski's sign is also indicative of the condition. Homans' sign indicates venous inflammation of the lower leg, not nuchal rigidity.
CN: Physiological integrity; CNS: Physiological adaptation; CL: Application

42. A nurse is caring for a child with spina bifida. The child's mother asks the nurse what she did to cause the birth defect. What is the <u>best</u> response by the nurse?
1. "Older age at conception is one of the major causes of the defect."
2. "It's a common complication of amniocentesis."
3. "It has been linked to maternal alcohol consumption during pregnancy."
4. "The cause is unknown, and there are many environmental factors that may contribute to it."

Check these signs carefully. They're critical for answering question 43.

42. 4. There is no known cause of spina bifida, but scientists believe that it's linked to hereditary and environmental factors; neural tube defects, including spina bifida, have been strongly linked to low dietary intake of folic acid. Maternal age doesn't have an impact on spina bifida. An amniocentesis is performed to help diagnose spina bifida in utero but doesn't cause the disorder. Maternal alcohol intake during pregnancy has been linked to mental retardation, craniofacial defects, and cardiac abnormalities, not spina bifida.
CN: Physiological integrity; CNS: Physiological adaptation; CL: Application

43. A child with a diagnosis of meningococcal meningitis develops signs of sepsis and a purpuric rash over both lower extremities. The primary health care provider should be notified immediately because these signs could be indicative of which complication?
1. A severe allergic reaction to the antibiotic regimen with impending anaphylaxis
2. Onset of the syndrome of inappropriate antidiuretic hormone (SIADH)
3. Fulminant (Waterhouse–Friderichsen syndrome) meningococcemia
4. Adhesive arachnoiditis

43. 3. Meningococcemia is a serious complication usually associated with meningococcal infection. When onset is severe, sudden, and rapid (fulminant), it's known as Waterhouse–Friderichsen syndrome. Anaphylactic shock would need to be differentiated from septic shock. SIADH can be an acute complication, but it wouldn't be accompanied by the purpuric rash. Adhesive arachnoiditis occurs in the chronic phase of the disease and leads to obstruction of the flow of cerebrospinal fluid.
CN: Physiological integrity; CNS: Reduction of risk potential; CL: Application

44. A 1-month-old infant is admitted to the pediatric unit and diagnosed with bacterial meningitis. Which assessment findings by the nurse support the diagnosis?
1. Hemorrhagic rash, first appearing as petechiae
2. Photophobia
3. Fever, change in feeding pattern, vomiting, or diarrhea
4. Fever, lethargy, and purpura or large necrotic patches

45. A child with an elevated temperature and change in behavior is scheduled for a lumbar puncture. To alleviate the child's pain and fear of lumbar puncture, which intervention should a nurse perform?
1. Sedate the child with fentanyl (Sublimaze).
2. Apply a topical anesthetic to the skin 5 to 10 minutes prepuncture.
3. Have a parent hold the child in his or her lap during the tap procedure.
4. Have the child inhale small amounts of nitrous oxide gas prepuncture.

46. The nurse is aware that antimicrobial therapy to treat meningitis should be instituted immediately <u>after</u> which event?
1. Admission to the nursing unit
2. Initiation of I.V. therapy
3. Identification of the causative organism
4. Collection of cerebrospinal fluid (CSF) and blood for culture

47. A nurse is teaching the parents of a child diagnosed with meningitis about the child's medications. Which statement by the nurse is the most accurate with respect to the use of steroid therapy (dexamethasone) in conjunction with antimicrobial therapy?
1. "It's the treatment of choice in aseptic meningitis."
2. "It's used for the prevention of GI hemorrhage."
3. "It's used for the management of problems related to blood pressure."
4. "It's used for the prevention of deafness with *Haemophilus influenzae* meningitis."

I see you've finished 44 questions. Super! Are you at least having "a little bit" of fun?

If you listen carefully, you can almost hear the answer to this question.

44. 3. Fever, change in feeding patterns, vomiting, and diarrhea are commonly observed in children with bacterial meningitis. Hemorrhagic rashes, petechiae, photophobia, fever, lethargy, and purpura are common manifestations in older children with meningitis.

CN: Physiological integrity; CNS: Physiological adaptation; CL: Application

45. 1. Sedation with fentanyl or other drugs can alleviate the pain and fear associated with a lumbar puncture. A topical anesthetic can be applied, but it should be done 1 hour before the procedure to be fully effective. A parent holding a child in his or her lap increases the risk of neurological injury due to the inability to assume and maintain the proper anatomic position required for a safe lumbar puncture. Use of nitrous oxide gas isn't recommended.

CN: Physiological integrity; CNS: Basic care and comfort; CL: Application

46. 4. Antibiotics are always begun immediately after the collection of CSF and blood cultures. Admission and initiation of I.V. therapy aren't, by themselves, appropriate times to begin antimicrobial therapy. After the specific organism is identified, bacteria-specific antibiotics can be administered if the organism isn't covered by the initial choice of antibiotic therapy.

CN: Physiological integrity; CNS: Pharmacological and parenteral therapies; CL: Analysis

47. 4. Dexamethasone may play a role in the prevention of bilateral deafness in children with *H. influenzae* type B meningitis, and its use is recommended by the American Academy of Pediatrics. Treatment of aseptic meningitis is primarily symptomatic with acetaminophen for headache and muscle pain and positioning for comfort. Use of dexamethasone could complicate rather than prevent GI bleeding and problems related to blood pressure.

CN: Physiological integrity; CNS: Pharmacological and parenteral therapies; CL: Application

48. Which description is accurate about the incidence of sequelae in a client with bacterial meningitis?
1. Occur during the first 2 months of life
2. Occur in children with meningococcal meningitis
3. Primarily involve the fourth ventricle of the brain
4. Tend to affect the ocular nerves, leading to retinal damage

49. Which goal of nursing care is the most difficult to accomplish in caring for a child with meningitis?
1. Protecting self and others from possible infection
2. Avoiding actions that increase discomfort such as lifting the head
3. Keeping environmental stimuli to a minimum, such as reduced light and noise
4. Maintaining I.V. infusion to administer adequate antimicrobial therapy

50. Which nursing assessment data should be given the <u>highest priority</u> for a child with clinical findings related to tubercular meningitis?
1. Onset and character of fever
2. Degree and extent of nuchal rigidity
3. Signs of increased intracranial pressure (ICP)
4. Occurrence of urine and fecal incontinence

51. The clinical manifestations of acute bacterial meningitis are dependent on which factor?
1. Age of the child
2. Length of the prodromal period
3. Time span from bacterial invasion to onset of symptoms
4. Degree of elevation of cerebrospinal fluid (CSF) glucose compared to serum glucose level

You're making great strides. Keep going.

All of the choices in question 50 may be correct. So you need to prioritize.

48. 1. In infants younger than age 2 months with bacterial meningitis, communicating hydrocephalus and the effects of cerebritis on the immature brain lead to the frequent occurrence of sequelae. Sequelae are least commonly seen in children experiencing meningococcal meningitis. Meningitis primarily affects the nerves for hearing rather than vision.
CN: Physiological integrity; CNS: Physiological adaptation; CL: Application

49. 4. One of the most difficult problems in the nursing care of children with meningitis is maintaining the I.V. infusion for the length of time needed to provide adequate therapy. All of the other options are important aspects in the provision of care to the child with meningitis, but they're secondary to antimicrobial therapy.
CN: Physiological integrity; CNS: Basic care and comfort; CL: Application

50. 3. Assessment of fever and evaluation of nuchal rigidity are important aspects of care, but assessment for signs of increasing ICP should be the highest priority due to the life-threatening implications. Urinary and fecal incontinence can occur in a child who is ill from nearly any cause but don't pose a great danger to life.
CN: Physiological integrity; CNS: Reduction of risk potential; CL: Analysis

51. 1. Clinical manifestations of acute bacterial meningitis depend largely on the age of the child. Clinical manifestations aren't dependent on the prodromal or initial period of the disease or the time from invasion of the host to the onset of the symptoms. The glucose level of the CSF is reduced, not elevated. A serum glucose level is drawn one-half hour before lumbar puncture so that the relationship between the CSF glucose and the serum glucose levels can be determined.
CN: Physiological integrity; CNS: Physiological adaptation; CL: Application

52. The mother of a child with a history of closed head injury asks the nurse why her son would begin having seizures without warning. Which response by the nurse is the <u>most</u> accurate?
1. "Clonic seizure activity is usually interpreted as falling."
2. "It's not unusual to develop seizures after a head injury because of brain trauma."
3. "Focal discharge in the brain may lead to absence seizures that go unnoticed."
4. "The epileptogenic focus in the brain needs multiple stimuli because it will discharge to cause a seizure."

53. A student nurse asks the nurse how anticonvulsant drugs work. Which statement by the nurse would be the most accurate?
1. Suppression of sodium influx through the gated pores in the cell membrane
2. Enhancement of calcium influx through the gated pores in the cell membrane
3. Potentiation of dopamine, facilitating passage across the neuronal cell membrane
4. Suppression of potassium removal from the neuronal intracellular compartment

54. The nurse is teaching the parents of a child who is scheduled to begin a trial period of anticonvulsant drug therapy. What is the most important information for the nurse to give the parents?
1. Plasma levels of the drug will be monitored on a daily basis.
2. Drug dosage will be adjusted depending on the frequency of seizure activity.
3. The drug must be discontinued immediately if even the slightest problem occurs.
4. The child shouldn't participate in activities that could be hazardous if a seizure occurs.

55. The nurse is planning care for a 4-year-old child hospitalized with meningitis. What is the most appropriate intervention by the nurse?
1. Avoid making noise when in the child's room.
2. Rock the child frequently.
3. Have the child's 2-year-old brother stay in the room.
4. Keep the lights on brightly so that he can see his mother.

I'm sorry! I didn't mean to steal your thunder.

Let the trial period begin!

52. 2. Stimuli from an earlier injury may eventually elicit seizure activity, a process known as kindling. Atonic seizures, not clonic, are frequently accompanied by falling. Focal seizures are partial seizures; absence seizures are generalized seizures. Focal seizures don't lead to absence seizures. The epileptogenic focus consists of a group of hyperexcitable neurons responsible for initiating synchronous, high-frequency discharges leading to a seizure rather than needing multiple stimuli.
CN: Physiological integrity; CNS: Physiological adaptation; CL: Application

53. 1. Anticonvulsant drugs, such as phenytoin (Dilantin), suppress the influx of sodium, thereby decreasing the ability of the neurons to fire. Some anticonvulsant drugs, such as valproate sodium (Depakene) used for absence seizures, suppress the influx of calcium. The role of potassium and dopamine in the generation of seizure activity hasn't been identified.
CN: Physiological integrity; CNS: Pharmacological and parenteral therapies; CL: Application

54. 4. Until seizure control is certain, clients shouldn't participate in activities (such as riding a bicycle) that could be hazardous if a seizure were to occur. Plasma levels need to be monitored periodically over the course of drug therapy; daily monitoring isn't necessary. Dosage changes are usually based on plasma drug levels as well as seizure control. Anticonvulsant drugs should be withdrawn over a period of 6 weeks to several months, never immediately, as this could precipitate status epilepticus.
CN: Physiological integrity; CNS: Pharmacological and parenteral therapies; CL: Analysis

55. 1. Meningeal irritation may cause seizures and heightens a child's sensitivity to all stimuli, including noise, lights, movement, and touch. Frequent rocking, presence of a younger sibling, and bright lights would increase stimulation.
CN: Physiological integrity; CNS: Basic care and comfort; CL: Application

56. The parents of a child with a history of seizures who has been taking phenytoin (Dilantin) ask the nurse why it's difficult to maintain therapeutic levels of this medication. Which statement by the nurse would be the <u>most</u> accurate?
1. "A drop in the plasma drug level will lead to a toxic state."
2. "The capacity to metabolize the drug becomes overwhelmed in time."
3. "Small increments in dosage lead to sharp increases in plasma drug levels."
4. "Large increases in dosage lead to more rapid stabilizing therapeutic effect."

57. Client teaching should stress which rule in relation to the differences in bioavailability of different forms of phenytoin?
1. Use the cheapest formulation the pharmacy has on hand at the time of refill.
2. Shop around to get the least expensive formulation.
3. There's no difference in one formulation from another, regardless of price.
4. Avoid switching formulations without the primary health care provider's approval.

58. A child diagnosed with meningitis is admitted to the hospital and started on I.V. fluids. The nurse is aware that the child is at risk for which condition?
1. Cerebral edema
2. Renal failure
3. Left-sided heart failure
4. Cardiogenic shock

59. The nurse determines that teaching was effective when a client taking an anticonvulsant drug states the importance of:
1. wearing a medical identification bracelet.
2. maintaining a seizure frequency chart.
3. avoiding potentially hazardous activities.
4. discontinuing the drug immediately if adverse effects are suspected.

A little bit of me goes a long way.

I'll give you this one...just because you've worked so hard.

EDEMA

56. 3. Within the therapeutic range for phenytoin, small increments in dosage produce sharp increases in plasma drug levels. The capacity of the liver to metabolize phenytoin is affected by slight changes in the dosage of the drug, not necessarily the length of time the client has been taking the drug. Large increments in dosage will greatly increase plasma levels leading to drug toxicity.
CN: Physiological integrity; CNS: Pharmacological and parenteral therapies; CL: Application

57. 4. Differences in bioavailability exist among different formulations (tablets and capsules) and among the same formulations produced by different manufacturers. Clients shouldn't switch from one formulation to another or from one brand to another without primary health care provider approval and supervision.
CN: Physiological integrity; CNS: Pharmacological and parenteral therapies; CL: Application

58. 1. Because the child with meningitis is already at increased risk of cerebral edema and increased intracranial pressure due to inflammation of the meningeal membranes, the nurse should monitor fluid intake and output to avoid fluid volume overload. Renal failure and cardiogenic shock aren't complications of I.V. therapy. The child with a healthy heart wouldn't be expected to develop left-sided heart failure.
CN: Physiological integrity; CNS: Pharmacological and parenteral therapies; CL: Application

59. 2. Ongoing evaluation of the therapeutic effects can be accomplished by maintaining a seizure frequency chart that indicates the date, time, and nature of all seizure activity. These data may be helpful in making dosage alterations and specific drug selection. Avoidance of hazardous activities and wearing a medical identification bracelet are ways to minimize danger related to seizure activity, but these factors don't affect drug efficacy. Anticonvulsant drugs should never be discontinued abruptly due to the potential for the development of status epilepticus.
CN: Physiological integrity; CNS: Pharmacological and parenteral therapies; CL: Application

60. The nurse is reviewing assessment data and the admission orders of a client. The doctor has ordered the I.V. administration of phenytoin. The nurse determines further intervention is required when the admission assessment includes which of the following?
1. Episodic nosebleeds
2. History of Stokes-Adams syndrome
3. History of bone marrow depression
4. Attention deficit hyperactivity disorder (ADHD)

You should be able to answer this question with your eyes closed.

60. 2. I.V. administration of phenytoin can lead to arrhythmia and hypotension and is contraindicated in a history of sinus bradycardia, sinoatrial block, second- or third-degree heart block, or Stokes-Adams syndrome. Phenytoin would be administered cautiously in clients with episodic nosebleeds or bone marrow depression due to its adverse effects of leukopenia, anemia, and thrombocytopenia. Phenytoin has no known effect on ADHD but can interfere with cognitive function in excessive doses.

CN: Physiological integrity; CNS: Pharmacological and parenteral therapies; CL: Analysis

61. The parents of a child newly diagnosed with seizures ask the nurse at what time seizure activity is most likely to occur. Which response by the nurse would be the most accurate?
1. During the rapid eye movement (REM) stage of sleep
2. During long periods of excitement
3. While falling asleep and on awakening
4. While eating, particularly if the client is hurried

61. 3. Falling asleep and awakening from sleep are periods of functional instability of the brain; seizure activity is more likely to occur during these times. Eating quickly, excitement without undue fatigue, and REM sleep haven't been identified as contributing factors.

CN: Physiological integrity; CNS: Physiological adaptation; CL: Application

62. When educating the family of a child with seizures, it's appropriate to tell them to call emergency medical services in the event of a seizure if which complication occurs?
1. Continuous vomiting for 30 minutes after the seizure
2. Stereotypic or automatous body movements during the onset
3. Lack of expression, pallor, or flushing of the face during the seizure
4. Unilateral or bilateral posturing of one or more extremities during the onset

I'm afraid no one will like this pattern or am I being too sensitive?

62. 1. Continuous vomiting after a seizure has ended can be a sign of an acute problem and indicates that the child requires an immediate medical evaluation. All of the other manifestations are normally present in various types of seizure activity and don't indicate a need for immediate medical evaluation.

CN: Physiological integrity; CNS: Reduction of risk potential; CL: Analysis

63. Identifying factors that trigger seizure activity could lead to which alteration in the child's environment or activities of daily living?
1. Avoiding striped wallpaper and ceiling fans
2. Having the child sleep alone to prevent sleep interruption
3. Including extended periods of intense physical activity daily
4. Allowing the child to drink soda only between noon and 5 p.m.

63. 1. Striped wallpaper, ceiling fans, and blinking lights on a Christmas tree can all be triggers to seizure activity if the child is photosensitive. Sleep interruption hasn't been identified as a triggering factor. Avoidance of fatigue can reduce seizure activity; therefore, intense physical activity for extended periods should be avoided. Restricting caffeine intake by using caffeine-free soda is a dietary modification that may prevent seizures.

CN: Physiological integrity; CNS: Physiological adaptation; CL: Application

64. Which nursing intervention should be included to support the goal of avoiding injury, respiratory distress, or aspiration during a seizure?
1. Positioning the child with the head hyperextended
2. Placing a hand under the child's head for support
3. Using pillows to prop the child into the sitting position
4. Working a padded tongue blade or small plastic airway between the teeth

65. Which diagnostic measure is the <u>most</u> accurate in detecting neural tube defects?
1. Flat plate of the lower abdomen after the 23rd week of gestation
2. Significant level of alpha-fetoprotein present in the amniotic fluid
3. Amniocentesis for lecithin-sphingomyelin (L/S) ratio
4. Presence of high maternal levels of albumin after 12th week of gestation

66. A nurse is teaching the parents of a child who has been diagnosed with spina bifida. Which statement by the nurse would be the <u>most</u> accurate description of spina bifida?
1. "It has little influence on the intellectual and perceptual abilities of the child."
2. "It's a simple neurological defect that's completely corrected surgically within 1 to 2 days after birth."
3. "Its presence means that many areas of the central nervous system (CNS) may not develop or function adequately."
4. "It's a complex neurological disability that involves a collaborative health care team effort for the entire first year of life."

67. Common deformities occurring in the child with spina bifida are related to the muscles of the lower extremities that are active or inactive. These may include which complication?
1. Club feet
2. Hip extension
3. Ankylosis of the knee
4. Abduction and external rotation of the hip

Hang on! You've reached question 65!

Checking your feet will tell me all about you!

64. 2. Placing a hand or a small cushion or blanket under the child's head will help prevent injury. Position the child with the head in midline, not hyperextended, to promote a good airway and adequate ventilation. Don't attempt to prop the child up into a sitting position but ease him to the floor to prevent falling and unnecessary injury. Don't put anything in the child's mouth because it could cause infection or obstruct the airway.
CN: Physiological integrity; CNS: Reduction of risk potential; CL: Application

65. 2. Significant levels of alpha-fetoprotein have been effective in detecting neural tube defects. Prenatal screening includes a combination of maternal serum and amniotic fluid levels, amniocentesis, amniography, and ultrasonography and has been relatively successful in diagnosing the defect. Flat plate X-rays of the abdomen, L/S ratio, and maternal serum albumin levels aren't diagnostic for the defect.
CN: Health promotion and maintenance; CNS: None; CL: Application

66. 3. When a spinal cord lesion exists at birth, it commonly leads to altered development or function of other areas of the CNS. Spina bifida is a complex neurological defect that heavily impacts the physical, cognitive, and psychosocial development of the child and involves a collaborative, lifelong management due to the chronicity and multiplicity of the problems involved.
CN: Physiological integrity; CNS: Physiological adaptation; CL: Application

67. 1. The type and extent of deformity in the lower extremities depends on the muscles that are active or inactive. Passive positioning *in utero* may result in deformities of the feet such as equinovarus (club foot), knee flexion and extension contractures, and hip flexion with adduction and internal rotation leading to subluxation or dislocation of the hip.
CN: Physiological integrity; CNS: Physiological adaptation; CL: Analysis

68. What is the nurse's priority when caring for a 10-month-old infant with meningitis?
1. Maintaining an adequate airway
2. Maintaining fluid and electrolyte balance
3. Controlling seizures
4. Controlling hyperthermia

69. The nurse is caring for an infant with myelomeningocele and notices a change in the assessment that may indicate the infant has a Chiari II malformation. Which change was noted in the assessment?
1. Rapidly progressing scoliosis
2. Changes in urological functioning
3. Back pain below the site of the sac closure
4. Respiratory stridor

70. A child with myelomeningocele and hydrocephalus may demonstrate problems related to damage of the white matter caused by ventricular enlargement. This damage may manifest itself in which condition?
1. Inability to speak
2. Early hand dominance
3. Impaired intellectual functions
4. Flaccid paralysis of the lower extremities

For question 70, it helps to know that my white matter is also known as the "association area."

68. 1. Maintaining an adequate airway is always a top priority. Maintaining fluid and electrolyte balance and controlling seizures and hyperthermia are all important but not as important as an adequate airway.

CN: Physiological integrity; CNS: Reduction of risk potential; CL: Application

69. 4. Children with a myelomeningocele have a 90% chance of having a Chiari II malformation. This may lead to a possibility of respiratory function problems, such as respiratory stridor associated with paralysis of the vocal cords, apneic episodes of unknown cause, difficulty swallowing, and an abnormal gag reflex. Urological function changes and scoliosis occur with myelomeningocele, but these complications aren't specifically related to Chiari II malformation. Lower back pain doesn't occur due to the loss of sensory function related to the cord defect.

CN: Physiological integrity; CNS: Reduction of risk potential; CL: Analysis

70. 3. Damage to the white matter (association area) caused by ventricular enlargement has been linked to impairment of intellectual and perceptual abilities often seen in children with spina bifida. It hasn't been related to hand dominance development, flaccid paralysis of the lower extremities, or the ability to speak, although it may affect the semantics of speech dependent upon the association areas.

CN: Physiological integrity; CNS: Physiological adaptation; CL: Analysis

71. The parents of a child newly diagnosed with myelomeningocele ask the nurse why surgical repair needs to be done immediately. Which response would be the most accurate?
1. "It's done for rapid restoration of the neural pathways to the legs."
2. "It's done to decrease the possibility of infection and further cord damage."
3. "It's done to expose the spinal cord defect to individualize the therapeutic strategy."
4. "It's done for removal of excess nerve tissue from the vertebral canal to decrease pressure on the cord."

72. The nurse is providing preoperative care for an infant with a myelomeningocele. The nurse is aware that <u>most appropriate</u> position for the nurse to place the client in is:
1. prone position with head turned to the side for feeding.
2. side-lying position with the head at a 30-degree angle to the feet.
3. prone position with a nasogastric (NG) tube inserted for feedings.
4. supported by diaper rolls, both anterior and posterior, in the side-lying position.

73. Large body areas of sensory and motor impairment associated with myelomeningocele necessitate which nursing intervention?
1. Gentle stretching of contractures
2. Vigorous active range-of-motion exercises
3. Frequent turning side-to-side and prone-to-supine
4. Keeping skin dry and avoiding the use of emollients and lubricants

Don't sweat it! Just choose the most appropriate response.

Sometimes it helps to stretch.

71. 2. The myelomeningocele sac presents a dynamic disability and is treated as a life-threatening situation with sac closure taking place within the first 24 to 48 hours after birth. This early management decreases the possibility of infection and further injury to the exposed neural cord. There's complete loss of nervous function below the level of the spinal cord lesion. The aim of surgery is to replace the nerve tissue into the vertebral canal, cover the spinal defect, and achieve a watertight sac closure.

CN: Physiological integrity; CNS: Reduction of risk potential; CL: Application

72. 1. Prone position is used preoperatively because it minimizes tension on the sac and the risk of trauma. The head is turned to one side for feeding. There's no advantage to positioning the body with a 30-degree head elevation. Although feeding can be a problem in the prone position, it can be accomplished without the need for an NG tube. Side-lying or partial side-lying positions are better used after the repair has been accomplished unless it permits undesirable hip flexion.

CN: Physiological integrity; CNS: Reduction of risk potential; CL: Application

73. 1. Areas of sensory and motor impairment require meticulous care, including gentle range-of-motion exercises to prevent contractures as well as stretching of contractures when indicated. Vigorous exercise is avoided in contrast to the gentle range of motion that is recommended. Frequent turning is indicated in order to maintain skin integrity, but the supine position shouldn't be used to avoid pressure on the surgical site. Skin should be kept clean and dry, but lubrication can be used to facilitate massage, which increases circulation to the areas involved.

CN: Physiological integrity; CNS: Basic care and comfort; CL: Application

74. Children with spina bifida are at high risk for developing intraoperative anaphylaxis linked to an allergic response to latex. Which risk factor leads to this allergic response?
1. Weakened immune response
2. Need for lifelong steroid therapy
3. Need for numerous bladder catheterizations
4. Use of large amounts of adhesive tape to attach sac dressings

Taking folic acid before conception reduces certain risks in infants.

75. Which explanation about how to avoid the incidence of a second child with spina bifida is most accurate?
1. There's no known way to avoid it; adoption is recommended.
2. A previous pregnancy affected by a neural tube defect isn't a factor.
3. Prepregnancy intake of 4 mg of folic acid daily reduces the recurrence rate.
4. Aerobic exercise in the first trimester decreases the chance of a positive alpha-fetoprotein (AFP).

76. A school-age child with a diagnosis of epilepsy is admitted to the pediatric unit of a local hospital for evaluation of his anticonvulsant medications. As a nurse enters the child's room, the child begins to have a seizure. Which nursing action should the nurse do first?
1. Push the call bell and ask for help.
2. Hold the child down so he doesn't injure himself.
3. Loosen any restrictive clothing.
4. Force the jaw open to maintain an open airway.

74. 3. Children with spina bifida are at high risk for developing a latex allergy because of repeated exposure to latex products during multiple surgeries and from numerous bladder catheterizations related to lack of bladder function. A weakened immune response wouldn't elicit an anaphylactic reaction due to the reduced functioning of the immune response. Steroid therapy isn't indicated in the management of spina bifida and also wouldn't support an anaphylactic reaction. Sac removal is accomplished as quickly as possible after birth, and the sac usually isn't covered with any type of dressing because it may contribute to trauma to the sac.
CN: Physiological integrity; CNS: Reduction of risk potential; CL: Application

75. 3. Studies have shown that women at high risk for having an infant with a neural tube defect, demonstrated by a previously delivered infant or fetus with spina bifida, significantly reduced the recurrence rate by taking supplements of folic acid before conception. The chances of having a second affected child are low (between 1% and 2%) but still greater than the chances of the general population. Aerobic exercise won't decrease the chance of a positive AFP.
CN: Health promotion and maintenance; CNS: None; CL: Analysis

76. 3. The primary nursing goal during a seizure is to protect the client from physical injury and maintain a patent airway. Loosening clothing will allow free movement and aid in keeping the airway open. After making sure the client is safe from injury, the nurse should push the call bell only if further assistance is needed. The nurse should never forcibly hold a client down and shouldn't force the jaw open; the jaw could be injured or break.
CN: Physiological integrity; CNS: Reduction of risk potential; CL: Application

77. A nurse is planning care for a 9-year-old boy with Down syndrome. What is the most appropriate statement regarding nursing intervention?
1. Nursing interventions should be planned at a 9-year-old developmental level.
2. Nursing interventions should be planned at a 7-year-old developmental level.
3. The nurse should assess the child's developmental level before planning interventions.
4. The developmental level of the child is not important in planning care.

78. A 6-year-old child is unconscious with a head injury from a bicycle accident. A nurse is assessing him for increased intracranial pressure (ICP). His baseline vital signs are respirations 20 breaths/minute, blood pressure 100/56 mm Hg, and pulse 100 beats/minute. The nurse continues to monitor the child and is most concerned with which assessment?
1. Respirations 12 breaths/minute; blood pressure 90/45 mm Hg; pulse 80 beats/minute
2. Respirations 14 breaths/minute; blood pressure 130/40 mm Hg; pulse 70 beats/minute
3. Respirations 30 breaths/minute; blood pressure 80/45 mm Hg; pulse 130 beats/minute
4. Respirations 14 breaths/minute; blood pressure 70/58 mm Hg; pulse 102 beats/minute

79. When assessing an infant for changes in intracranial pressure (ICP), it's important to palpate the fontanels. Identify the area where a nurse should palpate to assess the anterior fontanel.

77. 3. Before developing a care plan, the nurse should assess the child's developmental level and plan care at that level. The nurse shouldn't plan care geared toward the child's chronological age without first assessing the child. The nurse also shouldn't assume that the child is at a lower developmental level without assessing the child. The child's developmental age is important in planning age-appropriate care and teaching.

CN: Health promotion and maintenance; CNS: None; CL: Application

78. 2. Classic signs of increased ICP are a decrease in respirations, an increase in blood pressure, and a decrease in pulse rate. Option 1 may indicate normal vital signs. Options 3 and 4 may indicate shock.

CN: Physiological integrity; CNS: Physiological adaptation; CL: Analysis

79. The anterior fontanel is formed by the junction of the sagittal, frontal, and coronal sutures. It's shaped like a diamond and normally measures 4 to 5 cm at its widest point. A widened, bulging fontanel is a sign of increased ICP.

CN: Health promotion and maintenance; CNS: None; CL: Application

80. A nurse is preparing a dose of amoxicillin for a 3-year old with acute otitis media. The child weighs 33 lb. The dosage prescribed is 50 mg/kg/day in divided doses every 8 hours. The concentration of the drug is 250 mg/5 ml. How many milliliters should the nurse administer? Record your answer using a whole number.

_____ milliliters

81. A nurse is caring for a 3-year old with viral meningitis. Which signs and symptoms should the nurse expect to find during the initial assessment? Select all that apply.
1. Bulging anterior fontanel
2. Fever
3. Nuchal rigidity
4. Petechiae
5. Irritability
6. Photophobia
7. Hypothermia

82. The nurse is assessing the primitive reflexes of a 1-month-old infant. Which of the reflexes shown in the photos below should not be present after the age of 2 months?

1.
2.
3.
4.

Congratulations! You finished! Give yourself a pat on the back.

80. 5. To calculate the child's weight in kilograms, the nurse should use the following formula: $1 \text{ kg}/2.2 \text{ lb} = X \text{ kg}/33 \text{ lb}$; $2.2X = 33$; $X = 15 \text{ kg}$. Next, the nurse should calculate the daily dosage for the child: $50 \text{ mg/kg/day} \times 15 \text{ kg} = 750 \text{ mg/day}$. To determine divided daily dosage, the nurse should know that "every 8 hours" means three times per day. So, she should perform the calculation in this way: Total daily dosage ÷ 3 times per day = divided daily dosage; $750 \text{ mg/day} ÷ 3 = 250 \text{ mg}$. The drug's concentration is 250 mg/5 ml, so the nurse should administer 5 ml.

CN: Physiological integrity; CNS: Pharmacological and parenteral therapies; CL: Application

81. **2, 3, 5,** and **6.** Common signs and symptoms of viral meningitis include fever, nuchal rigidity, irritability, and photophobia. A bulging anterior fontanel is a sign of hydrocephalus, which isn't likely to occur in a toddler because the anterior fontanel typically closes by age 18 months. A petechial, purpuric rash may be seen with bacterial meningitis. Hypothermia is a common sign of bacterial meningitis in an infant younger than age 3 months.

CN: Physiological integrity; CNS: Physiological adaptation; CL: Application

82. **4.** Option 4 shows the tonic neck reflex. Persistence of this reflex beyond 2 months suggests asymmetric central nervous system development. Option 1 shows the palmer grasp reflex. This reflex disappears around age 3 to 4 months. Option 2 shows the plantar grasp reflex. This reflex disappears at age 6 to 8 months. Option 3 shows the Moro reflex. This reflex disappears around age 4 months.

CN: Physiological integrity; CNS: Reduction of risk potential; CL: Analysis

Chapter 31
Musculoskeletal disorders

1. A nurse is caring for a 10-year old in Buck's traction for a fractured femur following a bicycle accident. The child complains of increasing pain 1 hour after receiving an I.V. opioid analgesic. What is the most appropriate action by the nurse?
1. Tell the child that he needs to give the analgesic time to work.
2. Perform a neurovascular assessment.
3. Make sure the weights are hanging freely.
4. Administer more analgesics.

We know you are going to do well on this chapter.

2. Which observation by a nurse indicates that an 18-month-old in Bryant's traction is properly positioned?
1. The hips are resting on the bed.
2. The hips are slightly elevated off the bed.
3. The hips are elevated above the level of the heart.
4. The hips are resting on a pillow.

3. A mother of a neonate with clubfoot feels guilty because she believes she did something to cause the condition and asks the nurse how this happened to her baby. The nurse should explain that the cause of clubfoot is:
1. unknown.
2. hereditary.
3. due to restricted movement in utero.
4. an anomalous embryonic development.

1. 2. Pain, unrelieved by analgesics, in a client with a dressing or cast may be a sign of compartment syndrome if pressure develops within the muscle and its surrounding structures due to the constrictive ace wrap dressing used in Buck's traction. The nurse should immediately perform a neurovascular assessment to detect signs of impaired circulation and nerve function. The findings should then immediately be reported to the physician and the pressure dressing loosened or removed. The child who has received an I.V. opioid should have had pain relief 1 hour after administration. While the weights in Buck's traction should hang freely, the child should be assessed first. More analgesics may be administered as ordered but only after the neurovascular status is assessed.

CN: Physiological integrity; CNS: Reduction of risk potential; CL: Analysis

2. 2. In Bryant's traction, the child's hips should be slightly elevated off the bed at a 15-degree angle. They shouldn't be resting on the bed or a pillow and shouldn't be elevated above the level of the heart.

CN: Physiological integrity; CNS: Basic care and comfort; CL: Application

3. 1. The definitive cause of clubfoot is unknown. In some families, there's an increased incidence. Some postulate that anomalous embryonic development or restricted fetal movement is the cause. Currently, there's no way to predict the occurrence of clubfoot.

CN: Psychosocial integrity; CNS: None; CL: Application

4. Which nursing diagnosis has the <u>highest priority</u> in a 6-year-old child who had a plaster cast applied 6 hours ago to the left leg for a fracture of the tibia?
1. Deficient knowledge
2. Impaired physical mobility
3. Risk for peripheral neurovascular dysfunction
4. Dressing self-care deficit

5. Which statement by the father of an 8-year-old boy with Duchenne's muscular dystrophy indicates that he has realistic expectations about the course of the disease?
1. "My son will gradually lose his ability to walk."
2. "Corticosteroids will help prevent muscle degeneration."
3. "Surgery will help my son walk."
4. "My son will have a normal lifespan."

6. A nurse is teaching the parents of a 3-month-old infant with severe torticollis who has presented with the head rotated to the left and the side bent to the right. The nurse determines that teaching has been effective when the parents identify which muscle as being shortened?
1. Left upper trapezius
2. Right middle trapezius
3. Left sternocleidomastoid
4. Right sternocleidomastoid

7. A 9-month-old infant has torticollis with rotation of the head to the left and side bending to the right. The nurse is aware that placing the infant in which position would be most effective for developing muscle lengthening?
1. Prone
2. Supine
3. Left side-lying
4. Right side-lying

I've heard of muscle strengthening, but what's muscle lengthening?

4. 3. The highest priority in a client with a newly applied cast is to assess for and prevent circulatory complications, which can lead to loss of function. The other nursing diagnoses are important for a client in a cast but only after adequate circulation has been assured.
CN: Safe, effective care environment; CNS: Management of care; CL: Analysis

5. 1. Duchenne's muscular dystrophy is a progressive muscular degenerative disorder in which children lose their ability to walk independently by age 12. Corticosteroids may slow muscle degeneration but won't stop its progression. Surgery may be done to correct contractures, but it doesn't change the course of the disease. Death occurs by early adulthood, usually from respiratory failure.
CN: Physiological integrity; CNS: Physiological adaptation; CL: Application

6. 4. The right sternocleidomastoid is shortened with the head in this position. The left upper trapezius isn't shortened; the right one is. The middle trapezius isn't affected, and the left sternocleidomastoid is in a lengthened position.
CN: Physiological integrity; CNS: Physiological adaptation; CL: Application

7. 3. The left side-lying position will help assist with lengthening of the muscles because this position will make it easier to stretch the sternocleidomastoid and upper trapezius. No other positions will assist in increasing muscle length.
CN: Physiological integrity; CNS: Reduction of risk potential; CL: Application

8. A nurse is teaching a 13-year-old girl diagnosed with scoliosis and her parents how to apply a Milwaukee brace. Which action should the nurse do first?
1. Refer them to a scoliosis support group.
2. Ask them to read the brochure that comes with the brace and then answer their questions.
3. Ask them what they already know about the brace and answer their questions.
4. Develop learning objectives and then explain them to the parents and teen.

9. A nurse is caring for a child who received a hip-spica cast 24 hours ago for hip dysplasia. Which nursing diagnosis should the nurse give the highest priority?
1. Impaired gas exchange
2. Risk for peripheral neurovascular dysfunction
3. Risk for impaired skin integrity
4. Urinary retention

Does this mean the brace was made in Milwaukee?

10. The nurse is caring for a child with a newly applied wet hip-spica cast. What is the most important nursing intervention?
1. Use the abductor bar to help move the child.
2. Cover the cast in plastic to keep it clean.
3. Reposition the child every 1 to 2 hours.
4. Use the fingertips when handling the cast.

Congratulations! You've finished the first 10 questions!

11. The parents of an infant born with clubfoot express feelings of guilt and anxiety about their child's condition to the nurse. What is the most appropriate intervention by the nurse?
1. Teach them about their child's condition.
2. Introduce them to other parents whose children have the same condition.
3. Ask if they would like to speak with the chaplain.
4. Encourage discussion of their feelings.

12. The Milwaukee brace is commonly used in the treatment of scoliosis. Which position best describes the placement of the pressure rods?
1. Laterally on convex portion of the curve
2. Laterally on concave portion of the curve
3. Posteriorly on convex portion of the curve
4. Posteriorly along the spinal column at the exact level of the curve

8. 3. The first step in teaching this teen and her parents is to assess what they already know about the brace and answer their questions. This allows the nurse to clear up misconceptions and address their concerns. A support group is helpful but isn't the initial step the nurse should take. Written instructions should reinforce the teaching done by the nurse, not take the place of the nurse's teaching. Learning objectives should be developed with the teen and her parents.
CN: Health promotion and maintenance; CNS: None; CL: Application

9. 2. After cast application, a client is at risk for peripheral neurovascular dysfunction due to swelling within the confined space of the cast. Impaired gas exchange isn't a high risk since the cast was applied for hip dysplasia and not a fracture of a long bone, which would increase the risk of pulmonary embolism. Risk for impaired skin integrity and urinary retention are important, but neurovascular impairment is a higher priority.
CN: Safe, effective care environment; CNS: Management of care; CL: Analysis

10. 3. The child in a wet hip-spica cast should be turned every 1 to 2 hours to help dry all sides of the cast and prevent skin breakdown. The abductor bar shouldn't be used for turning the child, even with a dry cast. A wet cast shouldn't be covered with plastic because this impairs the drying of the cast. A wet cast should be handled using the palms because fingers may cause indentations and pressure points.
CN: Physiological integrity; CNS: Basic care and comfort; CL: Application

11. 4. While all the options are appropriate interventions for the nurse to implement, the first step is to encourage the parents to verbalize their concerns and feelings about their child's condition. This helps alleviate anxiety and to develop a trusting therapeutic relationship.
CN: Physiological integrity; CNS: None; CL: Analysis

12. 1. Lateral pressure applied to the convex portion of the curve will help best in reducing the curvature. Pressure pads applied posteriorly will help maintain erect posture. Pressure applied to the concave portion of the curve will increase the lordosis.
CN: Physiological integrity; CNS: Reduction of risk potential; CL: Application

13. The nurse is aware that the strengthening of which muscle group is important for a client diagnosed with talipes equinovarus?
1. Evertors
2. Invertors
3. Plantar flexors
4. Plantar fascia musculature

All this studying is strengthening my muscle groups. Oh, goody.

14. A nurse is caring for a 15-year old who sustained a fracture of the femur 24 hours ago. Which finding would alert the nurse to an early complication?
1. Pain
2. Local swelling
3. Loss of function
4. Dyspnea

15. The nurse determines that an adolescent client with scoliosis understands the treatment plan when the client makes which statement?
1. "I will have to wear a brace for several years."
2. "I can put on the brace after I get home from school."
3. "I should avoid any exercise that will stretch my spine."
4. "I can remove the brace at night."

Brace yourself. Question 15 requires a long-term solution.

16. A child has just returned to his room with a cast on his leg after open reduction of a fractured femur. The nurse assesses the child and notes a 6 cm by 10 cm area of blood on the cast. What is the most important action for the nurse to take?
1. Tape gauze pads over the bloody area.
2. Mark the bloody drainage and monitor hourly.
3. Assess vital signs.
4. Call the physician.

17. Which observation by a nurse indicates proper fit of crutches in a 9-year-old boy?
1. The crutches fit snugly under the axilla.
2. The crutches end 2 in. (5 cm) below the axilla.
3. The elbow is flexed 60 degrees.
4. The elbow is flexed 90 degrees.

13. 1. Because the foot is held in inversion, it's important to strengthen the evertors to counter the inversion present in the foot. Inversion is incorrect because the foot is already held in this position. Plantar musculature and plantar flexors aren't important because the foot is already in a plantar flexed position.

CN: Physiological integrity; CNS: Reduction of risk potential; CL: Analysis

14. 4. After the fracture of a long bone, such as the femur, the client is at risk for fat embolism. Clinical manifestations include dyspnea, hypoxia, tachypnea, tachycardia, and chest pain. Pain, local swelling, and loss of function are all typical findings after a fracture.

CN: Physiological integrity; CNS: Reduction of risk potential; CL: Analysis

15. 1. A brace worn to correct scoliosis must be worn for several years to correct the spinal deformity. The child must wear the brace all day, even during school and sleep. Exercises are commonly prescribed to be performed several times per day to stretch and strengthen back muscles. It should only be removed for 1 hour each day while bathing.

CN: Physiological integrity; CNS: Basic care and comfort; CL: Analysis

16. 3. The most appropriate action for the nurse to take is to assess the client's vital signs for evidence of hemorrhage, such as tachycardia and hypotension. After the nurse has assessed the client, the physician should be notified with the findings. Gauze pads may be placed over the bloody drainage after the client is assessed and the physician notified. The size of the bloody drainage should be monitored after the client is assessed and the physician notified.

CN: Physiological integrity; CNS: Reduction of risk potential; CL: Application

17. 2. The crutches should end 2 in. below the axilla, and the elbow should be flexed 20 to 30 degrees.

CN: Physiological integrity; CNS: Basic care and comfort; CL: Application

18. Which technique may assist a 3-month-old client diagnosed with torticollis?
1. Lying supine
2. Gentle massage
3. Range-of-motion (ROM) exercises
4. Lying on the side

19. A physical therapist has instructed the nursing staff in range-of-motion (ROM) exercises for an infant with torticollis. The nurse is uncomfortable performing the exercises that result in crying and grimacing of the client. What is the most important action for the nurse to take?
1. Check the primary health care provider's orders.
2. Call the primary health care provider.
3. Call the physical therapist.
4. Discontinue the exercises.

20. A client has developed a right torticollis with side bending to the right and rotation to the left. The nurse is aware that which exercises may assist in reduction of the torticollis?
1. Rotation exercises to the right
2. Rotation exercises to the left
3. Cervical extension exercises
4. Cervical flexion exercises

21. The nurse is caring for a client with severe scoliosis. The nurse determines that the client is at risk for which of the following?
1. Increased vital capacity
2. Increased oxygen uptake
3. Diminished vital capacity
4. Decreased residual volume

22. The parents of a 4-year-old child diagnosed with cerebral palsy and resultant thoracic scoliosis ask the nurse what caused the scoliosis. What is the best response by the nurse?
1. Hypotonia
2. Mental retardation
3. Autonomic dysreflexia
4. Increased thoracic kyphosis

18. 4. Side-lying opposite the affected side may help elongate shortened muscles. Lying supine won't assist with elongation of muscles. Gentle massage won't assist with elongation of muscles. ROM exercises won't assist with shortened muscles unless in specific patterns and with stretching.
CN: Health promotion and maintenance; CNS: None; CL: Application

19. 3. The only cure for the torticollis is exercise or surgery. The physical therapist is the expert in exercise and should be called for assistance in this situation. The primary health care provider would be called only if there was concern over the orders written or an abnormal development in the child.
CN: Physiological integrity; CNS: Physiological adaptation; CL: Analysis

20. 1. Performing rotation exercises to the right will help increase the length of the shortened right sternocleidomastoid. Rotation to the left will just add to the torticollis because the head is already rotated in that direction. Cervical extension exercises won't lengthen tightened muscles. Cervical flexion will add to shortening of the muscles.
CN: Physiological integrity; CNS: Reduction of risk potential; CL: Application

21. 3. Scoliosis of greater than 60 degrees can cause shifting of organs and decreased ability for the ribs to expand, thus decreasing vital capacity. An increase in vital capacity also won't occur secondary to a decrease in chest expansion. An increase in oxygen uptake won't occur secondary to a decrease in chest expansion. Residual volume will increase secondary to decreased ability of the lungs to expel air.
CN: Physiological integrity; CNS: Physiological adaptation; CL: Analysis

22. 1. Cerebral palsy is usually associated with some degree of hypotonia or hypertonia. Poor muscle tone may result in scoliosis. Mental retardation isn't a cause of scoliosis. Autonomic dysreflexia is described in spinal cord injury and involves abnormal muscle spasms secondary to abnormal inhibitory neurons present during stretch reflexes. Increased thoracic kyphosis won't result in scoliosis.
CN: Physiological integrity; CNS: Physiological adaptation; CL: Application

23. Which statement by the parents of a child with crutches indicates understanding of how to safely walk down stairs?
1. "First, place the crutches on the lower step."
2. "Advance the fractured leg first."
3. "Advance the strong leg first."
4. "First, place the crutch on the fractured side on the lower step."

24. During a scoliosis screening, a school nurse notices a raised iliac crest height. She should suspect which condition?
1. Forward head posture
2. Leg length discrepancy
3. Increased lumbar lordosis
4. Increased thoracic kyphosis

25. A school nurse is performing a scoliosis screening on a group of students. Which student would most commonly develop this condition?
1. A 7-year-old girl
2. A 7-year-old boy
3. A 13-year-old girl
4. A 13-year old boy

26. The nurse is caring for a child with a Harrington instrumentation rod placement. While assessing the child on the second postoperative day, the nurse is most concerned when the data include which finding?
1. Fever of 99.5° F (37.5° C)
2. Pain along the incision
3. Decreased urinary output
4. Hypoactive bowel sounds

27. The school nurse is providing instructions on scoliosis screening for the student nurses. The nurse explains that which structure is best to observe when screening a child?
1. Iliac crests
2. Spinous processes
3. Acromion processes
4. Posterior superior iliac spines

28. Which intervention may be a possible treatment choice for talipes equinovarus?
1. Traction
2. Serial casting
3. Short leg braces
4. Inversion range-of-motion exercises

Read question 23 carefully and take it one step at a time.

In question 26, you've got to determine the symptom that causes the most concern.

No bones about it. You're doing great!

23. 1. To walk down the stairs with crutches, the crutches are first placed on the lower step. Then the fractured or weaker leg is lowered, followed by the unaffected or stronger leg. This way the arms and unaffected leg share the work of carrying the body weight.
CN: Safe, effective care environment; CNS: Safety and infection control; CL: Application

24. 2. A raised iliac crest may be indicative of a leg length discrepancy or a curvature in the lumbar spine. It isn't indicative of forward head posture, lumbar lordosis, or thoracic kyphosis.
CN: Health promotion and maintenance; CNS: None; CL: Application

25. 3. Scoliosis is eight times more prominent in adolescent girls than boys. Peak incidence is between ages 8 and 15. Therefore, a 13-year-old girl is at the highest risk. Seven-year-old boys and girls are at lower risk.
CN: Health promotion and maintenance; CNS: None; CL: Analysis

26. 3. Because of extensive blood loss during surgery and possible renal hypoperfusion, decreased urinary output could indicate decreased renal function. A fever of 99.5° F is of concern, but it may be due to decreased chest expansion secondary to anesthesia, surgery, and pain. Pain along the incision site is expected. A paralytic ileus is common after this surgery, and the client may have a nasogastric tube for the first 48 hours.
CN: Physiological integrity; CNS: Reduction of risk potential; CL: Analysis

27. 2. Spinous processes are the best bony landmark to identify when attempting to screen for scoliosis because this will show lateral deviation of the column. Abnormalities in the acromion process, iliac crests, and posterior superior iliac spines may not be indicative of scoliosis.
CN: Health promotion and maintenance; CNS: None; CL: Application

28. 2. Serial casting is a treatment choice in attempts to change the length of soft tissue. Traction isn't an option. Corrective shoes are used instead of short leg braces. Inversion exercises won't help; eversion exercise will.
CN: Physiological integrity; CNS: Reduction of risk potential; CL: Application

29. When performing stretches with a child who has scoliosis, which technique should be used by the nurse?
1. Slow and sustained
2. Until a change in muscle length is seen
3. Quick movements to the end range of pain
4. Slow movements for brief, 3- to 4-second periods

30. Which observation by a nurse indicates that the parent of a neonate with developmental dysplasia of the hip understands the discharge teaching?
1. A folded towel is placed between the infant's legs.
2. The infant is wearing three diapers.
3. The infant is tightly swaddled in a blanket.
4. The infant is placed in a prone position to sleep.

31. A nurse is caring for an infant with suspected developmental dysplasia of the hip (DDH). Which information should the nurse give the parents about diagnostic testing?
1. A diagnosis can't be confirmed until the child begins to walk.
2. Diagnostic testing is performed at 6 months if the dysplasia hasn't resolved by then.
3. A radiopaque dye will be injected into the subarachnoid space of the spine.
4. An X-ray confirms the diagnosis.

32. Which hip position should be avoided in an 8-month-old infant who has been diagnosed with developmental dysplasia of the hip?
1. Extension
2. Abduction
3. Internal rotation
4. External rotation

33. Which activity in a client with muscular dystrophy should a nurse anticipate the client having difficulty with <u>first</u>?
1. Breathing
2. Sitting
3. Standing
4. Swallowing

> You might need a stretch right now. Why not take a brief one and then get right back to work?

> It's all about stability and, in this case, instability.

29. 1. Stretches should be slow and sustained. It's difficult to see changes in muscle length. Stretches shouldn't be performed with quick movements. Stretches should be performed for longer than a few seconds.
CN: Health promotion and maintenance; CNS: None; CL: Application

30. 2. Placing several diapers on the infant will keep the hips and knees flexed and the hips abducted. A towel placed between the legs is not enough to keep the hips abducted. Swaddling the infant tightly straightens the legs and doesn't allow the hips to be abducted. Placing the infant in a prone position won't keep the hips abducted and isn't recommended due to the increased risk of sudden infant death syndrome.
CN: Physiological integrity; CNS: Basic care and comfort; CL: Application

31. 4. X-rays show the location of the femur head and a shallow acetabulum, confirming the diagnosis DDH. The diagnosis can be made in the neonate and should be made as soon as possible since it becomes more difficult to correct as the child ages. Myelography is an invasive procedure used to evaluate abnormalities of the spinal canal and cord. It isn't used in the diagnosis of congenital hip dysplasia.
CN: Physiological integrity; CNS: Physiological adaptation; CL: Application

32. 3. Internal rotation of the hip is an unstable position and should be avoided in infants with hip instability. Hip extension is a relatively stable position. Typically, the child is placed in slight abduction while in a hip-spica cast. External rotation isn't necessarily an unstable position, as long as it isn't externally rotated too far.
CN: Physiological integrity; CNS: Reduction of risk potential; CL: Application

33. 3. Muscular dystrophy usually affects postural muscles of the hip and shoulder first. Sitting may be affected, but a client would have difficulty standing before having difficulty sitting. Swallowing and breathing are usually affected last.
CN: Physiological integrity; CNS: Physiological adaptation; CL: Application

34. The nurse would expect her client's suspected developmental dysplasia of the hip (DDH) to be confirmed by which diagnostic technique?
1. X-ray
2. Positive Ortolani's sign
3. Positive Trendelenburg gait
4. Audible clicking with adduction

35. Which finding should a nurse expect when assessing a neonate with a positive Galeazzi sign?
1. Raised iliac crest
2. Pelvic downward tilt on weight bearing
3. Knees are flexed to 90 degrees, one knee higher
4. Involved leg flexed to 90 degrees, audible click with external rotation

36. A young child sustains a dislocated hip as well as a subcapital fracture. The nurse is aware that the client is at <u>greatest risk</u> for which of the following?
1. Avascular necrosis
2. Postsurgical infection
3. Hemorrhage during surgery
4. Poor postsurgical ambulation

Question 36? Another chance to prioritize.

37. Which position of the femur is accurate in relation to the acetabulum in a child with developmental dysplasia of the hip (DDH)?
1. Anterior
2. Inferior
3. Posterior
4. Superior

I'm not the muscle I used to be.

38. The nurse is planning to teach the parents of a child with newly diagnosed muscular dystrophy about the disease. Which description accurately describes this condition?
1. A demyelinating disease
2. Lesions of the brain cortex
3. Upper motor neuron lesions
4. Degeneration of muscle fibers

39. When a child is suspected of having muscular dystrophy, a nurse should expect which muscles to be affected <u>first</u>?
1. Hip muscles
2. Foot muscles
3. Hand muscles
4. Respiration muscles

34. 1. X-ray will confirm the diagnosis of DDH. All of the options are positive signs of DDH, but only the X-ray will confirm the diagnosis.
CN: Physiological integrity; CNS: Physiological adaptation; CL: Application

35. 3. A positive Galeazzi sign is used to help diagnose hip dislocation. It's exhibited as one knee being higher than the other. Raised iliac crest isn't indicative of specific hip pathology. A downward pelvic tilt with weight bearing is Trendelenburg gait. External rotation of the hip with audible click is Ortolani-Barlow test.
CN: Health promotion and maintenance; CNS: None; CL: Application

36. 1. Avascular necrosis is common with fractures to the subcapital region secondary to possible compromise of blood supply to the femoral head. Postsurgical infection is always a concern but not a priority at first. Hemorrhage shouldn't occur. Poor postsurgical ambulation is of concern but not as much as the possibility of avascular necrosis.
CN: Physiological integrity; CNS: Reduction of risk potential; CL: Application

37. 1. The head of the femur is anterior to the acetabulum in developmental dysplasia of the hip. All other positions are inaccurate.
CN: Physiological integrity; CNS: Physiological adaptation; CL: Application

38. 4. Degeneration of muscle fibers with progressive weakness and wasting best describes muscular dystrophy. Demyelination of myelin sheaths is a description of multiple sclerosis. Lesions within the cortex and in upper motor neurons suggest a neurological, not a muscular, disease.
CN: Physiological integrity; CNS: Physiological adaptation; CL: Application

39. 1. Positional muscles of the hip and shoulder are affected first. Progression advances to muscles of the foot and hand. Involuntary muscles, such as the muscles of respiration, are affected last.
CN: Physiological integrity; CNS: Physiological adaptation; CL: Application

40. Which information should a nurse provide to the parents of child undergoing testing for the diagnosis of muscular dystrophy?
1. The genitals will be covered by a lead apron.
2. A local anesthetic will be used for the test.
3. Electrode wires will be attached to the scalp.
4. A fiber-optic endoscope will be inserted into a joint.

Question 41 asks which lab test helps in diagnosing the condition.

41. The nurse is reviewing the laboratory tests of a child diagnosed with muscular dystrophy. Which laboratory test would aid in the diagnosis of this condition?
1. Bilirubin
2. Creatinine
3. Serum potassium
4. Sodium

42. The nurse is teaching the student nurse about muscular dystrophy. The student nurse asks which form of muscular dystrophy is most common. Which response is most accurate?
1. Duchenne's
2. Becker's
3. Limb girdle
4. Myotonic

43. Which condition would alert the nurse that a child might be suffering from muscular dystrophy?
1. Hypertonia of extremities
2. Increased lumbar lordosis
3. Upper extremity spasticity
4. Hyperactive lower extremity reflexes

It's all in the jeans...I mean the genes.

44. The parents of a child with Duchenne's muscular dystrophy want to know how it is acquired. What is the most accurate response by the nurse?
1. Virus
2. Hereditary
3. Autoimmune factors
4. Environmental toxins

40. 2. A muscle biopsy, used to confirm the diagnosis of muscular dystrophy, shows the degeneration of muscle fibers and infiltration of fatty tissue. It's typically performed using a local anesthetic. Genitals are covered by a lead apron during an X-ray examination, which is used to detect osseous, not muscular, problems. Electrode wires are attached to the scalp during EEG to observe brain wave activity. It isn't used to diagnose muscular dystrophy. Arthroscopy involves the insertion of a fiber-optic scope into a joint and isn't used to diagnose muscular dystrophy.
CN: Physiological integrity; CNS: Basic care and comfort; CL: Application

41. 2. Creatinine values would aid in the diagnosis of muscular dystrophy. Creatinine is a by-product of muscle metabolism as it hypertrophies. Bilirubin is a by-product of liver function. Potassium and sodium levels can change due to various factors and aren't indicators of muscular dystrophy.
CN: Health promotion and maintenance; CNS: None; CL: Application

42. 1. Duchenne's, also known as pseudohypertrophic, muscular dystrophy accounts for 50% of all cases of muscular dystrophy. It affects cardiac and respiratory muscles as well as all voluntary muscles.
CN: Physiological integrity; CNS: Physiological adaptation; CL: Application

43. 2. An increased lumbar lordosis would be seen in a child suffering from muscular dystrophy secondary to paralysis of lower lumbar postural muscles; it also occurs to increase lower extremity support. Hypertonia isn't seen in this disease. Upper extremity spasticity isn't seen because this disease isn't due to upper motor neuron lesions. Hyperactive reflexes aren't indications of muscular dystrophy.
CN: Physiological integrity; CNS: Physiological adaptation; CL: Analysis

44. 2. Muscular dystrophy is hereditary and acquired through a recessive sex-linked trait. Therefore, it isn't viral, autoimmune, or caused by toxins.
CN: Physiological integrity; CNS: Physiological adaptation; CL: Application

45. A client with muscular dystrophy has lost complete control of his lower extremities. He has some strength bilaterally in the upper extremities but poor trunk control. Which mechanism would be the most important to have on the wheelchair?
1. Antitip device
2. Extended breaks
3. Headrest support
4. Wheelchair belt

46. A 2-year-old toddler has muscular dystrophy. His legs are held together with the knees touching. Which muscles are contracted?
1. Hip abductors
2. Hip adductors
3. Hip extensors
4. Hip flexors

47. A 12-year-old child diagnosed with muscular dystrophy is hospitalized secondary to a fall. Surgery is necessary as well as skeletal traction. Which complication should be of <u>greatest concern</u> to the nursing staff?
1. Skin integrity
2. Infection of pin sites
3. Respiratory infection
4. Nonunion healing of the fracture

48. A nurse is talking with a 12-year-old boy and his parents about his osteogenesis imperfecta. The client tells the nurse he likes to swim. What is the most appropriate response by the nurse?
1. He should also add a weight-bearing exercise.
2. Swimming isn't safe since he can slip on the wet area around the pool.
3. He should restrict his exercise to only swimming.
4. Any form of exercises isn't safe.

49. Which problem is most commonly encountered by adolescent females with scoliosis?
1. Respiratory distress
2. Poor self-esteem
3. Poor appetite
4. Renal difficulty

Question 45 tests your ability to ensure the client's safety.

Prioritize? What a surprise!

45. 4. This client has poor trunk control; a belt will prevent him from falling out of the wheelchair. Antitip devices, head rest supports, and extended breaks are all important options but aren't the best choice in this situation.

CN: Safe, effective care environment; CNS: Safety and infection control; CL: Application

46. 2. The hip adductors are in a shortened position. The abductors are in a lengthened position. This position isn't indicative of hip flexor or hip extensor shortening.

CN: Health promotion and maintenance; CNS: None; CL: Application

47. 3. Respiratory infection can be fatal for clients with muscular dystrophy due to poor chest expansion and decreased ability to mobilize secretions. Skin integrity, infection of pin sites, and nonunion healing are important but not as important as prevention of respiratory infection.

CN: Physiological integrity; CNS: Reduction of risk potential; CL: Analysis

48. 1. Swimming is a beneficial form of exercise for people with osteogenesis imperfecta, but since it does little to prevent bone loss, the client should add a weight-bearing exercise. Although wet areas around the pool are a risk for the person with osteogenesis imperfecta, the risk can be minimized by walking carefully and wearing nonskid footwear. In the past, clients with osteogenesis imperfecta were told that exercise increased the risk of bone fractures. Mild forms of exercise are encouraged to promote bone density and cardiovascular conditioning and to maintain joint mobility.

CN: Health promotion and maintenance; CNS: None; CL: Application

49. 2. Poor self-esteem is a major issue with many adolescents. The use of orthopedic appliances, such as those used to treat scoliosis, make this issue much more significant for adolescents with scoliosis. Although respiratory distress and poor appetite may surface, they aren't as common as self-esteem problems. Renal problems aren't usually an issue in adolescents with scoliosis.

CN: Health promotion and maintenance; CNS: None; CL: Application

50. A child has developed difficulty ambulating and tends to walk on his toes. Which surgical technique may benefit the client?
1. Adductor release
2. Hamstring release
3. Plantar fascia release
4. Achilles tendon release

51. The parents of a child with muscular dystrophy ask the nurse what causes this condition. What is the best response by the nurse?
1. Gene mutation
2. Chromosomal aberration
3. Unknown nongenetic origin
4. Environmental factors

52. The nurse is assessing a child suspected of having muscular dystrophy for muscle weakness. At what age would evidence of muscle weakness associated with muscular dystrophy appear?
1. Age 1
2. Age 2
3. Age 3
4. Age 4

53. To promote safe transfers in a client with muscular dystrophy, a nurse should teach exercises to maintain which muscles?
1. Gastrocnemius
2. Gluteus maximus
3. Hamstrings
4. Quadriceps

54. Which of the following strategies would be the first choice in attempting to maximize function in a child with muscular dystrophy?
1. Long leg braces
2. Motorized wheelchair
3. Manual wheelchair
4. Walker

55. A child is having increased difficulty getting out of his chair at school. Which recommendation should the nurse make to assist the child?
1. A seat cushion
2. Long leg braces
3. Powered wheelchair
4. Removable armrests on wheelchair

Hooray! You've reached question 50!

The words *first choice* can help you focus on the answer to question 54.

50. 4. A shortened Achilles tendon may cause a child to walk on his toes. A release of the tendon may assist the child in walking. An adductor release is commonly performed if the legs are held together. A plantar fascia release won't help, and a hamstring release is done only when there's a knee flexion contracture.
CN: Physiological integrity; CNS: Reduction of risk potential; CL: Application

51. 1. Muscular dystrophy is a result of a gene mutation. It isn't from a chromosome aberration or environmental factors. It's genetic, and there's a known origin of the disease.
CN: Physiological integrity; CNS: Physiological adaptation; CL: Application

52. 3. Studies have shown that children diagnosed with muscular dystrophy usually show some form of weakness around age 3.
CN: Health promotion and maintenance; CNS: None; CL: Application

53. 2. Gluteus maximus is the strongest muscle in the body and is important for standing as well as for transfers. All of the named muscles are important, but the maintenance of the gluteus maximus will enable maximum function.
CN: Health promotion and maintenance; CNS: None; CL: Application

54. 1. Long leg braces are functional assistive devices that provide increased independence and increased use of upper and lower body strength. Wheelchairs, both motorized and manual, provide less independence and less use of upper and lower body strength. Walkers are functional assistive devices that provide less independence than braces.
CN: Physiological integrity; CNS: Basic care and comfort; CL: Application

55. 1. A seat cushion will put the hip extensors at an advantage and make it somewhat easier to get up. Long leg braces wouldn't be the first choice. A powered wheelchair wouldn't be important in assisting with the transfer. Removable armrests have no bearing on assisting the client.
CN: Physiological integrity; CNS: Basic care and comfort; CL: Application

56. What findings would the nurse expect when palpating the muscles of a child with muscular dystrophy?
1. Soft on palpation
2. Firm or woody on palpation
3. Extremely hard on palpation
4. No muscle consistency on palpation

56. 2. Muscles will commonly be firm on palpation secondary to the infiltration of fatty tissue and connective tissue into the muscle. The muscles won't be soft secondary to the infiltration and won't be hard upon palpation. There's some consistency to the muscle, although in advanced stages, atrophy is present.

CN: Physiological integrity; CNS: Physiological adaptation; CL: Analysis

57. A nurse is instructing a wheelchair-bound client with muscular dystrophy on exercises to best prevent skin breakdown. What is the best information for the nurse to provide?
1. Wheelchair push-ups
2. Leaning side to side
3. Leaning forward
4. Gluteal sets

To remember Gowers' sign, think going somewhere—that's a description of what the child is trying to do.

57. 1. A wheelchair push-up will alleviate the most pressure off the buttocks. Leaning side to side and leaning forward will help but not as much as wheelchair push-ups. Gluteal sets won't help with pressure relief.

CN: Health promotion and maintenance; CNS: None; CL: Application

58. How would the nurse best describe <u>Gowers' sign</u> to the parents of a child with muscular dystrophy?
1. A transfer technique
2. A waddling-type gait
3. The pelvis position during gait
4. Muscle twitching present during a quick stretch

58. 1. Gowers' sign is a description of a transfer technique present during some phases of muscular dystrophy. The child turns on the side or abdomen, extends the knees, and pushes on the torso to an upright position by walking his hands up the legs. Waddling-type gait doesn't describe Gowers' sign. The position of the pelvis during gait isn't described by Gowers' sign. Muscle twitching present after a quick stretch is described as clonus.

CN: Physiological integrity; CNS: Physiological adaptation; CL: Analysis

59. A 13-year-old boy admitted with a fractured femur had an open reduction and internal fixation 2 days ago and currently is in traction. He asks the nurse what would happen to him if a terrorist decided to bomb the hospital. What's the nurse's best response?
1. "I wouldn't worry about that. Spend your energy on getting well and going home."
2. "We have plans to call your parents and take care of you if there's a problem."
3. "What do you think might happen if terrorists attack?"
4. "That's silly thinking. Why would anyone bomb a hospital?"

Focus on what response is best.

59. 3. Something prompted the child to ask such a question, and the nurse needs to take advantage of this opportunity to further explore his concerns and fears. Option 1 discounts the boy's feelings and may actually increase his anxiety. Although option 2 may be technically correct, it doesn't provide reassurance or help build a therapeutic relationship that can promote health and wellness. Option 4 is dismissive and childes the boy for asking the question.

CN: Physiological integrity; CNS: None; CL: Analysis

60. A client with bilateral fractured femurs is scheduled for a double–hip-spica cast. She says to the nurse, "Only 3 more months and I can go home." Further investigation reveals that the client and her family believe she'll be hospitalized until the cast comes off. The nurse should explain to the client and her family that the client:
1. may be hospitalized 2 to 4 months.
2. will go home 2 to 4 days after casting.
3. will go home 1 week after casting.
4. will go home as soon as she can move.

61. Which observation by a nurse indicates that an infant in a hip-spica cast is properly positioned?
1. The infant's upper body and cast are at a 180-degree angle.
2. The infant's hips are higher than the head.
3. The infant's upper body and the cast are at a 45-degree angle.
4. The infant is flat in bed.

62. The nurse receives a report on a child admitted with the most severe form of muscular dystrophy. The nurse knows this means the child has which type of muscular dystrophy?
1. Duchenne's
2. Facioscapulohumeral
3. Limb girdle
4. Myotonic

63. The nurse assesses a client with a cast following a fracture of the radius and is most concerned about which finding?
1. Discomfort occurs at the site of the break.
2. Fingers are pink and warm.
3. Swelling is reduced with cast elevation.
4. Pain occurs over a bony prominence.

64. The parents of a child with newly diagnosed developmental dysplasia of the hip (DDH) ask the nurse how their child developed this condition. The nurse explains that the <u>greatest number</u> of cases is caused by which condition?
1. Dislocation
2. Subluxation
3. Acetabular dysplasia
4. Dislocation with fracture

I know all about pain over a bony prominence.

The greatest number of cases? This is getting complicated.

60. 2. The cast will dry fairly rapidly with the use of fiberglass casting material. The time spent in the hospital after casting, typically 2 to 4 days, will be for teaching the client and her family how to care for her at home and evaluating the client's skin integrity and neurovascular status before discharge. The time frames in the other options given are inaccurate for a double–hip-spica cast.
CN: Health promotion and maintenance; CNS: None; CL: Application

61. 1. The infant's body and cast should be at a 180-degree angle. While the cast should be kept level with the body, it should be on a slant with the head of the bed elevated so that urine and stool can drain downward and not soil the cast.
CN: Physiological integrity; CNS: Basic care and comfort; CL: Application

62. 1. Studies have shown that Duchenne's is the most severe form of muscular dystrophy, affecting all voluntary muscles as well as cardiac and respiratory muscles.
CN: Physiological integrity; CNS: Physiological adaptation; CL: Analysis

63. 4. Pain over a bony prominence, such as in the wrist or elbow, signals an impending pressure ulcer and requires prompt attention. Pain or discomfort at the site of the fracture is expected and is relieved by analgesics. Warm and pink fingers are an expected finding. Swelling may be relieved by elevation of the extremity. Swelling that isn't relieved by elevation of the affected limb should be reported to the physician.
CN: Physiological integrity; CNS: Reduction of risk potential; CL: Application

64. 2. Studies show that subluxation accounts for the greatest number of cases of DDH.
CN: Physiological integrity; CNS: Physiological adaptation; CL: Application

65. Which finding would the nurse expect in a client with developmental dysplasia of the hip (DDH)?
1. Ligamentum teres is shortened.
2. Femoral head loses contact with acetabulum and is displaced inferiorly.
3. Femoral head loses contact with the acetabulum and is displaced posteriorly.
4. Femoral head maintains contact with acetabulum, but there's noted capsular rupture.

66. A toddler is immobilized with traction to the legs. Which play activity would be appropriate for the nurse to include in the plan of care for this child?
1. Pounding board
2. Tinker toys
3. Pull toy
4. Board games

67. An unlicensed assistive personnel (UAP) asks the nurse how to care for a client's hip-spica cast that has been soiled. What is the best response by the nurse?
1. Clean with damp cloth and dry cleanser.
2. Clean with soap and water.
3. Don't do anything.
4. Change the cast.

68. A child in a hip-spica cast needs to be toileted. How should the nurse position the child?
1. Supine
2. Sitting in a toilet chair
3. Shoulder lower than buttocks
4. Buttocks lower than shoulder

69. Which intervention should a nurse perform in a 4-year-old child in Buck's traction?
1. Provide daily pin site care.
2. Release weights for 1 hour each day.
3. Change the child's position every 4 hours.
4. Unwrap the elastic bandage every shift to assess the skin.

Knowing the shape of a hip-spica cast can help answer this question.

Pulling and pins? This doesn't sound like fun.

65. 3. In DDH, the femoral head loses contact with the acetabulum and is displaced posteriorly, not inferiorly. Ligamentum teres is lengthened.
CN: Physiological integrity; CNS: Physiological adaptation; CL: Application

66. 1. A pounding board is appropriate for an immobilized toddler because it promotes physical development and provides an acceptable energy outlet. Toys with small parts, such as tinker toys, aren't suitable because a toddler may swallow the parts. A pull toy is suitable for most toddlers but not for one who is immobilized. Board games are usually too advanced for the developmental skills of a toddler.
CN: Health promotion and maintenance; CNS: None; CL: Application

67. 1. A damp cloth is best to use rather than water. Water will break the cast down. If nothing is done, the cast will give off an odor. Changing the cast isn't an option.
CN: Physiological integrity; CNS: Basic care and comfort; CL: Application

68. 4. The buttocks need to be lowered to toilet the child. This will keep the cast from being soiled. Supine will cause soiling of the cast. The child isn't able to use a toilet chair.
CN: Physiological integrity; CNS: Basic care and comfort; CL: Application

69. 1. Buck's traction is a form of skeletal traction that pulls directly on the skeleton using a pin placed into the bone. Pin site care involves cleaning the insertion sites to reduce the risk of infection and observing the site for signs and symptoms of infection. Weights should hang freely and shouldn't be released. The child's position should be changed every 2 hours to prevent skin breakdown. Elastic bandages are used in skin, not skeletal, traction.
CN: Physiological integrity; CNS: Basic care and comfort; CL: Application

70. The nurse observes a client who has a positive Trendelenburg gait. Which characteristic would indicate this gait?
1. Pelvis tilts downward upon weight bearing
2. Pelvis tilts upward upon weight bearing
3. Abnormal height of the iliac crests
4. Leg length discrepancy

71. Which complication involving leg length should a nurse anticipate in a client with developmental dysplasia of the hip?
1. Increased hip abduction
2. Increased leg length on the affected side
3. Decreased leg length on the affected side
4. No change in muscle length or leg length

72. A nurse recognizes that the parent of a child with developmental hip dysplasia needs more teaching when the parent places the child in a position that encourages:
1. hip abduction.
2. knee extension.
3. external rotation.
4. internal rotation.

73. Immediately after a spinal fusion, which restriction is usually put on the child's activity?
1. Supine bed rest
2. Non–weight bearing
3. No restriction
4. Limited weight bearing

74. Which intervention should a nurse expect to use to prevent venous stasis after skeletal traction application?
1. Bed rest only
2. Convoluted foam mattress
3. Vigorous pulmonary care
4. Antiembolism stockings or an intermittent compression device

75. A 13-year-old girl is suspected of having structural scoliosis by her school nurse. What should the nurse ask the girl to do to help confirm her suspicion?
1. Bend over and touch her toes while the nurse observes from the back.
2. Stand sideways while the nurse observes her profile.
3. Assume a knee-chest position on the examination table.
4. Arch her back while the nurse observes her from the back.

Easy does it.

70. 1. The pelvis will tilt downward upon weight bearing secondary to a weakness of the abductors on the affected side. The pelvis doesn't tilt upward. Leg length and iliac crest height aren't indicative of Trendelenburg gait.

CN: Physiological integrity; CNS: Physiological adaptation; CL: Application

71. 3. The internal rotation with subsequent dislocation will cause the leg to be shorter, not longer. There's usually decreased abduction as well as muscle and leg length changes.

CN: Physiological integrity; CNS: Physiological adaptation; CL: Analysis

72. 4. Internal rotation increases the risk of hip dislocation. Abduction, external rotation, and knee extension won't increase the risk of dislocation.

CN: Health promotion and maintenance; CNS: None; CL: Application

73. 1. After a spinal fusion, the child is usually placed on bed rest and ordered to lie flat. In 2 to 4 days, the child is allowed to sit up in and get out of bed. Other activities are gradually reintroduced.

CN: Physiological integrity; CNS: Basic care and comfort; CL: Application

74. 4. To prevent venous stasis after skeletal traction application, antiembolism stockings or an intermittent compression device is used on the unaffected leg. Bed rest can cause venous stasis. Convoluted foam mattresses and pulmonary care don't prevent venous stasis.

CN: Health promotion and maintenance; CNS: None; CL: Application

75. 1. As the child bends over, the curvature of the spine is more apparent. The scapula on one side becomes more prominent, and the opposite side hollows. The knee-chest position is used for lumbar puncture. Scoliosis can't be properly assessed from the side or the front.

CN: Health promotion and maintenance; CNS: None; CL: Application

76. At the scene of a trauma, which nursing intervention is appropriate for a child with a <u>suspected fracture</u>?
1. Never move the child.
2. Sit the child up to facilitate breathing.
3. Move the child to a safe place immediately.
4. Immobilize the extremity and then move the child to a safe place.

77. A nurse is assessing an 18-month-old infant who's in Bryant's traction for a fractured left femur. The infant is properly positioned when:
1. the left leg is extended 90 degrees off the bed.
2. the right leg is extended 90 degrees off the bed.
3. both legs are extended 90 degrees off the bed.
4. both legs are extended at 180 degrees with the upper body.

78. A child in skeletal traction for a fracture of the right femur exhibits a positive Homans' sign, complains of left-sided leg pain, and has edema in the left leg. A nurse should further assess the child for which condition?
1. A fat emboli
2. An infection
3. A pulmonary embolism
4. Deep vein thrombosis (DVT)

79. Nursing care for a client in traction may include which intervention?
1. Assessing pin sites every shift and as needed
2. Ensuring that the rope knots catch on the pulley
3. Adding and removing weights per client's request
4. Placing all joints through range of motion (ROM) every shift

80. After assisting the primary health care provider in applying a cast, a nurse should include which intervention in the immediate cast care?
1. Rest the cast on the bedside table.
2. Dispose of the plaster water in the sink.
3. Support the cast with her palms.
4. Wait until the cast dries before cleaning surrounding skin.

At a trauma scene, think safety first!

Is Homans' sign an astrological sign?

Your performance has been Oscar winning so far. Good luck!!

76. 4. At the scene of a trauma, the nurse should immobilize the extremity of a child with a suspected fracture and then move him to a safe place. If the child is already in a safe place, don't attempt to move him. Never try to sit the child up; this could make the fracture worse.
CN: Safe, effective care environment; CNS: Safety and infection control; CL: Application

77. 3. Bryant's traction, a type of skin traction, is for lower extremity fractures in children younger than age 2 years. Both legs are suspended at 90 degrees off the bed, even though only one is fractured, with the child's body weight providing the countertraction.
CN: Physiological integrity; CNS: Basic care and comfort; CL: Application

78. 4. Unilateral leg pain and edema with a positive Homans' sign (not always present) should lead you to suspect DVT. Symptoms of fat emboli include restlessness, tachypnea, and tachycardia and are more common in long bone injuries. It's unlikely that an infection would occur on the opposite side of the fracture without cause. Tachycardia, chest pain, and shortness of breath may be symptoms of a pulmonary embolism.
CN: Physiological integrity; CNS: Reduction of risk potential; CL: Analysis

79. 1. Nursing care for a client in traction may include assessing pin sites every shift and as needed and ensuring that the knots in the rope don't catch on the pulley. Weights should be added and removed per the primary health care provider's order, and all joints, except those immediately proximal and distal to the fracture, should be placed through ROM every shift.
CN: Physiological integrity; CNS: Basic care and comfort; CL: Application

80. 3. After a cast has been applied, it should be immediately supported with the palms of the nurse's hands. Later, the nurse should dispose of the plaster water in a sink with a plaster trap or in a garbage bag, clean the surrounding skin before the cast dries, and make sure that the cast isn't resting on a hard or sharp surface.
CN: Physiological integrity; CNS: Reduction of risk potential; CL: Application

81. A school-age child tells a nurse that he's experiencing intense itching from under his cast. What is the most appropriate response by the nurse?
1. "Toughen up; there's nothing that can be done."
2. "Place the eraser end of a new pencil under the cast to scratch."
3. "Elevate the cast above the level of your heart."
4. "Aim cool air from a hair dryer under the cast."

82. Which nursing intervention should be taken if, while a cast is drying, the client complains of heat from the cast?
1. Remove the cast immediately.
2. Notify the primary health care provider.
3. Assess the client for other signs of infection.
4. Explain to the client that this is a normal sensation.

83. Which nursing intervention can be implemented to <u>prevent</u> foot drop in a casted leg?
1. Encourage bed rest.
2. Support the foot with 45 degrees of flexion.
3. Support the foot with 90 degrees of flexion.
4. Place a stocking on the foot to provide warmth.

84. The nurse instructs a client with a hip-spica cast to avoid gas-forming foods. The client asks the nurse what can happen if the food is consumed. What is the best response by the nurse?
1. Flatus
2. Diarrhea
3. Constipation
4. Abdominal distention

85. A nurse determines that a client with a fractured left femur understands the instructions for touch-down weight bearing when the client makes which statement?
1. "I will place full weight on my left leg."
2. "I will place about 30% to 50% of my weight on my left leg."
3. "I will keep my left leg off the floor."
4. "I will allow my left leg to touch the floor without placing weight on it."

Can you help me prevent foot drop?

My eyes are bigger than my stomach...or not.

81. 4. Cool air from a hair dryer may soothe the itchiness. Telling the child to toughen up isn't therapeutic, erodes the nurse–client relationship, and isn't true since cool air may relieve itchiness. Nothing should be placed under a cast because this can cause skin irritation and breakdown. Elevating the cast above the heart doesn't relieve itching. This position is used to reduce swelling.
CN: Physiological integrity; CNS: Basic care and comfort; CL: Application

82. 4. Normally, as the cast is drying, the client may complain of heat from the cast. The nurse should offer reassurance but doesn't need to notify the primary health care provider or remove the cast. Heat from the cast isn't a sign of infection.
CN: Physiological integrity; CNS: Reduction of risk potential; CL: Application

83. 3. To prevent foot drop in a casted leg, the foot should be supported with 90 degrees of flexion. Bed rest can cause foot drop. Keeping the extremity warm won't prevent foot drop.
CN: Health promotion and maintenance; CNS: None; CL: Application

84. 4. A client with a hip-spica cast should avoid gas-forming foods to prevent abdominal distention. Gas-forming foods may cause flatus, but that isn't a reason to avoid them. Gas-forming foods don't generally cause diarrhea or constipation.
CN: Physiological integrity; CNS: Reduction of risk potential; CL: Application

85. 4. Touch-down weight bearing allows the client to put no weight on the extremity, but the client may touch the floor with the affected extremity. Full weight bearing allows for full weight bearing on the affected extremity. Partial weight bearing allows for only 30% to 50% weight bearing on the affected extremity. Non–weight bearing is no weight on the extremity, and the extremity must remain elevated.
CN: Physiological integrity; CNS: Basic care and comfort; CL: Application

86. Which strategy should a nurse teach an adolescent to prevent sports-related injuries?
1. Warming up
2. Pacing activity
3. Building strength
4. Moderating intensity

87. Which activity may be most helpful for a child who's allowed full activity after repair of a clubfoot?
1. Playing catch
2. Standing
3. Swimming
4. Walking

88. The parent of an infant diagnosed with clubfoot is discussing the casting treatment regimen with the nurse. The nurse determines further instruction is not needed when the parent states that the cast will be changed:
1. in 8 weeks.
2. in 2 weeks.
3. when his child starts to walk.
4. when his child starts to crawl.

89. The X-ray result for a child who experienced a fall on the basketball court indicates a greenstick fracture of the tibia. Which graphic represents a greenstick fracture?

This warming-up activity should keep me awake for the rest of the test.

1.

2.

3.

4.

86. 1. To prevent sports-related injuries, instruct your client that the best prevention is warming up. Pacing activity, building strength, and using moderate intensity are also prevention measures.
CN: Health promotion and maintenance; CNS: None; CL: Application

87. 4. Walking will stimulate all of the involved muscles and help with strengthening. All of the options are good exercises, but walking is the best choice.
CN: Health promotion and maintenance; CNS: None; CL: Application

88. 2. Because an infant grows quickly, a series of casts will be needed as often as every 2 weeks to correct the deformity as the child grows. Eight weeks is too long to leave a cast on the rapidly growing child. Casting should be complete by the time the child is crawling and walking.
CN: Physiological integrity; CNS: Reduction of risk potential; CL: Analysis

89. 3. A greenstick fracture occurs when the bone is bent beyond its limits, causing an incomplete fracture. The first graphic is a plastic deformation or bend, where there is a microscopic fracture line where the bone bends. The second graphic shows a buckle fracture, which occurs due to compression of the porous bone, causing a raised area or bulge at the fracture site. The fourth graphic is of a complete fracture in which the bone is broken into separate pieces.
CN: Physiological integrity; CNS: Physiological adaptation; CL: Application

90. Which instruction should the nurse include in the teaching plan for a 10-year-old child with a fracture of the radial bone?
1. Report capillary refill less than 3 seconds.
2. Report warmth under the cast during the first 24 hours after application.
3. Report foul odors coming from the cast.
4. Report cool fingers that warm within 20 minutes of being covered.

The nose knows the answer to this question.

90. 3. Foul odors from the cast may be a sign of infection and should be reported to the physician immediately. Capillary refill less than 3 seconds is a normal finding. During the first 24 hours, the client may feel warmth under the cast as it dries. After 24 hours, warmth may be a sign of infection and should be reported. Cool fingers that warm up within 20 minutes of being covered are normal; cool fingers that don't warm up after 20 minutes of being covered should be reported because the client may have circulatory impairment under the cast.

CN: Physiological integrity; CNS: Reduction of risk potential; CL: Application

91. Which history finding is the <u>most significant</u> related to developmental dysplasia of the hip (DDH)?
1. Mother's activity during the third trimester
2. Breech presentation at birth
3. Infant's serum calcium level at birth
4. Apgar score of 4 at 1 minute and 6 at 5 minutes

91. 2. Breech presentation is a factor commonly associated with DDH. The mother's activity during the third trimester, the infant's serum calcium level at birth, and Apgar scores have no bearing on DDH.

CN: Health promotion and maintenance; CNS: None; CL: Application

92. A 13-year old with structural scoliosis has Harrington rods inserted. Which position would be best during the postoperative period?
1. Supine in bed
2. Side-lying
3. Semi-Fowler's
4. High Fowler's

92. 1. After placement of Harrington rods, the client must remain flat in bed. The gatch on a manual bed should be taped, and electric beds should be unplugged to prevent the client from raising the head or foot of the bed. Other positions, such as side-lying, semi-Fowler's, or high Fowler's, could prove damaging because the rods may not be able to maintain the spine in a straight position.

CN: Physiological integrity; CNS: Reduction of risk potential; CL: Application

Remember you're looking for the nursing diagnosis with the highest priority.

93. A nurse notes dyspnea and calf pain in a 14-year-old client 48 hours after open reduction of a fractured femur. Which nursing diagnosis has the <u>highest priority</u>?
1. Impaired gas exchange
2. Acute pain
3. Impaired physical mobility
4. Deficient knowledge

93. 1. Immobility, a fractured femur, and orthopedic surgery all increase the risk of deep vein thrombosis (DVT). The client who complains of calf pain and dyspnea should be promptly assessed for a pulmonary embolism. While all these nursing diagnoses are appropriate, assessing for impaired gas exchange has the highest priority.

CN: Physiological integrity; CNS: Reduction of risk potential; CL: Analysis

94. A 6-month-old male with developmental dysplasia of the hip has been treated for the past 6 weeks with a Frejka splint, which maintains abduction through padding of the diaper area. At his follow-up visit, the child's mother reports that she removes the splint when he gets too fussy and that he settles down and sleeps well for several hours after the padding is removed. Which response by the nurse would be most appropriate?
  1. "I can tell you're concerned about his comfort, but he must wear the padded splint except during the three times per day when you perform range-of-motion exercises on his legs."
  2. "I'm pleased that you recognize that the padding is too thick and have adjusted it so he can sleep comfortably."
  3. "I realize that seeing him uncomfortable is difficult for you, but he needs to keep his splint on except when you bathe him or change his diaper."
  4. "If he seems uncomfortable while wearing the splint, it's important that you call us immediately."

95. The nurse is caring for an 8-month-old child in Bryant's traction for a congenital abnormality of the hips. Which of the following are potential complications of traction that the nurse should be aware of? Select all that apply.
  1. Muscle strain
  2. Decubitus ulcers
  3. Diarrhea
  4. Respiratory infection
  5. Constipation

94. 3. Soft abduction devices, such as the Frejka splint, must be worn continually except for diaper changes and skin care. The abduction position must be maintained to establish a deep hip socket. Discomfort is anticipated; appropriate responses include changing position, holding, cuddling, and providing diversion.
CN: Physiological integrity; CNS: Physiological adaptation; CL: Application

95. 1, 2, 4, and 5. Muscle strain is a potential complication of Bryant's traction, and nurses should use safe handling techniques when working with the child when it is necessary to change or rebandage the traction. The weights should be inspected often to make sure they are hanging freely. Skin integrity can also be compromised, and nurses should assess skin integrity for presence of skin breakdown. Respiratory infections are a potential complication due to immobility. Part of client care should include coughing and deep breathing exercises. Constipation is a potential complication due to immobility. Client care should include adequate fluid and fiber intake.
CN: Physiological integrity; CNS: Reduction of risk potential; CL: Analysis

Remember to always be aware of "potential" complications.

96. A 14-year-old client sustained a femoral fracture and is in a hip-spica cast. The client has been on bed rest and has not had a bowel movement for 3 days. The physician has ordered Colace (docusate) 100 mg by mouth twice daily. The client asks the nurse, "What is this medication for?" What is the best response by the nurse?
  1. "It causes retention of fluid in the intestinal lumen by osmotic effect."
  2. "It increases peristalsis by irritating the colon wall and stimulates the enteric nerves."
  3. "It absorbs water, increasing bulk, which stimulates peristalsis."
  4. "It lubricates the intestinal tract and softens the feces, making hard stools easier to pass."

96. 4. A client with a hip-spica cast is at risk for constipation due to decreased physical activity and use of pain medications. While the first line of defense is a diet high in bulk and roughage, if these measures are not effective, the physician may order a stool softener to promote bowel movements. Answer choice 1 is incorrect; this is the effect of saline or osmotic solutions. Answer choice 2 is incorrect; this is caused by stimulants. Answer choice 3 is incorrect; this is the effect of bulk-forming medications.
CN: Physiological adaptation; CNS: Pharmacology; CL: Application

97. A nurse is explaining discharge instructions to a client with a fractured right femur who lives alone. The nurse determines that the client understands the instructions when he makes which of the following statements? Select all that apply.
1. "I can get the cast wet and allow it to air dry."
2. "I will move the joints above and below the cast regularly."
3. "I can remove the padding at the top of the cast to scratch underneath it if it is bothering me."
4. "I will report any foul odor under the cast to my physician."
5. "I can use a hair dryer on the cool setting for any itching."
6. "I will apply ice directly over the fracture site for 20 minutes a day."

98. A 15-year-old male with structural scoliosis has Harrington rods inserted. Following routine postoperative care, the nurse monitors the following laboratory values. Three days after the operation, which of the following lab values would the nurse report to the physician?
1. Hemoglobin (Hgb) 14 gm/dL; hematocrit (Hct) 41%
2. Na 135; K+ 4.0 mEq/L
3. White blood cells (WBC) 17,000 × 10³/mm³
4. Platelet count 400.00/cu/mm

99. A 7-year-old boy is admitted to the pediatric unit following a car accident and treatment of a fractured femur of the right leg. The physician orders morphine 0.02 mg/kg I.V. for severe pain control. The client weighs 52 lb and is experiencing pain of 9 out of 10 on the pain scale. What is the dosage of morphine that the nurse will administer to this client?
_____ milligrams

97. 2, 4, and 5. To offset some of the potential problems associated with prolonged immobility, the client should use range-of-motion exercises on the uninvolved joints. Foul odor can be a sign of a potential infection or complication and should be reported to the physician for further assessment. The client can use a hair dryer set on a cool setting and directed under the cast for itching. The client should not get the cast wet, but if the client has a fiberglass cast, the client can dry the cast thoroughly after exposure to water by blotting it dry with a towel and using a hair dryer on a low setting until the cast is thoroughly dry. The client should not remove any of the protective padding from the cast or scratch underneath the cast with any object; this predisposes the client to skin breakdown and infection. Ice should be applied during the first 24 hours postoperatively by placing the ice in a plastic bag, with the cast covered with a cloth for protection.

CN: Physiological integrity; CNS: Basic care and comfort; CL: Application

98. 3. A WBC of 17,000 is indicative of an infection and should be reported to the physician. The other answers are normal laboratory values for 13- to 18-year olds include the following: Hgb: 12.0 to 15.2 gm/dL, Hct: 36% to 47%, Platelets: 150.00 to 450.00/cu/mm.

CN: Physiological integrity; CNS: Reduction of risk potential; CL: Analysis

99. 0.47. Convert the weight from pounds to kilograms. (One kilogram equals 2.2 lb).

52 (lb) ÷ 2.2 (kg) = 23.6 kg

Dosage calculation

23.6 kg × 0.02 mg = 0.47 mg

Morphine dosage (http://www.drugs.com/dosage/morphine.html#Usual_Pediatric_Dose_for_Pain):

Age: ≥ 1 month but < 12 years: I.V./subcutaneous continuous: 0.025 to 0.206 mg/kg/hour (sickle cell or cancer pain) or 0.01 to 0.04 mg/kg/hour (postoperative pain); maximum per 24 hours: 5 mg.

CN: Physiological integrity; CNS: Pharmacological therapies; CL: Application

100. The nurse is caring for a 15-year-old female client whose mother and grandmother both have osteoporosis. The client asks the nurse if there are any foods that she could include in her diet to help prevent osteoporosis. The best response by the nurse is: Select all that apply.
1. American cheese.
2. 8 oz container of yogurt.
3. potatoes.
4. sardines.
5. eggs.
6. spinach.

101. The nurse is managing the care of a client with osteoarthritis (OA). Appropriate interventions for osteoarthritis include which of the following? Select all that apply.
1. Continuous complete bed rest
2. Administration of muscle relaxants such as Flexeril
3. Administration of herbals and nutritional supplements
4. Use of nonsteroidal anti-inflammatory drugs (NSAIDs)
5. Daily strenuous physical therapy to involved joints
6. Weight reduction

102. A nurse is caring for a 2-year-old child who weighs 25 lb (11.3 kg) and has a simple fracture of his femur. For this client, which <u>initial</u> treatment is <u>most</u> likely?
1. Setting the fracture with a pin during surgery
2. Placing the child in skeletal traction
3. Immediately setting and casting the fractured leg
4. Putting the child in Bryant's traction

103. A female client, age 15 months, has just had a hip-spica cast applied. Which nursing intervention is a <u>priority</u> for this client?
1. Limit fluids so she won't urinate often and won't risk getting the cast wet.
2. Instruct the parents on how to get their child home in the car.
3. Assess sensation, circulation, and motion of her feet and toes.
4. Avoid giving her pain medication so she won't become constipated.

100. 1, 2, 4, and 6. American cheese, yogurt, sardines, and spinach are all good sources of calcium. Potatoes and eggs are considered poor sources of calcium.
CN: Physiological integrity; CNS: Reduction of risk potential; CL: Analysis

101. 3, 4, and 6. Nutritional supplements such as glucosamine and chondroitin sulfate may be helpful for some clients in improving joint mobility and relieving moderate to severe arthritis pain in the knees. NSAIDS can be used for clients who are not getting adequate pain relief with acetaminophen. If the client is overweight, a plan to reduce the client's weight is an important part of the total treatment plan.
CN: Physiological integrity; CNS: Reduction of risk potential; CL: Analysis

102. 4. Bryant's traction is the usual method for treating a child younger than age 3 and weighing less than 35 lb (15.9 kg). Surgery and pin placement is an invasive treatment that isn't usually needed. Skeletal traction is used for older children. For a femur fracture to heal properly, it usually requires traction before casting.
CN: Physiological integrity; CNS: Reduction of risk potential; CL: Application

103. 3. Assessing sensation, circulation, and motion is necessary in all children with a cast. Fluids should be encouraged; careful diapering and padding will keep the cast dry. Instructions about discharge can be shared with the parents at a later date. Children experiencing pain should receive medication as needed.
CN: Safe, effective care environment; CNS: Management of care; CL: Application

104. A 16-year-old male client was injured in a motorcycle accident and fractured his left tibia and fibula. He's in a long leg cast and complains of deep pain unrelieved by analgesics. The nurse suspects this client may be developing which condition?
1. Volkmann's contracture
2. Dupuytren's contracture
3. Compartment syndrome
4. Peroneal nerve compression

105. A 6-year-old boy is admitted to a pediatric unit for treatment of osteomyelitis. The nurse knows that osteomyelitis is most commonly caused by which organism?
1. *Staphylococcus epidermidis*
2. *Escherichia coli* O157.H7
3. *Pneumocystis carinii*
4. *Staphylococcus aureus*

I admit it! I'm the common cause.

106. A 14-year-old girl was recently fitted with a full back brace for scoliosis. Which response by the girl indicates she understands when she must wear the brace?
1. "I can leave the brace off for school parties."
2. "I have to wear the brace all the time, except when bathing."
3. "I can take the brace off for a couple of hours if my back starts to hurt."
4. "I only have to wear the brace for a couple of weeks."

107. A 16-year-old client had a full body cast applied 3 days ago. She's diaphoretic, tachycardic, and tachypneic. Which condition is the client <u>most likely</u> experiencing?
1. Pneumonia
2. Compartment syndrome
3. Anxiety
4. Decreased intestinal motility

104. 3. Deep pain unrelieved by analgesics is an important sign of compartment syndrome, which may occur with a crush injury or when a fracture is reduced. Compartment syndrome occurs when swelling associated with inflammation reduces blood flow to the affected areas; casting causes additional constriction of blood flow. Volkmann's contracture is a contraction of the fingers and sometimes the wrist that occurs after severe injury or improper use of a tourniquet or cast. Dupuytren's contracture is a flexion deformity of the fingers or toes caused by shortening, thickening, and fibrosis of the palmar or plantar fascia. Peroneal nerve compression is compression of the nerve that innervates the calf and foot.
CN: Physiological integrity; CNS: Physiological adaptation; CL: Analysis

105. 4. *S. aureus* is the most common causative pathogen of osteomyelitis; the usual source of the infection is an upper respiratory infection. *S. epidermidis* is a microorganism found on the skin of healthy individuals. *E. coli* O157.H7, which is in uncooked meat, can cause a severe case of diarrhea. *P. carinii* causes pneumonia in clients with human immunodeficiency virus or acquired immunodeficiency syndrome but doesn't normally cause healthy individuals to become ill.
CN: Physiological integrity; CNS: Physiological adaptation; CL: Application

106. 2. A brace must be worn at all times except for bathing. It can't be removed for other reasons including parties and discomfort. Most braces must be worn for several months to 1 year.
CN: Physiological integrity; CNS: Reduction of risk potential; CL: Analysis

107. 3. The client is exhibiting signs and symptoms of anxiety most likely caused by the feeling of being claustrophobic. Pneumonia usually presents with fever and coughing. A client with compartment syndrome would exhibit signs of intense pain unrelieved by analgesics. Compression of the mesenteric blood supply can cause constipation, but the symptoms don't indicate that constipation is the most likely condition.
CN: Psychological integrity; CNS: Psychological adaptation; CL: Analysis

108. A nurse is preparing to give an I.M. injection into the left leg of a 2-year-old client. Identify the area where the nurse would give the injection.

109. A nurse is caring for a 5-year-old client who's in the terminal stages of cancer. Which statements are true? Select all that apply.
1. The parents may be at different stages in dealing with the child's impending death.
2. The child is thinking about the future and knows he may not be able to participate.
3. The dying child may become clingy and act like a toddler.
4. Whispering in the child's room will help the child cope.
5. The death of a child may have long-term disruptive effects on the family.
6. The child doesn't fully understand the concept of death.

108. The vastus lateralis muscle, located in the thigh, is the muscle into which the nurse should administer an I.M. injection for a toddler. To give the injection, the nurse should first divide the distance between the greater trochanter and the knee joints into quadrants and then inject in the center of the upper quadrant.

CN: Physiological integrity; CNS: Pharmacological and parenteral therapies; CL: Application

109. 1, 3, 5, and 6. When dealing with a dying child, parents may be at different stages of grief at different times. The child may regress in his behaviors. The stress of a child's death commonly results in divorce and behavioral problems in siblings. Preschoolers see death as temporary, a type of sleep or separation. They recognize the word "dead" but don't fully understand its meaning. Thinking about the future is typical of an adolescent facing death, not a preschooler. Whispering in front of the child only increases his fear of death.

CN: Psychosocial integrity; CNS: None; CL: Analysis

Congratulations!
You finished!
Great job!

Chapter 32
Gastrointestinal disorders

1. The nurse determines further teaching is not needed when the mother of a child with celiac disease makes which statement?
1. "I won't serve wheat, rye, oats, or barley."
2. "I will provide a diet high in gluten."
3. "I won't serve potatoes, rice, or corn bread."
4. "I can safely serve any frozen or packaged food."

2. Which goal is <u>most important</u> when teaching the parents of a child diagnosed with celiac disease?
1. Promote a normal life for the child.
2. Stress the importance of good health in preventing infection.
3. Introduce the parents and child to a peer with celiac disease.
4. Help the parents and child follow the prescribed dietary restrictions.

In question 2, the words *most important* guide you to the right answer.

3. The nurse is assessing the stool of a child with celiac disease. How would the nurse expect the stool to appear?
1. Constipated hard stool
2. Clay-colored stool
3. Red currant jelly stool
4. Foul-smelling, fatty, frothy stool

4. A client with celiac disease is being discharged from the hospital. The nurse determines that the client understands discharge instructions when the client states she can eat which foods? Select all that apply.
1. Oatmeal raisin cookie
2. Bologna sandwich
3. Pepperoni and cheese pizza made with rice flour
4. Rice cakes
5. Apple juice

1. 1. The child with celiac disease should consume a gluten-free diet, thus eliminating foods containing wheat, rye, oats, and barley. Foods containing potatoes, rice, and corn flour are permissible. The mother should read the packages of all foods carefully to ensure that they're gluten-free.
CN: Physiological integrity; CNS: Basic care and comfort; CL: Application

2. 4. It takes a long time to describe the disease process, the specific role of gluten, and the foods that must be restricted. Gluten is added to many foods but is obscurely listed on labels. To avoid hidden sources of gluten, parents need to read labels carefully. Promoting a normal life for the child, stressing good health in preventing infection, and meeting a peer with celiac disease are also important nursing considerations, but they would come after the dietary means of dealing with this chronic disease.
CN: Physiological integrity; CNS: Reduction of risk potential; CL: Analysis

3. 4. Steatorrhea (fatty, foul-smelling, frothy, bulky stools) is common because of the inability to absorb fat. Profuse and watery diarrhea, not constipated hard stool, is usually a sign of celiac crisis. Clay-colored stools are characteristic of a decrease or absence of conjugated bilirubin. Red currant jelly-type stool is an indication of intussusception.
CN: Physiological integrity; CNS: Physiological adaptation; CL: Application

4. 4 and 5. Sources of gluten found in wheat, rye, barley, and oats should be avoided. Rice and corn are suitable substitutes because they don't contain gluten. Pepperoni pizza, luncheon meat, and oatmeal cookies contain gluten and, when broken down, can't be digested by people with celiac disease. Rice cakes and apple juice do not contain gluten.
CN: Physiological integrity; CNS: Basic care and comfort; CL: Application

CN: Client needs category   CNS: Client needs subcategory   CL: Cognitive level

5. The parents of a child with celiac disease ask the nurse how they can help promote a normal life for their child. What is the best response by the nurse?
1. Treat the child differently from other siblings.
2. Focus on restrictions that make him feel different.
3. Introduce the child to another peer with celiac disease.
4. Don't allow the child to express doubt in keeping with dietary restrictions.

6. The nurse is evaluating the effectiveness of nutritional therapy for a child with celiac disease. What is the most important assessment?
1. Vital signs
2. Appearance, size, and number of stools
3. Blood urea nitrogen (BUN) and serum creatinine levels
4. Intake and output

7. The nurse is caring for a child with celiac disease who has been started on the prescribed diet. The nurse expects that 1 or 2 days after starting the diet the child will have which of the following?
1. Diarrhea
2. Foul-smelling stools
3. Improved appetite
4. Weight loss

8. The nurse is planning care for a neonate with cleft lip and palate. Which issue is a <u>priority</u> of care?
1. Feeding difficulties
2. Operative care
3. Pain management
4. Parental reaction

You'll be finished before you know it!

Here's a key word to consider.

5. 3. Introducing the child to another child with celiac disease will let him know he isn't alone. It will show him how other people live a normal life with similar restrictions. Treat the child no differently from other siblings, but stress appropriate limit setting. Instead of focusing on restrictions that make him feel different, the nurse should encourage the parents to focus on ways he can be normal. Allow the child with celiac disease to express his feelings about dietary restrictions.
CN: Psychosocial integrity; CNS: None; CL: Application

6. 2. The fat, bulky, foul-smelling stools should be gone when a child with celiac disease follows a gluten-free diet. Vital signs, BUN and serum creatinine levels, and intake and output aren't affected by a gluten-free diet.
CN: Physiological integrity; CNS: Basic care and comfort; CL: Analysis

7. 3. Within a day or two of starting their diet, most children with celiac disease show improved appetite, disappearance of diarrhea, and weight gain. It takes longer than 2 days for steatorrhea (fatty, oily, foul-smelling stools) to subside.
CN: Physiological integrity; CNS: Physiological adaptation; CL: Application

8. 4. Parents typically show strong negative responses to this deformity. They may mourn the loss of the perfect child. Helping the parents cope with their child's condition is the first step. Feeding issues are important, but parents must first cope with the reality of their neonate's condition. Surgical repair is usually delayed until 6 to 12 weeks of age. This deformity isn't painful.
CN: Psychosocial integrity; CNS: None; CL: Analysis

9. The nurse is assessing an infant who has just returned to the pediatric unit after undergoing a cleft lip repair. The nurse is aware of the potential for trauma to the suture line and determines that which of the following is the best intervention?
1. Placing mittens on the infant's hands
2. Maintaining arm restraints
3. Not allowing the parents to touch the infant
4. Removing the lip device from the infant after surgery

10. To prevent tissue infection and breakdown after cleft palate or lip repair, a nurse should use which intervention?
1. Keep the suture line moist at all times.
2. Allow the infant to suck on his pacifier.
3. Rinse the infant's mouth with water after each feeding.
4. Follow orders from the physician to not feed the infant by mouth.

11. Which nursing intervention has the highest priority for an infant during the first 24 hours after surgery for cleft lip repair?
1. Carefully clean the suture line using sterile technique after feedings to reduce the risk of infection.
2. Position the infant in the prone position after feedings to promote drainage.
3. Allow the infant to cry to promote lung expansion.
4. Encourage the infant to use a pacifier to satisfy the urge to suck.

12. The nurse is teaching parents how to feed their infant who has a cleft palate. The nurse teaches the parents to apply gentle steady pressure to the base of the bottle. The nurse explains that this will:
1. reduce the risk of choking or coughing.
2. prevent further damage to the affected area.
3. decrease the amount of formula lost while eating.
4. decrease the amount of noise the infant makes when eating.

You're off to a great start.

9. 2. Arm restraints are used to prevent the infant from rubbing the sutures. Placing mittens alone won't prevent the infant from rubbing the suture line. Parental contact will increase the infant's comfort. The lip device shouldn't be removed.
CN: Physiological integrity; CNS: Reduction of risk potential; CL: Analysis

10. 3. To prevent formula buildup around the suture line, the mouth is usually rinsed. The sutures should be kept dry at all times. Placing objects in the mouth is generally avoided after surgery. Infants are fed by mouth using the syringe technique.
CN: Physiological integrity; CNS: Physiological adaptation; CL: Analysis

11. 1. The suture line must be cleaned after each feeding to reduce the risk of infection, which could adversely affect the healing and cosmetic results. The incision should be cleaned carefully so the sutures are not disrupted. A sterile solution should be used to reduce the risk of infection. The infant shouldn't be placed on his abdomen in the prone position because this puts pressure on the incision and may affect healing. Anticipatory care should be provided to reduce the risk of the infant crying, which puts pressure on the incision. Pacifiers and other firm objects shouldn't be placed in the infant's mouth because they can disrupt the suture line.
CN: Physiological integrity; CNS: Reduction of risk potential; CL: Application

12. 1. Children with cleft palate or lip have a greater risk of choking while eating, so all measures are used to reduce this risk. Steady pressure creates a seal when the nipple is against the cleft palate or lip, reducing the risk of aspiration. The nurse can't cause more damage to an infant's cleft lip or palate unless proper precautions aren't followed postoperatively. If the nipple is cut correctly and proper procedures are followed, the infant won't lose a lot of formula during a feeding. Infants with cleft palate or lip usually make more noise while eating.
CN: Physiological integrity; CNS: Reduction of risk potential; CL: Application

CN: Client needs category   CNS: Client needs subcategory   CL: Cognitive level

13. The pediatric unit has just been notified that they will be admitting an infant with cleft lip and palate. What is the best nursing intervention to implement when feeding the infant?
1. Burp the infant often.
2. Limit the amount the infant eats.
3. Feed the infant at scheduled times.
4. Remove the nipple if the infant is making loud noises.

14. Which intervention is essential in the nursing care of an infant with cleft lip or palate?
1. Discourage breastfeeding.
2. Hold the infant flat while feeding.
3. Involve the parents as soon as possible.
4. Use a normal nursery nipple for feedings.

15. The parents of an infant born with cleft lip and palate are seeing the infant for the first time. The nurse caring for the infant should focus on which area?
1. The infant's positive features
2. Irritation with how the infant eats
3. Ambivalence in caring for an infant with this defect
4. Dissatisfaction with the infant's physical appearance

16. Following repair of a cleft lip in a 3-month-old infant, the mother asks the nurse what would be the most appropriate toy to bring the infant. What is the best response by the nurse?
1. A plastic teething ring
2. A stuffed animal
3. A mobile to hang over the crib
4. Children's books

I'll bet you feel better now.

Here's where to show your compassion.

13. 1. Infants with cleft lip and palate have a tendency to swallow an excessive amount of air and need to be burped frequently during feedings. The amount of formula they eat at each feeding is the same as an infant without cleft lip or palate. Loud noises are common when these infants eat, and scheduled feedings aren't necessary.
CN: Physiological integrity; CNS: Physiological adaptation; CL: Application

14. 3. The sooner the parents become involved, the quicker they're able to determine the method of feeding best suited for them and the infant. Breastfeeding, like bottle feeding, may be difficult but can be facilitated if the mother intends to breastfeed. Feedings are usually given in the upright position to prevent formula from coming through the nose. Various special nipples have been devised for infants with cleft lip or palate; a normal nursery nipple isn't effective. Sometimes, especially if the cleft isn't severe, breastfeeding may be easier because the human nipple conforms to the shape of the infant's mouth.
CN: Physiological integrity; CNS: Physiological adaptation; CL: Application

15. 1. To relieve the parents' anxiety, positive aspects of the infant's physical appearance need to be emphasized. Showing optimism toward surgical correction and showing a photograph of possible cosmetic improvements may be helpful. Because this is the parents' first encounter with the infant, there isn't any indication of irritation, ambivalence, or dissatisfaction.
CN: Psychosocial integrity; CNS: None; CL: Application

16. 3. Given the infant's age, a mobile would be the most appropriate toy because he doesn't have the manual dexterity to play with a stuffed animal. The mobile would provide the infant with visual stimulation. A plastic teething ring and a stuffed animal should be avoided because they can disrupt the suture line if the infant sucks on them. The infant wouldn't be able to understand children's stories but may enjoy the sound of another person's voice. A mobile, however, could be used when no one was around to read.
CN: Physiological integrity; CNS: None; CL: Analysis

17. The mother of a neonate born with a cleft lip and palate is preparing to feed the baby for the first time. The most important information for the nurse to give the mother is:
1. burp the neonate.
2. clean the mouth.
3. hold the neonate in an upright position.
4. prepare the bottle using a normal nursery nipple.

18. An infant returns from surgery after repair of a cleft palate. What is the priority nursing intervention?
1. Offer a pacifier for comfort.
2. Position the infant on his side.
3. Suction the mouth and nose of all secretions.
4. Remove the arm restraints placed on the infant after surgery.

19. A small child has undergone surgical repair of a cleft palate and is ready for discharge. What is the most important information for the nurse to tell the parents?
1. Continue a normal diet.
2. Continue using arm restraints at home.
3. Don't allow the child to drink from a cup.
4. Establish good mouth care and proper brushing.

20. What is the best position for the nurse to place an infant in following cleft lip and palate repair to irrigate the mouth after feeding?
1. Supine with the head to the side
2. Fowler's position with the head to the side
3. Upright with the head tilted forward
4. Prone with the head over the side of the bed

21. The parents of an infant who had cleft lip repair ask the nurse how the area will appear when it is healed. What is the best response by the nurse?
1. A large scar on the lip
2. An abnormally large upper lip
3. A distorted jaw
4. Minimal scarring

There are many things to teach this mother, so what do you teach her *first*?

Client teaching includes the family.

17. 3. When neonates are held in the upright position, the formula is less likely to leak out of the nose or mouth. Neonates need to be burped frequently but not before a feeding. There's no need to clean the mouth before eating. After surgical repair, the mouth is cleaned at the suture site to prevent infection. The bottle should be prepared using a special nipple or feeding device.
CN: Physiological integrity; CNS: Physiological adaptation; CL: Application

18. 2. The infant should be positioned on his side to allow oral secretions to drain from the mouth and avoid suctioning. Pacifiers shouldn't be used because they can damage the suture line. Arm restraints should be kept on to protect the suture line. The restraints should be removed periodically to allow for full range of motion during this time. Only one restraint should be removed at a time, and the infant should be closely supervised.
CN: Physiological integrity; CNS: Reduction of risk potential; CL: Analysis

19. 2. Arm restraints are also used at home to keep the child's hands away from the mouth until the palate is healed. A soft diet is recommended; no food harder than mashed potatoes can be eaten. Fluids are best taken from a cup. Proper mouth care is encouraged after the palate is healed.
CN: Physiological integrity; CNS: Physiological adaptation; CL: Application

20. 3. Following repair of a cleft palate, the nurse should irrigate the infant's mouth with the infant in an upright position and head tilted forward to prevent aspiration. A supine or Fowler's position with the head to the side won't prevent aspiration. The prone position isn't appropriate following cleft lip repair because this may put pressure on the suture line.
CN: Physiological integrity; CNS: Reduction of risk potential; CL: Application

21. 4. If there's no trauma or infection to the site, healing occurs with little scar formation. There may be some inflammation right after surgery, but after healing, the lip is a normal size. No jaw malformation occurs with cleft lip repair.
CN: Physiological integrity; CNS: Physiological adaptation; CL: Application

22. The nurse would explain to the parents of a newborn with a cleft lip and palate that they will need to schedule an appointment with which specialist?
1. Cardiologist
2. Neurologist
3. Nutritionist
4. Otolaryngologist

23. The nurse is most concerned when a neonate with esophageal atresia and tracheoesophageal fistula presents with:
1. bulging eyeballs.
2. sunken anterior fontanelle.
3. skin that returns briskly when pinched.
4. fluctuating weight gain.

24. Feedings are being withheld in a neonate with esophageal atresia and tracheoesophageal fistula until a gastrostomy tube can be placed. What is the most appropriate nursing intervention to implement when the neonate is irritable and crying?
1. Offer him a pacifier.
2. Encourage his parents to talk to him.
3. Encourage his parents to hold him.
4. Distract him by placing a mobile over the crib.

25. Which assessment finding indicates to a nurse that a neonate born with esophageal atresia needs suctioning?
1. Cyanosis
2. Decreased production of saliva
3. Inability to cough
4. Inadequate swallow

26. A neonate is suspected of having esophageal atresia. The nurse is aware that a definitive diagnostic evaluation would include which factor?
1. Decreased breath sounds
2. Absence of bowel sounds
3. How the neonate tolerates eating
4. Ability to pass a catheter down the esophagus

This will help satisfy the infant's need to suck.

It's time to take action.

CYANOSIS

22. **4.** An otolaryngologist is used because ear infections are common, along with hearing loss. Cardiac and brain function is usually normal. A nutritionist isn't needed unless the neonate becomes malnourished.
CN: Safe, effective care environment; CNS: Management of care; CL: Application

23. **2.** A sunken anterior fontanelle is a sign of dehydration in the neonate whose fontanelle hasn't yet closed. Bulging eyeballs are sign of overhydration. Fluctuating weight gain is not a sign of dehydration. Skin that returns quickly when pinched is a sign of adequate hydration.
CN: Physiological integrity; CNS: Reduction of risk potential; CL: Application

24. **1.** A neonate who's unable to suck to obtain nutrition may be comforted if given a pacifier to satisfy his need to suck. Encouraging his parents to hold and talk to him and placing a mobile over the crib are appropriate interventions but won't satisfy a newborn as much as a pacifier.
CN: Physiological integrity; CNS: Basic care and comfort; CL: Analysis

25. **1.** Cyanosis occurs when fluid from the blind pouch is aspirated into the trachea, requiring suctioning. Increased saliva production is common, along with choking, coughing, and sneezing. The ability to swallow isn't affected by this disorder.
CN: Physiological integrity; CNS: Physiological adaptation; CL: Analysis

26. **4.** A moderately stiff catheter will meet resistance if the esophagus is blocked and will pass unobstructed if the esophagus is patent. Breath sounds are normal unless aspiration occurs. The intestinal tract isn't affected with this anomaly, so bowel sounds are present. If a neonate doesn't tolerate eating, it doesn't mean he has an esophageal atresia.
CN: Physiological integrity; CNS: Physiological adaptation; CL: Analysis

27. A neonate has been diagnosed with a tracheoesophageal fistula. The nurse is aware that the treatment plan will include which measure?
1. Starting antibiotic therapy
2. Keeping the neonate lying flat
3. Continuing feedings
4. Removing the diagnostic catheter from the esophagus

28. A nurse suspects an infant may have a tracheoesophageal fistula or esophageal atresia. What is the <u>most important</u> intervention by the nurse?
1. Give oxygen.
2. Tell the parents.
3. Put the neonate in an Isolette or on a radiant warmer.
4. Report the suspicion to the physician.

Question 28 asks you to prioritize your care.

29. The nurse is aware that an infant who had surgical repair of a tracheoesophageal fistula is most at risk for which of the following?
1. Atelectasis
2. Choking during feeding attempts
3. Damaged vocal cords
4. Infection

I feel so bloated!

30. The nurse is caring for an infant suspected of having esophageal atresia and tracheoesophageal fistula. Which sign would the nurse <u>initially</u> observe?
1. Abdominal distention
2. Decreased oral secretions
3. Normal respiratory effort
4. Scaphoid abdomen

27. 1. Antibiotic therapy is started because aspiration pneumonia is inevitable and appears early. The neonate's head is usually kept in an upright position to prevent aspiration. I.V. fluids are started, and the neonate isn't allowed oral intake. The catheter is left in the upper esophageal pouch to easily remove fluid that collects there.
CN: Physiological integrity; CNS: Pharmacological and parenteral therapies; CL: Analysis

28. 4. The physician needs to be told so that immediate diagnostic tests can be done for a definitive diagnosis and surgical correction. Oxygen should be given only after notifying the physician, except in the case of an emergency. It isn't the nurse's responsibility to inform the parents of the suspected finding. By the time tracheoesophageal fistula or esophageal atresia is suspected, the neonate would have already been placed in an Isolette or a radiant warmer.
CN: Physiological integrity; CNS: Physiological adaptation; CL: Analysis

29. 1. Respiratory complications (atelectasis) are a threat to the neonate's life preoperatively and postoperatively because of the continual risk of aspiration. Choking is more likely to occur preoperatively, although careful attention is paid postoperatively when neonates begin to eat to make sure they can swallow without choking. Vocal cord damage isn't common after this repair. The neonate is generally given antibiotics preoperatively to prevent infection.
CN: Physiological integrity; CNS: Physiological adaptation; CL: Analysis

30. 1. Crying may force air into the stomach, causing distention. Secretions in a client with this condition may be more visible, although normal in quantity, because of the client's inability to swallow effectively. Respiratory effort is usually more difficult. When no distal fistula is present, the abdomen will appear scaphoid.
CN: Physiological integrity; CNS: Physiological adaptation; CL: Application

31. The nurse is providing information on dietary management to a child diagnosed with ulcerative colitis. The nurse should teach the child the importance of which diet?
1. High-calorie diet
2. High-residue diet
3. Low-protein diet
4. Low-salt diet

32. A neonate returns from the operating room after surgical repair of a tracheoesophageal fistula and esophageal atresia. Which nursing intervention should be performed <u>immediately</u>?
1. Maintain a patent airway.
2. Start feedings right away.
3. Let the parents hold the neonate right away.
4. Suction the endotracheal tube, stopping when resistance is met.

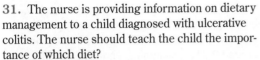

Immediately means, you know, right away!

33. The nurse is providing discharge instructions to the parents of a neonate who has undergone repair of a tracheoesophageal fistula and esophageal atresia. What is the most important information for the nurse to tell the parents?
1. Give antibiotics through the feeding tube.
2. Maintain proper care of a chest tube.
3. Maintain proper positioning for feedings.
4. Utilize tips for preventing crying.

34. Which nursing intervention should be done postoperatively for a neonate after the repair of a tracheoesophageal fistula and esophageal atresia?
1. Withhold mouth care.
2. Offer a pacifier frequently.
3. Decrease tactile stimulation.
4. Use restraints to prevent injury to the repair.

35. A client is admitted with a history of tracheoesophageal fistula and esophageal atresia repair. The nurse is aware that the client is at risk for which of the following?
1. Oral aversion
2. Gastroesophageal reflux
3. Inability to tolerate feedings
4. Strictures

Hmmm. Now I have to think what are you at risk for???

31. 1. A high-calorie diet is given to combat weight loss and restore nitrogen balance. A low-residue or residue-free diet is encouraged to decrease bowel irritation. A high-protein diet is also encouraged. Salt reduction isn't a factor in this disease.
CN: Physiological integrity; CNS: Basic care and comfort; CL: Analysis

32. 1. Maintaining a patent airway is essential until sedation from surgery wears off. Feedings usually aren't started for at least 48 hours after surgery. Parents are encouraged to participate in the neonate's care but not immediately after surgery. The catheter should be measured before suctioning so the tube doesn't meet resistance, which could cause damage.
CN: Safe, effective care environment; CNS: Management of care; CL: Application

33. 3. The neonate should be kept in an upright position after feeding to reduce the risk of refluxed stomach contents and aspiration pneumonia. Although antibiotics are given after surgery, they're discontinued before discharge. Because the chest cavity is entered during surgery, the neonate may have a chest tube inserted that's removed prior to discharge. Because lung expansion is important following chest surgery, vigorous crying helps expand the lungs and shouldn't be discouraged.
CN: Physiological integrity; CNS: Basic care and comfort; CL: Application

34. 2. Meeting the neonate's oral needs, such as by offering him a pacifier, is important because he can't drink from a bottle. The nurse should give mouth care to this neonate. The nurse should provide tactile stimulation. Restraints should be avoided, if possible.
CN: Physiological integrity; CNS: Physiological adaptation; CL: Application

35. 4. Strictures of the anastomosis occur in 40% to 50% of the cases. Oral aversion can be a problem, but it occurs quickly after surgery. Reflux is a common complication but appears when feedings are started. If the neonate is having problems tolerating feedings, it's quickly noted.
CN: Physiological integrity; CNS: Physiological adaptation; CL: Application

36. The nurse observes a neonate who is having excessive salivation and drooling, accompanied by coughing, choking, and sneezing. The nurse suspects the neonate has which condition?
1. Cleft lip
2. Cleft palate
3. Gastroschisis
4. Tracheoesophageal fistula and esophageal atresia

37. Which nursing diagnosis takes the highest priority during the first 24 hours following surgical repair of esophageal atresia and tracheoesophageal fistula?
1. Ineffective airway clearance
2. Imbalanced nutrition: Less than body requirements
3. Risk for impaired parenting
4. Ineffective infant feeding pattern

38. An infant was born with a portion of an organ protruding through an abnormal opening. The nurse explains to the parents that this structural defect is called what?
1. Omphalocele
2. Meckel's diverticulum
3. Gastroschisis
4. Tracheoesophageal fistula

39. When an infant is diagnosed with a diaphragmatic hernia on the <u>left side</u>, which abdominal organ may be found in the thorax?
1. Appendix
2. Descending colon
3. Right kidney
4. Spleen

40. When assessing an infant diagnosed with a diaphragmatic hernia, the nurse would expect the mediastinum to:
1. not shift.
2. shift to the affected side.
3. shift to the unaffected side.
4. partially shift to the affected or unaffected sides.

Think surgery for an esophageal disorder, and then prioritize.

Hmmm, which way did that mediastinum go?

36. 4. Because tracheoesophageal fistula and esophageal atresia cause an ineffective swallow, saliva and secretions appear in the mouth and around the lips. Coughing, choking, and sneezing occur for the same reason and usually after an attempt at eating. Cleft lip and palate don't produce excessive salivation. None of these symptoms occurs with gastroschisis.
CN: Physiological integrity; CNS: Physiological adaptation; CL: Application

37. 1. The priority nursing diagnosis for the first postoperative day is ineffective airway clearance. The nurse must assess the infant's airway for the buildup of mucus and other secretions. The nurse must also perform a respiratory assessment and keep suction equipment, a laryngoscope, and endotracheal suction equipment immediately available. The other nursing diagnoses are all important in the infant in the immediate postoperative period, but assessing and maintaining a patent airway is the greatest priority.
CN: Physiological integrity; CNS: Reduction or risk potential; CL: Analysis

38. 3. Gastroschisis is a herniation of the bowel through an abnormal opening in the abdominal wall with no covering membrane. An omphalocele is an abdominal wall defect with herniated viscera with covering membrane. Meckel's diverticulum is a pouch on the wall of the lower intestine. Tracheoesophageal fistula is a malformation of the trachea and esophagus.
CN: Physiological integrity; CNS: Physiological adaptation; CL: Application

39. 4. The spleen has commonly been seen in the thorax of infants with this defect. The appendix and descending colon usually don't protrude into the thorax because of limited space from the other organs present. The right kidney wouldn't be seen with a left-sided defect.
CN: Physiological integrity; CNS: Physiological adaptation; CL: Analysis

40. 3. The increased volume in the chest cavity from the abdominal organs causes the mediastinum to shift to the unaffected side, which causes a partial collapse of that lung. Because of the increased volume on the affected side, the mediastinum can't shift that way.
CN: Physiological integrity; CNS: Physiological adaptation; CL: Analysis

41. What is the <u>best</u> way for a nurse to position an infant with a diaphragmatic hernia before surgery?
1. On the affected side
2. On the unaffected side
3. Supine
4. Trendelenburg's position

Which position would help us expand?

42. Before surgery, which nursing intervention should be used for an infant with a diaphragmatic hernia?
1. Feed the infant.
2. Provide tactile stimulation.
3. Prevent the infant from crying.
4. Place the infant on the unaffected side.

43. What is the <u>most important</u> intervention for the nurse to implement when caring for a neonate with an omphalocele?
1. Keep the omphalocele dry.
2. Don't let the parents see the omphalocele.
3. Carefully position and handle the omphalocele.
4. Touch the omphalocele often to assess any changes.

44. What is the most appropriate toy for a nurse to give to an 8-month-old infant admitted for repair of a diaphragmatic hernia?
1. Large building blocks
2. Colorful, plastic, multitextured rattle
3. Black-and-white mobile
4. Colorful pull toys

Shake, rattle, and roll!

41. 1. Positioning the infant on the affected side lets the lung on the unaffected side expand, making breathing easier. Positioning the infant on the unaffected side or in Trendelenburg's position would further diminish respiration and would increase pressure in the chest cavity, compromising respirations. Supine position doesn't facilitate lung expansion.
CN: Physiological integrity; CNS: Basic care and comfort; CL: Analysis

42. 3. To prevent the intestines from being pulled into the chest cavity by the negative pressure caused by crying, it should be avoided. The stomach and intestine in the chest cavity may also become distended with swallowed air from crying. The infant usually isn't fed until after surgery. Tactile stimulation is limited because it may disturb the infant's fragile condition. The infant is always placed on the affected side.
CN: Physiological integrity; CNS: Physiological adaptation; CL: Application

43. 3. Careful positioning and handling prevent infection and rupture of the omphalocele. The omphalocele is kept moist until the neonate is taken to the operating room. The parents can see the defect if they so choose. Touching it often increases the risk of infection.
CN: Physiological integrity; CNS: Physiological adaptation; CL: Application

44. 2. By 8 months old, an infant can transfer toys and enjoys different textures, making a colorful plastic rattle with different textures an age-appropriate toy. Newborns enjoy the visual stimulation of black-and-white mobiles. Large building blocks and pull toys are appropriate for toddlers.
CN: Health promotion and maintenance; CNS: None; CL: Analysis

45. An adolescent who has a nasogastric (NG) tube in place following surgery for a ruptured appendix reports feeling nauseated. What is the most appropriate action by the nurse?
1. Provide oral hygiene.
2. Measure the gastric drainage.
3. Assess serum electrolytes.
4. Irrigate the tube.

45. 4. When a client with an NG tube complains of nausea, the nurse should first determine the position of the tube and then irrigate it to check for patency. A clogged tube allows contents to accumulate in the stomach, contributing to nausea. Oral hygiene is important to promote comfort but isn't the most appropriate intervention here. Measuring the gastric drainage is important but won't relieve nausea. Serum electrolytes should be monitored in the client with an NG tube. Although an electrolyte imbalance may cause nausea, the tube should first be checked for patency.
CN: Physiological integrity; CNS: Reduction of risk potential; CL: Application

46. What is the most appropriate nursing intervention for an infant with pyloric stenosis who is vomiting?
1. Place the infant in a supine position to sleep.
2. Weigh the infant every 8 hours.
3. Assess for signs of dehydration.
4. Assess vital signs every 8 hours.

46. 3. Because the infant is vomiting, the nurse should assess for signs and symptoms of dehydration. The infant should be placed on the right side to sleep to prevent aspiration of vomitus. The infant should be weighed daily, not every 8 hours. Vital signs should be assessed every 4 hours until stable.
CN: Physiological integrity; CNS: Reduction of risk potential; CL: Application

A 6-month-old should have no Moro of this reflex... get it?

47. The nurse is performing an admission assessment on a 6-month-old infant being admitted for intestinal obstruction. The nurse is most concerned when the assessment reveals which finding?
1. Moro reflex
2. Positive Babinski reflex
3. Eruption of the first tooth
4. Rolling from stomach to back

47. 1. By 6 months of age, the Moro reflex should no longer be observed. Positive Babinski reflex, eruption of the first tooth, and rolling from stomach to back are all normal for a 6-month-old infant.
CN: Health promotion and maintenance; CNS: None; CL: Analysis

48. The nurse explains to an infant's parents that the pyloric canal narrows in clients with pyloric stenosis at:
1. the stomach and esophagus.
2. the stomach and duodenum.
3. both the stomach and esophagus and the stomach and duodenum.
4. the duodenum and jejunum.

48. 2. The narrowing of the pyloric canal occurs between the stomach and duodenum, where the pyloric sphincter is located. Hyperplasia and hypertrophy cause narrowing and, possibly, obstruction of the circular muscle of the pylorus.
CN: Physiological integrity; CNS: Physiological adaptation; CL: Application

49. The nurse is caring for an infant with pyloric stenosis. What is a priority assessment for this infant?
1. Loss of appetite
2. Explosive diarrhea
3. Projectile vomiting
4. Coffee ground emesis

49. 3. The obstruction doesn't allow food to pass through to the duodenum. When the stomach becomes full, the infant vomits for relief. Chronic hunger is commonly seen. There's no diarrhea because food doesn't pass the stomach. Coffee ground emesis is a result of partially digested blood in the stomach.
CN: Physiological integrity; CNS: Physiological adaptation; CL: Analysis

50. When assessing a neonate, the nurse notes visible peristaltic waves across the epigastrium. This characteristic is indicative of which disorder?
1. Hypertrophic pyloric stenosis
2. Imperforate anus
3. Intussusception
4. Short-gut syndrome

51. After surgical repair of pyloric stenosis, the nurse should expect an infant's <u>normal</u> feeding regimen to resume after what time frame?
1. 4 to 6 hours after surgery
2. 24 hours after surgery
3. 48 hours after surgery
4. 1 week after surgery

Not this kind of wave!

52. A nurse admits an infant diagnosed with pyloric stenosis. Which nursing intervention would be a <u>priority</u>?
1. Weigh the infant.
2. Check urine specific gravity.
3. Place an I.V. catheter.
4. Change the infant and weigh the diaper.

53. A nurse is caring for an infant with pyloric stenosis. After feeding the infant, the nurse should place him in which position?
1. Prone in Fowler's position
2. On his back without elevation
3. On the left side in Fowler's position
4. Slightly on the right side in high semi-Fowler's position

54. The nurse is preparing to feed an infant with pyloric stenosis prior to surgical repair. What is the most important intervention?
1. Give feedings quickly.
2. Burp the infant frequently.
3. Encourage parental participation.
4. Don't give more feedings if the infant vomits.

Here's that important positioning again!

50. 1. The diagnosis of pyloric stenosis can be established from a finding of hypertrophic pyloric stenosis. Imperforate anus, intussusception, and short-gut syndrome are each diagnosed by other characteristics.
CN: Physiological integrity; CNS: Physiological adaptation; CL: Analysis

51. 3. Small, frequent feedings of clear fluids are usually started 4 to 6 hours after surgery. If clear fluids are tolerated, formula feedings are started 24 hours after surgery, in gradually increasing amounts. It usually takes 48 hours to reach a normal full feeding regimen in this manner. The infant usually goes home on the fourth postoperative day.
CN: Physiological integrity; CNS: Physiological adaptation; CL: Application

52. 1. Weighing the infant would be done first so a baseline weight can be established and weight changes can be assessed. After a baseline weight is obtained, an I.V. catheter can be placed because oral feedings generally aren't given. These infants are usually dehydrated, so although specific gravity and checking the diaper are important tools to help assess their status, they aren't the first priority.
CN: Physiological integrity; CNS: Physiological adaptation; CL: Analysis

53. 4. Positioning the infant slightly on the right side in high semi-Fowler's position will help facilitate gastric emptying. The other positions won't facilitate gastric emptying and may cause the infant to vomit.
CN: Physiological integrity; CNS: Physiological adaptation; CL: Application

54. 2. These infants usually swallow a lot of air from sucking on their hands and fingers because of their intensive hunger (feedings aren't easily tolerated). Burping frequently will lessen gastric distention and increase the likelihood that the infant will retain the feeding. Feedings are given slowly with the infant lying in a semiupright position. Parental participation should be encouraged and allowed to the extent possible, but it does not increase the likelihood that the feeding will be retained. Record the type, amount, and character of the vomit as well as its relation to the feeding. The amount of feeding volume lost is usually refed to the infant.
CN: Physiological adaptation; CNS: Physiological adaptation; CL: Application

55. A nurse should expect which finding up to 48 hours after the surgical repair of pyloric stenosis?
1. Oliguria
2. Oral aversion
3. Scaphoid abdomen
4. Vomiting

56. Which nursing intervention will help prevent vomiting in an infant diagnosed with pyloric stenosis?
1. Hold the infant for 1 hour after feeding.
2. Handle the infant minimally after feedings.
3. Space the feedings out and give them in large amounts.
4. Lay the infant prone with the head of the bed elevated

Encourage parents to be involved with their infant's care.

57. The nurse determines that the best intervention to provide support to the parents of an infant diagnosed with pyloric stenosis would be?
1. Keep the parents informed of their infant's progress.
2. Provide all care for the infant during the parents visit.
3. Encourage the parents to minimize handling their infant while awake.
4. Ask the physician to keep the parents informed of the infant's progress.

58. An infant has been diagnosed with pyloric stenosis. The nurse would assess the infant for which symptom?
1. Apathy
2. Bradycardia
3. Dry lips and skin
4. Hypothermia

Question 59 asks what's normally found with a disease, not what's normal in a healthy infant.

59. When assessing an infant diagnosed with pyloric stenosis, the nurse would determine that which of the following is a <u>normal</u> finding?
1. Decreased or diminished bowel sounds
2. Heart murmur
3. Normal respiratory effort
4. Hyperactive bowel sounds

55. 4. Even with successful surgery, most infants have some vomiting during the first 24 to 48 hours afterward. Oliguria isn't a complication with this surgical procedure. Oral aversion doesn't occur because these infants may be fed up until surgery. Scaphoid abdomen isn't characteristic of this condition; the abdomen may appear distended, not scaphoid.
CN: Physiological integrity; CNS: Physiological adaptation; CL: Application

56. 2. Minimal handling, especially after a feeding, will help prevent vomiting. Holding the infant would provide too much stimulation, which might increase the risk of vomiting. Feedings are given frequently and slowly in small amounts. An infant should be positioned in a semi-Fowler's position and slightly on the right side after a feeding.
CN: Physiological integrity; CNS: Physiological adaptation; CL: Application

57. 1. Keeping the parents informed will decrease their anxiety. The nurse should encourage the parents to be involved with the infant's care. Telling the parents to minimize handling of the infant isn't appropriate because parent–child contact is important. The physician is responsible for updating the parents on the infant's medical condition, and the nurse is responsible for updating the parents on the day-to-day activities of the infant and his improvement with the day's activities.
CN: Psychosocial integrity; CNS: None; CL: Analysis

58. 3. Dry lips and skin are signs of dehydration, which is common in infants with pyloric stenosis. These infants are constantly hungry because of their inability to retain feedings. Apathy, bradycardia, and hypothermia aren't clinical findings with pyloric stenosis.
CN: Physiological integrity; CNS: Physiological adaptation; CL: Application

59. 1. Bowel sounds decrease because food can't pass into the intestines. Heart murmurs may be present but aren't directly associated with pyloric stenosis. Normal respiratory effort is affected by the abdominal distention that pushes the diaphragm up into the pleural cavity.
CN: Physiological integrity; CNS: Physiological adaptation; CL: Analysis

60. The nurse explains to the parents of a child with hypertrophied pylorus that the defect is located between:
1. the duodenum and jejunum.
2. the stomach and duodenum.
3. the stomach and esophagus.
4. the liver and bile ducts.

61. What is the <u>most important</u> nursing intervention when dealing with a child who has been poisoned?
1. Stabilize the child.
2. Notify the parents.
3. Identify the poison.
4. Determine when the poisoning took place.

Practice setting priorities because it's part of nursing practice.

62. A child has ingested a poisonous substance. What is the priority intervention?
1. Make the child vomit.
2. Call 911 as soon as possible.
3. Give large amounts of water to flush the system.
4. Empty the mouth of pills, plant parts, or other material.

Would you know what to do first in this emergency situation?

EMERGENCY

63. The nurse is caring for a child in the recovery phase following an ingestion of drain cleaner. The nurse is aware that the child is at risk for which of the following?
1. Esophageal strictures
2. Esophageal diverticula
3. Tracheal stenosis
4. Tracheal varices

60. **2.** This defect occurs at the pyloric sphincter, which is located between the stomach and duodenum. The jejunum, esophagus, liver, and bile ducts aren't affected by this obstructive disorder.
CN: Physiological integrity; CNS: Physiological adaptation; CL: Application

61. **1.** Stabilization and the initial emergency treatment of the child (such as respiratory assistance, circulatory support, or control of seizures) will prevent further damage to the body from the poison. If the parents didn't bring the child in, they can be notified as soon as the child is stabilized or treated. Identification of the poison is crucial and should begin at the same time as the stabilization of the child, although the initial ABCs (airway, breathing, and circulation) should be assessed first. Determining when the poisoning took place is an important consideration, but emergency stabilization and treatment are priorities.
CN: Physiological integrity; CNS: Physiological adaptation; CL: Analysis

62. **4.** Emptying the mouth of pills, plant parts, or other material will stop exposure to the poison. Making the child vomit won't remove exposure to the substance; it's also contraindicated with some poisons. Calling 911 is important, but removing any further sources of the poison would come first. Only small amounts of water are recommended so the poison is confined to the smallest volume. Large amounts of water will let the poison pass the pylorus. The small intestines will then absorb fluid rapidly, increasing the potential toxicity.
CN: Physiological integrity; CNS: Physiological adaptation; CL: Analysis

63. **1.** Scar tissue develops as the burn from the drain cleaner ingestion heals, leading to esophageal strictures. The formation of esophageal diverticula is rare. Tracheal stenosis may occur but only if the child vomited and aspirated. Tracheal varices don't commonly occur after drain cleaner ingestion.
CN: Physiological integrity; CNS: Physiological adaptation; CL: Analysis

64. A preschooler is brought to the emergency department after ingesting kerosene. The nurse is aware the child is at risk for which condition?
1. Pneumonitis
2. Carditis
3. Uremia
4. Hepatitis

65. What is the most important information for a nurse to tell parents if their child ingests a poison?
1. Administer syrup of ipecac.
2. Call the poison control center.
3. Transport the child to the emergency department.
4. Watch the child for adverse effects.

You're moving right along!

66. A child has ingested poisonous hydrocarbons. What is the most important nursing intervention?
1. Induce vomiting.
2. Keep the child calm and relaxed.
3. Administer activated charcoal.
4. Monitor the parent–child interactions for possible child abuse.

67. Shock is a complication of several types of poisoning. Which measure would help reduce the risk of shock?
1. Keep the child on his right side.
2. Let the child maintain normal activity as possible.
3. Elevate the head and legs to the level of the heart.
4. Keep the head flat and raise the legs to the level of the heart.

The right position helps!

64. 1. Chemical pneumonitis is the most common complication following ingestion of a hydrocarbon, such as kerosene. The pneumonitis is caused by irritation from the hydrocarbon aspirated into the lungs. The other options aren't complications of kerosene ingestion.
CN: Physiological integrity; CNS: Physiological adaptation; CL: Analysis

65. 2. The first step parents should take if their child has ingested a poisonous substance is to call the poison control center for instructions. Home administration of syrup of ipecac is no longer recommended by the American Academy of Pediatrics. The parents should contact poison control before transporting their child since valuable time may be lost if poison control recommends a specific action to take to remove the poisonous substance from the body. If the child needs to be taken to the emergency department, the parents should call emergency services to transport the child. Poison control may recommend watching the child for adverse effects, but parents shouldn't make this decision without consulting with poison control.
CN: Physiological integrity; CNS: Reduction of risk potential; CL: Analysis

66. 2. Keeping the child calm and relaxed will help prevent vomiting. If vomiting is induced, there's a strong chance the esophagus will be damaged from regurgitation of the gastric poison. Additionally, the risk of chemical pneumonitis exists if vomiting occurs. Activated charcoal poorly absorbs hydrocarbons, and it tends to distend the stomach and cause vomiting. The parents should remain with the child to help keep him calm. It is not necessary to monitor the parent–child interactions for possible child abuse.
CN: Physiological integrity; CNS: Physiological adaptation; CL: Analysis

67. 3. Elevating the head and legs to the level of the heart will promote venous drainage and decrease the chance of the child going into shock. The child may safely lie on the side he prefers. The child should be encouraged to get plenty of rest.
CN: Physiological integrity; CNS: Physiological adaptation; CL: Application

CN: Client needs category   CNS: Client needs subcategory   CL: Cognitive level

68. A 7-year-old child who ingested several leaves of a poinsettia plant has arrived in the emergency department. What is the priority nursing intervention?
1. Begin teaching accident prevention.
2. Provide emotional support to the child.
3. Be prepared for immediate intervention.
4. Provide emotional support to the parents.

69. A child is being admitted through the emergency department with a diagnosis of suspected accidental poisoning by medication. The nurse is aware that the most common cause of accidental poisoning in children is which of the following?
1. Pain medications
2. Vitamins
3. Laxatives
4. Antibiotics

70. A client is undergoing testing for a diagnosis of ulcerative colitis. Which symptom would the nurse most likely identify during this initial diagnosis?
1. Constipation
2. Diarrhea
3. Vomiting
4. Weight loss

71. A child arrives in the emergency department after ingesting poisonous amounts of salicylates. The nurse is aware that obvious signs of toxicity will be evident when?
1. Immediately
2. 2 to 4 hours after ingestion
3. 6 hours after ingestion
4. 18 hours after ingestion

72. The nurse is caring for a client with an extreme case of salicylate poisoning. The nurse anticipates the client will receive which treatment?
1. Gastric lavage
2. Hypothermia blankets
3. Peritoneal dialysis
4. Vitamin K injection

I'm just a common, run-of-the-mill guy.

There's more on the next page. Hooray!

68. 3. Time and speed are critical factors in recovery from poisonings. The remaining three answers are important nursing functions but don't require the immediate attention that first stabilizing the child does.
CN: Health promotion and maintenance; CNS: None; CL: Analysis

69. 1. According to the Centers for Disease Control and Prevention, the most common accidentally ingested class of drugs is pain medications. The most common pain medications ingested are acetaminophen-containing (Tylenol-containing) drugs, nonsteroidal anti-inflammatory drugs, and opioids. The other classes of drugs are less commonly ingested.
CN: Health promotion and maintenance; CNS: None; CL: Analysis

70. 2. Recurrent or persistent diarrhea is a common feature of ulcerative colitis. Constipation doesn't occur because the bowel becomes smooth and inflexible. Vomiting isn't common in this disease. Weight loss will occur after or during the episode but not initially.
CN: Physiological integrity; CNS: Physiological adaptation; CL: Analysis

71. 3. There's usually a delay of 6 hours before evidence of toxicity is noted. Toxic evidence is rarely immediate. Aspirin will exert its peak effect in 2 to 4 hours. The effect of aspirin may last as long as 18 hours.
CN: Health promotion and maintenance; CNS: None; CL: Application

72. 3. Peritoneal dialysis is usually reserved for cases of life-threatening salicylism. Gastric lavage is used in the immediate treatment for salicylate poisoning because the stomach contents and salicylates will move from the stomach to the remainder of the GI tract, where vomiting will no longer result in the removal of the poison. Hyperthermia blankets may be used to reduce the possibility of seizures. Vitamin K may be used to decrease bleeding tendencies but only if evidence of this exists.
CN: Physiological integrity; CNS: Physiological adaptation; CL: Analysis

73. When a child has been poisoned, it is important for the nurse to identify the ingested poison. What is the most appropriate intervention to identify the poison?
1. Call the local poison control center.
2. Ask the child.
3. Ask the parents.
4. Save all evidence of poison.

Know your nursing responsibilities.

74. One of the most important nursing responsibilities to help prevent salicylate poisoning should include which action?
1. Identify salicylate overdose.
2. Teach children the hazards of ingesting non-food items.
3. Decrease children's curiosity by teaching parents to keep aspirin and drugs in clear view.
4. Teach parents that the bottles must be kept out of reach of their children.

75. The nurse is evaluating the effectiveness of therapy with acetylcysteine (Mucomyst) in a child with acetaminophen poisoning. It is <u>most</u> important for the nurse to monitor which value?
1. Serum alanine aminotransferase and aspartate aminotransferase
2. Serum calcium levels
3. Prothrombin time (PT)
4. Serum glucose levels

Don't sweat it! You know the answer.

76. A client is diagnosed with acetaminophen poisoning. Which signs would the nurse expect when assessing the client 12 to 24 hours after ingestion? Select all that apply.
1. Hyperthermia
2. Nausea and vomiting
3. Sweating
4. Diarrhea
5. Irritability

73. 4. Saving all evidence of poison (container, vomitus, urine) will help determine which drug was ingested and how much. Calling the local poison control center may help get information on specific poisons or if a certain household placed a call, although rarely can they help determine which poison has been ingested. Asking the child may help, but the child may fear punishment and may not be honest about the incident. The parent may be helpful in some instances, although the parent may not have been home or with the child when the ingestion occurred.
CN: Health promotion and maintenance; CNS: None; CL: Analysis

74. 2. Teaching children the hazards of ingesting nonfood items will help prevent ingestion of poisonous substances. Identifying the overdose won't prevent it from occurring. Aspirin and drugs should be kept out of the sight of children. Parents should be warned about keeping large quantities of drugs on hand.
CN: Health promotion and maintenance; CNS: None; CL: Application

75. 1. Acetaminophen poisoning damages the liver, leading to elevated serum alanine aminotransferase and aspartate aminotransferase levels. After therapy with acetylcysteine is started, these liver enzymes should begin to fall. Serum calcium levels may fall following chelation therapy in clients with lead poisoning. Because PT is elevated and blood glucose levels are reduced with salicylate poisoning, after treatment is initiated, the nurse should observe the PT and blood glucose levels return to normal.
CN: Physiological integrity; CNS: Reduction of risk potential; CL: Analysis

76. 2, 3, 4, and 5. The signs and symptoms observed during the first 12 to 24 hours or first phase of acetaminophen poisoning are: sweating, anorexia, nausea, vomiting, diarrhea, and irritability. Hyperthermia is not a sign.
CN: Physiological integrity; CNS: Physiological adaptation; CL: Analysis

CN: Client needs category   CNS: Client needs subcategory   CL: Cognitive level

77. A client ingested a large amount of acetaminophen at 1:00 a.m. Two hours later, the client comes to the emergency department and is diagnosed with acetaminophen poisoning. What is the priority intervention for this client?
1. Perform gastric lavage.
2. Obtain blood work.
3. Administer I.V. fluid.
4. Administer activated charcoal.

78. The mother of a child admitted for ingesting a caustic cleaning product tells the nurse she feels guilty. What is the best response by the nurse?
1. "Now you'll know to keep all cleaning products locked up."
2. "Luckily, your child is going to be fine."
3. "You'll need to watch your child more carefully."
4. "Tell me more about your guilty feelings."

79. The ingestion of lead-containing substances is <u>mostly</u> influenced by which risk factor?
1. Child's age
2. Child's gender
3. Child's race
4. A parent with the same habit

80. The nurse explains to the mother of a child with lead poisoning that X-rays are necessary, as lead retained in the body is initially stored in the:
1. bone.
2. brain.
3. kidney.
4. liver.

81. Which condition is one of the <u>initial</u> signs of lead poisoning?
1. Anemia
2. Constipation
3. Anorexia
4. Paralysis

Everything tastes good to me!

Be aware of the initial signs of lead poisoning.

77. 4. If the client is seen within 4 hours, activated charcoal should be given to prevent absorption of acetaminophen. Gastric lavage is recommended only if the client is seen within 1 hour of ingestion. Blood work would be obtained but wouldn't be the first priority. I.V. fluids would also be administered, but administering activated charcoal is the priority.
CN: Physiological integrity; CNS: Physiological adaptation; CL: Analysis

78. 4. Encouraging the mother to talk about her feelings shows the nurse accepts the mother's feelings and that she's prepared to listen. This also helps establish a trusting nurse–client relationship. Telling the mother she should keep all cleaning products locked up and that she needs to watch her child more carefully acknowledges that the mother was at fault and may block further communication. Telling the mother that the child will be fine dismisses the mother's feelings and may be giving false reassurances.
CN: Psychosocial integrity; CNS: None; CL: Analysis

79. 1. The highest risk of lead poisoning occurs in young children who have a tendency to put things in their mouth. In older homes that contain lead-based paint, paint chips may be eaten directly by the child or they may cling to toys or hands that are then put into the child's mouth. Poisoning isn't gender-related. African Americans have a higher incidence of lead poisoning, but it can happen in any race. Most parents don't eat lead-based paint on purpose.
CN: Health promotion and maintenance; CNS: None; CL: Application

80. 1. Ingested lead is initially absorbed by bone; X-rays reveal a characteristic "lead line" at the epiphyseal line. If chronic ingestion occurs, then the central nervous, renal, and hematologic systems are affected.
CN: Physiological integrity; CNS: Physiological adaptation; CL: Application

81. 1. Lead is dangerously toxic to the biosynthesis of heme, and the reduced heme molecule in red blood cells causes anemia. Constipation and anorexia are vague, nonspecific symptoms. Paralysis may occur as toxic damage to the brain progresses.
CN: Physiological integrity; CNS: Physiological adaptation; CL: Analysis

82. The most serious and irreversible adverse effects of lead intoxication affect which system?
1. Central nervous system (CNS)
2. Hematologic system
3. Renal system
4. Respiratory system

83. A mother of a recently admitted child asks the nurse about the bluish black lines along her child's gums. The nurse would respond that the bluish black lines indicate which of the following types of poisoning?
1. Acetaminophen
2. Lead
3. Plants
4. Salicylates

84. The parents of a child with lead poisoning ask the nurse which procedure is the main treatment for lead poisoning. What is the best response by the nurse?
1. Exchange transfusion
2. Bone marrow transplant
3. Chelation therapy
4. Dialysis

Watch for these two words—most important.

85. What is the <u>most important</u> nursing intervention for a child with lead poisoning who must undergo chelation therapy with edetate calcium disodium?
1. Prepare the child for complete bed rest.
2. Prepare the child for I.V. fluid therapy.
3. Prepare the child for an extended hospital stay.
4. Prepare the child for a large number of injections.

86. The nurse is aware that a child receiving chelation therapy for the treatment of lead poisoning is at risk for which condition?
1. Hypercalcemia
2. Hypocalcemia
3. Hyperglycemia
4. Hypoglycemia

You know the routine; keep on teachin'.

87. A nurse is aware that the best way to prevent lead poisoning in children is to do which of the following?
1. Educate the child about the dangers of chewing on pencils.
2. Educate the public about imported toys containing lead.
3. Identify high-risk groups.
4. Provide home chelation kits.

82. 1. Damage that occurs to the CNS is difficult to repair. Damage to the hematologic and renal systems can be reversed if treated early. The respiratory system isn't affected until coma and death occur.
CN: Physiological integrity; CNS: Physiological adaptation; CL: Analysis

83. 2. One diagnostic characteristic of lead poisoning is bluish black lines along the gums. Bluish black lines don't occur along the gums with acetaminophen, plant, or salicylate poisoning.
CN: Physiological integrity; CNS: Physiological adaptation; CL: Application

84. 3. Chelation therapy is the main treatment for lead poisoning and involves the removal of metal by combining it with another substance. Sometimes, exchange transfusions are used to rid the blood of lead quickly. Bone marrow transplants usually aren't needed. Dialysis usually isn't part of the treatment.
CN: Physiological integrity; CNS: Physiological adaptation; CL: Application

85. 4. Chelation therapy for symptomatic children most commonly involves getting a large number of injections in a relatively short period of time. It's traumatic to the majority of children, and they need some preparation for the treatment. Edetate calcium disodium can be given I.V. The other components of the treatment plan are important but aren't as likely to cause the same anxiety as multiple injections. Allowing adequate rest to not aggravate the painful injection sites is important. Receiving I.V. fluid isn't as traumatizing as multiple injections. Physical activity is usually limited.
CN: Physiological integrity; CNS: Physiological adaptation; CL: Analysis

86. 2. A calcium chelating agent is used for the treatment of lead poisoning, so calcium is removed from the body with the lead. Hypocalcemia, not hypercalcemia, occurs. Hyperglycemia and hypoglycemia don't occur as a result of this therapy.
CN: Physiological integrity; CNS: Physiological adaptation; CL: Analysis

87. 2. By educating others about lead poisoning, including the danger signs, symptoms, and treatment, identification can be determined quickly. Very young children may not understand the dangers of lead poisoning. Identifying high-risk groups will help but won't prevent the poisoning. Home chelation kits currently aren't available.
CN: Health promotion and maintenance; CNS: None; CL: Analysis

CN: Client needs category   CNS: Client needs subcategory   CL: Cognitive level

88. A nurse is planning care for a 14-year-old client following surgical repair of a ruptured appendix. What is the most important intervention?
1. Reduce conflict between the client and his parents.
2. Promote the development of an identity and independence.
3. Encourage the development of trust.
4. Confirm plans for the future.

89. Certain forms of pica are caused by a deficiency. Which nutrient is most commonly deficient?
1. Minerals
2. Vitamins
3. Electrolytes
4. Protein

90. A child with appendicitis reports a sudden cessation of abdominal pain to the nurse. What is the most appropriate intervention by the nurse?
1. Prepare the child and parents for discharge.
2. Begin feeding the child, as tolerated.
3. Prepare the child for emergency surgery.
4. Begin ambulation, as tolerated.

91. Which advice should a nurse give over the telephone to the mother of a 7-year-old child with abdominal pain, a low-grade fever, and vomiting?
1. Give prune juice to relieve constipation.
2. Test for rebound tenderness in the left lower quadrant of the abdomen.
3. Encourage fluids to prevent dehydration.
4. Seek immediate emergency medical care.

92. Which symptom is the most common for acute appendicitis?
1. Bradycardia
2. Fever
3. Pain descending to the lower left quadrant
4. Pain radiating into the rectum

88. 2. Since adolescents are in Erikson's stage of identity versus role confusion, the nursing care plan should include interventions that promote a sense of identity and independence. During adolescence, conflict is usually intensified, not reduced. Trust is a developmental task of infancy. Plans for the future aren't confirmed at age 14.
CN: Health promotion and maintenance; CNS: None; CL: Analysis

89. 1. Eating clay is related to zinc deficiency; eating chalk, to calcium deficiency; and eating ice, to iron deficiency. Vitamin, electrolyte, and protein deficiencies aren't related to pica.
CN: Health promotion and maintenance; CNS: None; CL: Analysis

90. 3. The sudden cessation of abdominal pain in the client with appendicitis may indicate perforation or infarction of the appendix requiring emergency surgery. Therefore, the child shouldn't be prepared for discharge or given oral feedings. The child with a ruptured appendix should be on complete bed rest and be prepared for surgery.
CN: Physiological integrity; CNS: Reduction of risk potential; CL: Application

91. 4. The client with abdominal pain, fever, and vomiting (the cardinal signs of appendicitis) should seek immediate emergency care to reduce the risk of complications if the appendix should rupture. Prune juice has laxative effects and shouldn't be given because laxatives increase the risk of rupture of the appendix. The nurse shouldn't rely on the mother's findings when testing for rebound tenderness. The client should be given nothing by mouth in case surgery is needed.
CN: Physiological integrity; CNS: Reduction of risk potential; CL: Application

92. 2. Fever, abdominal pain, and tenderness are the first signs of appendicitis. Tachycardia, not bradycardia, is seen. Pain can be generalized or periumbilical. It usually descends to the lower right quadrant, not the left.
CN: Physiological integrity; CNS: Physiological adaptation; CL: Analysis

Keep up the good work!

93. The nurse is providing preoperative care for a child diagnosed with appendicitis. What is the most appropriate intervention?
1. Give clear fluids.
2. Apply heat to the abdomen.
3. Maintain complete bed rest.
4. Administer an enema, if ordered.

94. Postoperative care of a child with a ruptured appendix should include which treatment or intervention?
1. Liquid diet
2. Oral antibiotics for 7 to 10 days
3. Positioning the child on the left side
4. Parenteral antibiotics for 7 to 10 days

Believe me, position counts.

95. After surgical repair of a ruptured appendix, which position would be the <u>most appropriate</u>?
1. High Fowler's position
2. Left side
3. Semi-Fowler's position
4. Supine

96. Which statement by the parent of a child being treated for pinworms indicates to the nurse that further teaching is necessary?
1. "I will make my child wash his hands well before meals."
2. "I will tell my child not to share hairbrushes or hats."
3. "I will give my child only one dose of medication."
4. "I will keep my child's nails short."

97. During an initial nursing assessment, a nurse determines that an 8-year-old child has right lower quadrant pain, a low-grade fever, nausea, rebound tenderness, and a positive psoas sign. The nurse suspects that the client has which condition?
1. Appendicitis
2. Gastroenteritis
3. Pancreatitis
4. Cholecystitis

93. 3. Bed rest will prevent aggravating the condition. Clients with appendicitis aren't allowed anything by mouth. Cold applications are placed on the abdomen because heat would increase blood flow to the area and possibly spread any infectious disease. Enemas may aggravate the condition.
CN: Physiological integrity; CNS: Reduction of risk potential; CL: Analysis

94. 4. Parenteral antibiotics are used for 7 to 10 days postoperatively to help prevent the spread of infection. The child is kept on I.V. fluids and isn't allowed anything by mouth. Oral antibiotics may continue after the parenteral antibiotics are discontinued. The child is positioned on the right side after surgery.
CN: Physiological integrity; CNS: Reduction of risk potential; CL: Analysis

95. 3. Using the semi-Fowler's or right side-lying positions will facilitate drainage from the peritoneal cavity and prevent the formation of a subdiaphragmatic abscess. High Fowler's, left side, and prone positions won't facilitate drainage from the peritoneal cavity.
CN: Physiological integrity; CNS: Physiological adaptation; CL: Analysis

96. 2. Sharing hairbrushes and hats reduces the spread of lice, not pinworms. Hands should be washed well before food preparation and eating to avoid ingesting eggs that may be under the fingernails from scratching the itchy, infested perianal area. Only a single dose of medication, such as mebendazole, is needed to treat pinworms. Keeping the fingernails short reduces the risk of carrying the eggs under the nails.
CN: Safe, effective care environment; CNS: Safety and infection control; CL: Application

97. 1. Right lower quadrant pain, a low-grade fever, nausea, rebound tenderness, and a positive psoas sign are all consistent with appendicitis. Gastroenteritis is characterized by generalized abdominal tenderness. Pancreatitis is characterized by pain in the left abdominal quadrant. Cholecystitis is characterized by pain in the right upper abdominal quadrant.
CN: Physiological integrity; CNS: Physiological adaptation; CL: Analysis

98. A neonate has been diagnosed with a unilateral complete cleft lip and cleft palate. The nurse formulating the care plan for this neonate will have which nursing diagnosis as a priority?
1. Risk for infection
2. Impaired skin integrity
3. Risk for aspiration
4. Delayed growth and development

99. A neonate is suspected of having a tracheoesophageal fistula (type III/C). Which symptom would be seen on the <u>initial</u> assessment?
1. Excessive drooling
2. Excessive vomiting
3. Mottling
4. Polyhydramnios

100. When assessing a client suspected of having pyloric stenosis, which finding should the nurse expect?
1. An "olive" mass in the right upper quadrant
2. An "olive" mass in the left upper quadrant
3. A "sausage" mass in the right upper quadrant
4. A "sausage" mass in the left upper quadrant

101. A nurse caring for an infant with pyloric stenosis should expect to observe which laboratory values?
1. pH, 7.30; chloride, 120 mEq/L
2. pH, 7.38; chloride, 110 mEq/L
3. pH, 7.43; chloride, 100 mEq/L
4. pH, 7.49; chloride, 90 mEq/L

98. 3. Although all of these diagnoses are important for the neonate with a cleft lip and cleft palate, the most important diagnosis relates to the airway. Neonates with a cleft lip and a cleft palate may have an excessive amount of saliva and usually have a difficult time with feedings. Special feeding techniques, such as using a flanged nipple, may be necessary to prevent aspiration.
CN: Physiological integrity; CNS: Reduction of risk potential; CL: Analysis

99. 1. In type III/C tracheoesophageal fistula, the proximal end of the esophagus ends in a blind pouch and a fistula connects the distal end of the esophagus to the trachea. Saliva will pool in this pouch and cause the child to drool. Because the distal end of the esophagus is connected to the trachea, the neonate can't vomit, but he can aspirate and stomach acid may go into the lungs through this fistula, causing pneumonitis. Mottling is a netlike, reddish blue discoloration of the skin usually due to vascular contraction in response to hypothermia. The mother of a neonate with tracheoesophageal fistula may have had polyhydramnios.
CN: Physiological integrity; CNS: Reduction of risk potential; CL: Analysis

100. 1. Pyloric stenosis involves hypertrophy of the circular (or olive-shaped) muscle fibers of the pylorus. This hypertrophy is palpable in the right upper quadrant of the abdomen. A "sausage" mass is palpable in the right upper quadrant in children with intussusception. A "sausage" mass in the left upper quadrant wouldn't indicate pyloric stenosis.
CN: Physiological integrity; CNS: Physiological adaptation; CL: Analysis

101. 4. Infants with pyloric stenosis vomit hydrochloric acid. This causes them to become alkalotic and hypochloremic. Normal serum pH is 7.35 to 7.45; levels above 7.45 represent alkalosis. The normal serum chloride level is 99 to 111 mEq/L; levels below 99 mEq/L represent hypochloremia.
CN: Physiological integrity; CNS: Physiological adaptation; CL: Analysis

102. Which nursing diagnosis has the highest priority in a 1-month-old infant admitted with projectile vomiting after feeding?
1. Deficient fluid volume
2. Risk for impaired parenting
3. Interrupted breastfeeding
4. Risk for infection

I see the highest priority nursing diagnosis for this infant.

103. Which findings would the nurse assess in a premature neonate who may have necrotizing enterocolitis?
1. Abdominal distention and gastric retention
2. Gastric retention and guaiac-negative stools
3. Metabolic alkalosis and abdominal distention
4. Guaiac-negative stools and metabolic alkalosis

104. An infant has been admitted to the hospital with gastroenteritis. What is the priority nursing diagnosis?
1. Acute pain
2. Diarrhea
3. Deficient fluid volume
4. Imbalanced nutrition: Less than body requirements

The nursing diagnosis is so important.

105. Nursing assessments in an infant with gastroenteritis should be directed toward detecting which potential problem?
1. Urinary retention
2. Heart failure
3. Electrolyte imbalance
4. Hyperactive reflexes

102. 1. Projectile vomiting in an infant is a sign of pyloric stenosis, a condition that requires surgical intervention to correct. Because the infant has been vomiting, he is at risk for fluid and electrolyte imbalances that must be corrected before surgery. Whenever an infant is hospitalized, there's the risk for impaired parenting and interrupted breastfeeding; however, correcting fluid and electrolyte imbalances is a priority. Following surgery, the infant is at risk for infection because the incision is near the diaper area.
CN: Physiological integrity; CNS: Reduction of risk potential; CL: Analysis

103. 1. Necrotizing enterocolitis is an ischemic disorder of the gut. The cause is unknown, but it's more common in premature neonates who had a hypoxic episode. The neonate's intestines become dilated and necrotic, and the abdomen becomes very distended. Paralytic ileus develops, causing the neonate to have gastric retention. These retained gastric contents, along with any passed stool, will be guaiac-positive. The neonate also develops metabolic acidosis.
CN: Physiological integrity; CNS: Physiological adaptation; CL: Analysis

104. 3. Young children with gastroenteritis are at high risk for developing a fluid volume deficit. Their intestinal mucosa allows for more fluid and electrolytes to be lost when they have gastroenteritis. The main goal of the health care team should be to rehydrate the infant. The other nursing diagnoses are important, but deficient fluid volume is more life threatening.
CN: Physiological integrity; CNS: Physiological adaptation; CL: Application

105. 3. Diarrhea in infants can rapidly lead to dehydration and electrolyte imbalances, especially hyponatremia and hypokalemia. Urinary retention isn't a sign of dehydration; however, it should be distinguished from kidney failure, which may occur with severe dehydration. Heart failure occurs with fluid volume overload, not fluid volume deficit. Reflexes are typically diminished or absent with hypokalemia.
CN: Physiological integrity; CNS: Reduction of risk potential; CL: Application

106. A mother calls the children's clinic and tells the nurse she found her toddler with an open and empty bottle of acetaminophen (Tylenol) and wants to know what to do. What is the <u>priority</u> nursing intervention?
1. Ask the mother whether she has any syrup of ipecac.
2. Ask the mother to give the child a large glass of milk.
3. Ask the mother to bring the child to the emergency department (ED).
4. Ask the mother whether she knows cardiopulmonary resuscitation (CPR).

107. The nurse is preparing a teaching plan for the parents of a child with celiac disease. What is the most important information for the nurse to include?
1. The gluten-free diet alterations must be continued for a lifetime.
2. The diet needs to be free of lactose because the child is intolerant.
3. Diet alterations are necessary when the child reports cramping and bloating.
4. The diet needs to be low in fats because of the malabsorption problem in the intestines.

108. A pediatrician suspects that a child has pinworms and instructs the nurse to assess the child for their presence. The nurse determines that which method is <u>most reliable</u> for assessing for pinworms?
1. A history of itching at the anal area and of restlessness at night
2. A blood culture
3. Eggs retrieved from the anal edge on a piece of cellophane tape
4. A stool culture

109. A 1-month-old infant is brought to the pediatrician's office. His mother states that he's fussy and cries as if in pain. He's tolerating normal amounts of formula, gaining weight, and having episodes of paroxysmal abdominal cramping after feedings. These signs and symptoms indicate that the infant <u>most likely</u> has which condition?
1. Intussusception
2. Meconium ileus
3. Colic
4. Pyloric stenosis

Do you know the priority intervention for this toddler?

What's all the fuss about?

106. 3. The child should be brought to the ED for evaluation and possible acetylcysteine administration. Home administration of syrup of ipecac is no longer recommended. Milk isn't an antidote for acetaminophen toxicity. Asking about CPR isn't appropriate as the priority intervention; it would distract from the immediate interventions needed.

CN: Safe, effective care environment; CNS: Safety and infection control; CL: Analysis

107. 1. Celiac disease is the inability to digest gluten. The treatment is a gluten-free diet for life. It's important the diet is continued to avoid symptoms and the associated risk of colon cancer. The disease isn't caused by lactose intolerance or a problem digesting fats.

CN: Health promotion and maintenance; CNS: None; CL: Application

108. 3. Cellophane tape placed near the anal edge will capture the eggs. A history of itching and of restlessness isn't enough to definitely diagnose pinworms. Neither a blood culture nor a stool culture would be helpful.

CN: Physiological integrity; CNS: Reduction of risk potential; CL: Application

109. 3. An infant with colic exhibits symptoms of abdominal cramping after feedings, cries as if in pain, and is fussy. An intussusception begins suddenly and leads to bloody stools and vomiting. A meconium ileus is nonpassage of meconium by 24 hours of age. Signs of pyloric stenosis include projectile vomiting and weight loss.

CN: Physiological integrity; CNS: Physiological adaptation; CL: Analysis

110. A 16-year-old African-American student visits a school nurse with complaints of nausea and fatigue. The nurse determines a need to check for jaundice. Which area of the body should the nurse examine?
1. Sclera of the eye
2. Overall skin color
3. Outer ears and back of the neck
4. Tongue and inside the cheek area

111. A mother brings her 4-week-old child to the clinic. She states that he hasn't been eating well and is lethargic when she holds and cuddles him. He has lost 7 oz (198.5 g) since birth. He's otherwise healthy and has no congenital defects. Which condition is the pediatrician <u>most likely</u> to diagnose?
1. Celiac disease
2. Failure to thrive
3. Hirschsprung's disease
4. Imperforate anus

112. A 15-year-old client needs a nasogastric tube inserted because of peritonitis caused by a ruptured appendix. The client is afraid that the procedure will hurt. Which statement by the nurse is <u>most appropriate</u> to help decrease the client's anxiety?
1. "Breathe deeply through your mouth and relax. It will be over soon."
2. "This is a simple procedure, and it won't hurt."
3. "You'll feel pressure and be uncomfortable for a few minutes, but it shouldn't be painful."
4. "You're old enough now and should be able to handle pain."

113. A mother brings her 18-month-old child to the emergency department and tells a nurse that he has been ill for the past 2 days. He has a fever of 104.8° F (40.8° C), is irritable, has had diarrhea, and hasn't been wetting his diaper much in the past 24 hours. The child is admitted to the pediatric unit for treatment of moderate dehydration and gastroenteritis. I.V. therapy and strict intake and output are ordered. As rehydration occurs, the child is started on oral feedings of a rehydration fluid. When caring for this child during the <u>later stage</u> of rehydration, the nurse should take which action?
1. Force fluids.
2. Allow the client to drink as much as he wants.
3. Monitor the client's intake and output.
4. Monitor the client's ability to retain fluids.

"Eye" think you know the answer to this one.

Just a little more to go and you're done with this chapter.

You're being asked for the later stage in question 113.

110. 1. The sclera is the best place to check for jaundice, especially in a person of darker color. The outer ears and back of the neck as well as the tongue and inside of the cheek aren't appropriate places to check for jaundice.

CN: Physiological integrity; CNS: Physiological adaptation; CL: Application

111. 2. These signs and symptoms are classic of the condition failure to thrive. Celiac disease presents with steatorrhea, weight loss, and inability to digest gluten foods. Hirschsprung's disease and imperforate anus present with abdominal distention and absence of stool; no anal opening is present in imperforate anus.

CN: Physiological integrity; CNS: Physiological adaptation; CL: Application

112. 3. Discussing the procedure will help the client understand the extent of discomfort. Breathing deeply will help relieve discomfort, but the statement may also imply that the procedure will be painful and will, thus, increase the client's anxiety. By saying the procedure is simple, the nurse isn't acknowledging the client's concerns. Telling the client that he is old enough now and should be able to handle pain is condescending. No matter what the client's age, he has a right to express his fears and to have those fears acknowledged.

CN: Psychosocial integrity; CNS: None; CL: Analysis

113. 4. The GI tract may not tolerate a full liquid diet immediately. Allowing only clear liquids gives the intestine time to heal, but the fluids should be reintroduced slowly to determine the child's ability to tolerate and retain them. The GI tract won't tolerate forcing fluids. Don't allow the client to drink as much as he wants; instead, offer small amounts of fluid every couple of hours. Monitoring intake and output is important and was initially ordered; it will continue until discharge.

CN: Physiological integrity; CNS: Basic care and comfort; CL: Analysis

114. A nurse is conducting an infant nutrition class for parents. Which foods should the nurse tell the parents it's okay to introduce during the first year of life? Select all that apply.
1. Sliced beef
2. Pureed fruits
3. Whole milk
4. Rice cereal
5. Strained vegetables
6. Fruit juice

115. A nurse is teaching a female adolescent with inflammatory bowel disease about treatment with corticosteroids. Which adverse effects are concerns for this client? Select all that apply.
1. Acne
2. Hirsutism
3. Mood swings
4. Osteoporosis
5. Growth spurts
6. Adrenal suppression

116. A mother brings her child to the pediatrician's office for evaluation of chronic stomach pain. The mother states that the pain seems to go away when she tells the child he can stay home from school. The physician diagnoses school phobia. Which other behaviors or symptoms may be present in the child with school phobia? Select all that apply.
1. Nausea
2. Headaches
3. Weight loss
4. Dizziness
5. Fever

114. 2, 4, and 5. The first food provided to a neonate is breast milk or formula. Between ages 4 and 6 months, rice cereal can be introduced, followed by pureed or strained fruits and vegetables, and then strained or ground meat. Meats must be chopped or ground prior to feeding them to an infant to prevent choking. Infants shouldn't be given whole milk until they're at least 1 year old. Fruit drinks provide no nutritional benefit and shouldn't be encouraged.

CN: Health promotion and maintenance; CNS: None; CL: Application

115. 1, 2, 3, 4, and 6. Adverse effects of corticosteroids include acne, hirsutism, mood swings, osteoporosis, and adrenal suppression. Steroid use in children and adolescents may cause delayed growth, not growth spurts.

CN: Physiological integrity; CNS: Pharmacological and parenteral therapies; CL: Application

116. 1, 2, and 4. Children with school phobia commonly complain of vague symptoms, such as stomachaches, nausea, headaches, and dizziness, to avoid going to school. Typically, these symptoms don't occur on weekends. A careful history must be taken to identify a pattern of school avoidance. Such signs as weight loss and fever are more likely to have a physiological cause and are uncommon in the child with school phobia.

CN: Psychosocial integrity; CNS: None; CL: Analysis

You're done with all those questions? I knew you could do it!

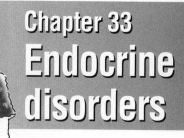

Chapter 33
Endocrine disorders

1. When explaining the causes of hypothyroidism to the parents of a newly diagnosed infant, a nurse should recognize that further education is needed when the parents ask which question?
 1. "Hypothyroidism can be only temporary, right?"
 2. "Are you saying that hypothyroidism is caused by a problem in the way the thyroid gland develops?"
 3. "Do you mean that hypothyroidism may be caused by a problem in the way the body makes thyroxine?"
 4. "Hypothyroidism can be treated by exposing our baby to a special light, right?"

2. An infant with hypothyroidism is receiving oral thyroid hormone. The nurse is most concerned about which assessment findings?
 1. Tachycardia, irritability, and diaphoresis
 2. Bradycardia, excessive sleepiness, and dry scaly skin
 3. Bradycardia, irritability, and cool extremities
 4. Tachycardia, cool extremities, and irritability

3. The nurse is teaching the parents of a neonate newly diagnosed with hypothyroidism about the condition. What is the most important information for the nurse to provide?
 1. "A large goiter in a neonate doesn't present a problem."
 2. "Preterm neonates usually aren't affected by hypothyroidism."
 3. "Usually, the neonate exhibits obvious signs of hypothyroidism."
 4. "The severity of the disorder depends on the amount of thyroid tissue present."

You're off to a good start.

1. 4. Congenital hypothyroidism can be permanent or transient and may result from a defective thyroid gland or an enzymatic defect in thyroxine synthesis. Only the last question, which refers to phototherapy for physiological jaundice, indicates that the parents need more information.
CN: Health promotion and maintenance; CNS: None; CL: Application

2. 1. Clinical manifestations of thyroid hormone overdose in an infant include tachycardia, irritability, and diaphoresis. Bradycardia, excessive sleepiness, dry scaly skin, and cool extremities are manifestations of hypothyroidism.
CN: Physiological integrity; CNS: Pharmacological and parenteral therapies; CL: Application

3. 4. The severity of the disorder depends on the amount of thyroid tissue present. The more thyroid tissue present, the less severe is the disorder. A large goiter in a neonate could possibly occlude the airway and lead to obstruction. Preterm neonates are usually affected by hypothyroidism due to hypothalamic and pituitary immaturity. Usually, the neonate doesn't exhibit obvious signs of the disorder because of maternal circulation.
CN: Health promotion and maintenance; CNS: None; CL: Application

4. The nurse is assessing an infant with a suspected diagnosis of hypothyroidism. The nurse would assess the infant for which sign?
1. Diarrhea
2. Lethargy
3. Severe jaundice
4. Tachycardia

5. A nurse is assessing a toddler with hypothyroidism. During the assessment, the nurse is most concerned when the toddler presents with which finding?
1. Low hemoglobin and hematocrit
2. Cyanosis
3. Bone and muscle dystrophy
4. Mental retardation

6. The nurse is counseling the parents of a neonate with congenital hypothyroidism. The parents tell the nurse that they are concerned about the severity of the intellectual deficit. The nurse explains that the deficit is related to which factor?
1. Duration of condition before treatment
2. Degree of hypothermia
3. Cranial malformations
4. Thyroxine (T_4) level at diagnosis

7. What is the most important statement for the nurse to include when explaining the diagnostic evaluation of neonates for congenital hypothyroidism?
1. "Tests are mandatory in all states."
2. "An arterial blood test is preferred."
3. "Tests shouldn't be performed until after discharge."
4. "Blood tests should be done after the first month of life."

The diagnostic evaluation of a neonate may include tests that are mandated by the state.

4. 2. Subtle signs of this disorder that may be seen shortly after birth include lethargy, poor feeding, prolonged jaundice, respiratory difficulty, cyanosis, constipation, and bradycardia. Diarrhea in the neonate isn't normal and isn't associated with this disorder. Severe jaundice needs immediate attention by the primary health care provider and isn't a subtle sign. Tachycardia typically occurs in hyperthyroidism, not hypothyroidism.
CN: Health promotion and maintenance; CNS: None; CL: Application

5. 4. The most serious consequence of congenital hypothyroidism is delayed development of the central nervous system, which leads to severe mental retardation. The other choices occur but aren't the most serious consequences.
CN: Physiological integrity; CNS: Physiological adaptation; CL: Analysis

6. 1. The severity of the intellectual deficit is related to the degree of hypothyroidism and the duration of the condition before treatment. Cranial malformations don't affect the severity of the intellectual deficit nor does the degree of hypothermia as it relates to hypothyroidism. It isn't the specific T_4 level at diagnosis that affects the intellect but how long the client has been hospitalized.
CN: Health promotion and maintenance; CNS: None; CL: Application

7. 1. Heelstick blood tests are mandatory in all states and are usually performed on neonates between 2 and 6 days of age. Typically, specimens are taken before the neonate is discharged from the hospital; the test is included with other tests that screen the neonate for errors of metabolism.
CN: Health promotion and maintenance; CNS: None; CL: Application

8. The nurse is reviewing lab results of a neonate who has the possible diagnosis of congenital hypothyroidism. The nurse is most concerned by which results?
1. High level of thyroxine (T_4) and low level of thyroid-stimulating hormone (TSH)
2. Low level of T_4 and high level of TSH
3. Normal TSH and high level of T_4
4. Normal T_4 and low level of TSH

9. A nurse is teaching parents about therapeutic management of their neonate diagnosed with congenital hypothyroidism. Which response by a parent would indicate the need for further teaching?
1. "My baby will need regular measurements of his thyroxine (T_4) levels."
2. "Treatment involves lifelong thyroid hormone replacement therapy."
3. "Treatment should begin as soon as possible after diagnosis is made."
4. "As my baby grows, his thyroid gland will mature and he won't need medications."

In question 9, the phrase *further teaching* indicates that you're looking for an *incorrect* statement.

10. The nurse asks the mother of a neonate at her 2-week office visit how the baby is doing. Which statement should the nurse be most concerned about?
1. "My baby is unusually quiet and good."
2. "My baby seems to be a yellowish color."
3. "After feedings, my baby pulls her legs up and cries."
4. "My baby seems to really look at my face during feeding time."

You've finished 10 questions already! Congratulations

11. The nurse is providing instruction to a single parent about administering levothyroxine (Synthroid) to her neonate. What is the most important information for the nurse to provide?
1. The drug has a bitter taste.
2. The pill shouldn't be crushed.
3. Never put the medication in formula or juice.
4. If a dose is missed, double the dose the next day.

8. 2. Screening results that show a low level of T_4 and a high level of TSH indicate congenital hypothyroidism and the need for further tests to determine the cause of the disease.
CN: Physiological integrity; CNS: Reduction of risk potential; CL: Application

9. 4. Treatment involves lifelong thyroid hormone replacement therapy that begins as soon as possible after diagnosis to abolish all signs of hypothyroidism and to reestablish normal physical and mental development. The drug of choice is synthetic levothyroxine (Synthroid or Levothroid). Regular measurements of T_4 levels are important in ensuring optimum treatment.
CN: Health promotion and maintenance; CNS: None; CL: Application

10. 1. Parental remarks about an unusually "quiet and good" neonate together with any of the early physical manifestations should lead to a suspicion of hypothyroidism, which requires a referral for specific tests. If a neonate begins to look yellow in color, hyperbilirubinemia may be the cause. If the neonate is pulling her legs up and crying after feedings, she might be showing signs of colic. The neonate likes looking at the human face and should show interest in this at age 2 weeks.
CN: Health promotion and maintenance; CNS: None; CL: Application

11. 4. If a dose is missed, twice the dose should be given the next day. The importance of compliance with the drug regimen for the neonate to achieve normal growth and development must be stressed. Because the drug is tasteless, it can be crushed and added to a small amount of water.
CN: Physiological integrity; CNS: Pharmacological and parenteral therapies; CL: Application

12. When teaching parents about signs that indicate levothyroxine (Synthroid) overdose, which comment from a parent indicates the need for further teaching?
1. "Irritability is a sign of overdose."
2. "If my baby's heartbeat is fast, I should count it."
3. "If my baby loses weight, I should be concerned."
4. "I shouldn't worry if my baby does not sleep very much."

13. A nurse should recognize that exophthalmos (protruding eyeballs) may occur in children with which condition?
1. Hypothyroidism
2. Hyperthyroidism
3. Hypoparathyroidism
4. Hyperparathyroidism

14. A nurse is assessing a child with juvenile hypothyroidism. The nurse documents which assessment finding?
1. Accelerated growth
2. Diarrhea
3. Dry skin
4. Insomnia

15. A nurse is observing an infant with thyroid hormone deficiency. Which signs would the nurse commonly observe?
1. Tachycardia, profuse perspiration, and diarrhea
2. Lethargy, feeding difficulties, and constipation
3. Hypertonia, small fontanels, and moist skin
4. Dermatitis, dry skin, and round face

16. When counseling parents of a neonate with congenital hypothyroidism, the nurse should encourage which behavior?
1. Seeking professional genetic counseling
2. Retracing the family tree for others born with this condition
3. Talking to relatives who have gone through a similar experience
4. Seeking alternative therapies for this condition

Watch out! Question 12 is another *further teaching* question.

Question 16 is asking for the most *appropriate* behavior. In other words, *prioritize!*

12. 4. Parents need to be aware of signs indicating overdose, such as rapid pulse, dyspnea, irritability, insomnia, fever, sweating, and weight loss. The parents would be given acceptable parameters for the heart rate and weight loss or gain. If the baby is experiencing a heart rate or weight loss outside of the acceptable parameters, the physician should be called.
CN: Physiological integrity; CNS: Pharmacological and parenteral therapies; CL: Analysis

13. 2. Exophthalmos occurs when there's an overproduction of thyroid hormone, or hyperthyroidism. This sign should alert the physician to follow up with further testing.
CN: Health promotion and maintenance; CNS: None; CL: Application

14. 3. Children with hypothyroidism will have dry skin. The other choices aren't evident in children with juvenile hypothyroidism.
CN: Health promotion and maintenance; CNS: None; CL: Application

15. 2. Hypothyroidism results from inadequate thyroid production to meet an infant's needs. Clinical signs include feeding difficulties, prolonged physiological jaundice, lethargy, and constipation.
CN: Health promotion and maintenance; CNS: None; CL: Analysis

16. 1. Seeking professional genetic counseling is the best option for parents who have a neonate with a genetic disorder. Education about the disorder should occur as soon as the parents are ready, so they'll understand the genetic implications for future children. Retracing the family tree and talking to relatives won't help the parents to become better educated about the disorder. Seeking alternative therapies should be discouraged to prevent possible complications.
CN: Health promotion and maintenance; CNS: None; CL: Application

17. While receiving teaching about giving insulin injections, an adolescent questions the nurse about the reuse of disposable needles and syringes. What is the best response by the nurse?
1. "This is an unsafe practice."
2. "This is acceptable for up to 7 days."
3. "This is acceptable for only 48 hours."
4. "This is acceptable only if the family has very limited resources."

I'm becoming quite acceptable!

18. When children are more physically active, which change in the management of the child with diabetes should the nurse expect?
1. Increased food intake
2. Decreased food intake
3. Decreased risk of insulin shock
4. Increased risk of hyperglycemia

19. The nurse is helping an adolescent deal with diabetes. What is the most important factor about the adolescent for the nurse to consider in her approach?
1. Wanting to be an individual
2. Needing to be like peers
3. Being preoccupied with future plans
4. Teaching peers that this is a serious disease

20. An adolescent with diabetes tells the community nurse that he has recently started drinking alcohol on the weekends. What is the most appropriate intervention by the nurse?
1. Recommend referral to counseling.
2. Make the adolescent promise to stop drinking.
3. Discuss with the adolescent why he has started drinking.
4. Teach the adolescent about the effects of alcohol on diabetes.

20 questions completed? That's cause for celebration!

17. **2.** It has become acceptable practice for clients to reuse their own disposable needles and syringes for up to 7 days. Bacteria counts are unaffected, and there are considerable cost savings. If this method is approved, it's imperative to stress the importance of vigorous hand washing before handling equipment as well as capping the syringe immediately after use and storing it in the refrigerator to decrease the growth of organisms.
CN: Safe, effective care environment; CNS: Safety and infection control; CL: Application

18. **1.** If a child is more active at one time of the day than another, food or insulin can be altered to meet the activity pattern of the individual. Food should be increased when children are more physically active. The child has an increased risk of insulin shock and a decreased risk of hyperglycemia when he's more physically active.
CN: Physiological integrity; CNS: Reduction of risk potential; CL: Application

19. **2.** Adolescents appear to have the most difficulty in adjusting to diabetes. Adolescence is a time when there's much stress on being "perfect" and being like one's peers, and to adolescents, having diabetes is being different.
CN: Health promotion and maintenance; CNS: None; CL: Application

20. **4.** Confusion about the effects of alcohol on blood glucose is common. Teenagers may believe that alcohol will increase blood glucose levels, when in fact, the opposite occurs. Ingestion of alcohol inhibits the release of glycogen from the liver, resulting in hypoglycemia. Teens who drink alcohol may become hypoglycemic, but they are then treated as if they were intoxicated. Behaviors may be similar, such as shakiness, combativeness, slurred speech, and loss of consciousness. Finding out why the adolescent has started drinking and recommending counseling may be appropriate but only after education is provided. An adolescent may promise to stop drinking but not follow through.
CN: Health promotion and maintenance; CNS: None; CL: Application

21. A child has experienced symptoms of hypoglycemia and has eaten sugar cubes. The priority intervention by the nurse would be to have the client ingest which of the following?
1. Fruit juices
2. Six glasses of water
3. Foods that are high in protein
4. Complex carbohydrates and protein

22. The nurse is teaching the parents of a child newly diagnosed with diabetes to identify the signs and symptoms of hypoglycemia. Which response by the parents indicates the teaching has been effective?
1. "Irritability, shakiness, hunger, headache, and dizziness are signs to look for."
2. "Drowsiness, lethargy, and decreased urine output need to be reported."
3. "Abdominal pain, nausea and vomiting, and constipation are the most common findings."
4. "We will report immediately any signs of urinary frequency."

23. The nurse is assessing a child recently admitted with diabetes who has developed ketoacidosis. Which statement is the most accurate?
1. This is a normal outcome of diabetes.
2. This is a life-threatening situation.
3. This is a situation that can easily be treated at home.
4. This is a situation best treated in the pediatrician's office.

24. Which guideline would be appropriate for the nurse to implement when teaching an 11-year-old child who was recently diagnosed with diabetes about insulin injections?
1. The parents don't need to be involved in learning this procedure.
2. Self-injection techniques aren't usually taught until the child reaches age 16.
3. At age 11, the child should be old enough to give most of his own injections.
4. Self-injection techniques should be taught only when the child can reach all injection sites.

If you know the definitions of hypo and hyper, it can help you with a bunch of questions.

21. 4. When a child exhibits signs of hypoglycemia, the majority of cases can be treated with a simple concentrated sugar, such as honey, that can be held in the mouth for a short time. A complex carbohydrate and protein, such as a slice of bread or a cracker spread with peanut butter, should follow the rapid-releasing sugar or the client may become hypoglycemic again.
CN: Health promotion and maintenance; CNS: None; CL: Application

22. 1. Signs of hypoglycemia include irritability, shaky feeling, hunger, headache, and dizziness. Drowsiness, abdominal pain, polyuria, nausea, and vomiting are signs of hyperglycemia.
CN: Physiological integrity; CNS: Physiological adaptation; CL: Application

23. 2. Diabetic ketoacidosis, the most complete state of insulin deficiency, is a life-threatening situation. The child should be admitted to an intensive care facility for management, which consists of rapid assessment, adequate insulin to reduce the elevated blood glucose level, fluids to overcome dehydration, and electrolyte replacement (especially potassium).
CN: Physiological integrity; CNS: Physiological adaptation; CL: Application

24. 3. The parents must supervise and manage the child's therapeutic program, but the child should assume responsibility for self-management as soon as he's capable. Children can learn to collect their own blood for glucose testing at a relatively young age (4 to 5 years), and most are able to check their blood glucose level and administer insulin at about age 9 years. Some children may be able to do it earlier.
CN: Health promotion and maintenance; CNS: None; CL: Application

25. The nurse suspects a client of having diabetic ketoacidosis. Which blood glucose value would be observed with this condition?
1. 50 mg/dl
2. 90 mg/dl
3. 150 mg/dl
4. 300 mg/dl

26. The nurse has just admitted a 2-year-old child with a diagnosis of diabetes mellitus. Which cardinal sign would support the diagnosis?
1. Nausea
2. Seizure
3. Hyperactivity
4. Frequent urination

27. The parent of a child with diabetes asks a nurse why blood glucose monitoring is needed. What is the best response by the nurse?
1. "This is an easier method of testing."
2. "This is a less expensive method of testing."
3. "This allows children the ability to better manage their diabetes."
4. "This gives children a greater sense of control over their diabetes."

28. What is the best intervention by a nurse to increase an adolescent's compliance with treatment for diabetes mellitus?
1. Provide for a special diet in the high school cafeteria.
2. Clarify the adolescent's values to promote involvement in care.
3. Identify energy requirements for participation in sports activities.
4. Educate the adolescent about long-term consequences of poor metabolic control.

29. A child with diabetes type 1 tells the nurse he feels shaky. The nurse assesses the child's skin to be pale and sweaty. What is the <u>most important</u> intervention by the nurse?
1. Give supplemental insulin.
2. Have the child eat a glucose tablet.
3. Administer glucagon subcutaneously.
4. Offer the child a complex carbohydrate snack.

Knowing blood glucose values is a must for the NCLEX.

Teaching clients how to help manage their own conditions is a common subject on the NCLEX.

The words *most important* signals a need for you to prioritize.

25. 4. Diabetic ketoacidosis is determined by the presence of hyperglycemia (blood glucose measurement of 300 mg/dl or higher), accompanied by acetone breath, dehydration, weak and rapid pulse, and a decreased level of consciousness.
CN: Physiological integrity; CNS: Physiological adaptation; CL: Analysis

26. 4. Polyphagia, polyuria (frequent urination), polydipsia, and weight loss are cardinal signs of diabetes mellitus. Other signs include irritability, shortened attention span, lowered frustration tolerance, fatigue, dry skin, blurred vision, sores that are slow to heal, and flushed skin.
CN: Health promotion and maintenance; CNS: None; CL: Application

27. 3. Blood glucose monitoring improves diabetes management and is used successfully by children from the onset of their diabetes. By testing their own blood, children are able to change their insulin regimen to maintain their glucose level in the normoglycemic range of 80 to 120 mg/dl. This allows them to better manage their diabetes.
CN: Health promotion and maintenance; CNS: None; CL: Application

28. 2. Adolescent compliance with diabetes management may be hampered by dependence versus independence conflicts and ego development. Attempts to have the adolescent clarify personal values promote involvement in his care and foster compliance.
CN: Health promotion and maintenance; CNS: None; CL: Application

29. 2. These are symptoms of hypoglycemia. Rapid treatment involves giving the alert child a glucose tablet (4 mg of dextrose) or, if unavailable, a glass of glucose-containing liquid. It would be followed by a complex carbohydrate snack and protein. Giving supplemental insulin would be contraindicated because that would lower the blood glucose even more. Glucagon would be given only if there was a risk of aspiration with oral glucose, such as if the child was semiconscious.
CN: Safe, effective care environment; CNS: Management of care; CL: Application

30. The parents of a child diagnosed with diabetes ask the nurse about maintaining metabolic control during a minor illness with loss of appetite. What is the best response by the nurse?
1. "Decrease the child's insulin by half the usual dose during the course of the illness."
2. "Call your physician to arrange hospitalization."
3. "Give increased amounts of clear liquids to prevent dehydration."
4. "Substitute calorie-containing liquids for uneaten solid food."

31. A parent asks the nurse what criteria are used to measure good metabolic control in a child with diabetes mellitus. What is the best response by the nurse?
1. "Fewer than eight episodes of severe hyperglycemia in a month"
2. "Infrequent occurrences of mild hypoglycemic reactions"
3. "Hemoglobin A values less than 12%"
4. "Growth below the 15th percentile"

32. In the neonatal intensive care unit, the nurse is assessing the neonate of a mother with poorly controlled diabetes. The nurse would assess the neonate for which condition?
1. Cataracts
2. Low-set ears
3. Cardiac malformations
4. Cleft lip and palate deformities

30. 4. Calorie-containing liquids can help to maintain more normal blood sugar levels as well as decrease the danger of dehydration. The child with diabetes should always take at least the usual dose of insulin during an illness based on more frequent blood sugar checks. During an illness where there's vomiting or loss of appetite, NPH insulin may be lowered by 25% to 30% to avoid hyperglycemia, and regular insulin is given according to home glucose monitoring results.
CN: Safe, effective care environment; CNS: Management of care; CL: Application

31. 2. Criteria for good metabolic control generally include few episodes of hypoglycemia or hyperglycemia, hemoglobin A values less than 8%, and normal growth and development.
CN: Health promotion and maintenance; CNS: None; CL: Application

32. 3. Cardiac and central nervous system anomalies, along with neural tube defects and skeletal and GI anomalies, are most likely to occur as a result of uncontrolled maternal diabetes.
CN: Health promotion and maintenance; CNS: None; CL: Application

33. A client with diabetes mellitus asks the nurse what condition could possibly cause <u>hypoglycemia</u>. What is the best response by the nurse?
1. Too little insulin
2. Mild illness with fever
3. Excessive exercise without a carbohydrate snack
4. Eating ice cream and cake to celebrate a birthday

34. A client tells the nurse that he has not been following his prescribed diabetes management program and is concerned because he is visiting his doctor for his routine 3-month assessment. He asks if the doctor will be able to determine his lack of compliance from the blood work. The nurse is aware that the <u>best</u> indicator of a client's diabetic control over the past 2 or 3 months is which measure?
1. Fasting glucose level
2. Oral glucose tolerance level
3. Glycosylated hemoglobin test
4. A client's record of glucose monitoring

35. A client has received diet instruction as part of his treatment plan for diabetes type 1. Which statement by the client indicates to the nurse that he needs <u>additional instructions</u>?
1. "I'll need a bedtime snack because I take an evening dose of NPH insulin."
2. "I can eat whatever I want as long as I cover the calories with sufficient insulin."
3. "I can have an occasional low-calorie drink as long as I include it in my meal plan."
4. "I should eat meals as scheduled, even if I'm not hungry, to prevent hypoglycemia."

36. The nurse suspects that a 10-year-old client with diabetes is hyperglycemic. What symptom would indicate hyperglycemia?
1. Rapid heart rate
2. Headache
3. Hunger
4. Thirst

I'm glad I had a snack before I started to race.

All this studying makes me thirsty.

33. 3. Excessive exercise without a carbohydrate snack could cause hypoglycemia. The other options describe situations that cause hyperglycemia.
CN: Health promotion and maintenance; CNS: None; CL: Application

34. 3. A glycosylated hemoglobin level provides an overview of a person's blood glucose level over the previous 2 to 3 months. Glycosylated hemoglobin values are reported as a percentage of the total hemoglobin within an erythrocyte. The time frame is based on the fact that the usual life span of an erythrocyte is 2 to 3 months; a random blood sample, therefore, will theoretically give samples of erythrocytes for this same period. The other options won't indicate a true picture of the person's blood glucose level over the previous 2 to 3 months.
CN: Health promotion and maintenance; CNS: None; CL: Application

35. 2. The goal of diet therapy in diabetes mellitus is to attain and maintain ideal body weight. Each client will be prescribed a specific caloric intake and insulin regimen to help accomplish this goal.
CN: Physiological integrity; CNS: Basic care and comfort; CL: Analysis

36. 4. Thirst (polydipsia) is one of the symptoms of hyperglycemia. Rapid heart rate, headache, and hunger are signs and symptoms of hypoglycemia.
CN: Physiological integrity; CNS: Physiological adaptation; CL: Application

37. A client is learning to mix regular insulin and NPH insulin in the same syringe. Which action, if performed by the client, would indicate the need for <u>further teaching</u>?
1. Withdrawing the NPH insulin first
2. Injecting air into the NPH insulin bottle first
3. After drawing up first insulin, removing air bubbles
4. Injecting an amount of air equal to the desired dose of insulin

37. 1. Regular insulin is always withdrawn first so it won't become contaminated with NPH insulin. The client is instructed to inject air into the NPH insulin bottle equal to the amount of insulin to be withdrawn, because there will be regular insulin in the syringe and he won't be able to inject air when he needs to withdraw the NPH. It's necessary to remove the air bubbles to ensure a correct dosage before drawing up the second insulin.
CN: Physiological integrity; CNS: Pharmacological and parenteral therapies; CL: Application

38. A client is diagnosed with diabetes type 1. The nurse reviews the prescribed insulin regimen of regular insulin and NPH insulin with the client to be administered subcutaneously each morning. The nurse determines that teaching was effective when the client states that the onset of regular insulin begins at what point after administration?
1. Within 5 minutes
2. ½ to 1 hour
3. 1 to 1½ hours
4. 4 to 8 hours

It's important to know how and when different types of insulin react.

38. 2. Regular insulin's onset is ½ to 1 hour, peak is 2 to 4 hours, and duration is 3 to 6 hours. Lispro insulin has an onset within 5 minutes. NPH insulin has an onset within 2 to 4 hours, and Ultralente insulin is the longest acting, with an onset of 6 to 10 hours.
CN: Physiological integrity; CNS: Pharmacological and parenteral therapies; CL: Application

39. When assessing a neonate for signs of diabetes insipidus, a nurse should recognize which symptom as a sign of this disorder?
1. Hyponatremia
2. Jaundice
3. Polyuria
4. Hypochloremia

39. 3. The cardinal sign of diabetes insipidus is polyuria, along with polydipsia. Hypernatremia, not hyponatremia, occurs with diabetes insipidus. Jaundice occurs because of abnormal bilirubin metabolism, not diabetes insipidus. Hyperchloremia, not hypochloremia, occurs with diabetes insipidus.
CN: Physiological integrity; CNS: Physiological adaptation; CL: Application

40. The nurse is assessing an infant with diabetes insipidus. What initial observation would the nurse would expect?
1. Dehydration
2. Inability to be aroused
3. Extreme hunger relieved by frequent feedings of milk
4. Irritability relieved with feedings of water but not milk

You've reached question 40. How cool is that?

40. 4. One initial symptom of diabetes insipidus in an infant is irritability relieved with feedings of water but not milk. Dehydration and the inability to be aroused are late symptoms.
CN: Health promotion and maintenance; CNS: None; CL: Application

41. A nurse is helping parents understand when treatments of growth hormone replacement will end. What is the most important statement for the nurse to include?
1. The dosage of growth hormone will decrease as the child's age increases.
2. The dosage of growth hormone will increase as the time of epiphyseal closure nears.
3. After giving growth hormone replacement for 1 year, the dose will be tapered down.
4. Growth hormone replacement can't be abruptly stopped; it must be spread out over several months.

42. A nurse is explaining diabetes insipidus to the parents of an infant with the disease. When explaining the diagnostic test that's used, which comment by a parent would indicate an understanding of the diagnostic test?
1. "Fluids will be offered every 2 hours."
2. "My infant's fluid intake will be restricted."
3. "I won't change anything about my infant's intake."
4. "Formula will be restricted, but glucose water is okay."

43. A nurse should anticipate which physiological response in an infant being tested for diabetes insipidus?
1. Increase in urine output
2. Decrease in urine output
3. No effect on urine output
4. Increase in urine specific gravity

44. An infant has a positive test result for diabetes insipidus. The nurse should anticipate the physician ordering a test dose of which medication?
1. Antidiuretic hormone
2. Biosynthetic growth hormone
3. Adrenocorticotropic hormone
4. Aqueous vasopressin (Pitressin Synthetic)

Question 42 asks you to identify a knowledgeable response.

Poly this and poly that. Hypo this and hyper that. I'm confused.

41. 2. Dosage of growth hormone is increased as the time of epiphyseal closure nears to gain the best advantage of the growth hormone. The medication is then stopped. There's no tapering off of the dose.
CN: Physiological integrity; CNS: Pharmacological and parenteral therapies; CL: Application

42. 2. The simplest test used to diagnose diabetes insipidus is restriction of oral fluids and observation of consequent changes in urine volume and concentration. A weight loss of 3% to 5% indicates severe dehydration, and the test should be terminated at this point. This is done in the hospital, and the infant is watched closely.
CN: Health promotion and maintenance; CNS: None; CL: Application

43. 3. In diabetes insipidus, fluid restriction for diagnostic testing has little or no effect on urine formation but causes weight loss from dehydration.
CN: Physiological integrity; CNS: Physiological adaptation; CL: Application

44. 4. If the fluid restriction test is positive, the child should be given a test dose of injected aqueous vasopressin, which should alleviate the polyuria and polydipsia. Unresponsiveness to exogenous vasopressin usually indicates nephrogenic diabetes insipidus. The other choices are used to determine other types of endocrine disorders.
CN: Physiological integrity; CNS: Pharmacological and parenteral therapies; CL: Application

45. The nurse is teaching the parents of an infant diagnosed with diabetes insipidus. What is the most important treatment for the nurse to include in teaching?
1. Antihypertensive medications
2. The need for blood products
3. Hormone replacement
4. Fluid restrictions

46. When providing information about treatments for diabetes insipidus to parents, a nurse explains the use of nasal spray and injections. Which indication might <u>deter</u> a parent from choosing nasal spray treatment?
1. Applications must be repeated every 8 to 12 hours.
2. Applications must be repeated every 2 to 4 hours.
3. Nasal sprays can't be used in infants.
4. Measurements are too difficult.

47. A nurse is teaching the parents of an infant with diabetes insipidus about an injectable drug used to treat the disorder. Which statement made by a parent would indicate the need for <u>further teaching</u>?
1. "I must hold the medication under warm running water for 10 to 15 minutes before administering it."
2. "The medication must be shaken vigorously before being drawn up into the syringe."
3. "Small brown particles must be seen in the suspension."
4. "I will store this medication in the refrigerator."

48. When teaching parents of an infant newly diagnosed with diabetes insipidus, which statement by a parent indicates an <u>understanding</u> of this condition?
1. "When my infant stabilizes, I won't have to worry about giving hormone medication."
2. "I don't have to measure the amount of fluid intake that I give my infant."
3. "I realize that treatment for diabetes insipidus is lifelong."
4. "My infant will outgrow this condition."

Although the word *deter* sounds like a negative, question 46 actually asks you to identify a *true* characteristic of nasal sprays.

Which of these statements is true?

45. 3. The usual treatment for diabetes insipidus is hormone replacement with vasopressin or desmopressin acetate (DDAVP). No problem with hypertension is associated with this condition, and fluids shouldn't be restricted. Blood products shouldn't be needed.

CN: Health promotion and maintenance; CNS: None; CL: Application

46. 1. Applications of nasal spray used to treat diabetes insipidus must be repeated every 8 to 12 hours; injections last for 48 to 72 hours. The nasal spray must be timed for adequate night sleep. However, the injections are oil-based and quite painful. Nasal sprays have been used in infants with diabetes insipidus and are dispensed in premeasured intranasal inhalers, eliminating the need for measuring doses.

CN: Physiological integrity; CNS: Pharmacological and parenteral therapies CL: Analysis

47. 4. The medication should be stored at room temperature. When giving injectable vasopressin, it must be thoroughly resuspended in the oil by being held under warm running water for 10 to 15 minutes and shaken vigorously before being drawn into the syringe. If this isn't done, the oil may be injected minus the drug. Small brown particles, which indicate drug dispersion, must be seen in the suspension.

CN: Physiological integrity; CNS: Pharmacological and parenteral therapies; CL: Application

48. 3. Diabetes insipidus is a condition that will need lifelong treatment. The amount of fluid intake is very important and must be measured with the infant's output to monitor the medication regimen. The infant won't outgrow this condition.

CN: Safe, effective care environment; CNS: Management of care; CL: Application

49. A child is admitted with diabetes insipidus. The nurse asks the parents if they know about this condition. Which statement tells the nurse that the parents understand the condition?
1. "We know that our child's thyroid is working too much."
2. "We know that our child's pituitary gland is not working hard enough."
3. "Our child's pituitary gland is working overtime."
4. "Our child's parathyroid gland is not doing a good job. It is acting very lazy."

50. After a nurse has explained the causes of diabetes insipidus to the parents, which statement made by a parent indicates the need for further teaching?
1. "This condition could be familial or congenital."
2. "Drinking alcohol during my pregnancy caused this condition."
3. "My child might have a tumor that's causing these symptoms."
4. "An infection such as meningitis may be the reason my child has diabetes insipidus."

51. Which assessment finding would alert a nurse to <u>change</u> the intranasal route for vasopressin administration that has been prescribed for a client?
1. Mucous membrane irritation
2. Severe coughing
3. Nosebleeds
4. Pneumonia

52. A nurse is providing in-home management instruction for a child who is receiving desmopressin acetate (DDAVP) for symptomatic control of diabetes insipidus. What is the most important instruction the nurse to include?
1. Give DDAVP only when urine output begins to decrease.
2. Cleanse skin with alcohol before application of the DDAVP dermal patch.
3. Increase the DDAVP dose if polyuria occurs just before the next scheduled dose.
4. Call the physician for an alternate route of DDAVP when the child has an upper respiratory infection (URI) or allergic rhinitis.

> Question 51 asks for a common adverse effect of vasopressin administration.

49. 2. The principal disorder of posterior pituitary hypofunction is diabetes insipidus. The disorder results form hyposecretion of antidiuretic hormone, producing a state of uncontrolled diuresis. It is not caused by the thyroid gland or parathyroid gland.

CN: Health promotion and maintenance; CNS: None; CL: Application

50. 2. Drinking alcohol during pregnancy can lead to a neonate born with fetal alcohol syndrome but has no known correlation to diabetes insipidus. The other options are possible causes of diabetes insipidus.

CN: Health promotion and maintenance; CNS: None; CL: Application

51. 1. Mucous membrane irritation caused by a cold or allergy renders the intranasal route unreliable. Severe coughing, pneumonia, and nosebleeds shouldn't interfere with the intranasal route.

CN: Physiological integrity; CNS: Pharmacological and parenteral therapies; CL: Application

52. 4. Excessive nasal mucus associated with URI or allergic rhinitis may interfere with DDAVP absorption because it's given intranasally. Parents should be instructed to contact the physician for advice in altering the hormone dose during times when nasal mucus may be increased. The DDAVP dose should remain unchanged, even if there's polyuria just before the next dose. This is to avoid overmedicating the child.

CN: Safe, effective care environment; CNS: Management of care; CL: Application

53. A nurse is assessing a client with suspected hypopituitarism. The nurse would observe the client for which of the following?
1. Sleep disturbance
2. Polyuria
3. Polydipsia
4. Short stature

54. Which statement made to a nurse by the parents of a child with idiopathic growth hormone deficiency would indicate the need for <u>further teaching</u>?
1. "This disorder may be familial."
2. "There's no genetic basis for this disorder."
3. "This disorder might be secondary to hypothalamic deficiency."
4. "There may be other disorders related to pituitary hormone deficiencies."

55. A nurse is teaching health to a class of fifth graders. Which information is most important for the nurse to include?
1. "There's nothing that you can do to influence your growth."
2. "Excessive physical activity that begins before puberty might stunt growth."
3. "All children who are short in stature also have parents who are short in stature."
4. "Because this is a time of tremendous growth, being concerned about calorie intake isn't important."

56. While teaching the parents of a child with short stature, the nurse discusses familial short stature. What is the <u>most</u> appropriate information for the nurse to include in the discussion?
1. "It occurs in children who are members of a very large family with limited resources."
2. "It occurs in children who have no siblings and who moved a great deal during their early childhood."
3. "It occurs in children with delayed linear growth and skeletal and sexual maturation that's behind that of age mates."
4. "It occurs in children who have ancestors with adult height in the lower percentiles and whose height during childhood is appropriate."

A nurse's responsibility to teach never ends.

Let's see how you measure up.

53. 4. The most common sign in most instances of hypopituitarism is short stature. Sleep disturbance may indicate thyrotoxicosis. Polydipsia and polyuria may be indications of diabetes mellitus or diabetes insipidus.
CN: Physiological integrity; CNS: Physiological adaptation; CL: Application

54. 2. The cause of idiopathic growth hormone deficiency is unknown. There's a higher-than-average occurrence of the disorder in some families, which indicates a possible genetic cause. The condition is commonly associated with other pituitary hormone deficiencies, such as deficiencies of thyroid-stimulating hormone and corticotropin, and may be secondary to hypothalamic deficiency.
CN: Psychosocial integrity; CNS: None; CL: Application

55. 2. Intensive physical activity (greater than 18 hours per week) that begins before puberty may stunt growth so that the child doesn't reach full adult height. Nutrition and environment influence a child's growth. All children who are short in stature don't necessarily have parents who are short in stature. During the school-age years, growth slows and doesn't accelerate again until adolescence.
CN: Health promotion and maintenance; CNS: None; CL: Application

56. 4. Familial short stature refers to otherwise healthy children who have ancestors with adult height in the lower percentiles and whose height during childhood is appropriate for genetic background. Children who are members of very large families with limited resources or who have no siblings don't fit the description of familial short stature. Children with delayed linear growth and skeletal and sexual maturation that's behind that of age mates are considered to have constitutional growth delay.
CN: Physiological integrity; CNS: Physiological adaptation; CL: Application

57. The nurse is assessing a 2-year-old toddler during a routine well-child visit. The nurse suspects the possibility of growth hormone deficiency when the assessment shows which finding?
1. The child had normal growth during the first year of life but showed a slowed growth curve below the 3rd percentile for the second year of life.
2. The child fell below the 5th percentile for growth during the first year of life but, at this check-up, falls below only the 50th percentile.
3. There has been a steady decline in growth over the 2 years of this toddler's life that has accelerated during the past 6 months.
4. There was delayed growth below the 5th percentile for the first and second years of life.

58. A nurse is assessing a child with growth hormone deficiency. The nurse documents the assessment data as:
1. decreased weight with no change in height.
2. decreased weight with increased height.
3. increased weight with decreased height.
4. increased weight with increased height.

59. During the assessment of a child with growth hormone deficiency, the nurse would expect to observe which finding?
1. Normal skeletal proportions
2. Abnormal skeletal proportions
3. Child appearing older than his age
4. Longer than normal upper extremities

60. The parents of a child with growth hormone deficiency ask the nurse what sport would be best for their child to participate in. What is the most appropriate response by the nurse?
1. Basketball
2. Field hockey
3. Football
4. Gymnastics

Which of these sports would be best for a child with growth hormone deficiency?

57. 1. Children with growth hormone deficiency generally grow normally during the first year and then follow a slowed growth curve that's below the 3rd percentile. If growth is consistently below the 5th percentile, it may be an indication of failure to thrive.

CN: Health promotion and maintenance; CNS: None; CL: Application

58. 3. Height may be retarded more than weight because, with good nutrition, children with growth hormone deficiency can become overweight or even obese. Their well-nourished appearance is an important diagnostic clue to differentiation from other disorders such as failure to thrive.

CN: Health promotion and maintenance; CNS: None; CL: Application

59. 1. Skeletal proportions are normal for the age, but these children appear younger than their chronological age. However, later in life, premature aging is evident.

CN: Physiological integrity; CNS: Physiological adaptation; CL: Application

60. 4. Children with growth hormone deficiency can be no less active than other children if directed to size-appropriate sports, such as gymnastics, swimming, wrestling, or soccer.

CN: Health promotion and maintenance; CNS: None; CL: Application

61. The nurse is explaining to parents the social behavior of children with hypopituitarism. The nurse determines further teaching is necessary when a parent makes which statement?
1. "I realize that my child might have school anxiety and a low self-esteem."
2. "Because my child is short in stature, people expect less of him than his peers."
3. "Because of my child's short stature, he may not be pushed to perform at his chronological age by others."
4. "My child's vocabulary is very well developed, so even though he's short in stature, no one will treat him differently."

62. The mother of a child diagnosed with hypopituitarism states to the nurse that she feels guilty because she should have recognized this disorder. What is the best response by the nurse about children with hypopituitarism?
1. "They're usually large for gestational age at birth."
2. "They're usually small for gestational age at birth."
3. "They usually exhibit signs of this disorder soon after birth."
4. "They're usually of normal size for gestational age at birth."

63. Which observation when plotting height and weight on a growth chart would indicate that a 4-year-old child has a growth hormone deficiency?
1. Upward shift of 1 percentile or more
2. Upward shift of 5 percentiles or more
3. Downward shift of 2 percentiles or more
4. Downward shift of 5 percentiles or more

64. When reviewing the results of radiographic examinations of a child with hypopituitarism, which characteristic should the nurse expect to observe?
1. Bone age near normal
2. Epiphyseal maturation normal
3. Epiphyseal maturation retarded
4. Bone maturation greatly retarded

It's important that parents have realistic expectations about their child's disorder.

It's important to pay attention to abnormal growth in a child.

61. 4. Height discrepancy has been significantly correlated with emotional adjustment problems and may be a valuable predictor of the extent to which growth hormone–delayed children will have trouble with anxiety, social skills, and positive self-esteem. Also, academic problems aren't uncommon. These children aren't usually pushed to perform at their chronological age but are commonly subjected to juvenilization (related to in an infantile or childish manner).
CN: Psychosocial integrity; CNS: None; CL: Application

62. 4. Children with hypopituitarism are usually of normal size for gestational age at birth. Clinical features develop slowly and vary with the severity of the disorder and the number of deficient hormones.
CN: Psychosocial integrity; CNS: None; CL: Application

63. 3. When the physician evaluates the results of plotting height and weight, upward or downward shifts of 2 percentiles or more in children older than 3 years may indicate a growth abnormality.
CN: Health promotion and maintenance; CNS: None; CL: Analysis

64. 3. Epiphyseal maturation is retarded in hypopituitarism consistent with retardation in height. This is in contrast to hypothyroidism, in which bone maturation is greatly retarded, or Turner's syndrome, in which bone age is near normal.
CN: Health promotion and maintenance; CNS: None; CL: Application

65. A child has been brought to a pediatrician's office for concerns about growth. The physician suspects hypopituitarism. The mother asks the nurse which test will be done to determine the diagnosis. Which response by the nurse would be appropriate?
1. Hypersecretion of thyroid hormone
2. Increased reserves of growth hormone
3. Hyposecretion of antidiuretic hormone (ADH)
4. Decreased reserves of growth hormone

66. The parents of a child who's going through testing for hypopituitarism ask the nurse what type of test results they should expect. The nurse's response should be based on which factor?
1. Measurement of growth hormone will occur only one time.
2. Growth hormone levels are decreased after strenuous exercise.
3. There will be increased overnight urine growth hormone concentration.
4. Growth hormone levels are elevated 45 to 90 minutes following the onset of sleep.

67. Which method is considered the <u>definitive</u> treatment for hypopituitarism due to growth hormone deficiency?
1. Treatment with desmopressin acetate (DDAVP)
2. Replacement of antidiuretic hormone (ADH)
3. Treatment with testosterone or estrogen
4. Replacement with biosynthetic growth hormone

All of these treatments may be used, but only one is definitive.

68. When obtaining information about a child, which comment made by a parent to the nurse would indicate the possibility of hypopituitarism in a child?
1. "I can pass down my child's clothes to his younger brother."
2. "Usually, my child wears out his clothes before his size changes."
3. "I have to buy bigger size clothes for my child about every 2 months."
4. "I have to buy larger shirts more frequently than larger pants for my child."

65. 4. Definitive diagnosis is based on absent or subnormal reserves of pituitary growth hormone. ADH and thyroid hormone levels aren't affected.
CN: Health promotion and maintenance; CNS: None; CL: Application

66. 4. Growth hormone levels are elevated 45 to 90 minutes following the onset of sleep. Low growth hormone levels following the onset of sleep would indicate the need for further evaluation. Exercise is a natural and benign stimulus for growth hormone release, and elevated levels can be detected after 20 minutes of strenuous exercise in normal children. Also, growth hormone levels will need to be checked frequently related to the type of therapy instituted.
CN: Physiological integrity; CNS: Physiological adaptation; CL: Application

67. 4. The definitive treatment of growth hormone deficiency is replacement of growth hormone and is successful in 80% of affected children. DDAVP is used to treat diabetes insipidus. ADH deficiency causes diabetes insipidus and isn't related to hypopituitarism. Testosterone or estrogen may be given during adolescence for normal sexual maturation, but neither is the definitive treatment for hypopituitarism.
CN: Physiological integrity; CNS: Pharmacological and parenteral therapies; CL: Application

68. 2. Parents of children with hypopituitarism frequently comment that the child wears out clothes before growing out of them or that, if the clothing fits the body, it's commonly too long in the sleeves or legs.
CN: Health promotion and maintenance; CNS: None; CL: Application

69. The nurse is providing teaching for parents who are planning to administer prescribed growth hormone to their child at home. The parents ask the nurse what the best time is to give the medication. What is the best response by the nurse?
1. At bedtime
2. After dinner
3. In the middle of the day
4. First thing in the morning

70. The nurse is educating parents of a child with hypopituitarism about realistic expectations of height for their child who is successfully responding to growth hormone replacement. What is the best information for the nurse to include?
1. "Your child will never reach a normal adult height."
2. "Your child will attain his eventual adult height at a faster rate."
3. "Your child will attain his eventual adult height at a slower rate."
4. "The rate of your child's growth will be the same as children without this disorder."

71. Which statement made by a parent of a child with short stature would indicate to the nurse the need for further teaching?
1. "Obtaining blood studies won't aid in proper diagnosis."
2. "A history of my child's growth patterns should be discussed."
3. "X-rays should be included in my child's diagnostic procedures."
4. "A family history is important information for me to share with my child's physician."

72. Which signs and symptoms would the health care team most commonly use as a basis for determining appropriate priorities and interventions for a child with type 1 diabetes mellitus? Select all that apply.
1. Polyuria
2. Weakness
3. Abdominal pain
4. Weight loss
5. Postprandial nausea
6. Orthostatic hypertension

All I can think about is optimum dozing.

Careful—here's another further teaching question.

69. 1. Optimum dosing is typically achieved when growth hormone is administered at bedtime. Pituitary release of growth hormone occurs during the first 45 to 90 minutes after the onset of sleep, so normal physiological release is mimicked with bedtime dosing.

CN: Physiological integrity; CNS: Pharmacological and parenteral therapies; CL: Application

70. 3. Even when hormone replacement is successful, these children attain their eventual adult height at a slower rate than their peers do; therefore, they need assistance in setting realistic expectations regarding improvement.

CN: Psychosocial integrity; CNS: None; CL: Application

71. 1. A complete diagnostic evaluation should include a family history, a history of the child's growth patterns and previous health status, physical examination, physical evaluation, radiographic survey, and endocrine studies that may involve blood samples.

CN: Health promotion and maintenance; CNS: None; CL: Application

72. 1, 2, 4, and 5. Polyuria, weakness, weight loss, and postprandial nausea are commonly seen in diabetes mellitus. The health care team would plan care to manage these signs and symptoms. Abdominal pain isn't a symptom in this disease, and orthostatic hypotension, rather than orthostatic hypertension, would be a significant finding.

CN: Safe, effective care environment; CNS: Management of care; CL: Analysis

73. Which metabolic alteration characteristic might be associated with growth hormone deficiency?
1. Galactosemia
2. Homocystinuria
3. Hyperglycemia
4. Hypoglycemia

74. When providing information to the parents of a child who's receiving growth hormone replacement therapy for hypopituitarism, the nurse should include which intervention?
1. Explaining that growth in height and weight won't begin until puberty
2. Teaching how to perform venipuncture for administration of the growth hormone
3. Helping parents recognize the importance of interacting with the child according to age rather than size
4. Advising parents to hold the child back in school until linear growth begins to approximate the normal patterns

75. When caring for a neonate diagnosed with diabetes insipidus, the nurse determines further intervention is necessary when the assessment identifies:
1. edema.
2. increased head circumference.
3. weight gain.
4. weight loss.

76. In a client with diabetes insipidus, a nurse could expect which characteristics of the urine?
1. Pale in color; specific gravity less than 1.006
2. Concentrated; specific gravity less than 1.006
3. Concentrated; specific gravity less than 1.03
4. Pale in color; specific gravity more than 1.03

73. 4. The development of hypoglycemia is a characteristic finding related to growth hormone deficiency. Galactosemia is a rare autosomal recessive disorder with an inborn error of carbohydrate metabolism. Homocystinuria is an indication of amino acid transport or metabolism problems. Hyperglycemia isn't a problem in hypopituitarism.
CN: Health promotion and maintenance; CNS: None; CL: Application

74. 3. To promote self-esteem and healthy development of a child with growth hormone deficiency, parents should be encouraged to interact with the child according to age, not size. Growth in height and weight will begin soon after treatment with growth hormone begins. Growth hormone administration is subcutaneous, and a child shouldn't be held back in school because of his size.
CN: Psychosocial integrity; CNS: None; CL: Application

75. 4. Diabetes insipidus usually presents gradually. Weight loss from a large loss of fluid occurs. Edema isn't evident in the neonate with diabetes insipidus. There should be an increase in his head circumference with treatment. A normal neonate should gain weight as he grows.
CN: Physiological integrity; CNS: Reduction of risk potential; CL: Application

76. 1. With diabetes insipidus, the client has difficulty with excessive urine output; therefore, the urine will be pale in color, and the specific gravity will fall below the low normal of 1.01.
CN: Physiological integrity; CNS: Reduction of risk potential; CL: Analysis

77. The nurse is obtaining the health history of a child with diabetes insipidus. The nurse expects the history to include which findings?
1. Delayed closure of the fontanels, coarse hair, and hypoglycemia in the morning
2. Gradual onset of personality changes, lethargy, and blurred vision
3. Vomiting early in the morning, headache, and decreased thirst
4. Abrupt onset of polyuria, nocturia, and polydipsia

78. The nurse is reviewing assessment data of a client on fluid restriction for diabetes insipidus diagnostic testing. The nurse determines further intervention is necessary when the assessment identifies which finding?
1. Weight gain of 3% to 5%
2. Weight loss of 3% to 5%
3. Increase in urine output
4. Generalized edema

79. A child with diabetes insipidus has a viral illness that includes congestion, nausea, and vomiting. What is the most important information for the nurse to tell the parents?
1. Make no changes in the medication regimen.
2. Give medications only once per day.
3. Obtain an alternate route for desmopressin acetate (DDAVP) administration.
4. Give medication 1 hour after vomiting has occurred.

80. A child with diabetes insipidus will be receiving injectable vasopressin when discharged from the hospital. What is the most important information for the nurse to provide when teaching injection techniques?
1. Teach injection techniques to the primary caregiver.
2. Teach injection techniques to anyone who will provide care for the child.
3. Teach injection techniques to anyone who will provide care for the child as well as to the child if he's old enough to understand.
4. Provide information about the nearest home health agency so the parents can arrange for the home health nurse to come and give the injection.

Do you know the symptoms of diabetes insipidus?

Good work! You're flying through this test!

77. 4. Diabetes insipidus is characterized by deficient secretion of antidiuretic hormone leading to diuresis. Most children with this disorder experience an abrupt onset of symptoms, including polyuria, nocturia, and polydipsia. The other choices reflect symptoms of pituitary hyperfunction.
CN: Health promotion and maintenance; CNS: None; CL: Application

78. 2. A weight loss between 3% and 5% indicates significant dehydration and requires termination of the fluid restriction. Weight gain would be a good sign. Generalized edema wouldn't occur with fluid restriction, nor would increased urine output.
CN: Physiological integrity; CNS: Physiological adaptation; CL: Analysis

79. 3. An alternate route for administration of DDAVP would be needed for absorption because of nasal congestion. The other options reflect actions that need to be covered by a physician's order.
CN: Health promotion and maintenance; CNS: None; CL: Application

80. 3. The best response is to teach all those who will provide care for the child. The child should be included if age-appropriate. It's unrealistic to arrange for home health nurses to give injections that are required throughout the life span.
CN: Physiological integrity; CNS: Pharmacological and parenteral therapies; CL: Application

81. When providing care for a school-age client with diabetes insipidus, the nurse understands that which behavior might be difficult related to this child's growth and development?
1. Taking desmopressin acetate (DDAVP) at school
2. Taking DDAVP before bedtime
3. Letting his mother administer the vasopressin injection
4. Giving himself a vasopressin injection before school starts

82. A client newly diagnosed with diabetes insipidus asks the nurse about what method is <u>best</u> to monitor the condition. What is the best response by the nurse?
1. Measuring abdominal girths every day
2. Measuring intake, output, and urine specific gravity
3. Checking daily weights and measuring intake
4. Checking for pitting edema in the lower extremities

83. A nurse is caring for a neonate with congenital hypothyroidism. The nurse observes the client for which finding?
1. Hyperreflexia
2. Long forehead
3. Puffy eyelids
4. Small tongue

84. A child is admitted with complaints of weight loss and lack of energy. The child's ears and cheeks are flushed, and the nurse observes an acetone odor to the child's breath. The child's blood glucose level is 325 mg/dl, his blood pressure is 104/60 mm Hg, his pulse is 88 beats/minute, and respirations are 16 breaths/minute. Which does the nurse expect the physician to order <u>first</u>?
1. Subcutaneous administration of glucagon
2. Administration of I.V. regular insulin by continuous infusion pump
3. Administration of regular insulin subcutaneously every 4 hours as needed by sliding scale insulin
4. Administration of I.V. fluids in boluses of 20 ml/kg

Question 82 asks you to rank monitoring methods for appropriateness. I know you can do it!

You're making great strides! Good job!

81. 1. Anything that singles a child out and makes him feel different from his peers will result in possible noncompliance with the medical regimen. It's important for the nurse to help the client schedule the need for medications around the times he will be in school.
CN: Health promotion and maintenance; CNS: None; CL: Application

82. 2. Measuring intake and output with related specific gravity results will enable the nurse to closely monitor the client's condition along with daily weights. All of the other options aren't as accurate for a child with diabetes insipidus.
CN: Physiological integrity; CNS: Reduction of risk potential; CL: Application

83. 3. Assessment findings would include depressed nasal bridge, short forehead, puffy eyelids, and large tongue; thick, dry, mottled skin that feels cold to the touch; coarse, dry, lusterless hair; abdominal distention; umbilical hernia; hyporeflexia; bradycardia; hypothermia; hypotension; anemia; and wide cranial sutures.
CN: Physiological integrity; CNS: Physiological adaptation; CL: Application

84. 2. Weight loss, lack of energy, acetone odor to breath, and a blood glucose level of 325 mg/dl indicate diabetic ketoacidosis. Insulin is given I.V. by continuous infusion pump. Glucagon is administered for mild hypoglycemia. Sliding scale insulin isn't as effective as the administration of insulin by continuous infusion pump. Administration of I.V. fluids in boluses of 20 ml/kg is recommended for the treatment of shock.
CN: Physiological integrity; CNS: Physiological adaptation; CL: Application

85. Which nursing objective is <u>most important</u> when working with neonates who are suspected of having congenital hypothyroidism?
1. Identifying the disorder early
2. Promoting bonding
3. Allowing rooming in
4. Encouraging fluid intake

What's the most important nursing objective?

85. 1. The most important nursing objective is early identification of the disorder. Nurses caring for neonates must be certain that screening is performed, especially in neonates who are preterm, discharged early, or born at home. Promoting bonding, allowing rooming in, and encouraging fluid intake are all important but are less important than early identification.
CN: Physiological integrity; CNS: Basic care and comfort; CL: Application

86. The nurse instructs the parents of an infant diagnosed with hypothyroidism on how to count the infant's pulse. The parents ask the nurse what they should do if the pulse rate is above the provided parameters. What is the best response by the nurse?
1. "Allow the infant to take a nap and then give the medication."
2. "Withhold the medication and give a double dose the next day."
3. "Hold the medication and call the physician."
4. "Give the medication and then consult the physician."

86. 3. If parents have been taught to count the infant's pulse, they should be instructed to withhold the dose and consult their physician if the pulse rate is above a certain value.
CN: Health promotion and maintenance; CNS: None; CL: Application

87. In an infant receiving inadequate treatment for congenital hypothyroidism, the nurse should expect to observe which symptom(s)?
1. Irritability and jitteriness
2. Fatigue and sleepiness
3. Increased appetite
4. Diarrhea

87. 2. Signs of inadequate treatment are fatigue, sleepiness, decreased appetite, and constipation.
CN: Health promotion and maintenance; CNS: None; CL: Application

88. When collecting data from a child with Cushing's syndrome, which would the nurse be <u>most</u> likely to find? Select all that apply.
1. Obesity
2. Moon-shaped face
3. Hypotension
4. Emotional instability
5. Quickened healing
6. Loss of hair

Question 90 is just around the corner.

88. 1, 2, and 4. Cushing's syndrome occurs as a result of excessive cortisol exposure (through corticosteroid medications or production by the adrenal glands). Common findings include obesity, moon-shaped face, and emotional instability. Hypertension, excessive hair growth, and slower healing are additional findings, making the other options incorrect.
CN: Physiological integrity; CNS: Physiological adaptation; CL: Analysis

89. An adolescent with type 1 diabetes tells the nurse he will be playing football for his school this year. He asks the nurse what he can do to prevent hypoglycemia. What is the best response by the nurse?
1. Limit participation in planned exercise activities that involve competition.
2. Carry crackers or fruit to eat before or during periods of increased activity.
3. Increase the insulin dosage before planned or unplanned strenuous exercise.
4. Check blood sugar before exercising and eat a protein snack if the level is elevated.

90. A child with diabetic ketoacidosis is to receive a continuous infusion of insulin for a blood glucose level of 780 mg/dl. The nurse reviews the orders and would administer which solution?
1. Normal saline with regular insulin
2. Normal saline with Ultralente insulin
3. 5% dextrose in water with NPH insulin
4. 5% dextrose in water with PZI insulin

Let's discuss some steps for preventing hypoglycemia.

91. An adolescent female client is admitted to the hospital with type 1 diabetes and unstable blood glucose levels. What is the <u>most important</u> question for the nurse to include in the health history?
1. Does she play any team sports?
2. Does she refrigerate her insulin?
3. Is she satisfied with her weight?
4. Does she use recreational drugs?

The answer to this question should be a slam dunk.

92. A 14-year-old male client with type 1 diabetes mellitus plans to join the basketball team at his school. The practices are twice a week with games on Saturdays. He calls the nurse at his clinic for advice. The nurse should respond with which statement?
1. "Delay eating a meal until after practice or a game."
2. "Time your insulin to peak at the time of practice and games."
3. "Monitor your blood sugar before, during, and after exercise."
4. "Increase your daily calorie intake by 10% and up your insulin dose by 10%."

89. 2. Hypoglycemia can usually be prevented if an adolescent with diabetes eats more food before or during exercise. Because exercise with adolescents isn't commonly planned, carrying additional carbohydrate foods is a good preventative measure.
CN: Health promotion and maintenance; CNS: None; CL: Application

90. 1. Short-acting regular insulin is the only insulin that should be used for insulin infusions. Initially, normal saline is used until blood glucose levels are reduced. Then a dextrose solution may be used to prevent hypoglycemia. Ultralente, NPH, and PZI insulins have a longer duration of action and shouldn't be used for continuous infusions.
CN: Physiological integrity; CNS: Pharmacological and parenteral therapies; CL: Application

91. 3. It's important to ascertain the adolescent's feelings about her body, in particular her weight. Some female adolescents skip their insulin because they know doing so will result in weight loss. The other issues of sports, drug use, and technique of administering insulin are all relevant but not as important as knowing what the client is thinking about her own body.
CN: Psychosocial integrity; CNS: None; CL: Application

92. 3. For increases in activity, a client with type 1 diabetes would require a snack before the activity and increased insulin. The amount of insulin is the most difficult determination. Monitoring is required for accurate regulation before, during, and after the activity. The client shouldn't delay eating until afterward because the body needs the calories to provide energy to the muscles and tissues. Extreme hypoglycemia may occur if the insulin peaks without extra calories. There's no standard of 10% increase in calories and insulin; every person would require individualization of the insulin and calories needed.
CN: Health promotion and maintenance; CNS: None; CL: Application

93. A nurse is collecting a health history from the parents of a 12-month-old infant being evaluated for possible hypopituitarism. What is the most important question for the nurse to ask?
1. Did the mother drink alcohol while pregnant?
2. Does the infant receive multivitamins?
3. What's the infant's growth pattern?
4. Was the infant premature?

94. A nurse has just completed teaching a family about hypothyroidism. Which actions would indicate the parents understand their child's diagnosis?
1. Providing a diet including whole grains, produce, and water
2. Anticipating their child outgrowing hypothyroidism
3. Providing a white diet for their child
4. Providing a diet high in fat for their child to encourage growth

95. A child with diabetes is receiving a continuous insulin infusion for diabetic ketoacidosis. When assessing the child, the nurse should be alert for signs and symptoms of which complication?
1. Hypercalcemia
2. Hyperphosphatemia
3. Hypokalemia
4. Hypernatremia

96. A nurse is caring for a client with pheochromocytoma. What is the most important intervention by the nurse?
1. Promoting an environment free from emotional distress
2. Avoiding analgesia administration
3. Advising a low-calorie, high-nutrient diet
4. Avoiding parents rooming in because they make the client less dependent on staff

I can see the finish line! You're doing great!

I feel the stress fading away.

93. 3. Hypopituitarism presents with a retarded growth pattern, appearance younger than chronological age, and normal skeletal proportions and intelligence. It's related to tumors, irradiation, infection, and head trauma. Therefore, serial growth patterns will be crucial to the diagnosis process. It isn't related to fetal alcoholism, use of multivitamins, or prematurity.
CN: Physiological integrity; CNS: Physiological adaptation; CL: Application

94. 1. A diet including fruits, vegetables, whole grains, and water will help counteract the trend toward obstinate constipation, the result of a slowed metabolism and hypotonic bowel. Congenital hypothyroidism isn't outgrown, and thyroid replacement is necessary throughout the life span. A white diet involves foods low in fiber, which leads to constipation. Hypothyroid individuals tend to have elevated cholesterol and triglyceride levels; therefore, a diet high in fat is contraindicated.
CN: Health promotion and maintenance; CNS: None; CL: Application

95. 3. Hypokalemia occurs as insulin causes potassium and glucose to move into the cells. Insulin administration doesn't affect calcium or sodium levels. Insulin administration may lead to hypophosphatemia, not hyperphosphatemia, as phosphorus enters the cells with insulin and potassium.
CN: Physiological integrity; CNS: Physiological adaptation; CL: Analysis

96. 1. The child experiencing hyperfunctioning of the adrenal gland, or pheochromocytoma, is in a chronic state of "fight or flight" related to excessive exogenous epinephrine. Therefore, the child has an accelerated metabolism. Symptoms include hypertension, headaches, hyperglycemia with weight loss, diaphoresis, and hyperventilation. Through provision of a low-stress environment, analgesia as needed, a high-calorie diet, and supportive parents, the child will be able to prepare for surgery to eliminate the tumor causing the hypersecretion of epinephrine.
CN: Physiological integrity; CNS: Physiological adaptation; CL: Application

97. A nurse is instructing parents about promoting the health of their child with diabetes. What is the most important information for the nurse to include?
1. Avoid daily bathing so the skin doesn't become too dry.
2. Cuts and scratches on the playground are of little concern.
3. Children with diabetes need few immunizations.
4. Regular dental care and annual ophthalmologic appointments should be kept.

98. A 10-year-old child monitors and adjusts his own insulin. Which response reflects an understanding of dosage adjustment when the child is ill?
1. "I withhold all insulin because I'm not eating."
2. "I'll take my usual dose of regular and NPH insulin."
3. "I'll perform fingerstick blood sugar testing and adjust my insulin according to results."
4. "I'll perform fingerstick blood sugar testing and record the results."

99. The nurse is teaching the parents of a child with hypopituitary dwarfism about the diagnosis. What is the most appropriate information for the nurse to provide?
1. Children with hypopituitary dwarfism are usually low-birth-weight babies.
2. Symptoms aren't apparent until puberty.
3. Symptoms include early primary dentition.
4. Children with hypopituitary dwarfism grow normally during the first 2 years and then fall below the 3rd percentile.

100. A 10-year-old child has been experiencing insatiable thirst and urinating excessively; his serum glucose is <u>normal</u>. Which condition is the client probably experiencing?
1. Type 2 diabetes mellitus
2. Type 1 diabetes mellitus
3. Hyperthyroidism
4. Diabetes insipidus

Adjusting insulin reflects that your client understands his disorder.

97. 4. Regular dental care will preserve oral health, and ophthalmologic examinations will ensure visual acuity for reading. Because of their impaired immune system, children with diabetes need to maintain a high level of health to avoid infection. Daily bathing and application of lotion, cleaning minor playground scrapes and applying antibiotic ointments, and keeping immunizations up-to-date are all important.

CN: Health promotion and maintenance; CNS: None; CL: Application

98. 3. Because of the stress of illness, serum glucose will likely be elevated during an episode of the flu. Appropriate adjustment of insulin dosage will help prevent the child from becoming hypoglycemic or ketoacidotic.

CN: Physiological integrity; CNS: Physiological adaptation; CL: Analysis

99. 4. Generally, hypopituitary children are of average birth weight and grow at a normal pace for the first 2 or 3 years and then fall behind their peers in height, usually below the 3rd percentile. Dentition of primary teeth is normal; permanent teeth are delayed.

CN: Health promotion and maintenance; CNS: None; CL: Application

100. 4. Polydipsia and polyuria with normal serum glucose may be indicative of diabetes insipidus. Interview and laboratory results can determine whether the origin is neurogenic or nephrogenic. Type 1 or 2 diabetes mellitus requires an elevated serum glucose. A child with hyperthyroidism may present as dehydrated from the excessive sweating and rapid respirations that accompany this hypermetabolic state.

CN: Physiological integrity; CNS: Physiological adaptation; CL: Analysis

101. A 4.5-year-old child with diabetes is ordered to receive 25 ml/hour of I.V. solution. The nurse is using a pediatric microdrip chamber to administer the medication. The microdrip chamber should be set for how many drops per minute? Record your answer using a whole number.

_____ gtt/minute

102. The nurse is preparing to administer I.V. methylprednisolone sodium succinate (Solu-Medrol) to a child who weighs 44 lb. The order is for 0.03 mg/kg I.V. daily. How many milligrams should the nurse prepare? Record your answer using one decimal point.

_____ milligrams

Hooray! Another chapter finished! Good job!

101. 25. When using a pediatric microdrip chamber, the number of milliliters per hour equals the number of drops per minute. If 25 ml/hour is ordered, the I.V. should infuse at 25 drops/minute.

CN: Physiological integrity; CNS: Pharmacological and parenteral therapies; CL: Application

102. 0.6. To perform this dosage calculation, the nurse should first convert the child's weight to kilograms: 44 lb ÷ 2.2 kg/lb = 20 kg. Then she should use this formula to determine the dose: 20 kg × 0.03 mg/kg = X mg. X = 0.6 mg.

CN: Physiological integrity; CNS: Pharmacological and parenteral therapies; CL: Application

Chapter 34
Genitourinary disorders

1. A child with acute glomerulonephritis has a nursing diagnosis of impaired urinary elimination related to fluid retention and impaired glomerular filtration. Which client goal best addresses the expected outcome for this diagnosis?
1. Exhibits no evidence of infection
2. Engages in activities appropriate to capabilities
3. Demonstrates no periorbital, facial, or body edema
4. Maintains a fluid intake of more than 2,000 ml in 24 hours

2. An important nursing intervention to support the therapeutic management of a child with acute glomerulonephritis should include which action?
1. Measuring daily weight
2. Increasing oral fluid intake
3. Providing sodium supplements
4. Monitoring the client for signs of hypokalemia

3. A nurse is taking frequent blood pressure readings on a child diagnosed with acute glomerulonephritis. The parents ask the nurse why this is necessary. Which statement by the nurse <u>most</u> accurately addresses their concerns?
1. "Blood pressure fluctuations are a sign that the condition has become chronic."
2. "Blood pressure fluctuations are a common adverse effect of the antibiotic therapy your child is on."
3. "Hypotension can lead to sudden shock and can develop at any time as part of the disease process."
4. "Acute hypertension must be anticipated and identified."

1. 3. The goal of this diagnosis involves interventions, such as decreased fluid and salt intake, designed to minimize or prevent fluid retention and edema. These interventions may be evaluated through observations for edema. The other options are appropriate outcomes for other nursing diagnoses, not the diagnosis in question.

CN: Health promotion and maintenance; CNS: None; CL: Analysis

If you're having trouble deciding on an answer, begin by eliminating the ones you *know* are incorrect.

2. 1. The child with acute glomerulonephritis should be monitored for fluid imbalance, which is done through daily weights. Increasing oral intake, monitoring for hypokalemia, and providing sodium supplements aren't part of the therapeutic management of acute glomerulonephritis.

CN: Physiological integrity; CNS: Basic care and comfort; CL: Application

3. 4. Regular measurement of vital signs, body weight, and intake and output is essential to monitor the progress of the disease and to detect complications that may appear at any time during the course of the disease. Blood pressure fluctuations don't indicate that the condition has become chronic and aren't common adverse reactions to antibiotic therapy. Hypertension is more likely than hypotension to occur with glomerulonephritis.

CN: Physiological integrity; CNS: Physiological adaptation; CL: Application

4. A nurse is reviewing the urine results of a child diagnosed with acute glomerulonephritis. Based on the results of the routine urinalysis, which component best supports this diagnosis?
   1. Specific gravity of 1.032
   2. Protein of 10 mg/100 cc
   3. Gross hematuria
   4. Urine crystals

5. When evaluating the urinalysis report of a child with acute glomerulonephritis, the nurse should expect which result?
   1. Proteinuria and decreased specific gravity
   2. Bacteriuria and increased specific gravity
   3. Hematuria and proteinuria
   4. Bacteriuria and hematuria

6. Which statement by a nurse would be the best response to a mother who wants to know what the first indication will be that her child's acute glomerulonephritis is improving?
   1. "The child's urine output will increase."
   2. "The child's urine will be free from protein."
   3. "The child's blood pressure will stabilize."
   4. "The child's energy will notably increase."

More than one answer may seem correct. It's your job to choose the best answer.

7. Which statement by the parents of a child with acute glomerulonephritis indicates that they understand the teaching provided by the nurse regarding the diagnosis?
   1. "This disease occurs after a urinary tract infection."
   2. "This disease is associated with renal vascular disorders."
   3. "This disease occurs after a streptococcal infection."
   4. "This disease is associated with structural anomalies of the genitourinary tract."

8. When obtaining a child's daily weights, the nurse notes that he has lost 6 lb (2.7 kg) after 3 days of hospitalization for acute glomerulonephritis. The nurse determines that this is most likely the result of which factor?
   1. Poor appetite
   2. Reduction of edema
   3. Decreased salt intake
   4. Restriction to bed rest

4. 3. Urinalysis findings consistent with acute glomerulonephritis would include a specific gravity less than 1.030, mild to moderate proteinuria, gross hematuria, and the presence of RBC casts. The presence of crystals in the urine typically indicates a congenital metabolic problem.
CN: Physiological integrity; CNS: Physiological adaptation; CL: Analysis

5. 3. Urinalysis during the acute phase of this disease characteristically shows hematuria, proteinuria, and increased specific gravity.
CN: Physiological integrity; CNS: Physiological adaptation; CL: Analysis

6. 1. One of the first signs of improvement during the acute phase of glomerulonephritis is an increase in urine output. It will take time for the urine to be free from protein. Antihypertensive drugs may be needed to stabilize the blood pressure. Children generally don't have much energy during the acute phase of this disease.
CN: Health promotion and maintenance; CNS: None; CL: Analysis

7. 3. Acute glomerulonephritis is an immune-complex disease that occurs as a by-product of a streptococcal infection. Certain strains of the infection are usually a beta-hemolytic *Streptococcus*. Other options are not applicable to this disease.
CN: Health promotion and maintenance; CNS: None; CL: Analysis

8. 2. When there's reduction of edema, the client will lose weight. This should normally occur after treatment for acute glomerulonephritis has been followed for several days. A poor appetite, decreased salt intake, or restriction to bed rest wouldn't lead to such a dramatic weight loss in a child this age.
CN: Physiological integrity; CNS: Basic care and comfort; CL: Application

9. A nurse is teaching the parents of a child who has been newly diagnosed with acute glomerulo-nephritis about nutrition. The nurse determines teaching was effective when the parents state the need to do what?
1. Decrease calories being consumed.
2. Increase the child's potassium intake.
3. Severely limit all sodium intake.
4. Moderately restrict sodium intake.

10. A nurse is evaluating a group of children for the potential development of acute glomerulonephritis. Which client would be most likely to develop the disease?
1. A client who had pneumonia a month ago
2. A client who was bitten by a brown spider
3. A client who has a history of cardiac disease
4. A client who had a streptococcal infection 2 weeks ago

Ten questions down! That's a good start!

11. A nurse is questioned by a student nurse about the long-term consequences of poststrepto-coccal acute glomerulonephritis. What is the most accurate response by the nurse?
1. "Children up to age 2 with this disease have the worst outcomes."
2. "Approximately 95% of children affected by acute glomerulonephritis will recover without problems."
3. "Chronic hypertension is a common long-term problem seen in children with this diagnosis."
4. "The higher the level of hematuria and pro-teinuria, the more likely it is the child will go into renal failure."

12. The nurse understands the reoccurrence of glomerulonephritis and is aware that:
1. second attacks are quite common.
2. a recessive gene transfers this disease.
3. multiple cases tend to occur in families.
4. overcrowding in the schoolroom leads to higher incidence.

9. 4. Moderate sodium restriction with a diet that has no added salt after cooking is usually effective. Calorie consumption doesn't need to decrease and is often encouraged to counterbalance the decreased appetite. Potassium consumption shouldn't increase because of the decrease in urinary output. Severe sodium restriction isn't needed and will make it more difficult to ensure adequate nutrition. It will also result in hyponatremia.
CN: Physiological integrity; CNS: Basic care and comfort; CL: Application

10. 4. A latent period of 10 to 14 days occurs between the streptococcal infection of the throat or skin and the onset of clinical manifestations. The peak incidence of disease corresponds to the incidence of streptococcal infections. Pneumonia isn't a precursor to glomerulonephritis, nor is a bite from a brown spider. Cardiac disease does not contribute to acute glomerulonephritis.
CN: Health promotion and maintenance; CNS: None; CL: Analysis

11. 2. Most children diagnosed with acute glomerulonephritis recover without any long-term sequelae. Acute glomerulonephritis is uncommon in children younger than age 2. Hypertension normally resolves within a few weeks of diagnosis. The level of blood in the urine and the protein spill-age within the kidneys have no correlation to the severity of problems seen with this disease.
CN: Health promotion and maintenance; CNS: None; CL: Application

12. 3. Multiple cases tend to occur in families. Second attacks are rare. Acute glomerulonephritis isn't transmitted through a recessive gene, and overcrowding in the schoolroom should have no influence on this disease.
CN: Health promotion and maintenance; CNS: None; CL: Application

CN: Client needs category   CNS: Client needs subcategory   CL: Cognitive level

13. A nurse is explaining enuresis to a child's parents. What is the most important information for the nurse to include? Select all that apply.
1. "Your child may experience involuntary urination after age 5."
2. "Episodes primarily occur when your child is awake and playing."
3. "Your child may suffer deep feelings of shame and may withdraw from peers because of ridicule."
4. "The condition may respond to tricyclic antidepressants and antidiuretics."
5. "The condition may become permanent without appropriate intervention."

14. Which comment made by a parent would indicate to the nurse the need for <u>further education</u> about acute glomerulonephritis complications?
1. "Dizziness is expected, and I should have my child lie down when he feels it."
2. "I should let the nurse know every time my child urinates."
3. "I need to ask my child whether he has a headache."
4. "I should encourage quiet play activities in the room."

15. The nurse is teaching parents of a 3-year-old child how to obtain a clean-catch urine specimen. What is the most appropriate statement by the nurse?
1. "Collect the specimen right after a nap."
2. "Never use the first voided specimen of the day."
3. "Collect the specimen at the beginning of urination."
4. "There is no need to wash the perineal area before collecting the specimen."

16. Which therapy should a nurse expect to incorporate into the care of a child with acute glomerulonephritis?
1. Antibiotic therapy
2. Dialysis therapy
3. Sodium therapy
4. Play therapy

The phrase *further education* indicates that question 14 is looking for an inaccurate statement.

Don't a-void this question. You're doing great!

13. 1, 3, and 4. Enuresis is a condition in which there's involuntary urination after age 5. It generally occurs while the child is sleeping. There can be long-lasting emotional trauma resulting from peer ridicule and feelings of shame and embarrassment. The condition may be treated with the use of tricyclic antidepressants and antidiuretics. With support and understanding, the condition generally resolves in time.
CN: Physiological integrity; CNS: Physiological adaptation; CL: Analysis

14. 1. Dizziness and headache are signs of encephalopathy and must be reported to the nurse. Hypertensive encephalopathy, acute cardiac decompensation, and acute renal failure are the major complications that tend to develop during the acute phase of glomerulonephritis. In order to maintain an accurate intake and output record, the parent should let the nurse know when the child urinates. Quiet play is encouraged to avoid overstressing the kidneys.
CN: Physiological integrity; CNS: Reduction of risk potential; CL: Application

15. 2. When collecting a clean-catch urine specimen, the first voided specimen of the day should never be used because of urinary stasis; this also applies after a nap. The specimen should be collected midstream, not at the beginning or end of urination. Washing the perineal area before collecting a specimen is very important to make sure there are no contaminants from the skin in the specimen.
CN: Physiological integrity; CNS: Reduction of risk potential; CL: Application

16. 4. Play therapy is an important aspect of care to help the child understand what's happening to him. Unless the child has the ability to express concerns and fears, he may have night terrors and regress in his stage of growth and development. Antibiotic therapy is indicated for an infectious process. Dialysis therapy is appropriate for renal failure. Administration of additional sodium is inappropriate.
CN: Health promotion and maintenance; CNS: None; CL: Application

17. A nurse is explaining the expected treatment for glomerulonephritis. What is the most important information for the nurse to include?
1. All children who have signs of glomerulonephritis are hospitalized for approximately 1 week.
2. Parents should expect children to have a normal energy level during the acute phase.
3. Children who have normal blood pressure and a satisfactory urinary output can generally be treated at home.
4. Children with gross hematuria and significant oliguria should be brought to the physician's office every 2 days for monitoring.

18. What is a priority nursing intervention for a school-age child with acute glomerulonephritis?
1. Assess blood pressure every 4 hours.
2. Check urine specific gravity every 8 hours.
3. Encourage daily fluid intake of 100 ml/kg/day.
4. Provide a 2,500-mg sodium diet.

19. A child with acute glomerulonephritis is selecting his menu. The nurse determines further teaching is necessary when the child selects which food?
1. Turkey sandwich with mayonnaise and celery sticks
2. Hot dog with ketchup and mustard and chips
3. Chocolate cake with white icing and ice cream
4. Apple slices with peanut butter and milk

20. A mother of a child with hypospadias asks the nurse what is wrong with her son's penis. What is the most appropriate response by the nurse?
1. "It is the absence of a urethral opening in the penis."
2. "It is a penis that is shorter than usual for the child's age."
3. "It is a urethral opening along the dorsal or top surface of the penis."
4. "It is a urethral opening along the ventral or underside surface of the penis."

Hypertension is a complication of glomerulonephritis.

What do you mean I'm being eliminated?

17. 3. Children who have normal blood pressure and a satisfactory urinary output can generally be treated at home. Parents should expect children to have a decrease in energy levels during the acute phase of the disease. Those with gross hematuria and significant oliguria will probably be hospitalized for monitoring. There is no set time frame of hospitalization, and not all clients need to be hospitalized.

CN: Health promotion and maintenance; CNS: None; CL: Application

18. 1. Because hypertension is a complication of acute glomerulonephritis, the nurse should check the child's blood pressure every 4 hours. The urine specific gravity should also be monitored, but it isn't as high a priority as monitoring the blood pressure. The child may be placed on fluid or sodium restrictions, and fluid intake of 100 ml/kg/day is too much for even a healthy child with normal renal function.

CN: Physiological integrity; CNS: Reduction of risk potential; CL: Application

19. 2. Foods that are high in sodium content, such as hot dogs, should be eliminated from the child's diet. Snacks such as pretzels and potato chips should also be discouraged. Any other foods that the child likes should be encouraged.

CN: Physiological integrity; CNS: Basic care and comfort; CL: Application

20. 4. Hypospadias refers to a condition in which the urethral opening is located below the glans penis or anywhere along the ventral surface of the penile shaft.

CN: Health promotion and maintenance; CNS: None; CL: Application

21. After the acute phase of glomerulonephritis is resolved, which discharge instruction should a nurse include?
1. Every 6 months, a cystogram will be needed for evaluation of progress.
2. Weekly visits to the physician may be needed for evaluation.
3. It will be acceptable to keep the regular yearly checkup appointment for the next evaluation.
4. There's no need for further evaluations by the physician related to this disease.

22. The mother of a newborn tells the nurse that she was told that her infant has chordee but does not understand what that means. What is the most appropriate response by the nurse?
1. "It is a ventral curvature of the penis."
2. "It is a dorsal curvature of the penis."
3. "It is a slit along the top of the penis."
4. "It is a misshapen penis."

23. The nurse is caring for an infant with hypospadias. The nurse understands that which anomaly commonly accompanies this condition?
1. Undescended testicles
2. Ambiguous genitalia
3. Umbilical hernias
4. Inguinal hernias

24. A nurse is explaining the rationale for timing of surgical repair of a hypospadias to the parents of a child with the disorder. Which best explains why it is done as early as possible?
1. To prevent separation anxiety
2. To prevent urinary complications
3. To promote acceptance of hospitalization
4. To promote development of a normal body image

25. A nurse would counsel parents to postpone which action until after their son's hypospadias has been repaired?
1. Circumcising the infant
2. Baptizing the infant
3. Getting hepatitis B vaccine
4. Checking blood for inborn errors of metabolism

Twenty-one questions done! Keep plugging along!

Knowing common accompanying conditions is important for taking the NCLEX.

21. 2. Weekly or monthly visits to the physician will be needed for evaluation of improvement and will usually involve the collection of a urine specimen for urinalysis. A cystogram isn't helpful in determining the progression of this disease; it's used to review the anatomic structures of the urinary tract.
CN: Physiological integrity; CNS: Reduction of risk potential; CL: Application

22. 1. Chordee, or ventral curvature of the penis, results from the replacement of normal skin with a fibrous band of tissue and usually accompanies more severe forms of hypospadias.
CN: Health promotion and maintenance; CNS: None; CL: Application

23. 1. Because undescended testes may also be present, the small penis may appear to be an enlarged clitoris. This shouldn't be mistaken for ambiguous genitalia. If there's any doubt, more tests should be performed. Hernias don't generally accompany hypospadias.
CN: Health promotion and maintenance; CNS: None; CL: Application

24. 4. Whenever there are defects of the genitourinary tract, surgery should be performed early to promote development of a normal body image. The older the child, the more likely he will be traumatized by the surgery. A child with normal emotional development shows separation anxiety at 7 to 9 months. Within a few months, he understands the mother's permanence, and separation anxiety diminishes. Hypospadias doesn't put the child at a greater risk for urinary complications.
CN: Health promotion and maintenance; CNS: None; CL: Application

25. 1. Circumcision shouldn't be performed until after the hypospadias has been repaired. The foreskin might be needed to help in the repair of the hypospadias. None of the other choices has any bearing on the repair of the hypospadias.
CN: Health promotion and maintenance; CNS: None; CL: Application

26. Which statement made by the parents of a child undergoing hypospadias repair implies a need for <u>further teaching</u> about the primary objective of surgical correction?
1. "The purpose is to improve the physical appearance of the genitalia for psychological reasons."
2. "The purpose is to enhance the child's ability to void in the standing position."
3. "The purpose is to decrease the chance of developing urinary tract infections."
4. "The purpose is to preserve a sexually adequate organ."

I'm looking for the one inaccurate statement.

27. What is the most important intervention for the nurse to include in the care plan for a male infant following surgical repair of hypospadias?
1. Sterile dressing changes every 4 hours
2. Frequent assessment of the tip of the penis
3. Removal of the suprapubic catheter on the second postoperative day
4. Urethral catheterization if voiding doesn't occur over an 8-hour period

28. The nurse is caring for an infant newly admitted with the diagnosis of exstrophy of the bladder. What are the most appropriate interventions? Select all that apply.
1. Gather supplies in anticipation of insertion of a Foley catheter.
2. Implement a latex-free environment for the infant.
3. Maintain the infant in a prone position.
4. Cover the defect with a nonadherent dressing.
5. Place the infant in a thermo-controlled environment.
6. Place a diaper snugly over the genitalia to ensure accurate output monitoring.

29. The nurse is providing discharge information to the parents of a child with a hypospadias repair. Which instructions would be most <u>appropriate</u>? Select all that apply.
1. Care of the circumcision
2. Techniques for providing tub baths
3. Care for the indwelling catheter or stent
4. Encouragement of voiding every 2 hours
5. Avoid penis-harmful items like straddle toys

You're almost at question 30 and you're doing great.

26. 3. A child with hypospadias isn't at greater risk for urinary tract infections. The principal objectives of surgical corrections are to enhance the child's ability to void in the standing position with a straight stream, to improve the physical appearance of the genitalia for psychological reasons, and to preserve a sexually adequate organ.
CN: Health promotion and maintenance; CNS: None; CL: Application

27. 2. Following hypospadias repair, a pressure dressing is applied to the penis to reduce bleeding and tissue swelling. The penile tip should then be assessed frequently for signs of circulatory impairment. The dressing around the penis shouldn't be changed as frequently as every 4 hours and is normally done by the surgeon initially. The physician will determine when the suprapubic catheter will be removed. Urethral catheterization should be avoided after repair of hypospadias to prevent trauma to the repaired urethra.
CN: Physiological integrity; CNS: Basic care and comfort; CL: Application

28. 2, 4, and 5. Exstrophy of the bladder is a congenital defect whereby the bladder is externalized on the abdomen and requires specialized care, including a latex-free environment, supine positioning, covering of the defect with a nonadherent dressing, and maintaining a thermoneutral environment. Catheterization is not performed for these clients, and the bladder defect is never covered up with a diaper.
CN: Health promotion and maintenance; CNS: None; CL: Application

29. 3 and 5. Parents are taught to care for the indwelling catheter or stent and irrigation techniques, if indicated. They are also told to avoid any toy that will put pressure or irritate the genital area until it is healed. The child with hypospadias shouldn't be circumcised because the foreskin may be needed during surgical repair. A tub bath should be avoided to prevent infection until the catheter or stent has been removed. Following surgical repair, the child will have an indwelling urinary catheter, so encouraging the child to void isn't appropriate.
CN: Physiological integrity; CNS: Reduction of risk potential; CL: Analysis

30. The nurse is providing discharge instructions to the parents of an older child who has had hypospadias repair. Which activity should be encouraged?
1. Riding a bicycle
2. Playing in sandboxes
3. Increased fluid intake
4. Playing with the family pet

31. The mother of a neonate born with hypospadias is sharing her feelings of guilt about this anomaly with a nurse. The nurse should explain which fact about the defect?
1. It occurs around the third month of fetal development and has nothing to do with anything the mother did.
2. It occurs around the sixth month of fetal development and often results from smoking or drinking while pregnant.
3. It's carried by an autosomal recessive gene and may occur with future children.
4. It's hereditary and is usually passed on as an X-linked problem from mother to son.

32. A mother reports that her 6-year-old daughter recently began wetting the bed and running a low-grade fever. A urinalysis is positive for bacteria and protein. A diagnosis of a urinary tract infection (UTI) is made, and the child is prescribed antibiotics. What are the most appropriate nursing interventions? Select all that apply.
1. Limit fluids for the next few days to decrease the frequency of urination.
2. Assess the mother's understanding of UTI and its causes.
3. Instruct the mother to administer the antibiotic as prescribed—even if the symptoms diminish.
4. Provide instruction solely to the mother, not the child.
5. Discourage the taking of bubble baths.
6. Advise wiping from back to the front after voiding and defecation.

33. A 3-year-old child who had a hypospadias repair yesterday has a suprapubic catheter in place and an I.V. The nurse is aware that which is the rationale for administering propantheline bromide (Pro-Banthine) on an as-needed basis?
1. To decrease the risk of infection at the suture line
2. To decrease the number of organisms in the urine
3. To prevent bladder spasms while the catheter is present
4. To increase urine flow from the kidney to the ureters

30. 3. The family is advised to encourage the child to increase fluid intake. Sandboxes, straddle toys, swimming, and rough activities are avoided until allowed by the surgeon.
CN: Physiological integrity; CNS: Physiological adaptation; CL: Application

31. 1. The defect of hypospadias occurs around the end of the third month of fetal development. Many women don't even know that they're pregnant at this time. This defect is not carried by an autosomal recessive gene. It is also not X-linked or related to smoking or ingestion of alcohol.
CN: Health promotion and maintenance; CNS: None; CL: Application

32. 2, 3, and 5. Assessing the mother's understanding of UTI and its causes provides the nurse with a baseline for teaching. The full course of antibiotics must be given to eradicate the organism and prevent recurrence, even if the child's signs and symptoms decrease. Bubble baths can irritate the vulva and urethra and contribute to the development of a UTI. Fluids should be encouraged, not limited, in order to prevent urinary stasis and help flush the organism out of the urinary tract. Instructions should be given to the child at her level of understanding to help her better understand the treatment and promote compliance. The child should wipe from front to the back, not back to front, to minimize the risk of contamination after elimination.
CN: Health promotion and maintenance; CNS: None; CL: Application

33. 3. Propantheline bromide is an antispasmodic that works effectively on children. It isn't an antibiotic and therefore won't decrease the chance of infection or the number of organisms in the urine. The drug has no diuretic effect and won't increase urine flow.
CN: Physiological integrity; CNS: Pharmacological and parenteral therapies; CL: Application

34. What is the <u>initial</u> intervention for a nurse to implement when discussing hypospadias with the parents of an infant with this defect?
1. Refer the parents to a counselor.
2. Be there to listen to the parents' concerns.
3. Notify the physician and have him talk to the parents.
4. Suggest a support group of other parents who have gone through this experience.

You can almost hear the answer to this question.

35. A nurse should understand that hypospadias defects take the greatest emotional toll on which person?
1. The father
2. The mother
3. The grandfather
4. The grandmother

36. A nurse is questioned by a student nurse about the difference between hypospadias and epispadias. Which response by the nurse is best?
1. Epispadias defects can only occur in males and affect sterility.
2. The difference between the defects is the length of the urethra and size of the urethral meatus.
3. Hypospadias is an abnormal opening on the ventral side of the penis; epispadias is an abnormal opening on the dorsal side.
4. Hypospadias is an abnormal opening on the dorsal side of the penis; epispadias is an abnormal opening on the ventral side.

Question 36 is asking you to differentiate between two conditions.

37. Which nursing diagnosis would be most appropriate for an infant with hypospadias?
1. Impaired body image
2. Impaired urinary elimination
3. Delayed growth and development
4. Risk for infection

34. 2. The nurse must recognize that parents are going to grieve the loss of the "normal" child when they have a neonate born with a birth defect. Initially, the parents need to have a nurse who will listen to their concerns for their neonate's health. Suggesting a support group or referring the parents to a counselor might be good actions but not initially. The physician will need to spend time with the parents, but again, the nurse is in the best position to allow the parents to vent their grief and anger.
CN: Psychosocial integrity; CNS: None; CL: Application

35. 1. Because the penis is involved, studies have shown that fathers have a great deal of difficulty dealing with a birth defect like hypospadias.
CN: Psychosocial integrity; CNS: None; CL: Application

36. 3. Hypospadias results from the incomplete closure of the urethral folds along the ventral surface of the developing penis. Epispadias results when the urinary meatus is on the dorsal surface of the penis. Epispadias defects can occur in males and females, although it is very rare in females. The difference is where the opening of the urinary meatus is located, not the length of the urethra or meatus size.
CN: Health promotion and maintenance; CNS: None; CL: Application

37. 2. The most appropriate diagnosis for a client with hypospadias is impaired urinary elimination. An infant with hypospadias should have no problems with body image. The child's growth and development aren't affected by this defect, and he doesn't have any problem with infection until possibly after a repair of the hypospadias is performed.
CN: Health promotion and maintenance; CNS: None; CL: Analysis

38. A nurse is teaching a parent how to care for the penis after a hypospadias repair with a skin graft. Which statement made by the parent would indicate the need for further teaching?
1. "My infant won't be able to take tub baths until healing has occurred."
2. "I will change the dressing around the penis daily."
3. "I will make sure I change my infant's diaper often."
4. "If there's a color change in the penis, I will notify my child's physician."

39. A nurse is preparing the parents of an infant born with hypospadias for upcoming surgery. The nurse determines further teaching is necessary when a parent makes which statement?
1. "Skin grafting might be involved in my infant's repair."
2. "After surgery, my infant's penis will look perfectly normal."
3. "Surgical repair may need to be performed in several stages."
4. "My infant will probably be in some pain after the surgery and might need to take some medication for relief."

40. Which assessment data collected by a nurse would indicate to the physician the need for a staged repair of a hypospadias rather than a single repair?
1. There's chordee present with the hypospadias.
2. The urinary meatus opens between the scrotum.
3. The urinary meatus is just below the tip of the penis.
4. The infant had been circumcised before the defect was discovered.

Stay alert for further teaching opportunities.

38. 2. Dressing changes after a hypospadias repair with a skin graft are generally performed by the physician and aren't performed every day because the skin graft needs time to heal and adhere to the penis. Baths aren't given until postoperative healing has taken place. Changing the infant's diapers typically helps keep the penis dry. If the penis color changes, it might be evidence of circulation problems and should be reported.

CN: Health promotion and maintenance; CNS: None; CL: Analysis

39. 2. It's important to stress to the parents that, even after a repair of hypospadias, the outcome isn't a completely "normal-looking" penis. The goals of surgery are to allow the child to void from the tip of his penis, void with a straight stream, and stand up while voiding.

CN: Psychosocial integrity; CNS: None; CL: Application

40. 2. Increased surgical experience and improvements in technique have reduced the number of staged procedures applied to hypospadias defects; however, a staged procedure is indicated in particularly severe defects with marked deficits of available skin for mobilization of flaps and inadequate urethral length. Having a chordee present doesn't require a staged hypospadias repair. If an infant has been circumcised but has a relatively minor hypospadias, the repair can still occur in one stage.

CN: Physiological integrity; CNS: Physiological adaptation; CL: Analysis

41. Which teaching statement by a nurse <u>best</u> reflects accurate reproductive education for a female adolescent in the prevention of pelvic inflammatory disease (PID)?
1. Poor hygiene practices will increase the risk of PID.
2. The use of hormonal contraceptives decreases the risk of PID.
3. There are long-term complications related to reproductive tract infections.
4. There are risks of defects in future infants born to adolescents with PID.

42. The nurse has completed discharge teaching to a teenage client who was treated for a sexually transmitted disease (STD). The nurse determines that teaching was effective when the client states:
1. "I don't need condoms because I'm not allergic to penicillin and I'll come for a shot at the first sign of infection."
2. "I will notify my sex partners of my infection and not have unprotected sex from now on."
3. "I will be careful not to have intercourse with someone who has an STD."
4. "If I am going to get it, there is not much I can do to prevent it."

43. A nurse is preparing an educational seminar for a local clinic directed at adolescent clientele. Which information regarding chlamydial infections would be most important to include in the presentation?
1. Females infected with chlamydia will have intense pelvic pain and irregular menstrual cycles.
2. Chlamydia can be treated with oral penicillin for 1 week and will be completely cured.
3. Clinical manifestations often include dysuria and urethral itching in males.
4. Most clients with chlamydia will exhibit genital vesicles that are highly contagious.

44. Before a client with syphilis can be treated, the nurse must determine which factor?
1. Portal of entry
2. Size of the chancre
3. Names of sexual contacts
4. Existence of medication allergies

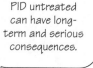

PID untreated can have long-term and serious consequences.

Some people are just hypersensitive— to me, that is.

41. 3. Long-term complications of PID include abscess formation in the fallopian tubes and adhesion formation leading to increased risk of ectopic pregnancy or infertility. It isn't prevented by proper personal hygiene or any form of contraception; some forms of contraception, such as the male or female condom, do help to decrease the incidence of PID. PID does not increase the risk of birth defects in infants born to adolescents with PID.
CN: Health promotion and maintenance; CNS: None; CL: Application

42. 2. Goal achievement is indicated by the client's ability to describe preventive behaviors and health practices. The other options indicate that the client doesn't understand the need to take preventive measures.
CN: Health promotion and maintenance; CNS: None; CL: Analysis

43. 3. Clinical manifestations of chlamydia include meatal erythema, tenderness, itching, dysuria, and urethral discharge in the male and mucopurulent cervical exudate with erythema, edema, and congestion in the female. Menstrual cycles are not affected. The treatment of choice is doxycycline or azithromycin. Vesicles in the genital area are more consistent with herpes simplex virus.
CN: Health promotion and maintenance; CNS: None; CL: Application

44. 4. The treatment of choice for syphilis is penicillin; clients allergic to penicillin must be given another antibiotic. The other choices aren't necessary before treatment can begin.
CN: Health promotion and maintenance; CNS: None; CL: Analysis

45. A nurse wants to provide an open environment for a discussion on sex and sexual activities with adolescents. Which technique would best meet the desired outcome?
1. Break down all the information into scientific terminology.
2. Refer the adolescents to their parents for sexual information.
3. Answer only questions that are asked; don't present any other content.
4. Present sexual information using the proper terminology and in a straightforward manner.

The NCLEX tests your ability to teach clients at different life stages.

46. Without proper treatment, anogenital warts caused by the human papillomavirus (HPV) increase the risk of which illness in adolescent females?
1. Gonorrhea
2. Cervical cancer
3. Chlamydial infections
4. Urinary tract infections (UTIs)

47. Which statement by a nurse most accurately addresses an adolescent's questions about gonorrhea treatment at his or her developmental level?
1. "It's treated with a 2-week dose of penicillin given orally, so you should have no problem curing your disease and no one will ever know."
2. "Gonorrhea can be spread easily, so you need to be sure that you notify anyone you had sex with that they need to be tested and treated too."
3. "I know you hate shots, but you will need to come into the clinic for multiple injections of penicillin given over several weeks to treat your sexually transmitted disease."
4. "You probably contracted the disease from using tampons and not changing them often enough."

48. A nurse is planning sex education and contraceptive instruction for adolescents. It is most important for the nurse to consider which factor?
1. Neither sexual activity nor contraception requires planning.
2. Most teenagers today are knowledgeable about reproduction.
3. Most teenagers use pregnancy as a way to rebel against their parents.
4. Most teenagers are open about contraception but inconsistently use birth control.

45. 4. Although many adolescents have received sex education from parents and school throughout childhood, they aren't always adequately prepared for the impact of puberty. A large portion of their knowledge is acquired from peers, television, movies, and magazines. Consequently, much of the sex information they have is incomplete, inaccurate, riddled with cultural and moral values, and not very helpful. The public perceives nurses as having authoritative information and being willing to take time with parents. To be effective teachers, nurses need to be honest and open with sexual information.
CN: Health promotion and maintenance; CNS: None; CL: Application

46. 2. All external lesions are treated because of concern regarding the relationship of HPV to cancer. HPV doesn't increase the risk of gonorrhea, chlamydia, or UTIs.
CN: Health promotion and maintenance; CNS: None; CL: Application

47. 2. Adolescents should be taught that treatment is needed for all sexual partners. Gonorrhea is treated by a one-time dose of antibiotics, not long-term oral ones. The medication of choice is a single dose of I.M. ceftriaxone sodium (Rocephin) in males and a single oral dose of cefixime (Suprax) in females. Gonorrhea can't be contracted from the use of tampons.
CN: Health promotion and maintenance; CNS: None; CL: Application

48. 4. Most teenagers today are open about discussing contraception and sexuality but may get caught up in the heat of sexuality and forget about birth control measures. Very few teenagers use pregnancy as a way to rebel against their parents. A good deal of the information adolescents have related to reproduction and sexuality may have come from their peers and may not be very reliable.
CN: Health promotion and maintenance; CNS: None; CL: Analysis

49. A sexually active adolescent is discussing prevention of sexually transmitted diseases (STDs) with the school nurse. Which statement by the adolescent best demonstrates accurate understanding of prevention?
1. "My girlfriend is on the pill, so we are not worried about contracting any diseases from each other."
2. "We practice the rhythm method of birth control, so we don't have sex when we could catch anything."
3. "I always use a condom and a spermicide whenever I have sex to prevent any chance of catching a disease."
4. "My friends tell me that if I use the withdrawal method, I am never going to get an STD."

50. A nurse understands that which developmental rationale explains risk-taking behavior in adolescents?
1. Adolescents are concrete thinkers and concentrate only on what's happening at the time.
2. Belief in their own invulnerability persuades adolescents that they can take risks safely.
3. Risk of parents' anger and disappointment usually deters adolescents from risky behavior.
4. Peer pressure usually doesn't play an important part in an adolescent's decision to become sexually active.

51. Statistics about sexually transmitted diseases (STDs) may not be reliable for which reason?
1. Most adolescents seek out treatment for their STD.
2. Adolescents are usually honest with their parents about their sexual behavior.
3. All STDs must be reported to the Centers for Disease Control and Prevention (CDC).
4. Chlamydial infections and human papillomavirus (HPV) infections aren't required to be reported to the CDC.

52. It's important for a nurse to include which statement in discharge education for the client who's taking metronidazole (Flagyl) to treat trichomoniasis?
1. Sexual intercourse should stop until the medication is completed.
2. Alcohol shouldn't be consumed while on the medication.
3. Milk products should be avoided since they reduce the effectiveness of the medicine.
4. Exposure to sunlight should be limited to only 1 hour per day.

Nice work! You've finished nearly 50 questions already!

Adolescents may engage in sex as part of risky behavior.

49. 3. Prevention of STDs is the primary concern of health care professionals. Barrier contraceptive methods, such as condoms with the addition of spermicide, seem to offer the best protection for preventing STDs and their serious complications. The other contraceptive choices don't prevent the transmission of an STD but only reduce the chance of pregnancy.

CN: Health promotion and maintenance; CNS: None; CL: Analysis

50. 2. Understanding the growth and development of adolescents helps the nurse see that they feel they're invulnerable. Adolescents think about the future and can formally operate in their thought process. Peer pressure plays an important role in risk-taking behaviors, more so than fear of parents' anger or disappointment.

CN: Health promotion and maintenance; CNS: None; CL: Analysis

51. 4. Chlamydial infections and HPV infections aren't required to be reported to the CDC. Most teenagers are afraid to seek out health care for sexual diseases or are unaware of the signs and symptoms of STDs. Teenagers find this a very difficult topic to discuss with their parents and will usually seek out a peer or another adult to obtain information.

CN: Safe, effective care environment; CNS: Safety and infection control; CL: Application

52. 2. While taking metronidazole to treat trichomoniasis, clients shouldn't consume alcohol for at least 48 hours following the last dose. The other choices have no effect on the client taking this medication.

CN: Physiological integrity; CNS: Pharmacological and parenteral therapies; CL: Application

CN: Client needs category   CNS: Client needs subcategory   CL: Cognitive level

53. The nurse determines that <u>more education</u> about sexually transmitted diseases (STDs) is needed when an adolescent makes which statement?
1. "You always know when you've got gonorrhea."
2. "The most common STD in kids my age is chlamydia infection."
3. "Most of the girls who have chlamydia don't even know it."
4. "If you have symptoms of gonorrhea, they can show up a day or a couple of weeks after you got the infection to begin with."

54. A school nurse is developing a new sexually transmitted disease (STD) prevention program. Which preventative behaviors should be addressed in the program? Select all that apply.
1. Delaying first sexual intercourse
2. Increased use of rhythm method
3. Reducing the number of sexual partners
4. Encouraging adolescents to not talk about sex with others
5. Increasing use of condoms

55. A nurse determines that which client is at greatest risk for developing acquired immunodeficiency syndrome (AIDS)?
1. A client who lives in crowded housing with poor ventilation
2. A young sexually active client with multiple partners
3. An adolescent who's homeless and lives in shelters
4. A young sexually active client with one partner

56. An adolescent client complains of a low-grade fever, lower abdominal pain, and painful urination with frequency. The nurse realizes that this client is exhibiting symptoms of which genitourinary problem?
1. Pelvic inflammatory infection (PID)
2. Chlamydia
3. Herpes genitalis
4. Syphilis

Some sexually transmitted diseases can occur with or without symptoms.

Questions about basic assessment skills are common on the NCLEX.

53. 1. Gonorrhea can occur with or without symptoms. There are four main forms of the disease: asymptomatic, uncomplicated symptomatic, complicated symptomatic, and disseminated disease. All of the other statements are accurate.

CN: Health promotion and maintenance; CNS: None; CL: Application

54. 1, 3, and 5. By addressing the importance of reducing the number of sexual partners of adolescents, delaying the initial sexual contact, and using condoms, STD prevention programs have had a significant impact on reducing sexual risk behaviors. The rhythm method has no impact on prevention of STDs, and adolescents are less likely to adhere to what is taught if they are not encouraged to discuss sex with other people.

CN: Health promotion and maintenance; CNS: Safety and infection control; CL: Application

55. 2. The younger the client when sexual activity begins, the higher the incidence is of HIV and AIDS. Also, the more sexual partners he or she has, the higher the incidence of these diseases. Neither crowded living environments nor homeless environments by themselves lead to an increase in the incidence of AIDS.

CN: Health promotion and maintenance; CNS: None; CL: Analysis

56. 1. PID is an infection of the upper female genital tract most commonly caused by sexually transmitted diseases. Presenting symptoms in the adolescent may be generalized, with fever, abdominal pain, urinary tract symptoms, and vague, influenza-like symptoms. A hard, painless, red, defined lesion indicates syphilis. Small vesicles on the genital area with itching indicate herpes genitalis. Cervical discharge with redness and edema indicates chlamydia.

CN: Health promotion and maintenance; CNS: None; CL: Analysis

57. A nurse should include which fact when teaching an adolescent group about the human immunodeficiency virus (HIV)?
1. The incidence of HIV in the adolescent population has declined since 1995.
2. The virus can be spread through many routes, including sexual contact.
3. Knowledge about HIV spread and transmission has led to a decrease in the spread of the virus among adolescents.
4. About 50% of all new HIV infections in the United States occur in people under age 22.

58. A nurse is planning a program to teach adolescents about human immunodeficiency virus (HIV) infection. Which action might lead to better program success?
1. Surveying the community to evaluate the level of education
2. Obtaining peer educators to provide information about HIV
3. Setting up clinics in community centers and having condoms readily available
4. Having primary health care providers host workshops in community centers

59. The nurse has completed her teaching about syphilis to an adolescent. The nurse determines further teaching is necessary when the adolescent makes which statement?
1. "The disease is divided into four stages: primary, secondary, latent, and tertiary."
2. "Affected persons are least infectious during the first year."
3. "Syphilis is easily treated with penicillin or doxycycline."
4. "Syphilis is usually transmitted sexually."

60. In teaching a group of parents about monitoring for urinary tract infection (UTI) in preschoolers, which symptom would indicate that a child should be evaluated?
1. Voids only twice in any 6-hour period
2. Exhibits incontinence after being toilet trained
3. Has difficulty sitting still for more than a 30-minute period of time
4. Urine smells strongly of ammonia after standing for more than 2 hours

Hey! I think I finally get genitourinary disorders.

Sixty questions down. You deserve a break.

57. 2. HIV can be spread through many routes, including sexual contact and contact with infected blood or other body fluids. The incidence of HIV in the adolescent population has increased since 1995, even though more information about the virus is targeted to reach the adolescent population. Only about 25% of all new HIV infections in the United States occur in people under age 22.
CN: Health promotion and maintenance; CNS: None; CL: Application

58. 2. Peer education programs have noted that teens are more likely to ask questions of peer educators than of adults and that peer education can change personal attitudes and the perception of risk of HIV infection. The other approaches would be helpful but wouldn't necessarily make the outreach program more successful.
CN: Health promotion and maintenance; CNS: None; CL: Analysis

59. 2. Affected persons are most contagious in the first year of the disease, not later. About 95% of syphilis cases are transmitted sexually. There are four stages to syphilis, although some people may only experience the first three stages. The drug of choice for treating syphilis is penicillin or doxycycline.
CN: Health promotion and maintenance; CNS: None; CL: Analysis

60. 2. A child who exhibits incontinence after being toilet trained should be evaluated for UTI. Most urine smells strongly of ammonia after standing for more than 2 hours, so this doesn't necessarily indicate UTI. The other options aren't reasons for parents to suspect problems with their child's urinary system.
CN: Health promotion and maintenance; CNS: None; CL: Application

61. Which instruction should a nurse include in the teaching plan for a client receiving co-trimoxazole (Septra) for a repeated urinary tract infection with *Escherichia coli*?
1. "For the drug to be effective, keep your urine acidic by drinking at least a quart of cranberry juice a day."
2. "Take the medication for 10 days, even if your symptoms improve in a few days."
3. "Return to the clinic in 3 days for another urine culture."
4. "Take two of the pills a day now but keep the rest of the pills to take if the symptoms reappear within the next 2 weeks."

62. A nurse should include which fact when teaching parents about managing a child with recurrent urinary tract infection (UTI)?
1. Antibiotics should be discontinued 48 hours after symptoms subside.
2. Recurrent symptoms should be treated by renewing the antibiotic prescription.
3. Complicated UTIs are related to poor perineal hygiene practice.
4. Follow-up urine cultures are necessary to detect recurrent infections and antibiotic effectiveness.

63. A nurse is reviewing a child's clean-voided urine specimen results. The nurse understands that which result best indicates a urinary tract infection (UTI)?
1. A specific gravity of 1.020
2. Cloudy color without odor
3. A large amount of casts present
4. 100,000 bacterial colonies per milliliter

64. The nurse is providing teaching to the parents of a child with a urinary tract infection. Which factor should the nurse recognize as predisposing the child to urinary tract infections?
1. Increased fluid intake
2. Short urethra
3. Ingestion of highly acidic juices
4. Frequent emptying of the bladder

Teaching about medications— that's another common NCLEX subject.

Multiplication is my favorite pastime.

61. **2.** Discharge instructions for clients receiving an anti-infective medication should include taking all of the prescribed medication for the prescribed time, regardless of whether symptoms continue. Drinking highly acidic juices, such as cranberry juice, may help maintain urinary health but won't get rid of an already present infection. Returning after only 3 days of medication will not accurately evaluate the medication's effectiveness. Taking medication for too brief of a period will not eliminate the infection.
CN: Physiological integrity; CNS: Pharmacological and parenteral therapies; CL: Application

62. **4.** A routine follow-up urine specimen is usually obtained 2 or 3 days after the completion of the antibiotic treatment. All of the antibiotic should be taken as ordered and not stopped when symptoms disappear. If recurrent symptoms appear, a urine culture should be obtained to see whether the infection is resistant to antibiotics prior to beginning a new regimen of antibiotics. Simple, not complicated, UTIs are generally caused by poor perineal hygiene.
CN: Health promotion and maintenance; CNS: None; CL: Application

63. **4.** The diagnosis of UTI is determined by the detection of bacteria in the urine. Infected urine usually contains more than 100,000 colonies per milliliter, usually of a single organism. The urine is often cloudy and hazy and may have strands of mucus. It also has a foul, fishy odor even when fresh. Casts and increased specific gravity aren't specific to UTI.
CN: Physiological integrity; CNS: Reduction of risk potential; CL: Application

64. **2.** A short urethra contributes to infection because bacteria have a shorter distance to travel to the urinary tract. The risk of infection is higher in women because women have shorter urethras than men (3/4″ [1.9 cm] in young women, 1″ [3.8 cm] in mature women, 7″ [19.7 cm] in adult men). Increased fluid intake would help flush the urinary tract system, and frequent emptying of the bladder would decrease the risk of urinary tract infection. Drinking highly acidic juices, such as cranberry juice, may help maintain urinary health.
CN: Health promotion and maintenance; CNS: None; CL: Application

65. A nurse is assessing a child with vesicoure-teral reflux. Which condition should the nurse be alert for as a potential complication?
1. Glomerulonephritis
2. Hemolytic uremia syndrome
3. Nephrotic syndrome
4. Renal infection

66. The mother of a female child asks the nurse why her child seems to have so many urinary tract infections (UTIs). Which response by the nurse would be the most accurate?
1. Vaginal secretions are too acidic.
2. Girls aren't protected by circumcision.
3. The urethra is in close proximity to the anus.
4. Girls touch their genitalia more often than boys do.

All this studying just to learn that girls are different from boys.

67. A child has been sent to the school nurse's office for wetting her pants three times in the past 2 days. The nurse should recommend that this child be evaluated for which problem?
1. School phobia
2. Emotional trauma
3. Urinary tract infection
4. Structural defect of the urinary tract

Sometimes, simple hygienic habits offer the best preventative measure.

68. A nurse is teaching parents of children about recurrent urinary tract infections (UTIs). Which goal should be recognized as having the <u>highest priority</u>?
1. Detection
2. Education
3. Prevention
4. Treatment

65. 4. Reflux of urine into the ureters and then back into the bladder after voiding sets up the client for a urinary tract infection due to urinary stasis. This can lead to renal damage due to scarring of the parenchyma. Glomerulonephritis is an autoimmune reaction to a beta-hemolytic strep infection. Hemolytic uremia syndrome may be the result of genetic factors. Eighty percent of nephrotic syndrome cases are idiopathic.
CN: Health promotion and maintenance; CNS: None; CL: Analysis

66. 3. Girls are especially at risk for bacterial invasion of the urinary tract because of basic anatomical differences; the urethra is short and in close proximity to the anus. Vaginal secretions are normally acidic, which decreases the risk of infection. Circumcision doesn't protect girls or boys from UTIs. There's no documented research that supports that girls touch their genitalia more often than boys do.
CN: Health promotion and maintenance; CNS: None; CL: Application

67. 3. Frequent urinary incontinence should be evaluated by the physician, with the first action being checking the urine for infection. Structural defects may be the cause of the urinary tract infection, but this is not the first consideration. Children exhibit signs of school phobia by complaining of an ailment before school starts and getting better after they're allowed to miss school. After infection, structural defect, and diabetes mellitus have been ruled out, emotional trauma should be investigated.
CN: Health promotion and maintenance; CNS: None; CL: Application

68. 3. Prevention is the most important goal in teaching about primary and recurrent UTIs; most preventive measures are simple, ordinary hygienic habits that should be a routine part of daily care. Treatment, detection, and education are all important, but none is the most important goal.
CN: Physiological integrity; CNS: Reduction of risk potential; CL: Analysis

69. Which intervention should a nurse recommend to parents of young girls to help prevent urinary tract infections (UTIs)?
1. Limit tub bathing as much as possible.
2. Increase fluids and decrease salt intake.
3. Have the child wear cotton underpants.
4. Have the child clean her perineum from back to front.

70. A nurse understands that which characteristic is the <u>single most important</u> factor influencing the occurrence of urinary tract infections (UTIs)?
1. Urinary stasis
2. Frequency of baths
3. Uncircumcised penis (in males)
4. Amount of fluid intake

71. When evaluating infants and young toddlers for signs of urinary tract infections (UTIs), a nurse recognizes that which symptom would be <u>most common</u> in this age group?
1. Abdominal pain
2. Feeding problems
3. Frequency
4. Urgency

72. When obtaining a urine specimen for culture and sensitivity, a nurse should understand that which method of collection provides the most accurate results?
1. Bagged urine specimen
2. Clean-catch urine specimen
3. First-voided urine specimen
4. Catheterized urine specimen

Hmmm... the single most important factor; I need to think about that.

If I'm not eating, something must be wrong!

69. 3. Cotton is a more breathable fabric and allows for dampness to be absorbed from the perineum. Bathing shouldn't be limited; however, the use of bubble bath or whirlpool baths should be minimized. However, if the child has frequent UTIs, taking a tub bath should be discouraged and taking a shower encouraged. Increasing fluids would be helpful, but decreasing salt isn't necessary. The perineum should always be cleaned from front to back.
CN: Health promotion and maintenance; CNS: None; CL: Application

70. 1. Ordinarily, urine is sterile. However, at 98.6° F (37° C), it provides an excellent culture medium. Under normal conditions, the act of completely and repeatedly emptying the bladder flushes away any organisms before they have an opportunity to multiply and invade surrounding tissue. By retaining urine or having urinary stasis, a child is much more likely to develop a UTI. Baths and fluid intake are factors in the development of UTIs but aren't the most important. There's an increased incidence of UTI in uncircumcised infants under 1 year but not after that age.
CN: Physiological integrity; CNS: Reduction of risk potential; CL: Application

71. 2. In infants and children less than 2 years old, the signs are characteristically nonspecific, and feeding problems are often the first indication. Symptoms more nearly resemble GI tract disorders. Abdominal pain, urgency, and frequency are signs that would be observed in the older child with a UTI but are very difficult to determine in a young child.
CN: Physiological integrity; CNS: Physiological adaptation; CL: Application

72. 4. The most accurate tests of bacterial content are suprapubic aspiration (for children less than 2 years old) and properly performed bladder catheterization. The other methods of obtaining a specimen have a high incidence of contamination not related to infection, which provides false positives.
CN: Physiological integrity; CNS: Basic care and comfort; CL: Application

73. After collecting a urine specimen, which action by a nurse is the most appropriate?
  1. Taking the specimen to the laboratory immediately
  2. Sending the specimen to the laboratory on the next scheduled run
  3. Taking the specimen to the laboratory during the nurse's next break
  4. Keeping the specimen in the refrigerator until it can be taken to the laboratory

This question calls for immediate action.

73. 1. Care of urine specimens obtained for culture is an important nursing aspect related to diagnosis. Specimens should be taken to the laboratory for culture immediately. If the culture is delayed, the specimen can be placed in the refrigerator, but storage can result in a loss of formed elements, such as blood cells and casts.

CN: Physiological integrity; CNS: Basic care and comfort; CL: Application

74. When teaching parents of a child with a urinary tract infection (UTI) about fluid intake, which statement by a parent would indicate the need for further teaching?
  1. "I should encourage my child to drink about 50 ml/lb of body weight daily."
  2. "Clear liquids should be the primary liquids that my child should drink."
  3. "I should offer my child carbonated beverages about every 2 hours."
  4. "My child should avoid drinking caffeinated beverages."

74. 3. Caffeinated or carbonated beverages are avoided because of their potentially irritating effect on the bladder mucosa. Adequate fluid intake is always indicated during an acute UTI. It is recommended that a person drink approximately 50 ml/lb of body weight daily. The client should primarily drink clear liquids.

CN: Physiological integrity; CNS: Basic care and comfort; CL: Analysis

75. Which treatment should a nurse anticipate for a child who has a history of recurrent urinary tract infections (UTIs)?
  1. Frequent catheterizations
  2. Prophylactic antibiotics
  3. Limited activities
  4. Surgical intervention

75. 2. Children who experience recurrent UTIs may require ongoing antibiotic therapy for months or years. Recurrent UTIs would be investigated for anatomic abnormalities, and surgical intervention may be indicated, but the client would also be placed on antibiotics before the tests. The child's activities aren't limited, and frequent catheterization predisposes a child to infection.

CN: Physiological integrity; CNS: Pharmacological and parenteral therapies; CL: Application

76. When teaching parents about giving medications to children for recurrent urinary tract infections (UTIs), which instruction should be included?
  1. The medication should be given first thing in the morning.
  2. The medication should be given right before bedtime.
  3. The medication is generally given four times a day.
  4. It doesn't matter when the medication is given.

Why do I feel like I'm forgetting something?

76. 2. Medication is commonly administered once a day, and the client and parents are advised to give the antibiotic before sleep because this represents the longest period without voiding, increasing the benefits of the medication.

CN: Physiological integrity; CNS: Pharmacological and parenteral therapies; CL: Application

77. The nurse is providing education to a group of parents about urinary tract infections (UTIs). The nurse knows that teaching has been effective when the parents state that which situation has the <u>greatest</u> impact on the potential for progressive renal injury following UTIs?
1. A school-age child who must get permission to go to the bathroom
2. An adolescent female who has started menstruation
3. Children who compete in competitive sports
4. Being a young infant or toddler

78. Which statement should a nurse make to help parents understand the recovery period after a child has had surgery to remove a Wilms' tumor?
1. "Children will easily lie in bed and restrict their activities."
2. "Recovery is usually fast despite the abdominal incision."
3. "Recovery usually takes a great deal of time because of the large incision."
4. "Parents need to perform activities of daily living for about 2 weeks after surgery."

79. The nurse is teaching parents about administering co-trimoxazole (Septra) to a child for treatment of a urinary tract infection (UTI). The nurse should include which instruction?
1. Give the medication with food.
2. Give the medication with water.
3. Give the medication with a cola beverage.
4. Give the medication 2 hours after a meal.

80. The nurse is questioned by a student nurse about the incidence of Wilms' tumor in children. Which response by the nurse is the most accurate?
1. Peak incidence occurs at 10 years of age.
2. It is the least common type of renal cancer.
3. It is the most common type of renal cancer.
4. It has a decreased incidence among siblings.

You've gotten this far. Hang in there!

Question 80 is looking for accurate information about a condition.

77. 4. The hazard of progressive renal injury is greatest when infection occurs in young children, especially those under 2 years old. The first two options might lead to a simple UTI that would need to be treated. Competitive sports have no bearing on a UTI.

CN: Safe, effective care environment; CNS: Safety and infection control; CL: Application

78. 2. Children generally recover very quickly from surgery to remove a Wilms' tumor, even though they may have a large abdominal incision. Children like to get back into the normalcy of being a child, which is through play. Parents need to encourage their children to do as much for themselves as possible, although some regression is expected.

CN: Psychosocial integrity; CNS: None; CL: Analysis

79. 2. When giving co-trimoxazole, the medication should be administered with a full glass of water on an empty stomach. If nausea and vomiting occur, giving the drug with food may decrease gastric distress. Carbonated beverages should be avoided because they irritate the bladder.

CN: Physiological integrity; CNS: Pharmacological and parenteral therapies; CL: Application

80. 3. Wilms' tumor is the most frequent intra-abdominal tumor of childhood and the most common type of renal cancer. The peak incidence is 3 years, and there's an increased incidence among siblings and identical twins.

CN: Health promotion and maintenance; CNS: None; CL: Application

81. A child presents at the emergency room with abdominal pain, blood in the urine, hypertension, and a palpable abdominal mass. The nurse would suspect which problem in this client?
 1. Urinary tract infection
 2. Wilms' tumor
 3. Acute glomerulonephritis
 4. Nephrotic syndrome

82. A nurse is explaining the diagnosis of Wilms' tumor to the parents of a child. The nurse determines the need for further teaching when a parent makes which statement?
 1. "Wilms' tumor usually involves both kidneys."
 2. "Wilms' tumor occurs slightly more commonly in the left kidney."
 3. "Wilms' tumor is staged during surgery for treatment planning."
 4. "Wilms' tumor stays encapsulated for an extended period of time."

83. A parent asks a nurse about the prognosis of her child who has been diagnosed with Wilms' tumor. The nurse should base her response on which factor?
 1. Usually, children with Wilms' tumor need only surgical intervention.
 2. Survival rates for Wilms' tumor are based on the tumor's location.
 3. Survival rates for Wilms' tumor are the highest among childhood cancers.
 4. Children with localized tumor have only a 30% chance of cure with multimodal therapy.

84. If <u>both kidneys</u> are involved in a child with Wilms' tumor, the nurse should anticipate that treatment prior to surgery might include which method?
 1. Peritoneal dialysis
 2. Abdominal gavage
 3. Radiation and chemotherapy
 4. Antibiotics and I.V. fluid therapy

Let me see what I can learn about Wilms' tumor.

Hmmm, might the treatment for both kidneys differ from that for one?

81. 2. The most common presenting sign of Wilms' tumor is a swelling or mass within the abdomen. The mass is characteristically firm, nontender, confined to one side, and deep within the flank. A urinary tract infection may cause bloody urine but none of the other symptoms. Acute glomerulonephritis will cause hypertension but has no abdominal mass associated with it. A child with nephrotic syndrome will have gross proteinuria and some hematuria but no abdominal mass.
CN: Health promotion and maintenance; CNS: None; CL: Analysis

82. 1. Wilms' tumor usually involves only one kidney and is usually staged during surgery so that an effective course of treatment can be established. Wilms' tumor has a slightly higher occurrence in the left kidney, and it stays encapsulated for an extended period of time.
CN: Health promotion and maintenance; CNS: None; CL: Application

83. 3. Survival rates for Wilms' tumor are the highest among childhood cancers. Usually, children with Wilms' tumor who have stage I or II localized tumor have a 90% chance of cure with multimodal therapy. The tumor size does not correlate to survival rates.
CN: Health promotion and maintenance; CNS: None; CL: Application

84. 3. If both kidneys are involved, the child may be treated with radiation therapy or chemotherapy preoperatively to shrink the tumor, allowing more conservative therapy. Peritoneal dialysis would be needed only if the kidneys aren't functioning. Abdominal gavage wouldn't be indicated. Antibiotics aren't needed because Wilms' tumor isn't an infection.
CN: Physiological integrity; CNS: Reduction of risk potential; CL: Application

85. A nurse is planning <u>preoperative</u> care for a child diagnosed with Wilms' tumor. What is the most important intervention for the nurse to implement?
1. Prepare the family for the initiation of chemotherapy and radiation.
2. Avoid abdominal palpation or manipulation.
3. Insert a nasogastric tube for enteral feedings.
4. Begin I.V. therapy of hyperalimentation and lipids.

Note the word preoperative in question 85.

86. A child is scheduled for surgery to remove a Wilms' tumor from one kidney. The parents ask the nurse what treatment, if any, they should expect after their child recovers from surgery. Which response would be most accurate?
1. "Chemotherapy may be necessary."
2. "Kidney transplant is indicated eventually."
3. "No additional treatments are usually necessary."
4. "Chemotherapy with or without radiation therapy is usually indicated."

87. When assessing the abdomen of a child with a potential diagnosis of Wilms' tumor, which factor would be most suggestive of a different diagnosis?
1. The mass is on one side of the abdomen.
2. There is a mass on both sides of the abdomen.
3. The mass crosses the midline of the abdomen.
4. There's no pain associated with palpation of the mass.

88. A parent of a child with Wilms' tumor asks the nurse about surgery. Which statement concerning the type of surgery for Wilms' tumor is <u>most accurate</u>?
1. Surgery is only done if chemotherapy and radiation fail.
2. Surgery is usually performed within 24 to 48 hours of admission.
3. Surgery is the least favorable therapy for the treatment of Wilms' tumor.
4. Surgery will be delayed until the client's overall health status improves.

Do you know the preferred treatment for Wilms' tumor?

85. 2. After the diagnosis of Wilms' tumor is made, the abdomen shouldn't be palpated. Palpation of the tumor might lead to rupture, which will cause the cancerous cells to spread throughout the abdomen. If surgery is successful, there won't be a need for long-term radiation and chemotherapy. Enteral feedings and total parenteral nutrition are not needed preoperatively in the treatment of Wilms' tumor. Radiation and chemotherapy are not routinely started preoperatively.
CN: Physiological integrity; CNS: Reduction of risk potential; CL: Analysis

86. 4. Because radiation therapy and chemotherapy are usually begun immediately after surgery, parents need an explanation of what to expect, such as major benefits and adverse effects. Kidney transplant isn't usually necessary.
CN: Physiological integrity; CNS: Physiological adaptation; CL: Application

87. 3. When an abdominal mass crosses the midline, a neuroblastoma should be suspected—not a Wilms' tumor. A Wilms' tumor arises off the kidneys and can be on one side or both sides of the abdomen but doesn't cross the midline. Pain isn't usually associated with Wilms' tumor.
CN: Health promotion and maintenance; CNS: None; CL: Analysis

88. 2. Surgery is the preferred treatment and is scheduled as soon as possible after confirmation of a renal mass, usually within 24 to 48 hours of admission, to be sure the encapsulated tumor remains intact.
CN: Physiological integrity; CNS: Physiological adaptation; CL: Application

89. A nurse is caring for a 3-year-old child following removal of a Wilms' tumor. The mother states that the child is in pain and requests pain medication. Which nursing action has the highest priority in response to the mother's request?
1. Assess the child's pain by asking the child to rate his pain on a 1 to 10 scale.
2. Prepare the ordered pain medication and administer it.
3. Use the Faces Pain Scale to assess the degree of pain the child is experiencing.
4. Document the pain complaint and note when the last pain medication was given.

90. A child has been diagnosed with Wilms' tumor. Because of the parents' religious beliefs, they choose not to treat the child. Which statement by the nurse indicates a lack of understanding of the parent's decision?
1. "I know they have received a lot of information in a short period of time."
2. "I don't think parents have the legal right to make these kinds of decisions."
3. "These parents don't understand how easily a Wilms' tumor can be treated."
4. "I think the parents are in shock and don't understand the situation well."

91. A child with a Wilms' tumor has had surgery to remove a kidney and has received chemotherapy. The nurse should include which instruction at the time of discharge?
1. Avoid contact sports.
2. Decrease fluid intake.
3. Decrease sodium intake.
4. Avoid contact with other children.

92. When caring for a child after removal of a Wilms' tumor, which assessment finding would indicate the need to notify the physician?
1. Fever of 101° F (38.3° C)
2. Absence of bowel sounds
3. Slight congestion in the lungs
4. Complaints of pain when moving

Remember to respect the parents' religious beliefs.

Which finding suggests the need to notify the physician?

89. 3. The highest priority of the nurse should be to assess the client for pain. A 3-year-old child is too young to use a pain scale from 1 to 10 but can easily use the Faces Pain Scale. After assessing the pain, the nurse should then investigate the time the pain medication was last given and administer the medication accordingly.
CN: Physiological integrity; CNS: Pharmacological and parenteral therapies; CL: Analysis

90. 2. Parents do have the legal right to make decisions regarding the health issues for their child. Religion plays an important role in many people's lives, and decisions about surgery and treatment for cancer are sometimes made that scientifically don't make sense to the health care provider. The parents are probably in a state of shock because a lot of information has been given, and this is a cancer that requires decisions to be made quickly, especially surgical intervention.
CN: Safe, effective care environment; CNS: Management of care; CL: Analysis

91. 1. Because the child is left with only one kidney, certain precautions, such as avoiding contact sports, are recommended to prevent injury to the remaining kidney. Decreasing fluid intake wouldn't be indicated; fluid intake is essential for renal function. The child's sodium intake shouldn't be reduced. Avoiding other children is unnecessary, will make the child feel self-conscious, and may lead to regressive behavior.
CN: Health promotion and maintenance; CNS: None; CL: Application

92. 2. This child is at risk for intestinal obstruction. GI abnormalities require notification of the physician. A slight fever following surgery isn't uncommon, nor are slight congestion in the lungs and complaints of pain.
CN: Physiological integrity; CNS: Reduction of risk potential; CL: Application

93. Because surgery is performed for a Wilms' tumor within 24 to 48 hours of admission, a nurse must prepare a family and child quickly for procedures. Which information should guide the nurse in her preparation of the family?
1. Because the parents are in a state of shock, they don't need explanations right now.
2. Explanations should be kept simple and should be repeated often.
3. Scientific terminology should be used with drawings and models to increase the family's understanding.
4. The play therapist is the best person to prepare this family.

94. Which statement made by the physician to the parents of a child who has had a Wilms' tumor removed would be the most difficult for the parents to hear and might require nursing intervention?
1. "We will start chemotherapy within the next 24 to 48 hours."
2. "The tumor was a stage IV, which indicates other organ involvement."
3. "We were able to remove all of the tumor, but we had to take the kidney as well."
4. "The incision is long, and the dressing will need to be changed daily."

95. In providing psychosocial care to a 6-year-old child who has had abdominal surgery for Wilms' tumor, which activity would be the <u>most appropriate</u>?
1. Allowing the child to watch a 2-hour movie without interruptions
2. Giving the child a puzzle with five pieces to encourage him to remain in bed
3. Telling the child that you can give him enough medication so that he feels no pain
4. Providing the child with puppets and supplies and asking him to draw how he feels

96. The nurse is teaching the parents of a child with Wilms' tumor about staging. The nurse knows the teaching has been effective when the parents provide which response?
1. Tumor size has no bearing on my child's stage of cancer or outcome.
2. Staging is done to help in determining how best to treat the tumor.
3. Even if the tumor has spread to other organs, staging is usually the same.
4. In stage IV, the scar may be larger since the tumor is larger.

Be sensitive to the needs of a client's family when delivering bad news.

Can you show me how you feel?

93. 2. Decisions are made rapidly after the diagnosis of Wilms' tumor is made. Parents are typically in shock at this time. Explanations should be kept simple and repeated often. The play therapist might become involved with this family, especially postoperatively, but is not the primary source of information. There's generally no time to prepare the play therapist for the role of educator in this situation.
CN: Health promotion and maintenance; CNS: None; CL: Application

94. 2. Surgery is an anxiety-producing event to parents. It also marks the confirmation of the stage of the tumor. A stage IV tumor has a poor prognosis because other organs are involved. This statement, above all others, would be the most difficult for the parents to hear.
CN: Psychosocial integrity; CNS: None; CL: Analysis

95. 4. A movie is a good diversion, but giving puppets and encouraging the child to draw his feelings is a better outlet. A puzzle with only five pieces is too basic for a 6-year-old child and wouldn't hold his interest. You probably can't give enough pain medication so that a person who has had surgery will feel no pain.
CN: Psychosocial integrity; CNS: None; CL: Application

96. 2. Staging of the tumor helps to determine the level of treatment because it provides information about the level of involvement. The other choices are inaccurate or irrelevant in staging of the tumor.
CN: Health promotion and maintenance; CNS: None; CL: Application

97. A nurse is educating parents about Wilms' tumor. Which statement made by a parent would indicate the need for <u>further teaching</u>?
1. "My child could have inherited this disease."
2. "Wilms' tumor can be associated with other congenital anomalies."
3. "This disease could have been a result of trauma to the baby in utero."
4. "There's no method of identification of gene carriers of Wilms' tumor."

98. Which assessment finding will aid in the differentiation of a Wilms' tumor from the liver when doing an abdominal assessment?
1. The liver moves with respiration.
2. The liver is a more encapsulated organ.
3. A Wilms' tumor isn't as deep as the liver.
4. A Wilms' tumor usually isn't well defined.

99. Which action by a nurse would be appropriate to take for a child diagnosed with a Wilms' tumor?
1. Take blood pressure in the right arm only.
2. Offer only clear liquids at room temperature.
3. Post a sign over the bed that reads, "Don't palpate abdomen."
4. Encourage the child to participate in group activities in the playroom.

100. Which is the most important instruction for a nurse to communicate to the parent of a 24-month-old child when the parent asks about when to start toilet-training?
1. The child must be developmentally ready.
2. Be consistent in your approach.
3. Maintain a positive attitude.
4. Start at the same age siblings were trained.

101. A previously toilet-trained 4-year-old child begins wetting the bed after being hospitalized, and the parents are concerned. Which statement by the nurse to the parents best addresses this situation?
1. "Children commonly show regressive behavior when hospitalized."
2. "Your child is just acting out to make you feel bad."
3. "Sometimes, 4-year-olds still have accidents."
4. "Let's try cutting back on fluids and see whether that helps."

Further teaching is so important that you'll see similar questions more than once.

Sometimes, you just have to spell it out.

Caution

97. 3. Wilms' tumor isn't a result of trauma to the fetus in utero. Wilms' tumor can be genetically inherited and is associated with other congenital anomalies. However, there's no method for identifying gene carriers of Wilms' tumor at this time.
CN: Health promotion and maintenance; CNS: None; CL: Application

98. 1. It's difficult to distinguish a Wilms' tumor from the liver if the tumor is on the right side of the body. One difference is that the liver will move with respirations and a Wilms' tumor won't. A Wilms' tumor is deep in the abdomen and is usually well defined and encapsulated.
CN: Health promotion and maintenance; CNS: None; CL: Application

99. 3. To reinforce the need for caution, it may be necessary to post a sign over the bed that reads, "Don't palpate abdomen." The blood pressure could be taken in any extremity; prior to surgery, there are usually no dietary restrictions. Careful bathing and handling are also important in preventing trauma to the tumor site; thus, group activities should be discouraged.
CN: Health promotion and maintenance; CNS: None; CL: Application

100. 1. Toilet training should begin when the child is developmentally ready. After training is started, a consistent approach and a positive attitude should be used. Each child's readiness for toilet training is individual, and the child shouldn't be compared to his siblings.
CN: Health promotion and maintenance; CNS: None; CL: Application

101. 1. Young children may exhibit regressive behaviors when they're under stress, such as occurs with hospitalization. The child may be acting out, but more likely this is not voluntary bed-wetting. Four-year-olds should be fully toilet trained. Restricting fluids as a first step in a hospitalized child isn't appropriate; other causes of bed-wetting should be considered first.
CN: Physiological integrity; CNS: None; CL: Application

102. A preschooler is scheduled to have a Wilms' tumor removed. Identify the area of the urinary system where this type of tumor is located.

102. Wilms' tumor, also known as nephroblastoma, is a tumor located in the area of the kidney, most commonly on the left side. It's most commonly found in children ages 2 to 4.

CN: Physiological integrity; CNS: Physiological adaptation; CL: Application

103. A 3-year-old child weighing 15.5 kg is to receive 5 ml/kg/hour of dextrose 5% in normal saline solution. At what rate (in ml/hour) should the nurse set the infusion pump? Round your answer to a whole number.

_____ ml/hour

103. 78. To calculate the rate per hour for the infusion, the nurse should multiply 15.5 kg by 5 ml, which equals 77.5 ml/hour, which should be rounded to 78 ml/hour.

CN: Physiological integrity; CNS: Pharmacological and parenteral therapies; CL: Application

Congratulations! You finished all 103 questions! Fantastic!

Skin diseases in children and teens are common and varied. This chapter covers common and uncommon skin disorders among these populations.

Chapter 35
Integumentary disorders

1. A 12-year-old child with burns over 40% of his body is ordered to receive 1,500 ml of I.V. fluid over 6 hours. At what rate should the nurse set the infusion pump?
  1. 125 ml/hour
  2. 150 ml/hour
  3. 175 ml/hour
  4. 250 ml/hour

2. The nurse is caring for a child with burns. Which statement by the nurse best describes the nutritional needs of a child who has burns?
  1. A child needs 100 cal/kg during hospitalization.
  2. The hypermetabolic state after a burn injury leads to poor healing.
  3. Caloric needs can be lowered by controlling environmental temperature.
  4. Maintaining a hypermetabolic rate will lower the child's risk for infection.

Measuring burns in children is different than measuring burns in adults.

3. A 1-year-old child is treated in the clinic for a burn to the anterior surface of the left hand. What is the most accurate way for the nurse to measure burn size?
  1. The rule of nines
  2. Percentage based on the child's weight
  3. The child's hand equals 1.25% of the child's body surface area
  4. Percentage can't be determined without knowing the type of burn

1. 4. 1,500 ml divided by 6 hours equals 250 ml/hour.

CN: Physiological integrity; CNS: Pharmacological and parenteral therapies; CL: Application

2. 2. A burn injury causes a hypermetabolic state leading to protein and lipid catabolism, which affects wound healing. Caloric intake should be 1.5 to 2 times the basal metabolic rate, with a minimum of 1.5 to 2 g/kg of body weight of protein daily. Keeping the temperature within a normal range lets the body function efficiently and use calories for healing and normal physiological processes. If the temperature is too warm or cold, energy must be used for warming or cooling, taking energy away from tissue repair. High metabolic rates increase the risk for infection.

CN: Physiological integrity; CNS: Basic care and comfort; CL: Analysis

3. 3. The anterior surface of a child's hand is equal to 1.25% of that child's body surface. The rule of nines is used for children aged 14 years and older. The child's weight is important to calculate fluid replacement for extensive burns, not to estimate total body surface area. Burn type doesn't determine the percentage of body surface involved.

CN: Physiological integrity; CNS: Physiological adaptation; CL: Application

4. An 18-month-old child is admitted to the hospital for full-thickness burns to the anterior chest. The mother asks the nurse how the burn will heal. What is the best response by the nurse?
1. Surgical closure and grafting are usually needed.
2. Healing takes 10 to 12 days with little or no scarring.
3. Pigment in a black client will return to the injured area.
4. Healing can take up to 6 weeks with a high incidence of scarring.

5. A 9-year-old child is admitted to the hospital with deep partial-thickness burns to 25% of his body. Which assessment finding would the nurse associate with a deep partial-thickness burn?
1. Erythema and pain
2. Minimal damage to the epidermis
3. Necrosis through all layers of skin
4. Tissue necrosis through most of the dermis

6. A 4-year-old child is admitted to the burn unit with a <u>circumferential</u> burn to the left forearm. Which finding should be reported to the physician?
1. Numbness of fingers
2. +2 radial and ulnar pulses
3. Full range of motion (ROM) and no pain
4. Bilateral capillary refill less than 2 seconds

7. What is the most important information for the nurse to give the parents of a child with fifth disease?
1. There is a possible reappearance of the rash for up to 1 week.
2. Isolation of high-risk contacts should be avoided for 4 to 10 days.
3. Pregnant clients are at risk for fetal death if infected with fifth disease.
4. Children with fifth disease are contagious only while the rash is present.

Do you remember what you learned about full-thickness burns?

The word circumferential is a clue, right?

4. 1. Full-thickness burns usually need surgical closure and grafting for complete healing. Healing in 10 to 12 days with little or no scarring is associated with superficial partial-thickness burns. With superficial partial-thickness burns, pigment is expected to return to the injured area after healing. Deep partial-thickness burns heal in 6 weeks, with scarring.
CN: Physiological integrity; CNS: Physiological adaptation; CL: Analysis

5. 4. A client with a deep partial-thickness burn will have tissue necrosis to the epidermis and dermis layers. Erythema and pain are characteristic of superficial injury. With deep burns, the nerve fibers are destroyed and the client won't feel pain in the affected area. Superficial burns are characteristic of slight epidermal damage. Necrosis through all skin layers is seen with full-thickness injuries.
CN: Physiological integrity; CNS: Physiological adaptation; CL: Application

6. 1. Circumferential burns can compromise blood flow to an extremity, causing numbness. +2 Pulses indicate normal circulation. Absence of pain and full ROM implies good tissue oxygenation from intact circulation. Capillary refill less than 2 seconds indicates a normal vascular blood flow.
CN: Physiological integrity; CNS: Physiological adaptation; CL: Application

7. 3. There's a 3% to 5% risk for fetal death from hydrops fetalis if a pregnant client is exposed during the first trimester. The cutaneous eruption of fifth disease can reappear for up to 4 months. The child should be isolated from pregnant women, immunocompromised clients, and clients with chronic anemia for up to 2 weeks. A child with fifth disease is contagious during the first stage, when symptoms of headache, body aches, fever, and chills are present, not after the rash.
CN: Safe, effective care environment; CNS: Safety and infection control; CL: Application

8. A mother is concerned that her 3-year-old child has been exposed to erythema infectiosum (fifth disease) and asks the nurse what symptoms to look for. What is the best response by the nurse?
   1. A fine, erythematous rash with a sandpaper-like texture
   2. Intense redness of both cheeks that may spread to the extremities
   3. Low-grade fever, followed by vesicular lesions of the trunk, face, and scalp
   4. Three- to 5-day history of sustained fever, followed by a diffuse erythematous maculopapular rash

9. A family that recently went camping brings their child to the clinic with a complaint of a rash after a tick bite. Lyme disease is suspected. The nurse would assess the child for which finding?
   1. Erythematous rash surrounding a necrotic lesion
   2. Bright rash with red outer border circling the bite site
   3. Onset of a diffuse rash over the entire body 2 months after exposure
   4. A linear rash of papules and vesicles that occur 1 to 3 days after exposure

10. A Mantoux test is ordered for a 6-year-old child. What is the most important action by the nurse?
   1. Read results within 24 hours.
   2. Read results 48 to 72 hours later.
   3. Use the large muscle of the upper leg.
   4. Massage the site to increase absorption.

11. The nurse is teaching the parents of a child with Kawasaki disease. What is the most accurate statement by the nurse?
   1. "It's a highly contagious condition that requires isolation."
   2. "It's an afebrile condition with cardiac involvement."
   3. "It usually occurs in children older than 5 years."
   4. "Prolonged fever, with peeling of the fingers and toes, is the initial symptom."

Different symptoms indicate different diagnoses.

8. **2.** The classic symptoms of erythema infectiosum begin with intense redness of both cheeks. An erythematous rash with a sandpaper-like texture is associated with scarlet fever, which is a bacterial infection. Children with varicella typically have vesicular lesions of the trunk, face, and scalp after a low-grade fever. An erythematous rash after a fever is characteristic of roseola.
CN: Physiological integrity; CNS: Physiological adaptation; CL: Application

9. **2.** A bull's-eye rash is a classic symptom of Lyme disease. Necrotic, painful rashes are associated with the bite of a brown recluse spider. In Lyme disease, the rash is located primarily at the site of the bite. A linear, papular, vesicular rash indicates exposure to the leaves of poison ivy.
CN: Physiological integrity; CNS: Physiological adaptation; CL: Application

Read the results at the right time!

10. **2.** The test should be read 48 to 72 hours after placement by measuring the diameter of the induration that develops at the site. The purified protein derivative is injected intradermally on the volar surface of the forearm. Massaging the site could cause leakage from the injection site.
CN: Physiological integrity; CNS: Reduction of risk potential; CL: Application

11. **4.** To be diagnosed with Kawasaki syndrome, the child must have a fever for 5 days or more, plus four of the following five symptoms: bilateral conjunctivitis, changes in the oral mucosa, dermatitis of the peripheral extremities, rash, and lymphadenopathy. The syndrome isn't contagious and doesn't require isolation. Kawasaki syndrome is more likely to occur in children younger than age 5 years.
CN: Physiological integrity; CNS: Physiological adaptation; CL: Application

CN: Client needs category   CNS: Client needs subcategory   CL: Cognitive level

12. A 22-lb child is diagnosed with Kawasaki syndrome and started on gamma globulin therapy. The physician orders an I.V. infusion of gamma globulin, 2 g/kg, to run over 12 hours. The nurse calculates the correct dose as:
1. 11 g.
2. 20 g.
3. 22 g.
4. 44 g.

13. A mother is concerned because her child was exposed to varicella in day care. Which statement by the nurse would be the most accurate?
1. "The rash is nonvesicular."
2. "The treatment of choice is aspirin."
3. "Varicella has an incubation period of 5 to 10 days."
4. "A child is no longer contagious once the rash has crusted over."

14. The nurse is discussing the appearance of a rash associated with varicella-zoster virus on a child in the pediatric unit with a student nurse. Which explanation about the rash would be correct?
1. It's diagnostic in the presence of Koplik's spots in the oral mucosa.
2. It's a macular papular rash starting on the scalp and hairline and spreading downward.
3. It's a vesicular macular papular rash that appears abruptly on the trunk, face, and scalp.
4. It appears as yellow ulcers surrounded by red halos on the surface of the hands and feet.

15. A child is brought to the emergency department after an extended period of sledding with suspected frostbite of the hands. The nurse assesses the skin on the hands and documents it as:
1. white.
2. deeply flushed and red.
3. cyanotic.
4. blistered.

Should I multiply or divide to calculate this dose?

I'm glad I dressed warmly!

12. 2. First, convert the weight from pounds to kilograms. One kilogram equals 2.2 lb. Convert the weight using the calculation:

$$22 \text{ (lb)} \div 2.2 = 10 \text{ (kg)}$$

Then, calculate the dose:

$$2 \text{ g} \times 10 = 20 \text{ g}$$

CN: Physiological integrity; CNS: Pharmacological and parenteral therapies; CL: Application

13. 4. Once every varicella lesion is crusted over, the child is no longer considered contagious. The rash is typically a maculopapular vesicular rash. Use of aspirin has been associated with Reye's syndrome and is contraindicated in varicella. The incubation period is 10 to 20 days.

CN: Physiological integrity; CNS: Physiological adaptation; CL: Application

14. 3. Teardrop vesicles on an erythematous base generally begin on the trunk, face, and scalp, with minimal involvement of the extremities. Koplik's spots are diagnostic of rubeola. A descending macular papular rash is characteristic of rubeola. Yellow ulcers of the hands and feet are associated with hand-foot-and-mouth disease caused by the coxsackievirus.

CN: Physiological integrity; CNS: Physiological adaptation; CL: Application

15. 1. Signs and symptoms of frostbite include tingling, numbness, burning sensation, and white skin.

CN: Physiological integrity; CNS: Physiological adaptation; CL: Application

16.   A mother brings her child to the physician's office because he complains of pain, redness, and tenderness of the left index finger. The child is diagnosed with a paronychia. The nurse suspects that which organism is the most likely cause?
1. *Borrelia burgdorferi*
2. *Escherichia coli*
3. *Pseudomonas* species
4. *Staphylococcus* species

17.   Which treatment for paronychia would be the most appropriate?
1. Give warm soaks.
2. Splint and put ice on the affected finger.
3. Allow the infection to resolve without treatment.
4. Admit the child to the hospital for I.V. antibiotic therapy.

18.   A mother is concerned that her 9-month-old infant has scabies and brings her to the pediatric clinic. The nurse assesses the infant for which findings?
1. Diffuse pruritic wheals
2. Oval white dots stuck to the hair shafts
3. Pain, erythema, and edema with an embedded stinger
4. Pruritic papules, pustules, and linear burrows of the finger and toe webs

19.   After treating her 16-month-old child with permethrin (Elimite) for scabies, the mother is concerned the cream didn't work because the child is still scratching. What is the best information for the nurse to give the mother?
1. Continue the application daily until the rash disappears.
2. Pruritus caused by secondary reactions of the mites can be present for weeks.
3. Stop treatment because the cream is unsafe for children younger than age 2 years.
4. Pruritus caused by permethrin is usually present in children younger than age 5 years.

I'm tough!

Stop and assess the symptoms.

16. 4. A paronychia is a localized infection of the nail bed caused by either staphylococci or streptococci. *Borrelia burgdorferi* is responsible for Lyme disease. *Escherichia coli* is associated with urinary tract infections. *Pseudomonas* species are associated with ecthyma.
CN: Physiological integrity; CNS: Physiological adaptation; CL: Application

17. 1. Giving warm soaks is the treatment of choice for paronychia. Splinting and icing aren't indicated. Untreated, the local abscess can spread beneath the nail bed, called secondary lymphangitis. I.V. antibiotic therapy isn't needed if the abscess is kept from spreading.
CN: Physiological integrity; CNS: Physiological adaptation; CL: Analysis

18. 4. Pruritic papules, vesicles, and linear burrows are diagnostic for scabies. Diffuse pruritic wheals are associated with an allergic reaction. Nits, seen as white oval dots, are characteristic of head lice. Bites from honeybees are associated with a stinger, pain, and erythema.
CN: Physiological integrity; CNS: Physiological adaptation; CL: Application

19. 2. Sensitization of the host is the cause of the intense itching and can last for weeks. Permethrin is the recommended treatment for scabies in infants as young as 2 months. It can safely be repeated after 2 weeks.
CN: Physiological integrity; CNS: Pharmacological and parenteral therapies; CL: Application

20. A mother of a 5-month-old infant is planning a trip to the beach and asks for advice about sunscreen for her child. Which instruction should the nurse give the mother?
1. The sunscreen protection factor (SPF) of the sunscreen should be at least 10.
2. Apply sunscreen to the exposed areas of the skin.
3. Sunscreen shouldn't be applied to infants younger than 6 months of age.
4. Sunscreen needs to be applied heavily only once one-half hour before going out in the sun.

Know the do's and don'ts about sunscreen and its application.

21. An infant is being treated with antibiotic therapy for otitis media and develops an erythematous, fine, raised rash in the groin and suprapubic area. Which instruction or explanation will most likely be given to the mother?
1. The infant has candidiasis.
2. Change the brand of diapers.
3. Use an over-the-counter diaper remedy.
4. Stop the antibiotic therapy immediately.

22. A parent tells the nurse that the skin in the diaper area of their 6-month-old infant is excoriated and red. What is the most appropriate information for the nurse to tell the parent?
1. Change the diaper more often.
2. Apply talcum powder with diaper changes.
3. Wash the area vigorously with each diaper change.
4. Decrease the infant's fluid intake to decrease saturating diapers.

Teaching parents helps keep their children healthy.

23. A 9-year-old child is being discharged from the hospital after severe urticaria caused by an allergy to nuts. What is the most important instruction for the nurse to give the parents?
1. Use emollient lotions and baths.
2. Apply topical steroids to the lesions as needed.
3. Apply over-the-counter products such as diphenhydramine (Benadryl).
4. Instruct the parents and child on how and when to use an epinephrine administration kit (Epi-Pen).

20. 3. Sunscreen isn't recommended for use in infants younger than 6 months of age. These children should be dressed in cool light clothes and kept in the shade. The SPF for children should be 15 or greater. Sunscreen should be applied to all areas of the skin. Sunscreen should be applied evenly throughout the day and each time the child is in the water.
CN: Health promotion and maintenance; CNS: None; CL: Application

21. 1. Candidiasis, caused by yeastlike fungi, can occur with the use of antibiotics. The treatment for candidiasis is topical nystatin ointment. Changing the brand of diapers or suggesting that the parent use an over-the-counter remedy would be appropriate for treating diaper rash, not candidiasis. Antibiotic therapy shouldn't be stopped.
CN: Physiological integrity; CNS: Physiological adaptation; CL: Analysis

22. 1. Simply decreasing the amount of time the skin comes in contact with wet soiled diapers will help heal the irritation. Talc is contraindicated in children because of the risks of inhaling the fine powder. Gentle cleaning of the irritated skin should be encouraged. Infants shouldn't have fluid intake restrictions.
CN: Safe, effective care environment; CNS: Safety and infection control; CL: Application

23. 4. Children who have urticaria in response to nuts, seafood, or bee stings should be warned about the possibility of anaphylactic reactions to future exposure. The use of epinephrine pens should be taught to the parents and older children. Other treatment choices, such as diphenhydramine hydrochloride, topical steroids, and emollients, are for the treatment of mild urticaria.
CN: Physiological integrity; CNS: Reduction of risk potential; CL: Application

24. When examining a nursery school–age child, the nurse finds multiple contusions over the body. Child abuse is suspected. Which statement indicates which findings should be documented?
1. Contusions confined to one body area are typically suspicious.
2. All lesions, including location, shape, and color, should be documented.
3. Natural injuries usually have straight linear lines, while injuries from abuse have multiple curved lines.
4. The depth, location, and amount of bleeding that initially occurs are constant, but the sequence of color change is variable.

25. A 7-year-old child is diagnosed with head lice. The mother asks what nits are. What is the most accurate response by the nurse?
1. Adult lice
2. Empty egg shells
3. Newly laid eggs
4. Nymphs

26. The nurse is teaching the mother of a child with lice about treatment options. What is the most important information for the nurse to include when discussing lindane (Kwell) shampoo?
1. Lindane causes alopecia.
2. Lindane causes hypertension.
3. Lindane is associated with seizures.
4. Lindane increases liver function test (LFT) results.

27. The nurse is providing instructions to the parents about the treatment of head lice. What is the most important information for the nurse to provide?
1. The treatment should be repeated in 7 to 12 days.
2. Treatment should be repeated every day for 1 week.
3. If treated with a shampoo, combing to remove eggs isn't necessary.
4. All contacts with the infested child should be treated even without evidence of infestation.

Question 24 already, and you're doing great!

There's nothing nice about head lice.

24. 2. An accurate precise examination of all lesions must be properly documented as a legal document. Contusions that result from falls are typically confined to a single body area and are considered a reasonable finding of a child still learning to walk. Injuries from normal falls are usually not linear in nature. The bleeding can cause variations, but the color change is consistent.
CN: Psychosocial integrity; CNS: None; CL: Application

25. 2. The mother is finding empty eggshells in the child's hair. Adults are the last stage of development, living about 30 days. Newly laid eggs are small, translucent, and difficult to see. Nymphs are the newly hatched lice and become adults in 8 to 9 days.
CN: Physiological integrity; CNS: Physiological adaptation; CL: Application

26. 3. Lindane is associated with seizures after absorption with topical use. Alopecia, increased LFT results, and hypertension aren't associated with the use of lindane.
CN: Physiological integrity; CNS: Pharmacological and parenteral therapies; CL: Application

27. 1. Treatment should be repeated in 7 to 12 days to ensure that all eggs are killed. Combing the hair thoroughly is necessary to remove the lice eggs. People exposed to head lice should be examined to assess the presence of infestation before treatment.
CN: Physiological integrity; CNS: Physiological adaptation; CL: Application

28. A mother reports that her 4-year-old child has been scratching at his rectum recently. Which infestation or condition should the nurse suspect?
1. Anal fissure
2. Lice
3. Pinworms
4. Scabies

29. The nurse is providing instructions on the diagnosing of pinworms to a parent. The parent asks how many clear cellophane tape tests are necessary to detect infestations at 100% accuracy. What is the best response by the nurse?
1. One
2. Three
3. Five
4. Ten

30. Each member of the family of a child diagnosed with pinworms is prescribed a single dose of pyrantel pamoate (Antiminth). What is the most important information for the nurse to tell the family?
1. The drug may stain the feces red.
2. The dose may be repeated in 2 weeks.
3. Fever and rash are common adverse effects.
4. The medicine will kill the eggs in about 48 hours.

31. A child received a bite to the hand from a large dog. The nurse would expect to assess which type of injury?
1. Abrasion
2. Crush injury
3. Fracture
4. Puncture wound

32. A nurse is working in her garden when a neighbor frantically comes over and states her child has been bitten by the new neighbor's dog. What is the most important intervention by the nurse?
1. Give the rabies vaccine.
2. Give antibiotics immediately.
3. Clean and irrigate the wounds.
4. Nothing; bites from dogs have a low incidence of infection.

You've finished 30 questions! Good for you!

If I come from a dog, grrrr, watch out!

28. 3. The clinical sign of pinworms is perianal itching that increases at night. Anal fissures are associated with rectal bleeding and pain with bowel movements. Lice are infestations of the hair. Scabies are associated with a pruritic rash characterized as linear burrows of the webs of the fingers and toes.
CN: Physiological integrity; CNS: Physiological adaptation; CL: Analysis

29. 3. Detection is virtually 100% accurate with five tests. One test is only 50% accurate. Three tests should detect infestations at about 90% accuracy. Ten tests aren't necessary.
CN: Physiological integrity; CNS: Reduction of risk potential; CL: Application

30. 2. Pyrantel is effective against the adult worms only (not eggs), so treatment can be repeated to eradicate any emerging parasites in 2 weeks. Staining the feces is associated with pyrvinium pamoate. Common adverse effects are headaches and abdominal complaints.
CN: Physiological integrity; CNS: Pharmacological and parenteral therapies; CL: Application

31. 2. Although the bite of a large dog can exert pressure of 150 to 400 psi, the bite causes crush injuries, not fractures. Abrasions are associated with friction injuries. Puncture wounds are associated with smaller animals, such as cats.
CN: Physiological integrity; CNS: Physiological adaptation; CL: Application

32. 3. Not every dog bite requires antibiotic therapy, but cleaning the wound is necessary for all injuries involving a break in the skin. Rabies vaccine is used if there is a suspicion the dog has rabies. The infection rate for dog bites has been reported to be as high as 50%.
CN: Physiological integrity; CNS: Reduction of risk potential; CL: Application

33. The nurse is reviewing the wound culture report from a child's infected wound caused by a dog bite. Which organism would the nurse suspect to be responsible for the infection?
1. *Escherichia coli*
2. *Francisella tularensis*
3. *Pasteurella multocida*
4. *Bartonella henselae*

Me and the pooch here are pals.

33. 3. *Pasteurella multocida* is associated with infection in up to 50% of the bites from dogs. *E. coli* is more likely to cause infections of the urinary tract. *Francisella tularensis* is found in such animals as rabbits, hares, and muskrats. *Bartonella henselae*, a gram-negative rickettsial bacterium, is associated with cat-scratch disease.

CN: Physiological integrity; CNS: Physiological adaptation; CL: Application

34. A child is brought to a physician's office for multiple scratches and bites from a kitten. The nurse would assess the child for which finding?
1. Abdominal pain
2. Adenitis
3. Fever
4. Pruritus

34. 2. Adenitis is the primary feature of cat-scratch disease. Although low-grade fever has been associated with cat-scratch disease, it's only present 25% of the time. Pruritus and abdominal pain aren't symptoms of cat-scratch disease.

CN: Physiological integrity; CNS: Physiological adaptation; CL: Analysis

35. The school nurse is discussing giardiasis, a parasitic intestinal infection, with a group of parents. Many parents ask the nurse what group is most at risk for developing this infection. What is the most accurate response by the nurse?
1. Children riding a school bus
2. Children playing on a playground
3. Children attending a sporting event
4. Children attending group day care or nursery school

You need to know the correct terms to share information with clients and other health care providers.

35. 4. The most common intestinal parasitic infection in the United States is giardiasis, prevalent among children attending group day care or nursery school. Playgrounds, sporting events, and school buses don't present unusual risk of giardiasis.

CN: Physiological integrity; CNS: Physiological adaptation; CL: Application

36. Which finding should the nurse expect to observe if a child has papules?
1. Palpable elevated masses
2. Loss of the epidermis layer
3. Fluid-filled elevations of the skin
4. Nonpalpable flat changes in skin color

36. 1. Papules are elevated up to 0.5 cm. Nodules and tumors are elevated more than 0.5 cm. Erosions are characterized as loss of the epidermis layer. Fluid-filled lesions are vesicles and pustules. Macules and patches are described as nonpalpable flat changes in skin color.

CN: Health promotion and maintenance; CNS: None; CL: Application

37. A child presents with pustules and is diagnosed with impetigo. The nurse documents which assessment findings?
1. Lesions filled with pus
2. Superficial areas of localized edema
3. Serous-filled lesions less than 0.5 cm
4. Serous-filled lesions greater than 0.5 cm

37. 1. Pustules are pus-filled lesions, such as acne and impetigo. A wheal is a superficial area of localized edema. Vesicles are serous-filled lesions up to 0.5 cm in diameter. Bullae are serous-filled lesions greater than 0.5 cm in diameter.

CN: Physiological integrity; CNS: Physiological adaptation; CL: Application

38. A 3-month-old infant is noted to have café-au-lait spots on examination. The presence of six or more of these lesions with a diameter greater than 1.5 cm is suggestive of which disorder?
1. Meningococcemia
2. Neurofibromatosis
3. Tinea versicolor
4. Vitiligo

39. A child is brought to the physician's office for treatment of a rash. Many petechiae are seen over his entire body. The nurse would suspect which condition?
1. Bleeding disorder
2. Scabies
3. Varicella
4. Vomiting

40. A child fell at camp and sustained a bruise to his thigh. Which description would accurately describe the bruise after 1 week?
1. Resolved
2. Reddish blue
3. Greenish yellow
4. Dark blue to bluish brown

41. Which assessment finding would lead the nurse to suspect child abuse?
1. Multiple contusions of the shins
2. Contusions of the back and buttocks
3. Contusions at the same stages of healing
4. Large contusion and hematoma of the forehead

42. Which statement would the nurse include when teaching a new mother about salmon patches (stork bites)?
1. They're benign and usually fade in adult life.
2. They're usually associated with syndromes of the neonate.
3. They can cause mild hypertrophy of the muscle associated with the lesion.
4. They're treatable with laser pulse surgery in late adolescence and adulthood.

Assessment is an enormously important skill.

38. 2. Six or more uniformly pigmented patches with irregular borders, known as café-au-lait spots, with diameters greater than 1.5 cm are associated with neurofibromatosis. Meningococcemia has petechiae, not café-au-lait spots. Tinea versicolor is a superficial fungus infection. Depigmented areas are signs of vitiligo.
CN: Health promotion and maintenance; CNS: None; CL: Analysis

39. 1. Petechiae are caused by blood outside a vessel, associated with low platelet counts and bleeding disorders. Petechiae aren't found with varicella disease or scabies. Petechiae can be associated with vomiting, but in that case, they'd be present on the face, not the entire body.
CN: Physiological integrity; CNS: Physiological adaptation; CL: Analysis

40. 3. After 7 to 10 days, the bruise becomes greenish yellow. Resolution can take up to 2 weeks. Initially after the fall, there's a reddish blue discoloration followed by a dark blue to bluish brown color at days 1 to 3.
CN: Physiological integrity; CNS: Physiological adaptation; CL: Application

41. 2. Contusions of the back and buttocks are highly suspicious of abuse related to punishment. Contusions at various stages of healing are red flags to potential abuse. Contusions of the shins and forehead are usually related to an active toddler falling and bumping into objects.
CN: Psychosocial integrity; CNS: None; CL: Analysis

42. 1. Salmon patches occur over the back of the neck in 40% of neonates and are harmless, needing no intervention. Port wine stains are associated with syndromes of the neonate such as Sturge-Weber syndrome. Port wine stains found on the face or extremities may be associated with soft tissue and bone hypertrophy. Laser pulse surgery isn't recommended for salmon patches because they typically fade on their own in adulthood.
CN: Health promotion and maintenance; CNS: None; CL: Application

43. A neonate is born with a blue-black macular lesion over the lower lumbar sacral region. Which term should the nurse use when teaching the parents about this lesion?
1. Café-au-lait spots
2. Mongolian spots
3. Nevus of Ota spot
4. Stork bites

44. A child is admitted with <u>severe</u> dehydration. The nurse would assess the child for which finding?
1. Gray skin and decreased tears
2. Capillary refill less than 2 seconds
3. Mottling and tenting of the skin
4. Pale skin with dry mucous membranes

45. A client is prescribed isotretinoin (Accutane). Which adverse effect should the nurse include in her teaching?
1. Diarrhea
2. Gram-negative folliculitis
3. Teratogenicity
4. Vaginal candidiasis

46. The nurse is developing a teaching plan for adolescents about acne. The nurse incorporates which characteristic as commonly responsible for the failure of treatment of acne in teenagers?
1. Topical treatment
2. Systemic treatment
3. A dominant parent who wants treatment and a passive teenager who doesn't
4. A dominant teenager who wants treatment and a passive uninterested parent

47. A teenager tells the nurse that he has heard many myths about what causes acne and asks the nurse what the real cause is. The nurse explains that acne is caused by:
1. diet.
2. gender.
3. poor hygiene.
4. hormonal changes.

The word *severe* is a clue to the correct answer.

I need to follow the treatment plan.

43. 2. Mongolian spots are large blue-black macular lesions generally located over the lumbo-sacral areas, buttocks, and limbs. Café-au-lait spots occur between ages 2 and 16 years, not in infancy. Nevus of Ota is found surrounding the eyes. Stork bites or salmon patches occur at the neck and hairline area.

CN: Health promotion and maintenance; CNS: None; CL: Application

44. 3. Severe dehydration is associated with mottling and tenting of the skin. Malnutrition is characterized by gray skin and tenting of the skin. Capillary refill less than 2 seconds is normal. Pale skin with dry mucous membranes is a sign of mild dehydration.

CN: Health promotion and maintenance; CNS: None; CL: Analysis

45. 3. The use of even small amounts of isotretinoin has been associated with severe birth defects. Most female clients taking this medication are prescribed hormonal contraceptives. Cleocin T (clindamycin), another medicine used in the treatment of acne, is associated with both diarrhea and gram-negative folliculitis. Tetracycline (Achromycin) is associated with yeast infections (vaginal candidiasis).

CN: Physiological integrity; CNS: Pharmacological and parenteral therapies; CL: Application

46. 3. The active participation of a teenager is needed for the successful treatment of acne. Systemic and topical therapies are needed in most acne treatment.

CN: Health promotion and maintenance; CNS: None; CL: Application

47. 4. Acne is caused by hormonal changes in sebaceous gland anatomy and the biochemistry of the glands. These changes lead to a blockage in the follicular canal and cause an inflammatory response. Diet, hygiene, and the client's gender don't cause acne.

CN: Health promotion and maintenance; CNS: None; CL: Application

48. The nurse is reviewing information with a client about tetracycline (Achromycin) that has been prescribed for severe inflammatory acne. It is most important for the nurse to instruct the client to take the medication:
1. with or without meals.
2. with milk and milk products.
3. on an empty stomach with small amounts of water.
4. 1 hour before or 2 hours after meals with large amounts of water.

49. The nurse is advising parents about the prevention of burns to their child from tap water. What is the most important instruction for the nurse to include?
1. Set the water heater temperature at 130° F (54.4° C) or less.
2. Run the hot water first and then adjust the temperature with cold water.
3. Before you put your infant in the tub, first test the water with your hand.
4. Supervise an infant in the bathroom, only leaving him for a few seconds, if needed.

50. While caring for a 2-day-old neonate, a nurse notices the left side of the neonate becomes reddened for 2 to 3 minutes. The nurse interprets this finding as suggestive of which condition?
1. Contact dermatitis
2. Environmental conditions
3. Harlequin color change
4. Tet spells

51. A 15-month-old child is diagnosed with pediculosis of the eyebrows. Which intervention is included in the treatment?
1. Use lindane.
2. Use petroleum jelly.
3. Shave the eyebrows.
4. No treatment is needed.

52. A 14-year-old male client is brought to the hospital with smoke inhalation because of a house fire. What is the priority intervention by the nurse?
1. Check the oral mucous membranes.
2. Check for any burned areas.
3. Obtain a medical history.
4. Ensure a patent airway.

It's hard to study on an empty stomach.

You've reached question 50 and your goal is in sight.

48. 4. Tetracycline must be taken on an empty stomach to increase absorption and with ample water to avoid esophageal irritation. Milk products impede absorption.
CN: Physiological integrity; CNS: Pharmacological and parenteral therapies; CL: Application

49. 3. Instruct the parents to fill the tub with water first and then test all of the water in the tub with their hand for hot spots. Water heaters should be set at 120° F. The cold water should be run first and then adjusted with hot water. Never leave an infant alone in the bathroom, even for a second.
CN: Health promotion and maintenance; CNS: None; CL: Application

50. 3. Harlequin color change is a benign disorder related to the immaturity of hypothalamic centers that control the tone of peripheral blood vessels. A newborn who has been lying on his side may appear reddened on the dependent side. The color fades on position change. Contact dermatitis isn't short lived. Changes in environmental conditions can cause diffuse bilateral mottling of the skin. Tet spells are associated with tetralogy of Fallot and cause cyanotic changes.
CN: Health promotion and maintenance; CNS: None; CL: Analysis

51. 2. Petroleum jelly should be applied twice daily for 8 days, followed by manual removal of nits. Lindane is contraindicated because of the risk for seizures. The eyebrow should never be shaved because of the uncertainty of hair return.
CN: Physiological integrity; CNS: Physiological adaptation; CL: Analysis

52. 4. The nurse's top priority is to make sure the airway is open and the client is breathing. Checking the mucous membranes and burned areas is important but not as vital as maintaining a patent airway. Obtaining a medical history can be pursued after ensuring a patent airway.
CN: Physiological integrity; CNS: Physiological adaptation; CL: Application

53. The nurse is assessing a child suspected of having Kawasaki syndrome. The nurse would assess the mouth for which finding?
1. Koplik's spots
2. Tonsillar exudate
3. Vesicular lesions
4. Strawberry tongue

Which symptom goes with which diagnosis?

53. 4. Oral changes associated with Kawasaki syndrome include reddened pharynx, red, dry fissured lips, and strawberry tongue. Koplik's spots are consistent with measles. Tonsillar exudate is consistent with pharyngitis caused by group A beta-hemolytic streptococci. Vesicular lesions are associated with coxsackievirus.
CN: Physiological integrity; CNS: Physiological adaptation; CL: Application

54. A 3-year-old child has palpable purpura of the buttocks and lower extremities. Which condition would the nurse suspect with these symptoms?
1. Child abuse
2. Henoch-Schönlein purpura (HSP)
3. Idiopathic thrombocytopenic purpura (ITP)
4. Rocky Mountain spotted fever

54. 2. The rash associated with HSP is believed to occur in every client and allows for a definitive diagnosis. It begins as petechiae and progresses to purpuric lesions of the buttocks and lower extremities. The lesions of child abuse are painful and nonraised. Petechiae or purpura associated with ITP are distributed over the entire body. The rash in Rocky Mountain spotted fever is a nonraised macular papular rash spread over the body.
CN: Physiological integrity; CNS: Physiological adaptation; CL: Application

55. Topical treatment with 2.5% hydrocortisone (Cortane) is prescribed for a 6-month-old infant with eczema. The nurse instructs the mother not to use the cream for longer than 1 week. The mother asks the nurse why there is a time limit. What is the best response by the nurse?
1. The drug loses its efficacy after prolonged use.
2. This reduces adverse effects, such as skin atrophy and fragility.
3. If no improvement is seen, a stronger concentration will be prescribed.
4. If no improvement is seen after 1 week, an antibiotic will be prescribed.

Adverse effects can result from prolonged use of certain medications.

55. 2. Hydrocortisone cream should be used for brief periods to decrease such adverse effects as atrophy of the skin. The drug doesn't lose efficacy after prolonged use, a stronger concentration may not be prescribed if no improvement is seen, and an antibiotic would be inappropriate in this instance.
CN: Physiological integrity; CNS: Pharmacological and parenteral therapies; CL: Application.

56. A 9-year-old child is examined because his mother noticed lesions on his tongue. Painless, slightly depressed, red lesions bordered with white bands are seen on assessment. The mother reports that the patterns were different yesterday. Which condition would the nurse suspect?
1. Geographic tongue
2. Koplik's spots
3. Scald burns
4. Stomatitis

56. 1. Geographic tongue is a benign disorder caused by loss of filiform papules. The configuration is known to change from day to day. Koplik's spots and stomatitis lesions don't change patterns. Scald burns are painful lesions from hot liquids.
CN: Physiological integrity; CNS: Physiological adaptation; CL: Application

57. A 4-year-old child had a subungual hemorrhage of the toe after a jar fell on his foot. Electrocautery is performed. The nurse explains to the parents that electrocautery is done to:
1. prevent loss of nail growth.
2. prevent spread of the infection.
3. relieve pain and reduce the risk for infection.
4. prevent permanent discoloration of the nail bed.

58. The nurse is caring for a 12-year-old child with a diagnosis of eczema. Which nursing intervention is appropriate for a child with eczema?
1. Antibiotics as prescribed
2. Antifungals as ordered
3. Tepid baths and application of moisturizers to the skin
4. Hot baths and vigorous drying of the skin

59. A 9-year-old child is brought to the emergency department with extensive burns received in a restaurant fire. What is the <u>most important</u> intervention by the nurse?
1. Administering antibiotics to prevent superimposed infections
2. Conducting wound management
3. Administering liquids orally to replace fluid
4. Administering frequent, small meals to support nutritional requirements

60. A mother of a 4-month-old infant asks about the strawberry hemangioma on his cheek. What information should the nurse provide to the mother?
1. The lesion will continue to grow for 3 years and then need surgical removal.
2. If the lesion continues to enlarge, referral to a pediatric oncologist is warranted.
3. Surgery is indicated before age 12 months if the diameter of the lesion is greater than 3 cm.
4. The lesion will continue to grow until age 1 year and then begin to resolve by age 2 to 3 years.

57. 3. The hematoma is treated with electrocautery to relieve pain and reduce risk for infection. Electrocautery doesn't prevent the loss of the nail. The discoloration seen with subungual hemorrhage is from the collection of blood under the nail bed. It isn't permanent and doesn't affect nail growth.
CN: Physiological integrity; CNS: Physiological adaptation; CL: Application

58. 3. Tepid baths and moisturizers are indicated to keep the infected areas clean and minimize itching. Antibiotics are given only when superimposed infection is present. Antifungals aren't usually administered in the treatment of eczema. Hot baths can exacerbate the condition and increase itching.
CN: Physiological integrity; CNS: Physiological adaptation; CL: Application

59. 2. The most important aspect of caring for a burned child is wound management. The goals of wound care are to speed debridement, protect granulation tissue and new grafts, and conserve body heat and fluids. Antibiotics aren't always administered prophylactically. Fluids are administered I.V. according to the child's body weight to replace volume. Enteral feedings, rather than meals, are initiated within the first 24 hours after the burn to support the child's increased nutritional requirements.
CN: Physiological integrity; CNS: Physiological adaptation; CL: Application

60. 4. These rapidly growing vascular lesions reach maximum growth by age 1 year. The growth period is then followed by an involution period of 6 to 12 months. Lesions show complete involution by age 2 or 3 years. These benign lesions don't need surgical or oncologic referrals.
CN: Health promotion and maintenance; CNS: None; CL: Application

61. A 3-year-old child is being discharged from the emergency department after receiving three sutures for a scalp laceration. The nurse determines discharge teaching was effective when the parents tell the nurse they will return for suture removal in:
1. 1 to 3 days.
2. 5 to 7 days.
3. 8 to 10 days.
4. 10 to 14 days.

62. Which symptom is an <u>early sign</u> of infection of a laceration?
1. Fever
2. Copious drainage
3. Excessive discomfort
4. Local nodal enlargement

63. The nurse is teaching a 17-year-old client how to change a sterile dressing on the right leg. During the teaching session, the nurse notices redness, swelling, and induration at the wound site, interpreting these as suggesting:
1. infection.
2. dehiscence.
3. hemorrhage.
4. evisceration.

64. A 6-year-old child is diagnosed with herpes zoster of the left anterior chest. Which assessment finding should the nurse expect to find?
1. Bruising and swelling
2. Papulovesicular eruption with complaints of pain and tenderness of the lesion
3. Linear burrows on the fingers and toes
4. Papulovesicular lesions on the chest, trunk, face, and scalp

65. During an examination of a 5-month-old infant, a flat, dull pink, macular lesion is noted on the infant's forehead. The nurse suspects which condition?
1. Cavernous hemangioma
2. Nevus flammeus
3. Salmon patch
4. Strawberry hemangioma

61. 2. The recommended healing time for this type of laceration is 5 to 7 days. Sutures need longer than 1 to 3 days to form an effective bond. Eight to 10 days is needed for sutures of the fingertips and feet, and 10 to 14 days is the recommended time for extensor surfaces of the knees and elbows.

CN: Physiological integrity; CNS: Physiological adaptation; CL: Application

62. 3. The first sign of infection is usually excessive discomfort. Nodal enlargement, fever, and copious drainage are advanced signs of infection.

CN: Health promotion and maintenance; CNS: None; CL: Analysis

63. 1. Infection produces such signs as redness, swelling, induration, warmth, and possible drainage. Dehiscence may cause unexplained fever and tachycardia, unusual wound pain, prolonged paralytic ileus, and separation of the surgical incision. Hemorrhage can result in increased pulse and respiratory rate, decreased blood pressure, restlessness, thirst, and cold, clammy skin. Evisceration produces visible protrusion of organs, usually through an incision.

CN: Physiological integrity; CNS: Physiological adaptation; CL: Analysis

64. 2. Herpes zoster is caused by the varicella-zoster virus. It has papulovesicular lesions that erupt along a dermatome, usually with hyperesthesia, pain, and tenderness. Contusions are present with bruising and swelling. Scabies appear as linear burrows of the fingers and toes caused by a mite. The papulovesicular lesions of varicella are distributed over the entire trunk, face, and scalp and don't follow a dermatome.

CN: Physiological integrity; CNS: Physiological adaptation; CL: Analysis

65. 3. Salmon patches are common vascular lesions in infants. They appear as flat, dull pink, macular lesions in various regions of the face and head. When they appear on the nape of the neck, they're commonly called "stork bites." These lesions fade by the first year of life. Both strawberry and cavernous hemangiomas are raised lesions. Nevus flammeus, or port wine stains, are reddish-purple lesions that don't fade.

CN: Physiological integrity; CNS: Physiological adaptation; CL: Analysis

66. A young child's parents ask for advice on the use of an insect repellent that contains DEET. Which statement by the nurse would be correct?
1. "Spray the child's clothing instead of the skin."
2. "The repellent works better as the temperature increases."
3. "The repellent isn't effective against the ticks responsible for Lyme disease."
4. "Apply insect repellent as you would sunscreen, with frequent applications during the day."

67. A nurse is teaching a parent about which DEET-containing insect repellent to use on his child. Which concentration should she instruct him to use on the child's skin for optimal results?
1. 10%
2. 15%
3. 20%
4. 30%

68. Which statement about warts would the nurse incorporate when assisting with a community health teaching program on common skin problems?
1. Cutting the wart is the preferred treatment for children.
2. No treatment exists that specifically kills the wart virus.
3. Warts are caused by a virus affecting the inner layer of skin.
4. Warts are harmless and usually last 2 to 4 years if untreated.

69. The nurse is assisting with a teaching program for new parents that focuses on oral hygiene promotion. Which factor would the nurse include as causing tooth decay and gum disease when allowed to remain on the teeth for prolonged periods?
1. Breast milk
2. Pacifiers
3. Thumb or other fingers
4. Formula

You're almost at question 70. That was quick!

You need to brush those carbs away.

66. 1. DEET spray has been approved for use on children. It should be used sparingly on all skin surfaces. By concentrating spray on clothing and camping equipment, the adverse effects and potential toxic buildup are significantly reduced. Repellent is lost to evaporation, wind, heat, and perspiration. Each 10° F increase in temperature leads to as much as a 50% reduction in protection time. DEET is very effective as a tick repellent.
CN: Physiological integrity; CNS: Reduction of risk potential; CL: Application

67. 1. The highest concentration approved by the Food and Drug Administration for children is 10%. Because of thinner skin and greater surface area to mass ratio in children, parents should use DEET products sparingly.
CN: Physiological integrity; CNS: Reduction of risk potential; CL: Application

68. 2. The goal of treatment is to kill the skin that contains the wart virus. Cutting the wart is likely to spread the virus. The virus that causes warts affects the outer layer of the skin. Warts are harmless and last 1 to 2 years if untreated.
CN: Health promotion and maintenance; CNS: None; CL: Application

69. 4. Tooth decay and gum disease result when the carbohydrates in formula, cow's milk, and fruit juices are allowed to remain on the teeth for a prolonged period. Studies have shown that breast milk only contributes to dental caries when sugar is already present on the teeth. Breast milk alone actually promotes enamel growth. Pacifiers and fingers don't cause tooth decay and gum disease, although they may contribute to malocclusion.
CN: Health promotion and maintenance; CNS: None; CL: Application

70. A child is suspected of having cellulitis. What classic signs should the nurse expect to see in a child?
1. Pale, irritated, cold to touch
2. Vesicular blisters at the site of the injury
3. Fever, edema, tenderness, warmth at the site
4. Swelling, redness, with well-defined borders

71. A 2-year-old child has cellulitis of the finger. Which organism or condition is the <u>most likely</u> cause of the infection?
1. Parainfluenza virus
2. Respiratory syncytial virus
3. *Escherichia coli*
4. *Streptococcus*

72. A child has a desquamation rash of the hands and feet. Which additional findings should the nurse expect to observe with this rash?
1. Peeling skin
2. Thin, reddened layers of epidermis
3. Thick skin with deep visible burrows
4. Thinning skin that may appear translucent

Note that this question asks about the most likely cause, not the only one.

73. Which instruction would the nurse include for the parents of a child who is to receive nystatin oral solution?
1. Give the solution immediately after feedings.
2. Give the solution immediately before feedings.
3. Mix the solution with small amounts of the feeding.
4. Give half the solution before and half the solution after the feeding.

74. An infant is examined and found to have a petechial rash. The nurse documents a description of this rash as:
1. a purple macular lesion larger than 1 cm in diameter.
2. purple to brown bruises, macular or papular, of various sizes.
3. a collection of blood from ruptured blood vessels larger than 1 cm in diameter.
4. a pinpoint, pink to purple, nonblanching macular lesion 1 to 3 mm in diameter.

Where are those petechiae?

70. 3. Cellulitis is a deep, locally diffuse infection of the skin. It's associated with redness, fever, edema, tenderness, and warmth at the site of the injury. Vesicular blisters suggest impetigo. Cellulitis has no well-defined borders.
CN: Physiological integrity; CNS: Physiological adaptation; CL: Application

71. 4. *Streptococcus* cause most cases of cellulitis. Parainfluenza and respiratory syncytial virus cause infections of the respiratory tract. *E. coli* is a cause of bladder infections.
CN: Physiological integrity; CNS: Physiological adaptation; CL: Analysis

72. 1. Desquamation is characteristic in diseases such as Stevens–Johnson syndrome. Scaling is thin, reddened layers of epidermis. Thickening of the skin with burrows is defined as lichenification. Thinning skin is best described as atrophy of the skin.
CN: Physiological integrity; CNS: Physiological adaptation; CL: Application

73. 1. Nystatin oral solution should be swabbed onto the mouth after feedings to allow for optimal contact with mucous membranes. Before meals and with meals doesn't give the best contact with the mucous membranes.
CN: Physiological integrity; CNS: Pharmacological and parenteral therapies; CL: Application

74. 4. Petechiae are small 1- to 3-mm macular lesions. Purple macular lesions greater than 1 cm are defined as purpura. A bruise is defined as ecchymosis. A hematoma is a collection of blood.
CN: Physiological integrity; CNS: Physiological adaptation; CL: Application

75. When inspecting the <u>palms</u> of a child, with which rash would the nurse expect to find no changes?
1. Coxsackie virus
2. Measles
3. Rocky Mountain spotted fever
4. Syphilis

76. A mother reports that her teenager is losing hair in small round areas on the scalp. The nurse interprets this as suggesting which condition?
1. Alopecia
2. Amblyopia
3. Exotropia
4. Seborrhea dermatitis

77. A topical corticosteroid cream is prescribed for a child with eczema. The nurse should instruct the mother to apply the cream:
1. over the entire body.
2. in a thin layer to the affected area and rub it in.
3. to the infected area without washing the area first.
4. in a thick layer and allow it to absorb.

78. A mother of a toddler diagnosed with atopic dermatitis is concerned about how her child acquired the disease. The best response by the nurse is:
1. fungal infection.
2. hereditary disorder.
3. sex-linked disorder.
4. viral infection.

79. A mother of a 6-month-old infant with atopic dermatitis asks the nurse for advice on bathing the child. What is the best response by the nurse?
1. Bathe the infant twice daily.
2. Bathe the infant every other day.
3. Use bubble baths to decrease itching.
4. The frequency of the infant's baths isn't important in atopic dermatitis.

What is the correct term for ready to "pull" your hair out?

75. 2. The rash in measles occurs on the face, trunk, and extremities. Rocky Mountain spotted fever, syphilis, and coxsackie virus show changes on the palms and soles.
CN: Physiological integrity; CNS: Physiological adaptation; CL: Analysis

76. 1. Alopecia is the correct term for thinning hair loss. Exotropia and amblyopia are eye disorders. Seborrhea dermatitis is cradle cap and occurs in infants.
CN: Physiological integrity; CNS: Physiological adaptation; CL: Application

77. 2. After gently cleansing the affected area, corticosteroid cream should be applied in a thin, not thick, layer and rubbed into the area thoroughly. It shouldn't be applied to the entire body.
CN: Physiological integrity; CNS: Pharmacological and parenteral therapies; CL: Analysis

78. 2. Atopic dermatitis is a hereditary disorder that isn't sex-linked and is associated with a family history of asthma, allergic rhinitis, or atopic dermatitis. Viral and fungal infections don't cause atopic dermatitis.
CN: Physiological integrity; CNS: Physiological adaptation; CL: Application

79. 2. Bathing removes lipoprotein complexes that hold water in the stratum corneum and increase water loss. Decreasing bathing to every other day can help prevent the removal of lipoprotein complexes. Soap and bubble bath should be used sparingly while bathing the child.
CN: Physiological integrity; CNS: Basic care and comfort; CL: Application

80. Discharge instructions for a child with atopic dermatitis include keeping the fingernails cut short. Which rationale should the nurse give for this intervention?
1. To prevent infection of the nail bed
2. To prevent the spread of the disorder
3. To prevent the child from causing a corneal abrasion
4. To reduce breaks in skin from scratching that may lead to secondary bacterial infections

81. A 10-year-old child being treated for common warts asks the nurse about the cause. What is the most appropriate response by the nurse?
1. Coxsackievirus
2. Human herpesvirus (HHV)
3. Human immunodeficiency virus (HIV)
4. Human papillomavirus (HPV)

82. The nurse is assessing a 6-year-old child with a spiny projection from the skin suspended from a narrow stalk on the forehead. Which condition would the nurse suspect?
1. Filiform wart
2. Flat wart
3. Plantar wart
4. Venereal warts

83. An adolescent says his feet itch, sweat a lot, and have a foul odor. The nurse suspects which condition?
1. Candidiasis
2. Tinea corporis
3. Tinea pedis
4. Molluscum contagiosum

84. A nurse is explaining treatments to the parents of a child with hypertrophic scarring. Which method would be the <u>best</u> for controlling this condition?
1. Compression garments
2. Moisturizing creams
3. Physiotherapy
4. Splints

Here's another question pointing out the importance of client teaching.

You know what they say about frogs and warts.

I can almost see the last question.

80. 4. Keeping fingernails cut short will prevent breaks in the skin when a child scratches. Cutting fingernails too short or cutting the skin around the nail can increase the risk of infection. Atopic dermatitis can be found in various areas of the skin but isn't spread from one area to another. Keeping fingernails short is a good way to reduce corneal abrasions but doesn't apply to atopic dermatitis.
CN: Physiological integrity; CNS: Physiological adaptation; CL: Application

81. 4. HPV is responsible for various forms of warts. Coxsackievirus is associated with hand-foot-and-mouth disease. HHV is associated with varicella and herpes zoster. HIV infections aren't associated with epithelial tumors known as warts.
CN: Physiological integrity; CNS: Physiological adaptation; CL: Application

82. 1. Filiform warts are long spiny projections from the skin surface. Flat warts are flat-topped, smooth-surfaced lesions. Plantar warts are rough papules, commonly found on the soles of the feet. Venereal warts appear on the genital mucosa and are confluent papules with rough surfaces.
CN: Physiological integrity; CNS: Physiological adaptation; CL: Application

83. 3. Tinea pedis is a superficial fungal infection on the feet, commonly called athletes' foot. Candidiasis is a fungal infection of the skin or mucous membranes commonly found in the oral, vaginal, and intestinal mucosal tissue. Tinea corporis, or ringworm, is a flat scaling papular lesion with raised borders. Molluscum contagiosum is a viral skin infection with lesions that are small red papules.
CN: Physiological integrity; CNS: Physiological adaptation; CL: Analysis

84. 1. Compression garments are worn for up to 1 year to control hypertrophic scarring. Moisturizing creams help decrease hyperpigmentation. Physiotherapy and splints help keep joints and limbs supple.
CN: Physiological integrity; CNS: Physiological adaptation; CL: Application

CN: Client needs category CNS: Client needs subcategory CL: Cognitive level

85. During a physical examination, a child is noted to have nails with "ice-pick" pits and ridges. The nails are thick and discolored and have splintered hemorrhages easily separated from the nail bed. Which condition would cause this to occur?
1. Paronychia
2. Psoriasis
3. Scabies
4. Seborrhea

86. A neonate is examined and noted to have bruising on the scalp, along with diffuse swelling of the soft tissue that crosses over the suture line. The nurse <u>most accurately</u> interprets these findings as:
1. caput succedaneum.
2. cephalhematoma.
3. craniotabes.
4. hydrocephalus.

What is the most accurate assessment?

87. A child has a healed wound from a traumatic injury. His mother is concerned because a lesion formed over the wound is pink, thickened, smooth, and rubbery in nature. The nurse should use what term to discuss this condition with the mother?
1. Erosion
2. Fissure
3. Keloids
4. Striae

Hmmm, white plaques with an erythematous base. What could that mean?

88. The mother of an infant gives a history of poor feeding for a few days. A complete physical examination shows white plaques in the mouth with an erythematous base. The plaques stick to the mucous membranes tightly and bleed when scraped. The nurse would suspect which condition?
1. Chickenpox
2. Herpes lesions
3. Measles
4. Oral candidiasis

85. 2. Psoriasis is a chronic skin disorder with an unknown cause that shows these characteristic skin changes. A paronychia is a bacterial infection of the nail bed. Scabies are mites that burrow under the skin, usually between the webbing of the fingers and toes. Seborrhea is a chronic inflammatory dermatitis or cradle cap.
CN: Physiological integrity; CNS: Physiological adaptation; CL: Application

86. 1. Caput succedaneum originates from trauma to the neonate while descending through the birth canal. It's usually a benign injury that spontaneously resolves over time. Cephalhematoma is a collection of blood in the periosteum of the scalp that doesn't cross over the suture line. Craniotabes is the thinning of the bone of the scalp. Hydrocephalus is an increased volume of cerebrospinal fluid (CSF) or the obstruction of the flow of the CSF and isn't related to soft tissue swelling.
CN: Physiological integrity; CNS: Physiological adaptation; CL: Analysis

87. 3. Keloids are an exaggerated connective tissue response to skin injury. An erosion is a depressed vesicular lesion. A fissure is a cleavage in the surface of skin. Striae are linear depressions of the skin.
CN: Physiological integrity; CNS: Physiological adaptation; CL: Application

88. 4. Oral candidiasis, or thrush, is a painful inflammation that can affect the tongue, soft and hard palates, and buccal mucosa. Chickenpox, or varicella, causes open ulcerations of the mucous membranes. Herpes lesions are usually vesicular ulcerations of the oral mucosa around the lips. Measles that form Koplik's spots can be identified as pinpoint white elevated lesions.
CN: Physiological integrity; CNS: Physiological adaptation; CL: Application

89. A child was found unconscious at home and brought to the emergency department by the fire and rescue unit. Physical examination showed cherry-red mucous membranes, nail beds, and skin. The nurse suspects the child's condition was the result of which of the following?
1. Aspirin ingestion
2. Carbon monoxide poisoning
3. Hydrocarbon ingestion
4. Spider bite

90. A 14-year-old diagnosed with acne vulgaris asks what causes it. Which factor(s) should the nurse identify for this client? Select all that apply.
1. Chocolates and sweets
2. Increased hormone levels
3. Growth of anaerobic bacteria
4. Caffeine
5. Heredity
6. Fatty foods

91. Which term describes a fungal infection found on the upper arm?
1. Tinea capitis
2. Tinea corporis
3. Tinea cruris
4. Tinea pedis

92. A 15-kg infant is started on amoxicillin/ clavulanate potassium (Augmentin) therapy, 200 mg/5 ml, for cellulitis. The dose is 40 mg/kg over 24 hours given three times daily. How many milliliters would be given for each dose?
1. 2.5 ml
2. 5 ml
3. 15 ml
4. 20 ml

93. A 5-year-old male sustained third-degree burns to the right upper extremity after tipping over a frying pan. Which skin structures would the nurse include when explaining a third-degree burn to the child's mother?
1. Epidermis only
2. Epidermis and dermis
3. All skin layers and nerve endings
4. Skin layers, nerve endings, muscles, tendons, and bones

Be careful! There may be more than one correct answer to this question.

Practice with numbers makes perfect.

89. **2.** Cherry-red skin changes are seen when a child has been exposed to high levels of carbon monoxide. Nausea and vomiting and pale skin are symptoms of aspirin ingestion. A hydrocarbon or petroleum ingestion usually results in respiratory symptoms and tachycardia. Spider bite reactions are usually localized to the area of the bite.
CN: Physiological integrity; CNS: Physiological adaptation; CL: Analysis

90. **2, 3, and 5.** Acne vulgaris is characterized by the appearance of comedones (blackheads and whiteheads). Comedones develop for various reasons, including increased hormone levels, heredity, irritation or application of irritating substances (such as cosmetics), and growth of anaerobic bacteria. A direct relationship between acne vulgaris and consumption of chocolates, caffeine, or fatty foods hasn't been established.
CN: Physiological integrity; CNS: Physiological adaptation; CL: Application

91. **2.** Tinea corporis describes fungal infections of the body. Tinea capitis describes fungal infections of the scalp. Tinea cruris is used to describe fungal infections of the inner thigh and inguinal creases. Tinea pedis is the term for fungal infections of the foot.
CN: Physiological integrity; CNS: Physiological adaptation; CL: Application

92. **2.** For each dose, 5 ml should be given. The dose is first calculated by multiplying the weight times the milligrams. It's then divided by three even doses. The milligrams are then used to determine the milliliters based on the concentration of the medicine. 40 mg $\times$ 15 kg = 600/3 doses = 200 mg/dose. The concentration is 200 mg in every 5 ml.
CN: Physiological integrity; CNS: Pharmacological and parenteral therapies; CL: Application

93. **3.** A third-degree burn involves all of the skin layers and the nerve endings. First-degree burns involve only the epidermis. Second-degree burns affect the epidermis and dermis. Fourth-degree burns involve all skin layers, nerve endings, muscles, tendons, and bone.
CN: Physiological integrity; CNS: Physiological adaptation; CL: Application

CN: Client needs category   CNS: Client needs subcategory   CL: Cognitive level

94. A 4-year-old child has a tick embedded in the scalp. Which method should the nurse use to remove the tick?
1. Burning the tick at the skin surface
2. Surgically removing the tick
3. Grasping the tick with tweezers and applying slow, outward pressure
4. Grasping the tick with tweezers and quickly pulling the tick out

95. A child with hives is prescribed diphenhydramine (Benadryl) 5 mg/kg over 24 hours in divided doses every 6 hours. The child weighs 8 kg. How many milligrams should be given with each dose?
1. 4.5 mg
2. 10 mg
3. 22 mg
4. 40 mg

96. The nurse is caring for an 8-year-old child who arrived at the emergency department with chemical burns to both legs. What is the <u>priority</u> intervention for this child?
1. Dilute the burns.
2. Apply sterile dressings.
3. Apply topical antibiotics.
4. Debride and graft the burns.

97. A 12-year-old child with full-thickness, circumferential burns to the chest has difficulty breathing. The nurse is aware that which is the priority intervention?
1. Chest tube insertion
2. Escharotomy
3. Intubation
4. Needle thoracocentesis

98. A 6-year-old child is evaluated after sustaining burns to his left shoulder. After the parents are instructed to use moisturizing cream and protect the burn from sunlight, they question the nurse about the purpose of the treatment. The nurse explains that the treatment will decrease:
1. keloids.
2. scarring.
3. hypopigmentation.
4. hyperpigmentation.

Not another math question!

Knowing why something happens allows you to teach more effectively.

94. 3. Applying gentle outward pressure prevents injury to the skin and the retention of tick parts. Burning the tick and quickly pulling the tick out may cause injury to the skin and should be avoided. Surgical removal is indicated when tick parts have been retained.
CN: Physiological integrity; CNS: Physiological adaptation; CL: Application

95. 2. For each dose, 10 mg should be given. Multiplying 5 mg by the weight (8 kg) gives the amount of milligrams for 24 hours (40 mg). Divide this by the number of doses per day (4), giving 10 mg/dose. 5 mg × 8 kg = 40 mg/4 doses = 10 mg/dose.
CN: Physiological integrity; CNS: Pharmacological and parenteral therapies; CL: Application

96. 1. Diluting the chemical is the first treatment. It will help remove the chemical and stop the burning process. The remaining treatments are initiated after dilution.
CN: Physiological integrity; CNS: Physiological adaptation; CL: Analysis

97. 2. Escharotomy is a surgical incision used to relieve pressure from edema. It's needed with circumferential burns that prevent chest expansion or cause circulatory compromise. Insertion of a chest tube and needle thoracocentesis are performed to relieve a pneumothorax. Intubation is performed to maintain a patent airway.
CN: Physiological integrity; CNS: Physiological adaptation; CL: Analysis

98. 4. Healed or grafted burns would require creams and protection from the sun to decrease hyperpigmentation. Scarring, hypopigmentation, and keloids aren't treated with moisturizing creams and avoidance of sunlight.
CN: Physiological integrity; CNS: Physiological adaptation; CL: Analysis

99. A child arrives in the emergency department 20 minutes after sustaining a major burn injury to 40% of his body. After initiating an I.V. line, which intervention should the nurse perform <u>next</u>?
1. Insert an indwelling catheter.
2. Apply Silvadene cream to the burn.
3. Shave the hair around the burn wound.
4. Obtain cultures from the deepest burn area.

100. A 12-year-old child sustains a moderate burn injury. The mother reports that the child last received a tetanus injection when he was 5 years old. An appropriate nursing intervention would be to administer which immunization?
1. 0.5 ml of tetanus toxoid I.M.
2. 0.5 ml of tetanus toxoid I.V.
3. 250 units of Hyper-Tet I.M.
4. 250 units of Hyper-Tet I.V.

101. A child arrives in the emergency department after sustaining a major burn injury. During the first 8 hours of admission, it is most important for the nurse to assess the child for which conditions?
1. Hyponatremia and hypokalemia
2. Hyponatremia and hyperkalemia
3. Hypernatremia and hypokalemia
4. Hypernatremia and hyperkalemia

102. A child weighing 10 kg has a deep partial-thickness burn to 40% of his body surface area. The nurse will titrate the child's I.V. fluids to achieve which hourly urinary outputs?
1. 5 ml
2. 10 ml
3. 30 ml
4. 50 ml

103. A team of nurses is preparing a trauma room for the arrival of a child with partial-thickness burns to both lower extremities and portions of the trunk. Which fluid should be ready for immediate use?
1. Albumin
2. Dextrose 5% and half-normal saline
3. Lactated Ringer's solution
4. Normal saline with 2 mEq KCl/100 ml

What's the magic urinary output number here?

99. 1. I.V. fluids must be started immediately on all children who sustain a major burn injury to prevent the child from going into hypovolemic shock. The fluids are titrated based on urine output. To monitor this output exactly, an indwelling urinary catheter must be inserted. The other interventions will be performed but not immediately.

CN: Physiological integrity; CNS: Reduction of risk potential; CL: Application

100. 1. Tetanus prophylaxis is given to all clients with moderate to severe burn injuries if it has been longer than 5 years since the last immunization or if there is no history of immunization. The correct dosage is 0.5 ml I.M. one time if the child was immunized within 10 years. If it has been more than 10 years or the child hasn't received tetanus immunization, the dosage is 250 units of Hyper-Tet one time. There is no I.V. form of tetanus available.

CN: Physiological integrity; CNS: Pharmacological and parenteral therapies; CL: Analysis

101. 2. Capillary permeability increases during the first 48 hours postburn, allowing fluids to shift from the plasma to the interstitial spaces. This fluid is high in sodium, causing the client's serum sodium level to decrease. Potassium also leaks from the cells into the plasma, causing hyperkalemia.

CN: Physiological integrity; CNS: Physiological adaptation; CL: Analysis

102. 2. Fluid resuscitation should be started on all clients with burns over more than 20% of their body surface area. In children, an hourly urine output of 1 to 2 ml/kg of body weight shows adequate kidney perfusion and fluid resuscitation. Adults should have an hourly urine output of 30 to 50 ml.

CN: Physiological integrity; CNS: Physiological adaptation; CL: Application

103. 3. Lactated Ringer's solution is recommended because it replaces the lost sodium and corrects the metabolic acidosis. The use of albumin is controversial. If albumin is given, it's as adjunct therapy and not for primary fluid replacement. The stress from a burn injury affects the glucose metabolism. Dextrose shouldn't be given during the first 24 hours because it can put the client into pseudodiabetes. The client is hyperkalemic from the potassium shift from the intracellular spaces to the plasma, and additional potassium would be detrimental.

CN: Physiological integrity; CNS: Pharmacological and parenteral therapies; CL: Application

104. A mother states that she recently received information that hand-foot-and-mouth disease has been diagnosed in a few of her child's preschool classmates. The nurse should instruct the mother to observe her child for which symptoms?
1. Low-grade fever, followed by vesicular lesions on the trunk, face, and scalp
2. Mild, self-limited eruption of vesicles on the buccal mucosa, tongue, soft palate, hands, and feet
3. Purpuric, maculopapular lesions with GI symptoms and joint pain
4. Bright red rash with a red outer border circling a bite mark

105. A 27.5 lb child is receiving antibiotics for cellulitis. The order reads Pen-Vee K 40 mg/kg/day divided every 6 hours. Which dosage of antibiotics should this child receive with <u>each</u> dose?
1. 225 mg
2. 500 mg
3. 125 mg
4. 12.5 mg

106. While assessing a 2-year-old child brought into the clinic with an upper respiratory infection, the nurse notes some bruising on his arms, legs, and trunk. Which findings would prompt the nurse to suspect child abuse? Select all that apply.
1. Superficial scrapes on the lower legs
2. Welts or bruises in various stages of healing on the trunk
3. A deep blue-black patch on the buttocks
4. One large bruise on the thigh
5. Circular, symmetrical burns on the lower legs
6. A parent who is hypercritical of the child and pushes the frightened child away

107. A 44-lb preschooler is being treated for inflammation. The physician orders 0.2 mg/kg/day of dexamethasone by mouth to be administered every 6 hours. The elixir comes in a strength of 0.5 mg/5 ml. How many milliliters of dexamethasone should the nurse give this client per dose? Record your answer using a whole number.

_____ milliliters

You're being asked about characteristics in question 104.

You did it! You should be on top of the world!

104. 2. Hand-foot-and-mouth disease is caused by coxsackievirus and usually occurs in preschool children. Vesicular lesions accompanied by a low-grade fever are typically signs of varicella. Purpura, GI symptoms, and joint pain are symptoms of Henoch-Schönlein purpura. A bright-red bull's-eye rash is a classic symptom of Lyme disease.

CN: Physiological integrity; CNS: Physiological adaptation; CL: Application

105. 3. The dose is 125 mg. One kilogram equals 2.2 pounds, so a 27.5 lb child weighs 12.5 kg. 40 mg/kg/day equals a total of 500 mg given every 6 hours or 4 times in 24 hours. 500 mg divided by 4 equals 125 mg.

CN: Physiological integrity; CNS: Pharmacological and parenteral therapies; CL: Application

106. 2, 5, and 6. Injuries at various stages of healing in protected or padded areas can be signs of inflicted trauma, leading the nurse to suspect abuse. Burns that are bilateral as well as symmetrical are typical of child abuse. The shape of the burn may resemble the item used to create it, such as a cigarette. Pushing away the child and being hypercritical are typical behaviors of abusive parents. Superficial scrapes and bruises on the lower legs are normal in a healthy, active child. A deep blue-black macular patch on the buttocks is more consistent with a Mongolian spot rather than a traumatic injury.

CN: Psychosocial integrity; CNS: None; CL: Analysis

107. 10. To perform this dosage calculation, convert the child's weight from pounds to kilograms: 44 lb ÷ 2.2 lb/kg = 20 kg. Then calculate the total daily dose: 20 kg × 0.2 mg/kg/day = 4 mg. Next, calculate the amount to be given at each dose: 4 mg ÷ 4 doses = 1 mg/dose. The elixir contains 0.5 mg of drug per 5 ml. To give 1 mg of drug, administer 10 ml to the child at each dose.

CN: Physiological integrity; CNS: Pharmacological and parenteral therapies; CL: Analysis

Part VI

Issues in nursing

In this chapter, you'll be asked questions about management concepts and methods and coordination and supervision of care. Take your time here.

Chapter 36
Management & leadership

The nurse-manager is accountable 24/7.

1. The team leader notices at the beginning of the shift that all of the I.V. antibiotics for a client are still in the medication room. Which action should the team leader take first?
   1. Ask the client if the client received the medications on the previous shift.
   2. Return the medications to the pharmacy so the client does not get billed.
   3. Ask the nurse who cared for the client about the medications.
   4. Notify the nurse-manager of the unit.

2. Which is an example of tertiary prevention in disaster planning?
   1. Providing routine tetanus immunizations
   2. Instituting disaster drills
   3. Implementing biohazard precautions
   4. Counseling disaster victims about stress reactions

3. The nurse is triaging clients from a large disaster. Which client should receive care first?
   1. Client with large shard of glass piercing chest wall, respirations 32 breaths/minute
   2. Client with forearm disfigured with protruding bone, finger cap refill 2 seconds
   3. Child with 3-in. oozing laceration on leg
   4. Woman who is 2 months pregnant, partial-thickness burn on forearm

1. 3. The team leader should attempt to clarify with the involved staff first. The client would not be the accurate source to verify I.V. medications. Handling the supplies is a secondary priority to ensuring that the client received the required medications. The team leader should attempt to deal with problems directly first.

CN: Safe, effective care environment; CNS: Safety and infection control; CL: Analysis

2. 4. Tertiary prevention involves reducing the degree and quantity of injury, disability, and damage following a disaster or crisis. Primary prevention focuses on keeping the crisis or disaster from happening. The goal of secondary prevention is to reduce the duration and intensity of the disaster or crisis. The other options are incorrect because a disaster had not occurred.

CN: Safe, effective care environment; CNS: Management of care; CL: Application

3. 1. The integrity of the chest wall has been compromised and is becoming a "breathing" problem. The others can wait for up to 2 hours.

CN: Safe, effective care environment; CNS: Safety and infection control; CL: Analysis

4. There has been a large disaster, and nurses have been floated to help with the large influx of clients. Which client is <u>most</u> appropriate to assign to the nurse floated from the mother–baby unit?
1. 1 day post-op hemicolectomy male with a Foley catheter
2. Woman in pelvic traction who is 3 months pregnant
3. Elderly woman who has herpes zoster
4. Male admitted for hearing command voices to kill himself

5. Which is an example of a staff nurse functioning in the role of an informal leader?
1. Verifying adequate staff coverage for a shift
2. Filling out a discipline form on a nursing assistant
3. Encouraging a peer to join a committee
4. Attending a hospital-wide policy meeting

6. Staff from two different departments are disagreeing over the transfer process between their respective departments. Which is the best process to handle this disagreement?
1. Ask the director of nursing to establish a policy.
2. Allow the staff to handle the issue on their own without authoritative interference.
3. Arrange managers from the departments to determine a solution.
4. Set up a meeting of staff from the departments to identify key issues.

The hint is most appropriate.

In question 6, it's asking what is the best.

4. 1. Give the floated nurses clients with whom they can use the skills they would ordinarily use. The client who is 1 day post-op hemicolectomy with a Foley catheter is similar to a client with a cesarean section. Obstetric (OB) nurses do not handle traction; the woman does not have any issues related to the pregnancy. OB nurses should not take care of infectious clients to avoid inadvertent transmission. OB nurses are not experienced in managing suicidal clients.
CN: Safe, effective care environment; CNS: Safety and infection control; CL: Analysis

5. 3. A leader doesn't always have formal power and authority but influences the success of a unit by being an excellent role model and by guiding, encouraging, and facilitating professional growth and development. A manager has formal power and authority from the status within the organization, and such power and authority are detailed in the manager's job description. Authority, a characteristic of a managerial position, is given by virtue of position within an organization.
CN: Safe, effective care environment; CNS: Management of care; CL: Application

6. 4. In this situation, functioning as a democratic leader is best. The staff who deal with the day-to-day problems of direct client care have the best grasp of the situation and should have autonomy to solve problems. The manager, however, should be available to help. Option 1 reflects the style of an autocratic manager. Without staff input, the managers won't have the necessary information to identify the best solution. In option 2, the managers have abdicated responsibility for problem solving (laissez-faire manager), yet the problem still exists. The staff may not have the skills or resources to just solve the problem on their own. In option 3, there may be resentment and frustration from the fact that the actual decision made by the manager may not include input from the staff.
CN: Safe, effective care environment; CNS: Management of care; CL: Analysis

7. A staff nurse at the nurses' station answers the phone and is told there is a bomb in a client's room. What action should the nurse take at this time?

1. Put the call on hold and obtain the charge nurse.
2. Transfer the call to security.
3. Ask the caller for details about the bomb placement.
4. Signal to staff to close the client's doors.

8. What is the most important aspect to determine when deciding which nursing care delivery system should be used?

1. Staff preference
2. Staff licensure
3. Number of staff
4. Experience of staff

9. The nurse-manager is considering whether to change the unit's nursing care delivery system (NCDS) from team nursing to primary nursing. Which of the following is a key aspect to determine whether primary nursing is appropriate?

1. The most common diagnosis for the unit's clients
2. The amount of training available about primary nursing
3. The number of registered nurses
4. The type of documentation system being used

10. On a busy medical-surgical unit, a winter storm has prevented most of the staff members from getting to work. One registered nurse, two licensed practical nurses, and three nursing assistants have been able to get to work. What nursing care delivery system (NCDS) should be implemented in this situation?

1. Team nursing
2. Primary nursing
3. Functional nursing
4. Case management

Most important is the hint.

What system will work in a crisis?

7. 3. With a potential danger, it is important to determine as much information as possible. Any transferring/holding could cause a loss of the caller and important information. More information should be obtained first; clients may need to be evacuated.

CN: Safe, effective care environment; CNS: Safety and infection control; CL: Analysis

8. 2. Determining who has responsibility for making decisions regarding client care is an essential element of all client care delivery systems. The number of licensed staff and level of license (registered nurse versus licensed practical nurse) are the most important criteria.

CN: Safe, effective care environment; CNS: Management of care; CL: Application

9. 3. Primary nursing is used for higher acuity clients, with a high registered nurse-to-client ratio. The diagnosis is not directly related; case management tends to be used with long-term cases. Training is important, but primary nursing is related to the roles, division of labor, and staffing. Documentation systems are not related to type of nursing delivery system.

CN: Safe, effective care environment; CNS: Management of care; CL: Analysis

10. 3. Functional nursing best uses the skills of all staff in a timely manner during this crisis. This delivery system requires the least staff and delegates tasks to those who can best perform them. Team nursing doesn't allow for the best use of a limited number of staff who must care for a large number of clients. Primary nursing and case management require more registered nurses than are currently available.

CN: Safe, effective care environment; CNS: Management of care; CL: Analysis

11. A nursing student asked the instructor for the best example of an appropriate nursing care delivery system. The best response by the instructor would be?
1. Case management in the emergency department
2. Team nursing in the intensive care unit
3. Functional nursing when most registered nursing staff cannot report to duty
4. Primary nursing in a rehabilitation unit

12. The emergency department (ED) staff report not receiving enough information from long-term care (LTC) facilities that are transferring clients. What is the best approach?
1. Tell the ED staff to handle it with the LTC staff by calling for what is needed.
2. Realize the behavior of others cannot be controlled.
3. Organize a meeting between the facilities to develop a satisfactory process.
4. Call the director of the LTC facility and ask that nursing be more complete.

13. A new graduate nurse is completing the scheduled 4-week orientation to a medical-surgical unit. Which self-recognized need should prompt the new graduate nurse to request some additional time or training before ending orientation?
1. Uncomfortable if had to manage a cardiac arrest independently
2. Unclear how staffing assignments are made on the unit
3. Frequently unable to establish new I.V. access on the first attempt
4. Unable to manage more than two clients at a time

14. Which action can the nurse be legally liable for?
1. Administering 2 mg hydromorphone (Dilaudid) when the client is prescribed 1 to 2 mg every 4 hours
2. Withholding digoxin (Lanoxin) when the client's apical pulse is 56 beats/minute
3. Withholding mononitrate (Imdur) when the client's blood pressure is 80/40 mm Hg
4. Administering cephalosporin when the client has an allergy to penicillin

It's important to function and manage the workload and learn to delegate.

I think I need some help!

11. 3. Functional nursing best uses the skills of all staff in a timely manner during this crisis. This delivery system requires the least staff and delegates tasks to those who can best perform them. Team nursing doesn't allow for the best use of a limited number of staff who must care for a large number of clients. Primary nursing and case management require more registered nurses than are currently available.
CN: Safe, effective care environment; CNS: Management of care; CL: Analysis

12. 3. The best solution for quality, consistent client care is to have the affected departments discuss key issues and develop a consistent policy and process for all to follow.
CN: Safe, effective care environment; CNS: Safety and infection control; CL: Application

13. 4. Handling multiple clients and prioritization are skills new graduates commonly need to enhance. Additional time with the help of a preceptor is a need that should be dealt with before being independent. New graduates are rarely in charge of a client in cardiac arrest; this knowledge will come with experience. New graduates are not in charge of running the unit. A skill such as I.V. insertion will come with more experience and is not an essential skill to acquire from orientation.
CN: Safe, effective care environment; CNS: Management of care; CL: Analysis

14. 4. There is a cross-sensitivity between cephalosporin and penicillin, and the drug should not be given. When a range is ordered, any dose in the range is acceptable. Bradycardia is a sign of digoxin toxicity, and the drug should not ordinarily be given if the pulse is less the 60. Nitrates cause vasodilation and should not be given when hypotension is present.
CN: Safe, effective care environment; CNS: Management of care; CL: Analysis

15. The nursing team consists of one RN (registered nurse), one LPN (Licensed practical nurse), and one nursing assistant. What is the most appropriate assignment for the RN to delegate to the LPN?
1. Pass the dinner trays.
2. Empty the Foley catheter.
3. Administer the morning daily medication.
4. Suction a client who is 1 day postoperative after tracheostomy.

16. Which is the best instructional guidance for the nurse-manager to include for the staff nurses when delegating the responsibility to revise the unit's educational policies?
1. "Let me know if you need anything."
2. "Complete the task in 6 weeks."
3. "Give me your suggestions and I'll decide."
4. "Tell me what you think after looking at everything."

What guidance shall I give?

17. Which is proper delegation of a task from the registered nurse to the nursing assistant?
1. "Please see if Mrs. Jones's pain is better in Room 313."
2. "Advance the diet for Mrs. Smith in Room 212 for lunch."
3. "Get Mr. Grey in Room 414 up today. Thank you."
4. "Take a tympanic temperature for Mr. Green in Room 515 at 5 p.m."

18. The nurse-manager meets with a staff nurse to evaluate performance after the 6-month probationary period. As part of the evaluation process, the nurse-manager would ask the staff nurse to:
1. accept the nurse-manager's evaluation by signing in agreement.
2. contribute a self-evaluation and suggested areas for future growth.
3. have peers vouch for his or her performance.
4. give her perception of how the manager is performing.

15. 3. LPNs should be assigned higher level skills in stable, predictable situations. Lower level custodial skills should be assigned to unlicensed assistive personnel. The new tracheostomy is potentially unstable and should be retained by the RN.

CN: Safe, effective care environment; CNS: Management of care; CL: Analysis

16. 2. Delegation must be done clearly and precisely. The nurse-manager must assign responsibility, identify the task to be accomplished, explain what outcomes are needed, and identify the time frame for completing the work. The remaining options don't give clear explanations of work to be done, don't clearly assign responsibility or the specific outcomes desired, and don't establish a time frame for completion of the task.

CN: Safe, effective care environment; CNS: Management of care; CL: Application

17. 4. Option 4 is a specific task delegation. The other options involve judgment/evaluation or are too vague.

CN: Safe, effective care environment; CNS: Management of care; CL: Application

18. 2. Performance evaluation is a primary managerial function for nurse managers. Professional growth of staff requires a self-reflective approach and evaluation and goal setting. A performance evaluation need not be agreed to in full by staff. Peer evaluation is used in some settings but is done in a systematic way with clear criteria rather than informal "vouching." An evaluation should focus on the person who is being evaluated, not other factors.

CN: Safe, effective care environment; CNS: Management of care; CL: Application

19. A new nurse is not performing dressing changes satisfactorily. What is the best approach for the nurse-manager to use <u>first</u>?
1. Ask the new nurse how she perceives her performance.
2. Tell her there are deficiencies that must be rectified by a stated deadline.
3. Document the inadequacies in writing and have the new nurse sign the paper.
4. Tell the unit's nurse educator to schedule a class for the unit on the topic.

20. The nurse-manager implements new processes to decrease the incidence of central I.V. line infection. What is the best indicator that the measures have resulted in improved outcomes?
1. A survey of the unit's nurses indicates perceived improvement in results.
2. A total decrease in the number of central I.V. line infections on the unit has been identified.
3. Retrospective chart audits for infection rate show improvement in clients with central I.V. lines.
4. Comparison of total number of I.V. antibiotics used between the two time periods has shown a decrease in antibiotic use.

21. The nurse-manager notes an unacceptable rate of falls on the unit. Hourly rounds by nursing staff are initiated. What is the best method to determine that the change has made a difference?
1. Scores on client satisfaction surveys
2. Survey of staff's perception of the effectiveness
3. Comparing fall rates after the rounds are initiated.
4. Documentation that the rounds are completed as scheduled.

22. A nurse-manager appropriately behaves as an autocrat in which situation?
1. Planning vacation time for staff
2. Directing staff activities if a client has a cardiac arrest
3. Evaluating a new medication administration process
4. Identifying the strengths and weaknesses of a client education video

How do you think you are doing?

Congratulations! You're finished with this chapter. You're a natural-born leader!

19. **1.** Determining how the involved individual perceives his or her performance and what would help the person improve is the first step. If there is resistance or failure to improve after initial approaches, a more directive approach (such as in options 2 or 3) can be taken. There is no evidence that the entire unit needs educational help on this topic.
CN: Safe, effective care environment; CNS: Management of care; CL: Application

20. **3.** Compare results in the affected population. Opinions are useful but do not carry the same weight as evidence-based practice. The absolute number of infections may vary if the number of central I.V. lines varies (options 2 and 4). In addition, I.V. antibiotics are used for reasons other than central I.V. line infections.
CN: Safe, effective care environment; CNS: Management of care; CL: Application

21. **3.** The best method is to obtain objective evidence that the desired results have been achieved. This is more reliable than opinions or just determining that an action itself was completed.
CN: Safe, effective care environment; CNS: Management of care; CL: Application.

22. **2.** In a crisis situation, the nurse-manager should take command for the benefit of the client. Planning vacation time and evaluating procedures and client resources require staff input characteristic of a democratic or participative manager.
CN: Safe, effective care environment; CNS: Management of care; CL: Application

We saved the best, and most challenging, topic for last! Don't stress—you've done an excellent job!

Chapter 37
Ethical & legal issues

1. An elderly client has been admitted to the medical-surgical unit from the postanesthesia care unit. The client falls out of bed while the bed is in high position, with side rails down, and the client unattended. Which charge is the <u>most appropriate</u> for the nurse's actions?
1. Collective liability
2. Willful misconduct
3. Battery
4. Negligence

Make sure you choose the most appropriate answer.

2. Which client cannot sign out against medical advice?
1. A pregnant 15-year old with vaginal spotting
2. A client with ST elevation on the electrocardiogram
3. A client who drank a bottle of vodka 1 hour ago
4. An emancipated (mature) minor

3. Which circumstance would keep the nurse from being liable for professional negligence when the nurse made an error when administering a drug?
1. The nurse did not know the drug was contra-indicated for this client.
2. The excess drug administered did not cause any client harm.
3. A coworker confirmed that the drug dose was correct.
4. The amount of drug was dispensed by the pharmacy.

What are the 4 D's?

1. 4. Negligence is failure to do what a reasonable, prudent nurse of similar training would do in the same or similar circumstances. Negligence is a general term that denotes conduct lacking in due care. Carelessness is interpreted as a deviation from the standard of care that a reasonable person would use in a particular set of circumstances. Collective liability stems from cooperation by several manufacturers in a wrongful activity that by its nature requires group participation. Willful misconduct is a known violation of a reasonable and enforced rule or policy. It is not specific to nursing. Battery involves harmful or unwarranted contact with the client.

CN: Safe, effective care environment; CNS: Safety and infection control; CL: Analysis

2. 3. A client who is intoxicated is not competent to sign out. A pregnant woman is an "adult." A competent client can sign out against medical advice for any reason. An emancipated (mature) minor is the same as an "adult."

CN: Safe, effective care environment; CNS: Management of care; CL: Application

3. 2. The four essential components of a lawsuit are duty, breach of duty, injury, and negligent act caused the injury.

CN: Safe, effective care environment; CNS: Management of care; CL: Application

4. The nurse is unsure whether it is appropriate to delegate I.V. site observation to the licensed practical nurse. Which is the ultimate authority to consult to make this decision?
1. Professional association policy statement
2. Facility's policies and procedures
3. American Nurses Association Standards of Care
4. State Nurse Practice Act

Do you know your state's Nurse Practice Act?

4. 4. The Nurse Practice Act is a series of statutes, enacted by each state legislature, that outline the legal scope of nursing practice within a particular state. The act sets educational requirements for the nurse, distinguishes between nursing practice and medical practice, and defines the scope of nursing practice. Facility policies and procedures govern the practice in that particular facility. Facility policies/procedures can be stricter than the Nurse Practice Act but not more liberal. Standards of care and professional policy statements, which are criteria that serve as a basis for comparison when evaluating the quality of nursing practice, are established by federal, accreditation, state, and professional organizations.

CN: Safe, effective care environment; CNS: Management of care; CL: Application

5. An alert, oriented, adult Jehovah Witness client is refusing blood even though he realizes he could die. The wife, who is not a believer, asks that blood be given. How should the situation be handled?
1. Do not give blood, respecting the client's right to refuse.
2. Give blood as the wife wants because refusal would be suicidal.
3. Contact the hospital administrator and take protective custody of the client.
4. See if the client has an advanced directive prior to making the decision.

5. 1. The right to refuse treatment is an ethical principle of respect for the autonomy of the individual. The client can refuse treatment if he's competent and aware of the risks and complications associated with that refusal. The right to die involves whether to initiate or withhold life-sustaining treatment for a client who is irreversibly comatose, vegetative, or suffering with end-stage terminal illness. A competent adult can refuse treatment even if the spouse does not agree. Protective custody is invoked with a minor. A durable power of attorney for health care is done when a client is incapacitated and cannot speak for himself.

CN: Safe, effective care environment; CNS: Management of care; CL: Application

I've got to complete this incident report.

6. A nurse gives a client the wrong medication. After assessing the client, the nurse completes an incident report. Which statement describes what will occur <u>next</u>?
1. The incident will be reported to the state board of nursing.
2. The form will be used for an adverse drug reaction (ADR) report.
3. The medication error will result in the nurse being suspended at the facility.
4. The incident report will be used for risk management.

6. 4. Unusual occurrences and deviations from care are documented on incident reports. Incident reports are internal to the facility and are used to evaluate care and determine potential risks or system problems that could have contributed to the error. This type of error won't result in a report to the state board of nursing or in suspension of the nurse. Some facilities do track the number of errors by a nurse or on particular units; the purpose of tracking errors is to provide appropriate education and to improve the nursing process. Adverse drug reaction forms are used to report an individual's reaction to a medication, not errors.

CN: Safe, effective care environment; CNS: Management of care; CL: Analysis

CN: Client needs category   CNS: Client needs subcategory   CL: Cognitive level

7. While giving the change of shift report to the oncoming night shift nurse, the evening shift nurse smells alcohol on the night shift nurse's breath. The evening shift nurse should:
1. immediately report this finding to the nursing supervisor.
2. observe the nurse for other signs of intoxication.
3. leave a note for the nurse-manager to read in the morning.
4. ask the nurse if she has been drinking.

8. The nurse is administering medication, and the client states, "I've never seen this pill before." What should the nurse do next?
1. Check the medication orders.
2. Reassure the client that the physician must have ordered it.
3. Teach the client about the effects of the medication.
4. Inform the client that pills often look different because of different brands.

9. What is essential for an informed consent?
1. The client has been informed of the facts, consequences, and implications of the scheduled procedure.
2. The client is told the statistical rate of success.
3. The client is told the names of assisting health care professionals.
4. The client knows the time of the procedure.

My job is to prevent errors.

Caution

7. 1. The evening shift nurse is liable to report a situation that could cause an unsafe situation for clients. She should immediately report the situation to the nursing supervisor. Observing for other signs of intoxication isn't the nurse's responsibility. The situation requires immediate attention; leaving a note is inappropriate. The evening shift nurse should not confront the night shift nurse; the supervisor should.

CN: Safe, effective care environment; CNS: Management of care; CL: Analysis

8. 1. When a client indicates that something is different, check the order before assuming it is a correct medication for that client.

CN: Safe, effective care environment; CNS: Safety and infection control; CL: Application

9. 1. Informed consent involves informing the client of the treatment, tests, surgery, and risks/benefits. It often does not include statistical data. The assisting health care professionals are usually not named in the consent, only the main provider/surgeon. Although the client is often aware of the date and time of the procedure, these can change. What is essential is agreeing to the procedure, regardless of the time. When the professional nurse is involved in the informed consent process, the nurse is only witnessing the consent process and doesn't actually obtain the consent. Only a minor who is married or emancipated can give informed consent. Obtaining consent is the responsibility of the physician. Legally, the client must be mentally competent, regardless of age, to give consent for procedures.

CN: Safe, effective care environment; CNS: Management of care; CL: Application

10. Which statement is correct regarding government requirements about organ donation?
1. All families of clients who have died must be approached about organ donation.
2. The medical examiner should be notified of all potential organ donors.
3. A request must be made to the family regarding release of the donor's name.
4. Clients over the age of 70 are not eligible for organ donation.

11. A client learns she is pregnant and asks the nurse for names of abortion clinics. The nurse does not believe abortion is morally right. What is the nurse's best response?
1. Remind the client that abortion stops a beating heart.
2. Tell the client that she will have to ask the physician.
3. Encourage the client to wait and think about it.
4. Give the client the available preprinted list of clinics.

12. A client has terminal cancer. Which is a correct illustration of the associated grief stage?
1. The client says, "I've lived a good life and am ready to go." This is an example of denial.
2. The client says, "I need a better doctor so he can cure me!" This is an example of bargaining.
3. The client says, "I'm not taking any more chemotherapy because the cancer is resistant." This is an example of depression.
4. The client says, "I can't believe God would do this to me!" This is an example of anger.

10. 1. The federal Omnibus Reconciliation Act of 1986 mandates that all hospitals establish written protocols for the identification of potential organ and tissue donors. The act sets standards for organ procurement agencies. The medical examiner should be notified if the client is a potential organ or tissue donor only if the medical examiner is involved in the case. Requesters for donation are health care professionals who have received special training on properly approaching family members regarding organ or tissue donation. Although certain organs or tissues may not be useable, age is not an automatic disqualification from donation.

CN: Safe, effective care environment; CNS: Management of care; CL: Application

11. 4. Nurses should provide nonjudgmental care. A nurse cannot withhold care based on the nurse's personal religious beliefs. Another option would be to allow a colleague to meet the client's request.

CN: Safe, effective care environment; CNS: Management of care; CL: Analysis

12. 4. Anger, the most intense grief reaction, arises when people realize that death and loss will actually occur or has occurred for a family member. Denial is the avoidance of death's inevitability and is the first step of the grieving process. Bargaining happens when family members attempt to stall or manipulate the outcome or death. Depression is a response to loss that's expressed as profound sadness or deep suffering. Acceptance is the final stage, and it's the ability to overcome the grief and accept what has happened.

CN: Psychosocial integrity; CNS: None; CL: Application

13. While performing an assessment of a 75-year-old client in the emergency department, a nurse notes many ecchymotic areas in various stages of healing on his body. Which action should the nurse perform first?
1. Notify the nursing supervisor.
2. Notify the physician.
3. Obtain information as to how these bruises occurred.
4. Document the findings.

14. The client does not want chemotherapy, but the family says he should take it. What is the best response by the nurse?
1. Ask the client if he has discussed this with his religious advisor.
2. Help the client think about his family and their concerns.
3. Assert the client's right to make the ultimate decision.
4. Share with the client what the nurse would do in that situation.

15. What is the most important action for a nurse to take when caring for a client who had a liver biopsy?
1. Ask about the level of pain.
2. Monitor for rising pulse and falling blood pressure.
3. Assess for feelings about body image.
4. Teach about avoiding alcohol in the future.

13. 3. The nurse should first try to obtain more information from the client to complete the assessment. Without the information, she shouldn't assume that the bruises are from abuse, and she shouldn't notify her nursing supervisor until she has obtained additional facts. She should, however, inform the physician, so he can examine the client. She should follow the facility's policy and procedure for reporting abuse and document her findings.

CN: Psychosocial integrity; CNS: None; CL: Application

14. 3. The nurse who understands the advocacy role promotes, protects, and, thereby, advocates a client's interests and rights in an effort to make the client well. The nurse doesn't make decisions for clients but provides care for the acutely ill client with the consent of his significant other, a power of attorney, or his living will. Standards of care are the basis for providing safe competent nursing care and set minimum criteria for proficiency on the job, enabling the nurse and others to judge the quality of care provided. Paternalism violates self-determination and advocacy by acting for another.

CN: Safe, effective care environment; CNS: Management of care; CL: Application

15. 2. A risk of liver biopsy is internal bleeding, and watching for shock and alteration of circulation is most important (the C in the ABCs). Pain is part of disability (ABCD). Physical needs take priority over psychological needs. Present needs take priority over future needs.

CN: Safe, effective care environment; CNS: Management of care; CL: Application

16. In which circumstance may a nurse legally and ethically disclose confidential information about a client?
1. The human immunodeficiency virus (HIV) status of a single male client to his family members
2. The diagnosis of pancreatic cancer to the client's significant other
3. The diagnosis of an uncontrolled seizure disorder of a taxi driver to a state agency
4. The client is 32 weeks pregnant with twins and is legally separated

There are legal and ethical issues posed in question 16. Which circumstance can the nurse disclose?

17. A competent client in a long-term care facility refuses to take his oral diuretic. The nurse tells him that if the medication isn't taken, restraints will be applied and the medication will be given by injection. The nurse's statement constitutes which legal tort?
1. Assault
2. Battery
3. Negligence
4. Autonomy

The neonate's safety and protection is the first priority.

18. Entering a client's room to get a neonate for an examination by the physician, the nurse on the maternity unit sees the client holding the crying neonate and slapping his face. Which action is most appropriate?
1. Take the neonate to the nursery, tell the physician so he can examine the neonate for injuries, and notify social services.
2. Leave the room without the neonate and notify the nursing supervisor.
3. Confront the client by asking her what she's doing and why.
4. Take the neonate to the nursery and tell coworkers to observe the client for further incidents.

16. 3. The nurse may lawfully disclose confidential information about a client when the welfare of a person is at stake. The physician is required to inform the Department of Motor Vehicles that the taxi driver has an uncontrolled seizure disorder because it's in the best interest of the public's and client's safety. Confidentiality of HIV testing is required, but the client should be encouraged to share the information with others. A positive HIV test can mean the loss of a job, medical insurance, financial security, and even housing because family, friends, and the public may fear the HIV-positive person. Options 2 and 4 don't affect the welfare of a person.

CN: Safe, effective care environment; CNS: Management of care; CL: Application

17. 1. Assault occurs when a person puts another person in fear of harmful or threatening contact. Battery is the actual contact with one's body. If the nurse actually carried out the threat, battery would also apply. Negligence involves actions below the standard of care. Autonomy is an ethical principle of self-determination but does not constitute a legal issue. In this situation, the correct action is to try to calm the client, allow him time to talk, and then determine if he will take the medications. If the client still won't take the medications, the nurse should document his refusal, note the medications, and notify the physician.

CN: Safe, effective care environment; CNS: Management of care; CL: Application

18. 1. The neonate's safety and protection are the first priority. The nurse should immediately take the neonate to the nursery and inform the physician of the abuse. By being the neonate's advocate, the nurse allows the physician to examine him for injuries resulting from the incident. The nurse shouldn't confront the client. Although observing the client for further incidents may be part of the revised care plan, it requires immediate intervention, not simple notification of coworkers.

CN: Psychosocial integrity; CNS: None; CL: Analysis

19. The mother of an infant client appears anxious when the infant cries and says, "I can't handle this." Which strategy should the care plan include early in the client's hospital stay?
1. Anger management therapy
2. Proper care of a crying infant
3. Bedtime rituals to minimize infant crying
4. Overall coping mechanisms

It is important to know who has the power.

20. A male client with a terminal illness is unconscious. His wife wants him to be a full code; his sister who has papers as durable power of attorney for health care says to make him a "DNR" (do not resuscitate). How should the situation be handled legally?
1. Respect the wife's wishes as she is closest to the client.
2. Respect the sister's wishes due to the documentation.
3. Ask the ethicist to mediate between the two individuals.
4. Ask the chaplain to discuss the implications of their decisions.

21. A woman presents to the emergency department with a fractured arm. Her husband is constantly by her side, and the woman appears anxious. What action should the nurse initially take?
1. Escort the woman to the restroom and ask her if she is being abused.
2. Ask the woman during triage if she is in a safe environment.
3. Clarify that all clients are asked about abuse prior to any questions.
4. Provide a written pamphlet about domestic abuse to the woman.

19. 4. Assessment of the client's strengths and weaknesses in her coping mechanisms and the presence of support systems is important. Assessment will also help identify situations that the client perceives as stressors. It hasn't been established that the client is angry, so anger management therapy isn't necessary. Proper care of a crying infant or preventative measures are necessary, but assessing the client's coping will help provide the basis for teaching. Providing education about alternatives to expressing feelings and about crisis hotlines and community support systems should also be part of the care plan.
CN: Psychosocial integrity; CNS: None; CL: Analysis

20. 2. The durable power of attorney for health care that is documented legitimately takes precedent. In fact, it is often recommended not to have the emotionally closest individual in that role because someone else will be more objective. While mediation/discussion can be helpful as the individuals "live with each other" afterward, it is not required by law.
CN: Safe, effective care environment; CNS: Management of care; CL: Application

21. 1. Possible victims should be asked privately about abuse, away from a potential abuser. Similarly, any counseling/resources should be given privately. Clarifying that all clients are asked about abuse prior to any questions is a good idea but is not as essential as privacy. The nurse must carefully and adequately document the assessment of the abused victim. The documentation must include statements from the victim, physical and psychological assessment findings, and observations relative to the abuse situation. The victim should be provided with local community resources, social agencies, and legal services as necessary to prevent recurrence of physical abuse.
CN: Psychosocial integrity; CNS: None; CL: Analysis

22. A client was voluntarily admitted to the inpatient psychiatric admission for anxiety. He is alert, oriented, and denies suicidal ideation. He states that he wants to leave. The most appropriate action by the nurse would be?
  1. Inform the client that he is not able to leave AMA (Against medical advice).
  2. Contact the attending physician.
  3. Determine the current level of anxiety.
  4. Provide discharge instructions.

23. While providing care to a 26-year-old, married, female client, a nurse notes multiple ecchymotic areas on her arms and trunk. The color of the ecchymotic areas ranges from blue to purple to yellow. When asked by the nurse how she got these bruises, the client responds, "Oh, I tripped." How should the nurse respond? Select all that apply.
  1. Document the client's statement and injuries.
  2. Indicate that the bruises do not look characteristic of a one-time fall.
  3. Ask about current administration of antiplatelet medications.
  4. Call the client's husband to discuss the situation.
  5. Notify local authorities of domestic abuse.

22. **2.** The client was a voluntary admission and can leave, but the attending physician should be notified. Options 3 and 4 are important but not as essential.

CN: Psychosocial integrity; CNS: None; CL: Application

23. **1, 2, and 3.** The nurse should objectively document her assessment findings. A detailed description of physical findings of abuse in the medical record is essential if legal action is pursued. The potential causes should be asked about before determining if it is actual abuse. Contacting the client's husband without her consent violates confidentiality. The nurse should respond to the client in a nonthreatening manner that promotes trust rather than ordering her to break off her relationship. Notifying local authorities is not appropriate if domestic abuse is not certain.

CN: Psychosocial integrity; CNS: None; CL: Analysis

You did it! You finished the final chapter! Now, for more fun, try the six comprehensive tests that follow!

Appendices and index

COMPREHENSIVE
Test 1

1. The nurse is assessing a 43-year-old client who sustained blunt chest trauma from a motor vehicle collision. The assessment data include sinus tachycardia, hypotension, and muffled heart sounds. There are no obvious signs of bleeding. The nurse interprets this information as indicating which condition?
1. Heart failure
2. Pneumothorax
3. Cardiac tamponade
4. Myocardial infarction (MI)

2. The nurse is caring for a client experiencing cardiac tamponade. The nurse is aware that the client is at highest risk for developing which type of shock?
1. Anaphylactic shock
2. Cardiogenic shock
3. Hypovolemic shock
4. Septic shock

3. A nurse asks a nursing assistant to help admit an elderly client diagnosed with pneumonia. Delegation by the nurse is considered appropriate when the nursing assistant:
1. obtains the client's height and weight.
2. obtains a wound culture.
3. inserts a small-bore feeding tube.
4. assesses lung sounds.

1. 3. Cardiac tamponade results in signs of obvious shock and muffled heart sounds. Heart failure would result in inspiratory crackles, pulmonary edema, and jugular vein distention. Pneumothorax would result in diminished breath sounds in the affected lung, respiratory distress, and tracheal displacement. In an MI, the client may complain of chest pain. Also, an electrocardiogram could confirm changes consistent with an MI.
CN: Physiological integrity; CNS: Physiological adaptation; CL: Analysis

2. 2. Fluid accumulates in the pericardial sac, hindering motion of the heart muscle and causing it to pump inefficiently, resulting in signs of cardiogenic shock. Anaphylactic shock and septic shock are types of distributive shock in which fluid is displaced from the capillaries and leaks into surrounding tissues. Hypovolemic shock involves the actual loss of fluid.
CN: Physiological integrity; CNS: Physiological adaptation; CL: Application

3. 1. Obtaining the client's height and weight are appropriate actions for the nursing assistant to perform. The client should be assessed before ambulation is attempted. The other options are the responsibility of the registered nurse or other licensed person.
CN: Safe effective care environment; CNS: Management of care; CL: Application

CN: Client needs category   CNS: Client needs subcategory   CL: Cognitive level

4. A client is experiencing cardiac tamponade. The nurse reviews the physician's orders and determines further intervention is not required when the orders include which intervention?
1. Surgery
2. Dopamine
3. Blood transfusion
4. Pericardiocentesis

5. A nurse is teaching a 50-year-old client how to decrease risk factors for coronary artery disease. He's an executive who smokes, has a type A personality, and is hypertensive. The nurse identifies which of the following as the client's nonmodifiable risk factor?
1. Age
2. Hypertension
3. Personality
4. Smoking

6. A client tells the nurse that he is stressed by his job but enjoys the challenge. What is the most appropriate response by the nurse?
1. Switch job positions.
2. Take stress management classes.
3. Spend more time with your family.
4. Avoid working from home.

7. A nurse is teaching a client with glaucoma the proper technique for instilling eye drops. The nurse would instruct the client to instill the drops:
1. on the cornea.
2. in the outer canthus.
3. near the opening of the lacrimal duct.
4. in the lower conjunctival sac.

8. A 28-year-old client with human immunodeficiency virus (HIV) is admitted to the hospital with flulike symptoms, dyspnea, and a cough. He's placed on a 100% nonrebreather mask, and arterial blood gases (ABGs) are drawn. The nurse reviews the results of the ABGs and is most concerned about which finding?
1. Pao_2, 90 mm Hg; $Paco_2$, 40 mm Hg
2. Pao_2, 85 mm Hg; $Paco_2$, 45 mm Hg
3. Pao_2, 80 mm Hg; $Paco_2$, 45 mm Hg
4. Pao_2, 70 mm Hg; $Paco_2$, 55 mm Hg

4. 4. Pericardiocentesis, or needle aspiration of the pericardial cavity, is done to relieve tamponade. An opening is created surgically if the client continues to have recurrent episodes of tamponade. Dopamine is used to restore blood pressure in normovolemic individuals. Blood transfusions may be given if the client is hypovolemic from blood loss.
CN: Physiological integrity; CNS: Physiological adaptation; CL: Application

5. 1. Age is a risk factor that is nonmodifiable. Type A personality, hypertension, and smoking factors can be controlled.
CN: Health promotion and maintenance; CNS: None; CL: Application

6. 2. Stress management classes will teach the client how to better manage the stress in his life, after identifying the factors that contribute to it. Alternatives may be found to leaving his job, which he enjoys. Not spending enough time with his family and taking his job home with him haven't yet been identified as contributing factors.
CN: Physiological integrity; CNS: Reduction of risk potential; CL: Application

7. 4. Eye drops should be placed in the lower conjunctival sac starting at the inner, not outer, canthus. Placing eye drops on the cornea causes discomfort and should be avoided. Eye drops shouldn't be placed by the opening of the lacrimal ducts to avoid systemic absorption.
CN: Physiological integrity; CNS: Pharmacological and parenteral therapies; CL: Application

8. 4. An increasing $Paco_2$ and decreasing Pao_2 indicate poor oxygen perfusion. Normal Pao_2 levels are 80 to 100 mm Hg, and normal $Paco_2$ levels are 35 to 45 mm Hg.
CN: Physiological integrity; CNS: Reduction of risk potential; CL: Analysis

9. The nurse is instructing a client regarding transmission of human immunodeficiency virus (HIV). The nurse instructs the client that the most likely route of virus transmission is:
1. blood.
2. feces.
3. saliva.
4. urine.

10. A client with acquired immunodeficiency syndrome has developed a protozoa infection. Which opportunistic infection will the client most likely develop as a result of the protozoa infection?
1. Tuberculosis (TB)
2. Histoplasmosis
3. Kaposi's sarcoma
4. *Pneumocystis jiroveci* infection

11. The nurse is caring for an intubated client diagnosed with acquired immunodeficiency syndrome. What is the most important intervention by the nurse?
1. Use lubricant on the lips.
2. Provide oral care every 2 hours.
3. Suction the oral cavity every 2 hours.
4. Reposition the endotracheal (ET) tube every 24 hours.

Ten questions done! Are you having fun yet?

12. A client with acquired immunodeficiency syndrome has developed *Pneumocystis carinii* pneumonia and has begun treatment with pentamidine isethionate (Pentam). Based on the diagnosis and treatment, the nurse determines that treatment is appropriate when the physician's order includes which medication?
1. Amphotericin B
2. Co-trimoxazole (Bactrim)
3. Fluconazole (Diflucan)
4. Sulfadiazine

13. A client is receiving pentamidine isethionate (Pentam). What is the most important assessment by the nurse?
1. Heart rate
2. Electrolyte levels
3. Blood sugar levels
4. Complete blood count (CBC)

9. **1.** HIV is transmitted by contact with infected blood. It exists in all body fluids, but transmission through saliva, urine, and feces is much less likely to occur than through blood.
CN: Safe, effective care environment; CNS: Safety and infection control; CL: Application

10. **4.** *P. jiroveci* infection is caused by protozoa. TB is caused by a mycobacterium. Histoplasmosis is a fungal infection. Kaposi's sarcoma is a neoplasm that is associated with human immunodeficiency virus.
CN: Physiological integrity; CNS: Physiological adaptation; CL: Application

11. **4.** Pressure causes skin breakdown. However, repositioning the ET tube from one side of the mouth to the other or to the center of the mouth can relieve pressure in one area for a time. Extreme care must be taken to move the tube only laterally; it must not be pushed in or pulled out. The tape securing the tube must be changed daily. Two nurses should perform this procedure. Oral care, suctioning, and lubricant help keep skin clean and intact and reduce the risk of further infection.
CN: Physiological integrity; CNS: Basic care and comfort; CL: Application

12. **2.** Co-trimoxazole is given orally or I.V. for *P. carinii* pneumonia. Fluconazole and amphotericin B are used for coccidioidomycosis. Sulfadiazine is used to treat toxoplasmosis.
CN: Physiological integrity; CNS: Pharmacological and parenteral therapies; CL: Application

13. **3.** Pentamidine isethionate can cause permanent diabetes mellitus and requires monitoring of blood sugar levels. The client's electrolyte levels, heart rate, and CBC can be monitored less frequently.
CN: Physiological integrity; CNS: Pharmacological and parenteral therapies; CL: Application

14. A nurse caring for a client with acquired immunodeficiency syndrome is working with a nursing student. She notes that the student doesn't attempt to suction or assist with care of the client. What is the most appropriate action by the nurse?
1. Talk to the student regarding her feelings about the client.
2. Talk to the charge nurse about the student's lack of initiative.
3. Address a coworker with the concerns about the student.
4. Seek advice from the student's instructor about the student.

15. A client's significant other is tearful over the client's condition and lack of improvement. He says he feels powerless and unable to help his significant other. What is the most appropriate response by the nurse?
1. Agree with the person.
2. Tell him there's nothing he can do.
3. State she understands how he must feel.
4. Ask if he would like to help with some comfort measures.

16. A 31-year-old client is admitted to the hospital with respiratory failure. He is intubated in the emergency department, placed on 100% FIO_2, and is coughing up copious secretions. What is the most appropriate action by the nurse?
1. Get an X-ray.
2. Suction the client.
3. Restrain the client.
4. Obtain an arterial blood gas (ABG) analysis.

17. The nurse is caring for an intubated client who has copious, brown-tinged secretions. What is the most appropriate intervention by the nurse?
1. Use a trap to obtain a specimen.
2. Instill saline to break up secretions.
3. Culture the specimen with a culturette swab.
4. Obtain an order for a liquefying agent for the sputum.

18. An X-ray shows an endotracheal (ET) tube is 2 cm above the carina, and there are nodular lesions and patchy infiltrates in the upper lobe. How does the nurse interpret this X-ray result?
1. The X-ray is inconclusive.
2. The client has a disease process going on.
3. The ET tube needs to be advanced.
4. The ET tube needs to be pulled back.

14. 1. The nurse should approach the student to determine her feelings and experience in caring for this client. The charge nurse and coworkers aren't familiar with the student's abilities, but the instructor may be approached if the nurse can't communicate with the student.
CN: Safe, effective care environment; CNS: Management of care; CL: Analysis

15. 4. The significant other expresses a need to help, and the nurse can encourage him to do whatever he feels comfortable with, such as putting lubricant on lips, a moist cloth on forehead, or lotion on skin. The nurse may not understand his situation, and agreeing with a person doesn't diminish powerlessness. There are many ways the significant other can help if he wants to.
CN: Psychosocial integrity; CNS: None; CL: Analysis

16. 2. Secretions can cut off the oxygen supply to the client and result in hypoxia so suctioning the client is your first priority. X-rays are a priority to check placement of the endotracheal tube. Restraints are warranted if the client is a threat to his safety. After the client has acclimated to his ventilator settings, ABGs can be drawn.
CN: Physiological integrity; CNS: Reduction of risk potential; CL: Analysis

17. 1. Suspicious secretions should be sent for culture and sensitivity using a sterile technique such as a trap. Saline would dilute the specimen. Swab culturettes are useful for wound cultures, not endotracheal cultures. Various agents are available to help break up secretions, and respiratory therapists can usually help recommend the right agent, but this isn't a priority.
CN: Safe, effective care environment; CNS: Safety and infection control; CL: Analysis

18. 2. The X-ray is suggestive of tuberculosis. At 2 cm, the ET tube is at an adequate level in the trachea and doesn't have to be advanced or pulled back.
CN: Physiological integrity; CNS: Reduction of risk potential; CL: Analysis

CN: Client needs category   CNS: Client needs subcategory   CL: Cognitive level

19. A client has copious secretions. X-ray results indicate tuberculosis (TB). The nurse anticipates that the client will most likely have which procedure ordered?
1. Repeat X-ray
2. Tracheostomy
3. Bronchoscopy
4. Arterial blood gas (ABG) analysis

20. A nurse is aware that family members of a client diagnosed with tuberculosis may have been exposed to the disease. The nurse explains that a tuberculin skin test should be performed on each family member and may indicate:
1. active disease.
2. recent infection.
3. extent of the infection.
4. infection at some point.

21. A client is diagnosed with tuberculosis (TB). In addition to recommending skin testing of the family members, the public health nurse is aware that cases of TB should be reported to which of the following?
1. Centers for Disease Control and Prevention (CDC)
2. Local health department
3. Infection-control nurse
4. Client's physician

22. A client with tuberculosis (TB) is being treated with isoniazid (INH). The nurse anticipates that the client will also be placed on which treatment?
1. Theophylline inhaler
2. I.M. penicillin
3. Multiple antibacterial agents
4. Aerosol treatments with pentamidine (Pentam)

23. A nurse is teaching a client with tuberculosis (TB) about his medication treatment. The client asks the nurse how long medication will be necessary. What is the best response by the nurse?
1. 2 to 4 months
2. 9 to 12 months
3. 18 to 24 months
4. More than 2 years

Looking good! Keep at it!

19. 3. Bronchoscopy can help diagnose TB and obtain specimens while clearing the bronchial tree of secretions. X-rays may be repeated periodically to determine lung and endotracheal tube status. Tracheostomy may be done if the client remains on the ventilator for a prolonged period. A change in condition or treatment may require an ABG analysis.

CN: Physiological integrity; CNS: Reduction of risk potential; CL: Application

20. 4. A tuberculin skin test shows the presence of infection at some point; a positive skin test doesn't guarantee that an infection is currently present, however. Some people have false-positive results. Active disease may be viewed on a chest X-ray. Computed tomography or magnetic resonance imaging can evaluate the extent of lung damage.

CN: Safe, effective care environment; CNS: Safety and infection control; CL: Application

21. 2. The local health department must be informed of an outbreak of TB because it's a reportable disease. They, in turn, inform the CDC. The infection-control nurse or employee health department may request that staff be tested if exposed. Generally, the client's family can inform his physician.

CN: Safe, effective care environment; CNS: Safety and infection control; CL: Application

22. 3. Because TB has become resistant to many antibacterial agents, the initial treatment includes the use of multiple antituberculotic or antibacterial drugs. These may include rifampin, ethambutol hydrochloride, pyrazinamide, cycloserine, clofazimine, and streptomycin. Theophylline is a bronchodilator used to treat asthma and chronic obstructive pulmonary disease. Penicillins are used to treat *Staphylococcus aureus*—not TB. Pentamidine is used in the treatment of pneumonia caused by *Pneumocystis jiroveci*.

CN: Physiological integrity; CNS: Pharmacological and parenteral therapies; CL: Application

23. 2. Treatment for TB is usually continued for at least 9 to 12 months.

CN: Physiological integrity; CNS: Pharmacological and parenteral therapies; CL: Application

24. A nurse is teaching a client with tuberculosis about the disease process and the importance of medication compliance. The client asks the nurse how long he is considered to be infectious after the medication is started. What is the best response by the nurse?
1. 72 hours
2. 1 week
3. 2 weeks
4. 4 weeks

25. A client tells his nurse that his tuberculosis medications are so expensive that he can't afford to take them. What is the most appropriate intervention by the nurse?
1. Refer the client to social services.
2. Tell the client to apply for Medicaid.
3. Refer the client to the local or county health department.
4. Tell the client to follow his insurance rules and regulations.

26. A 62-year-old client is admitted to the hospital with pneumonia. He has a history of Parkinson's disease, which his family says is progressively worsening. Which symptom will the nurse most likely observe when assessing the client?
1. Impaired speech
2. Muscle flaccidity
3. Pleasant and smiling demeanor
4. Tremors in the fingers that increase with purposeful movement

27. Which nursing diagnosis describes a clinical judgment that an individual, family, or community is more vulnerable to developing a certain problem than others in the same or similar situation are?
1. Risk for compromised human dignity
2. Moral distress
3. Stress overload
4. Readiness for enhanced comfort

24. 4. After 4 weeks, the disease is no longer infectious, but the client must continue to take the medication.

CN: Safe, effective care environment; CNS: Safety and infection control; CL: Application

25. 3. The local and county health departments provide treatment and follow-up free of charge for all residents to ensure proper care. Social services can help seek alternative methods of payment and reimbursement but would probably first refer the client to the local and county health departments. Medicaid or medical assistance is another avenue for the client, if he qualifies. Insurance can be an alternative source to help pay for treatment, but the client may not be insured or the policy may not cover prescriptions.

CN: Safe, effective care environment; CNS: Management of care; CL: Analysis

26. 1. In Parkinson's disease, dysarthria, or impaired speech, is due to a disturbance in muscle control. Muscle rigidity results in resistance to passive muscle stretching. The client may have a masklike appearance. Tremors should decrease with purposeful movement and sleep.

CN: Physiological integrity; CNS: Physiological adaptation; CL: Application

27. 1. Risk for compromised human dignity is a risk nursing diagnosis that refers to the vulnerability of a client, family, or community to health problems. Moral distress and stress overload are nursing diagnoses that describe a human response to a health problem being manifested. Readiness for enhanced comfort is a diagnostic statement describing the human response to levels of wellness in an individual, family, or community that have a potential for enhancement to a higher state.

CN: Safe, effective care environment; CNS: Management of care; CL: Analysis

CN: Client needs category   CNS: Client needs subcategory   CL: Cognitive level

28. A client is ordered to receive 1,000 ml of 0.45% normal saline with 20 mEq of potassium chloride (KCl) over 6 hours. The infusion set administers 15 gtt/ml. At how many gtt/minute should the nurse set the flow rate?
1. 36
2. 40
3. 42
4. 45

29. The nurse is caring for an 82-year-old male client with Parkinson's disease who is frequently incontinent of urine. What is the most appropriate intervention by the nurse?
1. Diaper the client.
2. Apply a condom catheter.
3. Insert an indwelling urinary catheter.
4. Provide skin care every 4 hours.

30. Family members report exhaustion and difficulty taking care of a dependent family member. What is the most appropriate action by the nurse?
1. Ask the client what he wishes.
2. Have the family members discuss it among themselves.
3. Tell the family the client should go to a nursing care facility.
4. Call a family conference and ask social services for assistance.

31. The nurse is assessing a 30-year-old primigravida in her second trimester who has a history of rheumatic fever. The client tells the nurse that her fingers feel tight and sometimes she feels as though her heart skips a beat. The nurse is most concerned when the client has which assessment finding?
1. Clear lungs
2. Sinus tachycardia
3. Increased dyspnea on exertion
4. Runs of paroxysmal atrial tachycardia

28. 3. The flow rate is determined by the rate of infusion and the number of drops per milliliters of the fluid being administered:
gtt/ml × amount to be infused divided by the number of minutes = the I.V. flow rate
15 gtt/ml × 1,000 ml = 15,000
15,000 ml ÷ 360 minutes = 41.6 gtt/minute
Therefore, the flow rate should be 42 gtt/minute.
CN: Physiological integrity; CNS: Pharmacological and parenteral therapy; CL: Application

29. 2. A condom catheter uses a condom-type device to drain urine away from the client. Diapering the client may keep urine away from the body but may also be demeaning if the client is alert or the family objects. Because the client with Parkinson's disease is already prone to urinary tract infections, an indwelling urinary catheter should be avoided because it may promote this. Skin care must be provided as soon as the client is incontinent to prevent skin maceration and breakdown.
CN: Physiological integrity; CNS: Basic care and comfort; CL: Analysis

30. 4. A family conference with social services can enlighten the family to all prospects of care available to them. The client should supply input if he's able, but this may not help solve the problems of exhaustion and care difficulties. The family may not be aware of alternative care measures for the client, so a discussion among themselves may not be helpful. The client may not qualify for a nursing care facility because of stringent criteria.
CN: Safe, effective care environment; CNS: Management of care; CL: Analysis

31. 3. Increasing dyspnea on exertion should alert the nurse to cardiovascular compromise. Cardiac arrhythmias (other than sinus tachycardia or paroxysmal atrial tachycardia) and persistent crackles at the bases are also symptoms of cardiovascular disease.
CN: Health promotion and maintenance; CNS: None; CL: Analysis

32. The nurse is caring for a pregnant client who is suspected of having cardiovascular disease. Select the diagnostic test that may be performed to determine the extent of cardiovascular disease during pregnancy.
1. Stress test
2. Chest X-ray
3. Echocardiography
4. Cardiac catheterization

33. A 25-year-old primigravida has been in labor for 20 hours with little progress. The doctor prescribes oxytocin for her. The order reads 10 U oxytocin in 1,000 ml/NSS to infuse via pump at 1 mU/minute for 15 minutes; then increase flow rate to 2 mU/minute. What's the flow rate needed to deliver 1 mU/minute for 15 minutes?
1. 4 ml/hr
2. 6 ml/hr
3. 12 ml/hr
4. 16 ml/hr

34. Which statement by the nurse most accurately reflects subjective data in a nursing assessment?
1. "The client's red blood cell count is elevated."
2. "The client has a positive Babinski sign."
3. "The client's X-ray result showed a fracture present."
4. "The client reported that his pain is a 7 on a 1 to 10 scale."

35. The nurse is caring for a pregnant client who is suspected of having cardiovascular disease. The nurse is aware that which classification of medication may be used safely in a pregnant client with cardiovascular disease?
1. Antibiotics
2. Warfarin (Coumadin)
3. Cardiac glycosides
4. Diuretics

You're doing great! Keep up the good work!

32. 3. Echocardiography is less invasive than X-rays and other methods and provides the information needed to determine cardiovascular disease, especially valvular disorders. Cardiac catheterization and stress tests may be postponed until after delivery.
CN: Physiological integrity; CNS: Physiological adaptation; CL: Analysis

33. 2. First, determine the concentration of the solution with 10 U/1,000 ml as the known factor and X as the unknown factor:

$$\frac{10\ U}{1,000\ ml} = \frac{X}{1\ ml} \quad X = .01\ U/ml$$

Then, cross-multiply and solve for X. Next, convert to mU by multiplying by 1,000.

$$0.01 \times 1,000 = 10\ mU/ml$$

Determine flow rate using the following equation:

$$\frac{10\ mU}{1\ ml} = \frac{15\ mU}{X} \quad X = \frac{15\ ml}{10} = 1.5\ ml$$

Convert to an hourly rate by multiplying by 4 (60 minutes/15 minutes = 4):

$$1.5\ ml/15\ minutes \times 4 = 6\ ml/hr$$

CN: Physiological integrity; CNS: Pharmacological and parenteral therapies; CL: Application

34. 4. Subjective data, also known as *symptoms* or *covert cues*, include the client's own verbatim statements about the health problems. Laboratory study results, physical assessment data, and diagnostic procedure reports are observable, perceptible, and measurable and can be verified and validated by others.
CN: Safe, effective care environment; CNS: Management of care; CL: Application

35. 3. Cardiac glycosides and common antiarrhythmics, such as procainamide (Procanbid) and quinidine (Quinaglute), may be used. Prophylactic antibiotics are reserved for clients susceptible to endocarditis. If anticoagulants are needed, heparin is the drug of choice—not warfarin. Diuretics should be used with extreme caution, if at all, because of the potential for causing uterine contractions.
CN: Physiological integrity; CNS: Pharmacological and parenteral therapies; CL: Analysis

36. A client arrives at the emergency department in her third trimester with painless vaginal bleeding. Based on the assessment data, the nurse suspects that the client is experiencing which of the following?
1. Placenta previa
2. Preterm labor
3. Abruptio placentae
4. A sexually transmitted infection (STI)

37. The nurse is caring for a client who has been admitted with suspected placenta previa. After assessing vital signs and applying an external monitor, what is the most important action by the nurse?
1. Insert an indwelling urinary catheter.
2. Plan for an immediate cesarean delivery.
3. Place the client in Trendelenburg position.
4. Obtain blood work and start I.V. catheters.

38. A pregnant client with vaginal bleeding asks a nurse how the fetus is doing. What is the most appropriate response by the nurse?
1. "I don't know for sure."
2. "I can't answer that question."
3. "It's too early to tell anything."
4. "Here's what the monitor shows."

39. A client is hospitalized at 35 weeks' gestation with placenta previa and placed on strict bedrest. She states, "I lost my last baby at 24 weeks." What is the priority nursing diagnosis?
1. Risk for constipation related to immobility
2. Anxiety related to unknown fetal outcome
3. Impaired physical mobility related to bedrest
4. Ineffective coping related to inappropriate thinking

40. A neonate requires blood transfusions after birth. Which cannulation site is most appropriate for the nurse to select?
1. Scalp veins
2. Intraosseous
3. Umbilical cord
4. Subclavian cutdown

41. A nurse working in the triage area of an emergency department sees that several pediatric clients arrive simultaneously. Which client should be treated first?
1. A crying 4-year-old child with a laceration on his scalp
2. A 3-year-old child with a barking cough and flushed appearance
3. A 3-year-old child with Down syndrome who's pale and asleep
4. A 2-year-old child with stridorous breath sounds, sitting up and drooling

36. **1.** Placenta previa presents with painless vaginal bleeding. Abruptio placentae usually includes vague abdominal discomfort and tenderness. Preterm labor and STIs usually don't cause bleeding.
CN: Health promotion and maintenance; CNS: None; CL: Analysis

37. **4.** Blood for hemoglobin, hematocrit, type, and crossmatch should be collected and I.V. catheters inserted. The nurse shouldn't attempt Trendelenburg positioning or urinary catheterization. The client may be placed on her left side. Depending on the degree of bleeding and fetal maturity, a cesarean delivery may be required.
CN: Physiological integrity; CNS: Reduction of risk potential; CL: Application

38. **4.** The client deserves a truthful answer, and the nurse should be objective without giving opinions. Vague answers may be misleading and aren't therapeutic.
CN: Psychosocial integrity; CNS: None; CL: Analysis

39. **2.** The client's statement reflects concern for her fetus. Therefore the priority diagnosis is anxiety related to unknown fetal outcome. The client may be at risk for constipation and mobility is impaired, but these aren't the priority. There's no indication of a disturbed thought process.
CN: Safe, effective care environment; CNS: Management of care; CL: Analysis

40. **3.** The umbilical cord may be easily cannulated and is the preferred site. Scalp veins may also be used. Intraosseous cannulation is attempted if two attempts at other sites prove inaccessible. A subclavian cutdown takes a prolonged time and is the least desired.
CN: Health promotion and maintenance; CNS: None; CL: Analysis

41. **4.** The child with the airway emergency should be treated first because of the risk of epiglottitis. The 3-year-old with the barking cough and fever should be suspected of having croup and should be seen promptly, as should the child with the laceration. The nurse would need to gather information about the child with Down syndrome to determine the priority of care.
CN: Safe, effective care environment; CNS: Management of care; CL: Analysis

42. The nurse is assessing a 2-year-old child in the emergency department for epiglottitis. Which assessment finding would the nurse expect to document?
1. Mild fever
2. Clear speech
3. Tripod position
4. Gradual onset of symptoms

43. The nurse needs to auscultate a 2-year old breath sounds. Which method of approaching the child is most appropriate?
1. Tell the child it's time to listen to his lungs now.
2. Tell the child to lie down while the nurse listens to his lungs.
3. Ask the caregiver to wait outside while the nurse listens to his lungs.
4. Ask the child if he would like the nurse to listen to the front or the back of his chest first.

44. A mother says that her 2-year-old child is up to date with his immunizations. The nurse can most accurately determine that the client is up to date with his immunizations if they include which of the following?
1. Diphtheria-pertussis-tetanus (DTaP), inactivated polio (IPV), measles-mumps-rubella (MMR)
2. DTaP, IPV, MMR, *Haemophilus influenza* type B (Hib), varicella, pneumococcal, hepatitis B, rotavirus (Rota)
3. DTaP, hepatitis B, IPV
4. MMR, IPV, hepatitis B

45. The nurse is caring for a child with epiglottitis. The child is at greatest risk of develop which condition?
1. Airway obstruction
2. Dehydration
3. Malnutrition
4. Seizures

46. A client has been diagnosed with epiglottitis. The nurse recognizes that the client was diagnosed based on which of the following?
1. Lateral neck X-ray
2. Direct visualization
3. History of sudden onset
4. Presenting signs and symptoms

You're more than halfway; the rest should be a snap!

SNAP

42. 3. The tripod position (sitting up and leaning forward) facilitates breathing. Epiglottitis presents with a sudden onset of symptoms, high fever, and muffled speech. Additional symptoms are inspiratory stridor and drooling.

CN: Physiological integrity; CNS: Physiological adaptation; CL: Application

43. 4. The 2-year-old child needs to feel in control, and this approach best supports the child's independence. Giving the child no choice may make him uncooperative. The child should be allowed to remain in the tripod position to facilitate breathing. The caregiver should be allowed to remain with the child because fear of separation is common in 2-year-old children.

CN: Health promotion and maintenance; CNS: None; CL: Application

44. 2. By the age of 2 years, the DTaP, IPV, MMR, Hib, varicella, pneumococcal, hepatitis B, and rotavirus vaccines should have been received. The nurse should clarify this with the mother or caregiver.

CN: Safe, effective care environment; CNS: Safety and infection control; CL: Application

45. 1. The biggest threat to the child is airway obstruction because of the inflammation and swelling of the epiglottis and surrounding tissue. Dehydration can be prevented with I.V. therapy and seizures averted by decreasing the fever. Malnutrition is least likely to occur because epiglottitis is a short-lived situation.

CN: Physiological integrity; CNS: Reduction of risk potential; CL: Application

46. 4. The presenting symptoms are diagnostic of epiglottitis. Lateral neck X-rays aren't necessary. Only an anesthesiologist or physician skilled in intubation should do direct visualization. History of sudden onset helps support the assessment, but a history alone wouldn't be sufficient to make a diagnosis.

CN: Health promotion and maintenance; CNS: None; CL: Application

47. A student nurse working with a registered nurse is assessing a child with epiglottitis. The student tells the client she needs to look at his throat. Which intervention by the registered nurse is most appropriate?
1. Hand her a flashlight and tongue blade.
2. Give her a sterile tongue blade and culturette swab.
3. Tell the student that the registered nurse will visualize the child's throat.
4. Tell the student that visualization will be done by the anesthesiologist.

48. The mother of a 2-year-old child with epiglottitis says she needs to pick up her older child from school. The 2-year-old child begins to cry and appears more stridorous. What is the priority action by the nurse?
1. Ask the mother how long she may be gone.
2. Tell the 2-year-old child everything will be all right.
3. Tell the 2-year-old child the nurse will stay with him.
4. Ask the mother if there's anyone else who can meet the older child.

49. A father arrives in a busy emergency department and is upset with his wife for bringing their 2-year-old child with epiglottitis in for treatment. Which intervention by the nurse is most appropriate?
1. Leave the room while the couple talks together.
2. Call for security since the husband is becoming upset.
3. Recognize the father's behavior as his attempt to cope with the situation.
4. Tell both parents to leave because they're upsetting the child.

50. A 40-year-old client is being treated for GI bleeding. On his fifth day of hospitalization, he begins to have tremors, is agitated, and is experiencing hallucinations. The nurse is aware that these symptoms may indicate which condition?
1. Alcohol withdrawal
2. Allergic response
3. Alzheimer's disease
4. Hypoxia

51. A nurse suspects a client is experiencing alcohol withdrawal syndrome. What is the priority action by the nurse?
1. Verify it with family.
2. Inform social services.
3. Ask the client about his drinking.
4. Tell the client everything will be all right.

47. 4. Direct visualization of the epiglottis can trigger a complete airway obstruction and should only be done in a controlled environment by an anesthesiologist or a physician skilled in pediatric intubation.
CN: Safe, effective care environment; CNS: Management of care; CL: Application

48. 4. Increased anxiety and agitation should be avoided in the child to prevent airway obstruction. A 2-year-old child fears separation from parents, so the mother should be encouraged to stay. Other means of picking up the older child need to be found. Telling the child that everything will be all right may not decrease his agitation; the mother is the primary caregiver and important to the child for emotional and security reasons.
CN: Health promotion and maintenance; CNS: None; CL: Analysis

49. 3. Lack of control over his son's situation results in irrational behavior. The nurse should try to calm both parents and let them know they did the right thing due to the seriousness of their child's situation. Calling for security, sending the parents out, or leaving the room won't help the child nor will it reduce frustration or inappropriate behavior.
CN: Safe, effective care environment; CNS: Management of care; CL: Analysis

50. 1. These are signs of alcohol withdrawal syndrome, which can begin 5 to 7 days after the last drink. An allergic reaction would cause difficulty breathing, skin rash, or edema as primary symptoms. Alzheimer's disease occurs in older individuals and has other psychosocial signs, such as a masklike face and altered mentation. Hypoxia would cause symptoms of respiratory distress.
CN: Psychosocial integrity; CNS: None; CL: Analysis

51. 3. Confirming suspicions with the client is the most beneficial way to help in diagnosis and treatment. If the client isn't cooperative, verification can be sought from the family. Social services aren't required at this time but may be helpful in discharge planning. Giving false reassurance isn't therapeutic for the client.
CN: Psychosocial integrity; CNS: None; CL: Application

52. A client experiencing alcohol withdrawal syndrome says he sees cockroaches on the ceiling. What is the most appropriate response by the nurse?
1. Ask the client where he sees them.
2. Ask the client if the cockroaches are still there.
3. Tell the client there are no cockroaches on the ceiling.
4. Tell the client it's dim in the room and turn on the overhead lights.

53. A client experiencing alcohol withdrawal syndrome says he's itching everywhere from the bugs on his bed. What is the most appropriate action by the nurse?
1. Examine the client's skin.
2. Ask what kind of bugs he thinks they are.
3. Tell the client there are no bugs on his bed.
4. Tell the client he's having tactile hallucinations.

54. A client with alcohol withdrawal syndrome is pulling at his central venous catheter, saying he's swatting the spiders crawling over him. What is the priority action by the nurse?
1. Encourage the client to rest.
2. Protect the client from harm.
3. Tell the client there are no spiders.
4. Tell the client he's pulling the I.V. tubing.

55. A client who experienced alcohol withdrawal syndrome is no longer having hallucinations or tremors and says he would like to enter a rehabilitation facility to stop drinking. What is the most appropriate intervention by the nurse?
1. Ask about his insurance.
2. Tell him he should talk with his family.
3. Refer him to Alcoholics Anonymous (AA).
4. Promote participation in a treatment program.

56. A 72-year-old man with cirrhosis is admitted to the hospital in a hepatic coma. What is the most important nursing intervention?
1. Perform a neurological check.
2. Complete the client admission.
3. Orient the client to his environment.
4. Check airway, breathing, and circulation.

Only 20 more to go. You can do it, I know you can!

52. 4. Try to reorient the client to reality and minimize distortions. Don't support the client's hallucinations or place the client on the defensive, but try to present reality gently without agitating the client.
CN: Psychosocial integrity; CNS: None; CL: Application

53. 1. Make sure the client doesn't have a rash, skin allergy, or something on his skin (such as crumbs) causing his discomfort. Reality should then be presented to the client gently without being derogatory. The nurse shouldn't support the client's hallucinations.
CN: Psychosocial integrity; CNS: None; CL: Application

54. 2. During periods of alcohol withdrawal syndrome, the client needs to be protected from harm. If the client dislodges the central venous catheter, he may incur an air embolus, which can be life threatening. Although reality should be presented to the client, telling him that there are no spiders and that he's pulling the I.V. tubing may not make him stop; therefore, his safety is still at risk. The client may need to be restrained if continued observation during this time isn't available. The client should also be encouraged to rest; however, this intervention doesn't take priority over safety.
CN: Psychosocial integrity; CNS: None; CL: Analysis

55. 4. The client should be encouraged to enter a facility if that's in his best interest. Arrangements that are covered by his insurance can be made and discussed with the social service coordinator and his physician. The client can inform his family, and support should be encouraged. Referral to AA should be considered after rehabilitation takes place.
CN: Psychosocial integrity; CNS: None; CL: Application

56. 4. Priorities include airway, breathing, and circulation. Once these are ensured, a neurological check is needed to determine status. General orientation and completing the admission may require the help and affirmation of family members. Depending on the client's alertness, orientation to the environment may need to be kept simple (where he is, date, time).
CN: Physiological integrity; CNS: Reduction of risk potential; CL: Application

57. A client with cirrhosis is restless and at times tries to climb out of bed. What is the most appropriate intervention by the nurse?
1. Obtain a physician's order to use leather restraints.
2. Obtain a physician's order to use soft wrist restraints.
3. Obtain a physician's order to use a vest restraint device.
4. Obtain a physician's order to use a sheet tied across the client's chest.

58. The nurse is assessing a client with cirrhosis. Which assessment finding would be most indicative of late-stage cirrhosis?
1. Constipation
2. Diarrhea
3. Hypoxia
4. Vomiting

59. A client with cirrhosis is jaundiced and edematous. He's experiencing severe itching and dryness and asks the nurse if anything can be done for his skin. What is the best intervention by the nurse?
1. Put mitts on his hands.
2. Use alcohol-free body lotion.
3. Lubricate the skin with baby oil.
4. Wash the skin with soap and water.

60. The nurse is writing a plan of care for a 20-year-old client who sustained a spinal cord injury and is frequently hospitalized for kidney stones. What is the most appropriate intervention for the nurse to include in the plan?
1. Eat yogurt daily.
2. Drink cranberry juice.
3. Eat more fresh fruits and vegetables.
4. Increase the intake of dairy products.

61. A client with a spinal cord injury tells the nurse that he has difficulty recognizing the symptoms of urinary tract infection (UTI) before it's too late. The nurse explains to the client that an early symptom of UTI is:
1. lower back pain.
2. burning on urination.
3. frequency of urination.
4. fever and change in the clarity of urine.

57. 3. The client may require gentle reminders not to get out of bed to prevent a fall. The vest restraint would help in this endeavor. Leather restraints are only warranted for extremely combative and unsafe clients. Soft wrist restraints may not stop the client from sitting up or trying to swing his legs over the bed rails. A sheet tied across the client's chest can hamper breathing or may asphyxiate the client if he slides down in the bed.
CN: Safe, effective care environment; CNS: Management of care; CL: Analysis

58. 3. In late-stage cirrhosis, fluid in the lungs and weak chest expansion can lead to hypoxia. Diarrhea, vomiting, and constipation are early signs and symptoms of cirrhosis.
CN: Physiological integrity; CNS: Physiological adaptation; CL: Application

59. 2. Alcohol-free body lotion applied to the skin can help relieve dryness and is absorbed without oiliness. Mitts may help keep the client from scratching his skin open. Soap dries out the skin. Baby oil doesn't allow excretions through the skin and may block pores.
CN: Physiological integrity; CNS: Basic care and comfort; CL: Application

60. 2. Acid urine decreases the potential for kidney stones. The majority of renal calculi form in alkaline urine. Cranberries, prunes, and plums promote acidic urine. Yogurt helps restore pH balance to secretions in yeast infections. Fruits and vegetables increase fiber in the diet and promote alkaline urine. Dairy products may contribute to the formation of kidney stones.
CN: Physiological integrity; CNS: Reduction of risk potential; CL: Application

61. 4. The client with a spinal cord injury should recognize fever and change in the clarity of urine as early signs of UTI. Lower back pain is a late sign. The client with a spinal cord injury may not have burning or frequency of urination.
CN: Physiological integrity; CNS: Reduction of risk potential; CL: Application

62. A client tells a nurse he boils his urinary catheters to keep them sterile. What is the most appropriate question for the nurse to ask the client?
1. "What technique is used for catheterization?"
2. "At what temperature are the catheters boiled?"
3. "Why aren't prepackaged sterile catheters used?"
4. "Are the catheters dried and stored in a clean, dry place?"

63. A 60-year-old client had a colostomy 4 days ago due to rectal cancer and is having trouble adjusting to it. Which nursing diagnosis is most appropriate for this client?
1. Anxiety
2. Situational low self-esteem
3. Impaired comfort
4. Disturbed body image

64. A nurse approaches a client with a recent colostomy for a routine assessment and finds him tearful. What is the most appropriate intervention by the nurse?
1. State she'll come back another time.
2. Ask the client if he's having pain or discomfort.
3. Tell the client she needs to perform an assessment.
4. Sit down with the client and ask if he'd like to talk about anything.

65. After a review of colostomy care, a client tells the nurse he doesn't know if he'll be able to care for himself at home without help. What is the most appropriate intervention by the nurse?
1. Review care with the client again.
2. Provide written instructions for the client.
3. Ask the client if there's anyone who can help.
4. Arrange for home health care to visit the client.

66. A client is experiencing mild diarrhea through his colostomy. What is the most appropriate instruction to give the client?
1. Eat prunes.
2. Drink apple juice.
3. Increase lettuce intake.
4. Increase intake of bananas.

You're almost finished. Keep pluggin' away!

62. 1. The client should describe his procedure to make sure aseptic technique is used. Water boils at 212° F (100° C), but the nurse should make sure the client is boiling the catheters for an appropriate amount of time. Catheters should be boiled just before use and allowed to cool before using. Prepackaged sterile catheters aren't necessary if the proper sterilization techniques are used.
CN: Physiological integrity; CNS: Reduction of risk potential; CL: Analysis

63. 4. Disturbed body image is most common with a new colostomy and dealing with its care. The client shouldn't have signs of anxiety, but he may not be comfortable caring for the colostomy. Low self-esteem may also be a concern for the client but may not be as common as disturbed body image. The client should be having less discomfort postoperatively.
CN: Safe, effective care environment; CNS: Management of care; CL: Application

64. 4. Asking open-ended questions and appearing interested in what the client has to say will encourage verbalization of feelings. Leaving the client may make him feel unaccepted. Asking closed-ended questions won't encourage verbalization of feelings. Ignoring the client's present state isn't therapeutic for the client.
CN: Psychosocial integrity; CNS: None; CL: Application

65. 4. Although all of these interventions may benefit the client, arranging for home health care will best ensure continuity of care.
CN: Safe, effective care environment; CNS: Management of care; CL: Application

66. 4. Bananas help make formed stool and aren't irritating to the bowel. Apple juice and prunes can increase the frequency of diarrhea. Lettuce acts as a fiber and can increase the looseness of stools.
CN: Physiological integrity; CNS: Basic care and comfort; CL: Application

67. A client reports a lot of gas in his colostomy bag. What is the best intervention by the nurse?
1. Burp the bag.
2. Replace the bag.
3. Put a tiny hole in the top of the bag.
4. Tell the client to eat less beans.

67. 1. Letting air out of the bag by opening it and burping it is the best solution. Replacing the bag is costly. Putting a hole in the bag will also cause fluids to leak out. The client can be encouraged to note which foods are causing gas and to eat less gas-forming foods.
CN: Physiological integrity; CNS: Basic care and comfort; CL: Application

68. A client at a routine blood glucose screening for diabetes mellitus tells a nurse he has excessive urination and excessive thirst. The priority question by the nurse would address which of the following?
1. Weakness
2. Weight loss
3. Vision changes
4. Excessive hunger

68. 4. Polyuria, polydipsia, and polyphagia are the three hallmark signs of diabetes mellitus. Weight loss, weakness, and vision changes also occur with diabetes mellitus.
CN: Health promotion and maintenance; CNS: None; CL: Application

69. A client recently diagnosed with prediabetes asks the nurse about the risk factors for developing diabetes mellitus. The nurse is aware that the client's greatest risk factor is which of the following?
1. Obesity
2. Japanese descent
3. A great-grandparent with diabetes mellitus
4. Delivery of a neonate weighing more than 10 lb

69. 1. Obesity is a risk factor associated with diabetes mellitus. Delivery of a neonate weighing more than 9 lb, a family history of diabetes mellitus (mother, father, or sibling), and those of Native American, Black, Asian, or Hispanic descent are at high risk for developing diabetes mellitus, but obesity puts the client at greatest risk.
CN: Health promotion and maintenance; CNS: None; CL: Analysis

70. A 52-year-old client who had gastric bypass surgery is nothing by mouth (NPO) status and is in pain. The nurse administers meperidine (Demerol) 75 mg I.M. as ordered. The client complains of nausea 20 minutes after the injection. The nurse recognizes that the nausea is most likely the result of which factor?
1. The surgery itself
2. The client's NPO status
3. The meperidine that was given for his pain
4. Blood remaining in his mouth after extubation

Five more to go! Oooooh, I'm getting excited!

70. 3. Although gastric bypass surgery may precipitate some feelings of nausea, the timing of this symptom after the administration of meperidine is suspicious. Most likely, this client is experiencing a very common adverse effect of the analgesic meperidine. The status of being NPO wouldn't cause an increase in gastric secretions. It's possible that there may be some blood in his mouth after extubation, but the chances of this happening are minimal and less likely to be the cause of the client's complaint.
CN: Physiological integrity; CNS: Pharmacological and parenteral therapies; CL: Analysis

71. A client asks the nurse what complications can occur from diabetes mellitus. What is the best response by the nurse?
1. Multiple sclerosis
2. Diabetic ketoacidosis
3. Cardiovascular disease
4. Hyperosmolar hyperglycemic nonketotic syndrome (HHNS)

71. 3. Cardiovascular disease is a common chronic complication of diabetes mellitus. There's no known relationship between multiple sclerosis and diabetes mellitus. Diabetic ketoacidosis and HHNS are acute complications that can occur.
CN: Health promotion and maintenance; CNS: None; CL: Application

72. A client with a family history of diabetes mellitus asks the nurse how he might decrease his risk factors. What is the best response by the nurse?
1. "Eat only poultry and fish."
2. "Omit carbohydrates from your diet."
3. "Start a moderate exercise program."
4. "Check blood glucose levels every month."

73. The nurse is assessing a client's arterial pulses. Which graphic displays the appropriate site for palpating the dorsalis pedis pulse?

1.

2.

3.

4.

72. 3. Exercise and weight control are the goals in preventing and treating diabetes mellitus. Red meat can be eaten but should be limited because it contributes to cardiovascular disease. Complex carbohydrates account for a large portion of the diabetic diet and shouldn't be omitted. Checking blood glucose levels will help monitor the development of diabetes mellitus but won't prevent or decrease the chance of it occurring.
CN: Physiological integrity; CNS: Reduction of risk potential; CL: Application

73. 4. To palpate the dorsalis pedis pulse, the nurse places her fingers on the medial dorsum of the foot while the client points his toes down. The first graphic shows palpation of the brachial pulse. This pulse is palpated with the fingers placed medial to the biceps tendon. The second graphic shows palpation of the popliteal pulse in the popliteal fossa of the back of the knee. The third graphic shows palpation of the posterior tibial pulse, slightly below the malleolus of the ankle.
CN: Health promotion and maintenance; CNS: None; CL: Application

74. A nurse is having lunch in the hospital cafeteria when a visitor sitting at the next table begins to choke on his food. According to the American Heart Association (AHA), the nurse should intervene using the actions listed below. List the actions in the sequence in which she should perform them.

> 1. Administer abdominal thrusts until effective or until the client becomes unresponsive.

> 2. Activate the emergency response team.

> 3. Ask the client if he can speak.

> 4. Start cardiopulmonary resuscitation (CPR).

74.

> 3. Ask the client if he can speak.

> 1. Administer abdominal thrusts until effective or until the client becomes unresponsive.

> 2. Activate the emergency response team.

> 4. Start cardiopulmonary resuscitation (CPR).

According to the AHA, the nurse should ask the client if he's choking and if he can speak. Next, she should administer abdominal thrusts or chest thrusts (if the client is obese or pregnant). She should continue thrusts until they're effective or until the client becomes unresponsive, at which time she should activate the emergency response team and begin to administer CPR.

CN: Physiological integrity; CNS: Physiological adaptation; CL: Application

75. A nurse is performing a cardiac assessment on a client with a suspected murmur. Identify the area where the nurse should place the stethoscope to auscultate the area referred to as Erb's point.

75. Erb's point is located at the third left intercostal space, close to the sternum. Murmurs of both aortic and pulmonic origin may be heard at Erb's point.

CN: Health promotion and maintenance; CNS: None; CL: Application

What a performance! For your first comprehensive test, that was outstanding. Congratulations!

COMPREHENSIVE
Test 2

1. A newly hired graduate nurse (GN) is helping the charge nurse admit a client. The charge nurse wants to ensure that the GN understands the facility's rules of ethical conduct. Which statement by the GN indicates the need for further teaching by the charge nurse?
1. "I will make sure that I do everything in my client's best interest."
2. "I will maintain client confidentiality always."
3. "I'll support the Client's Bill of Rights."
4. "I won't discuss advance directives unless the client initiates the conversation."

2. A nurse suspects that an infant may have transposition of the great vessels (TGV) based on her assessment findings. Which diagnostic test would be performed first to detect this problem?
1. Blood cultures
2. Cardiac catheterization
3. Chest X-ray
4. Echocardiogram

3. Four 6-month-old children arrive at the clinic for diphtheria-pertussis-tetanus (DTaP) immunization. Which child can safely receive the immunization at this time?
1. The child with a temperature of 103° F (39.4° C)
2. The child with a runny nose
3. The child with uncontrolled epilepsy
4. The child with difficulty breathing after the last immunization

4. A nurse is giving discharge instructions to parents of a child who had a tonsillectomy. Which instruction would be most important to include?
1. The child should drink extra milk.
2. The child shouldn't drink from straws.
3. Orange juice should be given to provide pain control.
4. The child's mouth should be rinsed with salt water to provide pain relief.

1. 4. The law mandates that health care agencies ask all clients if they have an advance directive. Therefore, the nurse must address this question regardless of whether the client initiates a conversation about it. Nurses always need to act in the best interest of their clients, maintain confidentiality, and support the Client's Bill of Rights.
CN: Safe, effective care environment; CNS: Management of care; CL: Analysis

2. 3. Chest X-ray would be done first to visualize congenital heart diseases such as TGV. Blood cultures won't diagnose TGV. Cardiac catheterization and an echocardiogram would be done but would not be the initial diagnostic intervention.
CN: Health promotion and maintenance; CNS: None; CL: Application

3. 2. Children with mild acute illness without fever can safely receive DTaP immunization. Children with a temperature of more than 102° F (38.9° C), uncontrolled epilepsy, or serious reactions to previous immunizations shouldn't receive DTaP immunization.
CN: Health promotion and maintenance; CNS: None; CL: Analysis

4. 2. Straws and other sharp objects inserted into the mouth could disrupt the clot at the operative site. Extra milk wouldn't promote healing and may encourage mucus production. Drinking orange juice and rinsing with salt water will irritate the tissue at the operative site.
CN: Physiological adaptation; CNS: Reduction of risk potential; CL: Application

CN: Client needs category   CNS: Client needs subcategory   CL: Cognitive level

5. A 2-year-old child is diagnosed with bronchiolitis caused by respiratory syncytial virus (RSV). The child's family also includes an 8-year-old child. Which statement is correct?
1. RSV isn't highly communicable in infants and toddlers.
2. RSV isn't communicable to older children and adults.
3. The 2-year-old client must be admitted to the hospital for isolation.
4. The children should be separated to prevent the spread of the infection.

6. A child with asthma uses a peak expiratory flowmeter in school. The results indicate his peak flow is in the yellow zone. Which intervention by the school nurse is appropriate?
1. Follow the child's routine asthma treatment plan.
2. Monitor the child for signs and symptoms of an acute attack.
3. Call 911 and prepare for transport to the nearest emergency department.
4. Call the child's mother to take the child to the family physician immediately.

7. Parents of a child with asthma are trying to identify possible allergens in their household. Which inhaled allergen is the most common?
1. Perfume
2. Dust mites
3. Passive smoke
4. Dog or cat dander

8. The nurse is devising a meal plan for a child newly diagnosed with celiac disease. Which menu choices best meets the child's needs?
1. Hamburger with chips and chocolate milk
2. Cheese pizza with a fruit cup
3. Chicken nuggets, fries, and a soda
4. Spaghetti with meat sauce and a brownie

9. A client is undergoing a thoracentesis at the bedside. The nurse assists the client to an upright position with a table and pillow in front of him to support his arms. Which rationale for this intervention is correct?
1. There's easier access to the fluid from this approach.
2. There's less chance to injure lung tissue.
3. It prevents the formation of subcutaneous emphysema.
4. It's less painful for the client in this position.

5. 4. Toddlers easily transmit and contract RSV and so they should be separated from other children. RSV is also communicable to older children and adults, but these clients may exhibit only mild symptoms of the disorder. Hospitalization is indicated only for children who need oxygen and I.V. therapy.
CN: Safe, effective care environment; CNS: Safety and infection control; CL: Analysis

6. 2. The child should be monitored to determine if an asthma attack is imminent. The routine treatment plan may be insufficient when the peak flow is in the yellow zone (50% to 80% of personal best). This isn't an emergency situation. There's no immediate need to see the physician if the child is asymptomatic.
CN: Physiological integrity; CNS: Reduction of risk potential; CL: Application

7. 2. The household dust mite is the most commonly inhaled allergen that can cause an asthma attack. Animal dander, passive smoke, and perfume are sometimes allergens causing asthma attacks but aren't as common as dust mites.
CN: Safe, effective care environment; CNS: Safety and infection control; CL: Application

8. 3. The intestinal cells of individuals with celiac disease become inflamed when the child eats products containing gluten, such as bagels, bread, crackers, malted breakfast cereals, pasta, and pizza. The child with celiac disease needs normal amounts of fat and protein in the diet for growth and development. Parents just have to be attentive label readers, watching out for hidden gluten content.
CN: Safe, effective care environment; CNS: Safety and infection control; CL: Application

9. 1. The posterior approach is superior. The posterior gutter is deep and fluid tends to collect in this dependent area while the client is in an erect position. There's a risk for pneumothorax and subcutaneous emphysema formation regardless of the client's position. This procedure is done using local anesthesia, so it isn't painful.
CN: Physiological integrity; CNS: Physiological adaptation; CL: Analysis

10. Which leisure activity would the nurse recommend to parents for a school-age child with hemophilia?
1. Baseball
2. Cross-country running
3. Football
4. Swimming

11. Which assessment is important for a child in sickle cell crisis?
1. The child has no bruises.
2. The child has normal skin turgor.
3. The child is ambulatory around the room.
4. The child maintains bladder control.

12. The nurse suspects that a client is experiencing metabolic alkalosis based on laboratory and physical findings. Which findings best validate this condition?
1. A pH of 7.30; HCO_3^- of 20 mEq/L; tachypnea and poor skin turgor
2. A pH of 7.51, HCO_3^- of 29 mEq/L; muscle cramps and confusion
3. A pH of 7.32; HCO_3^- of 48 mEq/L; shortness of breath and lethargy
4. A pH of 7.46; HCO_3^- of 28 mEq/L; dizziness and numbness of hands and feet

You're doing great! Keep at it!

13. A client with chronic alcohol abuse is admitted to the hospital for detoxification. Later that day, his blood pressure increases and he's given lorazepam (Ativan) to prevent which complication?
1. Stroke
2. Seizure
3. Fainting
4. Anxiety reaction

14. An adolescent client ingests a large number of acetaminophen (Tylenol) tablets in an attempt to commit suicide. Which laboratory result is most consistent with acetaminophen overdose?
1. Metabolic acidosis
2. Elevated liver enzyme levels
3. Increased serum creatinine level
4. Increased white blood cell (WBC) count

10. 4. Swimming is a noncontact sport with low risk for traumatic injury. Baseball, cross-country running, and football all involve a risk for trauma from falling, sliding, or contact.
CN: Physiological integrity; CNS: Physiological adaptation; CL: Application

11. 2. Normal skin turgor indicates the child isn't severely dehydrated. Dehydration may cause sickle cell crisis or worsen a crisis. Bruising isn't associated with sickle cell crisis. Bed rest is preferable during a sickle cell crisis. Bladder control may be lost when oral or I.V. fluid intake is increased during a sickle cell crisis but has no bearing on the primary problem of sickling.
CN: Physiological integrity; CNS: Physiological adaptation; CL: Analysis

12. 2. A pH greater than 7.45 and a $Paco_2$ less than 35 mm Hg indicate respiratory alkalosis. A pH less than 7.35 and an HCO_3^- less than 22 mEq/L indicate metabolic acidosis. A pH greater than 7.45 and an HCO_3^- greater than 24 mEq/L indicate metabolic alkalosis. A pH less than 7.35 and a $Paco_2$ greater than 45 mm Hg indicate respiratory acidosis. Physical findings include muscle spasms and twitching and notable confusion for metabolic alkalosis; rapid breathing and confusion/lethargy for metabolic acidosis; dizziness and numbness of hands and feet for respiratory alkalosis; and confusion, lethargy, and shortness of breath for respiratory acidosis.
CN: Physiological integrity; CNS: Reduction of risk potential; CL: Analysis

13. 2. During detoxification from alcohol, changes in the client's physiological status, especially an increase in blood pressure, may indicate a possible seizure. Clients are treated with benzodiazepines to prevent this. Stroke, fainting, and anxiety aren't the primary concerns when withdrawing from alcohol.
CN: Physiological integrity; CNS: Pharmacological and parenteral therapies; CL: Application

14. 2. Elevated liver enzyme levels, which could indicate liver damage, are associated with acetaminophen overdose. Metabolic acidosis isn't associated with acetaminophen overdose. An increased serum creatinine level may indicate renal damage. An increased WBC count indicates infection.
CN: Physiological integrity; CNS: Pharmacological and parenteral therapies; CL: Application

15. A nurse is caring for a client recently diagnosed with acute pancreatitis. Which statement indicates that a short-term goal of nursing care has been met?
1. The client denies abdominal pain.
2. The client doesn't complain of thirst.
3. The client denies pain at McBurney's point.
4. The client swallows liquids without coughing.

16. A client is to take 8 oz of magnesium sulfate solution. The calibrations on the measuring device are in milliliters. How many milliliters should the nurse give?
1. 8 ml
2. 80 ml
3. 240 ml
4. 480 ml

17. A man stepped on a piece of sharp glass while walking barefoot. He comes to the emergency department with a deep laceration on the bottom of his foot. Which question is the most important for the nurse to ask?
1. "Was the glass dirty?"
2. "Are you immune to tetanus?"
3. "When did you have your last tetanus shot?"
4. "How many diphtheria-pertussis-tetanus (DTaP) shots did you receive as a child?"

18. A postmenopausal client asks a nurse how to prevent osteoporosis. What is the best response by the nurse?
1. "Take a multivitamin daily."
2. "After menopause, there's no way to prevent osteoporosis."
3. "Drink two glasses of milk each day and swim three times a week."
4. "Do weight-bearing exercises regularly."

19. A client diagnosed with cardiomyopathy saw a posting on the Internet describing research about a new herbal treatment for the disorder. When the client asks about this research, which response by the nurse is most appropriate?
1. "Herbs are often used to treat cardiomyopathy."
2. "Cardiomyopathy can be treated only by heart surgery."
3. "The Internet is a reliable source of research, so try this treatment."
4. "Any research found on the Internet should be verified with a physician."

15. 1. Pancreatitis is accompanied by acute pain from autodigestion by pancreatic enzymes. When the client denies abdominal pain, the short-term goal of pain control is met. Clients with acute pancreatitis receive I.V. fluids and may not have a sensation of thirst. Pain at McBurney's point accompanies appendicitis. Clients with acute pancreatitis receive nothing by mouth during initial therapy.

CN: Physiological integrity; CNS: Physiological adaptation; CL: Application

16. 3. To determine the amount of milliliters to give, use the following equation: One ounce equals 30 ml. 8 oz × 30 ml = 240 ml.

CN: Physiological integrity; CNS: Pharmacological and parenteral therapies; CL: Application

17. 3. Questioning the client about the date of his last tetanus immunization is important because the booster immunization should be received every 10 years in adulthood or at the time of the injury if the last booster immunization was given more than 5 years before the injury. Whether the client noticed dirt on the glass is immaterial because all deep lacerations require a tetanus immunization or booster. A client wouldn't know his tetanus immunity status. DTaP immunizations in childhood don't give lifelong immunization to tetanus.

CN: Safe, effective care environment; CNS: Safety and infection control; CL: Application

18. 4. Weight-bearing exercises are recommended for the prevention of osteoporosis. Telling the client that there's no way to prevent osteoporosis would be an incorrect statement. A multivitamin doesn't provide adequate calcium for a postmenopausal woman, and calcium alone won't prevent osteoporosis. Two glasses of milk per day don't provide the daily requirements for adult women, and swimming isn't a weight-bearing exercise.

CN: Health promotion and maintenance; CNS: None; CL: Application

19. 4. Although the Internet contains some valid medical research, there's no control over the validity of information posted on it. The research should be discussed with a physician who has access to medical research and can verify the accuracy of the information. Herbs aren't standard treatment for cardiomyopathy. Cardiomyopathy is treatable with drugs or surgery.

CN: Safe, effective care environment; CNS: Management of care; CL: Application

20. A young adult client received her first chemotherapy treatment for breast cancer. Which statement, if made by the client, requires further exploration by the nurse?
1. "I'm thinking about joining a dance club."
2. "I don't think I'm going to work tomorrow."
3. "I don't care about the side effects of the drugs."
4. "I want to return to school for a college degree."

You've finished 20 questions already? Wow, super!

21. A male client has been diagnosed with panhypopituitarism. Which hormone will be given to the client orally?
1. Estrogen
2. Levothyroxine (Synthroid)
3. Serotonin
4. Testosterone

22. Which nursing intervention is appropriate for an adult client with chronic renal failure?
1. Weigh the client daily before breakfast.
2. Offer foods high in calcium and phosphorous.
3. Serve the client large high-protein/high-fat meals and a bedtime snack.
4. Encourage the client to drink large amounts of fluids.

23. A physician prescribes acetaminophen (Tylenol) gr X (10 grains) as necessary every 4 hours for pain for a client in a long-term care facility. How many milligrams of acetaminophen should the nurse give? Record your answer using a whole number:

_____ milligrams

24. Which assessment finding by the nurse indicates an increased risk for skin cancer in a client?
1. A deep sunburn
2. A small café-au-lait spot on the client's back
3. An irregular scar on the client's abdomen
4. White irregular patches on the client's arm

25. Which behavior is consistent with the diagnosis of conduct disorder in a child?
1. Enuresis
2. Suicidal ideation
3. Cruelty to animals
4. Fear of going to school

20. 3. Adverse effects of chemotherapy may occur after treatment and should be discussed with the client because some can be treated, controlled, or prevented. The nurse needs to explore what the client means by this statement. Joining social clubs is typical behavior for a young adult. The client may feel poorly after chemotherapy and may want to take time off from work until feeling better. Returning to school is also typical of a young adult.
cn: Health promotion and maintenance; cns: None; cl: Analysis

21. 2. Thyroid hormone release depends on the release of thyroid-stimulating hormone (TSH) by the anterior pituitary. TSH is absent from the pituitary when panhypopituitarism exists, so levothyroxine should be given orally. Estrogen isn't indicated for a male client. Serotonin release isn't controlled by the pituitary gland. Testosterone is given by injection or topically by patch.
cn: Physiological integrity; cns: Pharmacological and parenteral therapies; cl: Application

22. 1. Daily weights are obtained to monitor fluid retention. Calcium intake is encouraged, but clients with chronic renal failure have difficulty excreting phosphorous. Therefore, phosphorous must be restricted. To improve food intake, meals and snacks should be given in small portions and fats and protein limited. Fluids should be restricted for the client with chronic renal failure.
cn: Physiological integrity; cns: Physiological adaptation; cl: Application

23. 650 mg. To determine the amount of milligrams to give, use the following equation:
    One grain = 65 mg, so 10 grains is
$65 \times 10 = 650$ mg.
cn: Physiological integrity; cns: Pharmacological and parenteral therapies; cl: Application

24. 1. A deep sunburn is a risk factor for skin cancer. An irregular scar is a benign finding, and café-au-lait spots are suggestive of neurofibromatosis, not cancer. White irregular patches are abnormal but aren't a risk factor for skin cancer.
cn: Health promotion and maintenance; cns: None; cl: Application

25. 3. Cruelty to animals is a symptom of conduct disorder. Enuresis and suicidal ideation aren't usually associated with conduct disorder. Fear of going to school is school phobia.
cn: Psychosocial integrity; cns: None; cl: Application

26. A client presents to the clinic and is diagnosed with a genital chlamydial infection. Which symptom would the nurse anticipate being reported by this client?
1. "Burning and itching down there," pointing to his penis
2. Visible fluid-filled lesions
3. Thick, purulent discharge from the penis
4. Genital warts

27. Which outcome is most appropriate for a client with a diagnosis of depression and attempted suicide?
1. The client will never feel suicidal again.
2. The client will find a group home to live in.
3. The client will remain hospitalized for at least 6 months.
4. The client will verbalize an absence of suicidal ideation, plan, and intent.

28. The nurse is reviewing the proper technique in obtaining a urine specimen from an indwelling urinary catheter. When collecting the urine, which would be the most appropriate technique to use?
1. Collect urine from the drainage collection bag.
2. Disconnect the catheter from the drainage tubing to collect urine.
3. Remove the indwelling catheter and insert a sterile straight catheter to collect urine.
4. Insert a sterile needle with syringe through a tubing drainage port after cleaning with alcohol to collect the specimen.

29. A registered nurse (RN) is supervising the care of a licensed practical nurse (LPN). The LPN is voicing concerns about a terminal client's end-of-life plan. Which statement by the LPN would indicate to the RN that further teaching is needed?
1. "Some clients write a living will indicating their end-of-life preferences."
2. "The law says you have to write a new living will each time you go to the hospital."
3. "You could designate another person to make end-of-life decisions when you can't make them yourself."
4. "Some people choose to tell their physician they don't want to have cardiopulmonary resuscitation."

26. 1. In men, one of the most common complaints with chlamydia is penile itching and burning, especially during urination. There may be a discharge, but it is usually clear or white in nature, not yellow or purulent. Genital warts are a sign of human papillomavirus. Fluid-filled blisters are a sign of herpes infection.
CN: Health promotion and maintenance; CNS: None; CL: Analysis

27. 4. An appropriate outcome is that the client will verbalize that he no longer feels suicidal. It's unrealistic to ask that he never feels suicidal again. There's no reason for a group home or 6 months of hospitalization.
CN: Psychosocial integrity; CNS: None; CL: Application

28. 4. Wearing clean gloves, cleaning the port with alcohol, and then obtaining the specimen with a sterile needle and syringe ensure that the specimen and closed drainage system won't be contaminated. A urine specimen must be new urine, and the urine in the drainage collection bag could be several hours old and growing bacteria. The urinary drainage system must be kept closed to prevent microorganisms from entering. It isn't necessary to remove an indwelling catheter to obtain a sterile urine specimen, unless the physician requests that the system be changed.
CN: Safe, effective care environment; CNS: Safety and infection control; CL: Application

29. 2. One living will is sufficient for all hospitalizations unless the client wishes to make changes. A living will explains a person's end-of-life preferences. A durable power of attorney for health care can be written to designate who will make health care decisions for the client in the event the client can't make decisions for himself. The "No-Code" or "Do-Not-Resuscitate" status is discussed with the physician, who then enters this in the client's chart.
CN: Safe, effective care environment; CNS: Management of care; CL: Analysis

30. An elderly client's husband tells a nurse he's concerned because his wife insists on talking about events that happened to her years in the past. The nurse assesses the client and finds her alert, oriented, and answering questions appropriately. Which response to the husband best addresses his concerns?
1. "Your wife is reviewing her life."
2. "A spiritual advisor should be notified."
3. "Your wife should be discouraged from talking about the past."
4. "Your wife is regressing to a more comfortable time in the past."

31. A client with a new colostomy asks a nurse how to avoid leakage from the ostomy bag. Which instruction is correct?
1. Limit fluid intake.
2. Eat more fruits and vegetables.
3. Empty the bag when it's about half full.
4. Tape the end of the bag to the surrounding skin.

32. A nurse must obtain the blood pressure of a client in airborne isolation. Which method is best to prevent transmission of infection to other clients by the equipment?
1. Dispose of the equipment after each use.
2. Wear gloves while handling the equipment.
3. Use the equipment only with other clients in airborne isolation.
4. Leave the equipment in the room for use only with that client.

33. To prevent circulatory impairment in an arm when applying an elastic bandage, which method is best?
1. Wrap the bandage around the arm loosely.
2. Apply the bandage while stretching it slightly.
3. Apply heavy pressure with each turn of the bandage.
4. Start applying the bandage at the upper arm and work toward the lower arm.

34. The physician's order reads 2 grams of cephalexin (Keflex) by mouth daily in equally divided doses of 500 mg each. The nurse would administer this medication at which frequency?
1. 3 times per day
2. 4 times per day
3. 6 times per day
4. 8 times per day

I'm so proud of you. Keep up the good work!

30. 1. Life review or reminiscing is characteristic of elderly people and the dying. A spiritual advisor might comfort the client but isn't necessary for a life review. Discouraging the client from talking would block communication. Regression occurs when a client returns to behaviors typical of another developmental stage.

CN: Health promotion and maintenance; CNS: None; CL: Application

31. 3. Emptying the bag when partially full will prevent the bag from becoming heavy and detaching from the skin or skin barrier. Limiting fluids may cause constipation but won't prevent leakage. Increasing fruits and vegetables in the diet will help prevent constipation, not leakage. Taping the bag to the skin will secure the bag to the skin but won't prevent leakage.

CN: Physiological integrity; CNS: Basic care and comfort; CL: Application

32. 4. Leaving equipment in the room is appropriate to avoid organism transmission by inanimate objects. Disposing of equipment after each use prevents the transmission of organisms but isn't cost-effective. Wearing gloves protects the nurse, not other clients. Using equipment for other clients spreads infectious organisms among clients.

CN: Safe, effective care environment; CNS: Safety and infection control; CL: Application

33. 2. Stretching the bandage slightly maintains uniform tension on the bandage. Wrapping the bandage loosely wouldn't secure the bandage on the arm, and it will come off. Using heavy pressure would cause circulatory impairment. Beginning the wrapping at the upper arm would cause uneven application of the bandage. For example, elastic stockings are applied distal to proximal to promote venous return.

CN: Physiological integrity; CNS: Reduction of risk potential; CL: Application

34. 2. 2 grams is equivalent to 2,000 mg (1 g = 1,000 mg). To give equally divided doses of 500 mg, divide the desired dose of 500 mg into the total daily dose of 2,000 mg. This gives an answer of 4, which is the number of times this dose of medication will be administered per day. This means giving 500 mg every 6 hours, for a total of 4 times per day.

CN: Physiological integrity; CNS: Pharmacological and parenteral therapies; CL: Analysis

CN: Client needs category   CNS: Client needs subcategory   CL: Cognitive level

35. A client complains of an inability to sleep while on the medical unit. Which intervention should the nurse perform first?
1. Offer a sedative routinely at bedtime.
2. Give the client a backrub before bedtime.
3. Question the client about sleeping habits.
4. Move the client to a bed farthest from the nurses' station.

36. In order to assess the function of a client's optic nerve, the nurse would be required to use which equipment?
1. Finger, to test the cardinal fields
2. Flashlight, to test corneal reflexes
3. Snellen's chart, to test visual acuity
4. Piece of cotton, to test corneal sensitivity

37. A nurse is caring for a client following surgery in the postanesthesia care unit. The nurse observes that the client is gagging on his airway and about to vomit. In which position would the nurse place the client?
1. Prone
2. Trendelenburg
3. Supine
4. Recovery

38. Which nursing intervention would best help prevent bladder infections for a client with an indwelling urinary catheter?
1. Recommend limiting fluid intake.
2. Encourage showers rather than tub baths.
3. Open the drainage system to obtain a urine specimen.
4. Irrigate the catheter twice daily with sterile saline solution.

Answer question 38 and you're halfway there.

39. A nurse wants to use a waist restraint for a client who wanders at night. Which factor should be considered before applying the restraint?
1. The nurse's convenience
2. The client's reason for getting out of bed
3. A sleeping medication ordered as needed at bedtime
4. The lack of nursing assistants on the night shift

35. 3. Interviewing the client about sleeping habits may give more information about the causes of the inability to sleep. Sedatives should be given as a last option. A backrub may promote sleep but may not address this client's problem. Moving the client may not address the client's specific problem.
CN: Physiological integrity; CNS: Basic care and comfort; CL: Application

36. 3. The Snellen's chart is used to test the function of the optic nerve. Testing the cardinal fields assesses the oculomotor, trochlear, and abducens nerves. Corneal light reflex reflects the function of the oculomotor nerve. Corneal sensitivity is controlled by the trigeminal and facial nerves.
CN: Health promotion and maintenance; CNS: None; CL: Application

37. 4. Unless contraindicated, the recovery position, or right- or left-side lying position, should be used. This position is commonly called the recovery position because it is used to prevent aspiration of secretions or vomitus during the postoperative phase. The prone position is face down and not appropriate. Trendelenburg position is used for shock, and supine position places the client flat on their back, making aspiration possible.
CN: Physiological integrity; CNS: Reduction of risk potential; CL: Application

38. 2. A shower would prevent bacteria in the bath water from sustaining contact with the urinary meatus and the catheter, while a tub bath is contraindicated for any client with an indwelling catheter to prevent transit of bacteria into the urinary tract. Increased—not limited—fluid intake is recommended for a client with an indwelling urinary catheter because concentrated urine is more likely to become infected. Opening the drainage system would provide a pathway for the entry of bacteria. Catheter irrigation is performed only with an order from the physician to keep the catheter patent and does not address infection prevention.
CN: Physiological integrity; CNS: Reduction of risk potential; CL: Application

39. 2. The nurse should question the client's reason for getting out of bed because the client may be looking for a bathroom. Lack of adequate staffing and convenience aren't reasons for applying restraints. Sleeping medications are chemical restraints that should be used only if the client is unable to go to sleep and stay asleep.
CN: Safe, effective care environment; CNS: Safety and infection control; CL: Application

40. Six months after the death of her infant son, a client is suspected of dysfunctional grieving. Which assessment would the nurse expect to find in this client?
1. She goes to the infant's grave weekly.
2. She cries when talking about the loss.
3. She's overactive without a sense of loss.
4. She states the infant will always be part of the family.

41. A nurse notices a hospitalized client has been crying. Which response is most therapeutic?
1. Do nothing; this is a private matter.
2. "You seem sad; would you like to talk?"
3. "Why are you crying and upsetting yourself?"
4. "It's hard being in the hospital, but you must keep your chin up."

42. A nurse gives the wrong medication to a client. The risk manager for the unit will expect to receive which communication?
1. Incident report
2. Oral report from the nurse
3. Copy of the medication Kardex
4. Order change signed by the physician

43. A student nurse (SN) witnesses a registered nurse (RN) performing a procedure on a client without obtaining informed consent for the procedure. The SN recognizes that the RN is guilty of committing which action?
1. Breach of confidentiality
2. Assault and battery
3. Harassment
4. Neglect of duty

44. A surgical client newly diagnosed with cancer tells a nurse she knows the laboratory made a mistake about her diagnosis. Which reaction is this client most likely experiencing?
1. Denial
2. Intellectualization
3. Regression
4. Repression

40. 3. One of the signs of dysfunctional grieving is overactivity without a sense of loss. Including the infant as a part of the family, going to the grave, and crying are all normal responses.
CN: Psychosocial integrity; CNS: None; CL: Application

41. 2. Therapeutic communication is a primary tool of nursing. The nurse must recognize that the client's nonverbal behaviors indicate a need to talk. Asking "why" is often interpreted as an accusation. Ignoring the client's nonverbal cues or giving opinions and advice are barriers to communication.
CN: Psychosocial integrity; CNS: None; CL: Application

42. 1. Incident reports are tools used by risk managers when a client might be harmed. They're used to determine how future problems can be avoided. An oral report won't serve as legal documentation. A copy of the medication Kardex wouldn't be sent with the incident report to the risk manager. A physician won't change an order to cover the nurse's mistake.
CN: Safe, effective care environment; CNS: Management of care; CL: Application

43. 2. Performing a procedure on a client without informed consent can be grounds for charges of assault and battery. Harassment means to annoy or disturb someone, and breach of confidentiality refers to conveying information about the client. Neglect of duty is failure to perform care that a prudent nurse would provide under similar circumstances.
CN: Safe, effective care environment; CNS: Management of care; CL: Application

44. 1. Cancer clients often deny this diagnosis when first made. Such a response may benefit the client in that it allows energy for surgical healing. Repression describes not remembering being diagnosed, regression describes childlike behavior, and intellectualization describes speaking of the disease as if reading a textbook.
CN: Psychosocial integrity; CNS: None; CL: Application

45. An unmarried client delivers a premature neonate. Which intervention would be included in her care plan?
  1. An early postpartum physician visit
  2. Referral to the health department
  3. Request for a social service visit in the hospital
  4. Request for a home health visit the day after discharge

46. Which statement made by a client about her neonate indicates the need for further teaching?
  1. "I'll trim the baby's nails when he's sleeping."
  2. "I'll remember to place the baby on his back when he sleeps."
  3. "Our infant car seat must be placed in the back seat of the car."
  4. "The first thing I'm going to do when we get home is give the baby a tub bath."

47. A client in labor is receiving oxytocin (Pitocin) to augment her labor. A nurse notes a change in her contraction pattern. The fetal heart monitor indicates that her contractions are lasting 2 minutes, with a notable rise in the baseline. Based on this finding, which action is the priority?
  1. Notify the physician.
  2. Give oxygen through a mask.
  3. Turn oxytocin to the lowest level.
  4. Turn the client on her left side.

48. A client who just gave birth is concerned about her neonate's Apgar scores of 7 and 8. She says she's been told scores lower than 9 are associated with learning difficulties in later life. Which response is best?
  1. "You shouldn't worry so much; your infant is perfectly fine."
  2. "I understand your concerns. You should ask about placing the infant in a follow-up diagnostic program."
  3. "You're right in being concerned, but there are good special education programs available."
  4. "Apgar scores are used to indicate a need for resuscitation at birth. Scores of 7 and above indicate that the baby has no problems."

45. 3. Due to the client's marital status and premature condition of the neonate, a social service visit is appropriate. The social service visit will determine if there's a need for a referral to the health department. The mother has no physical indications for an early postpartum visit or need for an early home visit.
CN: Safe, effective care environment; CNS: Management of care; CL: Analysis

46. 4. Neonates shouldn't be placed in a tub bath until after the cord falls off and is completely healed to prevent infection. It's correct to cut his nails while he sleeps, place a neonate on his back, and place the car seat in the back.
CN: Safe, effective care environment; CNS: Safety and infection control; CL: Analysis

47. 3. The first action must be to lower the oxytocin to prevent fetal hypoxia or possible rupture of the uterus. The client would then be placed on her left side and given oxygen to prevent fetal hypoxia, and the physician would be notified.
CN: Safe, effective care environment; CNS: Management of care; CL: Analysis

48. 4. Apgar scores don't indicate future learning difficulties; they're for rapid assessment of the need for resuscitation. It's inappropriate to just tell a client not to worry. Apgar scores of 7 and 8 are normal and don't indicate a need for intervention.
CN: Health promotion and maintenance; CNS: None; CL: Application

49. After delivering a neonate with a cleft palate and cleft lip, a client has minimal contact with her neonate. She asks the nurse to do most of the neonate's care. Which nursing diagnosis is appropriate?
1. Anxiety related to fear of harming the neonate
2. Deficient knowledge related to neonate's potential
3. Risk for impaired parenting related to birth defect
4. Altered family support related to lack of involvement

50. A breastfeeding client asks how she can do breast self-examination (BSE) while nursing. Which response would be the most accurate?
1. "You should do BSE after the infant has emptied the breast."
2. "You don't have to do BSE until after you stop breastfeeding."
3. "You should continue to do BSE the way you did before becoming pregnant."
4. "Your physician will examine your breasts until after you stop breastfeeding."

51. A prenatal client tells the nurse she can't believe she has such mixed feelings about being pregnant. She tried for 10 years to become pregnant and now she feels guilty for her conflicting reactions. Which response is best?
1. "You need to talk to your midwife about these unusual feelings."
2. "You're experiencing the normal ambivalence pregnant mothers feel."
3. "These feelings are expected only in women who have had difficulty becoming pregnant."
4. "Let's make an appointment with a counselor to help you sort through your feelings."

52. A maternity client tells the nurse her husband is behaving in strange ways since she became pregnant. He's having morning sickness, has put on weight, complains of intestinal pains, and is acting like he's pregnant. The nurse interprets this as indicating which of the following?
1. Extreme anxiety
2. Normal couvade
3. Signs of reaction formation
4. Abnormal, needing counseling

You've now completed 50 questions and are two-thirds finished. Super!

49. 3. Neonates born with birth defects are at risk for impaired parenting. The parents must work through issues of not producing the perfect child and guilt associated with this. There's nothing in the question that indicates the client felt anxious about caring for the neonate, had lack of family support, or a knowledge deficit.
CN: Safe, effective care environment; CNS: Management of care; CL: Analysis

50. 1. During breastfeeding, the client should examine each breast after the neonate has emptied the breast. Women must continue to examine their breasts, even if they're lactating. Contrary to how it's performed before pregnancy, BSE should be done on the same day of the month until the menstrual cycle returns. Breast examination shouldn't be done solely by the physician.
CN: Health promotion and maintenance; CNS: None; CL: Application

51. 2. Conflicting, ambivalent feelings regarding pregnancy are normal for all pregnant women. These feelings don't call for counseling or other professional interventions. Ambivalence is felt by most pregnant women, not only mothers who had difficulty becoming pregnant.
CN: Psychosocial integrity; CNS: None; CL: Application

52. 2. The father's adjustment may include behaviors referred to as couvade. Historically, there have been different cultural couvades. Today, the term is associated with the father developing pregnancy-like symptoms. Because the behavior is normal and isn't reaction formation or anxiety, there's no need for counseling.
CN: Psychosocial integrity; CNS: None; CL: Analysis

53. Three days after discharge, a client who is bottle feeding her neonate calls the postpartum floor and asks the nurse what she can do for breast engorgement. What is the best response by the nurse?
1. Put a tight binder around her breasts or use a snug-fitting bra.
2. Get under a warm shower and let the water flow on her breasts.
3. Stop drinking milk because it contributes to breast engorgement.
4. Contact her physician; she shouldn't be engorged at this late date.

54. A pregnant client complains of leg cramps that wake her from sleep. What is the best instruction by the nurse?
1. Dorsiflex the foot.
2. Elevate the legs at night.
3. Point the toes until the cramp releases.
4. Drink more than 1 qt of milk a day.

55. A client is being treated for premature labor with ritodrine (Yutopar). After receiving this medication for 12 hours, her blood pressure is slightly elevated, her chest is clear, and her pulse is 120 beats/minute. She complains of a little nausea, and the fetal heart rate is 145 beats/minute. Which intervention is correct?
1. Continue routine monitoring.
2. Contact the physician immediately.
3. Turn the client on her left side and give oxygen.
4. Increase the flow rate of the I.V. and give oxygen.

56. At 6 cm of dilation, the client in labor receives a lumbar epidural for pain control. Which nursing diagnosis is most appropriate?
1. Risk for injury related to rapid delivery
2. Acute pain related to wearing off of anesthesia
3. Hyperthermia related to effects of anesthesia
4. Ineffective peripheral tissue perfusion related to effects of anesthesia

57. When assessing a client who just delivered a neonate, a nurse finds the following: blood pressure, 110/70 mm Hg; pulse, 60 beats/minute; respirations, 16 breaths/minute; lochia, moderate rubra; fundus, above the umbilicus to the right; and negative Homans' sign. What is the most appropriate nursing intervention?
1. Nothing; all findings are normal.
2. Have the client void and recheck the fundus.
3. Turn the client on her left side to decrease the blood pressure.
4. Rub the fundus to decrease lochia flow and prevent hemorrhage.

53. 1. A tight binder or snug bra is recommended for the client bottle feeding her neonate to reduce engorgement. A warm shower will stimulate milk production. It's normal to become engorged during the first few days after delivery, and drinking milk isn't the cause.
CN: Physiological integrity; CNS: Basic care and comfort; CL: Application

54. 1. Dorsiflexion of the foot is the recommended intervention to relieve a leg cramp during pregnancy. Elevating the legs isn't a usual treatment. Drinking more than 1 qt of milk and pointing the toes are associated with causing leg cramps.
CN: Physiological integrity; CNS: Basic care and comfort; CL: Application

55. 1. These findings are normal adverse effects to the medication and don't call for interventions at this time except to continue routine monitoring. Contacting the physician, placing the client on her left side, changing the I.V. flow rate, and giving oxygen are all interventions for abnormal assessment findings.
CN: Physiological integrity; CNS: Pharmacological and parental therapies; CL: Analysis

56. 4. A disadvantage of a lumbar epidural is the risk for hypotension, which can lead to ineffective tissue perfusion. Epidurals are associated with a longer labor and hypothermia. There's no pain involved with the anesthesia wearing off.
CN: Safe, effective care environment; CNS: Management of care; CL: Application

57. 2. A fundus up and to the right indicates a full bladder. The client should empty her bladder and be reassessed. Lochia flow and blood pressure are normal.
CN: Physiological integrity; CNS: Reduction of risk potential; CL: Analysis

58. A client with gestational diabetes delivers an infant weighing 9 lb, 11 oz after a labor time of 8 hours and rupture of membranes 3 hours ago. Which interventions would be a priority for the neonate? Select all that apply.
1. Obtain blood cultures for prolonged ruptured membranes.
2. Obtain a serum glucose.
3. Maintain a thermoneutral environment.
4. Begin breastfeedings by mother in delivery room.
5. Monitor infant for respiratory distress.

58. 2, 3, and 5. Neonates of mothers with diabetes are at risk for hypoglycemia related to increased production of insulin by the neonate in utero, so blood glucose must be checked immediately after birth and interventions implemented if it is low. Maintaining the infant's body temperature will reduce the risk of hypothermia, which can cause increased metabolism and increased burning of glucose. These infants are at increased risk of developing respiratory distress shortly after birth due to decreased surfactant production secondary to increased insulin in the baby's system. Membranes ruptured for 3 hours is not considered prolonged. Although early feedings are important, beginning breastfeeding immediately will not prevent hypoglycemic episodes, and infants of diabetic mothers usually do not feed well. Providing a standardized glucose source is a better solution.
CN: Physiological integrity; CNS: Reduction of risk potential; CL: Application

59. A prenatal client, age 13, asks about getting fat while she's pregnant. A nurse tells her she needs to gain enough weight to be in the upper portions of her recommended weight due to her age to prevent which of the following?
1. Delivery of a premature neonate
2. A difficult delivery
3. Delivery of a low-birth-weight neonate
4. Preeclampsia

59. 3. Adolescent girls, especially those younger than age 15, are at higher risk for delivering low-birth-weight neonates unless they gain adequate weight during pregnancy. Gaining weight isn't associated with having an easier delivery, risk for preeclampsia, or risk of delivering a premature neonate.
CN: Physiological integrity; CNS: Reduction of risk potential; CL: Application

60. A mother of a neonate receiving phototherapy asks why her child has developed loose stools. Which response by the nurse would be accurate?
1. They're abnormal and may indicate an infection.
2. They're associated with an adverse reaction to formula.
3. They're common when receiving phototherapy treatments.
4. They're abnormal, and phototherapy should be discontinued.

60. 3. While receiving phototherapy, a breakdown of bilirubin often results in loose stools. The neonate must be monitored for diarrhea, skin irritation, and dehydration when under the lights. The loose stools wouldn't be considered related to infection or formula at this time.
CN: Physiological integrity; CNS: Physiological adaptation; CL: Application

61. A client at 36 weeks' gestation chokes on her food while eating at a restaurant. Which statement is correct about performing the Heimlich maneuver on a pregnant client?
1. Chest thrusts are used when the client is pregnant.
2. Only back thrusts are used when the client is pregnant.
3. The Heimlich maneuver is performed the same as when not pregnant.
4. The Heimlich maneuver can't be performed on a pregnant client.

61. 1. During pregnancy, chest thrusts are used instead of abdominal thrusts. Abdominal thrusts compress the abdomen, which would harm the fetus. Because of this, the Heimlich is adjusted for the pregnant woman. A fist is made with one hand, placing the thumb side against the center of the breastbone. The fist is grabbed with the other hand and thrust inward. Avoid the lower tip of the breastbone. Back thrusts aren't done because they may result in dislodgment of the obstruction, further obstructing the airway.
CN: Physiological integrity; CNS: Reduction of risk potential; CL: Application

62. A nurse is reviewing principles of good body mechanics with a student nurse. Which of the following techniques should be emphasized?
1. Bending from the waist
2. Pulling rather than pushing
3. Stretching to reach an object
4. Using large muscles in the legs for leverage

62. 4. Keeping one's back straight and using the large muscles in the legs will help avoid back injury, as the muscles in one's back are relatively small compared with the larger muscles of the thighs. Bending from the waist can cause stress on the back muscles, causing a potential injury. Pulling isn't the best option and may cause straining. When feasible, one should push an object rather than pull it. Stretching to reach an object increases the risk of injury.
CN: Safe, effective care environment; CNS: Safety and infection control; CL: Application

63. A client with a substance abuse problem is being discharged from the state treatment facility. The client's discharge plans should include which intervention?
1. Referral to Al-Anon
2. Weekly urine testing for drug use
3. Day hospital treatment for 6 months
4. Participation in a support group like Alcoholics Anonymous (AA)

63. 4. AA is a major support group for alcoholics after treatment. Membership in AA is associated with relapse prevention. Al-Anon is a support group for the family of the abuser of alcohol. Weekly urine testing or day hospital treatment isn't usual.
CN: Safe, effective care environment; CNS: Management of care; CL: Application

64. A community mental health nurse visits a client diagnosed with paranoid schizophrenia. When she arrives at his house, he calls her Satan, shouts at her, and proclaims "Away from me, Demon!" What is the most important intervention for the nurse to implement?
1. Use his phone and call the police.
2. Remain safe by leaving the house.
3. Talk to him in a calm voice to reduce his agitation.
4. Remind him who she is and that he has nothing to fear.

64. 2. Safety is the first priority during any home visit, so the nurse should leave. Attempting to talk with the client, reminding him who she is, or using the phone places the nurse at risk for harm. After the nurse has ensured her safety, arrangements should be made to provide help for the client.
CN: Safe, effective care environment; CNS: Safety and infection control; CL: Analysis

65. A client is scheduled to retire in the next month. He phones his nurse therapist and says he can't cope; his whole world is falling apart. The therapist recognizes this reaction as which of the following?
1. Panic reaction
2. Situational crisis
3. Normal separation anxiety
4. Maturational crisis

65. 4. A maturational (developmental) crisis is one that occurs at a predictable milestone during a life span; birth, marriage, and retirement are examples. A panic reaction would also involve physical symptoms. Situational crisis is caused by events such as an earthquake. Separation anxiety is a childhood disorder.
CN: Health promotion and maintenance; CNS: None; CL: Analysis

66. A client with a phobic condition is being treated with behavior modification therapy. Which intervention best addresses this technique?
1. Suggest she face the phobia head-on.
2. Talk to the client and have her identify why she has phobias.
3. Recommend gradual and repeated exposure to the source of the phobia.
4. Undergo electroconvulsive therapy (ECT) to jump-start the brain.

66. 3. Systematic desensitization is a behavior therapy used in the treatment of phobias. Forcing the client to face the phobia head-on and identifying a phobia do not help eliminate the problem and are not behavior modification methods. ECT is used with depression.
CN: Psychosocial integrity; CNS: None; CL: Analysis

Only 10 more to go! Oh my, I just can't wait!

67. A severely depressed client rarely leaves his chair. To prevent physiological complications associated with psychomotor retardation, which client goal is appropriate?
1. Limit television time.
2. Increase calcium intake.
3. Rest in bed three times per day.
4. Empty the bladder on a schedule.

67. 4. To prevent bladder infections associated with stasis of urine, the client should be encouraged to routinely empty his bladder. Calcium intake is not directly related to the psychological effects associated with this condition. Resting in bed is another form of psychomotor retardation. Watching television is merely a distraction and not beneficial to preventing physiological problems.
CN: Health promotion and maintenance; CNS: None; CL: Application

68. During the termination phase of a therapeutic nurse–client relationship, which intervention is avoided?
1. Refer the client to support groups.
2. Address new issues with the client.
3. Review what has been accomplished during this relationship.
4. Have the client express sadness that the relationship is ending.

68. 2. During the termination phase, new issues shouldn't be explored. It's appropriate to refer the client to support groups. To review what has been accomplished is a goal of this phase. Sadness is a normal response.
CN: Psychosocial integrity; CNS: None; CL: Application

69. The behavior of a client with borderline personality disorder causes a nurse to feel angry toward the client. Which response, if made by the nurse, is the most therapeutic?
1. Ignore the client's irritating behavior.
2. Restrict the client to her room until supper.
3. Report her feelings to the client's physician.
4. Tell the client how her behavior makes the nurse feel.

69. 4. A nursing intervention used with personality disorders is to help the client recognize how her behavior affects others. Restricting the client to her room, ignoring the client, and reporting feelings to the physician aren't appropriate interventions at this time.
CN: Psychosocial integrity; CNS: None; CL: Application

70. During a manic state, a client paced around the dayroom for 3 days. He talked to the furniture, proclaimed he was a king, and refused to partake in unit activities. Which nursing diagnosis has priority?
1. Impaired verbal communication related to hyperactivity
2. Risk for self-directed violence related to manic state
3. Imbalanced nutrition: Less than body requirements related to hyperactivity
4. Ineffective coping related to manic state

70. 3. During a manic state, clients are at risk for malnutrition due to not taking in enough calories for the energy they're expending. The client is not displaying impaired verbal communication. This client isn't showing self-directed violent behavior. Individual coping issues aren't the primary concern at this time.
CN: Safe, effective care environment; CNS: Management of care; CL: Application

71. A client with a panic disorder is having difficulty falling asleep. Which nursing intervention should be performed first?
1. Call the client's psychotherapist.
2. Teach the client progressive relaxation.
3. Allow the client to stay up and watch television.
4. Obtain an order for a sleeping medication as needed.

71. 2. Relaxation techniques work very well with a client showing anxiety. If this doesn't work, then contacting the psychotherapist, diversionary activities, and pharmacological interventions would be in order.
CN: Psychological integrity; CNS: None; CL: Application

72. Following electroconvulsive therapy (ECT), which nursing intervention would be implemented?
1. Assessing the client's vital signs
2. Leaving the client alone to sleep undisturbed
3. Allowing the family to visit immediately
4. Restraining the client until completely awake

73. A client diagnosed with bipolar disease is receiving a maintenance dosage of lithium carbonate (Lithobid). His wife calls the community mental health nurse to report that her husband is hyperactive and hyperverbal. Which intervention would be most important to implement?
1. Mental status examination
2. Measurement of lithium blood levels
3. Evaluation at the local emergency department (ED)
4. Admission to the hospital for observation

74. A nurse is caring for a client with emphysema. Which nursing interventions are appropriate? Select all that apply.
1. Reduce fluid intake to less than 2,500 ml/day.
2. Teach diaphragmatic, pursed-lip breathing.
3. Administer low-flow oxygen.
4. Keep the client in a supine position as much as possible.
5. Encourage alternating activity with rest periods.
6. Teach the family use of postural drainage and chest physiotherapy.

75. A nurse is assessing the abdomen of a client who was admitted to the emergency department with suspected appendicitis. Identify the area of the abdomen that the nurse should palpate last.

72. 1. Vital signs are monitored carefully for approximately 1 hour after ECT or until the client is stable. The client shouldn't be restrained or left alone. Visitors should not be allowed until the client is awake and ready.

CN: Physiological integrity; CNS: Reduction of risk potential; CL: Application

73. 2. Increased activity might indicate a need for an increased dose of lithium or that the client isn't taking his medications; blood levels will determine this. The client doesn't need to have a mental status examination, go to the ED, or be admitted to the hospital at this time.

CN: Physiological integrity; CNS: Pharmacological and parenteral therapies; CL: Analysis

74. 2, 3, 5, and 6. Diaphragmatic, pursed-lip breathing strengthens respiratory muscles and enhances oxygenation in clients with emphysema. Low-flow oxygen should be administered because a client with emphysema has chronic hypercapnia and a hypoxic respiratory drive. Alternating activity with rest allows the client to perform activities without excessive distress. If the client has copious secretions and has difficulty mobilizing them, the nurse should teach him and his family members how to perform postural drainage and chest physiotherapy. Fluid intake should be increased to 3,000 ml/day, if not contraindicated, to liquefy secretions and facilitate their removal. The client should be placed in high Fowler's position to improve ventilation.

CN: Physiological integrity; CNS: Basic care and comfort; CL: Application

75. An acute attack of appendicitis localizes as pain and tenderness in the lower right quadrant, midway between the umbilicus and the crest of the ilium. This area should be palpated last in order to determine if pain is also present in other areas of the abdomen.

CN: Health promotion and maintenance; CNS: None; CL: Application

I knew you could do it! Super job! You're well on your way to total confidence for the NCLEX.

COMPREHENSIVE Test 3

1. To meet the nutritional needs of a postoperative client who is tolerating clear liquids, the nursing priority is to:
1. check for bowel sounds.
2. advance to full liquids.
3. order a soft diet.
4. allow the client to select from the menu.

2. The nurse assesses the client's intake and output record at end of the 7 a.m. to 3 p.m. shift. The recorded intake is listed as follows: milk, 180 ml; orange juice, 60 ml; 1 serving scrambled eggs; 1 slice toast; 1 can Ensure oral nutritional supplement, 240 ml; I.V. dextrose 5% in water at 100 ml/hour; 50 ml water after twice daily medications. Medications are given at 9:00 a.m. and 9:00 p.m. The nurse totals the intake at the end of shift as:
1. 1,000 ml.
2. 1,250 ml.
3. 1,330 ml.
4. 1,380 ml.

3. The registered nurse is caring for a neonate diagnosed with a cardiac anomaly. The pediatrician orders digoxin (Lanoxin), 2.5 mg. The nurse questions the order with both the pharmacist and physician. The nurse demonstrates responsible professional practice according to which of the following?
1. American Medical Association
2. American Nurses Association (ANA)
3. American Pharmaceutical Association
4. Nurse Practice Act

1. 2. Clear liquid diets are nutritionally inadequate but minimally irritating to the stomach. Clients are advanced to the full liquid diet next, adding bland and protein foods. A soft diet comes next, which omits foods that are hard to chew or digest. A regular or general diet has no limitations. A fluid restriction is ordered in addition to the diet order for clients in renal failure or congestive heart failure. Although a correct assessment, assessing for bowel sounds does not respond to the question.
CN: Physiological integrity; CNS: Basic care and comfort; CL: Application

2. 3. The client's total intake is 1,330 ml. Use the following equation:
$180 + 60 + 240 + 800 + 50 = 1,330.$
CN: Physiological integrity; CNS: Basic care and comfort; CL: Application

3. 4. Each state has a Nurse Practice Act that dictates a nurse's scope of practice. Each nurse must practice competent standards based on her state's Nurse Practice Act. The ANA is an organization of nurses that offers credentialing and nursing education. The ANA has published *Nursing: Scope and Standards of Nursing Practice*, but this does not govern practice. Physicians and pharmacists must practice competency based on the standards established by their professional organizations.
CN: Safe, effective care environment; CNS: Management of care; CL: Application

CN: Client needs category   CNS: Client needs subcategory   CL: Cognitive level

4. When making rounds after returning from lunch, the nurse assesses a client's pain as 9 out of 10 on a 0 to 10 pain scale. There is no record of an opioid being given to the client, even though the previous nurse signed for one at 12:15 p.m. The client denies receiving anything for pain since the previous night. Which action should the nurse take next?
1. Notify the physician that an opioid is missing.
2. Notify the supervisor that the client didn't receive the prescribed pain medication.
3. Notify the pharmacist that the client didn't receive the prescribed pain medication.
4. Approach the nurse who signed out the opioid to seek clarification about the missing drug.

5. When the nurse is assessing a client admitted to the emergency room following a traumatic rape, the nurse has both client and legal responsibilities. Select all the responsibilities that apply.
1. Place client's clothing in a labeled bag.
2. Have a nurse of the same sex stay with the client.
3. Call for the nurse trained in evaluation of sexual assault victims.
4. Prepare client for complete physical examination including Pap smear.
5. Remind the client to return for follow-up for sexually transmitted disease (STD) testing in 6 weeks.
6. Recognize that assessment charting may be used in legal proceedings.

6. The nursing profession has a responsibility to provide quality cost-effective care. A priority nursing judgment is to recognize that financial reimbursement for care will be lost for certain hospital-acquired conditions if the:
1. client develops a pressure ulcer postoperatively.
2. client admitted with a urinary tract infection (UTI) has a positive urinary culture and sensitivity.
3. client's peripheral I.V. infiltrates at the insertion site in the arm.
4. client feels faint while walking with the nurse and is assisted to the floor.

7. A nurse finds a client crying after she was told by the physician that she is to start hemodialysis to treat her acute renal failure. Which nursing intervention is best?
1. Sit quietly with the client.
2. Refer the client to the hemodialysis team.
3. Remind the client this is a temporary situation.
4. Discuss with the client the other abilities she has.

4. **4.** The nurse needs to seek clarification in a nonthreatening manner. If the nurse who signed out the opioid can't give a plausible explanation, the nurse who discovered the error must then notify the supervisor. The nurse who signed out the opioid may have a drug problem. The appropriate line of communication is to the hospital supervisor. The physician needs to be notified if the client didn't receive the prescribed medication. The pharmacist needs to be notified of discrepancies in the opioid count.
CN: Safe, effective care environment; CNS: Management of care; CL: Application

5. **1, 2, 3, 4, and 6.** The nurse should recognize that clothing and physical evidence should be collected and preserved. The nurse should provide supportive care to the client victim of assault. A rape crisis nurse or nurse trained in caring for victims of sexual assault should be called to assess the client and collect and preserve evidence. Accurate charting of physical and emotional findings will be important. The client should be followed for possible STDs within 3 weeks or sooner if any symptoms appear.
CN: Safe, effective care environment; CNS: Management of care; CL: Application

6. **1.** In 2008, Medicare restricted or eliminated reimbursement for certain hospital-acquired events that could have reasonably been prevented; pressure ulcers are one such condition. The other events are not included in the Centers for Medicare and Medicaid Services guidelines.
CN: Safe, effective care environment; CNS: Management of care; CL: Application

7. **1.** Sitting with the client shows compassion and concern and may help the nurse establish therapeutic communication. Making a referral doesn't allow the client to explore feelings with the nurse. The nurse can't guarantee the acute renal failure is temporary. Discussing the client's other abilities is diverting the emphasis away from the primary issue for this client.
CN: Psychosocial integrity; CNS: None; CL: Analysis and application

8. A client is admitted to a mental health unit. While assessing the client, the nurse finds the client exhibiting signs of hyperexcitability, increasing agitation, and distractibility. Based on the assessment, which nursing intervention has priority?
1. Involve the client in a group activity.
2. Be direct and firm and set rules for the client.
3. Use a quiet room for the client away from others.
4. Channel the client's energy toward a planned activity.

9. A client is awake and alert following maxillo-facial surgery and complains of pain, rating it as a 9 on a scale of 1 to 10. He has orders for meperidine (Demerol) 50 mg and hydroxyzine (Vistaril) 50 mg, every 4 hours as needed. When assessing the client 20 minutes after the first dose, he reports his pain as 6. Two hours later, he reports his pain as 8. What is the priority nursing judgment?
1. The hydroxyzine has interfered with the analgesic effect of the meperidine.
2. The client has been moving too much.
3. The client may need a higher dose.
4. The prescription should be changed.

10. A public health nurse visiting a new postpartum client notices that the client has two children under age 4. The nurse notices one infant playing in the cabinet under the sink. Which instruction should the public health nurse give the client?
1. Keep a bottle of ipecac syrup in the house.
2. Make sure all liquid cleaners are labeled.
3. Tighten all cap tops on the bottles under the sink.
4. Remove all cleaners that could be ingested orally.

11. A nurse arrives at a motor vehicle collision involving a school bus and a large truck. The school bus is lying on its side. The nurse observes that several children have been thrown from the windows of the school bus. Which child should the nurse assess first?
1. A girl crying hysterically
2. A boy who is unconscious
3. A boy bleeding from a laceration of the scalp
4. A girl with an obvious open leg fracture

You've finished 10 questions already! Good job!

8. 3. Being in a quiet environment away from stimuli facilitates helping the client regain a sense of control. If the nurse attempts to be firm and set rules for this client, it will most likely heighten the agitation. The client is too excited to focus at this time; group activities or other activities may worsen the client's situation.

CN: Psychosocial integrity; CNS: None; CL: Application

9. 3. It is reasonable to assume that the dose is probably too low for the amount of pain, and it would be prudent to report the client's response to the physician and inquire if the physician feels it's appropriate to increase the dose. The hydroxyzine potentiates the effects of meperidine and doesn't interfere with its effectiveness. There's no evidence to suggest that the client has been moving around too much. It's beyond the nurse's scope of practice to determine that the current medication should be changed.

CN: Physiological integrity; CNS: Pharmacological and parenteral therapies; CL: Analysis and application

10. 4. All liquid cleaners must be removed to reduce the risk for poisoning. Safety locks should be placed on cabinets to prevent young children from opening the cabinets or the bottles. Infants can't read danger labels. Ipecac is no longer routinely used to induce vomiting in children.

CN: Safe, effective care environment; CNS: Safety and infection control; CL: Application

11. 2. The unconscious child should be assessed for breathing and circulation status. An unconscious or unresponsive client always needs assistance first. Once help arrives, emotional support can be given to the girl crying hysterically, pressure can be applied to the laceration of the scalp to stop the bleeding, and the girl's fracture can be stabilized.

CN: Safe, effective care environment; CNS: Management of care; CL: Application

12. The nurse is reviewing discharge teaching with a client newly diagnosed with diabetes. Which statement made by the client indicates further instruction is needed?
1. "I need to check my feet daily for sores."
2. "I need to store my insulin in the refrigerator."
3. "I can eat bread in exchange for rice."
4. "I will see my physician for follow-up examinations."

13. A client with terminal cancer is receiving large doses of opioids for pain control. He becomes agitated and continues trying to get out of bed but can't stand without two-person assistance. To reduce the risk of falling, which type of restraint would the nurse ask to be ordered for the client?
1. Leg restraints
2. Chemical restraints
3. Mechanical restraints
4. Jacket restraint

14. Your client is returned to his room following a stem cell transplant. The client requires reverse isolation. The nurse understands that implementing this isolation will protect:
1. the client from his own bacteria.
2. the hospital staff from the client.
3. the other clients on the nursing unit.
4. the client from outside infections from others.

15. A physician ordered a sterile dressing tray set up in a client's room to insert a subclavian central venous catheter and 500 ml of normal saline to be infused at 40 ml/hour. Place the nursing activities to set up the sterile field in order, omitting any if they are not appropriate.
1. Open sterile packs away from self.
2. Use correct handwashing technique.
3. Put on sterile gloves.
4. Place the sterile dressing tray on an overbed table.
5. Connect the I.V. to the subclavian line.

12. 2. Insulin only needs to be stored in the refrigerator if it won't be used within 6 weeks after being opened; it should be at room temperature when given to decrease pain and prevent lipodystrophy. The remaining statements show that the client understands his condition and the importance of preventing complications.
CN: Safe, effective care environment; CNS: Safety and infection control; CL: Analysis

13. 2. Antianxiety medication can be used to calm the client. Chemical restraints are effective, especially with highly agitated clients receiving large doses of opioids. Other forms of restraint will only increase the client's agitation and hostility, thus increasing the safety risk.
CN: Safe, effective care environment; CNS: Safety and infection control; CL: Application

14. 4. Immunosuppressed clients need to be protected from infections from others following a stem cell transplant. Infections can occur if strict handwashing techniques aren't observed, especially with hospital staff going from one room to the next. Protective isolation is used to protect the hospital staff and other clients from an infected client.
CN: Safe, effective care environment; CNS: Safety and infection control; CL: Application

15. 2, 4, 1, and 3. Use appropriate handwashing technique before participating in a sterile procedure. Clean the area with an appropriate antiseptic, place the tray in the center of the clean area, and open it away from the nurse. After the dressing tray and/or sterile packs are opened, put on sterile gloves to assist the physician. Connecting the I.V. line after the procedure is not part of setting up the sterile field.
CN: Safe, effective care environment; CNS: Safety and infection control; CL: Application

16. Which nursing action demonstrates the principle of medical asepsis?
1. Return unused linen to the linen supply cart.
2. Keep the environment as clean as possible.
3. Test for microorganisms in the environment.
4. Clean the client's equipment with alcohol as needed.

17. The nurse has compiled an admission assessment on an ex-military serviceman who has served two tours in Iraq and is now retired from military service. The assessment data include the following: The client is upset, continually fidgeting, makes no eye contact, and responds to questions with "yes" and "no" answers. What is the priority nursing intervention?
1. Determine his plans for civilian life.
2. Discuss how his family is adjusting to his return.
3. Explore what experiences cause him distress.
4. Ask if he is feeling suicidal.

18. The nurse is assigned to develop a care plan for a client admitted to the unit. The nurse is aware that the assessment will include which step?
1. Identifying actual or potential health problems specific to the individual client
2. Gathering information about the client's future plans
3. Identifying goals and interventions specific to the individualized needs of the client
4. Systematically collecting subjective and objective data with the goal of making a clinical nursing judgment

19. While caring for a terminally ill infant, the nurse asks the mother if she wants the baby to be baptized. The mother becomes upset and asks to speak to the nurse-manager. What is the best response by the nurse-manager?
1. Call the chaplain on duty to talk to the mother.
2. Explain that since the nurse is catholic, she is only trying to determine the mother's wishes.
3. Apologize for the nurse's behavior and assign another nurse to her care.
4. Let the mother express her own spiritual beliefs and wishes.

16. 2. Medical asepsis is the process of avoiding contamination from outside sources by keeping the environment clean. A clean environment has a reduced number of microorganisms but isn't necessarily sterile (the absence of all microorganisms). Testing for microorganisms or culturing isn't indicated in the promotion of asepsis. Alcohol is not an approved cleansing agent.
CN: Safe, effective care environment; CNS: Safety and infection control; CL: Application

17. 3. Explore with the client what causes him distress and anxiety. Many returning service personnel suffer from posttraumatic stress disorder. Sudden noises and not being able to see who is entering his space could cause him further anxiety and "flashbacks" to wartime experiences. Determining his plans for civilian life addresses the future and is not appropriate at this time; how the family is adjusting does not assess the client at admission; and although suicide is of concern, the priority is to gather more information about what causes him distress.
CN: Safe, effective care environment; CNS: Safety and infection control; CL: Application

18. 4. Assessment involves data collection, organization, and validation. The information related to the client's current status is more relevant at this time than future plans. The diagnosis step of the nursing process involves the identification of actual or potential health problems. The nurse and client work together to identify goals, outcomes, and intervention strategies that will reduce identified client problems in the planning step.
CN: Safe, effective care environment; CNS: Management of care; CL: Application

19. 4. The best response is to allow the mother to express her own feelings. The chaplain may or may not be an appropriate response later. Explaining and apologizing for another's behavior is not likely to diffuse the situation or help the mother.
CN: Safe, effective care environment; CNS: Management of care; CL: Application

20. The nurse is making a home health visit to an elderly blind client who is living with his daughter. While completing the visit, the daughter expresses concern about the cost of caring for her father. Which program could the client be referred to?
1. Medicare
2. Meals On Wheels
3. Supplemental Security Income
4. Aid to Families with Dependent Children

21. The school nurse provided vision and hearing screenings for elementary school children at the beginning of the school year. Later in the year, the nurse offers an immunization clinic during the evening hours. This is an example of which type of prevention strategy?
1. Primary
2. Secondary
3. Tertiary
4. None of the above

22. The nurse is caring for a hospice client in a holistic manner and has included complementary and alternative medicine aspects in the plan of care. Select all of the complementary measures that could be used.
1. Administering morphine sulphate for breakthrough pain
2. Asking a harpist to play in the client's room
3. Using aroma therapy
4. Assessing for impaction
5. Providing an air mattress
6. Allowing the family to give oral fluids as needed

23. A new graduate nurse has almost completed orientation on the assigned nursing unit; however, a skills checklist and performance test identify deficient skills. What is the most appropriate action for the nurse-manager to take?
1. Talk with the supervisor about terminating the new graduate.
2. Discuss with the graduate that a transfer to another unit is necessary.
3. Have the graduate's preceptor work with her to meet requirements.
4. Counsel the graduate that if performance doesn't improve, the graduate will be terminated.

Stay focused, now. You're nearly one-third finished!

20. 3. Supplemental Security Income is a governmental subsidy assisting the poor and medically disabled. Medicare is available to elderly individuals age 65 years and older and individuals younger than 65 years with long-term disabilities or end-stage renal disease. Meals On Wheels is a nonprofit organization that delivers food to the poor. Aid to Families with Dependent Children is a state subsidy given to poor families with dependent children.

CN: Safe, effective care environment; CNS: Management of care; CL: Application

21. 1. Primary prevention strategies are aimed at preventing the disease from the beginning by avoiding or modifying risk factors. Screening is a major secondary prevention strategy. Secondary prevention is aimed at early detection and treatment of illness. Tertiary prevention strategies focus on rehabilitation and prevention of complications arising from advanced disease.

CN: Health promotion and maintenance; CNS: None; CL: Application

22. 2 and 3. Hospice clients traditionally have increased pain relief measures and comfort measures such as air mattresses and family involvement in care. Maintaining the client free from constipation and impaction is not an alternative therapy. The use of music, massage, and aroma therapy are considered aspects of complementary medicine.

CN: Physiological integrity; CNS: Physiological adaptation; CL: Application

23. 3. The leader needs to assign a preceptor to work with the new graduate and provide opportunities for the graduate to grow and develop. The other responses wouldn't give the new graduate the opportunity and support needed for improvement.

CN: Safe, effective care environment; CNS: Management of care; CL: Application

24. A local community health nurse is asked to speak to a group of adolescent girls on the topic of preventing pregnancy. Which statement indicates the adolescents need more information on this topic?
1. "I can get pregnant even on the first time we have sex."
2. "I can get pregnant even though I don't have sex regularly."
3. "I can get pregnant only when my menstrual cycle becomes regular."
4. "I can get pregnant even if my boyfriend withdraws before he comes."

25. The nurse is caring for a 3-year-old child with acute lymphocytic leukemia and notes the child has a decreased appetite. What is the priority nursing intervention?
1. Provide oral hygiene after eating.
2. Serve snacks as requested.
3. Have the dietician meet with the child and family to provide foods he will eat.
4. Encourage the child to eat all his meal to get adequate nutrition.

26. A nurse working in a public health clinic is planning tuberculosis (TB) screening. The nurse understands that which is the priority group to screen for TB?
1. All clients coming into the clinic
2. People living in a homeless shelter
3. Clients who haven't received the TB vaccine
4. Clients suspected of having human immuno-deficiency virus (HIV)

27. A nurse who is working at the health department has been assigned to obtain a sputum culture for possible tuberculosis (TB) from a client. After collecting the specimen, the professional nurse should report positive TB smears or cultures to the health department within which time period?
1. 12 hours
2. 48 hours
3. 1 week
4. 10 to 14 days

24. 3. Many adolescents have misunderstandings related to risk periods and timing, including periods of susceptibility during the menstrual cycle, age-related susceptibility, and timing of male ejaculation.

CN: Health promotion and maintenance; CNS: None; CL: Analysis

25. 3. The dietician should be involved because it is important to provide foods appropriate to children in certain age groups. Involve the child and family in food selection of foods the child will eat. Assess the family's beliefs about food habits. Let the child eat all food that can be tolerated. Take advantage of a hungry period and serve small snacks. Encourage parents to relax pressures placed on eating by stressing the legitimate nature of loss of appetite. The other responses do not help to stimulate the child's appetite.

CN: Physiological integrity; CNS: Physiological adaptation; CL: Application

26. 4. Clients with HIV infection or suspected of having HIV are at greater risk for developing TB. A screening test should be done and, if positive, treatment with isoniazid (Nydrazid) given. Clients coming to the clinic don't need to be tested unless they're at high risk—for example, living with someone infected with TB, abusing I.V. drugs, or suffering from chronic health conditions, such as diabetes mellitus and end-stage renal disease. Clients living in a homeless shelter aren't necessarily at greater risk unless other residents in the shelter have TB. The TB vaccine isn't widely used in the United States.

CN: Health promotion and maintenance; CNS: None; CL: Application

27. 2. A client is considered contagious if he has a positive TB smear or culture, so the results must be reported within 24 to 48 hours. The smear or culture may not have grown an organism in 12 hours. One week or 10 to 14 days is too long to wait.

CN: Safe, effective care environment; CNS: Safety and infection control; CL: Application

28. A 62-year-old female client has been taking vitamin C 500 mg by mouth (P.O.) daily, multivitamins 1 tablet P.O. every day, and ibuprofen 400 mg every 6 hours as needed for arthritic pain for 4 days. The nurse notices that the client's stool is becoming darker and that a test for occult blood is positive. What is the most appropriate nursing judgment?
1. The combination of vitamin C and multivitamins are irritating the lining of the intestine.
2. The ibuprofen should be withheld because it may be causing gastric bleeding.
3. Vitamin C is acidic in nature and may be irritating the GI tissues.
4. From the appearance of the stool, the nurse suspects the client has hemorrhoids.

29. The home health nurse is assessing a client and determines that the client has an unsteady gait. The client tells the nurse that she has recently fallen. Which nursing action represents an advocacy role for the home health nurse?
1. Contacting the local church to borrow a walker for the client to use
2. Listening to a client express feelings of frustration over the client's increasing limitations
3. Instructing the client to contact the senior day care
4. Reassuring the client that using a walker will prevent falls in the future

30. Which of the following activities is an example of an indirect care function of a home health nurse?
1. Observing the home health aide
2. Participating in a team conference about a client
3. Confirming the client's condition at the time of the monitor reading.
4. Teaching the client's family how to read a food label for sodium content

31. A nurse at a prenatal clinic is assessing a young pregnant client who expresses behaviors related to drug and alcohol abuse. Which statement indicates the client's child is at high risk of fetal alcohol syndrome (FAS)?
1. "I just snort once or twice a day."
2. "I had one glass of wine with dinner last week."
3. "I drink a six pack of beer daily to settle my nerves."
4. "I smoke marijuana with my boyfriend and his friends."

28. 2. Nonsteroidal anti-inflammatory drugs such as ibuprofen may cause gastric irritation and bleeding. Vitamin C and multivitamins generally don't have an adverse effect in the GI tract. There may be hemorrhoids present, but bleeding from this source would generally be bright red.
CN: Physiological integrity; CNS: Pharmacological and parenteral therapies; CL: Analysis and application

29. 1. Referral to community agencies is an advocacy role for home health nurses. The role of the advocate implies the home care nurse is able to advise clients how to find alternative sources of care. Giving emotional support, giving therapies to clients, and instructing clients about other resources are direct care activities. Reassuring the client is superficial, and using a walker does not necessarily prevent falls in the future.
CN: Safe, effective care environment; CNS: Management of care; CL: Application

30. 2. Participating in a team conference is an example of indirect care. Direct care is defined as the actual nursing care given to clients in their homes. Direct care may involve assessment of physical or psychosocial status, performance of skilled interventions, supervision of other disciplines, and teaching.
CN: Safe, effective care environment; CNS: Management of care; CL: Application

31. 3. Ingestion of alcohol on a daily basis increases the risk of FAS. Other forms of addictive behavior, such as the ingestion of cocaine and smoking marijuana, increase the risk of fetal abuse—not fetal alcohol syndrome.
CN: Health promotion and maintenance; CNS: None; CL: Analysis and application

32. The nurse in the public health clinic would provide preventive therapy for tuberculosis (TB) to which of the following clients?
1. Clients with human immunodeficiency virus (HIV) infection
2. Clients with recent tuberculin skin tests and low risk
3. Persons with no contact with infectious TB clients
4. Clients with abnormal chest X-rays

Didn't I tell you all your hard work would pay off?

33. The nurse is assessing an elderly client in the emergency room and observes the client to be fearful and noncommunicative. The nurse suspects the client is intimidated by the presence of family members. What is the most appropriate intervention by the nurse?
1. Continue the assessment in private.
2. Be supportive and nonthreatening.
3. Ask the supervisor to talk to the family.
4. Call for the social worker to do a family assessment.

34. The mother of a middle school boy tells the school nurse she is concerned that her 13-year-old son may be depressed. Which behavior would the nurse expect the boy to exhibit?
1. Becomes angry at peers easily
2. Seeks out support from peers
3. Eats several small meals daily
4. Feels he can control everything in his life

35. The hospice bereavement nurse is conducting a family support group. During the session, a 56-year-old client, who recently lost his 82-year-old father to lung cancer, describes how he is responding to his loss. The bereavement nurse expects which sign of grief?
1. Decreased libido
2. Absence of anger and hostility
3. Difficulty crying or controlling crying
4. Clear dreams and imagery of the deceased

36. The home health nurse is visiting a 72-year-old client with severe osteoarthritis. During the visit, the client tells the nurse that his wife died a year ago. Which statement by the client requires further intervention?
1. "My children live close but are very busy."
2. "I really don't have anything to live for."
3. "My health isn't very good, and I don't like to have pain."
4. "I relied on my wife to remember where I placed things."

32. 1. Preventive therapy should be initiated for clients infected with HIV because latent TB can become active if the immune system is weakened. Clients with low risk and negative skin tests are unlikely to be infected with TB or to progress if infected. Clients with no contact with infectious TB cases aren't at high risk for developing TB. Although clients with active TB may have abnormal chest X-rays, many other conditions can cause abnormalities.
CN: Health promotion and maintenance; CNS: None; CL: Application

33. 2. It is most important to provide emotional support in a nonthreatening manner when dealing with the client who may experience family violence. It is also important to provide a private, secure environment for the client to establish trust and a therapeutic relationship. Approaches that may be interpreted as threatening, aggressive, or punitive can increase the anxiety of the perpetrator, increasing the risk of more violence for the victim.
CN: Psychosocial integrity; CNS: None; CL: Application

34. 1. Adolescents experiencing depression may experience and express anger at peers. Adolescents feel a lack of control over their current situation, so they isolate themselves from their peers. The adolescent often has an intake of nutrients insufficient to meet metabolic needs.
CN: Psychosocial integrity; CNS: None; CL: Analysis and application

35. 4. A grieving client usually has vivid, clear dreams and fantasies. He also has a good capacity for imagery, particularly involving the loss. Difficulty crying or controlling crying, absence of anger and hostility, and decreased libido are signs of depression.
CN: Psychosocial integrity; CNS: None; CL: Analysis and application

36. 2. Wishing for death is a sign of depression. Usually after a year, most individuals accept the death of their loved ones and begin restoring their lives. Expressing how he is adapting to his health and family situation may be a sign of the reality of his new life experiences after the loss of his wife. Memory loss can be a sign of dementia or depression.
CN: Psychosocial integrity; CNS: None; CL: Analysis and application

37. The nurse is assessing a laboring client. The client suddenly screams and states that the baby is coming. What is the priority action by the nurse?
1. Calm the mother.
2. Assess for crowning.
3. Take the fetal heart tones.
4. Administer pain medication.

38. The nurse explains the preparation for a bone marrow transplant to a client. Which statements are appropriate for the nurse to make? Select all that apply.
1. An arteriovenous shunt will be established.
2. A course of chemotherapy will be administered.
3. A suitable donor must be identified prior to final preparations for transplant.
4. Total-body radiation will be administered.
5. The donor bone marrow will be injected into the client's bone marrow.
6. The client will be placed in isolation to protect the family.

39. A client has developed oral ulcerations secondary to chemotherapy agents. What is the most appropriate nursing intervention?
1. Serve a high-calorie diet.
2. Use a soft bristle toothbrush to clean teeth.
3. Avoid taking oral temperatures.
4. Rinse the mouth with hydrogen peroxide and water.

40. The new graduate nurse on the cardiac rehabilitation unit is observed looking up a drug prior to administering morning medications. This behavior demonstrates which of the following professional nursing responsibilities? Select all that apply.
1. Continuing education
2. Quality care
3. Resource utilization
4. Ethical practice
5. Healthy environment

37. 2. The priority nursing action is to assess for crowning of the fetus's head and prepare for an imminent delivery. The other actions do not respond to a possible spontaneous delivery of the fetus.
CN: Health promotion and maintenance; CNS: Physiological adaptation; CL: Application

38. 2, 3, and 4. The identified donor's healthy bone marrow is infused intravenously, usually through a peripherally inserted central catheter. An arteriovenous shunt is not established. Chemotherapy and total-body radiation are necessary to prepare the recipient or the healthy bone marrow. Reverse isolation will protect the client from exposure to pathogens from others.
CN: Health promotion and maintenance; CNS: Physiological adaptation; CL: Application

39. 3. If oral ulcers are present, taking oral temperatures will be painful. Use the axillary region, rectum, or ear as sites for temperature readings. Serving a high-calorie diet won't reduce mouth pain and irritation. Use a soft-sponge applicator for oral hygiene, cotton-tipped applicator, or gauze-wrapped finger to clean teeth. Do not use a toothbrush. Give normal saline solution mouthwashes and rinses to reduce pain and inflammation. Hydrogen peroxide mixed with water is too irritating if oral ulcers are present.
CN: Physiological integrity; CNS: Basic care and comfort; CL: Application

40. 1, 2, and 4. The nurse is acting responsibly and continuing her learning. The nurse is practicing quality safe nursing care with integrity and nursing ethics. Resource utilization and maintaining a healthy environment do not apply in this situation.
CN: Safe, effective care environment; CNS: Management of care; CL: Application

41. The nurse is caring for an 8-year-old child diagnosed with attention deficit hyperactivity disorder (ADHD) who has been running around the playroom for the past 15 minutes. Which behavior is the nurse most likely to observe in this client?
1. Lethargy
2. Flight of ideas
3. Short attention span
4. Preoccupation with body parts

42. The nurse is caring for a burn client who is receiving total parenteral nutrition (TPN) at 75 ml/hour. The nurse is most concerned when the client experiences which symptom?
1. Pain
2. Absent bowel sounds
3. Abdominal cramping
4. Increased urine glucose

43. The nurse is admitting a 35-year-old client to an inpatient substance abuse unit with a diagnosis of alcohol dependence. Which comment by the client would the nurse interpret as supporting this diagnosis?
1. "I don't drink more than two beers when I'm out."
2. "I always remember what happens the next day."
3. "I always ask a friend to drive me home when I'm drinking."
4. "I had four tickets for driving while intoxicated last month."

44. A nurse is caring for a client who has been diagnosed with alcoholism in an acute care mental health unit. The client has been referred to Alcoholics Anonymous (AA). Which statement best indicates that the client is ready to begin the AA program?
1. "I know I need help since I can't control my drinking by myself."
2. "I think it will be interesting and helpful to join AA."
3. "I'd like to sponsor another alcoholic with this same problem."
4. "My family is very supportive and will attend meetings with me."

41. 3. Short attention span is a common characteristic of ADHD due to difficulty concentrating. These children show hyperexcitability, not lethargy. Children with this disorder are distracted by environmental stimuli, so they won't be concentrating on their body parts. Flight of ideas is a condition seen in manic states and schizophrenia.
CN: Psychosocial integrity; CNS: None; CL: Application

42. 4. Glycosuria, increased urine glucose, is associated with high blood glucose levels, a complication of TPN. Pain from major burns is expected. Absent bowel sounds are an indication to begin TPN. Abdominal cramping is associated with diarrhea or constipation.
CN: Physiological integrity; CNS: Basic care and comfort; CL: Application

43. 4. Driving while intoxicated can be seen as a symptom of alcohol dependence. Designating drivers and limiting alcohol consumption are self-responsible actions but don't address the underlying problem. The amount one drinks doesn't matter. An alcoholic experiences blackouts, which are periods of amnesia about experiences while intoxicated. By asking someone to drive them home, clients with alcohol dependence rationalize that it's okay to drink if they're responsible.
CN: Psychosocial integrity; CNS: None; CL: Analysis and application

44. 1. In step 1 of AA, a person admits his powerlessness over alcohol and is ready to accept help. This should occur before he begins AA. A supportive family and a desire to help others with the same problem are good for the client, but they don't necessarily indicate readiness to participate in the program.
CN: Psychosocial integrity; CNS: None; CL: Application

CN: Client needs category   CNS: Client needs subcategory   CL: Cognitive level

45. The psychiatric home health nurse is planning care for a client with paranoid schizophrenia who was recently discharged from a mental health facility. Which nursing action should be included in the plan of care?
  1. Confront the client about her hallucinations.
  2. Ask the minister to provide spiritual direction.
  3. Instruct family members to discourage delusions.
  4. Affirm when the client's perceptions and thinking are in touch with reality.

46. The psychiatric home health nurse arrives to visit a client with bipolar disorder. The client is swinging rapidly on the porch swing. She is wearing a red polka dot dress, large yellow hat, and heavy makeup with large gold jewelry. The nurse interprets the client's behavior as evidence of which of the following?
  1. Delusions
  2. Depression
  3. Mania
  4. Paranoia

47. A pediatric nurse is caring for a 4-week-old neonate with severe colic. Which assessment finding does the nurse interpret as a sign of acute pain?
  1. Whimpering
  2. Eyes opened wide
  3. Limp body posture
  4. Wanting to breastfeed frequently

48. A home health nurse is caring for a 4-year-old child diagnosed with juvenile rheumatoid arthritis (JRA). The mother tells the nurse she is concerned about the child's posture. What is the most important information for the nurse to give the mother?
  1. Use a soft mattress.
  2. Turn him prone several times a day.
  3. Support him with fluffy comfortable pillows.
  4. Let him sit in a semireclining position during the day.

45. 4. The nursing plan of care focuses on reinforcing perceptions and thinking that are in touch with reality. Confronting a client about her hallucinations and delusions isn't effective or therapeutic. Spiritual direction is important, but a client with paranoid schizophrenia may have issues surrounding her religious or spiritual orientation. Therefore, asking a minister to provide spiritual direction may not be effective or therapeutic. Using family members could create distrust between the client and the family.
CN: Psychosocial integrity; CNS: None; CL: Application

46. 3. Extreme labile moods are characteristic of clients in the manic phase of bipolar disorder. Hyperactivity, verbosity, and drawing attention to oneself through dress are typical of the manic phase. Delusions and suspiciousness may be seen in bipolar disorder but are more commonly seen in schizophrenia. In the depressive phase, clients are withdrawn, cry, and may not eat. Visual or auditory hallucinations, delusional thoughts, and extreme suspiciousness are behaviors seen in clients diagnosed with paranoid schizophrenia.
CN: Psychosocial integrity; CNS: None; CL: Application

47. 1. Crying, whimpering, and groaning are vocal expressions of acute pain in the neonate. Eyes tightly closed, changes in feeding behavior, and fist clenching with rigidity also are signs of acute pain in the neonate.
CN: Health promotion and maintenance; CNS: None; CL: Application

48. 2. Lying in the prone position is encouraged to straighten hips and knees. A firm mattress is needed to maintain good alignment of spine, hips, and knees, and no pillow or a very thin pillow should be used. Semi-Fowler's position in a recliner increases pressure on the hip joints and should be avoided.
CN: Physiological integrity; CNS: Basic care and comfort; CL: Application

49. The home health nurse is instructing the mother of a child diagnosed with juvenile rheumatoid arthritis (JRA) on interventions to reduce the child's pain and stiffness. What is the most appropriate intervention?
1. Hot packs
2. Alternating heat and cold applications
3. Cold compresses
4. A warm bath

50. The nurse documents an outcome for an elderly client with an indwelling catheter as "client will be free of urinary tract infection (UTI), with negative urine culture and sensitivity (C&S) on removal of catheter." If the client develops a nosocomial UTI, the nurse understands the impact may include which of the following? Select all that apply.
1. The hospital will have to absorb the cost of treatment.
2. The catheter will be reinserted for instillation of antibiotics.
3. Medicare identifies this as a hospital-acquired condition.
4. This outcome could negatively impact evaluation of nursing care.
5. The Joint Commission will note this as a failure to meet national goals.

51. The nurse is assessing a client during a home health visit. The client complains of severe burning on urination. What is the most important information for the nurse to give the client?
1. Drink some cranberry juice.
2. Take a sitz bath twice daily.
3. Avoid carbonated beverages.
4. Drink 2,500 to 3,000 ml of water per day.

52. The nurse is caring for a client with hearing loss on the rehabilitation unit. In planning care, the nurse documents ways to minimize the difficulty and frustration when communicating with the client. Select all that may apply.
1. Stand or sit in his line of vision.
2. Close the door to the client's room.
3. Talk loudly and slowly to the client.
4. Minimize distraction from television and visitors.
5. Check for use and function of hearing aid.
6. Get his attention before communicating.

You've finished 50 questions! The remaining 25 should be a snap!

SNAP

49. 4. Heat is beneficial to children with arthritis. Moist heat is best for relieving pain and stiffness. The most efficient and practical method is in the bathtub. Cold, cool, or lukewarm treatment isn't beneficial in relieving pain or stiffness in children with JRA. Hot packs and heating pads could burn the child.
CN: Physiological integrity; CNS: Basic care and comfort; CL: Application

50. 1, 3, 4, and 5. Urinary tract infection with an indwelling catheter is identified as a hospital-acquired condition that is not reimbursed by Medicare or insurance. The hospital will have to absorb the cost of treating the client. The Joint Commission has prevention of UTI with indwelling catheters as one of its national patient safety goals. Nursing care could be evaluated negatively when there is an adverse outcome. The client will not likely receive antibiotics through another indwelling catheter. Antibiotic therapy will be administered parenterally or orally.
CN: Physiological integrity; CNS: Reduction of risk potential; CL: Application

51. 4. Drinking large amounts of water will help flush bacteria from the urinary tract. Avoid tea, coffee, carbonated drinks, and alcoholic beverages because of bladder irritation. Avoid using bubble baths, perfumed soaps, or bath powders in the perineal area. A sitz bath may provide comfort but does not address the priority need.
CN: Physiological integrity; CNS: Basic care and comfort; CL: Application

52. 1, 2, 4, 5, and 6. It is essential to communicate appropriately with the hearing-impaired client. Face the client and get his attention before speaking to him. Eliminate distractions and background noises. Make sure the client has his hearing aid in and that the battery is working. Speaking loudly and slowly is not necessary and may interfere with comprehension, as loud sounds may reverberate.
CN: Physiological integrity; CNS: Basic care and comfort; CL: Application

CN: Client needs category   CNS: Client needs subcategory   CL: Cognitive level

53. A 72-year-old client is being discharged from outpatient surgery after having a cataract removed from his right eye. Prior to discharging the client, it is most important for the nurse to teach the client to:
1. resume all activities as before.
2. begin eye drops in 3 days.
3. not rub or place pressure on the eye.
4. wear eye shields on both eyes at night.

53. 3. Rubbing or placing pressure on the eye increases the risk of accidental injury to ocular structures. An eye shield should be worn on the operative eye at night. Eye drops should be instilled as ordered beginning the day of discharge. Additional teaching includes caution against lifting objects, straining, strenuous exercise, and sexual activity because such activities can increase intraocular pressure. Caution against sleeping on the operative side to reduce the risk of accidental injury to ocular structures. Glasses or shaded lenses should be worn to protect the eye during waking hours after the eye dressing is removed.

CN: Physiological integrity; CNS: Reduction of risk potential; CL: Application

54. The nurse is planning discharge instructions for the client going home on Coumadin (warfarin sodium). What is the priority teaching?
1. Avoid injury and watch for signs of bleeding.
2. Take the medication at the same time daily.
3. Injections may be given in the abdomen.
4. Dietary restrictions include tomatoes and cucumbers.

54. 1. Coumadin is an anticoagulant, so the priority teaching is to watch for signs of hemorrhage and prevent bleeding. It is administered orally. The client should have scheduled blood tests for prothrombin time. Leafy green vegetables are to be avoided.

CN: Physiological integrity; CNS: Pharmacological and parenteral therapies; CL: Application

55. The nurse and occupational therapist are planning an outdoor volleyball game and picnic for eight mental health clients. What action should the nurse take for the two clients taking nortriptyline (Pamelor) for depression?
1. Be aware that this drug can cause hypotension.
2. Recognize that these clients may experience excessive thirst.
3. Omit the morning dose on the day of the picnic.
4. Provide protective clothing and apply sunscreen before going out.

55. 4. A common adverse effect of this drug is sensitivity to the sun. Protective clothing and sunscreen are worn in the sun. Pamelor is a tricyclic antidepressant, often administered at night because it may cause drowsiness. This drug can cause hypertension. It doesn't work immediately but takes 2 to 3 weeks to achieve the desired effect.

CN: Physiological integrity; CNS: Pharmacological and parenteral therapies; CL: Application

56. The nurse preceptor is preparing to admit a postoperative thyroidectomy client who has just returned from surgery. Which instructions should the preceptor provide the new graduate nurse regarding specific preparations and observations for the postoperative client? Select all that apply.
1. Place bed in high Fowler's position.
2. Have emergency tracheotomy set on hand.
3. Check behind the neck for bleeding.
4. Monitor voice quality regularly.
5. Observe for sudden increase in temperature, respiratory distress, and tetany.

56. 2, 3, 4, and 5. Postoperative thyroidectomy clients may need humidified oxygen and to be placed in the semi-Fowler's position. Vital signs will need to be monitored for any changes, and the client should be observed for bleeding behind the neck and back of dressing. It is important to observe for signs of respiratory distress and to have tracheotomy equipment on hand. Monitor voice quality for injury to vocal chords. If the client develops thyroid storm/crisis postoperatively, the temperature could rise as high as 106° F, and tetany may develop if the parathyroid glands were injured or removed.

CN: Physiological integrity; CNS: Reduction of risk potential CL: Application

57. The emergency room team is caring for a 52-year-old client in cardiac arrest. After all emergency measures were administered, the client was pronounced dead after 1 hour and 40 minutes of resuscitation. At the end of the experience, the new graduate nurse reviews the activities that occurred during the arrest. Select all that apply.
1. Establishment of nasal oxygen
2. Removal of clothing
3. Application of electrodes for cardiac monitor
4. Drawing venous blood for blood gases
5. Establishing an I.V. line
6. Insertion of a Foley catheter
7. Cardiac defibrillation
8. Administration of I.V. medications
9. Call for chaplain and family privacy

57. 2, 3, 5, 6, 7, 8, and 9. In the emergency room, all of the listed activities could be employed during cardiac resuscitation, except that an endotracheal tube would be inserted for oxygenation and arterial blood is required for blood gas measurements.

CN: Physiological integrity; CNS: Reduction of risk potential; CL: Application

58. The nurse is teaching the client and family about the total parenteral nutrition (TPN) that the client is receiving. The nurse would include which of the following information? Select all that apply.
1. TPN is administered through a large central blood vessel.
2. The solution contains sugar, protein, and fat for increased calories.
3. The client may experience constipation.
4. Tests to monitor blood and urine glucose levels will be done.
5. The client will need insulin to prevent diabetes.

58. 1, 2, and 4. There is a possibility of abdominal cramping and diarrhea, not constipation, from TPN. Some clients may need insulin to regulate blood glucose levels during TPN, but the client will not develop diabetes from TPN.

CN: Physiological integrity; CNS: Pharmacological and parenteral therapies; CL: Application

59. The nurse is caring for a frail, elderly client. At the client care conference, the family asks if it is safe for him to receive narcotics for pain. The nurse is aware that the client is receiving hydromorphone hydrochloride (Dilaudid) for pain. What is the most appropriate response for the nurse to give the family?
1. The narcotic is safe because it does not accumulate in the body.
2. The drug does not cause any problems with breathing.
3. The drug is not as strong as morphine.
4. This drug is similar to methamphetamine.

59. 1. Hydromorphone is a fast-acting narcotic analgesic drug and is a useful alternative to morphine or meperidine due to its short half-life. Morphine and meperidine can increase the risk of confusion in the elderly. Hydromorphone is a synthetic drug similar to morphine with 8 to 10 times more potent analgesic effect. Respiratory depression may occur but is less frequent than with some other narcotics. Dilaudid is not a central nervous system stimulant as is methamphetamine.

CN: Physiological integrity; CNS: Pharmacological and parenteral therapies; CL: Application

60. The nurse is caring for a client who had a pacemaker inserted over 20 years ago. He has been admitted to the cardiac care unit with possible bacterial endocarditis. The nurse would expect which test to confirm the diagnosis of bacterial endocarditis?
1. Electrolytes
2. Blood cultures
3. Prothrombin time (PT)
4. Venereal Disease Research Laboratory (VDRL)

60. 2. Blood cultures are crucial in diagnosing bacterial endocarditis. Electrolyte levels indicate abnormalities that occur with drug therapy as well as with complications associated with heart failure. PT values are useful in monitoring anticoagulant therapy. A positive VDRL may be evidence of syphilitic heart disease.

CN: Physiological integrity; CNS: Reduction of risk potential; CL: Application

61. The nurse is preparing a client for cardiac catheterization. What is the priority nursing communication?
1. "Do you have allergies to shellfish or contrast dye?"
2. "Have you had this procedure before?"
3. "You will need to fast for 24 hours before the procedure."
4. "You'll be given medication to help you sleep during the procedure."

61. 1. The nurse must assess the client for allergies to iodine before the procedure because the dye used during catheterization contains iodine. Knowing the client's history and prior experience with this procedure would be helpful, but knowing the client's allergies is more important. The client is instructed to fast for 6 hours before the procedure. The client will be asked to empty his bladder before the procedure. The client needs to stay awake during the procedure to follow directions, such as taking a deep breath and holding it during injection of the dye, and to report chest, neck, or jaw discomfort.
CN: Physiological integrity; CNS: Reduction of risk potential; CL: Application

62. The nurse is caring for a 60-year-old male client suspected of having coronary artery disease. The physician has ordered a noninvasive diagnostic test to evaluate cardiac changes. The nurse prepares the client for which test?
1. Cardiac biopsy
2. Cardiac catheterization
3. Magnetic resonance imaging (MRI)
4. Pericardiocentesis

62. 3. MRI is a noninvasive procedure that aids in the diagnosis and detection of thoracic aortic aneurysm and evaluation of coronary artery disease, pericardial disease, and cardiac masses. Cardiac biopsy, cardiac catheterization, and pericardiocentesis are invasive techniques used to evaluate cardiac changes.
CN: Health promotion and maintenance; CNS: None; CL: Application

63. The nurse working in the telemetry unit notices a premature ventricular contraction (PVC) on the client's monitor. While assessing the client, he states that he felt something "flip flop" in his chest. There are no other PVCs noted in the following hour. The nurse would make which documentation?
1. One PVC occurred today between 1:00 and 2:00 p.m. There was no preceding P wave, and the QRS complex was wide and inverted.
2. One PVC was observed on monitor between 1:00 and 2:00 p.m. today. The client stated that he felt a "flip flop" in his chest. No changes in vital signs and no complaints of chest pain or shortness of breath.
3. Client had one PVC today, observed closely, no other PVCs noted.
4. Only one PVC was observed on monitor between 1:00 and 2:00 today.

63. 2. It is important to chart about the client and his condition and to note frequency and any abnormal symptoms with premature ventricular contractions (PVCs). Response 1 describes the PVC but not the client. Responses 3 and 4 are brief and incomplete. PVCs are caused by an ectopic cardiac pacemaker located in the ventricle. PVCs are characterized by premature and bizarrely shaped QRS complexes usually wider than 120 msec on the width of the electrocardiogram. These complexes are not preceded by a P wave, and the T wave is usually large, and its direction is opposite the major deflection of the QRS. The clinical significance of PVCs depends on their frequency, complexity, and hemodynamic response.
CN: Physiological integrity; CNS: Reduction of risk potential; CL: Application

64. The nurse is recording an electrocardiogram (ECG) for a client with a pacemaker in the cardiac clinic. He has had the fixed-rate pacemaker for many years and states that at times he feels funny and gets nauseated. The nurse interprets which ECG pattern as possible pacemaker malfunction?
1. Short T waves
2. Absence of P waves
3. Pacing spikes appearing at different times during a cardiac cycle
4. Pacing spike followed by a wide QRS complex

64. 3. When pacing spikes appear at different times during a cardiac cycle, it indicates a failure to capture. Failure to capture may result in inappropriate pacing; the ECG would show a pacing spike delivered on time but not followed by a wide QRS complex. Tall T waves or an irregular heart rate indicate a failure-to-sense malfunction. P waves are not expected. The pacemaker takes over for the sinoatrial node. A pacing spike followed by a QRS indicates a paced beat.
CN: Physiological integrity; CNS: Reduction of risk potential; CL: Application

65. The nurse is reviewing discharge teaching for an elderly client who was treated for arterial insufficiency and has undergone an endarterectomy. What is the most important information for the nurse to provide? Select all that apply.
1. You may leave your feet open to the air.
2. Sit and rest for several hours a day.
3. Avoid crossing your legs at the knees or ankles.
4. The physical therapist will come 3 times a week for 2 weeks.
5. Avoid constrictive clothing, such as tight elastic on socks.

66. The nurse is instructing the client who will be discharged on anticoagulant therapy. Which of the following is an appropriate instruction?
1. Do not shave with an electric razor.
2. You may take ibuprofen or aspirin for pain.
3. Take the anticoagulant at the same time each day.
4. It is important to eat green, leafy vegetables and salad daily.

67. The nurse on the rehabilitation unit is admitting a visually impaired elderly client for cardiac rehabilitation therapy. What plan should the nurse include to reduce sensory deprivation for a visually impaired client?
1. Keep the lights dimmed.
2. Close the curtains or blinds on windows to reduce glare.
3. Open the hospital door so bright light can shine in the room.
4. Open the curtains during the day so the sun can shine brightly.

68. The nurse is caring for a hearing-impaired client in the coronary care unit. To reduce sensory overload for the client, it is most important for the nurse to do what?
1. Reduce the overhead light to dim.
2. Draw bedside curtains so the client is less distracted.
3. Allow all family members to stay with the client.
4. Limit bedside conversation to that directed to the client.

Only 10 left. You're amazing!

65. 3, 4, and 5. Leg crossing should be avoided because it compresses the vessels in the legs. Feet and extremities must be protected to reduce the risk of trauma. Clients usually go home on physical therapy to improve mobility and circulation. Sitting for several hours isn't recommended. Constrictive clothing, such as tight elastic on socks, should be avoided to prevent compression of vessels in the legs.

CN: Physiological integrity; CNS: Reduction of risk potential; CL: Application

66. 3. It is important to take the anticoagulant at the same time each day to maintain an adequate blood level. An electric razor reduces the risk of cutting the skin. Avoid the use of standard razors. Avoid taking aspirin or ibuprofen because these drugs decrease clotting time. Eating a large amount of green, leafy vegetables, which contain vitamin K, increases the clotting time, thus requiring more anticoagulants.

CN: Physiological integrity; CNS: Pharmacological and parenteral therapies; CL: Application

67. 2. Closing curtains or blinds on windows can reduce glare and improve vision for the older client. Controlled lighting can help the older client see better in the hospital. Adequate background lighting helps the older client decrease visual accommodation when moving from brightly lit to dimly lit rooms and hallways.

CN: Physiological integrity; CNS: Reduction of risk potential; CL: Application

68. 4. It is most important to limit bedside conversation to that directed to the client to create fewer disturbances, thus reducing sensory overload. Conversations at the bedside that do not include the client may increase anxiety and heighten his senses as he tries to understand. Turning off or dimming the overhead lights further reduces visual stimulation and facilitates day and night light fluctuations. Although fostering family interaction with the client is necessary, only one or two family members should be allowed to visit with the client at one time. Crowding of people in the client's room may precipitate a loss of privacy and control for the client.

CN: Physiological integrity; CNS: Reduction of risk potential; CL: Application

69. The nurse is preparing a client for a total left knee replacement. Which of the following instructions are important to include preoperatively? Select all that apply.
1. You will be placed on a continuous passive motion (CPM) device.
2. You may actually experience little discomfort for the first day if the anesthesia includes a nerve block of the left leg.
3. You will be up walking within 24 hours.
4. Physical therapy will begin after you go home.
5. You should take what you need to be pain free.

70. A home care aide notified the agency that she found a client lying on the floor. When the home health nurse arrives, she quickly assesses the newly diagnosed diabetic client. The assessment includes the following: client is semicomatose, apical heart rate is 102 beats/minute, blood pressure is 84/30 mm Hg, and skin is warm and dry. The nurse instructs the home care aide to call for an ambulance because these are signs of which condition?
1. Hypoglycemia
2. Cardiogenic shock
3. Diabetic ketoacidosis (DKA)
4. Hyperosmolar hyperglycemic nonketotic syndrome (HHNS)

71. A nurse is standing next to a person eating fried shrimp at a parade. Suddenly, the man clutches at his throat and is unable to speak, cough, or breathe. The nurse asks the man if he's choking, and he nods yes. What action should the nurse take next?
1. Attempt rescue breathing.
2. Perform the Heimlich maneuver.
3. Deliver external chest compressions.
4. Use the head tilt-chin lift maneuver to establish the airway.

72. The nurse is caring for an unstable cardiac client and must be prepared for a possible cardiopulmonary emergency. What is the most important preparation the nurse should include?
1. Have nasal oxygen ready when needed.
2. Place an oropharyngeal airway at the bedside.
3. Alert the family that he is not stable.
4. Locate where the emergency cart is on the unit.

69. 1, 2, and 3. It is important to prepare the client for the use of the CPM device on the operative leg. Nerve blocks are commonly used along with general anesthesia, and clients may have little postoperative pain. Physical therapy begins in the hospital, and it is important for the client to walk. The use of analgesics is important for the client's comfort and to be able to cooperate with therapy. It is not realistic to expect to be free of pain.
CN: Physiological integrity; CNS: Reduction of risk potential; CL: Application

70. 3. DKA develops as a result of severe insulin deficiency. The incidence of DKA generally results from undiagnosed diabetes and inadequacy of prescribed medication and dietary therapies. Signs of DKA include flushed dry skin, restlessness, fruity odor of the breath, and confusion, and the client may become unconscious. Hypoglycemia involves episodes of low blood glucose levels caused by erratic or altered absorption of insulin. In cardiogenic shock, the client has pale, cool, and moist skin. HHNS is a deadly complication of diabetes distinguished by severe hyperglycemia, dehydration, and changed mental status.
CN: Physiological integrity; CNS: Physiological adaptation; CL: Application

71. 2. If a conscious victim acknowledges that he's choking, the best response is to perform the Heimlich maneuver to relieve the airway obstruction. The other options are used for an unresponsive victim with absent heart rate and breathing.
CN: Physiological integrity; CNS: Physiological adaptation; CL: Application

72. 2. A nurse should learn to anticipate clinical deterioration before overt signs and symptoms are apparent. If a client is having breathing difficulties, the nurse should place an oropharyngeal airway at the bedside while the client is monitored for deterioration. The emergency cart should be placed outside the client's room for easy access. If breathing stops, the client will need to be intubated and placed on a respirator, if necessary. The client should have a stable I.V. line for administration of emergency drugs. Alerting the family could cause anxiety that the client may respond to.
CN: Physiological integrity; CNS: Physiological adaptation; CL: Application

73. The nurse in the telemetry unit is preparing a client with sinus tachycardia for cardioversion. It is most important for the nurse to do what?
1. Keep the client awake and alert.
2. Keep the side rails up for client safety.
3. Set the machine on SYNC and charge at 200 watts.
4. Set the machine on DEFIB and charge at 400 watts.

74. The nurse is assessing a prenatal client who is at 37 weeks' gestation. The nurse performs Leopold's maneuvers to assess the position of the fetus. After performing the maneuvers, the nurse suspects that the physician will attempt external version because the head of the fetus is at the:
1. symphysis pubis.
2. top of the uterus.
3. on the mother's left side.
4. vertex position.

75. The pediatric nurse is caring for a 10-month-old infant. The physician orders an I.V. infusion of dextrose 5% in quarter-normal saline solution to be infused at 7 ml/kg/hour. The infant weighs 22 lb. How many ml/hour of the ordered solution should the nurse infuse? Record your answer using a whole number.

_____ ml/hour

73. **3.** If cardioversion is needed, the nurse should set the machine on SYNC and look for a marker on each QRS complex. The nurse should anticipate that the cardioversion will be started at a low energy level and increase as needed. The client will be sedated for the procedure. Lowering the side rails will make it easier to place paddle electrodes.

CN: Physiological integrity; CNS: Physiological adaptation; CL: Application

74. **2.** If the fetal head is palpated at the top of the uterus, the fetus is in the breech position. The physician may consider external version to convert the fetus to a vertex lie, or head-down position. This is accomplished by applying pressure on the maternal abdomen to turn the infant over, as in a somersault.

CN: Physiological integrity; CNS: Reduction of risk potential; CL: Application

75. 70. To perform this dosage calculation, the nurse should first convert the infant's weight to kilograms: 2.2 lb/kg; convert 22 lb to kg: 22 lb/2.2 = 10 kg. Next, the nurse should multiply the infant's weight by the ordered rate: 10 kg × 7 ml/kg/hour = 70 ml/hour.

CN: Physiological integrity; CNS: Pharmacological and parenteral therapies; CL: Application

Here's another comprehensive test to practice for the NCLEX. Check it out!

COMPREHENSIVE
Test 4

1. A nurse-manager has identified several interpersonal problems with a staff member. Which approach is best for the nurse-manager to take?
1. Map out a plan of action for each problem and discuss it.
2. Begin to solve the first problem and work through the list.
3. Ask the staff member to select the problem she would like to resolve.
4. Prioritize the problems with the staff member and begin to work on them together.

2. A team leader notes increasing unrest among the staff members. Which action is best for the team leader to take?
1. Discuss the problem with a coworker.
2. Report the problem to the nurse-manager.
3. Bring the group together and discuss the team leader's perception.
4. Ignore the problem and hope the attitude won't interfere with the functioning of the floor.

3. A physician ordered a urine specimen for culture and sensitivity stat. Which approach is best for a nurse to use in delegating this task?
1. "We need a stat urine culture on the client in room 101."
2. "Please get the urine for culture for the client in room 101."
3. "A stat urine was ordered for the client in room 101. Would you get it?"
4. "We need urine for culture stat on the client in room 101. Tell me when you send it to the lab."

1. 4. It's important for the nurse-manager and staff member to agree on which problem is a priority and work on its resolution together. Mapping out the problem without input from the staff member leaves the possibility that the staff member might not be committed to work on its resolution.
CN: Safe, effective care environment; CNS: Management of care; CL: Application

2. 3. The leader should comment to the group on the observed behavior. This is a firm approach but one that shows concern. Ignoring problems or discussing them with someone else doesn't confront the issue at hand.
CN: Safe, effective care environment; CNS: Management of care; CL: Application

3. 4. This option not only delegates the task but also provides a checkpoint. To effectively delegate, you need to follow up on what someone else is doing. The other options don't provide for feedback, which is essential for communication and delegation.
CN: Safe, effective care environment; CNS: Management of care; CL: Application

4. A 67-year-old client asks the nurse, "Do you think it's wrong to masturbate?" Which response by the nurse is best?
1. "How do you feel about that?"
2. "Do you really want to do that?"
3. "I think you're a little too old for that."
4. "Why don't you ask your physician?"

5. A nurse is assisting a client on a clear liquid diet in selecting his menu. The nurse determines further teaching is necessary when the client selects which of the following?
1. Gelatin dessert
2. Milkshake
3. Popsicle or similar frozen dessert
4. Tea

6. Which medication should a nurse withhold from a client 6 hours before a series of pulmonary function tests (PFTs)?
1. Azithromycin
2. Robitussin
3. Albuterol
4. Cefaclor

7. A client returns to a nursing unit after a bronchoscopy and is expectorating pink-tinged mucus. Which action by the nurse is most appropriate?
1. Notify the physician as soon as possible.
2. Take the client's vital signs and then call the physician.
3. Auscultate the client's lung fields for possible pulmonary edema.
4. Tell the client this is expected after the procedure but continue to monitor the client.

8. The assessment of a client on the first day after thoracotomy shows a temperature of 100° F (37.8° C); heart rate, 96 beats/minute; blood pressure, 136/86 mm Hg; and shallow respirations at 24 breaths/minute, with rhonchi at the bases. The client complains of incisional pain. Which nursing action is most important?
1. Medicate the client for pain.
2. Help the client get out of bed.
3. Give ibuprofen (Motrin) as ordered to reduce the fever.
4. Encourage the client to cough and deep-breathe.

4. 1. It's essential in communication to find out how the client thinks and feels. Telling the client that he's too old or asking him if he really wants to do that is biased and puts the client down. The last option tells the client the nurse isn't interested. The client might be too uncomfortable to discuss this topic with the physician.
CN: Psychosocial integrity; CNS: None; CL: Analysis

5. 2. Full-liquid diets contain milk, cereal, gruel, clear liquids, and plain frozen desserts. The clear liquid diet contains only foods that are clear and liquid at room or body temperature, such as gelatin, fat-free broth, bouillon, popsicles or similar frozen desserts, tea, and regular or decaffeinated coffee.
CN: Physiological integrity; CNS: Basic care and comfort; CL: Analysis

6. 3. PFTs measure the volume and capacity of air. If a bronchodilator is given, it will improve the bronchial airflow and alter the test results. The other drugs would have no effect on the bronchial tree with regard to PFT results.
CN: Physiological integrity; CNS: Pharmacological and parenteral therapies; CL: Application

7. 4. Pink-tinged mucus is an expected outcome after a bronchoscopy due to irritation of the bronchial tree. The client should be told this is common but that he'll be monitored. The physician doesn't need to be called with this finding. This symptom isn't related to pulmonary edema.
CN: Health promotion and maintenance; CNS: None; CL: Application

8. 1. Although all the interventions are incorporated in this client's care plan, the priority is to relieve pain and make the client comfortable. This would give the client the energy and stamina to achieve the other objectives.
CN: Physiological integrity; CNS: Basic care and comfort; CL: Application

9. Which nursing intervention is most important to include in a nursing care plan for a client with atelectasis?
1. Give oxygen continuously at 3 L/minute.
2. Cough and deep-breathe every 4 hours.
3. Use the incentive spirometer every hour.
4. Get the client out of bed to a chair every day.

10. Two hours after submucous resection, a client's nostrils are packed and a drip pad is anchored under the nose. Which assessment alerts the nurse that the surgical site is bleeding?
1. Frequent swallowing
2. Dry mucous membranes
3. Decrease in urine output
4. Temperature elevation

11. A bedridden client develops disuse osteoporosis. Which nursing intervention is most important for this client?
1. Turn, cough, and deep-breathe.
2. Increase fluids to 3,000 ml daily.
3. Promote venous return by elevating the legs.
4. Provide active and passive range-of-motion (ROM) exercises.

12. An elderly client on bed rest for a week after a bout of pneumonia is in a negative nitrogen balance. Which complication has highest priority?
1. Constipation
2. Renal calculi
3. Muscle wasting
4. Vitamin B$_6$ deficiency

13. The nurse reviews the arterial blood gas results of a client with asthma. The nurse is aware that the client's partial pressure of arterial oxygen (Pao$_2$) result will provide information about which of the following?
1. Respiratory status
2. Degree of dyspnea
3. Efficiency of gas exchange
4. Effectiveness of ventilation

You're off to a good start! Keep going!

9. **3.** Incentive spirometry is used to prevent or treat atelectasis. Done every hour, it will produce deep inhalations that help open the collapsed alveoli. Oxygen use doesn't encourage deep inhalation. Coughing and deep breathing are good interventions but rarely result in as deep an inspiratory effort as using an incentive spirometer and should be performed more frequently than every 4 hours. Getting the client out of bed will also help expand the lungs and stimulate deep breathing, but it's done less frequently than incentive spirometry.
CN: Safe, effective care environment; CNS: Management of care; CL: Application

10. **1.** Frequent swallowing is a sign of hemorrhage in this surgery. Decreased urine output and dry mucous membranes as well as temperature elevation are usually signs of dehydration.
CN: Physiological integrity; CNS: Reduction of risk potential; CL: Analysis

11. **4.** All the interventions listed are good for a bedridden client. However, active and passive ROM exercises provide the mechanical stresses of weight bearing that are absent and their absence can lead to disuse osteoporosis.
CN: Health promotion and maintenance; CNS: None; CL: Application

12. **3.** Negative nitrogen balance leads to muscle wasting. The body breaks down muscle tissue to use as energy. Renal calculi can be a complication of bed rest and demineralization of the bone, but treating a negative nitrogen balance takes priority. Constipation and vitamin B$_6$ deficiency also need to be corrected but aren't the highest priority.
CN: Physiological integrity; CNS: Physiological adaptation; CL: Application

13. **3.** The Pao$_2$ reflects the gas exchange ventilation and perfusion. It doesn't measure the respiratory status, degree of dyspnea, or effectiveness of ventilation.
CN: Physiological integrity; CNS: Reduction of risk potential; CL: Application

14. The nurse prepares to administer morphine to a client with an acute myocardial infarction for which reason?
1. To decrease cardiac output
2. To increase preload and afterload
3. To increase myocardial oxygen demand
4. To decrease myocardial oxygen demand

15. A toddler is ordered 350 mg of amoxicillin (Augmentin) by mouth, four times per day. The pharmacy supplies a bottle of amoxicillin with a concentration of 250 mg/5 ml. How many milliliters would the nurse give for each dose? Record the answer using a whole number:
_____ milliliters

16. A nurse is assessing a client and notes an increase in the tactile fremitus. Which condition would the nurse suspect with this client?
1. Atelectasis
2. Emphysema
3. Pneumonia
4. Pneumothorax

17. A client with an arm cast complains of severe pain in the affected extremity, and decreased sensation and motion are noted. Swelling in the fingers is also increased. What is the most important intervention?
1. Elevating the arm
2. Removing the cast
3. Giving an analgesic
4. Calling the physician

18. A client is hospitalized for 5 days with mononucleosis. Which assessment finding indicates a possibly serious consequence?
1. Vomiting
2. Dark brown urine
3. Temperature of 101° F (38.3° C)
4. Cervical lymphadenopathy

19. A nurse is teaching a client about lifestyle changes that need to be made after a myocardial infarction (MI). The diagnosis of ineffective coping is supported when the client is observed in which action?
1. Reading a book about meal planning
2. Pacing the floor of his room on occasion
3. Sitting quietly in his room for a short time
4. Telling his family he didn't have an MI

14. 4. Morphine will calm and relax the client and decrease respiratory rate, anxiety, and stress, thus decreasing myocardial oxygen demand. It doesn't have any effect on cardiac output or preload or afterload.
CN: Physiological integrity; CNS: Pharmacological and parenteral therapies; CL: Application

15. 7. The nurse would give 7 ml for each dose. Use the following equation:
dose on hand/quantity on hand = dose desired/X.
In this example, the equation is:
250 mg/5 ml = 350 mg/X.
$X = 7$ ml.
CN: Physiological integrity; CNS: Pharmacological and parenteral therapies; CL: Analysis

16. 3. Pneumonia produces a consolidation of mucus and debris. Mucus causes the lung field to have an increase in tactile fremitus. The other diseases involve air, which would decrease tactile fremitus.
CN: Health promotion and maintenance; CNS: None; CL: Analysis

17. 4. The cast may be too tight and may need to be split or removed by the physician. Notify the physician when circulation, sensation, or motion is impaired. The arm should already be elevated. Giving analgesics wouldn't be the first step, as it may mask the signs of a serious problem.
CN: Physiological integrity; CNS: Reduction of risk potential; CL: Application

18. 2. Dark brown urine could indicate the presence of bilirubin and implicate liver involvement. The other answers are typical findings for a client with this diagnosis.
CN: Physiological integrity; CNS: Physiological adaptation; CL: Analysis

19. 4. The client is showing the defense mechanism of denial. Reading a book on meal planning is a positive intervention. Pacing the floor on occasion is a form of anxiety that's normal for the client to experience. Sitting quietly is a normal behavior. The client needs time to come to terms with his diagnosis.
CN: Psychosocial integrity; CNS: None; CL: Analysis

20. A client with a history of myasthenia gravis is admitted to the emergency department with complaints of respiratory distress. The client's condition worsens, and arterial blood gases are drawn. The nurse anticipates that the client will develop which condition?
1. Metabolic acidosis
2. Metabolic alkalosis
3. Respiratory acidosis
4. Respiratory alkalosis

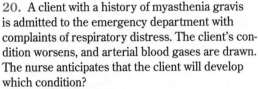

I'm impressed! Keep up the good work!

20. 3. The client has a restrictive lung problem because of myasthenia gravis. This is aggravated by respiratory distress. Because of the restrictive problem, the client won't be able to exhale efficiently and carbon dioxide will build up, causing respiratory acidosis. Metabolic acidosis is a metabolic condition that occurs with either accumulation of acids or excessive loss of bases in the body, such as in diarrhea or renal failure. Metabolic alkalosis occurs due to excessive acid loss or base retention, such as from vomiting. Respiratory alkalosis results from a decreased carbon dioxide level, which could occur if the client were hyperventilating.

CN: Physiological integrity; CNS: Physiological adaptation; CL: Analysis

21. A client who had a thoracotomy is using oxygen and having an arterial blood gas (ABG) analysis. What is the most appropriate information for the nurse to tell the client?
1. "I will shave the puncture site before the test."
2. "You need to keep the oxygen mask on for the entire test."
3. "You'll be suctioned immediately before the blood is drawn."
4. "You won't be allowed to drink anything for 2 hours before the blood is drawn."

21. 2. To determine the effectiveness of oxygen therapy, ABGs are drawn with the oxygen in use. This also needs to be written on the test form. No special preparations for the test with regard to skin preparation or diet are needed. Suctioning decreases available oxygen.

CN: Physiological integrity; CNS: Basic care and comfort; CL: Application

22. Which condition causes heart failure after a myocardial infarction (MI)?
1. Increased workload of the heart
2. Increased oxygen demands of the heart
3. Inability of the heart chambers to adequately fill
4. Impairment of contractile function of the damaged myocardium

22. 4. After an MI, the injured myocardium is replaced by scar tissue. This scar tissue causes the ventricle to pump less efficiently. After an MI has resolved, oxygen and workload demands should normalize and the heart's chambers should fill adequately.

CN: Physiological integrity; CNS: Physiological adaptation; CL: Application

23. A client is admitted to the emergency department with severe epistaxis. The physician inserts posterior packing. Later, the client is anxious and says he doesn't feel he's breathing right. Which nursing action is appropriate?
1. Cut the packing strings and remove the packing.
2. Reassure the client that what he's experiencing is normal.
3. Ask the client to fully explain what he means by "right."
4. Use a flashlight and inspect the posterior oral cavity of the client.

23. 4. The nurse must assess the patency of the airway. The packing might have become dislodged. The nurse shouldn't remove the packing or give the client false reassurance. The client is too anxious to explain what he means.

CN: Physiological integrity; CNS: Reduction of risk potential; CL: Analysis

24. The nurse is teaching another nurse about pulmonary capillary wedge pressure. Which response is the most accurate regarding this pressure?
1. "It reflects systemic vascular resistance."
2. "It reflects right ventricular end pressure."
3. "It reflects right atrial presystolic pressure."
4. "It reflects left ventricular end-diastolic pressure."

25. The nurse is teaching a student nurse about the purpose of diaphragmatic breathing exercises for a client with chronic obstructive pulmonary disease (COPD). Which statement by the nurse is correct?
1. "It dilates the bronchioles."
2. "It decreases vital capacity."
3. "It increases residual volume."
4. "It decreases alveolar ventilation."

26. A client with chronic obstructive pulmonary disease (COPD) is being discharged from the hospital. The nurse provided teaching on medications, diet, and exercise. Which statement by the client indicates further teaching is necessary?
1. "I'll eat six small meals a day."
2. "I'll get a flu shot every winter."
3. "I'll walk every morning before breakfast."
4. "I'll call my physician if I get cold symptoms."

27. The nurse is caring for a client showing symptoms of bronchial obstruction. Which assessment finding would the nurse expect to find?
1. Hacking cough
2. Diminished breath sounds
3. Production of rust-colored sputum
4. Decreased use of accessory muscles

28. A client has just started treatment with rifampin for tuberculosis. Which statement indicates the client has a good understanding of his medication?
1. "I won't go to family gatherings for 6 months."
2. "My urine will look orange because of the medication."
3. "Now, I don't need to cover my mouth or nose when I sneeze or cough."
4. "I told my wife to throw away all the spoons and forks before I come home."

24. 4. The pulmonary capillary wedge pressure is the reflection of the pressure in the left ventricle at rest, which is end diastole. Wedge pressure doesn't reflect pressures in the right side of the heart or systemic vascular resistance.
CN: Physiological integrity; CNS: Physiological adaptation; CL: Application

25. 1. In COPD, the bronchioles constrict during exhalation due to pressure changes in the lungs. Diaphragmatic breathing exercises keep the bronchioles open during exhalation. These exercises aren't performed for the other reasons stated.
CN: Physiological integrity; CNS: Reduction of risk potential; CL: Application

26. 3. The worst time of the day for a client with COPD is morning. Exercise is important but should be done later in the day. All other choices are appropriate for the client with COPD.
CN: Physiological integrity; CNS: Basic care and comfort; CL: Application

27. 2. Bronchial obstruction means no passage of air through the bronchi, so diminished or no breath sounds would be heard. A hacking cough is often associated with upper respiratory tract infection and dryness in the upper airways. Rust-colored sputum is a sign of pneumococcal pneumonia. There would be increased use of accessory muscles.
CN: Physiological integrity; CNS: Physiological adaptation; CL: Application

28. 2. Rifampin discolors body fluids, such as urine and tears. The client can go to family functions and eat with normal utensils. The client should cover his mouth and nose when coughing and sneezing until he has been on the medication at least 2 weeks.
CN: Physiological integrity; CNS: Pharmacological and parenteral therapies; CL: Application

29. Before feeding a client with Parkinson's disease, which nursing action is most important?
1. Sit the client upright.
2. Have suction available.
3. Order a clear liquid diet.
4. Have a speech therapist evaluate the client.

30. The nurse is caring for a pregnant client with cardiovascular disease. Which treatment would the nurse expect for this client?
1. Scheduled rest periods throughout the day
2. Hospitalization
3. Therapeutic abortion
4. Continuous cardiac monitoring

31. Which assessment finding most likely indicates a urinary tract infection (UTI) in a 5-year-old child?
1. Incontinence
2. Lack of thirst
3. Concentrated urine
4. Subnormal temperature

32. During a home health visit, a nurse assesses a client's medication and notes the client has two prescriptions for fluid retention. One prescription reads, "Lasix, 40 mg, one tablet daily." The next prescription reads, "Furosemide, 40 mg, one tablet daily." Which instruction is given to the client?
1. Take both medications as ordered.
2. Lasix and furosemide are the same drug.
3. Use Lasix one day and furosemide the next day.
4. Throw away one of the drugs to avoid confusing the client.

33. A school nurse is called to assess a preadolescent Vietnamese girl attending a new school. A teacher tells the nurse the student sits in the back of the class and won't speak when spoken to, although her parents confirmed the student speaks English. Which assessment finding is most likely?
1. The student is experiencing cultural shock.
2. The student is developing a peer support system.
3. The student is going through a socialization period.
4. The student is becoming acculturated to the new school.

29. 4. A speech therapist can evaluate the client's swallowing and make recommendations before the client is fed. Aspiration due to involuntary movement is common. Sitting the client upright and having suction available are helpful when feeding the client, but evaluation of the client's swallowing ability should come first. Clear liquids may be too difficult for the client; semisoft foods may be easier to swallow.
CN: Physiological integrity; CNS: Reduction of risk potential; CL: Analysis

30. 1. The goal of antepartum management is to prevent complications and minimize the strain on the client. This is done with rest. Hospitalization may be required in older women or those with previous decompensation. Therapeutic abortion is considered in severe dysfunction, especially in the first trimester. Continuous cardiac monitoring isn't necessary.
CN: Physiological integrity; CNS: Reduction of risk potential; CL: Application

31. 1. Incontinence in a toilet-trained child is associated with UTI. Lack of thirst wouldn't be expected in a child with UTI. Concentrated urine is a sign of dehydration. Subnormal temperature isn't a sign of UTI.
CN: Health promotion and maintenance; CNS: None; CL: Application

32. 2. Using generic names for medications is common, especially for home health clients. It's the responsibility of the nurse to teach the client both brand and generic names of drugs. Setting up medications in a medication tray, using only one pharmacy to dispense medications, and using all medications until the bottle is emptied will reduce medication errors.
CN: Physiological integrity; CNS: Pharmacological and parenteral therapies; CL: Analysis

33. 1. Cultural shock involves feelings of helplessness and discomfort and a state of disorientation when an outsider attempts to comprehend or adapt to a new cultural situation. Peer groups usually develop based on the background, interests, and capabilities of its members. Developing peer cultures is part of the socialization process. Acculturation occurs when there's a blending of cultural or ethnic backgrounds. This process takes time to develop.
CN: Health promotion and maintenance; CNS: None; CL: Application

You're doing sensationally! You really know your stuff!

34. A school nurse is screening for hearing and vision with a group of 11- to 13-year-old students. Which technique is used to communicate effectively with this age group?
1. Give undivided attention to each student.
2. Have the parents present during the screening.
3. Have several adolescents listen to each other's health histories.
4. Use puppets or dolls to show how the screening is going to take place.

34. 1. Give undivided attention to communicate effectively with adolescents. Respect their privacy. The presence of parents and use of puppets or dolls can be used to effectively communicate with younger children.

CN: Health promotion and maintenance; CNS: None; CL: Application

35. A nurse practitioner at a rural health clinic is screening an 18-month-old infant for developmental problems. Which developmental screening test is the most appropriate?
1. Goodenough-Harris Draw-a-Person Test
2. Denver Developmental Screening Test (DDST)
3. McCarthy Scales of Children's Abilities (MSCA)
4. Preschool readiness screening scales

35. 2. The DDST is applicable for children from birth through age 6. The Goodenough-Harris Draw-a-Person Test is used to assess intellectual ability in children ages 3 to 10. The MSCA is a developmental tool for children ages 2½ to 8½. Preschool readiness screening scales are designed for screening 5-year-old children for readiness for school.

CN: Health promotion and maintenance; CNS: None; CL: Application

36. In preparing an educational intervention for college students, a nurse understands that drinking alcoholic beverages is often used to relieve which condition?
1. Fatigue
2. Anxiety
3. Headache
4. Stomach pain

36. 2. Drinking alcoholic beverages is commonly thought to alleviate anxiety. These beverages aren't commonly used to relieve fatigue, headache, or stomach pain.

CN: Psychosocial integrity; CNS: None; CL: Application

37. An educational forum about relaxation techniques is provided for college students preparing for their final exams. Which relaxation technique is most effective to counteract anxiety?
1. Meditation
2. Music therapy
3. Dance therapy
4. Reality orientation

37. 1. Meditation is a relaxation therapy used to counteract anxiety related to stress-inducing internal and external stimuli. Music therapy, dance therapy, and reality orientation are used as adjuncts to psychiatric care.

CN: Psychosocial integrity; CNS: None; CL: Application

38. The parents of a 9-year-old child diagnosed with oppositional defiant disorder (ODD) are discussing treatment options with the nurse. Which action would the nurse expect to have the most positive impact on managing the child's behavior?
1. Daily administration of methylphenidate hydrochloride (Ritalin)
2. Providing praise to the child for positive behaviors
3. Including the child in group therapy with other children diagnosed with ODD
4. Assigning several household chores to the child for weekly completion

38. 2. Children with ODD consistently display negativity, defiance to authority, and hostility. ODD is best managed with consistent parenting and the establishment of a warm, positive home environment. Medication therapies aren't typically used for children with ODD. Methylphenidate is commonly used to manage attention deficit disorder. The focus of treatment for ODD is on the family unit, not on other children with similar problems. The child should be asked to participate in chores, but the parents need to be aware that overwhelming tasks may cause frustration and more defiance.

CN: Psychosocial integrity; CNS: None; CL: Analysis

39. A 40-year-old female client is admitted to a women's shelter after being raped by her estranged husband. The client describes the traumatic event. Which response by the nurse is best?
1. Change the subject to prevent the client from crying.
2. Listen attentively while the client describes the event.
3. Arrange for the client to tell her story in group therapy.
4. Medicate the client with a tranquilizer to prevent hysteria.

40. A nurse is assessing a client with manic-depressive disorder. The client tells the nurse his family physician prescribed lithium. Which symptom indicates the client is developing lithium toxicity?
1. Lethargy
2. Hypertension
3. Hyperexcitability
4. Low urine output

41. Which nursing intervention is used during assessment of a pediatric client?
1. Ask the parents to leave the room during health assessment.
2. Position the client on an examination table or bed at all times.
3. Organize the health assessment in the same way for every infant or child.
4. Identify the source (child, parent, caregiver, guardian) and indicate the reliability of the information obtained.

42. Which nursing intervention is used during assessment of an elderly client?
1. Ask the client to change positions quickly.
2. Keep the room temperature cool during health assessment.
3. Speak loudly and quickly to facilitate understanding of directions.
4. Change the height of the examination table or modify the client's position.

More than halfway home! Excellent!

39. 2. Retelling the event is part of the healing process. Giving medication and changing the subject don't allow the client to integrate the experience into her life. Group therapy may be helpful, but the best nursing response is to listen and convey empathy.
CN: Psychosocial integrity; CNS: None; CL: Application

40. 1. Nausea, vomiting, diarrhea, thirst, polyuria, lethargy, slurred speech, hypotension, muscle weakness, and fine hand tremors are signs of lithium toxicity.
CN: Physiological integrity; CNS: Pharmacological and parenteral therapies; CL: Application

41. 4. Document the source of information obtained for the nursing assessment of a child. Separation from the parent may cause anxiety and increase the child's fear and distrust. Depending on the child's age, parents may help position and hold the child, facilitating assessment. Organization of the assessment is changed to accommodate the individual child's age and development.
CN: Health promotion and maintenance; CNS: None; CL: Application

42. 4. You may need to change the height of the examination table or use a different position when assessing an elderly client. Physiologically, an older client is prone to falls and dizziness due to decreased ability to respond to sudden movements and position changes. The room temperature should be warm because older clients become hypothermic easily. Speak in a slow, normal tone of voice to facilitate communication.
CN: Health promotion and maintenance; CNS: None; CL: Application

43. Which nursing diagnosis is appropriate for a client with chronic obstructive pulmonary disease who is anxious, dyspneic, and hypoxic?
1. Ineffective breathing pattern related to anxiety
2. Risk for aspiration related to absence of protective mechanisms
3. Impaired gas exchange related to altered oxygen-carrying capacity of the blood
4. Ineffective airway clearance related to presence of tracheobronchial obstruction or secretions

44. Which statement is a wellness nursing diagnosis?
1. Readiness for enhanced spiritual well-being
2. Risk for activity intolerance related to prolonged bed rest
3. Bathing self-care deficit related to fatigue and muscular weakness
4. Constipation related to decreased activity and fluid intake as manifested by hard, formed stool every 3 days

45. A nurse observes that a client with a below-the-knee amputation on the third postoperative day refuses to look at the stump and changes the subject when the nurse attempts to discuss its care. Which nursing diagnosis should the nurse use to address this situation?
1. Hopelessness
2. Impaired physical mobility
3. Disturbed body image
4. Powerlessness

46. An intake nurse at a mental health facility is admitting a client with psychosis. Which assessment technique is most valuable to use when planning this client's care?
1. Rorschach test
2. Interview with the client
3. Mental Status Examination (MSE)
4. Review old records of the client

43. 3. The correct nursing diagnosis for this client is based on the impaired oxygenation at the cellular level. The first option applies to a client whose inhalation or exhalation pattern doesn't enable adequate pulmonary inflation or emptying. The second option applies if the client is at risk for aspirating gastric or pharyngeal secretions, food, or fluids into the tracheobronchial passages. The last option is appropriate for a client who's unable to clear secretions or obstructions from the respiratory tract.
CN: Safe, effective care environment; CNS: Management of care; CL: Application

44. 1. Wellness diagnoses are one-part statements containing the label only and begin with "Readiness for enhanced," followed by the higher level of wellness desired for the individual or group. The second option is a "risk for" nursing diagnosis. The third option describes a suspected problem for which additional data are needed for confirmation. The last option describes a manifested health problem validated by identifiable major defining characteristics.
CN: Safe, effective care environment; CNS: Management of care; CL: Application

45. 3. Refusing to look at the stump is a characteristic of disturbed body image. Other defining characteristics include having a missing body part, hiding a body part, and negative feelings about one's body. The other nursing diagnoses may also be appropriate for this client, but the data presented best reflects disturbed body image. Hopelessness occurs when a person sees limited or no alternatives and is unable to mobilize energy to act. Impaired physical mobility may also occur in the client following an amputation, but the data presented don't support this diagnosis. With powerlessness, the client doesn't believe his actions will have an effect. Again, the data presented don't support this diagnosis.
CN: Safe, effective care environment; CNS: Management of care; CL: Analysis

46. 3. The MSE is a basis for planning care with a mental health client, especially one who's psychotic. The Rorschach test is used for depression. An interview with a client with psychosis would be unreliable. Review of old records won't assess the current state on which interventions are planned.
CN: Psychosocial integrity; CNS: None; CL: Application

CN: Client needs category   CNS: Client needs subcategory   CL: Cognitive level

47. Which is a sign that a client with a new diagnosis of breast cancer is having difficulty coping?
1. The client cries when discussing her diagnosis.
2. The client asks questions about treatment.
3. The client is concerned about missing work during chemotherapy.
4. The client changes the topic when treatment is discussed.

48. Which patient outcome or goal should a nurse identify for a client with the nursing diagnosis of risk for disuse syndrome?
1. The client will be free of musculoskeletal complications.
2. The client will experience shorter periods of immobility and inactivity.
3. The nurse will stress the importance of maintaining adequate fluid intake.
4. The nurse will provide holistic care by collaborating with the health care team.

49. A 42-year-old client who underwent a right modified mastectomy with insertion of a Hemovac drain will be hospitalized overnight because of minor complications. Which goal statement should the nurse include in the plan of care?
1. Teach proper care of the incision site and drain by October 12.
2. The client will know how to care for the incision site and drain by October 12.
3. The client will show the proper care of the incision site and drain by October 12.
4. The client will care for the incision site and contend with psychological loss by October 12.

50. Which expected outcome or goal should a nurse identify for a client with the nursing diagnosis of risk for injury related to lack of awareness of environmental hazards?
1. Encourage the client to discuss safety rules with children.
2. Help the client learn safety precautions to take in the home.
3. The client will eliminate safety hazards in his surroundings.
4. The client will contact community resources for more information.

Your goal is in sight. Keep at it!

47. 4. By changing the topic when breast cancer treatment is discussed, the client may be denying her condition and having difficulty coping. It is normal to cry, ask questions, and be concerned about missing work when discussing a diagnosis such as breast cancer.
CN: Psychosocial integrity; CNS: None; CL: Application

48. 2. This is an appropriate outcome for a client with this nursing diagnosis. Disuse syndrome, a result of prolonged or unavoidable immobility or inactivity, can be prevented. Musculoskeletal complications indicate actual disuse or complications of immobility. Stressing the importance of adequate fluid intake and providing holistic care describe nursing goals, not patient outcomes.
CN: Safe, effective care environment; CNS: Management of care; CL: Application

49. 3. This statement contains a specific, measurable verb; clearly identifies the client behavior; and includes a date. Option 1 is a nursing goal as written, not a client-centered goal. The client goal of option 2 isn't measurable as stated. Option 4 includes two goals that need to be addressed separately under the appropriate nursing diagnosis, and it contains nonmeasurable verbs.
CN: Physiological integrity; CNS: Basic care and comfort; CL: Application

50. 3. This goal is appropriate and measurable as written and focuses on the client. The other options are nursing interventions as written.
CN: Safe, effective care environment; CNS: Management of care; CL: Application

51. What is the best action by a nurse when talking with a client diagnosed with prostate cancer who is tearful and having difficulty talking about his concerns?
1. Ask if he would like to speak with a chaplain.
2. Tell the client that she will be back once he has stopped crying.
3. Sit and ask him if he would like to talk about his concerns.
4. Tell the client that she knows how he is feeling.

52. A client with heart failure is given furosemide (Lasix) 40 mg I.V. daily. The morning serum potassium level is 2.8 mEq/L. Which nursing action is the most appropriate?
1. Question the physician about the dosage.
2. Give 20 mg of the ordered dose and recheck the laboratory test results.
3. Notify the physician, repeat the potassium as ordered, and obtain additional orders.
4. Give the furosemide and get an order for sodium polystyrene sulfonate.

53. Which client is at greatest risk for developing respiratory alkalosis?
1. A client in labor
2. A client with diabetes
3. A client with renal failure
4. An immediate postoperative client

54. Which condition indicates to a nurse that a sterile field has been contaminated?
1. Sterile objects are held above the waist of the nurse.
2. Sterile packages are opened with the first edge away from the nurse.
3. The outer inch of the sterile towel hangs over the side of the table.
4. Wetness on the sterile cloth on top of the nonsterile table has been noted.

51. 3. By sitting down, the nurse shows the client that he is important. Asking if he would like to talk about his concerns lets the client know that the nurse cares about him and wants to help. Calling a chaplain is appropriate after the nurse has assessed the situation and the client has verbalized his concerns. Telling the client that she will return after he stops crying does not show concern for his feelings and does not encourage verbalization. Telling the client that she understands how he feels doesn't help him verbalize his feelings.

CN: Psychosocial integrity; CNS: None; CL: Application

52. 3. Furosemide is a diuretic. As water is lost, so is potassium. Diuresis is a treatment for heart failure. Notifying the physician of the low potassium level and getting an order for potassium chloride are the appropriate actions before giving the furosemide. Furosemide, 40 mg, is an appropriate dose for the treatment of heart failure. The nurse shouldn't give half the dose without an order. Giving furosemide and sodium polystyrene sulfonate together would further lower the potassium level.

CN: Physiological integrity; CNS: Pharmacological and parenteral therapies; CL: Application

53. 1. A client's respirations at certain stages of labor increase in volume, causing the $Paco_2$ to decrease and increasing the pH. Diabetes often causes a metabolic imbalance, resulting in metabolic acidosis. In renal failure, the inability of the kidneys to eliminate wastes increases the risk of developing metabolic acidosis. The respirations of a postoperative client are usually shallow after anesthesia and, because of pain, often cause respiratory acidosis.

CN: Physiological integrity; CNS: Physiological adaptation; CL: Analysis

54. 4. Moisture outside the sterile package and field contaminates it because fluid can be wicked into the sterile field. Bacteria tend to settle, so there's less contamination above waist level and away from the nurse. The outer inch of the drape is considered contaminated but doesn't indicate that the sterile field itself has been contaminated.

CN: Safe, effective care environment; CNS: Safety and infection control; CL: Application

55. Which intervention should a nurse perform for a client with respiratory alkalosis?
1. Have the client breathe into a paper bag.
2. Give one ampule of bicarbonate as ordered.
3. Give oxygen at 3 L/minute through a nasal cannula.
4. Reposition the client in a high Fowler's position.

56. The nurse is reviewing the laboratory results from a female diabetic client admitted to the acute care facility with dehydration. Which laboratory result is consistent with a diagnosis of dehydration?
1. Serum hematocrit of 40%
2. Urine dipstick specific gravity of 1.035
3. Serum creatinine level of 0.8 mg/dl
4. HbA$_{1c}$ level of 4%

57. A client admitted with hypoparathyroidism is being monitored for hypocalcemia. Which finding would the nurse observe with hypocalcemia?
1. Battle's sign
2. Brudzinski's sign
3. Chvostek's sign
4. Homans' sign

58. A client is complaining of pain 1 day after a colostomy. The nurse gives morphine I.M. and, 30 minutes later, finds the respiratory rate at 8 breaths/minute, with the nasal cannula on the floor. Arterial blood gas (ABG) results are pH, 7.23; Pao$_2$, 58 mm Hg; Paco$_2$, 61 mm Hg; HCO$_3^-$, 24 mEq/L. Which group of factors contributes most to this client's ABG results?
1. Colostomy, pain, and morphine
2. Morphine, the nasal cannula on the floor, and the colostomy
3. Morphine, respiratory rate of 8 breaths/minute, and the nasal cannula on the floor
4. Pain, respiratory rate of 8 breaths/minute, and the nasal cannula on the floor

55. 1. By breathing into a paper bag, the client will rebreathe some of his own exhaled carbon dioxide and increase the carbon dioxide in his blood, which will correct his respiratory alkalosis. Giving one ampule of bicarbonate will worsen the alkalosis. Giving oxygen won't increase the carbon dioxide to correct the imbalance. Repositioning the client won't help him retain carbon dioxide.
CN: Physiological integrity; CNS: Physiological adaptation; CL: Analysis

56. 2. Urine specific gravity reflects the ability of the kidneys to concentrate urine. Normal urine specific gravity is 1.005 to 1.030. A higher urine specific gravity indicates that the urine is more concentrated, and this is consistent with dehydration. The normal hematocrit range for a female client is 36% to 48%, so this value is within normal limits. Dehydration would cause an increase in hematocrit. Serum creatinine is used to assess kidney function. The normal range for women is 0.6 to 0.9 mg/dl. HbA$_{1c}$ is used to monitor diabetes treatment and evaluate the average blood glucose over a period of months. The normal range for HbA$_{1c}$ is 4% to 6.7%.
CN: Physiological integrity; CNS: Physiological adaptation; CL: Analysis

57. 3. Hypocalcemia can cause Chvostek's sign, abnormal facial muscle and nerve spasms elicited when the facial nerve is tapped. Battle's sign is bruising over the temporal bone in the presence of a basilar skull fracture. Brudzinski's sign is the flexion of the hips and knees in response to flexion of the head and neck toward the chest, indicating meningeal irritation. A positive Homans' sign indicates deep vein thrombosis.
CN: Physiological integrity; CNS: Reduction of risk potential; CL: Application

58. 3. This client has respiratory acidosis. Opioids can suppress respirations, causing retention of carbon dioxide. A Pao$_2$ of 58 mm Hg indicates hypoxemia, which is caused by the removal of the client's supplementary oxygen and the decreased respiratory rate. Pain increases— not decreases—the respiratory rate, which causes a decrease in Paco$_2$. Colostomy drainage doesn't start until 2 to 3 days postoperatively, and this drainage would contribute to metabolic alkalosis.
CN: Physiological integrity; CNS: Physiological adaptation; CL: Analysis

59. Which arterial blood gas (ABG) results should a nurse expect to see in a client with emphysema?
1. pH, 7.52; $Paco_2$, 18 mm Hg; HCO_3^-, 22 mEq/L
2. pH, 7.50; $Paco_2$, 38 mm Hg; HCO_3^-, 38 mEq/L
3. pH, 7.30; $Paco_2$, 52 mm Hg; HCO_3^-, 30 mEq/L
4. pH, 7.30; $Paco_2$, 40 mm Hg; HCO_3^-, 18 mEq/L

60. Which factor does a nurse identify as a major cause of metabolic alkalosis in a client who had a colon resection?
1. Hyperventilation
2. Pain management
3. Nasogastric suction
4. I.V. therapy

61. Which nursing action should be included in the plan of care to prevent an increase in intracranial pressure (ICP) in a comatose client with a closed head injury?
1. Suction the airway every hour to maintain patency.
2. Elevate the head of the bed 20 degrees.
3. Place in a supine position with the head turned to the side.
4. Provide environmental stimulation.

62. After making the bed of a client with dementia, which action has priority?
1. Put the bed in the lowest position.
2. Put the call button within the client's reach.
3. Put the top side rails in the upright position.
4. Put soiled linen in a hamper or biohazard bag.

63. After emptying urine from the bedpan of a client whose urinary output is being monitored, which step should a nurse do next?
1. Wash hands thoroughly.
2. Apply a clean pair of gloves.
3. Report the amount of urine to the nurse in charge right away.
4. Document the amount and characteristics of urine in the chart.

Only 15 more to go!

59. 3. Clients with emphysema retain carbon dioxide due to air trapping, causing an elevated $Paco_2$ and respiratory acidosis. Because emphysema is a chronic disease, the kidneys compensate over time for the increased $Paco_2$ by retaining HCO_3^-, thus attempting to normalize the pH. The other ABG results aren't consistent with results found in a client with emphysema.
CN: Physiological integrity; CNS: Physiological adaptation; CL: Analysis

60. 3. Removing acidic gastric secretions from the stomach is a metabolic cause of alkalinization of the blood pH. Hyperventilation decreases carbon dioxide and increases the pH, causing respiratory alkalosis. Pain management may further decrease the respiratory rate. Most I.V. fluids don't influence pH.
CN: Physiological integrity; CNS: Physiological adaptation; CL: Analysis

61. 2. The head of the bed should be elevated between 15 and 30 degrees to promote venous drainage. Suctioning the airway may increase ICP and should only be performed when needed. Turning the head to the side may cause jugular venous compression and an elevation in ICP. Environmental stimulation should be minimized to reduce any rise in ICP.
CN: Physiological integrity; CNS: Reduction in risk potential; CL: Application

62. 1. To reduce the risk of injury due to falls, the bed should be placed in the lowest position. The call button should be in reach of the client, but the immediate safety of the client comes first. All four side rails should be up to prevent accidental falls and to remind clients to stay in bed. Soiled linens should be placed in a hamper or biohazard bag, but client safety is a priority.
CN: Safe, effective care environment; CNS: Management of care; CL: Application

63. 1. After any procedure is completed, the nurse must wash her hands to prevent transmission of microorganisms. The application of gloves is only necessary if the nurse must attend to another item of personal care before documenting urinary output; even so, hands should be washed first. Crucial information is reported to the charge nurse, not routine intake and output. Documentation should take place but following the handwashing.
CN: Safe, effective care environment; CNS: Safety and infection control; CL: Application

CN: Client needs category   CNS: Client needs subcategory   CL: Cognitive level

64. Which client should a nurse place in an orthopneic position?
1. A client with edema of the lower legs and ankles
2. A client with a pressure ulcer on the coccyx and buttocks
3. An immobilized client with calf tenderness due to a thrombus
4. An elderly client with difficulty breathing

65. A client preparing to transfer from the bed to a wheelchair complains of feeling light-headed and dizzy as he rises from a supine to a sitting position. Which action should the nurse take next?
1. Lift the client quickly into the wheelchair.
2. Return the client to the supine position and apply a safety vest.
3. Ask the client to dangle his legs at the bedside while leaving the room for a few seconds to get assistance.
4. Have the client sit at the side of the bed for a few minutes while supporting his back and shoulders.

66. Which nursing action is the most effective infection control measure for preventing the transmission of microorganisms?
1. Change a client's bed linen daily.
2. Wash hands before and after client contact.
3. Wear sterile gloves when touching a client's skin.
4. Wear a mask when in direct contact with infected clients.

67. The nurse is teaching a student nurse about standard precautions. Which action by the student nurse indicates that the teaching has been effective?
1. Wear eye goggles while giving a complete bed bath.
2. Recap a needle used for an injection before disposal.
3. Dispose of blood-contaminated materials in a biohazard container.
4. Use alcohol to decontaminate blood-contaminated steel instruments.

64. 4. The orthopneic position, which is appropriate for a client with breathing difficulty, is a sitting position with the arms leaning on a bedside table. Sitting with the legs elevated to decrease edema is appropriate for clients with ankle and lower leg swelling. A client with a pressure ulcer will need to be positioned on his side and turned every 2 hours. Fowler's or semi-Fowler's positions are most appropriate for a client on complete bed rest.
CN: Physiological integrity; CNS: Physiological adaptation; CL: Application

65. 4. A quick change in position will decrease the blood pressure, causing momentary light-headedness and dizziness. An additional change in position may further reduce the client's blood pressure to a level that may require emergency assistance. This can be avoided by waiting with the client in the sitting position until the blood pressure stabilizes. A safety vest isn't necessary. Leaving the room may put the client in danger if the blood pressure decreases further and the client needs emergency assistance. If the client continues to complain of dizziness and light-headedness, then return the client to bed.
CN: Physiological integrity; CNS: Reduction of risk potential; CL: Application

66. 2. Typically, the transmission of microorganisms occurs when health care personnel don't wash their hands before and after touching a client or contaminated objects. A daily linen change isn't the most effective method of controlling infection. Sterile gloves and a mask aren't needed during routine client care.
CN: Safe, effective care environment; CNS: Safety and infection control; CL: Application

67. 3. Blood-contaminated materials are disposed of in a biohazard container. Recapping needles puts the health care provider at risk for sticking himself. Standard precautions needn't be observed during a bath because of the low risk for exposure to blood. Blood-contaminated steel instruments are decontaminated in an autoclave.
CN: Safe, effective care environment; CNS: Safety and infection control; CL: Application

68. A team leader would instruct team members to wear a mask and protective eyewear or a face shield in which situation?
1. When strong odors are emitted from an infected wound
2. When the client has an oral temperature greater than 101° F (38.3° C)
3. If needles or other sharp instruments are to be used in the procedure
4. During a procedure where splashing of blood or body fluid is anticipated

69. A nurse is caring for a client on neutropenic precautions. At which point should the nurse remove the barrier protection when leaving the room?
1. Within the client's room, just inside the doorway
2. Out of the client's room, just outside the doorway
3. In the hallway, a significant distance from the client's room
4. At the bedside, immediately after completing work with the client

70. Which time frame is most appropriate for completing client teaching for a client undergoing an open cholecystectomy?
1. The day of discharge
2. A few weeks before the surgery
3. The first 12 hours after surgery
4. Before discharge, 1 to 2 days after the surgery

71. Which technique is appropriate for promoting proper breathing in a client experiencing pain or anxiety?
1. Rapid, light respirations
2. Rapid, deep respirations
3. In through the mouth and out through the nose
4. In through the nose and out through the mouth

Pat yourself on the back. Only five more to go.

68. 4. Wearing eye goggles or face shields prevents blood or body fluid splashes into the eyes. Odors don't transmit microorganisms. A client with a fever won't transmit microorganisms into the eyes any more frequently than a client without a fever. The use of needles or other sharp instruments doesn't mandate eye protection.

CN: Safe, effective environment; CNS: Management of care; CL: Application

69. 2. Disposing of gowns and gloves just outside the doorway provides sufficient distance from the client for all but airborne microorganisms. The client is protected from infection by airborne pathogens by keeping the door shut as much as possible to decrease the chance of exposure. Disposal of barriers at the bedside or inside the door negates the effectiveness of wearing barriers in the first place. It's unnecessary to wear the barriers away from the doorway as the door should remain closed.

CN: Safe, effective care environment; CNS: Safety and infection control; CL: Application

70. 4. Pain levels should have sufficiently subsided 1 to 2 days after the surgical procedure, allowing the client to concentrate on the information. The day of discharge is too late, because it doesn't give the client time to ask questions or practice procedures (such as syringe preparation) that may be necessary. Also, the individual may be anxious about returning home, which may interfere with learning. A few weeks before surgery is generally too early to retain information, and teaching within the first 12 hours after surgery isn't likely to produce retention of information, either.

CN: Physiological integrity; CNS: Physiological adaptation; CL: Application

71. 4. Air inhaled through the nose is warmed, humidified, and filtered for large particles with the nasal hairs, conditioning the air for delivery to the lungs. Exhaling through the mouth after inhaling through the nose requires some concentration and provides a focus to distract a client experiencing pain and anxiety. This method is used to control respiratory rates when clients are anxious or in pain and optimizes air exchange. Rapid, light, or deep respirations cause the client to lose oxygen exchange time while continuing to blow off carbon dioxide. This leads to hypoxemia and respiratory alkalosis.

CN: Physiological integrity; CNS: Physiological adaptation; CL; Application

CN: Client needs category   CNS: Client needs subcategory   CL: Cognitive level

72. The nurse is assessing a client who was admitted with a pressure ulcer. The nurse determines that the ulcer is at stage II. Which graphic represents stage II of a pressure ulcer?

1.
2.
3.
4.

73. A 46-year-old single female client is concerned about her 15-year-old son's behavior. He has suddenly decided his mother shouldn't date or have men in the house. He told his mother he was the "man of the house." Which disturbance is occurring in the internal dynamics of the family?
1. Age-appropriate behavior is occurring.
2. The son is powerful in the family system.
3. The son is trying to establish a role reversal.
4. It's culturally acceptable to be the man of the house at age 15.

74. A nurse is reviewing the causes of gastroesophageal reflux disease (GERD) with a client. What area of the GI tract should the nurse identify as the cause of reduced pressure associated with GERD?

75. A nurse is preparing a client with a tracheostomy for discharge. Which of the following statements by the client indicates that he understands the teaching regarding his tracheostomy care?
1. "I will need to cover the opening when I shower."
2. "I can swim as long as I keep my head above water."
3. "I will need to wash my hands after caring for my tracheostomy."
4. "I will need to take antibiotics to prevent infections."

You did a wonderful job! Only two more tests left!

72. 2. Stage II is marked by partial-thickness skin loss that involves the epidermis, dermis, or both, with an abrasion, blister, or shallow crater. The first graphic is stage III, which is a full-thickness wound that appears like a deep crater. The third graphic is of stage IV, which involves all thicknesses and involves the muscle, bone, and supporting structures. The fourth graphic is of stage I, which is a reddened area with intact skin, or in those with dark skin, there may be warmth, edema, discoloration, induration, or hardness.
CN: Physiological integrity; CNS: Physiological adaptation; CL; Analysis

73. 3. Role reversal occurs when the patterns of expected behavior aren't appropriate to age and ability. Males age 13 to 17 are developing their identities, and separation from parents becomes necessary for individuation to occur. Males have a better understanding of their roles in relationships and families if they're raised around strong male role models. In healthy families, power is shared appropriate to age until the children are independent.
CN: Psychosocial integrity; CNS: None; CL: Analysis

74. Normally, there is enough pressure around the lower esophageal sphincter (LES) to close it. Reflux occurs when LES pressure is deficient or when pressure in the stomach exceeds LES pressure.

CN: Health promotion and maintenance; CNS: None; CL: Application

75. 1. The opening will require protection when bathing. Swimming isn't recommended; drowning can occur even if the client's head isn't submerged. It's necessary to wash hands before and after caring for the tracheostomy. Prophylactic antibiotics aren't required for the client with a tracheostomy.
CN: Safe, effective care environment; CNS: Safety and infection control; CL: Application

This is the next to last comprehensive test. Go for it, and good luck!

COMPREHENSIVE Test 5

1. Which assessment data should a nurse report to the physician?
1. Blood pressure of 120/72 mm Hg in a healthy man
2. Pulse of 110 beats/minute on awakening in the morning
3. Blood pressure of 110/68 mm Hg in a healthy woman
4. Pulse of 120 beats/minute after 30 minutes of aerobic exercise

2. Immediately after a client's cardiac catheterization via the femoral artery, the client is being assessed by the nurse. Which assessment finding would the nurse report immediately to the physician?
1. Apical pulse of 98 beats/minute
2. Dressing with dime-sized red drainage
3. Absence of dorsalis pedis pulse
4. Blood pressure of 105/70 mm Hg

3. A nurse is preparing to bathe a client who is hospitalized for emphysema. What is the most important intervention by the nurse?
1. Remove the oxygen and proceed with the bath.
2. Increase the flow of oxygen to 6 L/minute by nasal cannula.
3. Keep the head of the bed slightly elevated during the procedure.
4. Lower the head of the bed and roll the client to his left side to increase oxygenation.

4. The nurse is assessing a 40-year-old client who is scheduled to have elective facial surgery later in the morning and notes a pulse rate of 130 beats/minute. The nurse suspects the increased pulse rate is the result of which of the following?
1. Age
2. Anxiety
3. Exercise
4. Pain

1. 2. The normal range for a pulse is 60 to 100 beats/minute, and in the morning, the rate is at its lowest. Blood pressures of 120/72 mm Hg for a healthy man and 110/68 mm Hg for a healthy woman are normal. Aerobic exercise increases the heart rate over the normal range of 60 to 100 beats/minute. The formula for maximum aerobic heart rate is: 210 − age × 80%. A person shouldn't go over the maximum heart rate during aerobic exercise.

CN: Physiological integrity; CNS: Physiological adaptation; CL: Analysis

2. 3. The dorsalis pedis is the pulse used to determine peripheral circulation to the lower extremities after a cardiac catheterization. Absence of this pulse should be reported immediately to the physician. An apical pulse of 98 beats/minute and a blood pressure of 105/70 mm Hg are within the normal range. A dressing with dime-sized, red drainage is normal after a catheterization but should continue to be monitored.

CN: Physiological integrity; CNS: Reduction of risk potential; CL: Application

3. 3. The elasticity of the lungs is lost for clients with emphysema, who can't tolerate lying flat because the abdominal organs compress the lungs. The best position is one with the head slightly elevated. The rate of oxygen delivery shouldn't be increased or decreased without an order from the physician. Increasing oxygen flow on a client with emphysema may also suppress the hypoxic drive to breathe. Positioning the client on his left side with the head of the bed flat would decrease oxygenation.

CN: Physiological integrity; CNS: Physiological adaptation; CL: Application

4. 2. Anxiety tends to increase heart rate, temperature, and respirations. The normal heart rate for a client this age is 60 to 100 beats/minute. Exercise will increase the heart rate but most likely won't occur preoperatively. The client shouldn't be in any pain preoperatively.

CN: Physiological integrity; CNS: Physiological adaptation; CL: Application

CN: Client needs category   CNS: Client needs subcategory   CL: Cognitive level

5. A thin client is sitting up in bed talking on the phone and has a blood pressure of 90/50 mm Hg. Which nursing action is correct?
1. Increase fluids.
2. Call the physician.
3. Document the blood pressure.
4. Suspect orthostatic hypotension.

6. Which assessment finding should alert a nurse to a potential problem in a client who has received morphine I.V. for postoperative pain?
1. Heart rate 124 beats/minute
2. Respiratory rate 8 breaths/minute
3. Sleeping but easily aroused
4. Blood pressure 90/62 mm Hg

7. A client arrives to the emergency department and the following assessments are made: active bleeding from three gunshot wounds to the abdominal area and complaints of pain and a headache. Which of the following would the nurse expect? Select all that apply.
1. Isotonic I.V. fluids
2. Pulse 44 beats/minute
3. Elevated oral temperature
4. Blood pressure 196/40 mm Hg
5. Biot's respirations

8. A client with type 1 diabetes mellitus is confused, weak, diaphoretic, and has palpitations. What action should the nurse take first?
1. Administer glucagon intramuscularly (I.M.) or subcutaneously (subQ).
2. Give an intravenous (I.V.) bolus of dextrose 50%.
3. Provide 15 to 20 g of a fast-acting oral carbohydrate.
4. Inject 10 units of fast-acting insulin subQ.

5. 3. A thin client can have a blood pressure as low as 88/68 mm Hg and remain asymptomatic. Calling the physician with this information is inappropriate, as is increasing fluids. Orthostatic hypotension is a decrease in blood pressure and increase in heart rate that occur with a sudden change in position from lying to sitting. It might indicate some dehydration, but this client had been sitting up without symptoms for a while.
CN: Health promotion and maintenance; CNS: None; CL: Analysis

6. 2. Since morphine depresses the respiratory center of the brain, the nurse should alert the physician of a respiratory rate less than 10 breaths/ minute. While a heart rate of 124 beats/minute is considered tachycardia, the nurse should further assess the client before calling the physician. Morphine shouldn't be given to a client who is sedated and not easily aroused. Morphine can cause hypotension, but the nurse should further assess the client before calling the physician because this may be the client's usual blood pressure.
CN: Physiological integrity; CNS: Pharmacological and parenteral therapies; CL: Analysis

7. 1 and 4. Fluid loss would require replacement of fluids rapidly, and isotonic fluids will not alter the fluid balance for this client. A decrease in blood pressure and an increase in pulse would occur as a response to the decreasing fluid volume in the body. The remaining options would not be present in this situation.
CN: Health promotion and maintenance; CNS: None; CL: Analysis

8. 3. The client is exhibiting signs of hypoglycemia. Since the client is conscious, the first intervention is to give a fast-acting oral carbohydrate, such as orange juice, hard candy, or honey. If the client becomes unconscious, the nurse would administer I.M. or subQ glucagon or I.V. dextrose 50%. Administering insulin wouldn't be appropriate because the client is experiencing hypoglycemia.
CN: Physiological integrity; CNS: Reduction of risk potential; CL: Analysis

9. Which nursing action is correct for performing tracheal suctioning?
1. Apply suction during insertion of the catheter.
2. Limit suctioning to 10 to 15 seconds in duration.
3. Resterilize the suction catheter in alcohol after use.
4. Repeat suctioning intervals every 15 minutes until clear.

10. While performing nasopharyngeal suction, a nurse notes a client's oxygen saturation reading is 86% by pulse oximeter. What is the most appropriate action by the nurse?
1. Stop suctioning and give oxygen to the client.
2. Withdraw the suction catheter and tell the client to cough several times.
3. Continue suctioning for 10 to 15 more seconds and then withdraw the suction catheter.
4. Keep the suction catheter inserted and wait a few seconds before beginning suctioning.

Ten done already! Good job!

11. Two hours after starting total enteral nutrition (TEN) through a nasogastric tube, a client starts to have abdominal distention. Which action should the nurse take first?
1. Aspirate stomach contents.
2. Reposition the tube.
3. Place client in supine position.
4. Stop the feeding.

12. What is the initial action of a nurse when preparing to insert a nasogastric (NG) tube?
1. Wash hands.
2. Apply sterile gloves.
3. Apply a mask and gown.
4. Open all necessary kits and tubing.

9. 2. The length of time a client should be able to tolerate the suction procedure is 10 to 15 seconds. Any longer may cause hypoxia. Suctioning during insertion can cause trauma to the mucosa and removes oxygen from the respiratory tract. Suctioning intervals with supplemental oxygen between suctions is performed after at least 1-minute intervals to allow the client to rest. Suction catheters are disposed of after each use and are cleansed in normal saline solution after each pass.

CN: Physiological integrity; CNS: Physiological adaptation; CL: Application

10. 1. The pulse oximeter reading indicates the client isn't oxygenating well, so the nurse must stop suctioning and give oxygen to increase the saturation. The normal range for oxygen saturation is 90% to 100%. Suctioning draws air as well as secretions from the lungs, reducing oxygen saturation in the blood. Withdrawing the suction catheter will stop the removal of oxygen, but coughing will delay an increase in saturation. Further suctioning will reduce the oxygen level even more. The suction catheter occupies space in the airway, making it harder for the client to breathe when it's left in place.

CN: Physiological integrity; CNS: Physiological adaptation; CL: Application

11. 4. Clients receiving TEN are at risk for abdominal distention due to rapid feeding or delayed emptying of the stomach contents. The first action would be to stop the feeding to prevent further distention and then continue to assess the distention's cause. Aspirating the stomach contents and repositioning the tube may be necessary but are not the priority. A client receiving a nasogastric tube feeding should be placed in an upright or Fowler's position, not supine, to prevent the risk of aspiration.

CN: Physiological integrity; CNS: Basic care and comfort; CL: Application

12. 1. The first intervention before a procedure is hand washing. Clean gloves are used because the mouth and nasopharynx aren't considered sterile. A mask and gown aren't required. Opening all the equipment is the next step before inserting the NG tube.

CN: Safe, effective care environment; CNS: Safety and infection control; CL: Application

13. As a nurse is inserting a nasogastric tube, the client begins to gag. Which action should the nurse take?
1. Remove the inserted tube and notify the physician of the client's status.
2. Stop the insertion, allow the client to rest, and then continue inserting the tube.
3. Encourage the client to take deep breaths through the mouth while the tube is being inserted.
4. Pause until the gagging stops and then tell the client to take a few sips of water and swallow as the tube is inserted.

14. Which step, if taken by a nurse after insertion of a nasogastric (NG) tube, could harm the client?
1. Affix the NG tube to the nose with tape.
2. Check tube placement by aspirating stomach contents using a piston syringe.
3. Check tube placement by instilling 100 ml of water into the tube to check for stomach filling.
4. Document in the chart the insertion, method used to check tube placement, and client's response to the procedure.

15. A new graduate nurse is assigned to a nursing unit. The nurse-manager notes that the graduate's skills are deficient. Which action is most appropriate for the nurse-manager to take?
1. Talk with the supervisor about terminating the new graduate.
2. Discuss with the graduate that a transfer to another unit is necessary.
3. Work with the graduate and develop a plan to improve the graduate's deficiencies.
4. Counsel the graduate that, if performance doesn't improve, the graduate will be terminated.

16. A client on a cardiac monitor has a heart rate of 170 beats/minute, with frequent premature contractions. Which nursing action is best?
1. Call the client's physician immediately.
2. Enter the client's room and complete a full assessment.
3. Delegate one of the nurses' assistants to take the client's vital signs.
4. Notify the supervisor about the change in the client's condition.

17. A client is hospitalized with an acute sinus infection. Which assessment made by the nurse indicates serious complications?
1. Orbital edema
2. Nuchal rigidity
3. Oral temperature 102° F (39° C)
4. Frontal headache

13. 4. Swallowing helps advance the tube by causing the epiglottis to cover the opening of the trachea, thus helping to eliminate gagging and coughing. Removing the tube or stopping the insertion is unnecessary because gagging is an expected response to this procedure. Deep breathing opens the trachea, allowing the tube to possibly advance into the lungs.
CN: Safe, effective care environment; CNS: Safety and infection control; CL: Analysis

14. 3. Should the tube be located in the lungs, instilling water would flood the lungs, precipitating choking, coughing, hypoxemia, and, possibly, pneumonia. Anchoring the tube after placement to the nose with tape or a manufactured device prevents the tube from becoming dislodged. Withdrawing stomach contents from the NG tube double-checks the correct placement. Documentation is required for any procedure.
CN: Safe, effective care environment; CNS: Management of care; CL: Application

15. 3. A principle of leadership involves mastery over ignorance by working with people. The leader needs to work with the new graduate and provide opportunities for the graduate to grow and develop. The other responses wouldn't give the new graduate the opportunity and support needed for improvement.
CN: Safe, effective care environment; CNS: Management of care; CL: Application

16. 2. Because a change has occurred in the client's status, the nurse must assess the client first. This shouldn't be delegated to unlicensed personnel. Before the physician or supervisor is notified, a full assessment must be made.
CN: Safe, effective care environment; CNS: Management of care; CL: Analysis

17. 2. Nuchal rigidity indicates neurological involvement, possibly meningitis. The other symptoms are typical of a sinus infection.
CN: Physiological integrity; CNS: Physiological adaptation; CL: Application

18. Which statement by a client who had nasal surgery indicates to the nurse that the client needs further teaching about postoperative care?
1. "I'll do frequent mouth care."
2. "I'll eat two oranges a day."
3. "I'll eat two bananas a day."
4. "I'll drink at least 8 glasses of fluid a day."

19. The nurse is collecting a urine specimen from a client's indwelling urinary catheter. Which action should the nurse take?
1. Collect urine from the drainage collection bag.
2. Disconnect the catheter from the drainage tubing to collect urine.
3. Remove the indwelling catheter and insert a sterile straight catheter to collect urine.
4. Insert a sterile needle with syringe through a tubing drainage port cleaned with alcohol to collect the specimen.

20. Which observation indicates to a nurse that a client understands his instructions on crutch walking?
1. The client's axillae rest on the crutches.
2. The client's hands bear the body weight.
3. Crutches are 12″ (30.5 cm) in front of the feet.
4. The client uses long strides when walking.

21. A client recovering from a knee replacement has normal saline solution ordered to run at 125 ml/hour I.V. The I.V. bag was hung at 8:00 a.m. It's now 3:00 p.m., and 300 ml have been infused. A nurse has just come on her shift at 3:00 p.m. Which action is correct?
1. Discontinue the I.V. infusion when the bag is complete.
2. Instruct the client to increase his fluid intake.
3. Speed up the rate of the I.V. fluids.
4. Assess the I.V. site.

Don't sweat it! You're doing great!

18. 3. After nasal surgery, the client shouldn't strain or bear down as this will increase the risk for bleeding. Bananas can cause severe constipation, which could lead to straining. The other interventions would be appropriate postoperative care for this client.
CN: Physiological integrity; CNS: Reduction of risk potential; CL: Analysis

19. 4. Wearing clean gloves, cleaning the port with alcohol, and then obtaining the specimen with a sterile needle ensures the specimen and the closed urinary drainage system won't be contaminated. A urine sample must be new urine, and the urine in the bag could be several hours old and growing bacteria. The urinary drainage system must be kept closed to prevent microorganisms from entering. A straight catheter is used to relieve urinary retention, obtain sterile urine specimens, measure the amount of postvoid residual urine, and empty the bladder for certain procedures. It isn't necessary to remove an indwelling catheter to obtain a sterile urine specimen unless the physician requests the whole system be changed.
CN: Safe, effective care environment; CNS: Safety and infection control; CL: Application

20. 2. When using crutches, the client should bear weight on his hands. The axillae shouldn't rest on the crutches; there should be 2″ (5 cm) between the crutch and axilla. Crutches should be placed 6″ (15 cm) in front of the feet for stability. A short stride provides maximum safety and mobility.
CN: Physiological integrity; CNS: Basic care and comfort; CL: Application

21. 4. At 125 ml/hour over 7 hours, 875 ml should have been infused. The I.V. fluid is 575 ml behind. The first action would be to make sure the site is not infiltrated before calling the physician for further fluid orders. The physician will determine how the I.V. fluids will be adjusted and will want to know why the client didn't get the prescribed fluids. The order is for I.V. fluids—not oral fluids—and the route change can only be authorized by a physician. Legally, the nurse can't change the rate of I.V. fluids.
CN: Safe, effective care environment; CNS: Management of care; CL: Application

22. A nurse is removing an indwelling urinary catheter from a client. Which action is appropriate?
1. Don sterile gloves.
2. Cut the lumen of the balloon.
3. Document the time of removal.
4. Position the client on the left side.

23. The nurse obtains a client's stool sample for occult blood. Which of the following diets can cause a false-positive test result?
1. Red meat, horseradish, and turnips
2. Dairy products, canned fruit, and pretzels
3. Cheese, raw fruits, and vegetables
4. Potatoes, orange juice, and decaffeinated coffee

24. A client complains of excessive flatulence. The nurse teaches the client about foods that may cause flatulence. Which selection of food, if made by the client, would indicate further teaching is needed?
1. Cauliflower
2. Ice cream
3. Steak
4. Potatoes

25. A nurse is teaching a client postoperative coughing and deep-breathing exercises. What is the most important information to include?
1. Splint the incision and cough.
2. Splint the incision, take a deep breath, and then cough.
3. Lie prone, splint the incision, take a deep breath, and then cough.
4. Lie supine, splint the incision, take a deep breath, and then cough.

26. Which care plan goal statement is written appropriately?
1. The nurse will perform the client's bath by 3:00 p.m.
2. The client will bathe with assistance.
3. The nurse will perform the client's bath.
4. The client will bathe with assistance by discharge.

22. 3. The client should void within 8 hours of the removal of an indwelling urinary catheter. Documenting the time of removal allows the nurse and physician to verify the duration of elapsed time since removal, thus contributing to continuity of care. Clean, disposable gloves are required because it isn't a sterile procedure. The catheter may retrograde into the bladder, requiring surgical removal, if the balloon is cut from the lumen and the catheter isn't secured. The client should be positioned comfortably on his back, and privacy should be provided.
CN: Safe, effective care environment; CNS: Safety and infection control; CL: Application

23. 1. Consumption of red meat has caused false-positive readings. The client should also avoid poultry, fish, turnips, and horseradish. Avoid foods that are high in iron. The other foods don't cause false-positive readings.
CN: Physiological integrity; CNS: Basic care and comfort; CL: Application

24. 1. Foods that cause flatulence in some people may not produce flatulence in others. It all depends on the amount consumed, but cauliflower is the only food listed that usually results in flatulence.
CN: Physiological integrity; CNS: Basic care and comfort; CL: Application

25. 2. Splinting the incision with a pillow will protect the incision while the client coughs. Taking a deep breath will help open the alveoli, which promotes oxygen exchange and prevents atelectasis. Coughing and deep-breathing exercises are best accomplished in a sitting or semi-sitting position. Expectoration of secretions will be facilitated in a sitting position, as will splinting and taking deep breaths.
CN: Physiological integrity; CNS: Reduction of risk potential; CL: Application

26. 4. All goals should be client focused, allowing the client to understand what needs to be accomplished. Specify a time limit for when this task should be achieved. Be realistic, so the client may be successful in reaching the goal. The goal must be measurable so all staff can evaluate the client's progress. Nurse flexibility is an important attribute and necessary for reassessing needs and approaches for the client's optimal recovery. However, in the actual goal, specific criteria must be identified to allow all staff to work from the same data for achieving client goals.
CN: Safe, effective care environment; CNS: Management of care; CL: Application

27. A client with acquired immunodeficiency syndrome (AIDS) requires assistance with oral care. What is the most appropriate intervention by the nurse?
1. Wear a mask, gown, and gloves.
2. Wear a gown and gloves.
3. Wear a mask with eye shield and gloves.
4. Wear gloves only.

28. A middle-age adult has been identified as being in the stagnation stage of developmental conflict. Which of the following would support this? Select all that apply.
1. Withdrawn from family obligations
2. Bought a new sports car
3. Started classes at the community college
4. Increased nap and sleeping hours
5. Recently became engaged

29. A nurse has identified ineffective airway clearance as a nursing diagnosis for a client with pneumonia. Which goal would be appropriate for this client?
1. The client will have clear breath sounds.
2. The client will have a respiratory rate of 32 breaths/minute.
3. The client will be pain free.
4. The client will have a normal body temperature.

30. A client on complete bed rest complains of excessive flatulence. What is the best position for the nurse to place the client in?
1. Fowler's
2. Knee-chest
3. Semi-Fowler's
4. Trendelenburg's

You're at question 30 and looking good!

27. 4. According to standard precautions, the nurse should wear gloves when coming in contact with a client's blood or body fluids. During oral care with a cooperative client, gloves are sufficient to protect the nurse. A mask is worn when airborne droplets of blood or body fluids are anticipated. A gown and mask with eye shield should be worn when splashing of body fluids is expected.
CN: Safe, effective care environment; CNS: Safety and infection control; CL: Application

28. 1 and 4. Clients in the stagnation stage of development have withdrawn from activities and relationships. The remaining responses do not express stagnation.
CN: Health promotion and maintenance; CNS: None; CL: Application

29. 1. Clear breath sounds in a client with pneumonia would indicate the airway is clear. Tachypnea would not indicate clear breath sounds and may occur when the client has difficulty clearing secretions. Being pain free and having a normal body temperature are appropriate goals for a client with pneumonia but are not an indication that the airway is clear.
CN: Safe, effective care environment; CNS: Management of care; CL: Analysis

30. 2. Because gas rises, the knee-chest position facilitates the passage of flatus. Semi-Fowler's and Fowler's positions inhibit gas passage. In Trendelenburg's position, the client lies flat with his head lower than his feet.
CN: Physiological integrity; CNS: Basic care and comfort; CL: Application

31. The nurse is assisting with the delivery of a fetus where the mentum is the presenting part. Which graphic illustrates that fetal presentation?

1.   2.

3.   4.

32. The nurse is performing percussion and postural drainage on the left lower lobe of a client diagnosed with pneumonia. The nurse is aware that the client should be placed in which position?
1. Supine with the foot of the bed elevated
2. On the left side with the foot of the bed elevated
3. On the left side with the head of the bed elevated
4. Prone with the head of the bed elevated

33. The client is complaining of moderate pain. Which assessment by the nurse indicates a physiological response to pain?
1. Restlessness
2. Decreased pulse rate
3. Increased blood pressure
4. Guarding of the painful area

34. A client with long-standing rheumatoid arthritis has frequent complaints of joint pain. The nurse's plan of treatment is based on the understanding that chronic pain is most effectively relieved when analgesics are administered in which way?
1. Conservatively
2. Intramuscular (I.M.) alternating with intravenous (I.V.)
3. On an as-needed basis
4. At regularly scheduled intervals

31. 1. In the cephalic, or head-down, presentation, the fetus' position may be classified by the presenting skull landmark: mentum or chin (option 1), brow (option 2), sinciput (option 3), or vertex (option 4).

CN: Health promotion and maintenance; CNS: None; CL: Application

32. 1. To mobilize secretions from the left lower lobe, the client should be positioned supine or on the right side. The foot of the bed should be elevated so that gravity can help mobilize secretions. Placing the client on the left side would put the left lobe in a low or dependent position. Elevating the head of the bed wouldn't use gravity to drain the lower lobes.

CN: Physiological integrity; CNS: Basic care and comfort; CL: Application

33. 3. Increased blood pressure is a physiological, or involuntary, response to moderate pain. Restlessness and guarding of the painful area are behavioral responses. Decreased pulse rate occurs when pain is severe and deep.

CN: Physiological integrity; CNS: Physiological adaptation; CL: Analysis

34. 4. To control chronic pain and prevent cycled pain, regularly scheduled intervals are most effective. As-needed and conservative methods aren't effective means to manage chronic pain because the pain isn't relieved regularly. I.M. administration isn't practical on a long-term basis.

CN: Physiological integrity; CNS: Pharmacological and parenteral therapies; CL: Application

35. A nurse notes crackles in the lung bases and pedal edema during a client assessment. Which factor is a common cause of fluid volume excess?
1. Prolonged fever
2. Hyperventilation
3. Excessive I.V. infusion
4. Fluid volume shifts secondary to vomiting

36. A client is to receive I.V. therapy. Place the following nursing actions in the correct order to ensure client safety.
1. Check the order.
2. Set the rate as ordered.
3. Label the site with the date.
4. Connect I.V. tubing to the insertion site.
5. Select a viable site distal to proximal.

37. A client is given instructions for a low-sodium diet. Which statement best shows the nurse that the client understands the diet instruction?
1. "Meat, fish, and chicken are high in sodium."
2. "I'll miss eating fruits."
3. "I'll enjoy eating at restaurants more often now."
4. "I'll avoid dairy products, potato chips, and carrots."

38. To prevent aspiration in a client with impaired swallowing, the nurse should:
1. provide a straw for drinking liquids.
2. remove dentures before eating.
3. position the client at a 90-degree angle.
4. place food on the paralyzed side of the mouth.

39. A client must choose a meal that follows his diet orders of a high-calorie, high-protein, low-sodium, and low-potassium diet. Which choice indicates to the nurse that the client understands the dietary guidelines?
1. Halibut, salad, rice, and instant coffee
2. Crab, beets, spinach, and baked potato
3. Salmon, rice, green beans, sourdough bread, coffee, and ice cream
4. Sirloin steak, salad, baked potato with butter, and chocolate ice cream

40. A client with terminal cancer tells the nurse, "I've given up. I have no hope left. I'm ready to die." What is the most appropriate response by the nurse?
1. "You've given up hope?"
2. "You should talk about dying to a social worker."
3. "You should talk to your physician about your fears of dying."
4. "You shouldn't give up hope. There are cures for cancer found every day."

You're more than halfway finished! You're amazing!

35. 3. Fluid volume excess can result from excess I.V. fluids, especially in a compromised client. Vomiting, fever, and hyperventilation will result in loss of body fluids, leading to a fluid volume deficit.
CN: Physiological integrity; CNS: Basic care and comfort; CL: Application

36. 1, 5, 4, 2, and 3. This would be the order the nurse would follow for the initiation of I.V. therapy.
CN: Physiological integrity; CNS: Pharmacological and parenteral therapy; CL: Analysis

37. 4. Dairy products, potato chips, carrots, and restaurant food are all high in sodium. Meat, fish, chicken, and fruits aren't.
CN: Physiological integrity; CNS: Basic care and comfort; CL: Application

38. 3. When feeding a client with impaired swallowing, the nurse should position the client at a 90-degree angle to reduce the risk of aspiration. Straws shouldn't be used because they increase the risk of aspiration by sending liquids directly to the back of the mouth. Dentures should be well-fitting and in place for eating. If one side of the mouth is paralyzed, food should be placed on the unaffected side.
CN: Physiological integrity; CNS: Basic care and comfort; CL: Application

39. 3. The best choice of these meals is salmon with rice and green beans, which is high in protein, and the sourdough bread and ice cream add calories. Halibut, instant coffee, and potatoes are high in potassium, and beets are high in sodium.
CN: Health promotion and maintenance; CNS: None; CL: Application

40. 1. The use of reflection invites the client to talk more about his concerns. Deferring the conversation to a social worker or physician closes the conversation. Telling the client the cure for cancer is right around the corner gives false hope.
CN: Psychosocial integrity; CNS: None; CL: Analysis

CN: Client needs category   CNS: Client needs subcategory   CL: Cognitive level

41. Which instruction should a nurse include in the teaching plan for a client with a platelet count of 25,000/mm³ and petechial rash on the legs, arms, and neck?
1. Take an iron supplement daily.
2. Take acetaminophen rather than aspirin for headache.
3. Stay away from crowds during the flu season.
4. Avoid fresh salads.

42. Which laboratory value for a newly diagnosed client with diabetes should the nurse report to the physician?
1. pH, 7.45
2. Sodium, 118 mEq/L
3. Glucose, 120 mg/dl
4. Potassium, 3.9 mEq/L

43. A client is 2 days postoperative from a femoral popliteal bypass. The nurse's assessment finds the client's left leg cold and pale. What is the most important action by the nurse?
1. Check distal pulses.
2. Notify the physician.
3. Elevate the foot of the bed.
4. Wrap the leg in a warm blanket.

44. The nurse can administer which mediation through a nasogastric (NG) tube?
1. Enteric-coated aspirin
2. Acetaminophen
3. Regular insulin
4. Sublingual nitroglycerine

45. The nurse knows that if a client requires oxygen delivery at a FIo₂ of 92%, the appropriate system would be a:
1. face tent.
2. Venturi mask.
3. nasal cannula.
4. mask with reservoir bag.

41. 2. The client with thrombocytopenia has a low platelet count and should avoid products containing aspirin since they may increase the risk of bleeding. Iron supplements would be helpful in the client with anemia. Staying away from crowds and avoiding fresh salads to reduce the risk of infection would be important for the client with leukopenia.
CN: Physiological integrity; CNS: Reduction of risk potential; CL: Analysis

42. 2. The normal range for sodium is 135 to 145 mEq/L. The rest of the results are within normal limits.
CN: Physiological integrity; CNS: Reduction of risk potential; CL: Analysis

43. 1. The client has arterial disease and had vascular surgery. The nurse must assess the client for complications. A potential problem would be a clot at the surgical site, so the nurse must assess circulation by checking for distal pulses. Before the physician is notified, the nurse should determine if distal pulses are present. Elevating the foot of the bed would promote venous return but decrease arterial blood flow and shouldn't be done. The leg can be covered lightly after circulation is assessed.
CN: Physiological integrity; CNS: Physiological adaptation; CL: Analysis

44. 2. Most oral medications can be given through an NG tube because they're intended for passage into the stomach. Some oral drugs have special coatings intended to keep the pill intact until it passes into the small intestine; these enteric-coated pills shouldn't be crushed and put through an NG tube. Some parenteral medications, such as insulin, may be destroyed by gastric juices. Sublingual means under the tongue, and parenteral means I.V., I.M., and subcutaneous.
CN: Physiological integrity; CNS: Pharmacological and parenteral therapies; CL: Application

45. 4. A mask with a reservoir bag administers 70% to 100% oxygen at flow rates of 8 to 10 L/minute. A face tent maximum delivery rate is 22% to 34%, the Venturi mask maximum rate is 24% to 55%, and the nasal cannula maximum rate is 44% at 6 L/minute.
CN: Physiological integrity; CNS: Pharmacological and parenteral therapies; CL: Analysis

46. The client has returned from the operating room with the nursing diagnosis of acute pain. The nurse knows the best means of providing comfort would be to administer:
1. morphine sulfate 10 mg intramuscularly.
2. morphine sulfate 0.2 mg/ml via patient-controlled analgesia.
3. Dilaudid 2 mg I.V. every 2 hours.
4. Percocet 5 mg orally every 4 to 6 hours.

47. A client with difficulty breathing has a respiratory rate of 34 breaths/minute and demonstrates anxious behaviors. He's refusing all his medications, claiming they're making him worse. Which nursing action is best?
1. Notify the physician of the status of this client.
2. Withhold the medication until the next scheduled dose.
3. Encourage the client to take some of his medications.
4. Put the medicine in applesauce to give it without the client's knowledge.

48. Which statement is an example of a key element in the nursing care plan?
1. Advance diet to regular as tolerated.
2. Ambulate 30′ (9 m) with walker by discharge.
3. Give furosemide (Lasix) 40 mg I.V. now.
4. Discontinue I.V. fluids when tolerating oral fluids.

49. A client who was recently hospitalized has a nursing diagnosis of constipation related to medical regimen. Which medication may contribute to this problem?
1. Folic acid
2. Iron
3. Potassium
4. Vitamin E

50. A client had an appendectomy 24 hours ago. Which nursing goal is appropriate for this client?
1. The client will be able to walk in the hallway.
2. The client will be able to attend physical therapy.
3. The client will be able to accomplish all activities of daily living.
4. The client will be able to state the rationale for all postoperative medications.

46. 2. Clients who have ready access to an analgesic are more likely to medicate themselves before the pain becomes severe and thus may require reduced amounts of medication. Having control over drug administration also reduces anxiety, which helps to relieve pain.
CN: Physiological integrity; CNS: Pharmacological and parenteral therapies; CL: Application

47. 1. Notifying the physician of the client's condition and his refusal to take his medications allows the physician to decide what alternatives should be instituted. Withholding a medication requires the physician to be notified. Even if the client takes some of the medications, the physician will still need to be notified. It needs to be explored why the client believes the medications are making him worse. Giving medications in applesauce destroys trust between the nurse and client.
CN: Physiological integrity; CNS: Pharmacological and parenteral therapies; CL: Application

48. 2. Ambulating 30′ with a walker by discharge is a measurable expected outcome or goal, a key element of a nursing care plan. Other key elements include nursing diagnoses and interventions. The other options are physician's orders, not key elements of care plans.
CN: Safe, effective care environment; CNS: Management of care; CL: Application

49. 2. Iron may cause constipation when supplements are taken at 100% of the Recommended Daily Allowance. Folic acid, potassium, and vitamin E don't increase the likelihood of constipation.
CN: Physiological integrity; CNS: Pharmacological and parenteral therapies; CL: Application

50. 1. A 24-hour postoperative client is expected to be able to walk in the hallway. A client who just had an appendectomy shouldn't need physical therapy unless deconditioning was evident. At 24 hours, a client should begin to assume responsibility for activities of daily living but shouldn't necessarily be responsible for all activities. It's too early to expect a client to state the rationale for all postoperative medications, especially if the client is elderly.
CN: Physiological integrity; CNS: Basic care and comfort; CL: Application

51. Which nursing discharge instruction has the highest priority for a client going home with a full leg cast?
1. Activity restrictions
2. Proper nutrition
3. Weight-bearing limitations
4. Reporting signs of impaired circulation

52. The nurse is performing an admission assessment. What is the best statement/question for the nurse to use to gather the most information about the reason for admission would be?
1. "Does your abdomen have sharp pains?"
2. "Are you noticing more gas with this condition?"
3. "Tell me how things have been going for you."
4. "I'd like to further question your pain."

53. A registered nurse (RN) is supervising an unlicensed care provider. Which principle would the nurse follow when delegating tasks?
1. The RN must directly supervise all delegated tasks.
2. After a task is delegated, it's no longer the RN's responsibility.
3. The RN is responsible for delegating tasks to adjunct personnel.
4. Follow-up with a delegated task is necessary only if the assistive personnel are untrustworthy.

54. An elderly client had recent surgery and is on bed rest. When planning care for the client, which nursing intervention is included in the care plan?
1. Daily assessment of the wound site
2. Foot and ankle range-of-motion (ROM) exercises
3. Wound cleaning with hydrogen peroxide
4. Coughing and deep breathing in the prone position

55. A client receiving phenothiazine has become restless and fidgety and has been pacing the hallway continuously for the past hour. This behavior suggests to the nurse that the client may be experiencing which adverse reaction to phenothiazine?
1. Dystonia
2. Akathisia
3. Parkinsonian effects
4. Tardive dyskinesia

51. 4. The nurse should include all these instructions in the teaching plan; however, the highest priority is teaching the signs of impaired circulation to prevent permanent neurovascular damage, including loss of the leg.
CN: Physiological integrity; CNS: Reduction of risk potential; CL: Analysis

52. 3. "Tell me how things have been going for you," is an open-ended question that will encourage the client to talk and express concerns. Options 1 and 2 are closed-ended questions and can be answered with a simple "yes" or "no," which will not give the most information necessary for an admission assessment. Option 4 is not asking for any information at this time but lends itself to future questions.
CN: Psychosocial integrity; CNS: None; CL: Application

53. 3. The RN must delegate tasks that are within the scope of practice of the unlicensed personnel. The RN need not directly supervise all delegated tasks as that would negate the benefits of delegation. Even when the task is delegated, the RN retains responsibility for the successful completion of the task. The RN must always follow up with the assistive personnel to ensure the task was completed appropriately, not only in instances of mistrust.
CN: Safe, effective care environment; CNS: Management of care; CL: Application

54. 2. Foot and ankle ROM exercises are standard protocol for clients who remain in bed for an extended period of time. ROM exercises promote blood flow to the area, prevent atrophy, and lessen the potential for edema. The wound site should be assessed every shift. Wound cleaning with hydrogen peroxide isn't generally recommended. Coughing and deep breathing aren't generally recommended in the prone position.
CN: Physiological integrity; CNS: Reduction of risk potential; CL: Application

55. 2. The client's behavior suggests akathisia—an adverse effect of phenothiazines. Dystonia appears as excessive salivation; difficulty speaking; and involuntary movements of the face, neck, arms, and legs. Parkinsonian effects include a shuffling gait, hand tremors, drooling, rigidity, and loose arm movements. Tardive dyskinesia is characterized by odd facial and tongue movements.
CN: Physiological integrity; CNS: Reduction of risk potential; CL: Application

56. A client who had his gallbladder removed 2 days ago now complains of pain in the right calf. Which nursing response has priority?
1. Assess the leg for swelling and redness.
2. Instruct the client to flex his knee and hip.
3. Apply a warm compress and call the physician.
4. Gently massage the calf and notify the physician.

56. 1. Pain in the calf is a symptom of possible deep vein thrombosis. The nurse must assess further. Assessing the client for redness and swelling would be the next intervention. Making the client flex his knee and hip won't help assess for the presence of a clot. Warm compresses may be ordered after a diagnosis of deep vein thrombosis is made. Never massage the calf muscle because the clot could be dislodged.

CN: Physiological integrity; CNS: Reduction of risk potential; CL: Analysis

57. Which goal will the nurse make the highest priority in a client with a new tracheostomy?
1. Developing an effective means of communication
2. Maintaining a patent airway
3. Preventing infection
4. Gaining independence in self-care

57. 2. Maintaining a patent airway has the highest priority in a client with a new tracheostomy since drainage and edema can obstruct the airway. The other goals are also important but only after airway patency has been assured.

CN: Physiological integrity; CNS: Reduction of risk potential; CL: Analysis

58. Which statement by a client with chronic arterial disease indicates to the nurse further teaching is needed?
1. "I'm going to stop smoking."
2. "I'm going to have the podiatrist check my feet."
3. "I'm going to keep the heat in my house at 80° F."
4. "I'm going to walk short distances every morning."

58. 3. Clients with peripheral vascular disease need to be at a comfortable temperature because of impaired circulation. Having the heat at 80° F is too warm. The other choices are all appropriate interventions for a client with peripheral vascular disease.

CN: Physiological integrity; CNS: Reduction of risk potential; CL: Application

59. A registered nurse is in charge of eight clients. The nurse has a licensed practical nurse (LPN) and a client care assistant working under her. Which activity should the nurse assign to herself rather than delegate to the staff?
1. Consoling a grieving visitor
2. Assessing a newly admitted client
3. Irrigating a Salem sump to continuous drainage
4. Giving a tap water enema to a preoperative client

59. 2. Assessment of a new admission can't be delegated to an LPN. Consoling a visitor and giving a tap water enema are within the scope of practice of an LPN and client care assistant. Irrigation of a Salem sump is under the scope of practice of an LPN.

CN: Safe, effective care environment; CNS: Management of care; CL: Application

You're almost there! Keep going!

60. A 6-year-old client needs diabetic teaching. Which factor is considered when the nurse plans the teaching?
1. Another child with diabetes can teach the client.
2. The child can teach his parents after the nurse teaches him.
3. The child and parents should be recipients of teaching.
4. Teaching should be directed to the parents, who then can teach the child.

60. 3. The parents and child should participate in the nurse's teaching to ensure accuracy of teaching and that the child has educated adult caregivers. The school-aged child shouldn't be the sole provider of teaching to the parents. Another school-aged child couldn't be entrusted to teach this child, although their input would be valuable. Parents should be included in the teaching plan but shouldn't be responsible for the teaching.

CN: Health promotion and maintenance; CNS: None; CL: Application

61. Parents of a toddler are having problems putting him to bed at night. Which recommendation by a nurse is most appropriate?
1. Stop the afternoon naps.
2. Allow the toddler to have a tantrum for ½ hour.
3. Encourage the parents to develop nighttime rituals.
4. Allow the toddler to have some control over bedtime.

62. After abdominal surgery for repair of an aortic aneurysm, a client may show maladaptive coping behavior in response to body changes related to the surgery. Which nursing intervention is best?
1. Let the client express his feelings.
2. Explain that a psychological referral would be beneficial.
3. Instruct the client on how to use positive coping strategies.
4. Encourage the client to participate in diversionary activities.

63. A new graduate nurse has started at the medical center and is assigned to a preceptor. The preceptor and other staff report that the nurse is uncooperative and unwilling to take direction. Which action by the preceptor is appropriate?
1. Explain the behavior won't be tolerated.
2. Ask the nurse why she wants to work here.
3. Reestablish goals with the nurse.
4. Begin the disciplinary process with this nurse.

64. A client with a history of bipolar disorder rushes into the mental health clinic waiting room scantily dressed and makes loud, obscene remarks to other clients. Which intervention by the nurse is most appropriate?
1. Encourage the other clients to ignore the behavior.
2. Confront the behavior and make the client take a seat.
3. Tell the client to sit down and stop upsetting the others.
4. Quietly escort the client to a private area and help put on a gown.

61. 3. Rituals are extremely important for toddlers to feel secure and relaxed. Allowing a toddler to make small decisions, such as choosing the order of the ritual and color of pajamas, will give him the feeling of some control. Stopping the naps may be helpful, depending on the toddler's needs. The toddler must clearly understand that tantrums won't get him what he wants.
CN: Health promotion and maintenance; CNS: None; CL: Application

62. 1. Allowing verbalization of feelings is the most therapeutic nursing intervention. Making a referral may help, but initially, the client should be allowed to express his feelings. Giving advice may stop therapeutic communication. Providing diversionary activities doesn't foster effective coping.
CN: Psychosocial integrity; CNS: None; CL: Analysis

63. 3. This is a new graduate in orientation, and the preceptor should help this nurse learn the responsibilities and routines and reestablish goals. If the behavior continues, the nurse may need career counseling. This person isn't experienced and therefore shouldn't be reprimanded. Asking the nurse "why" in relation to working is inappropriate; it's the behavior that's creating the problem. This nurse shouldn't be disciplined as an initial step.
CN: Safe, effective care environment; CNS: Management of care; CL: Application

64. 4. The client with bipolar disorder is highly excitable. The nurse needs to be firm yet distracting, and this is best done in a private area, which also preserves the client's dignity. Having the others ignore the client won't alter the problem. Confronting the behavior isn't desired as this client lacks judgment and insight. Telling the client to sit down may cause the client to be more resistive and even heighten the behavior.
CN: Psychosocial integrity; CNS: None; CL: Analysis

65. A nurse is reviewing treatment of hyper-cyanotic spells (tet spells) with the parents of a 4-month-old client being discharged from the hospital. What is the most important information for the nurse to tell the parents?
1. "Calm the baby down by holding her and placing her knees up to her chest."
2. "Call 911 immediately and begin cardiopulmonary resuscitation (CPR) on the baby."
3. "You'll need to administer four back blows to the baby if she begins having a tet spell."
4. "You don't need to worry about these spells yet because the baby is too young. You'll need to watch for them when she becomes more mobile."

66. A nurse is caring for a client with gout. Which nursing intervention should the nurse include in the plan of care?
1. Administer antibiotics.
2. Restrict fluid intake.
3. Encourage a low-purine diet.
4. Administer opioids.

67. The nurse is evaluating a client who is 2 days post-crush injury to his right leg. Which symptom is a late indicator of compartment syndrome?
1. Sudden decrease in pain
2. Swelling in toes or fingers
3. Inability to move fingers or toes
4. Diminished distal pulses

68. A client with an arm cast complains of severe pain in the affected extremity, and decreased sensation and motion are noted. Swelling in the fingers is also increased. Which nursing intervention has priority?
1. Elevate the arm.
2. Remove the cast.
3. Give an analgesic.
4. Call the physician.

65. **1.** Tet spells are acute episodes of cyanosis and hypoxia that occur when the infant's oxygen demand exceeds the available supply. They may occur when the infant is crying or eating. Tet spells are emergency situations that require immediate intervention. Begin by calming the infant down and placing the infant in the knee-chest position, which increases systemic vascular resistance by limiting venous return. This decreases the right to left shunting and improves oxygenation. CPR won't calm the infant down or improve oxygenation. Back blows are given to infants who have something lodged in their trachea.

CN: Physiological integrity; CNS: Reduction of risk potential; CL: Application

66. **3.** A low-purine diet decreases uric acid formation and should be encouraged. Antibiotics aren't used to treat gout. Fluid intake should be encouraged to flush out the uric acid. Anti-inflammatory medications are used during acute phases, but because this is a long-term condition, opioids aren't generally given.

CN: Physiological integrity; CNS: Reduction of risk potential; CL: Application

67. **4.** Compartment syndrome is a complication of a cast that places pressure on the blood vessels and nerves to the extremity. Symptoms include pain not relieved by analgesics and swelling of the extremity. A late symptom is a change in skin color with diminished distal pulses. After a fracture, some swelling and pain result, but pulses need to be monitored as well as color, sensation, and movement.

CN: Physiological integrity; CNS: Reduction of risk potential; CL: Analysis

68. **4.** The cast may be too tight and may need to be split or removed by the physician. The arm should already be elevated. Notify the physician when circulation, sensation, or motion is impaired. Giving analgesics wouldn't be the first step as they may mask the signs of a serious problem.

CN: Physiological integrity; CNS: Reduction of risk potential; CL: Application

CN: Client needs category   CNS: Client needs subcategory   CL: Cognitive level

69. The nurse is performing preoperative teaching on a 4-year-old child scheduled for cardiac catheterization. Which characteristic is correct for preoperative teaching?
1. Basic and performed close to the implementation of the procedure
2. Done several days before the procedure so the child will have time to prepare
3. Detailed in regard to the actual procedure so the child will know exactly what to expect
4. Directed at the child's parents because the child is too young to understand the procedure

70. A registered nurse is directing unlicensed personnel to draw the morning blood work for a 4-year-old child in the hospital. The nurse emphasizes the procedure is to be done in the treatment room. Which rationale is correct?
1. The procedure will be faster.
2. The child won't fear painful procedures done while he's in his bed.
3. The child can only be restrained on the examination table.
4. The parents won't observe the procedure and upset the child.

71. A client tells a nurse, "My medical illness is the result of something bad I did to someone in the past." Which response by the nurse is the most appropriate?
1. "What did you do wrong?"
2. "Let's talk about your concerns."
3. "That's silly! Don't believe that!"
4. "You're suffering from a psychiatric delusion. Relax, it will end soon."

72. A client on a psychiatric unit asks a nurse about the medications another client takes. Which response is best?
1. "How close are the two of you?"
2. "I can't give you that information; her privacy must be protected."
3. "Let me ask her if it's okay for me to tell you about her condition and medications."
4. "The client is taking insulin for her diabetes and digoxin for her heart condition."

Hooray! Only 5 more to go!

69. **1.** Four-year-old children are in Piaget's cognitive stage of preoperational thought. Their thinking is concrete and tangible, and they're unable to make deductions or generalizations and are egocentric. They don't have a concept for the future so explanations need to be done close to the time of the procedure, not days in advance. They need simple explanations of procedures in relationship to how the procedure will affect them. A 4-year-old child is old enough to understand basic teaching close to the implementation of the procedure.
CN: Health promotion and maintenance; CNS: None; CL: Application

70. **2.** This implementation is based on the concept of "atraumatic care" and growth and development principles. Small children need to have a safe zone in their beds to relax and rest in their rooms. The treatment room is used instead. It won't be faster to draw blood in the treatment room; it would take the same amount of time regardless of where it's done. The child could be restrained in his room, but it isn't appropriate. Parental support is important and needs to be encouraged during stressful and painful procedures.
CN: Psychosocial integrity; CNS: None; CL: Application

71. **2.** Asking the client to talk about his concerns allows an opportunity for the nurse to clarify issues. Calling the client silly or asking the client what he did wrong would likely escalate the client's concerns. Telling the client it will end soon gives false reassurance.
CN: Psychosocial integrity; CNS: None; CL: Application

72. **2.** Revealing one client's medication to another client is violating procedures of client confidentiality. Asking the client the nature of his relationship to the other client won't help the client understand the purpose of protecting confidentiality. Seeking the client's permission to release confidential information is an inappropriate action. Assuring the client that the hospital has an obligation to protect not only his confidentiality but also that of others will provide the client with a sense of comfort.
CN: Safe, effective care environment; CNS: Management of care; CL: Application

73. A client's goal is to interact verbally at least once in each group therapy session by a certain date. The client attended the group session, maintained eye contact with the group members, followed the conversation nonverbally as indicated by head nodding, and spoke once to the group leader by giving a one-word answer. Which judgment by a nurse about goal attainment is correct?
1. The goal was partially met.
2. The goal was completely met.
3. The goal was completely unmet.
4. New problems or nursing diagnoses have developed.

74. A client is prescribed heparin 6,000 units subcutaneously every 12 hours for deep vein thrombosis prophylaxis. The pharmacy dispenses a vial containing 10,000 units/ml. How many milliliters of heparin should a nurse administer? Record your answer using one decimal place.

_____ milliliters

75. A client is prescribed lisinopril (Zestril) for treatment of hypertension. He asks the nurse about possible adverse effects. The nurse should teach him about which common adverse effects of angiotensin-converting enzyme (ACE) inhibitors? Select all that apply.
1. Constipation
2. Dizziness
3. Headache
4. Hyperglycemia
5. Hypotension
6. Impotence

73. **1.** This goal was partially met because the client must verbally participate more in the group. For a goal to be completely met, the client must show the subjective and objective data indicating the goal has been clearly attained. A completely unmet goal indicates the client's complete lack of behavior change and absence of subjective and objective data to indicate the achievement of the goal. In this case, no new problems or new nursing diagnoses were evident.

CN: Psychosocial integrity; CNS: None; CL: Analysis

74. 0.6. The following formula is used to calculate drug dosages: Dose on hand/Quantity on hand = Dose desired/X. The dose dispensed by the pharmacy is 10,000 units/1 ml, and the desired dose is 6,000 units. The nurse should use the following equations: 10,000 units/1 ml = 6,000 units/X; 10,000 units (X) = 6,000 units (ml)/ 10,000 units; $X = 0.6$ ml.

CN: Physiological integrity; CNS: Pharmacological and parenteral therapies; CL: Analysis

75. **2, 3, and 5.** Dizziness, headache, and hypotension are all common adverse effects of lisinopril and other ACE inhibitors. Lisinopril may cause diarrhea, not constipation. It isn't known to cause hyperglycemia or impotence.

CN: Physiological integrity; CNS: Pharmacological and parenteral therapies; CL: Application

COMPREHENSIVE
Test 6

1. The nurse is teaching clients about hypertension and the importance of risk factors. Which client response identifying a nonmodifiable risk factor indicates that the teaching has been effective?
   1. High sodium intake
   2. Sedentary lifestyle
   3. Tobacco use
   4. Family history

2. A client experienced an acute inferior myocardial infarction at a community hospital. After antithrombolytic therapy fails, the physician wants to transfer the client to another hospital for emergency cardiac catheterization. Which member of the health care team must accompany the client?
   1. Physician
   2. Paramedic
   3. Registered nurse (RN)
   4. Licensed practical nurse (LPN)

3. A 56-year-old client with heart failure is allergic to sulfa-based medications. Which type of diuretic should be used cautiously?
   1. Osmotic diuretics
   2. Thiazide and thiazide-like diuretics
   3. Potassium-sparing diuretics
   4. Carbonic anhydrase inhibitors

4. A client with heart failure says he sleeps with two pillows because he experiences difficulty breathing when lying flat. The nurse would documents this as which condition?
   1. Bradypnea
   2. Dyspnea on exertion
   3. Paroxysmal nocturnal dyspnea
   4. Orthopnea

1. 4. Family history is a risk factor for hypertension that can't be modified. Risk factors that can be modified include high sodium intake, sedentary lifestyle, and tobacco use.
CN: Health promotion and maintenance; CNS: None; CL: Application

2. 3. During transfer, the client must receive the same level of care that he received in the hospital; therefore, an RN must accompany him. It isn't necessary for a physician to accompany the client. A paramedic, although not required, will most likely accompany the nurse. An LPN is below the standard of care for this situation.
CN: Safe, effective care environment; CNS: Management of care; CL: Application

3. 2. Thiazide and thiazide-like diuretics are sulfonamide derivatives, so their use should be used cautiously in clients allergic to sulfa-based medications. Osmotic, potassium-sparing, and carbonic anhydrase inhibitor diuretics can be safely administered to these clients.
CN: Physiological integrity; CNS: Pharmacological and parenteral therapies; CL: Application

4. 4. A client with orthopnea has shortness of breath when lying flat, so he prefers sleeping with the upper body elevated. Bradypnea is decreased but regular breathing. Dyspnea on exertion occurs when the client has difficulty breathing with activity. Paroxysmal nocturnal dyspnea occurs when the client awakens at night and feels short of breath.
CN: Health promotion and maintenance; CNS: None; CL: Application

5. During an initial assessment of a neonate, the nurse notes a respiratory rate of 52 breaths/minute. What is the most appropriate intervention by the nurse?
1. Notify the physician immediately.
2. Do nothing; this is a normal respiratory rate for a neonate.
3. Position the Isolette so the neonate's head is elevated.
4. Prepare for emergency endotracheal (ET) intubation.

6. During a neonate's 1-month checkup, the pediatrician flexes the neonate's legs to right angles at the hips and knees and abducts both hips until the knees touch the table. Which statement describes the purpose of this test?
1. To check the neonate's flexibility
2. To assess leg strength
3. To check for developmental dysplasia of the hip
4. To examine the neonate for a hydrocele

7. At which age should a nurse initially screen for idiopathic juvenile scoliosis?
1. 7 years
2. 10 years
3. 13 years
4. 16 years

8. The nurse is screening a 10-year-old client for scoliosis. How should the nurse place the client?
1. Facing away from the examiner, standing upright with his arms held out straight in front of his body
2. Facing away from the examiner, bending forward in 50% flexion with his arms and head dangling
3. Facing the examiner, standing upright with his arms held straight at his sides
4. Sitting in a chair with feet flat on the floor and his back at a 90-degree angle

9. Parents bring their infant to the clinic for a checkup after he was hospitalized with a new onset of type 1 diabetes mellitus. Which statement to the nurse indicates an understanding of their child's current situation?
1. "The physician was wrong about the diagnosis because all of my child's fingersticks have been normal."
2. "My child has experienced a honeymoon period, which could last 1 month to 1 year, and hasn't required any insulin injections."
3. "Nobody in our family has diabetes, so how can my child have it?"
4. "If our child lives a careful, sedentary lifestyle, she won't need as much insulin."

5. 2. A normal respiratory rate for a neonate is 30 to 60 breaths/minute, so notifying the physician or elevating the neonate's head isn't necessary. The nurse should prepare for ET intubation if the neonate has signs of imminent respiratory distress such as an expiratory grunt.
CN: Health promotion and maintenance; CNS: None; CL: Analysis

6. 3. This test assesses for developmental dysplasia of the hip. If dysplasia is present, the physician can see, feel, and, sometimes, hear a click. Although a neonate's flexibility and leg strength may be assessed at age 1 month, the examination techniques differ from those described here. To identify a hydrocele, the physician palpates the neonate's testes.
CN: Physiological integrity; CNS: Physiological adaptation; CL: Analysis

7. 2. Children should have initial screening at age 10—immediately before the adolescent growth spurt—when promontory signs of scoliosis may become apparent. By age 13, a child may have significantly developed scoliosis that requires surgery.
CN: Health promotion and maintenance; CNS: None; CL: Application

8. 2. Assessing a client's back for asymmetry, or a "razorback" hump, is best done with the client bending at the waist in 50% flexion with the arms and head dangling. This assessment can also be done with the arms hanging dependently at the sides so the examiner can check for asymmetry at the shoulders, waist folds, and space between the arms and waist.
CN: Health promotion and maintenance; CNS: None; CL: Application

9. 2. A honeymoon phase—in which injected insulin seems to wake up the islet cells and cause them to secrete insulin—is common with type 1 diabetes mellitus. This phase has given many parents false hope that their child has been cured. Type 1 diabetes isn't a genetic trait, and a sedentary lifestyle will increase the secondary effects of diabetes.
CN: Physiological integrity; CNS: Physiological adaptation; CL: Analysis

10. The nurse is preparing to administer an injection subcutaneously. Which graphic indicates the appropriate needle selection for this type of injection?

1.

2.

3.

4.

You've finished 10 questions! Cool!

11. Which intervention should a nurse include in the care plan for a 2-year-old child with Wilms' tumor?
1. Tell the parents that surgery will be within 24 to 48 hours.
2. Palpate the abdomen to monitor tumor size.
3. Massage the abdomen to relieve pain.
4. Place a tight binder around the abdomen for support.

12. Two days after undergoing a left thoracotomy, a client's temperature reaches 102° F (38.9° C). The nurse notifies the physician, who orders two sets of blood cultures. Which amount of blood would the nurse obtain for cultures?
1. 2 ml
2. 5 ml
3. 10 ml
4. 20 ml

13. A charge nurse is developing the client-care assignments for the shift. Which client is most appropriately assigned to a licensed practical nurse (LPN)?
1. A client who has experienced a cerebral vascular accident and has a do-not-resuscitate (DNR) status
2. A client who underwent cerebral arteriography 1 hour ago
3. A client who underwent carotid endarterectomy 4 hours ago
4. A client who underwent craniotomy 3 days ago and has just been transferred from the intensive care unit (ICU)

10. 2. When choosing a needle, consider its purpose as well as its gauge, bevel, and length. Graphic 2 indicates a subcutaneous needle which has a length of ½″ to ⅝″ long and medium bevel. The first graphic is of an intradermal needle, which has a length of ⅜″ to ⅝″ and short bevel. The third graphic is an intramuscular needle, which is 1″ to 3″ in length with a medium bevel. The fourth graphic is an intravenous needle, which is 1″ to 3″ long with a long bevel.

CN: Physiological integrity; CNS: Pharmacological and parenteral therapies; CL: Application

11. 1. The nurse tells the parents that the child will be scheduled for a nephrectomy within 24 to 48 hours because these tumors metastasize quickly. To reduce the risk of dissemination of cancer cells, the abdomen shouldn't be palpated or massaged. A tight binder may put pressure on the tumor, increasing the risk of dissemination, and should, therefore, be avoided.

CN: Safe, effective care environment; CNS: Management of care; CL: Application

12. 3. When an adult client requires blood cultures, the nurse should draw 10 ml of blood; 5 ml should be injected into an anaerobic (without oxygen) bottle and 5 ml injected into an aerobic (with oxygen) bottle.

CN: Physiological integrity; CNS: Reduction of risk potential; CL: Application

13. 1. The most appropriate client to assign to the LPN is the newly admitted client with DNR status; typically, a newly admitted client is assigned to a registered nurse (RN) because the client requires frequent assessments. The client who recently underwent cerebral arteriography and the client who recently underwent carotid endarterectomy require frequent assessments by an RN. The client just transferred from the ICU has the potential for becoming unstable; therefore, an RN should care for this client.

CN: Safe, effective care environment; CNS: Management of care; CL: Analysis

14. A physician prescribes carbamazepine (Tegretol) 1,200 mg by mouth twice daily for a client with trigeminal neuralgia. Which action should the nurse take first?
1. Administer the medication with meals.
2. Encourage the client to promptly report unusual bleeding, bruising, fever, or chills.
3. Question the order because the dose exceeds the recommended daily dose.
4. Store the drug in a cool, dry place.

15. Emergency medical system personnel have used the Cincinnati Prehospital Stroke Scale to assess a client and have alerted the hospital that they're transporting a client with a possible stroke. The nurse plans to administer fibrinolytics within which time period?
1. 4 hours of the onset of symptoms
2. 60 minutes of arrival in the emergency department (ED)
3. 2 hours of arrival in the ED
4. 25 minutes of arrival in the ED

16. A client with an above-the-knee amputation visits the orthopedic surgeon for a follow-up. Which comment to the nurse would indicate the client is properly caring for the stump and prosthetic leg?
1. "I inspect the stump weekly to look for signs of redness, blistering, or abrasions."
2. "I put my prosthesis on before I get out of bed."
3. "I wash the stump every day with an antiseptic soap."
4. "I wipe out the socket of my prosthesis with a damp, soapy cloth weekly."

14. 3. The first intervention by the nurse should be to question the order because it exceeds the recommended daily dose. Clients with trigeminal neuralgia should receive no more than 1,200 mg/day. After the nurse obtains an appropriate order, she should encourage the client to take the drug at equally spaced intervals with food to avoid GI distress. The nurse should also encourage the client to promptly report unusual bleeding; bruising; jaundice; dark urine; pale stools; abdominal pain; impotence; fever; chills; sore throat; mouth ulcers; edema; or disturbances in mood, alertness, or coordination. The drug should be stored in a cool, dry place.

CN: Physiological integrity; CNS: Pharmacological and parenteral therapies; CL: Analysis

15. 2. The goal for initiating fibrinolytic therapy is within 60 minutes of arrival in the ED. Fibrinolytics must be administered within 3 hours of the onset of symptoms.

CN: Physiological integrity; CNS: Pharmacological and parenteral therapies; CL: Application

16. 2. The prosthesis should be applied upon rising in the morning. The stump and prosthesis should be inspected daily and cleaned daily with a mild soap. The prosthesis should be kept clean to prevent irritation or pressure areas from dirt or bacteria.

CN: Health promotion and maintenance; CNS: None; CL: Analysis

17. A nurse is caring for a client after a total knee replacement. The extremity was placed in a continuous passive motion (CPM) machine. Which action is one of the nurse's responsibilities?
  1. Check the cycle and range-of-motion settings every morning.
  2. Increase the degrees of flexion daily guided by client level of tolerance.
  3. Decrease the degree of extension daily.
  4. Turn the machine off when the client is eating a meal.

18. A client has multiple myeloma. Which action should alert the nurse that he may be having difficulty coping with his prognosis?
  1. He becomes tearful when discussing his condition.
  2. He asks questions about his prognosis.
  3. He shows concerns about his family.
  4. He avoids any conversation concerning his health.

19. Which client is <u>most</u> likely to develop ankylosing spondylitis?
  1. White female, age 16, with knee pain
  2. Black male, age 50, with hip pain
  3. Asian female, age 70, with chest pain
  4. White male, age 23, with back pain

20. A client with pernicious anemia undergoes gastrectomy. Which route should the nurse use to administer cyanocobalamin (vitamin B_{12}) after the surgery?
  1. Buccal route
  2. Transdermal route
  3. Oral route
  4. Parenteral route

21. After a nurse teaches a client with diverticular disease about proper diet, he fills out his lunch menu. Which selection by the client demonstrates the need for further teaching?
  1. Tossed salad with tomatoes, sunflower seeds, and tuna
  2. Egg salad on whole-wheat bread and an apple
  3. Cottage cheese with apple, pear, and plum slices
  4. Ham salad served with whole-wheat crackers and a banana

17. 4. The CPM machine can be turned off during meals to improve client comfort. The cycle and degrees of flexion should be checked every shift, and either the physician or physical therapist determines how and when the degrees of flexion can be increased. Usually, extension—as well as flexion—is increased, not decreased, on a regular basis.
CN: Physiological integrity; CNS: Basic care and comfort; CL: Application

18. 4. A client who avoids conversation about his health may be denying his condition and not coping well with his prognosis. Crying is a normal response to his disease. Asking questions about his prognosis and showing concern for his family are normal coping responses.
CN: Psychological integrity; CNS: None; CL: Analysis

19. 4. Ankylosing spondylitis usually begins between ages 15 and 30 years, and the prevalence is highest in white males. Back pain is the characteristic feature.
CN: Health promotion and maintenance; CNS: None; CL: Analysis

20. 4. A client who has undergone gastrectomy is no longer able to produce the intrinsic factor necessary for vitamin B_{12} absorption through the GI tract; therefore, the parenteral route (intramuscular or deep subcutaneous injections) is required. This medication isn't available for buccal or transdermal routes.
CN: Physiological integrity; CNS: Pharmacological and parenteral therapies; CL: Application

21. 1. Clients with diverticular disease should avoid high-roughage foods, such as nuts, seeds, popcorn, and raw celery. They should, however, consume high-fiber foods, such as fresh fruit with skins (apples, pears, and plums), bananas, dried fruits, whole-wheat bread and crackers, and raw vegetables (lettuce, carrots, and cauliflower).
CN: Physiological integrity; CNS: Basic care and comfort; CL: Application

22. A nurse is teaching nursing students about maintaining a healthy liver. Which measure should the nurse include in her teaching?
1. Take over-the-counter (OTC) medication as needed.
2. Take prescribed medications according to instructions.
3. Add a nutritional supplement to the diet to ensure adequate nutrition.
4. Consume a low-protein diet that contains moderate carbohydrate and fat.

23. A 28-year-old male client complaining of a racing heart and nervousness is admitted to the telemetry floor. His telemetry shows a heart rate of 130 beats/minute in sinus tachycardia. His skin is very warm and dry, and his eyes appear to be bulging. Which nursing action is the most important upon admission?
1. Inserting a urinary catheter and assessing appearance of urine
2. Observing the client's gait
3. Reaching out and feeling the client's neck
4. Standing behind the client and gently palpating the cricothyroid area

24. A client is unemployed, has no health insurance, hasn't filled his levothyroxine (Synthroid) prescription for some time, and has been getting "sicker by the day." Which problem is probably related to him not taking his medication?
1. Diarrhea and vomiting
2. Rapid heart rate
3. Warm, dry, flushed skin
4. Rectal temperature of 94° F (34.4° C)

25. A child with chronic renal failure is scheduled for hemodialysis with an external shunt three times per week. As part of the discharge planning, the nurse should tell the family to perform which step?
1. Assess the site daily for symptoms of redness.
2. Wash the serum at the shunt site with normal saline.
3. Assess the child's blood pressure on the same side as the shunt.
4. Keep a clean dressing in place over the shunt site.

You're doing terrific! Keep going!

22. 2. Taking these measures will help maintain a healthy liver: take prescribed medications according to instructions; avoid taking unnecessary OTC medications; eat a balanced diet that's moderate to high in protein, moderate in carbohydrate and fat, and adequate in vitamins; and take a nutritional supplement only if advised to do so by a physician.
CN: Health promotion and maintenance; CNS: None; CL: Application

23. 4. The client shows signs of hyperthyroidism, and standing behind him and palpating the cricothyroid area is the correct way to assess for an enlarged thyroid gland. Inserting a catheter isn't necessary; assessing the client's urine, which would be concentrated because of dehydration, can be done after he voids. Observing the client's gait isn't necessary at this time.
CN: Physiological integrity; CNS: Physiological adaptation; CL: Analysis

24. 4. Hypothyroidism leads to a hypodynamic state, so a low body temperature is expected after the levothyroxine has been metabolized. Each of the other symptoms is indicative of a hypermetabolic state, and although the client may exhibit these problems, they're probably related to infection and dehydration.
CN: Physiological integrity; CNS: Physiological adaptation; CL: Application

25. 1. The child and parents should assess the shunt site for redness daily because a color change may indicate infection. Serum at the shunt site should be washed away with half-strength hydrogen peroxide and an antibiotic ointment applied. Blood pressure shouldn't be taken in the arm with the shunt. A sterile dressing should be placed over the shunt site.
CN: Safe, effective care environment; CNS: Safety and infection control; CL: Application

26. A 17-year-old client tells the nurse that she has vulvar itching and a thick, cream cheese–like vaginal discharge. The nurse anticipates treating the client with which medication?
1. Metronidazole (Flagyl)
2. Erythromycin (Ery-Tab)
3. Miconazole (Monistat)
4. Amoxicillin (Amoxil)

27. When assessing a 5-hour-old neonate born via vaginal delivery, which finding would prompt a nurse to call a physician?
1. Color is dusky, axillary temperature is 96.8° F (37° C), and the baby is spitting up mucus.
2. Hands and feet are cyanotic, abdomen is rounded, and the infant hasn't voided or passed meconium.
3. Anterior fontanel is ¾″ (2 cm) wide, head is molded, and sutures are overriding.
4. Irregular abdominal respirations and intermittent tremors in the extremities are present.

28. A mother calls the pediatrician because there's an outbreak of scabies at her child's school. The nurse would teach the mother to check for which finding?
1. Pain, erythema, and edema at the site of the bite
2. Oval white dots that adhere to hair shafts
3. Diffuse pruritic wheals
4. Pruritic papules, vesicles, and linear burrows on the finger and toe webs

29. The school nurse assesses a young child with a rash that's raised and has circumscribed areas filled with fluid. The nurse documents this finding as which type of rash?
1. Vesicular rash
2. Papular rash
3. Macular rash
4. Petechial rash

26. 3. The client most likely has candidiasis, which produces a thick cream cheese–like vaginal discharge and is treated with miconazole or nystatin (Mycostatin). Metronidazole is used to treat *Trichomonas vaginalis*. Erythromycin, amoxicillin, or other antibiotic therapy can contribute to candidiasis infections and isn't used to treat this infection.
CN: Physiological integrity; CNS: Pharmacological and parenteral therapies; CL: Application

27. 1. Skin color should be pink tinged or ruddy, and saliva should be scant. The normal axillary temperature ranges from 97.7° to 98.6° F (36.5° to 37° C). Acrocyanosis may be present for 2 to 6 hours. The neonate should pass meconium and void within 24 hours. Overriding sutures and molding, when present, may persist for a few days. Neonatal tremors are normal in the neonate; however, they must be evaluated to differentiate them from seizures.
CN: Safe, effective care environment; CNS: Management of care; CL: Application

28. 4. The mother should check her child for pruritic papules, vesicles, and linear burrows on the finger and toe webs. Oval white dots that adhere to the hair shaft can indicate head lice.
CN: Safe, effective care environment; CNS: Safety and infection control; CL: Application

29. 1. A vesicular rash contains small, raised, circumscribed lesions filled with clear fluid. A papular rash contains raised solid lesions with color changes in circumscribed areas. A macular rash is flat with color changes in circumscribed areas. Petechiae are pinpoint purple or red spots on the skin caused by multiple hemorrhages.
CN: Safe, effective care environment; CNS: Safety and infection control; CL: Application

30. A 20-month-old toddler has been treated with permethrin (Nix) for scabies. Because he continues to scratch, his mother wonders whether the drug is working. Which response by a nurse is most appropriate?
1. "Stop treatment because the drug isn't safe for children under age 2."
2. "Pruritus can be present for weeks after treatment."
3. "Apply the drug every day until the rash and itching disappear."
4. "Pruritus is common in children under age 5 treated with permethrin."

31. An 8-year-old child was sent home after the school reported the presence of head lice. Which information is most helpful to the parents?
1. The child should remain isolated for 1 week after treatment.
2. Lindane (Kwell) is the treatment of choice for head lice.
3. Treatment with a pediculicide followed by combing the hair with a fine-tooth comb will usually kill all lice and remove the nits. Retreatment in 7 to 10 days may be necessary to kill newly hatched lice.
4. The only way to get rid of head lice is to cut the hair.

32. Which assessment should a nurse do prior to administering disulfiram (Antabuse) to a client with a history of alcohol abuse?
1. Assess the client's commitment to attend Alcoholics Anonymous (AA) meetings.
2. Assess whether the client admits to a problem with alcohol.
3. Assess when the client's last alcoholic beverage was consumed.
4. Assess the client's nutritional status.

33. The nurse is assessing a client with schizophrenia who exhibits negativism, rigidity, excitement, stupor, and posturing. The nurse suspects that the client has which type of schizophrenia?
1. Catatonic
2. Undifferentiated
3. Disorganized
4. Paranoid

30. 2. Pruritus may be present for weeks in a child treated with permethrin for scabies. The drug is safe for use in infants as young as age 2 months. Treatment with permethrin can be safely repeated in 2 weeks. Pruritus is caused by secondary reactions of the mites.

CN: Physiological integrity; CNS: Pharmacological and parenteral therapies; CL: Application

31. 3. Treatment with a pediculicide followed by combing the hair with a fine-tooth comb will usually kill all lice and remove the nits. Retreatment in 7 to 10 days may be necessary to kill newly hatched lice. After the infestation has been appropriately treated, there's no reason to isolate the child. Lindane isn't the drug of choice because of its potential for neurotoxicity. The hair should be cut in severe cases only.

CN: Safe, effective care environment; CNS: Safety and infection control; CL: Application

32. 3. The client must be alcohol free for 12 hours before starting therapy with disulfiram. Assessing the client's commitment to attend AA meetings, the client's perception of his problem, and nutritional status are all important interventions, but they aren't necessary prior to starting disulfiram.

CN: Physiological integrity; CNS: Pharmacological and parenteral therapies; CL: Application

33. 1. Catatonic schizophrenia is a state of psychologically induced immobilization, which is, at times, interrupted by episodes of extreme agitation, such as negativism, rigidity, excitement, stupor, or posturing. Undifferentiated schizophrenia occurs when no single clinical presentation dominates (paranoid, disorganized, or catatonic). Disorganized schizophrenia is characterized by disorganized speech, disorganized behavior, and inappropriate affect. The dominant theme in paranoid schizophrenia is one of delusions and hallucinations.

CN: Psychosocial integrity; CNS: None; CL: Application

34. Which statement is an example of a key element in a nursing care plan?
 1. Advance diet to regular as tolerated.
 2. Ambulate 30 feet (9.1 m) with walker by discharge.
 3. Give furosemide (Lasix) 40 mg I.V. now.
 4. Discontinue I.V. fluids when tolerating oral fluids.

35. A client complains of chronic lower back pain and fatigue and has seen multiple care providers without relief of symptoms. The client insists that something is "terribly wrong." Which action should the nurse take first?
 1. Refer the client for a psychiatric evaluation.
 2. Initiate group therapy for behavior modification.
 3. Obtain a thorough health assessment to rule out physical illnesses.
 4. Refer the client to physical therapy.

36. Which sign alerts a nurse to a possible mild toxic reaction in a client receiving lithium for manic episodes of manic-depressive illness?
 1. Vomiting and diarrhea
 2. Hypertension
 3. Seizures
 4. Increased appetite

37. A client with bipolar disorder is taking lithium and tells the nurse, "I can stop taking the medicine when I feel better." Which response by the nurse is best?
 1. "That's correct. When you feel better, you can stop taking the medication."
 2. "Take the medication for 1 week after you feel better to be sure there's enough medication in your system."
 3. "Bipolar disorders may require lithium indefinitely to prevent relapses."
 4. "This medication is given as needed. That means that you can take it when you feel that you need it."

38. A client's condition is becoming stabilized after an episode of substance-induced delirium. During the initial recovery period, the nurse should assess the client for which psychosocial health problem?
 1. Flashbacks
 2. Depression
 3. Nightmares
 4. Dissociation

34. 2. Option 2 is a measurable expected outcome or goal, a key element of a nursing care plan. Other key elements include nursing diagnoses and interventions. The other options are physician's orders, not key elements of nursing care plans.
CN: Safe, effective care environment; CNS: Management of care; CL: Application

35. 3. The first action by the nurse should be to take a thorough health assessment including laboratory studies to rule out physical illnesses. The other actions aren't appropriate until a diagnosis is made.
CN: Safe, effective care environment; CNS: Management of care; CL: Application

36. 1. Vomiting and diarrhea are signs of mild to moderate lithium toxicity. Hypotension, not hypertension, and seizures occur with moderate to severe toxic reactions. Anorexia occurs with mild toxic reactions.
CN: Physiological integrity; CNS: Pharmacological and parenteral therapies; CL: Application

37. 3. Lithium, which helps clients with bipolar disorder stabilize their mood swings, is a long-term treatment. Blood measurements are taken regularly to monitor lithium levels in the client's body. He shouldn't stop taking lithium when he feels better because the therapeutic blood level will decrease. Stopping the medication 1 week after he feels better or taking it as needed will also decrease the therapeutic blood level of lithium.
CN: Physiological integrity; CNS: Pharmacological and parenteral therapies; CL: Analysis

38. 2. Depression and anxiety are common mental health problems seen immediately after substance withdrawal. Flashbacks and nightmares are commonly observed in clients with posttraumatic stress disorder. Dissociation occurs when a client undergoes prolonged physical and sexual abuse.
CN: Psychosocial integrity; CNS: None; CL: Analysis

39. A client with a history of depression demonstrates some inconsistent symptoms of cognitive impairment. The nurse should expect which situation when the depression is treated?
1. Delusional thinking ceases.
2. Recognition of objects improves.
3. Memory problems resolve.
4. Suicidal ideation is no longer a problem.

40. A client with borderline personality disorder has extreme views of himself and his situation. Which behavior indicates that the client is a candidate for medication?
1. Disorientation
2. Hyperactivity
3. Regression
4. Mood swings

41. A client has traits of an avoidant personality disorder. Which family intervention should the nurse give the highest priority in the care plan?
1. Explaining that the family should teach the client social skills
2. Recommending that the family recognize the client's high sensitivity to criticism
3. Exploring ways for the family to help the client express true feelings
4. Asking the family to keep a daily log of the client's adjustment difficulties

42. A client with a substance abuse disorder says the problem doesn't really exist. Which intervention should be the nurse's initial one?
1. Educating about the principles of mental health
2. Examining the use of defense mechanisms
3. Recognizing and discussing feelings of resentment
4. Discussing the need for a caretaker while in recovery

43. A nurse is evaluating drug therapy effectiveness in a client undergoing alcohol detoxification. Which finding indicates that drug therapy needs to be adjusted?
1. There are signs of toxicity from the drug.
2. The drug prevents the occurrence of further problems.
3. During the course of treatment, the dosage has increased.
4. The drug facilitates the client's interactions with staff.

You're making great strides!

39. 3. In a condition called pseudodementia, a client treated for depression will have a dramatic improvement in memory. Delusional thinking and object recognition problems aren't characteristic of pseudodementia. The nurse must assess all clients with depression for suicidal ideation because they're at some degree of risk for suicide.
CN: Psychosocial integrity; CNS: None; CL: Application

40. 4. Medications aren't typically given to clients with personality disorders. However, clients with mood swings, hallucinations, or psychotic behaviors are appropriate candidates for medications. Disorientation, hyperactivity, and regression aren't necessarily seen in clients with borderline personality disorders.
CN: Psychosocial integrity; CNS: None; CL: Application

41. 2. A client with traits of an avoidant personality disorder is very sensitive to criticism and disapproval but doesn't typically have learning or social skills problems. Such a client may have difficulty expressing feelings and may have few friends or only family members for interaction. Having the family keep a log of the client's adjustment difficulties isn't an appropriate intervention; the list may be interpreted as a statement of rejection.
CN: Safe, effective care environment; CNS: Management of care; CL: Analysis

42. 2. Defense mechanisms contribute to the client's denial. Education won't be well received unless the client recognizes the problem and determines that the nurse's teaching would be useful. The client can't recognize and discuss feelings of resentment when denying that a problem exists. The client needs to become responsible for his own behavior and take care of himself.
CN: Psychosocial integrity; CNS: None; CL: Application

43. 1. If signs of toxicity from drug therapy occur during the detoxification period, the drug therapy needs to be adjusted. The medication is working if it prevents further problems. Sometimes, the dosage must be adjusted to obtain the maximum benefit. If the drug enables the client to have therapeutic interactions with the staff, the client is benefiting from the therapy.
CN: Physiological integrity; CNS: Pharmacological and parenteral therapies; CL: Application

44. A nurse explains the unit's rules to a client with bulimia nervosa. Which action by the client indicates that learning has occurred?
1. The client asks to be accompanied to the bathroom after lunch.
2. The client writes down every food item eaten in the past 24 hours.
3. The client decides to help the dietitian plan the unit's meals.
4. The client discusses current problems with the nurse before mealtime.

45. A nurse is teaching a client with an eating disorder about cues that trigger unhealthy eating behaviors. Which example represents a social cue?
1. Diet advertisements
2. Troublesome memories
3. Interpersonal conflict
4. Frustration fatigue

46. A schizophrenic client states, "The voices keep talking to me. They're telling me that I have to leave here and that I shouldn't talk to you. Don't you hear what they're saying?" Which response is best?
1. "You didn't take your medicine this morning, did you?"
2. "The voices aren't real. You're sick and they're part of your illness."
3. "Are you hearing voices again?"
4. "I don't hear the voices, but I see that you are upset."

47. The nurse is teaching caregivers about the signs and symptoms of schizophrenia relapse. Which response by the caregivers about the signs and symptoms to report to a mental health professional indicates that the teaching has been effective?
1. Changes in appetite resulting in weight loss or gain
2. Loss of interest in sexual activities
3. Increased socialization
4. Feelings of tenseness and difficulty sleeping

48. A client with schizophrenia has been prescribed risperidone (Risperdal). The client's symptoms include hallucinations, delusions, and withdrawal. A nurse explains that the medication will help improve which symptoms?
1. Negative symptoms
2. Positive symptoms
3. Negative and positive symptoms
4. Paranoid symptoms

44. 1. When the client asks to be accompanied to the bathroom after a meal, the client is following protocol for restoring healthy eating and promoting adequate nutrition. This action indicates the client's commitment to not purging after a meal. Recording the food eaten in a 24-hour period would be appropriate for a client with anorexia nervosa, not a client with bulimia nervosa. It's inappropriate for a client to plan meals for the unit's clients. The client can discuss problems any time, not just before mealtimes.
CN: Psychosocial integrity; CNS: None; CL: Analysis

45. 3. Social cues that trigger maladaptive behavior include feelings of isolation and conflict with family or friends. Diet advertisements are considered situational cues. Troublesome memories are psychological cues. Frustration fatigue is an example of a physiological cue.
CN: Psychosocial integrity; CNS: None; CL: Application

46. 4. The nurse should be honest and tell the client that she doesn't hear the voices while acknowledging the client's feelings. Asking if the client took his medication or explaining his illness doesn't allow the client to feel valued by the nurse. Asking him if he hears voices makes him feel that the nurse wasn't listening.
CN: Psychosocial integrity; CNS: None; CL: Application

47. 4. Signs and symptoms of schizophrenia relapse include difficulty concentrating and sleeping, feelings of tenseness, and increased bizarre thinking and withdrawal. The other choices aren't signs and symptoms of schizophrenia.
CN: Psychosocial integrity; CNS: None; CL: Analysis

48. 3. Risperidone targets both negative and positive symptoms. Positive symptoms include delusions, hallucinations, and bizarre behaviors. Negative symptoms indicate a loss or lack of normal functioning such as lack of motivation and social withdrawal.
CN: Physiological integrity; CNS: Pharmacological and parenteral therapies; CL: Application

49. A newly graduated nurse is caring for a client recently diagnosed with dissociative identity disorder. The nurse asks the preceptor about discussing the client's traumatic childhood with the client. Which advice from the preceptor is best?
1. "Ask pointed questions and demand specific answers."
2. "If the client begins talking about it, just listen and be supportive."
3. "Tell the client that you suspect that much of his memory is exaggerated."
4. "Tell the client that those issues can be discussed with a physician only."

50. A client with dissociative identity disorder frequently switches from one personality to another. The nurse can identify the switch by which finding?
1. Episodes of orthostatic hypotension
2. Blinking or rolling the eyes frequently
3. Dystonic reactions
4. Episodes of tachycardia

51. A 38-year-old female client is scheduled to have a hysterectomy and is concerned about no longer being a "whole woman." Which intervention by the nurse is best?
1. Tell her to talk to her husband about the permanent changes that will be taking place with her body.
2. Refer her to group therapy.
3. Encourage her to discuss her concerns and feelings.
4. Give her information to read and leave the room.

52. A 23-year-old female client is seen in the emergency department for rape. The woman is very calm and appears emotionally unaffected by the event. Which assessment of the client's behavior is appropriate?
1. The client probably isn't telling the truth but is trying to get the perpetrator in trouble.
2. The client was a willing partner.
3. The client's initially deceptive calm may be masking distress, denial, or emotional shock.
4. The client is pregnant and is trying to blame the pregnancy on a rape.

49. 2. If the subject is painful, the client will discuss it when he feels comfortable and ready. Forcing him to talk about the subject will cause severe anxiety and result in distrust. The other choices don't facilitate a trusting relationship between the nurse and the client.
CN: Safe, effective care environment; CNS: Management of care; CL: Application

50. 2. Switching from one personality to another is manifested in a number of ways including blinking, facial movements, and changes in voice. Changes in blood pressure or pulse or dystonic reactions aren't indicative of switching from one personality to another.
CN: Psychosocial integrity; CNS: None; CL: Application

51. 3. The nurse should encourage the client to express her feelings. Telling her to talk to her husband will cause the client added concern and anxiety. Referring her to group therapy isn't an appropriate intervention at this time. Giving her information and leaving the room don't allow her to ask questions and express concerns.
CN: Psychosocial integrity; CNS: None; CL: Analysis

52. 3. One of the immediate consequences of rape is deceptive calmness. This behavior usually masks emotional shock, denial, or distress. The other responses are judgmental opinions. Nurses are to remain nonjudgmental in providing care.
CN: Psychosocial integrity; CNS: None; CL: Analysis

53. A full-term neonate was just admitted to the transitional nursery. He has a large meningomyelocele covered by an intact sac. The nurse knows immediately to place this neonate on his stomach with hips slightly elevated. Which statement describes the rationale for this position?
1. To prevent the sac covering the defect from rupturing
2. To preserve urine and bowel control
3. To assess neurological functioning more easily
4. To prevent further neurological damage

54. A nurse is teaching the mother of a neonate with a cleft palate how to feed him. Which instruction should the nurse give the mother?
1. Feed the neonate in a semireclining position with his head resting on the mother's curved elbow.
2. Feed the neonate in an upright position.
3. Feed the neonate lying on his stomach with his head turned toward his mother.
4. Feed the neonate in any position in which the mother and child are comfortable.

55. A nurse observes school-age children playing. Playing with which toy is typical of this age group?
1. Barbie dolls
2. The game of Operation
3. Sony Play Station video games
4. Hot Wheels cars

56. A nurse is assessing an infant's growth and development. Which action by the nurse indicates the best understanding of a 4-month old's stage of growth and development?
1. Eliciting a social smile
2. Allowing the infant to hold his own bottle
3. Playing peekaboo with the infant
4. Letting the infant sit without support

57. The nurse is caring for an 11-year-old client with cerebral palsy who has a pressure ulcer on the sacrum. When teaching the client's mother about dietary intake, which foods should the nurse plan to emphasize?
1. Legumes and cheese
2. Whole-grain products
3. Fruits and vegetables
4. Lean meats and low-fat milk

Keep moving along! You're almost finished!

53. 1. The sac covering the defect is the only barrier preventing bacteria from directly entering the neonate's central nervous system and causing meningitis and encephalitis. A large defect will result in loss of urine and bowel control. The nurse can assess neurological functioning when the child is on his back or stomach. The damage to the neurological system happened in utero, and the nurse should prevent further damage by placing the infant on his stomach until after surgery. Preventing neurological damage isn't the priority.
CN: Physiological integrity; CNS: Reduction of risk potential; CL: Analysis

54. 2. Feed the neonate with a cleft palate in an upright position. Incorrect feeding can allow formula to slip through the palate opening, enter the upper respiratory tract and lungs, and cause aspiration pneumonia. Any of the other positions is placing the neonate at risk for aspiration pneumonia.
CN: Physiological integrity; CNS: Reduction of risk potential; CL: Analysis

55. 2. School-age children engage in competitive play with established rules and goals. Operation is an excellent example of play that pulls these elements together. Playing with Barbie dolls is an example of associative play, which preschoolers engage in. Solitary play of video games is seen in adolescents. Playing with Hot Wheels cars is more indicative of toddlers' parallel play.
CN: Health promotion and maintenance; CNS: None; CL: Application

56. 1. A social smile should be seen in a 4-month old. An infant can't hold his own bottle until age 6 to 7 months, and he'll engage in peekaboo activity at age 10 to 12 months. He can sit without support at about age 8 months.
CN: Health promotion and maintenance; CNS: None; CL: Application

57. 4. Although the client should eat a balanced diet with foods from all food groups, the diet should emphasize foods that supply complete protein, such as lean meats and low-fat milk. Protein helps build and repair body tissue, which promotes healing. Legumes provide incomplete protein. Cheese contains complete protein but also fat, which should be limited to 30% or less of caloric intake. Whole-grain products supply incomplete proteins and carbohydrates. Fruits and vegetables mainly provide carbohydrates.
CN: Physiological integrity; CNS: Basic care and comfort; CL: Application

58. A client is diagnosed with pneumonia. Which nursing diagnosis would take <u>priority</u> for this client?
1. Excess fluid volume
2. Ineffective airway clearance
3. Activity intolerance
4. Deficient knowledge

58. 2. Pneumonia refers to inflammation of the lungs and can produce copious amounts of tracheobronchial secretions. These secretions interfere with airway patency and gas exchange. Therefore, airway clearance is a priority. The client may experience a decrease in fluid volume, not an excess, due to increased temperature and respiratory rate. The client also may experience activity intolerance and deficient knowledge, but neither is the priority diagnosis.
CN: Safe, effective care environment; CNS: Management of care; CL: Analysis

59. A nurse is caring for a client in active labor. Which observation would cause the nurse to suspect fetal distress?
1. Fetal heart rate of 144 beats/minute
2. Accelerations of the fetal heart rate with contractions
3. Fetal scalp pH of 7.14
4. Presence of long-term variability

59. 3. A scalp pH below 7.25 indicates acidosis and fetal hypoxia. A fetal heart rate of 144 beats/minute, acceleration of the fetal heartbeat with contractions, and the presence of long-term variability with contractions are normal responses of a healthy fetus to labor.
CN: Health promotion and maintenance; CNS: None; CL: Application

60. During a routine examination, the mother of a 3-month-old child asks the nurse, "How soon will she have her first tooth?" Which response by the nurse would be the most accurate as to the age by which the first tooth usually erupts?
1. 4 months
2. 5 months
3. 6 months
4. 7 months

60. 3. The first tooth typically erupts at age 6 months, although some infants do get their first tooth when a little younger or older.
CN: Health promotion and maintenance; CNS: None; CL: Application

61. A nurse assesses an 18-month-old toddler. Which activity would indicate to the nurse that the child is exhibiting normal growth and development patterns?
1. Running and jumping in place
2. Jumping down from a chair
3. Naming a specific color
4. Saying his full name

61. 1. An 18-month-old child should be able to run and jump in place. Typically, a child of 30 months is able to jump down from a chair, can name one color, and knows his full name.
CN: Health promotion and maintenance; CNS: None; CL: Application

62. A mother was diagnosed with polyhydramnios during her pregnancy and just delivered a preterm male neonate. In which manner should the nurse assess a neonate for tracheoesophageal atresia?
1. Observing the neonate during the first formula feeding
2. Determining if cyanosis is present at birth
3. Attempting to insert a catheter from the mouth to the stomach through the esophagus
4. Assessing lung sounds to determine if possible pneumonia is present

62. 3. Esophageal atresia is present if a catheter can't be passed through the neonate's mouth to the stomach. A barium swallow or a bronchial endoscopy examination will reveal the blind-end esophagus. The condition should be diagnosed before the infant is fed; otherwise, the infant will be unable to retain the feeding, and if a tracheoesophageal fistula is present, the infant may choke, gag, and become cyanotic during feeding. Immediately after birth, pneumonia should not be present if the infant has an esophageal atresia with a tracheoesophageal fistula. Emergency surgery will be essential to create a patent gastrointestinal tract.
CN: Health promotion and maintenance; CNS: None; CL: Analysis

63. Which instruction should be included in the care plan for a client following total hip replacement?
1. Keeping the legs adducted
2. Not bending at the hip more than 90 degrees
3. Keeping the hips lower than the knees when seated
4. Teaching how to bend forward to put on socks and shoes

63. 2. Following a total hip replacement, the client should be instructed not to bend more than 90 degrees at the hip. The legs should be kept abducted to prevent dislocation of the prosthesis. The hips should be kept higher than the knees when seated to minimize hip flexion. The client should be instructed not to bend forward at the hip to put on shoes and socks. Assistive devices can be used to help the client safely dress below the waist.
CN: Physiological integrity; CNS: Reduction of risk potential; CL: Application

64. Which cause of myocarditis is the most common?
1. Bacteria
2. Parasite
3. Fungus
4. Virus

64. 4. Myocarditis (inflammation of the myocardium) is usually caused by a virus. Of all the viruses, Coxsackie viruses and echoviruses are the most common agents. Bacteria, parasites, and fungi may cause myocarditis, but they aren't the most common causes.
CN: Physiological integrity; CNS: Physiological adaptation; CL: Analysis

65. A nurse is caring for a 7-year-old client receiving cyclophosphamide (Cytoxan). In addition to administering mesna (Mesnex), which action should the nurse take?
1. Transfusing platelets before administering the drug
2. Giving the child cranberry juice to drink
3. Encouraging the child to void frequently
4. Limiting the child's fluid intake

Only 10 more questions. Can you believe it?

65. 3. Hemorrhagic cystitis can result when the by-products of cyclophosphamide metabolism remain in the bladder; therefore, emptying the bladder at least every 2 hours when the child is awake can help prevent this painful condition. The child should be encouraged to void as soon as the urge is felt. Bacteria or low platelets don't cause the condition, so transfusing platelets and giving cranberry juice aren't correct. Limiting fluid is contraindicated. Instead, the child will be given fluids liberally, usually by I.V. infusion, and encouraged to drink; a high intake of fluids will increase elimination of the drug's toxic by-products.
CN: Physiological integrity; CNS: Pharmacological and parenteral therapies; CL: Analysis

66. When protective isolation isn't indicated, a nurse plans which activity for a child receiving chemotherapy?
1. Bed rest
2. Activity as tolerated
3. Walk to bathroom only
4. Out of bed for brief periods

66. 2. Children receiving chemotherapy should be able to engage in activities of interest and maintain as much independence and autonomy as possible; they'll limit their activity when they feel tired or ill. Limiting their activities to bed rest, walking to bathroom only, or only out of bed for brief periods isn't necessary and restricts activity unnecessarily. Whenever possible, include children in planning their care. These children should avoid adults and other children with infections.
CN: Health promotion and maintenance; CNS: None; CL: Application

67. A child is intubated and placed on a ventilator after a near drowning. The physician's order is to suction every 3 to 4 hours. The child's parents ask the nurse why the suctioning is necessary. Which response by the nurse is the most accurate?
1. To keep the client free of infection
2. To keep the client from experiencing cardiac arrhythmias
3. To keep the client's airway patent
4. To maintain fluid and electrolyte balance

68. A child with cystic fibrosis has a bronchodilator, steroids ordered by metered-dose inhaler, and chest physiotherapy. In which order should these medications and treatments be administered?
1. Perform chest physiotherapy first.
2. Administer the bronchodilator first.
3. Administer the steroid first.
4. Let the client eat lunch first and then perform chest physiotherapy.

69. A nurse is teaching a student nurse about ketogenic diet. The nurse knows that a ketogenic diet is sometimes used to treat which condition?
1. Anorexia nervosa
2. Nephrotic syndrome
3. Epilepsy
4. Ulcerative colitis

70. A child is unable to walk without assistance because of decreased oxygen at birth. Which disorder is characterized by a malfunction of the brain's motor center from hypoxia?
1. Down syndrome
2. Cerebral palsy
3. Sickle cell anemia
4. Osteogenesis imperfect

71. A 17-year-old client who injured his right knee during a basketball game is scheduled for an arthroscopy. The nurse teaches the client about the procedure. Which response by the nurse regarding arthroscopy would be accurate?
1. An X-ray using a contrast media
2. Visualization of the joint with a small instrument
3. Inserting a needle and withdrawing fluid for biopsy
4. Aspirating synovial fluid from the bursa

67. 3. Because of the increased secretions from drowning, the airway is more prone to obstruction, and suctioning is essential for maintaining patency. Suctioning won't prevent infection and may even cause it. Suctioning can cause bradycardia; therefore, preoxygenation is essential to prevent arrhythmias. Suctioning doesn't affect fluid and electrolyte balance.
CN: Physiological integrity; CNS: Reduction of risk potential; CL: Application

68. 2. Administer the bronchodilator to dilate the bronchi. The steroid can then reach further down the respiratory tract. After each medication is given, perform chest physiotherapy to expectorate secretions in the lower airways. Administer the medications and chest physiotherapy before meals to prevent aspiration.
CN: Physiological integrity; CNS: Pharmacological and parental therapies; CL: Application

69. 3. A ketogenic diet is typically suggested as a method of treatment for epilepsy. Anorexia nervosa is treated with counseling and slowly reintroducing food. Children with nephrotic syndrome are usually on a low-sodium diet. Ulcerative colitis is treated with a low-residue diet.
CN: Physiological integrity; CNS: Reduction of risk potential; CL: Application

70. 2. Cerebral palsy affects the motor center of the brain and is usually caused by brain trauma. Down syndrome is a chromosomal abnormality. Sickle cell anemia is a genetic disorder of red blood cells. Osteogenesis imperfecta is a congenital anomaly involving decreased calcium in the bones and leads to multiple fractures at birth.
CN: Physiological integrity; CNS: Physiological adaptation; CL: Application

71. 2. After a small incision is made in the knee, a small tube-shaped instrument is inserted for viewing the knee and surrounding cartilage, tendon, and ligaments. Contrast media is typically used for X-rays of joints. Biopsies are taken if cancer is a concern. Synovial fluid is collected for culture if an infection or inflammation is a concern.
CN: Physiological integrity; CNS: Physiological adaptation; CL: Application

72. A nurse is assessing a 13-year-old child 12 hours after surgery for a compound-fracture repair of the right arm. Which finding requires immediate attention?
1. Bruising of the fingers
2. Capillary refill of 3 seconds
3. Pallor of the nail beds
4. Edema of the extremity

73. A 3-year-old child has diarrhea, and the pediatrician has recommended a BRAT diet for the next 24 hours. The nurse teaches the parents about the diet. Which response by the parents about the diet indicates the teaching has been effective?
1. "The diet consists of bran, Rice Krispies, apple juice, and tomato juice."
2. "The diet consists of beans, red meat, apples, and tomatoes."
3. "The diet consists of bananas, rice, applesauce, and toast."
4. "The diet consists of broccoli, red ice pops, apple butter, and tacos."

74. After undergoing small-bowel resection, a client is prescribed metronidazole (Flagyl) 500 mg I.V. The mixed I.V. solution contains 100 ml. A nurse is to run the drug over 30 minutes. The drip factor of the available I.V. tubing is 15 gtt/ml. What is the drip rate? Record your answer using a whole number.

_____ gtt/minute

75. A nurse is caring for a client whose cultural background is different from her own. Which actions are appropriate? Select all that apply.
1. Consider that nonverbal cues, such as eye contact, may have different meanings in different cultures.
2. Respect the client's cultural beliefs.
3. Ask the client if he has cultural or religious requirements that should be considered in his care.
4. Explain your beliefs so that the client will understand the differences.
5. Understand that all cultures experience pain in the same way.

72. 3. Pallor suggests a decrease in circulation to the extremity, and the surgeon should be notified. Bruising can be expected with a compound fracture. The fingers should be observed for further discoloration indicating decreased circulation. Capillary refill of 3 seconds is normal. Edema is expected but should be watched; increased edema might impair circulation.
CN: Physiological integrity; CNS: Reduction of risk potential; CL: Application

73. 3. BRAT stands for bananas, rice, applesauce, and toast. This diet is commonly used for children with diarrhea because these foods add some form to the stool without further irritating the bowel. The other diet choices can cause gas, irritation, and inflammation in the already inflamed bowel.
CN: Physiological integrity; CNS: Basic care and comfort; CL: Application

74. 50. Use the following equation:
100 ml × 15 gtt/ml / 30 minutes = 50 gtt/minute.
CN: Physiological integrity; CNS: Pharmacological and parenteral therapies; CL: Application

75. 1, 2, and 3. Nonverbal cues may have different meanings in different cultures. In one culture, eye contact is a sign of disrespect; in another, eye contact shows respect and attentiveness. The nurse should always respect the client's cultural beliefs and ask if he has cultural or religious requirements. This may include food choices or restrictions, body coverings, or time for prayer. The nurse should attempt to understand the client's culture; it isn't the client's responsibility to understand the nurse's culture. The nurse should never impose her own beliefs on her clients. Culture influences a client's experience of pain. For example, in one culture pain may be openly expressed, whereas in another culture, it may be quietly endured.
CN: Psychosocial integrity; CNS: None; CL: Analysis

Congrats! You did it! You finished the last question!

Index